Essentials of
Aesthetic Surgery

Essentials of Aesthetic Surgery

Edited by

Jeffrey E. Janis, MD, FACS

Professor of Plastic Surgery, Neurosurgery,
Neurology, and Surgery;
Executive Vice Chairman, Department
of Plastic Surgery;
Chief of Plastic Surgery, University Hospitals;
President-Elect, American Society
of Plastic Surgeons;
The Ohio State University Wexner Medical Center,
Columbus, Ohio

With Illustrations by

Graeme Chambers
Amanda L. Tomasikiewicz, MA
Sarah J. Taylor, MS, BA
Jennifer N. Gentry, MA, CMI

 Thieme

Managing Editor: Haley Paskalides
Director, Editorial Services: Mary Jo Casey
Production Editor: Sean Woznicki
International Production Director: Andreas Schabert
Editorial Director: Sue Hodgson
International Marketing Director: Fiona Henderson
International Sales Director: Louisa Turrell
Director of Institutional Sales: Adam Bernacki
Senior Vice President and Chief Operating Officer:
Sarah Vanderbilt
President: Brian D. Scanlan

Library of Congress Cataloging-in-Publication Data

Names: Janis, Jeffrey E., editor.
Title: Essentials of aesthetic surgery / [edited by] Jeffrey
E. Janis, MD, FACS, Professor of Plastic Surgery,
Neurosurgery, Neurology, and Surgery Executive Vice
Chairman, Department of Plastic Surgery, Chief of
Plastic Surgery, University Hospitals, President-Elect,
American Society of Plastic Surgeons, Ohio State Uni-
versity Wexner Medical Center, Columbus, OH.
Description: New York : Thieme, [2018] | Includes biblio-
graphical references.
Identifiers: LCCN 2017054012 | ISBN 9781626236547
(paperback) | ISBN 9781626238671 (ebook)
Subjects: LCSH: Surgery, Plastic. | BISAC: MEDICAL /
Surgery / Plastic & Cosmetic. | MEDICAL / Surgery /
General.
Classification: LCC RD118 .E87 2018 | DDC 617.9/52—dc23
LC record available at https://lccn.loc.gov/2017054012

© 2018 Thieme Medical Publishers, Inc.
Thieme Publishers New York
333 Seventh Avenue, New York, NY 10001 USA
+1 800 782 3488, customerservice@thieme.com

Thieme Publishers Stuttgart
Rüdigerstrasse 14, 70469 Stuttgart, Germany
+49 [0]711 8931 421, customerservice@thieme.de

Thieme Publishers Delhi
A-12, Second Floor, Sector-2, Noida-201301
Uttar Pradesh, India
+91 120 45 566 00, customerservice@thieme.in

Thieme Publishers Rio, Thieme Publicações Ltda.
Edifício Rodolpho de Paoli, 25º andar
Av. Nilo Peçanha, 50 – Sala 2508
Rio de Janeiro 20020-906, Brasil
+55 21 3172 2297 / +55 21 3172-1896

Cover design: Thieme Publishing Group
Typesetting by Debra Clark

Printed in India by Replika Press, Pvt Ltd.   5 4 3 2 1

ISBN 978-1-62623-654-7

Also available as an e-book:
eISBN 978-1-62623-867-1

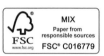

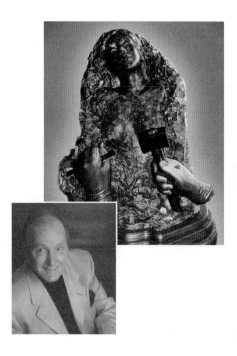

Cover photograph of the sculpture
"Surgical Aesthetic Art"
provided by the Ronadró Collection.
Additional sculptures by the artist can be found at
www.ronadro.com

To my wife, Emily, and my three children, Jackson, Brinkley, and Holden,

who are the center of my life and universe, and who give me the love, support,

understanding, and inspiration to do better, and be better, every day

Contributors

Paul N. Afrooz, MD
Aesthetic Surgery Fellow, Dallas Plastic Surgery Institute, Dallas, Texas

Patricia Aitson
Medical Photography Supervisor, Department of Plastic Surgery, University of Texas Southwestern Medical Center, Dallas, Texas

Amy Kathleen Alderman, MD, MPH
Private Practice, Alpharetta, Georgia

Tyler M. Angelos, MD, FACS
Columbus Aesthetic and Plastic Surgery, Columbus, Ohio

Molly Burns Austin, MD
Dermatologist, Dermatology Consultants of North Dallas, Dallas, Texas

James L. Baker, Jr., MD, FACS
Clinical Professor of Plastic Surgery, University of South Florida, Tampa; Professor of Surgery, College of Medicine, University of Central Florida, Orlando, Florida

Alfonso Barrera, MD, FACS
Clinical Assistant Professor of Plastic Surgery, Baylor College of Medicine, Houston, Texas

Daniel O. Beck, MD
Private Practice, Dallas Plastic Surgery Institute, Dallas, Texas

Amanda Behr, MA, CMI, CCA, FAMI
Interim Chair and Program Director, Clinic Director and Anaplastologist, Department of Medical Illustration, Augusta University; Augusta University Clinic for Prosthetic Restoration, Augusta, Georgia

J. Byers Bowen, MD, MS
Independent Resident, Department of Plastic and Reconstructive Surgery, The Ohio State University Wexner Medical Center, Columbus, Ohio

George Broughton II, MD, PhD, FACS
Regional Health Command Europe, Assistant Chief of Staff, Warrior Transition Faculty, Plastic and Reconstructive Surgery, Landstuhl Regional Medical Center, Landstuhl, Germany

Joseph M. Brown, MD
Plastic Surgeon and Medical Director, Tampa Aesthetic and Plastic Surgery, Lutz, Florida

Alton Jay Burns, MD
Dallas Plastic Surgery, Dallas, Texas

Michael R. Bykowski, MD
Resident, Department of Plastic Surgery, University of Pittsburgh Medical Center, Pittsburgh, Pennsylvania

Jeff Chang, MD
Resident, Division of Plastic and Reconstructive Surgery, Stanford University Medical Center, Palo Alto, California

Wendy Chen, MD, MS
Resident Physician, Department of Plastic Surgery, University of Pittsburgh Medical Center, Pittsburgh, Pennsylvania

William Pai-Dei Chen, MD
Clinical Professor of Ophthalmology, UCLA School of Medicine, Los Angeles; Harbor UCLA Medical Center, Irvine, California

Christopher T. Chia, MD
Surgical Director, bodySCULPT; Clinical
Attending, Manhattan Eye, Ear, and Throat
Hospital, New York, New York

Jeffrey R. Claiborne, MD
Plastic Surgeon, Private Practice,
Sieveking and Claiborne Plastic Surgery,
Nashville, Tennessee

Sydney R. Coleman, MD
Clinical Assistant Professor of Plastic
Surgery, Hansjörg Wyss Department
of Plastic Surgery, New York University
School of Medicine, New York University
Langone Medical Center, New York,
New York

Mark B. Constantian, MD, FACS
Adjunct Clinical Professor, Department
of Surgery, Division of Plastic and
Reconstructive Surgery, University of
Wisconsin School of Medicine, Madison,
Wisconsin; Visiting Professor, Department
of Plastic Surgery, University of Virginia
School of Medicine, Charlottesville,
Virginia

Michelle Coriddi, MD
Plastic Surgeon, Memorial Sloan Kettering
Cancer Center, Plastic and Reconstructive
Surgery Service, New York, New York

Melissa A. Crosby, MD, PLLC
Plastic Surgeon, Private Practice,
Sugar Land, Texas

Lily Daniali, MD
Burn and Reconstructive Centers of
Colorado, Englewood, Colorado

Edward H. Davidson, MA (Cantab), MD
Assistant Professor, Division of Plastic
Surgery, Montefiore Medical Center/Albert
Einstein, College of Medicine; The Atrium,
Montefiore Medical Center, New York,
New York

Zoe Diana Draelos, MD
Consulting Professor, Department of
Dermatology, Duke University School of
Medicine, Durham, North Carolina

Dino R. Elyassnia, MD, FACS
Marten Clinic of Plastic Surgery, San
Francisco, California

Maristella S. Evangelista, MD, MBA
Assistant Professor, The Ohio State
University, Columbus, Ohio

Steve Fagien, MD, PA
Physician, Private Practice, Boca Raton,
Florida

Jordan P. Farkas, MD
Plastic Surgeon, Private Practice, Paramus,
New Jersey

Darrell Wayne Freeman, MD
Department of Plastic Surgery, The Ohio
State University, Columbus, Ohio

Brian H. Gander, MD
Assistant Professor, Division of Plastic
Surgery, University of Wisconsin, Madison,
Wisconsin

Ashkan Ghavami, MD
Assistant Clinical Professor, David Geffen
UCLA School of Medicine, Los Angeles;
Private Practice, Ghavami Plastic Surgery,
Beverly Hills, California

Grant Gilliland, MD
Physician, Baylor University Medical
Center, Waco; Texas A&M College of
Medicine, Dallas, Texas

†Mark Gorney, MD
Plastic Surgeon, Napa, California

---

†Deceased.

Miles Graivier, MD
Plastic Surgeon, The Graivier Center for
Plastic Surgery, Roswell, Georgia

James Christian Grotting, MD, FACS
Clinical Adjunct Professor, The University
of Alabama at Birmingham; Private
Practice, Grotting Plastic Surgery
Birmingham, Alabama; The University of
Wisconsin, Madison, Wisconsin

Jeffrey A. Gusenoff, MD
Associate Professor of Plastic Surgery, Co-
Director, Life After Weight Loss Program,
Department of Plastic Surgery, University
of Pittsburgh School of Medicine,
Pittsburgh, Pennsylvania

Bahman Guyuron, MD, FACS
Emeritus Professor, School of Medicine,
Case Western Reserve University,
Lyndhurst, Ohio

Richard Y. Ha, MD
Dallas Plastic Surgery Institute, Dallas,
Texas

Elizabeth Hall-Findlay, MD
Private Practice, Banff Plastic Surgery,
Banff, Alberta, Canada

Adam H. Hamawy, MD, FACS
Plastic Surgeon, Princeton Plastic
Surgeons, Princeton, New Jersey

Dennis C. Hammond, MD
Partners in Plastic Surgery, Grand Rapids,
Michigan

Christine Hamori, MD
Cosmetic Surgery and Skin Spa, Duxbury,
Massachusetts

Bridget Harrison, MD
Hand Surgery Fellow, UCLA School of
Medicine, Los Angeles, California

Ahmed M. Hashem, MD
Professor of Plastic Surgery, Cairo
University, Kasr Al-Ainy, Faculty of
Medicine, Cairo University, El Manial,
Cairo, Egypt

William Y. Hoffman, MD
Professor and Chief, Division of Plastic and
Reconstructive Surgery, Stephen J. Mathes
Endowed Chair in Plastic Surgery, Division
of Plastic Surgery, University of California,
San Francisco, San Francisco, California

Ronald E. Hoxworth, MD, MBA, FACS
Chief of Plastic Surgery, University
Hospitals, University of Texas
Southwestern Medical Center, Dallas,
Texas

John H. Hulsen, MD
Plastic Surgeon, Associated Plastic
Surgeons, Leawood, Kansas

Joseph Hunstad, MD, FACS
President, The Hunstad Kortesis Center
for Cosmetic Plastic Sugergy; President,
The Internatonal Consortium of Aesthetic
Plastic Surgeons; Member, Board of
Directors, The American Society for
Aesthetic Plastic Surgery; Associate
Consulting Proessor, Division of Plastic
Surgery, The University of North Carolina,
Chapel Hill; Section Head of Plastic
Surgery, Department of Surgery, Carolinas
Medical Center, University Hospital,
Charlotte, North Carolina

Cedric L. Hunter, MD
Stanford University Medical Center, Palo
Alto, California

Jeffrey E. Janis, MD, FACS
Professor of Plastic Surgery, Neurosurgery, Neurology, and Surgery; Executive Vice Chairman, Department of Plastic Surgery; Chief of Plastic Surgery, University Hospitals; President-Elect, American Society of Plastic Surgeons; The Ohio State University Wexner Medical Center, Columbus, Ohio

Rishi Jindal, MD
Fellow, University of Pittsburgh Medical Center, Pittsburgh, Pennsylvania

Glyn Jones, MD, FRCS(Ed), FCS(SA), FACS
Visiting Professor of Surgery, Plastic and Reconstruction, Illinois Cosmetic and Plastic Surgery, Peoria, Illinois

Girish P. Joshi, MBBS, MD, FFARCSI
Professor of Anesthesiology and Pain Management, University of Texas Southwestern Medical Center, Dallas, Texas

Evan B. Katzel, MD
University of Pittsburgh Medical Center, Pittsburgh, Pennsylvania

Phillip D. Khan, MD
Plastic Surgeon, Lead Clinician, Coastal Plastic Surgery, Supply, North Carolina

Sami U. Khan, MD, FACS
Associate Professor of Plastic Surgery, Stony Brook Medicine, Stony Brook, New York

Ibrahim Khansa, MD
Resident, Department of Plastic Surgery, The Ohio State University Wexner Medical Center, Columbus, Ohio

Rohit K. Khosla, MD
Division of Plastic and Reconstructive Surgery, Stanford University, Palo Alto, California

Kuylhee Kim, MD
Aesthetic and Reconstructive Breast Surgery Fellow, Partners in Plastic Surgery in West Michigan, Grand Rapids, Michigan

Janae L. Kittinger, MD
One Health Plastic and Reconstructive Surgery, Owensboro, Kentucky

David M. Knize, MD
Associate Clinical Professor of Surgery, Department of Plastic Surgery, University of Colorado Health Sciences Center, Colorado Springs, Colorado

Michael Larsen, MD
Department of Plastic Surgery, The Ohio State University Medical Center, Columbus, Ohio

Michael R. Lee, MD
Assistant Professor, Department of Plastic Surgery, University of Texas Southwestern Medical Center, Dallas, Texas

Jason E. Leedy, MD
Cleveland Plastic Surgery Institute, Mayfield Heights, Ohio

Joshua Lemmon, MD
Private Practice, DFW Metroplex, Richardson, Texas

Jerome H. Liu, MD, MSHS
Liu Plastic Surgery, Los Gatos, California

Deborah Stahl Lowery, MD
Assistant Professor, Anesthesiology, The Ohio State University Wexner Medical Center; Ear and Eye Institute Outpatient Surgery Center, Columbus, Ohio

Raman C. Mahabir, MD
Chair, Division of Plastic, Reconstructive, and Cosmetic Surgery, Mayo Clinic Arizona, Phoenix, Arizona

Alexey M. Markelov MD
Private Practice, Coos Bay, Oregon;
Clinical Assistant Professor, The Ohio State
University, Columbus, Ohio

Constantino G. Mendieta, MD
Surgeon, Private Practice, Miami, Florida

Joseph Meyerson, MD
Resident, The Ohio State University
Wexner Medical Center, Columbus, Ohio

Cecilia Alejandra Garcia de Mitchell, MD
Division Chief, Plastic Surgeon, The
Children's Hospital of San Antonio; Affiliate
Faculty Department of Surgery, Baylor
College of Medicine; Adjunct Assistant
Professor, Department of Surgery, Division
of Plastic Surgery, University of Texas
Health Science Center, San Antonio, Texas

Girish S. Munavalli, MD, MHS
Medical Director, Dermatology, Laser, and
Vein Specialists of the Carolinas, Charlotte;
Assistant Professor, Department of
Dermatology, Wake Forest University
School of Medicine, Winston Salem, North
Carolina

Purushottam A. Nagarkar, MD
Assistant Professor, Department of Plastic
Surgery, University of Texas Southwestern
Medical Center, Dallas, Texas

Foad Nahai, MD, FACS
Maurice Jurkiewicz Chair in Plastic Surgery
and Professor of Surgery, Division of
Plastic and Reconstructive Surgery,
Department of Surgery, Emory University
School of Medicine, Atlanta, Georgia

Christopher J. Pannucci, MD, MS
Assistant Professor, Division of Plastic
Surgery, University of Utah, Salt Lake City,
Utah

Thornwell H. Parker III, MD
Volunteer Faculty, Department of Plastic
Surgery, University of Texas Southwestern
Medical Center; Staff, Department of
Plastic Surgery, Texas Health Presbyterian
Hospital of Dallas, Dallas, Texas

Harlan Pollock, MD, FACS
Instructor, Retired, University of Texas
Southwestern, Dallas, Texas

Todd A. Pollock, MD, FACS
Surgeon, University of Texas Southwestern
Medical Center, Dallas, Texas

Jason K. Potter, MD, DDS
Dallas Plastic Surgery Institute, Dallas,
Texas

Smita R. Ramanadham, MD
Attending Surgeon, Division of Plastic
Surgery, Boston Medical Center;
Assistant Professor of Surgery, Boston
University School of Medicine, Boston,
Massachusetts

Neal R. Reisman, MD, JD, FACS
Clinical Professor, Plastic Surgery, Baylor
College of Medicine, Houston, Texas

Juan L. Rendon, MD, PhD
Clinical Instructor Housestaff, The Ohio
State University Wexner Medical Center,
Columbus, Ohio

Luis M. Rios, Jr.
Adjunct Clinical Professor, Department of
Surgery, University of Texas Health Science
Center, Edinburg, Texas

Edward J. Ruane, Jr., MD
Resident, Department of Plastic Surgery,
University of Pittsburgh, Pittsburgh,
Pennsylvania

Christopher J. Salgado, MD
Professor of Surgery and Interim Chief,
Division of Plastic Surgery, Section Chief,
University of Miami Hospital; Medical
Director, LGBTQ Center for Wellness,
Gender and Sexual Health, University of
Miami/Miller School of Medicine, Miami,
Florida

Renato Saltz, MD
Saltz Plastic Surgery, Salt Lake City, Utah

Robert K. Sigal, MD
President, Austin-Weston, The Center for
Cosmetic Surgery, Inova Fairfax Hospital,
Reston, Virgnia

Sammy Sinno, MD
TLKM Plastic Surgery, Chicago, Illinois

Wesley N. Sivak, MD, PhD
Resident, Department of Plastic Surgery,
University of Pittsburgh, Pittsburgh,
Pennsylvania

Christopher Chase Surek, MD
Aesthetic Surgery Fellow, Department
of Plastic Surgery, Cleveland Clinic,
Cleveland, Ohio

Sumeet Sorel Teotia, MD
Associate Professor, Plastic Surgery,
University of Texas Southwestern Medical
Center, Dallas, Texas

Edward O. Terino, MD
CEO and President, Plastic Surgery
Institute, Agoura Hills, California

Spero J. Theodorou, MD
Instructor, Aesthetic Plastic Surgery
Fellowship, Manhattan Eye, Ear, and Throat
Hospital, New York, New York

Charles H. Thorne, MD
Chairman, Department of Plastic Surgery,
Lenox Hill Hospital; Manhattan Eye, Ear,
and Throat Hospital, New York, New York

Dean M. Toriumi, MD
Professor, Department of Otolaryngology,
University of Illinois at Chicago, Chicago,
Illinois

Derek Ulvila, MD
Aesthetic Plastic Surgery Fellow,
Manhattan Eye, Ear, and Throat Hospital,
New York, New York

Simeon H. Wall, Jr., MD, FACS
Private Practice, The Wall Center for Plastic
Surgery; Assistant Clinical Professor,
Department of Plastic Surgery, University
of Texas Southwestern Medical Center,
Dallas, Texas; Assistant Clinical Professor,
Division of Plastic Surgery, Louisiana State
University Health Sciences Center at
Shreveport, Shreveport, Louisiana

Ted H. Wojno, MD
Director, Oculoplastic and Orbital Surgery,
Department of Ophthalmology, The
Emory Clinic; Professor of Ophthalmology,
Emory University School of Medicine, The
Emory Clinic, Atlanta, Georgia

Vernon Leroy Young, MD
Private Practice, Washington, Missouri

James E. Zins, MD
Chairman, Department of Plastic Surgery,
Cleveland Clinic, Cleveland, Ohio

Terri A. Zomerlei, MD
Resident, Department of Plastic Surgery,
The Ohio State University, Columbus, Ohio

Foreword

I first met Dr. Janis when he was in training. We established a friendship and I have followed his career with interest and admiration ever since. It was clear to me immediately that he had leadership qualities, a commitment to teaching, and academics and most of all excellence as a clinician. He very quickly became a contributor, educator and innovator. His published works, his many international and national presentations attest to his commitment to teaching and his leadership qualities were recently recognized as he assumed the presidency of the American Society of Plastic Surgeons.

The idea behind *Essentials of Aesthetic Surgery* has been in gestation for many years and it is exciting to see the concept come to fruition. The intent is to provide a detailed guide to the field based on the same didactic, high-yield format of the best-selling book *Essentials of Plastic Surgery*, now in its second edition. Although there are some chapters in the *Essentials of Plastic Surgery* that cover aesthetic surgery, this new book has vastly deeper and wider, comprehensive coverage, offering 65 detailed chapters as opposed to the 16 offered in *Essentials* and covering the full spectrum of procedures in the face and body. The book has been thoughtfully structured to maximize learning with signature bulleted text and clear, memorable line drawings. It is published with an e-book version ideal for use by readers on-the-go and who may not wish to carry the print version with them.

A new concept, and unique to this text, is that most chapters are authored by a younger plastic surgeon working with one who has been in practice far longer. The younger author would be more aware of the needs of those in the early years in practice as well as those in training. The senior author with more years of experience has the long-term perspective of the procedures discussed. Specifically, which are efficacious, which are safe and which last longest. This blending of a young plastic surgeon's views and the experience of the senior surgeon brings valuable perspective to each chapter in the book and sets this book apart from the others in its class.

ASAPS statistics indicate the undiminished growth of aesthetic surgery, with patient procedures up 19% in the last decade.[1] More and more trainees aspiring to a career in aesthetic surgery, as evidenced by diplomates of the American Board of Plastic Surgery, overwhelmingly select the Aesthetic module for maintenance of certification. This book provides an invaluable educational resource, guide, and companion to those seeking the core facts—a treasure trove of knowledge distilled by Dr. Janis and his team of highly regarded contributors. It is my distinct pleasure to recommend this volume as the perfect first step into the world of aesthetic surgery and to congratulate Dr. Janis warmly for his dedication and skill in putting the volume together.

Foad Nahai, MD, FACS
Maurice Jurkiewicz Chair in Plastic Surgery
and Professor of Surgery, Division of Plastic
and Reconstructive Surgery, Department
of Surgery, Emory University School of Medicine,
Atlanta, Georgia

---

[1]Cosmetic Surgery National Data Bank Statistics. Aesthet Surg J 37(Suppl 2):1, 2017.

Preface

The idea for this book actually came right after the first edition of *Essentials of Plastic Surgery* was published in 2007. At the time, I thought it would be neat to carry the concept one step further by focusing on aesthetic surgery, dedicating a book to it in the same stylistic vein as the parent title—with high-point and high-impact information that was current and relevant, presented in bullet-point format with references to classic articles and best available data, richly illustrated and presented in a fit-in-your-coat-pocket format. The table of contents was created in 2008 and both junior and senior authors were invited to contribute. The concept was to present the information comprehensively but concisely and to supplement it with "color commentary" from experienced surgeons who can add a three-dimensionality to the work by adding decades of experience—things known, but not necessarily written down all the time. Ultimately, despite a decade in the making, the book is now in your hands as the culmination of so many hands and minds, hopefully as a valuable and practical guide to the world of cosmetic surgery.

The book comprises 65 chapters spanning the breadth of aesthetic surgery, organized into nine parts—from Skin Care to Noninvasive Modalities to Surgical Approaches and everything in between. Each chapter follows the same basic format for ease of familiarity and readability. The common topics are covered, of course, such as facelift, necklift, blepharoplasty, rhinoplasty, breast augmentation, liposuction, abdominoplasty, thigh lift, and beyond. However, deep dive chapters are provided to get into the detail required to truly master the content—such as correction of the tear trough deformity, lateral canthopexy, Asian blepharoplasty, secondary and ethnic rhinoplasty, the nasolabial fold, lip augmentation, nonsurgical rejuvenation, augmentation-mastopexy, gluteal augmentation, genital surgery, and transgender surgery. Furthermore, there are topics covered to round out the utility and comprehensive approach to cosmetic surgery, such as proper patient selection, safety considerations, the artistry of aesthetic surgery, anesthesia considerations, multimodal analgesia, and photography.

Rich, two-color figures and tables were added to help effectively illustrate and convey the information to the reader. An online version was developed to make it more universal, accessible, and current. Top Takeaways were added to the end of each chapter to summarize the content for the quick hit review.

The true test of its utility, however, will be whether it sits on your shelf or in your pocket. My sincere hope is that you find it to be an indispensable companion with you on rounds, in the clinic, in the operating room, in the conference room, or in the emergency department as you care for these patients. And although it took 10 years to create, my hope is that you find it to be current, relevant, and of the same highest level of quality you've come to expect from an *Essentials* book.

Jeffrey E. Janis

Acknowledgments

Without question, this book could not have been possible without a tremendous number of people who have contributed to it since 2008. Indeed, the book has actually seen three different publishers, originally Quality Medical Publishing, then CRC Press, and finally Thieme Publishers, so clearly there are many to acknowledge.

Without question, I owe a tremendous debt of gratitude to the authors across the country who have taken an incredible amount of time out of their busy practices and lives to carefully comb and review the literature in order to create and construct these high quality chapters. Their careful attention to detail was matched by their patience as they endured a lengthy and rigorous editing process where every word and illustration was carefully scrutinized. As they will clearly attest, meticulous attention to detail and emphasis on quality and accuracy demanded much energy, persistence and determination. To them, I am sincerely grateful for their time and for the fruit of their efforts.

Sincere appreciation also is owed to Karen Berger, Michelle Berger, Andrew Berger, and Amy Debrecht of Quality Medical Publishing, who originally signed the book back in 2008, and to Makalah Boyer and Suzanne Wakefield of CRC Press and subsequently Thieme Publishers for their significant contributions. Special recognition goes to Editorial Director Sue Hodgson, without whom this book would never be possible, and Judith Tomat who dedicated an incredible amount of effort in the editing process and who carried it across the finish line. Special gratitude also goes to Brenda Bunch and her team of illustrators, who deserve an amazing amount of credit for all of the graphics that were drawn from scratch, which makes this book pop alive with color, clarity, and flavor.

Most importantly, and with the deepest and most sincere appreciation, I would like to thank my wife, Emily, and our three children Jackson, Brinkley, and Holden, all of whom were born during the creation of this book, for their understanding and patience during the years, allowing the time and travel to complete this book, and above all else, for their unconditional love and support. Without them, this book would not be possible, and my life would be empty.

Contents

FOREWORD   XV
Foad Nahai

PART I ▪ BASIC CONSIDERATIONS

1 THE AESTHETIC SURGERY PATIENT   3
Adam H. Hamawy, Foad Nahai

2 THE ARTISTRY OF PLASTIC SURGERY   13
Sumeet Sorel Teotia, Mark B. Constantian

3 PHOTOGRAPHY FOR THE AESTHETIC SURGEON   21
Amanda Behr, Patricia Aitson, William Y. Hoffman

4 MEDICOLEGAL CONSIDERATIONS IN AESTHETIC SURGERY   43
Mark Gorney, Neal R. Reisman

PART II ▪ ANESTHESIA

5 BASICS OF ANESTHESIA FOR THE AESTHETIC SURGERY PATIENT   59
Deborah Stahl Lowery, Jeffrey E. Janis

6 PERIOPERATIVE ANESTHESIA CONSIDERATIONS FOR THE AESTHETIC SURGERY PATIENT   85
Deborah Stahl Lowery

7 PROCEDURE-SPECIFIC ANESTHESIA GUIDELINES FOR THE AESTHETIC SURGERY PATIENT   95
Deborah Stahl Lowery

8 MULTIMODAL ANALGESIA FOR THE AESTHETIC SURGERY PATIENT   107
Girish P. Joshi, Jeffrey E. Janis

Part III • Safety

9 Safety Considerations in Aesthetic Surgery   **119**
Jeffrey E. Janis, Sumeet Sorel Teotia, J. Byers Bowen, Girish P. Joshi, Vernon Leroy Young

10 Decreasing Complications in Aesthetic Surgery   **143**
Edward H. Davidson, Zoe Diana Draelos, Bridget Harrison, Ibrahim Khansa, Jeffrey E. Janis

11 Venous Thromboembolism and the Aesthetic Surgery Patient   **160**
Christopher J. Pannucci, Amy Kathleen Alderman

Part IV • Skin Care

12 The Medi Spa and Other Practice Considerations   **171**
Rishi Jindal, Renato Saltz

13 Anatomy, Physiology, and Disorders of the Skin   **181**
Thornwell H. Parker III, Molly Burns Austin, Alton Jay Burns

14 Cosmeceuticals and Other Office Products   **191**
Sammy Sinno, Zoe Diana Draelos

15 Ethnic Skin Care   **197**
Sammy Sinno, Zoe Diana Draelos

Part V • Noninvasive and Minimally Invasive Therapy

16 Basics of Laser Therapy   **205**
Darrell Wayne Freeman, Ibrahim Khansa, Molly Burns Austin, Alton Jay Burns

17 Ablative Laser Resurfacing   **212**
Darrell Wayne Freeman, Molly Burns Austin, Alton Jay Burns

18 Nonablative Laser Resurfacing   **223**
Ibrahim Khansa, Molly Burns Austin, Alton Jay Burns

19 Chemical Peels   **231**
George Broughton II, Ahmed M. Hashem, Christopher Chase Surek, James E. Zins

20 Dermabrasion   **259**
George Broughton II, James L. Baker, Jr.

21 Botulinum Toxin   **269**
Joshua Lemmon, Smita R. Ramanadham, Miles Graivier

22 Soft Tissue Fillers   **280**
Ashkan Ghavami, Miles Graivier

23 FAT GRAFTING   297
George Broughton II, Sydney R. Coleman

24 TREATMENT OF PROMINENT VEINS   313
Edward J. Ruane, Girish S. Munavalli

PART VI • ADJUNCTS TO AESTHETIC SURGERY

25 TISSUE GLUES   323
Joseph Meyerson, Renato Saltz

26 FIXATION DEVICES   329
Brian H. Gander, Renato Saltz

27 IMPLANTS AND ALLOPLASTS (NONBREAST)   335
Jason K. Potter, Edward O. Terino

28 PROGRESSIVE TENSION SUTURES   344
Terri A. Zomerlei, Todd A. Pollock, Harlan Pollock

PART VII • FACIAL SURGERY

29 PERIORBITAL ANATOMY   355
Jason K. Potter, Grant Gilliland

30 FACE AND NECK ANATOMY   372
John H. Hulsen, Jeffrey E. Janis

31 FACIAL ANALYSIS   390
Janae L. Kittinger, Raman C. Mahabir

32 HAIR TRANSPLANTATION   402
Michelle Coriddi, Jeffrey E. Janis, Alfonso Barrera

33 BROWLIFT   411
Joshua Lemmon, Michael R. Lee, David M. Knize

34 UPPER BLEPHAROPLASTY   429
Ashkan Ghavami, Foad Nahai

35 LOWER BLEPHAROPLASTY   451
Jason K. Potter, Ted H. Wojno

36 ASIAN BLEPHAROPLASTY   462
Jerome H. Liu, Richard Y. Ha, Lily Daniali, William Pai-Dei Chen

37 CORRECTION OF THE TEAR TROUGH DEFORMITY   482
Jason K. Potter, Grant Gilliland

38 LATERAL CANTHOPEXY   490
Jason K. Potter, Steve Fagien

39 BLEPHAROPTOSIS   498
Jason E. Leedy, Jordan P. Farkas

40 MIDFACE REJUVENATION   509
Sumeet Sorel Teotia, Sami U. Khan, Foad Nahai

41 PERIORAL REJUVENATION   528
Alexey M. Markelov, Molly Burns Austin, Alton Jay Burns

42 FACELIFT   540
Adam H. Hamawy, Dino R. Elyassnia

43 NASOLABIAL FOLD   551
Sumeet Sorel Teotia, Maristella S. Evangelista

44 NECKLIFT   565
Sumeet Sorel Teotia, Foad Nahai

45 RHINOPLASTY   581
Ashkan Ghavami, Jeffrey E. Janis, Bahman Guyuron

46 SECONDARY RHINOPLASTY   620
Richard Y. Ha, Lily Daniali, Cecilia Alejandra Garcia de Mitchell, Bahman Guyuron

47 ETHNIC RHINOPLASTY   634
Paul N. Afrooz, Dean M. Toriumi

48 LIP AUGMENTATION   645
Michael Larsen, Robert K. Sigal

49 GENIOPLASTY   676
Ashkan Ghavami, Bahman Guyuron

50 OTOPLASTY   691
Joseph M. Brown, Jeffrey E. Janis, Charles H. Thorne

PART VIII ▪ BREAST SURGERY

51 BREAST ANATOMY   711
Melissa A. Crosby, Glyn Jones

52 BREAST AUGMENTATION   723
Evan B. Katzel, Thornwell H. Parker III, Jeffrey E. Janis, Dennis C. Hammond

53 MASTOPEXY   751
Joshua Lemmon, Smita R. Ramanadham, James Christian Grotting

54 AUGMENTATION-MASTOPEXY   763
Purushottam A. Nagarkar

55 BREAST REDUCTION   769
Joshua Lemmon, Michael R. Lee, Daniel O. Beck, Elizabeth Hall-Findlay

56 GYNECOMASTIA   789
Ronald E. Hoxworth, Kuylhee Kim, Dennis C. Hammond

PART IX ▪ BODY CONTOURING

57 LIPOSUCTION   799
Cedric L. Hunter, Rohit K. Khosla, Jeffrey R. Claiborne, Simeon H. Wall, Jr.

58 BRACHIOPLASTY   818
Tyler M. Angelos, Jeffrey E. Janis, Constantino G. Mendieta

59 BUTTOCK AUGMENTATION   828
Sammy Sinno, Constantino G. Mendieta

60 ABDOMINOPLASTY   837
Wesley N. Sivak, Luis M. Rios, Jr., James Christian Grotting

61 MEDIAL THIGH LIFT   856
Wendy Chen, Jeffrey A. Gusenoff

62 BODY CONTOURING IN MASSIVE-WEIGHT-LOSS PATIENTS   869
Jeff Chang, Rohit K. Khosla, Joseph Hunstad

63 FEMALE GENITAL AESTHETIC SURGERY   887
Phillip D. Khan, Christine Hamori

64 NONINVASIVE BODY CONTOURING   927
Michael Bykowski, Derek Ulvila, Spero J. Theodorou, Christopher T. Chia

65 AESTHETICS OF GENDER AFFIRMATION SURGERY   934
Juan L. Rendon, Christopher J. Salgado

CREDITS   957

INDEX   965

Essentials of
Aesthetic Surgery

PART I

Basic Considerations

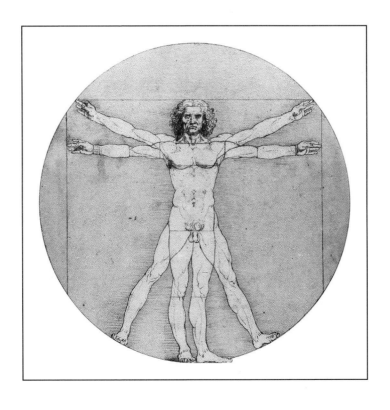

PART I

Basic Considerations

1. The Aesthetic Surgery Patient

Adam H. Hamawy, Foad Nahai

> **SENIOR AUTHOR TIP:** Cosmetic surgery is elective and rarely addresses medical conditions, but it restores or improves physical features that are concerning to patients. Although the request for aesthetic surgery is most commonly associated with aging, some patients seek improvement of normal anatomic structures to enhance their appearance.

DEMOGRAPHICS AND STATISTICS[1,2]

- Interest in cosmetic procedures continues to increase with over $15 million spent annually in the United States for combined surgical and nonsurgical procedures.
- 91% are women, and 9% are men.
- Approximately 25% of cosmetic patients are minorities.
- Approximately 40% of cosmetic patients are 35-55 years of age.
- Approximately 50% of patients have multiple procedures.
  - >50% of patients who have a cosmetic procedure will return for another one.
  - 47% of patients have multiple procedures performed simultaneously.

ROLE OF THE AESTHETIC SURGEON

- Is a **physician first** and an aesthetic surgeon second
- Acts as a physician, therapist, and artist:
  - **Physician:** Evaluates the patient to determine surgical feasibility and medical fitness
  - **Therapist:** Recognizes psychology that may be amplified by surgery
  - **Artist:** Considers aesthetic objectives. Will not go against aesthetic sense
- Must have a clear understanding of patient's motivation and expectations before surgery
- Ultimately concerned with the patient's welfare
- An experienced aesthetic surgeon should be able to recognize **body dysmorphic disorder** and **severe depression.** Many patients seeking aesthetic surgery are excellent candidates and do well postoperatively despite taking antidepressants.[3]
- A well-informed patient is a happy patient.

PATIENT CHARACTERISTICS

- **The shopper:** Consults several surgeons before making decision, compares factors such as prices, staff, availability, reputation, website, and online reputation
- **The talker:** Takes considerable time during consultation and may have many questions about multiple problems
- **The planner:** Has already decided exactly what he or she wants and is looking to see if surgeon can do it
- **The listener:** Does not talk much and wants surgeon to explain everything and make the decisions

PATIENT CONSULTATION

INTRODUCTION AND FIRST IMPRESSION
- Patients may be nervous and insecure about their appearance.
- Personal conversation at the beginning of the consultation helps to relax patients and establish rapport.
- The surgeon should begin immediately assessing the patient's general appearance, demeanor, and behavior during the initial interaction.
- The initial introduction should also establish why the patient is there to see the surgeon and what their aesthetic concerns are.
- Psychological and physical evaluation begins with the first impression.[4]

> **SENIOR AUTHOR TIP:**   Today most patients come in for a consultation having researched on the Internet and most likely consulted with other physicians. After an introduction and "small talk" designed to put patients at ease, I will ask how much they know about the procedure they are interested in. After they respond, I will add that I will provide them all the information I feel is important in making a decision.

HEALTH HISTORY
- Baseline health, comorbidities, tobacco use, prior surgeries, and prior pregnancies are determined.
- Surgical risk is carefully assessed based on medical history and desired procedure.
- Health criteria for aesthetic surgery should be at least as stringent as those for reconstructive cases because of the strictly elective nature.
- Surgery may be deemed inappropriate for unhealthy patients and those with a high risk of complications.

> **SENIOR AUTHOR TIP:**   Patients often ask me if they are too old for a facelift. I tell them there is no such thing as "too old for a procedure"; it is not age that counts but general health. The question should be, "Am I healthy enough for a facelift?" I am also asked, "Am I too young for a facelift." My answer is that there is no set age. If I think the patient will see an improvement, I will recommend a facelift regardless of age.

> **SENIOR AUTHOR TIP:**   I find some patients are not always forthcoming about health issues for fear of being turned down. For facial rejuvenation, I usually ask about smoking history. If they say, "I do not smoke," I will ask if they ever have in the past and, if so, for how long and how heavily. I repeatedly ask about high blood pressure, because I believe untreated and or unrecognized hypertension is the major contributing factor to hematoma after facial rejuvenation. When patients are asked about prior surgery, most may not list cosmetic surgery. I specifically ask every patient if they had previous aesthetic procedures.

PSYCHOLOGICAL EVALUATION[4]

- A significant proportion of patients desiring cosmetic surgery may have some psychopathology.
  - Cosmetic surgery may improve symptoms in some patients with psychological conditions like depression or neurosis.
  - Certain groups consistently are shown to do poorly after aesthetic procedures.
- Aesthetic surgeons should be able to identify psychologically unfit patients and make suitable recommendations.[5] *Psychiatric consultation should be obtained when appropriate.*
- Aesthetic surgeons determine how closely a patient's self-image matches the true image and decide if the patient's self-image can be improved with surgery performed on the true image.[6]

> **SENIOR AUTHOR TIP:**   I like to determine the motivation behind the desire for surgery. Is the patient doing this for himself or herself? Are there hidden agendas such as saving a failing marriage, wishing to please a partner or parent? I advise my patients they should do it for themselves and not for anyone else. An otherwise excellent surgical result may lead to patient disappointment if it does not meet the hidden agenda. A more youthful face or shapely body may not save a failing marriage or push a boyfriend or girlfriend into a proposal. Why patients seek a procedure and who they are trying to please may not always be readily apparent, but it is important for surgeons to know.

PSYCHOLOGICAL INDICATORS

- **Positive indicators (green light)**
  - Patient has anatomic flaw that is visible to both the patient and the surgeon.
  - Patient is not preoccupied with flaw and has been planning cosmetic surgery for a long time.
  - Patient generally feels good about himself or herself, is aging, and wants to look younger.
- **Negative indicators (red flags)**
  - Patient complains of anatomic flaws that the aesthetic surgeon does not perceive.
  - Patient is attempting to fix a social problem by surgically correcting appearance.
  - Patient impulsively decided on cosmetic surgery and has considered it for only a brief period of time.
  - Patient had multiple cosmetic procedures and is always dissatisfied with the results.
  - Patient has excessively "shopped" for surgeons. Patients who are still uncertain after meeting with three or more surgeons are often difficult and unhappy after surgery.
  - Patient is being treated for multiple psychiatric illnesses and/or history of numerous psychiatric admissions.

MOTIVATION

- Intensity of motivation positively correlates with satisfaction and shorter recovery and negatively correlates with postoperative pain.
- Patients seeking cosmetic surgery are motivated by **internal** or **external** pressures.
  - Patients with **internal motives** are generally better candidates than those with external motives.
  - Patients with internal motives desire change for themselves and usually feel vulnerable about deficits in appearance and a commitment to physical change.

- Psychological state is secondary to a definite physical defect. Correction of the defect alleviates the anxiety.
- Perceived physical deficit may not be easy to discern from genuine deficit.

CAUTION: If a perceived deficit is a major focus and is out of proportion with the genuine deficit, then the patient may find another focus to channel anxiety after surgical correction.

- Patients with **external motives** seek to please others who think that physical change will result in a social change (e.g., improve a relationship, save a marriage, advance a career).
  - ▶ Social goals are often not met, resulting in dissatisfaction with surgery.
  - ▶ May be pressured into the procedure and passive about surgery
  - ▶ Motivation levels are weaker if not also driven internally and may indicate a more difficult postoperative course.

PSYCHOLOGICAL CONDITIONS
- **Depression**[7-9]
  - The **most commonly** encountered psychological disorder in cosmetic patients
  - Can be transient as a reaction to grief or a persistent pathological process. Patients have minimal joy and poor motivation and consistently appear tired.
  - When treated and controlled, depressed patients make great surgical candidates and may show additional improvement of symptoms with cosmetic surgery.

SENIOR AUTHOR TIP: A significant number of my patients undergoing facial rejuvenation take antidepressants. They do well and recover as rapidly and are as pleased as those who do not take antidepressants. Though concerns have been raised that selective serotonin reuptake inhibitor (SSRI) antidepressants may increase the risk of hematoma, this has not been my experience.

- **Personality disorders**
  - *Personality disorders present usually with behavioral issues.* Some personality disorders are not well suited for cosmetic surgery, and psychiatric evaluations may be warranted before proceeding.
  - **Narcissistic patients** take good care of their appearance and are obsessed with subtle or unperceived imperfections. They have pompous opinions of themselves and are often "name droppers." They are prone to postoperative depression and dissatisfaction.
  - **Histrionic patients** are emotional and have an intense need for attention. They have volatile emotional responses and may laugh or cry easily. They use their emotional displays to control others. They are usually noncompliant with instructions and late to appointments and may be difficult for staff to work with. During evaluation, a histrionic patient will seek praise, approval, and reassurance.
  - **Schizoid patients** are socially withdrawn and eccentric. They are unable to maintain eye contact, have a flat affect, and are unable to relax during the evaluation. They make few comments and do not elaborate on their responses. They are vague and unable to give a specific goal for desiring cosmetic surgery. For example, a patient might explain the reason for desiring surgery as, "I just want to look that way."

- Patients with a **paranoid personality** are preoccupied with suspicion and have unjustifiable cynicism about others. They present themselves as victims and blame others for any misfortune. They usually are secretive and can be argumentative and moralistic. During evaluation they may be very guarded and businesslike with difficulty relaxing.
- **Neurotic patients** are characterized by being exceptionally concerned or anxious, having somatic complaints. They usually ask multiple, repetitive questions and expect detailed, technical responses. They are often obsessed and well read about all possible complications. A neurotic patient will get very defensive if not addressed seriously. But, with reassurance and proper preoperative counseling, they are usually good surgical candidates and are happy with the results.
- **Body dysmorphic disorder**
  - Characterized by:
    - Preoccupation with slight or imagined flaws in appearance
    - Excessively time consuming
    - Results in a significant disruption of their lives
  - Estimated incidence is 0.2% of the general population but **much higher (2%-7%) in patients requesting aesthetic surgery**
  - The body as a whole or specific anatomic areas, such as the face, nose, ears, breasts, or genitals perceived as flaws
  - Often think others are taking special notice of their imagined or slight deficits
  - Take constant precautions to hide their focus of concern with clothing, makeup, and body position
  - May accompany other disorders, including major depression, obsessive-compulsive disorder, and eating disorders

CAUTION: Patients with body dysmorphic disorder are rarely satisfied, and symptoms may be exacerbated with cosmetic surgery. Therefore cosmetic surgery is contraindicated, and patients should be referred for psychiatric care.

> **SENIOR AUTHOR TIP:**   A thorough evaluation of a patient's motivation and mental state, as described above, is essential and a predictor of patient behavior postoperatively. Turning down or referring patients for psychological evaluation is rare in my practice. Referral for evaluation has to be handled delicately so a patient does not have the impression that I think he or she is unstable. Turning down a patient also has to be handled with sensitivity. I tell the few patients I turn down that I am aware of their concerns but do not think I am able to address them to their satisfaction.

PHYSICAL EVALUATION

- A patient's physical appearance must correlate with the health history.
- A focused physical examination of the area of concern, with objective documentation of any deviation from the aesthetic norm, is performed and appropriate measurements are obtained when possible.
- Adjacent anatomic areas are examined to determine whether they contribute to the aesthetic flaw.
- Patients seeking cosmetic surgery of the breasts or body should disrobe appropriately to allow a complete examination. Surgeons should be cautious with patients who will not disrobe to allow proper examination.

> **TIP:** A chaperone should always be in the room during the physical examination of sensitive body areas.

- Any physical deformities, scars, flaws, or asymmetries are clearly identified to the patient and documented.

REJECTION
- After psychological and physical evaluation, surgical eligibility can be decided (Fig. 1-1).

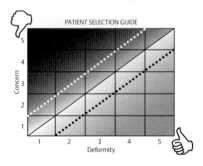

Fig. 1-1 Surgical eligibility guide. The vertical axis represents the degree of the patient's concern regarding the problem, from 1 (minimal) to 5 (maximal). The horizontal axis represents the surgeon's objective evaluation of the nature of the complaint, from 1 (minimal) to 5 (maximal). Most applicants are categorized within the area between the diagonal *dotted lines*. The closer to the upper left corner, the more likely the possibility of patient dissatisfaction regardless of quality of result. The converse is true of patients categorized in the lower right corner. From experience, we suggest keeping this scheme on the back page of each patient's record in simple diagrammatic form with no written explanation after the first visit. If a patient returns after researching other surgeons and websites, this record will help a surgeon or an associate remember original impressions. Experience shows that this helps to keep us out of trouble.

- **Aesthetic surgeons should refuse to proceed with surgery if:**
  - The aesthetic flaw is **not visible** to the surgeon.
  - The aesthetic flaw **cannot be corrected** by surgery.
  - The **risk of failure is greater than the risk of success.**
  - The **surgical goals are unclear.**
  - The patient has **unrealistic expectations.**
  - The patient's comorbidities deem them to be **unsafe** for elective surgery.
- Aesthetic surgeons should listen to their instincts and not proceed if they are uneasy about the patient or the surgery.
- For patients with unrealistic goals, surgeons should attempt to clarify that these results are not achievable.

> **TIP:** To prevent confrontation, if a persistent patient insists on proceeding with surgery, the surgeon can claim that he or she is not able to achieve the desired results.

PREPARING FOR SURGERY

- **Effective communication** is critical in preventing disappointment postoperatively.
- Surgical options for achieving desired goals specific recommendations are given in a language that patients can easily understand.
- Patients are informed about what to expect after surgery.
  - Thorough counseling on all risks of the procedure
  - Clear description of the location and length of expected scars
  - Realistic timeline for recovery and downtime
  - Express guarantees should *not* be made.
  - All discussions documented, with detailed informed consent forms
- **Photography is an essential tool** for preoperative planning and documentation of surgical alteration.
  - It is the only postoperative record of a patient's preoperative appearance for comparison.
  - Photographs can be used to demonstrate the aesthetic deformity to the patient from multiple views that are not possible to observe in a mirror.

CAUTION: Surgeons should be cautious of patients who will not allow preoperative photographs to be taken.

- Preoperative imaging, testing, and/or medical clearance are arranged, as indicated.
- If appropriate, it may be necessary to see the patient again before operating to ensure understanding, review preoperative testing and consultation results, and answer additional concerns or questions.

> **SENIOR AUTHOR TIP:**   Patients like to have lists of dos and don'ts before surgery. Video imaging has proved a useful tool in my practice, not only to show patients what the anticipated result might be, but also to indicate to me the patient's expectations.
>
> Most patients think that plastic surgery and cosmetic surgery in particular leave no scars! I emphasize the length and location of the scars while explaining that our goal is to place the scars to be least noticed.

OPERATIVE AND FOLLOW-UP CARE

THE DAY OF SURGERY

- **In the holding area**
  - The patient is examined and marked preoperatively.
    - ▶ Markings are made before patients are sedated.
    - ▶ Having a private room with a mirror where the patient can see and confirm the markings is helpful.
    - ▶ Additional photographs of the markings can be helpful.
  - Final questions about the procedure and recovery are answered.
  - The patient and accompanying family are reassured. It is normal for them to be nervous and have last-minute reservations.
  - All operative goals are restated.

> **SENIOR AUTHOR TIP:** After explaining the procedure again, describing the scars, and marking the patient, I always ask if we left anything out. Are we adding anything? Too many patients wake up thinking they had less performed than they had requested, and some ask, while being prepped preoperatively, that we remove moles or undertake separate aesthetic procedures.
>
> I always tell the family that I will personally come out and talk with or call them after the procedure. I also add that if we finish before the estimated time, it does not mean I rushed through the procedure, and if it takes longer, it does not mean that the patient or I had a problem. For long procedures or and those that take longer than scheduled, I ask the circulating nurse to call and update the family.

- **In the operating room**
  - The patient is covered to maintain modesty and provide warmth.
  - Soft music can have a calming effect and may help the patient relax before induction.
  - The waiting family is frequently given progress reports.
  - A clean and neat dressing is carefully applied to cover the surgical site.

> **SENIOR AUTHOR TIP:** I always like to be in the operating room and if appropriate hold the patient's hand as anesthesia is being induced. A time-out is mandatory for all surgeries, even cosmetic ones.

- **After surgery**
  - Reassuring and talking with the patient in the recovery room is important.
  - The surgeon should visit the waiting spouse or family or call them if they are not readily available.
  - The patient is seen again before discharge or that evening in the room if he or she is staying overnight.
  - **Specific written and oral instructions are given.** Being repetitive with the patient and family is essential.
  - The patient is called that evening at home or in the hospital room.

POSTOPERATIVE CARE
- Patients are seen within 1 or 2 days or called at home postoperatively for a progress report.
- Surgeons should be present and perform the first dressing change if possible.
- Patients are reassured that wounds are healing normally.
- Patients are typically seen at 1, 3, 6, and 12 months, then annually, assuming no complications.
- Photos are obtained at 6-12 months postoperatively.
- Progress of long-term results is explained.

RECOVERY AFTER COSMETIC SURGERY
- **The "Healing Curve"**
  - Patients will not see their final results immediately.
  - Depending on the procedure, results become apparent in a week (injecting fillers) or up to 1 year (rhinoplasty).
  - Patients are informed of the expected time course for resolution before surgery and at each follow-up visit (Figs. 1-2 and 1-3).

- Edema and ecchymosis are to be expected after any procedure.
- Surgeons should give reassurance that results will continue to improve over time, as appropriate.
- **Emotional response**
  - ▶ Patients can be expected to feel different emotions as they recover from cosmetic surgery.

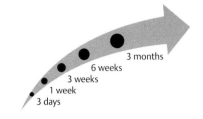

Fig. 1-2   Physical recovery. Times may vary depending on the procedure.

  - ▶ Listening to the patients' concerns and maintaining a calm demeanor to reassure them what is normal are essential.
  - ▶ Patients commonly feel a wide range of emotions in the postoperative period, characterized by the following commonly heard comments:
    - ◆ **Week 1:** "I wish it was a month from now."
      - – Days 1-3: "I'm beat." Patient is exhausted, sleepy.
      - – Days 4-7: "What did I do?" Patient is sad, irritated, angry.

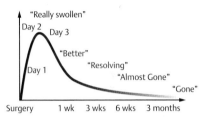

Fig. 1-3   Edema curve. The time range may vary depending on the procedure.

    - ◆ **Week 2:** "You should have told me about..." Patient is critical, nitpicky, scared, impatient, complaining.
    - ◆ **Week 3:** "Not too bad..." Patient begins to normalize and see results.
    - ◆ **Weeks 4-5:** "You look great." Patient notices others' reactions and compliments and begins to feel good about surgery.
    - ◆ **Weeks 6-8:** "But what about..." As most of the swelling and bruising resolve, some focal areas may lag in recovery or may not appear as expected.
    - ◆ **Weeks 8-12:** "Wow, I love it."
    - ◆ **After 3-6 months:** "What's next?"

SENIOR AUTHOR TIP: Surgeons should be supportive with patients who have a complication or delayed recovery, seeing and calling them often, and explaining the course of their care as the problem resolves. I reassure patients with complications that we will see them through it, and that in all likelihood it will not affect the final result.

MAINTENANCE COUNSELING
- **Maintenance counseling** will improve patient satisfaction in the long term and allow patients to be a partner in the aesthetic improvement process.
- Keeping a healthy lifestyle and sustaining good habits will augment the results of cosmetic procedures beyond what can be achieved surgically.
- Information for physical training and nutritional counseling is provided, if needed.
- **A skin care regimen for facial procedures is essential** in enhancing the results and preserving longevity.

REVISIONS

- A clear, documented revision policy should be agreed on **before surgery.**
- Adequate time for healing and resolution of edema is allowed before considering revision. The following timeframes are useful guidelines:
  - **Body contouring:** Wait at least 6 months
  - **Rhinoplasty:** Wait at least 12 months
  - **Blepharoplasty:** Wait 3-6 months
  - **Facelift:** Wait 6-12 months
  - **Breast:** Wait at least 3 months
- Surgeons should "see" and clearly understand what needs to be revised and the expected goals of revision.
- Patients should have **realistic expectations** of what can be achieved with a revision.

TOP TAKEAWAYS

➤ Contrary to the perception of most patients, aesthetic surgery and cosmetic medicine is not a commodity. It is a very personal service based on a professional relationship between the patient and surgeon—a partnership based on mutual trust, mutual respect, and a common goal.

➤ As surgeons, we have different personalities, bedside manners, experience, surgical skills, and aesthetic sense.

➤ Our patients are also as varied as we are, with different personalities and differing expectations.

➤ Most patients shop around and pick a surgeon based on price, reputation, bedside manner, and qualifications, usually in that order. In short, they choose a surgeon they are "comfortable" with. Similarly, operating on patients with whom we are not comfortable or have not established rapport preoperatively will lead to a difficult postoperative course if problems occur.

REFERENCES

1. 2016 Cosmetic Surgery National Databank Statistics. American Society for Aesthetic Plastic Surgery. Available at *http://www.surgery.org/sites/default/files/ASAPS-Stats2016.pdf.*
2. 2015 Plastic Surgery Statistics Report. American Society of Plastic Surgeons. Available at *https://d2wirczt3b6wjm.cloudfront.net/News/Statistics/2015/plastic-surgery-statistics-full-report-2015.pdf.*
3. Rohrich RJ. Streamlining cosmetic surgery patient selection—just say no! Plast Reconstr Surg 104:220, 1999.
4. Rohrich RJ. The who, what, when, and why of cosmetic surgery: do our patients need a preoperative psychiatric evaluation? Plast Reconstr Surg 106:1605, 2000.
5. Gorney M. Recognition and management of the patient unsuitable for aesthetic surgery. Plast Reconstr Surg 126:2268, 2010.
6. Ferraro GA, Rossano F, D'Andrea F. Self-perception and self-esteem of patients seeking cosmetic surgery. Aesthetic Plast Surg 29:184, 2005.
7. Nahai F. Evaluating the cosmetic patient on antidepressants. Aesthet Surg J 34:326, 2014.
8. Nahai F. What is aesthetic surgery, anyway? Aesthet Surg J 30:874, 2010.
9. Nahai F, ed. The Art of Aesthetic Surgery: Principles and Techniques, ed 2. New York: Thieme Publishers, 2010.

2.   The Artistry of Plastic Surgery

Sumeet Sorel Teotia, Mark B. Constantian

Nature's paradigm for survival relies to a great extent on the concept of *beauty*. Ultimately, evolution requires successful survival of a species, animal or plant, through nature's own rules of beauty: harmony, balance, and symmetry. An overarching study of beauty lends itself to the philosophical comprehension of *aesthetics*—a field dedicated to the art and understanding of beauty and good taste. Thus the study of beauty through scientific methods is an effort toward explaining aesthetics.

AESTHETICS AND ITS ASSOCIATION

- Often refers to the study and philosophy of **beauty** and **taste**
- Origin from Greek word, *aisthetikos,* implying "sensitive, relating to perception of the sense," which in turn derives from *aisthánomai,* implying "I sense and feel."
- The field of aesthetics—thus our understanding of beauty—changes in each stage of human civilization and evolution.
  - What is acceptable as the "ideal" beauty has evolved.
  - Classical female beauty is much different from the "cover girl" concepts of beauty of the modern world, which influence aesthetic medicine.
- **Aesthetic medicine** comprises several disciplines whose goal is **to improve the cosmetic appearance of patients.**
  - The rise of aesthetic medicine and surgery in modern times has an increasing relationship to the science of aesthetic medicine and the safety of invasive and noninvasive procedures.
  - Social acceptance of aesthetic procedures continues to evolve among the sexes and various cultures.
  - Clinical and psychological studies have shown an **overall sense of well-being** of patients who seek aesthetic procedures.[1-3]

BEAUTY AND ITS CONCEPTS

ANCIENT CONCEPTS IN BEAUTY

- Symbols of ancient beauty can be found in early civilizations such as Egypt and Troy and are unavoidable when we study Western beauty.
  - Arguably, some modern concepts of beauty were influenced by what we think was considered beautiful in ancient Egypt.
  - Two most powerful and ubiquitous symbols of Western beauty originate from two queens of antiquity: Cleopatra and Nefertiti.
    - ▶ **Cleopatra** has been known as the paragon of beauty, ever since Roman conquest of Egypt.

► **Nefertiti's** emergence came after her painted bust was discovered in 1912.
  ♦ She was the little-known wife of Pharaoh Akhenaten.
  ♦ The logo for the American Society for Aesthetic Plastic Surgery (ASAPS) is Nefertiti (Fig. 2-1).
• Ancient Egyptians provided vast information indicating that both sexes went to great lengths to improve their appearance.
  ► Based on ubiquitous beauty products left by ancient Egyptians in burial and around mummies
    ♦ Use of **kohl** as eye makeup in ancient Egypt perhaps gave rise to the smoky eye makeup worn today.
    ♦ Kohl, a mineral base composed of lead, may have antibacterial properties.
    ♦ Perhaps the use of kohl by both sexes was to reduce glare from the sun, thus providing not only a function, but also beauty.

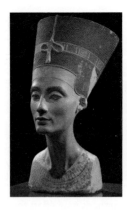

Fig. 2-1 Bust of Nefertiti.

• The **symbolism** of beauty perhaps is even more powerful than the subject itself, even when we consider "beauty" in ancient terms.
  ► Plutarch (ancient Greek philosopher) described Cleopatra as having a strong voice and vivacity, and not necessarily beauty.
  ► On ancient coins, Cleopatra is depicted as having a big nose, protruding chin, and wrinkled face—hardly what one would call *beautiful* in any era.
  ► Yet we have decided that "Cleopatra" represents a powerful message for beauty.
■ Ancient Greeks described what we know as earliest Western theories of beauty:
  • Pre-Socratic philosophers such as **Pythagorus** offered concepts of beauty in mathematical terms.
  • Pythagoreans saw an innate connection between beauty and mathematics.
    ► They noted that the **"golden ratio"** embodied proportions considered to be beautiful.
  • Early Greek architecture relied on establishing **symmetry** and **proportion,** thereby evoking harmony and beauty, and Aristotle saw that the goal of virtue was to obtain beauty.
  • **Euclid,** a Greek mathematician, recorded in his treatise, *Elements,* the definition of *golden ratio:*
    ► He described cutting a line "in extreme and mean ratio"—what we now call the *golden ratio.*

GOLDEN RATIO
■ Also known as the *golden mean* or *golden proportion*
■ Mathematically, two quantities are in the **golden ratio** if their **ratio** is the same as the ratio of their **sum** to the larger of the two quantities.
  • In algebra, for any numbers *a* and *b* with a>b>0, the golden ratio is:

$$(a + b)/a = a/b = \phi$$

  • The golden ratio can be geometrically described using the golden rectangle, and thus is easier to understand (Fig. 2-2).

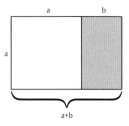

Fig. 2-2   The golden rectangle generates the golden ratio, phi (Φ). A golden rectangle consists of a square and a rectangle. The square (white) has four sides with a length of 'a.' The rectangle (red) has two sides with lengths of 'a' and two sides with lengths of 'b.' When the rectangle is placed next to the square with both 'a' lengths adjacent, the two shapes together generate a golden rectangle. In the golden rectangle, side 'a+b' and side 'a' generate phi (Φ).

- In decimal system, the golden ratio is represented by 1.6180339887498948482...
- Mark Barr, a twentieth-century mathematician, proposed φ to designate the golden mean, based on Greek sculptor **Phidias**, who is credited as having built the Parthenon.
- The **platonic solids** (cube, tetrahedron, octahedron, dodecahedron, and icosahedron) have some correlation to the golden ratio.
- **Fibonacci numbers** also reflect and are intimately connected with the golden ratio
  ▶ Fibonacci, also known as *Leonardo of Pisa,* was an Italian mathematician, who in 1202 in his book *Liber Abaci* introduced the number sequence named after him.
  ▶ The Fibonacci numbers are integers in the following sequence, known as *the Fibonacci sequence:*
    ◆ 0, 1, 1, 2, 3, 5, 8, 13, 21, 34, 55, 89, 144...
    ◆ These numbers are defined by the following recurrence relation:
    $$F_n = F_{n-1} + F_{n-2}$$
  ▶ Besides use in theoretical mathematics, Fibonacci numbers, in conjunction with golden ratio, are extremely popular and have been used in various fields, including art, music, sculpture, and architecture.
  ▶ Fibonacci sequences appear in nature (Fig. 2-3):
    ◆ Leaf arrangement on a stem
    ◆ Pineapple fruitlets
    ◆ Artichoke flowering
    ◆ Pine cone arrangement

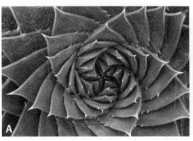
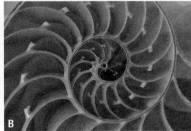

Fig. 2-3   Fibonacci sequences in nature. **A,** Fibonacci leaf pattern in nature. **B,** Cross section of nautilus depicting Fibonacci spiral.

- Luca Pacioli, Italian mathematician of Renaissance period and a colleague of Leonardo da Vinci, explored the mathematics of golden ratio as it related to art.
  ▶ Published *De Divina Proportione* (The Divine Proportion) in 1509; defined *golden ratio* as the "divine proportion"[4]

▸ Leonardo da Vinci was the illustrator of the book
▸ Description of golden ratio was tied to Vitruvian explanation of proportion (see Fig. 2-4).

THE VITRUVIAN MAN

■ The *Vitruvian Man*, by Leonardo da Vinci, was inspired by writings of **Marcus Vitruvius Pollio**, an ancient Roman architect and engineer.
• Pen and ink drawing interpreting Vitruvius' work on proportions of human body, created circa 1490 (Fig. 2-4)
• da Vinci drew various drawings for Pacioli's book, and they often collaborated.

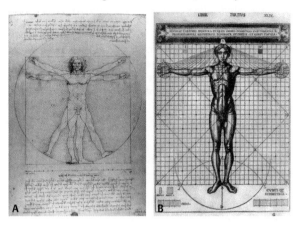

Fig. 2-4   Vitruvian Man.

■ Many refer to this drawing as "the proportion of man."
■ Even though the drawing has been connected with the golden ratio, the proportions of the figure in reality do not match 1.618033 . . . and da Vinci only mentioned whole number ratios.
■ The drawing is based on ideal geometric human proportions as related to geometric principles outlined by Vitruvius in his extensive treatise, *De Architectura.*[5]
■ He determined that the **human body** is the principle source of proportion among the classical order of architecture.
• Vitruvius asserted that a structure must have qualities of *firmitas, utilitas,* and *venustas*—solidness, usefulness, and beauty, known as **Vitruvian Triad.**
• Vitruvius defined the Vitruvian Man to have the ideal proportions, because the Greeks thought the human form was the greatest work of art.
• Vitruvius wrote about the proportion of man:
▸ *"Just so the parts of Temples should correspond with each other, and with the whole. The navel is naturally placed in the centre of the human body, and, if in a man lying with his face upward, and his hands and feet extended, from his navel as the centre, a circle be described, it will touch his fingers and toes. It is not alone by a circle, that the human body is thus circumscribed, as may be seen by placing it within a square. For measuring from the feet to the crown of the head, and then across the arms fully extended, we find the latter measure equal to the former; so that lines at right angles to each other, enclosing the figure, will form a square."*

■ The following text is stated above and below da Vinci's drawing:
- Above: *"Vetruvio, architect, puts in his work on architecture that the measurements of man are in nature distributed in this manner, that is:*
  - ▶ *A palm is four fingers*
  - ▶ *A foot is four palms*
  - ▶ *A cubit is six palms*
  - ▶ *Four cubits make a man*
  - ▶ *A pace is four cubits*
  - ▶ *A man is 24 palms*
  - ▶ *And these measurements are in his buildings"*
- Below:
  - ▶ *The length of the outspread arms is equal to the height of a man.*
  - ▶ *From the hairline to the bottom of the chin is one tenth the height of a man.*
  - ▶ *From below the chin to the top of the head is one eighth the height of a man.*
  - ▶ *From above the chest to the top of the head is one sixth the height of a man*
  - ▶ *From above the chest to the hairline is one seventh the height of a man.*
  - ▶ *The maximum width of the shoulders is a fourth the height of a man.*
  - ▶ *From the breasts to the top of the head is a fourth the height of a man.*
  - ▶ *The distance from the elbow to the tip of the hand is a fourth the height of a man.*
  - ▶ *The distance from the elbow to the armpit is an eighth the height of a man.*
  - ▶ *The length of the hand is a tenth the height of a man.*
  - ▶ *The root of the penis is at half the height of a man.*
  - ▶ *The foot is a seventh the height of a man.*
  - ▶ *From below the foot to below the knee is a fourth the height of a man.*
  - ▶ *From below the knee to the root of the penis is a fourth the height of a man.*
  - ▶ *The distances from below the chin to the nose and the eyebrows and the hairline are equal to the ears and to a third of the face.*

■ da Vinci's figure and interpretation of Vitruvius' work set the tone for future classical painters who were inspired by representing nature's perfection in proportion. The often-idealized figures of Renaissance painters represented the Greek ideals of symmetry, harmony, and form as they related to the human figure.

CLASSICAL CONCEPTS IN BEAUTY

■ The ideals of human beauty described by ancient Greek philosophers were rediscovered during the Renaissance.
■ The definition of *classical beauty* arose from this reemergence.
■ The "classical ideal" refers to readoption of ancient Greek idealism and the study of nature.
- Studied and redefined through imitating ancient Greek sculptures of men and women
■ "Classical beauty" is a woman who conforms to the standard Greek classical ideal, with proportion and symmetry as it relates to nature's ideal, and not necessarily "mankind's ideal."
■ One such female classical ideal was the famous statue, **Venus de Milo** (Fig. 2-5).
- The statue of Venus de Milo is marble and exhibited in Paris, France, at the Louvre.

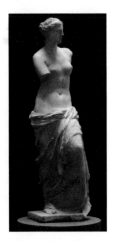

Fig. 2-5 Venus de Milo.

- Also known as *Aphrodite of Milo* in Greek; thought to be sculpted around 100 BC by Alexandros of Antioch
  - ▶ *Aphrodite:* Greek goddess of love and beauty
- Discovered by a peasant in the island of Milos in 1820
- Formerly, logo of the journal **Plastic and Reconstructive Surgery** and the seal of **American Society of Plastic Surgeons (ASPS)**[6]:
  - ▶ Designed by Charles Liedl, an artist and friend to Gustave Aufricht
  - ▶ Venus de Milo became part of ASPS during Aufricht's presidency of the Society (1944-1946).

SENIOR AUTHOR COMMENTARY: *"Just so the parts of Temples should correspond with each other, and with the whole."*

This principle articulated by Vitruvius and quoted above is key because it relies on internal aesthetics (i.e., the relationship of one part to another) rather than external ones (i.e., the relationship of one part to an external absolute). In practice, the surgeon may be guided by each of the principles described above, but at some point a compromise has to be made between what is desired and what is achievable. We never work with the anatomy that we would like, but rather the anatomy that we have been given. Rarely do neoclassical canons follow the surgeon into the operating room.

Actually, most evidence indicates that these canons do not even apply very often outside the arts. Farkas and his co-authors[7-10] assessed these ideals in white, black, and Chinese populations, and found that they rarely existed.[11] When Farkas tested "attractive" and "average" faces in North American populations against the canons, none conformed to them.

It actually appears that three components of facial attractiveness are critical: *averageness, symmetry,* and *neoteny* (juvenile features in an adult).

Averageness indicates similarity to a typical phenotype for a group and therefore signals genetic diversity (and presumably greater health and disease resistance).

Symmetry seems obvious as a characteristic of attractiveness; in fact, studies across a number of species have shown that less fluctuating asymmetry (that is, greater symmetry) is associated with both fitness and fertility.

Interestingly, it is not simple youthfulness but *neoteny* that is particularly associated with facial attractiveness. A baby's features (large eyes, small nose, round cheeks, smooth skin, glossy hair, and lighter skin tones) correlate with greater perceived attractiveness, more paternal attention, and even a lower incidence of childhood abuse. The preference for childlike facial features appears consistently across ethnic populations, regardless of sexual orientation.[9,10]

Attractiveness is also related to sexual dimorphism—that is, the degree to which a particular face resembles the prototype of his or her sex. In men, this means larger jaws and supraorbital ridges; more prominent cheekbones; smaller eyes; thinner lips; and wider, larger noses. In women, dimorphism implies prominent cheekbones; smooth, hairless skin; wider eyes; higher, thinner eyebrows; smaller jaws; fuller lips; and shorter, smaller noses. Therefore, although facial attractiveness may not always conform to *phi* or other mathematical proportions, it still derives from species-specific psychological adaptations.[11]

One of my favorite neoclassical canons not mentioned above dictates that, "the distance between the eyes equals the width of the nose." Farkas and co-authors[7,8] determined that this ideal actually occurs in only 41% of whites, 35% of Han Chinese, and only 3% of blacks. I have treated many patients in whom well-meaning surgeons tried to follow this rule and instead produced lower noses that were now disproportionately narrow for the widths of the patients' tips or bony vaults.

Therefore, when confronted with a patient whose interalar width exceeds his or her intercanthal distance and in whom narrowing would produce an unaesthetic result, these are the surgeon's practical choices:

Reduce the alar base anyway and accept a distorted result;
Move the orbits laterally; or
Ignore the rule.

I always choose the last one.

Ideal proportions and indices are harmonious and lovely—for painters and sculptors. Individual human anatomy gives much less room for surgeons to follow—and it should be our patients themselves who dictate what is normal and what they wish to change, not us. Surgeons' right brains can still guide them to optimal proportions and shapes that fit the patient's canons, the only ones that really count.

Top Takeaways
➤ Concept of beauty exists within nature's paradigm for survival
➤ Aesthetics is the field of understanding beauty.
➤ Historical scholars have given us the golden ratio as a means to study patterns in nature, art, mathematics and beauty.
➤ Plastic surgeons adapt themselves to study form and function of the human body and dedicate their careers to refine aesthetic results in both cosmetic and reconstructive surgery.
➤ Artistry in plastic surgery comes from a lifetime of dedication, education, and immersion in improving results that produce harmony.

References
1. Saariniemi KM, Helle MH, Salmi AM, et al. The effects of aesthetic breast augmentation on quality of life, psychological distress, and eating disorder symptoms: a prospective study. Aesthetic Plast Surg 36:1090, 2012.
2. Saariniemi KM, Salmi AM, Peltoniemi HH, et al. Does liposuction improve body image and symptoms of eating disorders? Plast Reconstr Surg Glob Open 3:e461, 2015.
3. Saariniemi KM, Salmi AM, Peltoniemi HH, et al. Abdominoplasty improves quality of life, psychological distress, and eating disorder symptoms: a prospective study. Plast Surg Int 2014:197232, 2014.
4. O'Connor JJ, Robertson EF. "Luca Pacioli." School of Mathematics and Statistics. University of St Andrews, 1999.
5. Rowland I, Howe TN, eds. Vitruvius. Ten Books on Architecture. Cambridge, UK: Cambridge University Press, 1999.

6. Brent B. The reconstruction of Venus: following our legacy. Plast Reconstr Surg 121:2170, 2008.
7. Farkas LG, Forrest CR, Litsas L. Revision of neoclassical facial canons in young adult Afro-Americans. Aesthetic Plast Surg 24:179, 2000.
8. Farkas LG, Hreczko TA, Kolar JC, et al. Vertical and horizontal proportions of the face in young adult North American Caucasians: revision of neoclassical canons. Plast Reconstr Surg 75:328, 1985.
9. Bashour M. History and current concepts in the analysis of facial attractiveness. Plast Reconstr Surg 118:741, 2006.
10. Bashour M. An objective system for measuring facial attractiveness. Plast Reconstr Surg 118:757, 2006.
11. Constantian MB. Rhinoplasty: Craft and Magic. New York: Thieme Publishers, 2009.

3. Photography for the Aesthetic Surgeon

Amanda Behr, Patricia Aitson, William Y. Hoffman

STANDARDIZED CLINICAL PHOTOGRAPHY

Photography is one of the most useful tools to plastic surgeons, but it can also be one of the most fallible tools. Quality clinical photography requires organization and adherence to a standard set of protocols. Lens magnification, lighting, patient preparation and positioning must all be consistent to ensure the accuracy of comparative photography. The following guidelines can help maintain consistency in photographic documentation.

> **TIP:** A standardized procedure saves time: decisions are largely predetermined by an existing set of rules.[1] Standardization requires planning, a systematic approach, adherence to protocols, and attention to detail.[2,3]

ELEMENTS OF STANDARDIZED CLINICAL PATIENT PHOTOGRAPHY

- **Consistent focal lengths and distances**
  - **Focal length** (measured in millimeters) determines how the lens brings an object into focus.
    - ▶ Longer focal length = higher magnification
    - ▶ Shorter focal length = lower magnification
  - **Focal distance** is the distance from the camera lens to the object being photographed.
  - Reference the **Cardiff Scales of Reproduction**[4] for guidelines.
- **Consistent lighting**
  - Use of dual strobe flashes in clinical setting
- **Standardized series** (a predetermined set of photographs per procedure)
  - Ensures patients will have the same views photographed each time
- Attention to detail
  - Remove jewelry, glasses, heavy makeup
  - Keep area clean
  - Use of background
- **Informed consent** is necessary before photographs can be taken.

FOCAL LENGTHS AND DISTANCES

> **NOTE:** In traditional film photography, a 35 mm image plane was a constant. In digital photography, a variety of different sizes of sensors in cameras are available. Most sensors are smaller than the size of 35 mm film, so the standards used to determine distances and magnifications in the past need to be adjusted for a digital camera.

- **Cardiff Scales of Reproduction**[2] advocate the use of lens with a focal length equal to at least **twice the diagonal of the image plane** to prevent unwanted distortion of the image.
  - Use of Cardiff Scales controls the magnification and perspective of patient photography.
  - Ensures standardization between photographs taken by different physicians and/or photographers
- Table 3-1 provides examples of the different-sized sensors and the recommended focal lengths to prevent distortion.
  - The manufacturer will supply the size of the sensor in the manual.

Table 3-1   *Sensors and Recommended Focal Lengths*

Sensor Type	Width (mm)	Height (mm)	Diagonal (mm)	Lens (mm)
1/2.7 inch	5.270	3.960	5.270	10
½ inch	6.400	4.800	8.000	20
⅔ inch	8.800	6.600	11.000	20
⅓ inch	18.000	13.500	22.500	50
35 mm film	36.000	24.000	43.300	50

- Disparities in focal lengths can make dramatic differences, especially in comparative views (Fig. 3-1).
  - Correcting for this difference to prevent unwanted distortions is essential.[4]

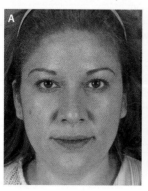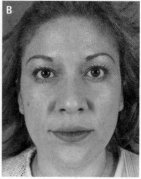

Fig. 3-1   Focal length distortion in facial features. **A,** Photograph taken using a 105 mm lens 1:10. **B,** Photograph taken with a 50 mm lens 1:10, which caused a lens distortion called a *barrel distortion.*

- A **digital SLR** (single-lens reflex) camera is recommended for clinical patient photography. These have better-quality lenses and sensors than "point-and-shoot" consumer cameras.
- The magnification of focal lengths and distances provided throughout the standardized series in this chapter are intended for photographing with a high-end, digital SLR camera with a ⅔-inch charge-coupled device (CCD) sensor.

> **SENIOR AUTHOR TIP:** For an average digital SLR camera, the multiplication factor for focal length is about 1.5×; therefore I recommend a 50-60 mm lens for facial photos and a wider one for body photos.

VARIABLES TO CONSIDER IN FACE OR NECK SERIES

All of the facial series in this chapter are intended to be photographed in addition to the standardized facelift and necklift series. There are, however, variables that exist in each face series depending on the surgical procedure. These variables are noted in each section. The following possible variations should be considered for standardized facelift and necklift series:
- Head positioning
- Oblique variables
- True lateral

HEAD POSITIONING (Fig. 3-2)
- The **Frankfort plane** is used as a reference line for correct head positioning in radiographs.
  - Some physicians have used it as a standard for head alignment when photographing the face.
  - Horizontal plane that traverses the top of the tragus (external auditory canal) across the infraorbital rim[5]
  - Can cause noticeable changes in jaw definition and submental soft tissue[6]

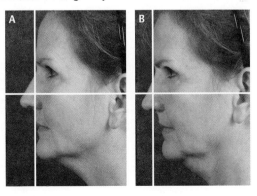

Fig. 3-2 Head positioning. **A,** Patient shown in the Frankfort plane. Neck retraction can overemphasize the degree of submental soft tissue. **B,** Patient shown in the natural horizontal facial plane.

- Some physicians choose to use the **natural horizontal facial plane** for alignment.[5]
  - Achieved when patients look straight ahead as if looking into a mirror at eye level[7]
  - Preferred for photographing plastic surgery
  - Used in patients with low-set ears[7]

OBLIQUE VARIABLES

- Preferences vary for photographing oblique views.
  - Some prefer the nasal tip to touch the opposite side of the cheek for the rhinoplasty series.
  - Some prefer the dorsum to visually touch the medial eye.
- Both views are shown in Fig. 3-3, but one may be excluded once the preferred view is chosen.

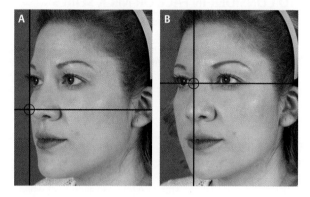

Fig. 3-3   Options for oblique views. **A,** Tip of the nose touching the side of the far cheek for a rhinoplasty series. **B,** Dorsum touching the medial eye.

TRUE LATERAL (Fig. 3-4)

■ Photographing an underrotated or overrotated head in lateral views is a common mistake.

■ Error can be corrected by viewing **straight across the two oral commissures.**[8]

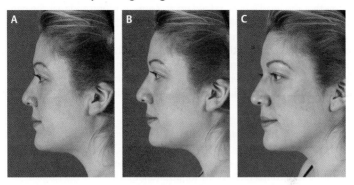

Fig. 3-4   Lateral view. **A,** Underrotation. **B,** True lateral. **C,** Overrotation.

STANDARD FACE/NECK SERIES

■ Series is photographed with a digital camera with a ⅔-inch sensor in a vertical position at a 1 m distance with an 80 mm focal length.

■ Face is typically photographed with the patient in a seated position.

TIP: Place a target on the wall for the patient to view while in the lateral position to help with standardizing the eye to radix alignment.

OBJECTIVES

■ Basis for all cosmetic procedures

■ Show anatomic relationship of whole face

■ Show anatomic bone/muscle/skin structure

■ Show skin laxity around mandible and neck

■ Show volume loss/depletion in malar area

KEY POINTS (Fig. 3-5)

- The contour of the neck can vary greatly according to the head and shoulder position.
  - Any degree of neck flexion or head retraction can greatly enhance the effect of submental fat/jowl line or, conversely, neck extension can improve the jowl line.[6]
- Make sure that the head is in the standard anatomic position and that the patient is sitting straight and not slumping.
- Have patients relax and not smile.
- Have patients remove distracting jewelry and/or heavily applied makeup.
- Fold down turtlenecks and turn collars away from the neck.
- Have patients pull hair back with neutral-colored headband.
- For oblique views, line the radix of the nose to touch the medial part of the opposite eye (see Fig. 3-3, A).
- Any slight tilting of the head can sometimes distort the view. Check the earlobe symmetry from the anterior view to determine the straightness of the head before photographing.[7]
  - Check true lateral through oral commissure alignment.
  - Use natural horizontal facial plane for positioning.

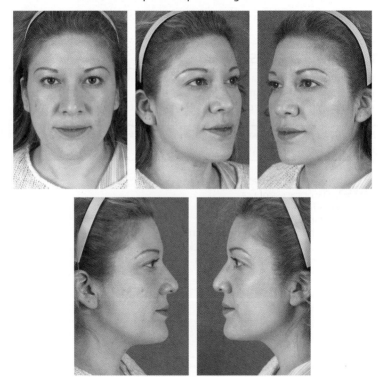

Fig. 3-5   Overview of standard face series and set distances. Some of the photographs can be eliminated, depending on the particular procedure performed.

SUPPLEMENTAL FACE/NECK VIEWS (Fig. 3-6)

- When photographing for a neck and/or face series, views can be added to show specific conditions.
  - Platysmal banding (teeth gritting)
  - Reading view (head down) which accentuates submental fat.[1]

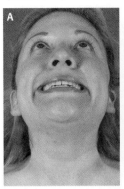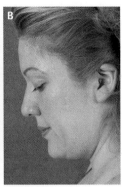

Fig. 3-6   A, View to show platysmal banding (teeth gritting). **B,** A reading view accentuates submental fat.

STANDARD BROW AND EYELID SERIES

- This series taken in addition to the standard face series.
- Patient photographed using a horizontally positioned digital camera with a ⅔-inch sensor at a 0.5 m distance with an 80 mm focal length.

OBJECTIVES

- Show brow-eye anatomic relationship to face
- Show skin laxity or excess of upper and lower eyelids
- Show ectropion/upper lid hooding
- Show existing fat deposits
- Show wrinkles of the forehead and glabellar area

KEY POINTS (Fig. 3-7)

- Photograph horizontally.
- The closeup of brow should extend below the lower crease of the lower eyelids to slightly above the hairline.
- Have patients relax the brow while they gaze upward.
- Make sure interpupillary line is horizontal in all views.
- Have patients gaze downward to reveal any excess lower lid fat.

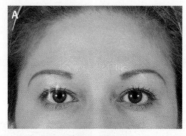

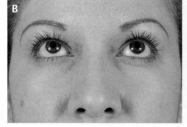 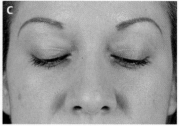

Fig. 3-7   Photographs of the eyes and brow are taken in addition to the standard facelift/necklift series. Image **A** was photographed at 0.8 m. Images **B** and **C** were photographed horizontally at 0.6 m with a 105 mm lens.

STANDARD LASER/CHEMICAL PEEL SERIES

- This series taken in addition to the standard face series.
- Patient photographed using a vertically positioned digital camera with a ⅔-inch sensor at a 0.5 m distance with an 80 mm focal length.

OBJECTIVES

- Show depth of creases and folds
- Show changes in skin coloration from area to area
- Show subtleties of skin texture

KEY POINTS (Fig. 3-8)

- Remove heavy makeup.
- Photograph closeup oblique views of cheeks in the vertical position and at jawline to slightly above eyebrow at 0.5 m.
- Photograph lateral views at 1 m to show the tonal changes in the skin, if any, from the cheek to the jaw to the neck.
- For a chemical peel of the chest area, obtain an additional view at 1 m horizontally.

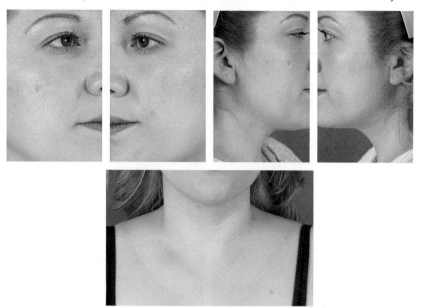

Fig. 3-8   Laser/chemical peel series. These photographs are taken in addition to the standard face/necklift series. Closeups are photographed at 0.6 m and 0.8 m with a 105 mm lens.

STANDARD LIP SERIES

- Patient photographed using a vertically and horizontally positioned digital camera with a ⅔-inch sensor at a 0.5 m distance for the closeups, and at a 1 m for the full-face view using an 80 mm focal length.

OBJECTIVES

- Show proportional relationship to face
- Show existing volume loss
- Show projection and dimension
- Show vermilion border irregularities/asymmetries
- Show philtral dimension
- Show loss of volume or excessive gum show from animated smiling view

KEY POINTS (Fig. 3-9)

- Have patients remove lipstick and liners.
- Inferior philtral column and tip of Cupid's bow should intersect opposite cheek in oblique view
- Have patients slightly part and relax the lips.

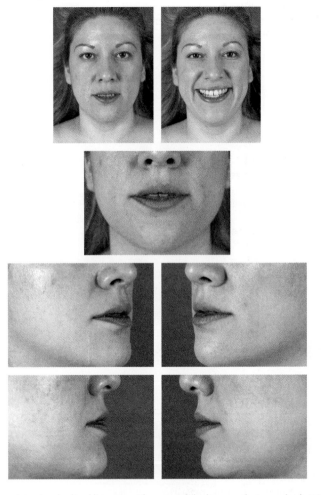

Fig. 3-9   Complete standardized lip series. Closeups of the lips are photographed at 0.7 m with a 105 mm lens, whereas the full face is photographed at 1 m.

STANDARD RHINOPLASTY SERIES

- This series taken in addition to the standard face series.
- Patient is photographed using a horizontally positioned digital camera with a ⅔-inch sensor at a 0.5 m distance with an 80 mm focal length.

- Rhinoplasty series is the most specialized photographic series.
- The nose is **frequently the most difficult series to photograph** due to the angles in the anatomy.
  - Depending on the type of nose, it is often necessary to make small adjustments to the series, as shown in the oblique view of Fig. 3-11.
  - The oblique preference must be decided before photographing.
- The series can also be used for facial fractures and Mohs reconstruction using forehead flaps and/or nasolabial folds.

OBJECTIVES
- Show proportional relationship of nose to face
- Show any existing deviation of the dorsal aesthetic lines in anterior view
- Show existing asymmetries
- Show projection of dorsal hump in lateral view
- Show radix position in lateral view

KEY POINTS (Fig. 3-10)
- Photograph closeup views horizontally.
- Make sure that the camera is parallel to the subject, focused on the midpoint (nose), and that a horizontal line is straight through the lower lateral eyes and perpendicular to the dorsum.
- Line the tip between the eyebrows in the full basal view. Adjustments for this view may be needed, especially if the patient has extremely low tip projection or large upper lip that may block the alar area.
- In the half-basal view (see Fig. 3-10, *B*), line the tip just below the eyes.
- Have patients relax their face and not smile.
- Have patients remove distracting jewelry.
- Have patients pull their hair back with neutral-colored headband.

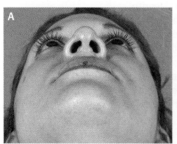
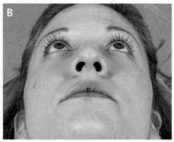
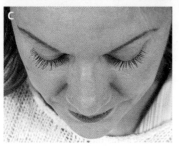

Fig. 3-10 Standardized rhinoplasty series. These photographs are taken in addition to the standard face/necklift series. Closeup views are photographed with a 105 mm lens at 0.8 and 0.6 m.

SUPPLEMENTAL RHINOPLASTY VIEWS (Fig. 3-11)

■ If a patient is having a depressor septi release, additional lateral and anterior views of the patient smiling are photographed.
■ Cephalic view (see Fig. 3-10, C) is also helpful to show nasal deviations.[9]

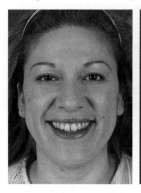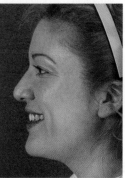

Fig. 3-11   Additional anterior and lateral views are needed if the patient is having a depressor septi release.

SENIOR AUTHOR TIP: I advocate always taking a lateral smiling photograph regardless of depressor septi release.

STANDARD BODY SERIES

■ Patient is photographed using a vertically positioned digital camera with a ⅔-inch sensor at 5-foot distance with a 35 mm focal length.
■ Body series is photographed vertically with the patient in a standing position.
   • Midpoint of the body should be centered in the frame
   • Position of the lens axis should be parallel to the patient at all times.
   • Photographing up or down should be avoided, because it can lead to distortion and difficultly producing standardized photographs.
■ **Pay close attention to the position of the feet.**
   • The contour of the body and muscle structure can vary greatly with positioning of the feet.
   • For ease of positioning, place cut-out feet or tape on the floor as a standing reference for patients, as shown in Fig. 3-12.

OBJECTIVES

■ Show proportional relationship of body
■ Show volume and dimension
■ Show skin laxity and muscle tone
■ Show contour irregularities/ asymmetries

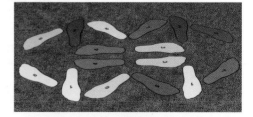

Fig. 3-12   For ease of positioning, place cut-out feet on the floor for the patient as a standing reference.

KEY POINTS (Fig. 3-13)

■ Feet are parallel to each other and separated a hip's distance.
■ Weight is distributed evenly.
■ Knees are facing straight ahead.
■ Camera should be parallel with subject and positioned at midpoint of body (usually the abdomen).
■ Have patients relax abdomen.
■ Have patients wear generic underwear, if any.

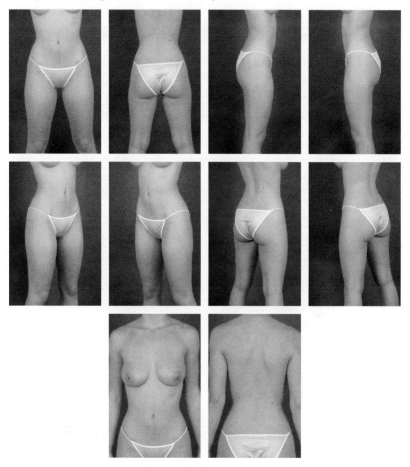

Fig. 3-13   Standard body series.

SUPPLEMENTAL VIEWS FOR THE BODY CONTOURING SERIES (Fig. 3-14)

■ A "diver's" view is sometimes photographed to evaluate skin laxity.[10]
   • An oblique view with the patient bending forward while relaxing the abdomen.
■ If the back is to be suctioned, an additional view is photographed from above the shoulders to below the hips.

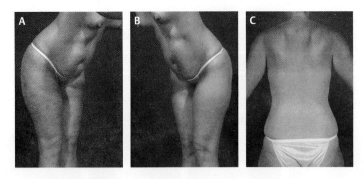

Fig. 3-14   Supplemental views for body contouring. **A** and **B,** A diver's view is an oblique view with the patient bending over while relaxing the abdomen. **C,** Back view.

SENIOR AUTHOR TIP: I prefer to have a lateral diver's view as well as an oblique view.

STANDARD ARM SERIES

KEY POINTS (Fig. 3-15)
■ Arms are photographed horizontally with elbows bent to 90 degrees with hands forward.
■ Have patients remove watches and/or jewelry.

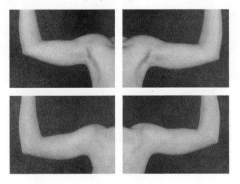

Fig. 3-15   Standard arm series.

STANDARD MALE BODY SERIES

■ Patient is photographed using a vertically positioned digital camera with a ⅔-inch sensor at a 5-foot distance with a 35 mm focal length.

OBJECTIVES
■ Show proportional relationship of body
■ Show volume and dimension
■ Show skin laxity and muscle tone
■ Show contour irregularities/asymmetries

KEY POINTS (Fig. 13-16)

- Photograph vertically.
- Photograph above shoulders to just above groin area.
- Position the camera parallel with subject and at midpoint of body.
- Have patients relax shoulders.
- Have patients position arms behind body in all views except the anterior and posterior.
- In posterior oblique views, have patients hold arms in front and away from body.
- Use a generic material/towel to cover undergarments.

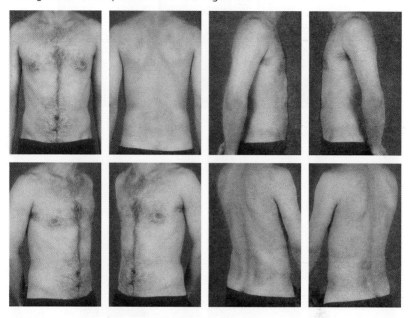

Fig. 3-16   The male body series.

STANDARD MASSIVE-WEIGHT-LOSS SERIES

- Patient is photographed using a vertically positioned digital camera with a ⅔-inch sensor at a 5-foot distance with a 35 mm focal length.

OBJECTIVES

- Show proportional relationship of body
- Show volume and dimension
- Show skin laxity and muscle tone
- Show contour irregularities/asymmetries
- Show skin irritations and/or worn grooves

KEY POINTS (Fig. 3-17)

- Feet are parallel to each other and separated a hip's distance. (If thighs touch, have patients separate feet slightly wider.)
- Weight is distributed evenly.

■ Knees face straight ahead.
■ Position the camera parallel with subject and at midpoint of body.
■ Have patients fold hands across breast area but no higher. (If breasts are large, have patient lift them to show abdomen.)
■ Have patient raise abdomen in anterior and lateral views to show the condition of skin.

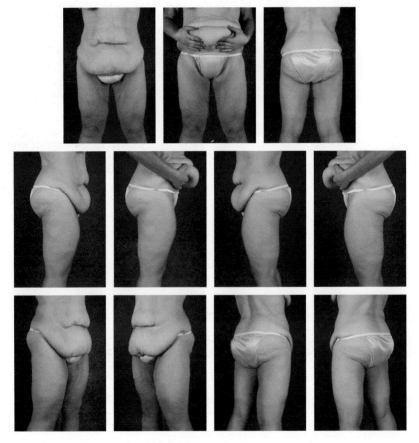

Fig. 3-17   Standard body contouring after weight-loss series, including view to document intertriginous areas.

STANDARD MASSIVE-WEIGHT-LOSS BRACHIOPLASTY AND LATERAL CHEST EXCISION SERIES

KEY POINTS (Fig. 3-18)
- Horizontally with elbows bent at 90 degrees and hands forward
- Arms straight out with palms facing down
- For lateral chest wall excision, photograph the patient's back as well as oblique views with the arms raised and bent to 90 degrees.
- Photograph below the breast area in oblique views.

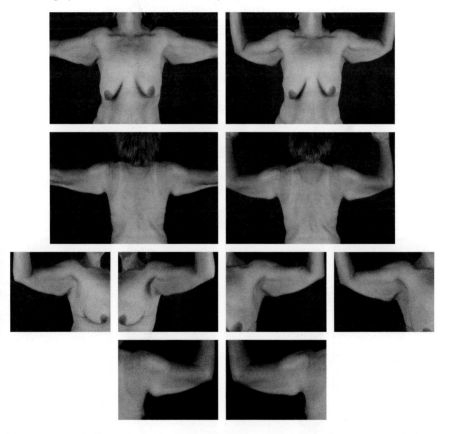

Fig. 3-18   Standard views for brachioplasty and/or lateral chest excision after massive weight loss.

STANDARD BREAST AUGMENTATION SERIES

■ Patients are photographed using a horizontally positioned digital camera with a ⅔-inch sensor at a 5-foot distance using a 35 mm focal length.

OBJECTIVES

■ Show proportional relationship of breasts to chest
■ Show breast laxity/skin tone
■ Show any asymmetries
■ Show nipple and areolar proportion and their relationship to breast

KEY POINTS (Fig. 3-19)

■ Photograph horizontally.
■ Photograph above shoulders and below navel for reference and proportion.
■ Position the camera parallel with subject and at midpoint of body.
■ Have patients relax shoulders.
■ Have patients remove jewelry, including wrist watch.

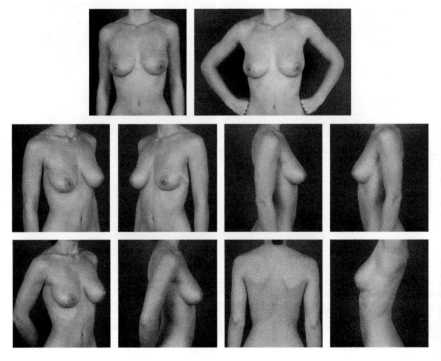

Fig. 3-19   Standard breast augmentation series.

SUPPLEMENTAL BREAST AUGMENTATION VIEWS

■ If a patient has a capsular contracture, photograph with arms up.
  • It is helpful to photograph the incisions after surgery, along with the standard series.

STANDARD BREAST REDUCTION/MASTOPEXY SERIES

KEY POINTS (Fig. 3-20)

- Photograph horizontally.
- Photograph above shoulders and below navel for reference and proportion.
- Arms are behind patient in oblique and lateral views.
- Position the camera parallel with subject and at midpoint of body.
- Have patients relax shoulders.
- Have patients remove all jewelry, including wrist watch.

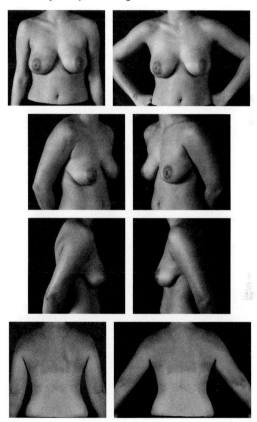

Fig. 3-20   Standard breast reduction series.

SUPPLEMENTAL BREAST REDUCTION/MASTOPEXY VIEWS

- Photograph the incisions after surgery, along with the standard series.

LIGHTING IN A CLINICAL SETTING

- Patients should be photographed using a **flash system** or **studio strobes.**
- **Dual flashes** are preferred.
  - Light from one source can produce harsh shadows and can wash out the details and texture of skin.
  - Additional lights can be used that are pointed toward the backdrop (away from the patient), which helps to eliminate shadow casts and separate the background from the patient.
  - To preserve a natural appearance, shadows should be cast *downward.*

PATIENT PREPARATION

- Have patients remove distracting items.
- Heavy makeup, glasses, and large jewelry can detract from patient results.
- Purchase disposable medical garments to ensure a "generic" patient appearance in photographs, as well as consistent standardization.

FACIAL EXPRESSION

- Slight animation can "pull" at facial anatomy, which can distort results.
- Patients should relax their face, with their eyes focused straight ahead.

BACKGROUND

- **Neutral-colored background** behind the patient is used to eliminate any unnecessary items that may detract from the scene.
  - Helps to produce a contour of the patient
  - Medium blue often used, because it contrasts with a variety of skin tones

INFORMED CONSENT[11-13]

The following are the basic guidelines for photographing patients and obtaining photographic consents that are the standards used for HIPAA (Health Insurance Portability and Accountability Act). Private and/or smaller entities may have different and/or additional requirements.

PHOTOGRAPHING FOR TREATMENT PURPOSES

- Health care providers may photograph and/or create audio or video recordings of patients for treatment purposes, without obtaining patients' written authorization.

PHOTOGRAPHING FOR NONTREATMENT PURPOSES

- If a patient agrees to be photographed or recorded for nontreatment purposes, the health care provider or staff must obtain the patient's written authorization. Some examples of "nontreatment" purposes that require patient authorization are:
  - Educational lectures and presentations for health care professionals (e.g., CME)

- Scientific publications, such as journals or books, for which another authorization is not already on file
- Patient education materials
- Use in broadcast, print, or Internet media for educational or public interest purposes
■ According to HIPAA, authorizations are not required if the photograph or recording will be fully de-identified of all patient information.
■ Full-face photographs and any comparable images cannot be de-identified and always require authorization.
■ *A photograph or electronic reproduction is considered to identify a patient if it shows the full face or comparable image of the patient, or if any of the 19 elements of Protected Health Information are not present. These elements are:*
- Name
- Date of birth
- Address
- Telephone number
- Fax number
- E-mail address
- Social Security number
- Medical record number
- Account number
- Driver's license number
- Credit card number
- Names of relatives
- Name of employer
- Health plan beneficiary number
- Vehicle or other device serial number
- Web Universal Resource Locator (URL)
- Internet Protocol (IP) address numbers
- Finger or voice prints
- Date and time of treatment
■ **Blacking out the eyes to de-identify a patient is not satisfactory.**
- Recognition of the patient not only applies to the eyes but also to other distinguishing features of the face.[1]
- HIPAA does not specifically address the use of masking the eyes, but obtaining a consent form when using any part of the face for purposes other than treatment is strongly recommended.
■ As standard practice, even if a patient has a "photographic consent for nontreatment purpose" on file, always contact the patient before potential use for publication in print or on the Internet.

TIP: Tattoos, scars, and birthmarks are also identifying landmarks in body shots and have been used successfully in lawsuits.

TOP TAKEAWAYS
➤ Uniformity and standardization are essential to producing accurate photographic documentation.
➤ Lack of quality can distort clinical findings and lead to misrepresentation of images.
➤ Special attention should be paid to obtaining photographic consent forms.
➤ A standardized camera, lens, distance, and views will produce photos that can be compared later.
➤ Understand the camera sensor's reproduction/magnification ratio; be sure to stand far enough from patients to prevent distortion (especially with facial photos).
➤ Digital photography requires good backup, with protection of HIPAA standards.
➤ Photos are legal records! Every patient should sign a consent form; additional consent should be obtained for publication or Internet use.

REFERENCES

1. Grom RM. Clinical and operating room photography. Biomed Photogr 20:251, 1992.
2. Roos O, Cederblom S. A standardized system for patient documentation. J Audiov Media Med 14:135, 1991.
3. DiBernadino BE, Adams RL, Krause J, et al. Photographic standards in plastic surgery. Plast Reconstr Surg 102:559, 1998.
4. Young S. Maintaining standard scales of reproduction in patient photography using digital camera. J Audiov Media Med 24:162, 2001.
5. Williams AR. Positioning and lighting for patient photography. J Biol Photogr 53:131, 1985.
6. Sommer D. Pitfalls of nonstandardized photography in facial plastic surgery patients. Plast Reconstr Surg 114:10, 2004.
7. Galdino GM, DaSilva D, Gunter JP. Digital photography for rhinoplasty. Plast Reconstr Surg 109:1421, 2002.
8. Davidson TM. Photography in facial plastic and reconstructive surgery. J Biol Photogr Assoc 47:59, 1979.
9. LaNasa JJ Jr, Smith O, Johnson CM Jr. The cephalic view in nasal photography. J Otolaryngol 20:443, 1991.
10. Gherardini G. Standardization in photography for body contour surgery and suction-assisted lipectomy. Plast Reconstr Surg 100:227, 1997.
11. Williams AR. Clinical and operating room photography. In Vetter JP, ed. Biomedical Photography. Boston: Focal Press, 1992.
12. Department of Health and Human Services. Standards for privacy of individually identifiable health information: final rule. 45 CFR Parts 160 and 164. Federal Register 65, no. 250 (December 28, 2000).
13. Roach WH Jr, Hoban RG, Broccolo BM, et al, eds. Medical Records and the Law. Gaithersburg, MD: Aspen Publishers, 1994.

4. Medicolegal Considerations in Aesthetic Surgery

Mark Gorney, Neal R. Reisman

- Aesthetic surgeons are the fifth most frequently sued physician, averaging one claim every 2½ years[1] (Fig. 4-1).
- Prevent medical lawsuits with good patient selection, strong patient relationships, and proper documentation.

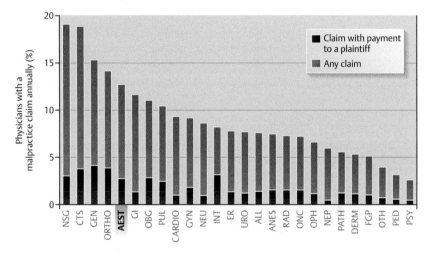

NSG	Neurosurgery	GYN	Gynecology	OPH	Ophthalmology
CTS	Cardiothoracic surgery	NEU	Neurology	NEP	Nephrology
GEN	General surgery	INT	Internal medicine	PATH	Pathology
ORTHO	Orthopedic surgery	ER	Emergency medicine	DERM	Dermatology
AEST	**Aesthetic surgery**	URO	Urology	FGP	Family general practice
GI	Gastroenterology	ALL	All physicians	OTH	Other specialities
OBG	Obstetrics and gynecology	ANES	Anesthesiology	PED	Pediatrics
PUL	Pulmonary medicine	RAD	Diagnostic radiology	PSY	Psychiatry
CARDIO	Cardiology	ONC	Oncology		

Fig. 4-1 Frequency of malpractice claims by specialty.

PATIENT SELECTION[2]

- More than half of the malpractice claims against aesthetic surgeons are preventable; the first step in preventing a claim is **patient selection.**

EXPECTATIONS TOO GREAT

- Patients with **unrealistic and idealized expectations,** or those who expect major life changes, are more likely to be disappointed with even a good surgery result.
  - Disappointed patients are more likely to seek legal counsel.
- Patients who **do not understand the risks** associated with major surgical procedures are more likely to be disappointed.
  - Patients must understand the possible inherent complications associated with surgery.

EXCESSIVELY DEMANDING PATIENTS

- Patients who bring photographs, drawings, and exact architectural specifications to a consultation should be managed with great caution. These patients demonstrate:
  - Little comprehension of the healing process vagaries
  - Little understanding of the natural margin of error inherent in elective surgery
  - Little flexibility in accepting failure

THE INDECISIVE PATIENT

> **SENIOR AUTHOR TIP:** I have always had a concern about defending a decision to perform completely elective surgery with, "The patient wanted this done." I think a patient cannot make a negligent decision. That is, the doctor has the responsibility to NOT accept patients for completely elective surgery if the choice of procedure does not reflect acceptable expectations and is achievable. Just because a patient asks for something does NOT mean it should be performed if inappropriate.
>
> *Question:* "Doctor, do you think I ought to have this done?"
>
> *Answer:* "I cannot make that decision for you; if you have any doubt whatsoever, I strongly encourage you to reconsider."

- The decision to undergo surgery is motivated from within:
  - **Strongly motivated patients** are more likely to be satisfied with the results.

CAUTION: Never "sell" a patient on a procedure.

- Selling the patient may lead to "buyer's remorse" ➤ lawsuit.

THE IMMATURE PATIENT

- Youthful and immature patients may have excessively romantic expectations.
- **Maturity** and **age** do not always correlate.

THE SECRETIVE PATIENT

- Be cautious of patients desiring secret surgery or requesting elaborate precautions to prevent knowledge of their surgery. This suggests guilt about the surgery.
  - **Guilty** patients are more likely to be **dissatisfied.**
  - **Dissatisfied** patients are more likely to **sue.**

FAMILY DISAPPROVAL
- Family approval is not necessary, but **family disapproval is a relative contraindication:**
  - Less optimal results may produce the "I told you so" familial reaction.
  - Such reaction may deepen patient's guilt and dissatisfaction.

PATIENTS PHYSICIANS DO NOT LIKE (OR WHO DO NOT LIKE THEM)
- **Surgeons should not accept patients they dislike.**
  - Clash of personalities may affect the case outcome and/or postoperative care.
- **Surgeons should not accept patients who do not like them.**
  - Perception of bad outcome is more likely, even with a good result.
  - Patients are much more likely to sue doctors they do not like.

THE "SURGIHOLIC"
- **WARNING:** Patients with multiple aesthetic surgeries are not good candidates because:
  - Personality problems: Patients are probably compensating for poor self-image.
  - Difficult anatomy from previous procedures
  - Risk of unfavorable comparison with previous surgeons

> **SENIOR AUTHOR TIP:**   Performing surgery on surgiholics is not worth the risk.

BODY DYSMORPHIC DISORDER
- Beware of patients who are occupied by physical traits that are hardly noticeable and within normal limits. Patients with body dysmorphic disorder never carry a diagnosis openly.
  - **Avoid the temptations of financial gain.**
    - ▶ A valid credit card is a poor criterion for elective aesthetic surgery.
  - **Practice good surgical judgment.**
    - ▶ Patients obsessed with a minor defect will probably continue to obsess, even with a good surgical result.

PATIENT COMMUNICATION[3]

- Busy doctors are less likely to listen effectively; ineffective listening can lead to the perception of arrogance and disinterest, which leads to lawsuits.
- Informed consent is a process and sometimes is never achieved, even after many visits.

TEN LISTENING BEHAVIORS TO AVOID[4]
1. **Dismissing the subject matter as uninteresting**
   - Surgeons must not become bored with the same complaints they have heard many times before; patience is a virtue: refuse the urge to "move the conversation along."
2. **Feigning attention**
   - More often than not, patients realize their doctor is merely "appearing engaged."
3. **Losing interest in verbose explanations**
   - Patients' explanations of their symptoms are often lengthy and unorganized.
   - Physicians must actively listen to their patients' explanations to appropriately synthesize the information that allows proper care.
   - A disorganized patient presentation is not a defense against a lawsuit.
   - Listening is a physician's duty.

4. **Allowing distractions**
   - Interruptions (phone, intercom, pager) should be avoided.
5. **Becoming distracted by the speaker**
   - Physicians should listen to patients, even those with distracting mannerisms or physical characteristics.
6. **Listening only for facts**
   - Physicians are scientifically trained to focus on objective observations and quantitative data. Human patients, however, are not objective or quantitative; physicians must comprehend the equally important patient emotional overtones and behavior.
7. **Becoming distracted by the presentation**
   - Surgeons should not become enamored with the patient's speaking style or mannerisms, because it may cause them to miss what the patient is saying.
8. **Allowing emotion-laden words that arouse antagonism**
   - Angry or defensive reactions to patient comments should be avoided.
   - "We" is used, instead of "you."
9. **Note-taking**
   - Note-taking is essential for documentation, but can be distracting.
   - Surgeons should listen to and make eye contact with patients, then jot down the key words needed to reconstruct the conversation *shortly after* the consultation.
10. **Wasting the advantage of thought-speech speed**
    - People can speak 150 words per minute but assimilate 500 spoken words per minute; thinking about something other than what the speaker is saying requires extra time and should not be done; active listening requires focus on the patient's words.

Employing Good Listening Skills
- **Reflective feedback**
  - Ask questions, make statements, and offer visual cues that indicate understanding.
- **Silence**
  - Silence is golden; focus on what the patient is saying.
- **Positioning**
  - Do not seem too relaxed (reflecting disinterest).
  - Do not cross your arms (appearing defensive).
  - Avoid sitting behind a desk (an ostensible barrier).
  - Try to **lean forward**—a nonverbal communication that says, "I am interested."

Employing Good Speaking Habits
- **Use calming speech tempo and voice tone.**
  - Speak slowly and clearly; use a voice tone that reflects calm and empathy.
- **Pause for assimilation and feedback**
  - Pause more often. Pausing during speaking gives the patient time to digest the words and ask for clarification.
  - Repeatedly invite questions; a good dialogue reinforces patients' beliefs that they are participating in their care.
  - Ask patients to repeat instructions; repetition adds reinforcement.
- **Do not talk medi-speak**
  - Use **simple terminology** (e.g., "cutting out" instead of "excise").
  - A surgeon's duty is not only to operate, but to ensure that their patients understand the surgery process; if they do not understand it, the surgeon has breached his or her duty.

- **Repetition**
  - The average patient retains only **35%** of what is said; repetition can increase patient comprehension, which can prevent inflated expectations and decrease litigations.
- **Request written questions**
  - After leaving the consultation, patients often remember questions they forgot to ask.
  - Encourage patients to write down questions they have before consultations. Answering their questions may avert a lawsuit.
- **Body language**
  - Start with a friendly handshake. Eye contact is critical and holds a patient's attention. A frown, raised eyebrow, sigh, or simple "hmmmm" can exacerbate patient anxiety. Alternatively, a gentle smile, combined with a confident caring attitude, will help to develop a solid doctor-patient relationship, which is essential for lawsuit avoidance.

DOCUMENTATION

TIP: Many lawsuits occur *not* because of bad doctoring, but because of *bad charting!*

Good doctors who chart poorly can still be sued—and lose.

Bad doctors can prevent lawsuits by charting well, and even if they are sued, they can win.

In today's litigious environment, being a good physician means not only practicing good medicine, but equally important, documenting the good medicine that is practiced.

TIP: Document defensively. The digital age poses many new problems. Interacting with a laptop or notebook and not with the patient interferes with the doctor-patient relationship. Developing a method by which the physician can create a healthy doctor-patient relationship AND have proper documentation is critical. Be aware also of "smart text" entries that default to a response. Check to make sure the entry is accurate.

- Plaintiff attorney premises: MURPHY'S LAW
  - If it is not in the chart, it was not done.
  - If the physician did not write it in the chart, then the physician did not consider it.
  - If the physician writes it in the chart wrong, then the physician did not understand it.
  - If the physician did not prescribe the right medications or treatment regimens, then the physician did not know what he or she was doing.

SENIOR AUTHOR TIP:

MYTH: Doctors should document as little as possible; if you document too much, the lawyer will just twist what you've written.

FACT: A lack of evidence is powerful evidence. A plaintiff attorney's dream is the surgeon's reality: Scant documentation because of a busy lifestyle. If documentation is scant or rushed, the plaintiff attorney will allege that patient care was equally scant and rushed. Remember, a physician's duty to patients includes not only good patient care, but documentation of such care.

Know the Legal Defenses!

> **TIP:**   Knowledge of the available legal defenses helps to better buttress these defenses with documentation. Below are three common legal defenses.

Defense No. 1: Standard of Care Defense
A doctor who gets an untoward result is not necessarily negligent if his or her care is within the standard of care applicable to the circumstances.
- This means that perfection is not required:
  - Doctors are human; they use judgment.
  - Judgment is not perfect; mistakes happen.
  - A mistake is not necessarily negligence.
- Translation: Physicians can make a reasonable mistake and not be negligent.
  - *Document reasoning.*

> **SENIOR AUTHOR TIP:**   Judges and juries do not like finding medical negligence against good, caring physicians. They know that hindsight is 20/20; they do not expect perfection. What they expect is a humane, concerned physician. Doctors win four of five jury trials: documenting good and compassionate care allows the jury to find for them.

Defense No. 2: Fork-in-the-Road Defense
Where there is more than one recognized method of diagnosis or treatment, and no one of them is used exclusively and uniformly by all practitioners of good standing, a practitioner is not negligent if in exercising his or her best judgment, he or she selects one of the approved methods, which later turns out to be a wrong selection, or one not approved by certain other practitioners.
- When physicians come to a fork in the medical road, they document why they go left instead of right. Generally, opposing counsel will easily find an expert witness to testify, with 20/20 hindsight, that left was the wrong choice, but physicians' counsel will just as easily find an expert to testify that left was reasonable. With offsetting expert testimony, the jury will look to whether a physician was kind and compassionate, trying to take good care of a patient.

Defense No. 3: Plaintiff's Fault Defense
Doctors are only as good as the information given to them.
- **Information provided by a patient should be documented *at the time of the event or shortly thereafter,* not later!**
  - Patients who have undergone psychological or physical trauma sometimes remember, and will so testify in court, conversations or events with their physician that never actually occurred.
  - Physicians need to protect themselves and immediately record the conversations and events they have with their patients.

> **TIP:** A picture is worth a thousand words. A medicolegal document made at the time of the event is PRICELESS!

IMPORTANCE OF LEGIBILITY

> **SENIOR AUTHOR TIP:**
>
> **MYTH:** Doctors should write illegibly; that way, the attorney won't be able to read the documentation, and thus won't sue.
>
> **FACT:** Physicians who write illegibly are more likely to be sued, and if they are sued, they are more likely to lose, even if not negligent.

- **Illegibility makes you susceptible to powerful theatrical ploys at trial**
  - **"Sloppy at documentation is sloppy at practice."**
    - ▶ Good trial attorneys have catchy themes or theatrical ploys that they run throughout their trials, e.g., "If the glove does not fit, you must acquit."
    - ▶ One such medical malpractice theme is: "Sloppy at documentation is sloppy at practice." Good plaintiffs' attorneys will have juries humming these words on their way to the jury room.

Box 4-1   *"SLOPPY AT DOCUMENTATION IS SLOPPY AT PRACTICE": HOW IT WORKS AT TRIAL*

Much of this is moot as we have entered the electronic health record era. However, "standard operative reports" may indicate a physician did everything the same and did not properly care for the patient. Or, if dictated, incorrect entries like "had no carcinoma" instead of "adenocarcinoma" may occur.

The duty is to read and correct everything entered before signing the document. The plaintiff attorney will delve through the records and find a physician's worst day—when he or she hurriedly scribbled and accidentally spilled coffee on the note. The attorney will then scan this note and project it on the courtroom wall opposite the jury, call on an unsuspecting nurse (or someone who commonly reads physician notes to care for patients), and ask him or her to read the note; inevitably, the nurse will not be able to read it. The plaintiff will point to the document on the wall, and say, "This chicken scratch is how that busy and rushed doctor" (pointing to the physician) "documents care of our poor, injured patient" (gesturing sympathetically toward the attorney's client). "If this doctor didn't have time to merely document patient care, she certainly didn't have time to properly care for our patient."

They will then project these words superimposed on the physician's notes:

 "SLOPPY AT DOCUMENTATION IS SLOPPY AT PRACTICE."

The attorney will repeat this theme over and over, and hammer it home in the closing statement.

DOCUMENT DEFENSIVELY!

> **TIP:** Documentation was originally required to protect the patient; in today's legal environment, however, documentation is to protect you! Protect yourself: document defensively.

- **Always perform a good history and physical examination!**
  - If physicians do not perform a good physical examination and history, the plaintiff will allege that they did not know their patient well enough to provide patient care.

> **TIP:** Physicians should not merely sign the bottom of each page, because the jury will not think they read everything.
>
> *Question:* Is template charting by a nurse or physician assistant acceptable, or do I have to perform a full history and physical examination myself for every patient?
>
> *Answer:* Template charting is acceptable, but physicians should circle, initial, and date any abnormal findings noted by their nurse or physician assistant.

- **Consults**
  - If in doubt, GET ONE.
    - ▶ It is easier to defend getting a consult than not getting one.

> **TIP:** In a practice, consults are easy because of financial incentives; in residency, however, consults are more difficult, because residents are not paid per consult and are barely paid at all. When a consulted resident physician avoids a consult, the physician must document the event properly; otherwise, he or she may be liable. The consult physician's name *and* the information relayed must be written down (e.g., "labs, path report, and MRI results reported in full"). If physicians do not record that they reported the information, at trial the consulted physicians will swear they did not: "She did not tell me about that laboratory value! If she had, I would have been there in a heartbeat!"

- Do **NOT** attack other physicians (especially in the medical record).
  - Fight lawsuits as a team if possible.
  - NEVER MISLEAD/COVER UP!!!
- Document troublesome patients!
  - Lawyers do not like troublesome clients any more than physicians like troublesome patients; professionally document the patient's troublesome nature, and good attorneys will get the picture:
    - ▶ "The patient was abusive and condescending to the nursing staff this a.m."
    - ▶ "The patient requests pain medication far in excess of what is reasonable, given the patient's circumstances."

- Never alter a chart.
  - Ink is like DNA: An expert can tell the year, make, and manufacturer of the ink on an original document. If a chart is altered, the attorney will know.
- Always document recommendations to see primary care!
  - Patients think that all doctors are generalists, not specialists; it is important to always tell patients to follow up with their primary care or OB-GYN physicians for all medical problems outside your area of expertise.

INFORMED CONSENT[2]

> **SENIOR AUTHOR TIP:** Doctors have an affirmative duty to disclose in detail the benefits, risks, alternatives, possible complications, and unpleasant side effects for any procedure or surgery.
>
> Without a consent, they risk legal liability for a complication, even if they are not negligent; theoretically, they could even be charged with "battery," the unlawful touching of another (remember, if it is not in the chart, it did not happen).
>
> A consent, however, provides proof that a patient has sufficient information to base an intelligent decision. The judge will inform the jury no liability attaches if a reasonable prudent person in the patient's position, armed with the consent information, would have accepted the treatment.

RIGHT OF REFUSAL

- Document a patient's refusal, and that the patient understood the consequences of such refusal.
  - Always time, date, and sign record entries.
- **Elements of a proper informed consent:**
  - The diagnosis or suspected diagnosis
  - The nature, purpose, and anticipated benefits of the proposed treatment or procedure
  - The risks, complications, or side effects
  - The probability of success, based on a patient's condition
  - Possible consequences if advice is not followed.

> **TIP:** Procedures that are cosmetic, experimental, or hazardous in nature, or which could potentially alter the patient's sexual capacity, all require more thorough documentation of foreseeable risks, possible untoward consequences, and potential unpleasant side effects. More than the average physician, aesthetic surgeons must document thoroughly their consents.

NO FORM IS "FOOLPROOF"

- Some consents are too long (incomprehensible); others are too short!
- Use a middle of the road consent form, and add to the form with handwritten notes.
- THINK! Use judgment as to what is and is not important when adding to the consent.

COMMON CLAIMS[2]

SCARRING IN GENERAL
- Something every patient should know: *Without a scar, there is no healing!*
  - Healing entails scar formation; without scarring, there is no healing.
  - Healing qualities are individual (genetically programmed) and cannot be predicted; everyone heals (scars) differently.
  - **Scar formation is a major genesis of patient dissatisfaction.**

BREAST REDUCTION
- Unsatisfactory scar
- Loss of nipple or breast skin
- Asymmetry or "disfigurement" too small or too large

BREAST AUGMENTATION: 44%
- Generally, discuss autoimmune diseases and their corresponding lawsuits.
- Encapsulation
- Wrong size (too little, too much)
- Infection
- Repetitive surgeries and attendant costs
- Nerve damage with sensory loss

FACELIFT AND BLEPHAROPLASTY: 11%
- Excessive skin removal (the "starey look")
- Dry eyes; inability to close
- Nerve damage, resulting in distorted expression
- Skin slough, resulting in excessive scarring and additional surgeries
- Blindness

> **TIP:**   A doctor's company survey on blepharoplasties complicated by blindness found two common traits: first, patients were released immediately after surgery; second, each patient at home performed a physical maneuver that generated a sudden rise in blood pressure (bowel movement, sudden coughing fit, bending over to tie their shoes, etc.).

> **TIP:**   The outpatient surgical facility should not discharge any patient until at minimum 3 hours after surgery and all evidence of local anesthetic effects have resolved.
>
> Physicians who undermine heavily vascularized tissues should strictly warn their patients to AVOID any sudden blood pressure elevating maneuvers.

SEPTORHINOPLASTY: 8%
- Unsatisfactory result: Improper performance allegations
- Continued breathing difficulties
- Asymmetry

> **TIP:** Rhinoplasty has the highest degree of unpredictability. Avoid inappropriate use of "brag books" containing only excellent results, or strictly counsel patients that these results cannot always be obtained.

ABDOMINOPLASTY: 3%

- Skin loss with poor scars (greater chance when preceded by suction-assisted liposuction)
- Nerve damage
- Inappropriate operation
- Infection with postoperative mismanagement

SKIN RESURFACING

- Blistering/burns with significant scarring
- Infection/postoperative mismanagement
- Permanent discoloration postoperatively

SUCTION-ASSISTED LIPECTOMY

- **Minor allegations**
  - Disfigurement and contour irregularities
  - Numbness
  - Disappointment/dissatisfaction
- **Major allegations**
  - Unrecognized abdominal perforation, resulting in disabling secondary surgery or death
  - Lidocaine overdose with fatal outcome
  - Pulmonary edema from overhydration
  - Pulmonary embolism and death

CAUTION: Liposuction is the most performed elective aesthetic procedure in the United States.[5,6] It is most commonly performed in the outpatient setting (outside regulatory control) and by a variety of practitioners (many of whom are unqualified).[2] Mortality increases significantly when lipoplasty is combined with other procedures,[5] or when a patient endures anesthesia for more than 6 hours.[2] Regardless of the number of procedures performed, restrict total aspirate to 5000 cc in office-based settings.[5] When using the "tumescent technique," be aware of fluid overload.[5] Limit lidocaine to 7 mg/kg.[5] Lidocaine toxicity presents with dizziness, agitation, lethargy, tinnitus, metallic taste, perioral anesthesia, and slurred speech.[5]

> **TIP:** Liposuction can have extremely high patient satisfaction rates (upward of 90%).[7] Patients who keep the weight off with diet and exercise are generally much happier with their surgery (and their surgeon). Inform patients that ultimately they, not you, control their surgery satisfaction. Use the handout in Fig. 4-2.

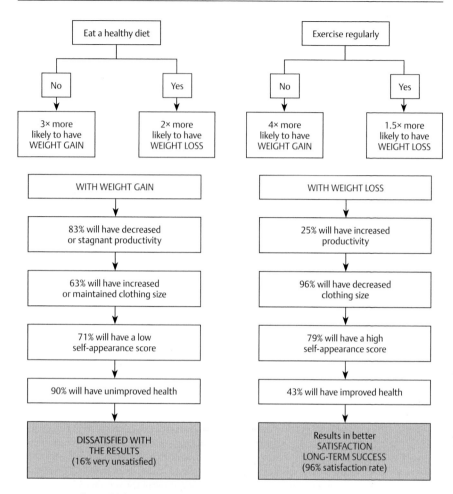

Fig. 4-2   Road map for long-term successful results, based on survey responses of 209 patients, given 6 months to more than 2 years postprocedure.

OTHER MISCELLANEOUS COMMON CLAIMS
- Untoward reaction to medications or anesthesia
- Improper use of preoperative or postoperative photos
- Sexual misconduct (doctor or employee)
- Lack of adequate disclosure (Tailor explanations to the patient's level of understanding.)
- General dissatisfaction (The patient's expectations were not met.)

Top Takeaways

➤ This chapter provides a good, broad road map to limit liability in the care of patients.

➤ The digital age brings new issues that can complicate and increase liability.

➤ The protection of patient privacy, especially with photographs must be addressed. If a photograph shows a physician for any advertising purpose, a specific HIPAA commercial consent should be used AND the photographs scrubbed of identifying metadata.

➤ A patient communication consent that indicates how to interact with the patient, such as cell phone, work phone, regular mail, texting, or social media is recommended. This should be reviewed periodically and updated appropriately.

➤ Electronic health records distract physicians from developing a good doctor-patient relationship. Often, the physician is focused on a laptop and not listening and interacting with the patient.

➤ Because patients usually do not bring litigation against doctors they like, it is wise to develop a behavior that involves interacting with the patient directly as well as entering information appropriately.

➤ An entry itself in an electronic health record may be problematic. Developing smart text that speeds data entry is recommended. The default entry must accurately reflect the examination and discussion. Electronic health records can be voluminous, and the physician's responsibility is to read, correct, and approve before digitally signing the document.

➤ Patient selection is a key aspect of a successful practice and avoiding additional risks.

➤ When possible, physicians should accept patients they like and in whom they can achieve reasonable goals and expectations.

➤ Doctors should know their limitations. Performing a procedure on a patient only because they asked for it is unacceptable.

➤ Physicians have the duty and responsibility to protect prospective patients and ensure that choices of procedure and care are reasonable and appropriate. This assumes that the physician has spent enough time listening to the patient and that the physician understands the patient's goals and expectations, answers all questions, and refines the choices discussed. This is difficult to achieve in one visit before surgery.

➤ Informed consent is a process that may require multiple visits and multiple discussions.

➤ It has been said that doctors earn their living by the patients they care for but develop their reputation based on those they do not.

REFERENCES

1. Jena AB, Seabury S, Lakdawalla D, et al. Malpractice risk according to physician specialty. N Engl J Med 365:629, 2011.
2. Gorney M. Medical liability in plastic and reconstructive surgery. In Anderson RE, ed. Medical Malpractice: A Physician's Sourcebook. Totowa, NJ: Humana Press, 2005.
3. Gorney M. Communication and patient safety. In Anderson RE, ed. Medical Malpractice: A Physician's Sourcebook. Totowa, NJ: Humana Press, 2005.
4. Nichols R. Are You Listening? New York: McGraw Hill, 1957.
5. Horton JB, Reece EM, Broughton G II, Janis JE, Thornton JF, Rohrich RJ. Patient safety in the office-based setting. Plast Reconstr Surg 117:61e, 2006.
6. Iverson RE. Patient safety in office-based surgery facilities: I. Procedures in the office-based surgery setting. Plast Reconstr Surg 110:1337; discussion 1343, 2002.
7. Rohrich RJ, Broughton G II, Horton B, et al. The key to long-term success in liposuction: a guide for plastic surgeons and patients. Plast Reconstr Surg 114:1945; discussion 1953, 2004.

PART II

Anesthesia

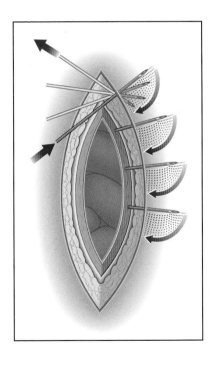

Part II

Anesthesia

5. Basics of Anesthesia for the Aesthetic Surgery Patient

Deborah Stahl Lowery, Jeffrey E. Janis

GENERAL PRINCIPLES[1,2]

- Anesthesia for patients undergoing *purely elective aesthetic procedures* presents specific challenges that encompass:
  - Patient selection
  - Surgical venue selection (ambulatory surgery centers, offices, hospital)
  - Choice of anesthetic technique(s)
  - Personnel requirements
  - Postoperative care and pain management
  - Discharge criteria
  - Patient satisfaction
- Requires high level of understanding, communication, and cooperation between surgeon and anesthesia provider to ensure optimal surgical outcome and patient experience
- Regulatory agencies establish minimum standards of care in aesthetic surgery environments.
  - Accreditation Association for Ambulatory Health Care (AAAHC)
  - The Joint Commission (TJC), formerly Joint Commission on Accreditation of Healthcare Organizations (JCAHO)
  - American Association for Accreditation of Ambulatory Surgery Facilities (AAAASF)
  - Regulations may vary with regard to state and type of facility.
- Professional societies provide consensus statements, guidelines, recommendations, practice parameters, and advisories for evidence-based best practices for ambulatory surgery centers (ASC) and office-based practices.
  - American Society of Anesthesiologists (ASA)
  - Society for Ambulatory Anesthesia (SAMBA)
  - American Society of Regional Anesthesia and Pain Medicine (ASRA)
  - American College of Cardiology and American Heart Association (ACC/AHA)
  - American College of Surgeons (ACS)
  - American Society of Plastic Surgeons (ASPS)
  - American Society for Aesthetic Plastic Surgery (ASAPS)

ANESTHETIC GOALS[3]

- Anxiolysis
- Amnesia
- Analgesia
- Sedation
- Unconsciousness or hypnosis
- Immobility, including muscle relaxation or paralysis
- Quiet, nondistracting operating milieu, if patient awake
- Attenuation of autonomic responses to noxious stimuli
- Preservation of vital functions

Objectives of Anesthesia in the Aesthetic Patient[2]
- Safe implementation of chosen technique
- Fast-track characteristics with rapid onset and emergence
- Predictable and reliable methodology
- Prevention of undesirable side effects
- Confidence in ability to meet accepted discharge criteria
- Patient satisfaction commensurate with entirely elective, often self-funded, procedures

Techniques[2-8]
General Anesthesia
- "Balanced" technique incorporates multiple classes of IV drugs (sedative-hypnotics, narcotics, muscle relaxants), along with the volatile/inhalational agents (desflurane, sevoflurane, less commonly isoflurane and nitrous oxide).
- Volatile agents
  - Easier titration of depth, faster emergence, and early recovery
  - Lesser risk of intraoperative awareness
  - Simple administration
  - Typically less expensive maintenance agent

Total Intravenous Anesthesia (TIVA)
- Component therapy involving sedative-hypnotic infusion (propofol, ketamine, dexmedetomidine)
  - Additional drugs such as midazolam, choice of narcotic, or muscle relaxant supplemented either by IV bolus or infusion
  - Aided by liberal surgical use of local anesthetic block or infiltration
- Reduced incidence of postoperative nausea and vomiting (PONV)
- High degree of patient satisfaction
- More complex administration
- Increased cost
- Avoids gas delivery systems and therefore need for scavenging equipment
- Avoids malignant hyperthermia (MH) triggers (see Malignant Hyperthermia section later in the chapter)
- Various well-described "recipes" for TIVA[5,6,8] commonly include:
  - Propofol: Sedation/hypnosis
  - Midazolam: Anxiolysis and amnesia
  - Ketamine: Dissociation and analgesia
  - Opioids (fentanyl, alfentanil, remifentanil): Analgesia
  - Rocuronium: Muscle relaxation
  - Dexmedetomidine: Anxiolysis, sedation, analgesia, decreased adrenergic output
  - Acetaminophen: Nonopioid analgesic
  - Ketorolac: NSAID
- Frequently accompanied by use of "depth of anesthesia" or "level of consciousness" monitoring
- Employs algorithm-driven surface EEG to calculate an "index" number that correlates with hypnotic level
- **Bispectral Index** (BIS; Medtronic) commonly used in the United States
  - Airway can be natural or controlled (endotracheal tube or supraglottic airway), with either mechanical or spontaneous ventilation.

Regional Anesthesia

- Neuraxial (spinal or epidural)
- **Nerve blocks:** Plexus, peripheral, paravertebral, intercostal, specific nerve branch, transversus abdominal plane (TAP), truncal, or other
- **IV sedation,** at multiple and varying levels
- **Local infiltration**
- Selection determined by
  - Type, extent, and duration of surgery
  - Patient or surgeon preference
  - Anesthesiologist experience
  - Patient's underlying medical status and/or any pertinent psychological aspects
- Can be isolated anesthetic technique or involve combinations listed previously

IMPORTANT CONSIDERATIONS WITH ADMINISTRATION OF ANESTHETICS[9]

- Standard of care for nonhospital locations should be equivalent to those of hospitals.
- ASA Standards for Basic Anesthetic Monitoring[10] (last amended 2011) must be met.
- Emergency protocols must be established, documented, and rehearsed.
- Transfer agreement with nearby/associated hospital for unplanned admission must be established.
- Preoperative risk assessment and evaluation are required, including laboratory tests and specialty consultation as needed.[11]
- Selection of anesthesia type with appropriate monitoring
- Selection of appropriate model of provider(s)
  - Anesthesiologist, alone or as part of anesthesia care team, with certified registered nurse anesthetist (CRNA) or, in some states, an anesthesia assistant (AA)
  - CRNA supervised by surgeon
  - Surgeon supervising RN whose *sole responsibility* is administration of ordered medication(s) and monitoring patient
- Appropriate education, training, and certification of staff involved in all phases of patient care
- Duration and complexity of procedure(s), *especially* if multiple procedures will be performed simultaneously or concurrently
- Preoperative medications and postoperative pain control plans
- Discharge criteria and postoperative follow-up

PREOPERATIVE SCREENING, EVALUATION, AND PATIENT SELECTION[12,13]

GOALS

- Identify and optimize comorbid conditions.
- Assess suitability for ASC or office.
- Align anesthetic needs and resources with proposed procedure and patient needs.
- Minimize perioperative risk.
- Reduce delays and cancellation.
- Assess ability for safe and timely discharge.
- Provide education and reassurance to patients to build confidence.

TOOLS
- Checklist-format patient questionnaire
- Primary care physician/practitioner evaluation
- Subspecialty consultations as needed
- Old anesthesia records
- In-person or phone interview with anesthesiologist or nurse
- Video chat, Skype, or telemedicine

TIMING[14]
- Process guided by
  - Patient demographics
  - Patients' clinical conditions
  - Invasiveness of procedure
  - Nature of the health care system
- Can be done day of surgery (DOS) if low severity of disease and procedure of low-medium surgical invasiveness, otherwise in advance

THINGS ANESTHESIOLOGISTS LIKE TO KNOW OR REVIEW
- Up-to-date history and physical examination
- Pertinent active medical conditions
- Current medications and therapies in place
- Status of optimization of current problems
- Pertinent subspecialty consultation
- Pertinent diagnostic studies of record
- Pertinent psychosocial conditions
- Surgical findings and operative plan
- History of difficult intubation
- History of PONV or postdischarge nausea and vomiting (PDNV) (discussed later in the chapter)
- History of other anesthetic complications like delayed emergence, unanticipated admission, or prolonged postanesthesia care unit (PACU) stay
- Personal or familial history suggestive of malignant hyperthermia
- **Intangibles, nuances, or needs that may affect patient's satisfaction or experience in this highly specialized, consumer-driven patient population**

IDENTIFYING RISK FACTORS
- **Red flags of unsuitability for general anesthesia in an ASC or office**[2, 5,9,12]
  - Unstable angina
  - Myocardial injury within 3-6 months
  - Severe cardiomyopathy
  - Uncompensated heart failure
  - Aortic stenosis (moderate to severe) or symptomatic mitral stenosis
  - Uncontrolled or poorly controlled hypertension
  - High-grade arrhythmias
  - Implantable cardiac devices (pacer-dependent or defibrillator)
  - Recent stroke within 3 months
  - End-stage renal disease (ESRD)/dialysis

- Severe liver disease
- Awaiting major organ transplant
- Sickle cell anemia
- Symptomatic or active multiple sclerosis
- Myasthenia gravis
- Severe chronic obstructive pulmonary disease (COPD)
- Abnormal/difficult airway
- Severe obstructive sleep apnea (OSA)
- Morbid obesity
- Psychiatric status unstable, dementia
- Acute substance intoxication
- Poor functional status <4 metabolic equivalents (METs) (discussed later in the chapter)
- **Mathis et al**[15] (2013) suggested **seven independent risk factors** associated with increased 72-hour morbidity and mortality in ambulatory surgery:
  1. Overweight BMI
  2. Obese BMI
  3. COPD
  4. History of transient ischemic attack/stroke
  5. Hypertension
  6. Previous cardiac surgical intervention
  7. Prolonged operative time

PREOPERATIVE TESTING[5,9,14,16]

- The culture shift is to NO routine testing.
- Tests should be for indication only, as per current medical conditions or per procedure.
- **Avoid baseline laboratory studies when:**
  - Patient is healthy
  - Patient has less than significant systemic disease (ASA I or II)
  - Blood loss expected to be minimal
  - Procedure is designated *low risk*
- Testing guidelines available from ASA, SAMBA, ACC/AHA

PREGNANCY (HCG) TEST

- Positive pregnancy tests have been reported in **0.3%-1.3% of premenopausal menstruating females,** which led to postponement, cancellation, or changes in management of 100% of the cases.[14]
- Routine testing of all females within childbearing years *remains controversial.*
- Evidence-based medicine is inadequate or unsupportive with regards to anesthetic exposure and teratogenic effects or other harmful effects, e.g., spontaneous abortion, stimulation of contractions, or premature birth.
- ASA provides no consensus on routine testing versus based on clinical menstrual history.
  - Recommends "offering" rather than "requiring" hCG testing
  - Affords "individual physicians and hospitals the opportunity to set their own practices and policies" according to ASA Choosing Wisely initiative[16]
- Many institutions perform routine point of care (POC) urine hCG on day of surgery.
- Some institutions perform rapid qualitative serum hCG testing should urine results be equivocal or contested by patient.

HEMOGLOBIN/HEMATOCRIT (HGB/HCT) AND COMPLETE BLOOD CELL COUNT (CBC)
- Significant blood loss anticipated (>500 ml)
- Patients with liver disease
- Extremes of age
- Preexisting anemia
- Hematologic disorders
- Factor deficiencies

CHEMISTRIES
- High-grade dysrhythmia, pacemaker, cardiac implantable electronic device (CIED), e.g., defibrillator
- H/O heart failure
- Diabetes
- Chronic renal insufficiency (CRI) or ESRD
- Hepatic disease
- Poorly controlled hypertension
- Malabsorption/malnutrition (note history of eating disorder or bariatric surgery)

BLOOD GLUCOSE
- In diabetics, obtain by blood draw as preadmission testing (PAT) or by point of care testing on day of surgery
- HbA1C is helpful in perioperative glucose interpretation and management

COAGULATION STUDIES (PT, PTT, INR)
- Bleeding disorders
- Liver disease
- Factor deficiencies
- Chemotherapy

ELECTROCARDIOGRAM (ECG)[14,17] (Box 5-1)

Box 5-1 *WHEN TO OBTAIN A PREOPERATIVE ELECTROCARDIOGRAM*

- Patient with known CAD or risk factors
- Patient for high risk (>1%) surgery
- Patient with known arrhythmias (helpful to have a baseline)
- Patient with known peripheral or cerebral vascular disease
- Patient with significant structural heart disease
- Patient with signs or symptoms of active cardiac conditions, e.g., chest pain, diaphoresis, shortness of breath (SOB), dyspnea on exertion (DOE)
- Patient with DM requiring insulin or end-organ damage
- Patient with renal insufficiency

- Based on cardiac risk
- **Not** indicated for **asymptomatic** patients undergoing **low-risk** surgery, **regardless of age** (ACC/AHA 2014)

- **Moderate-risk** cosmetic procedures (abdominoplasty, large-volume liposuction, or body contouring after massive weight loss) with at least **one clinical risk factor** supports obtaining baseline or current/updated ECG.
- ECGs valid for **6 months,** if patient clinically stable
- **Revised Cardiac Risk Index (RCRI)** clinical risk factors:
  - Coronary artery disease (CAD) with H/O myocardial infarction, coronary artery bypass graft (CABG) bypass, percutaneous coronary intervention (PCI), intracoronary stents
  - Cerebral vascular disease, with H/O stroke or transient ischemic events
  - Heart failure
  - Diabetes, requiring insulin, poorly controlled, or with end-organ damage
  - Renal insufficiency, serum creatinine >2.0 mg/dl or ESRD
- RCRI stratifies risk of major cardiac complications.
  - No risk factors: 0.4%
  - One risk factor: 1.0%
  - Two risk factors: 2.4%
  - Three or more risk factors: 5.4%

  Risk interpreted as:
  - Patients with **<1.0%** are **low risk** and need no further testing.
  - Patients with ≥**1.0%** are a **greater risk** and should be evaluated for optimization or further workup before elective surgery.
- **High-risk indicators** that should command attention and dissuade from elective surgery in anything but a hospital setting, or not at all, are:
  - Recent MI
  - Unstable angina
  - Uncompensated heart failure
  - High-grade arrhythmias
  - Hemodynamically significant valvular disease, e.g., aortic stenosis
- Additional considerations used as risk factors
  - Morbid obesity
  - Poorly controlled hypertension
  - High-grade arrhythmia, pacemaker, or implanted defibrillators
  - H/O significant peripheral arterial disease

CHEST RADIOGRAPH
- Not many indications in the elective aesthetic surgery patients
- Active symptomatic pulmonary disease

ADVANCED CARDIOVASCULAR TESTING
- Stress test, ECG, carotid duplex, vascular studies guided by subspecialty consultation

ASA PHYSICAL STATUS CLASSIFICATION (ASA PS)[5,18-20] (Table 5-1)
- Used as a global descriptor of a patient's clinical state based on history, physical examination, and laboratory data
- Most widely used and accepted method of describing preoperative health status
- Gross predictor of overall risk; does not assess surgical risk per se[9]
- Robust predictor of postoperative morbidity and mortality
- Validated by and incorporated in current risk assessment models[18]

- Other applications include allocation of resources and anesthesia reimbursement.[19]
- Limitations include subjectivity and interrater inconsistency.[18]
- Recently updated by ASA 2014
  - Definitions remain unchanged, but clinical examples reflect liberalization with some stable chronic severe diseases, e.g., ESRD with hemodialysis, moving from class IV to class III

Table 5-1   *American Society of Anesthesiologists Physical Status Classification*

Physical Status	Description
Class I	Normal, healthy patient
Class II	Mild systemic disease
Class III	Severe systemic disease
Class IV	Severe systemic disease that is a constant threat to life
Class V	Moribund patient not expected to survive without operation
Class VI	Patient declared brain dead for organ donation purposes

Emergency surgery (E) denotes any of the above patient classes requiring emergency operation (e.g., normal, healthy patient for surgery is class IE).

- Patients frequently present for aesthetic surgery with multiple medical problems that represent an ASA III status.
- ASA III patients are a widely disparate group with huge variations in pathophysiology.

NOTE: The presence of stable, optimized preexisting diseases consistent with an ASA III status is NOT a contraindication for elective surgery.

NPO FASTING GUIDELINES AND PREVENTION OF PULMONARY ASPIRATION (Table 5-2)[21]

FASTING

Table 5-2   *ASA Guidelines for Fasting (in adults, updated 2011)*

Ingested Material	Minimum Fasting Period (hours)
Clear liquids	2
Dairy, nonclear juices	6
Light meal (toast and clear liquid)	6
Heavy meal (fried, fatty foods; meat)	≥8

- Guidelines are limited to healthy patients undergoing elective procedures.
- Modification based on clinical indicators may be needed.
- Modification may be needed if difficult airway is anticipated.
- Patients need to be informed (verbal, written) and status verified on day of surgery.
- Following the guidelines does not guarantee sufficient gastric emptying.

NOTE: Allowing black coffee and plain tea as "clear liquid" intake per guidelines for healthy patients without aspiration concerns can have added benefit of preventing caffeine withdrawal headaches.

ACID ASPIRATION PROPHYLAXIS AND CONSIDERATIONS

- **Pulmonary aspiration:** Aspiration of gastric contents occurring after the induction of general anesthesia, during a procedure, or in the immediate period after surgery
- ASA and SAMBA recommend **NO ROUTINE** administration of preoperative acid aspiration prophylaxis medications.
- Clinical indications for use of medications, AS WELL AS EXTENDING OR MODIFYING NPO GUIDELINES, incorporate comorbidities that **affect or delay gastric emptying:**
  - Obesity
  - Pregnancy
  - Diabetes
  - Gastroesophageal reflux disease (GERD)
  - Hiatal hernia
  - After bariatric surgery (especially laparotomy band)
  - Ileus or bowel obstruction
  - Emergency surgery (e.g., return to OR for hematoma or wound dehiscence after PO intake in PACU)
- **Preoperative prophylactic medications include:**
  - Gastrointestinal stimulants (metoclopramide)
  - Gastric acid blockers
    - ▶ H2-receptor antagonists (cimetidine, ranitidine, famotidine)
    - ▶ Proton pump inhibitors (omeprazole, lansoprazole)
  - Antacid, nonparticulate (sodium citrate)
  - Antiemetics (ondansetron, prochlorperazine) used alone or in combination

FUNCTIONAL STATUS AND METABOLIC EQUIVALENTS (METS)

FUNCTIONAL STATUS OR FUNCTIONAL CAPACITY[9,17]

- Derived by estimating patient's abilities to perform various tasks and activities of daily living (ADLs)
- Expressed in **METs**
  - **1 MET = 3.5 ml O_2 uptake/kg/min** (resting oxygen uptake in sitting position)
- **Adjunct to assess cardiac risk**
- Although not a formal component of the ASAPS classification, it is part of the routine anesthetic preoperative evaluation described as:
  - <4 METs; = 4 METs; >4 METs
- Used as an indicator on Gupta Myocardial Infarction and Cardiac Arrest (MICA) Perioperative Cardiac Risk Calculator[22]
- Used as an indicator on ASC National Surgical Quality Improvement Program (NSQIP) Surgical Risk Calculator[11]
- Has been suggested as a useful adjunct in assessing ASA class II-IV patients and an independent predictor of outcome and mortality[23]
- Patient descriptors:
  - Totally independent
  - Partially dependent
  - Totally dependent

POOR FUNCTIONAL STATUS

- Has been suggested for use as an additional (downgrading) subset to the ASA PS criteria[24]
  - **<4 METs** is of concern and indicates **poor functional status** with **increased risk of cardiopulmonary complications.**

Assessment of METs (Fig. 5-1)

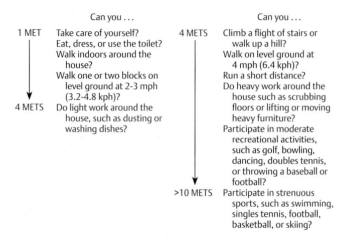

	Can you . . .		Can you . . .
1 MET	Take care of yourself?	4 METS	Climb a flight of stairs or
	Eat, dress, or use the toilet?		walk up a hill?
	Walk indoors around the		Walk on level ground at
	house?		4 mph (6.4 kph)?
	Walk one or two blocks on		Run a short distance?
	level ground at 2-3 mph		Do heavy work around the
	(3.2-4.8 kph)?		house such as scrubbing
4 METS	Do light work around the		floors or lifting or moving
	house, such as dusting or		heavy furniture?
	washing dishes?		Participate in moderate
			recreational activities,
			such as golf, bowling,
			dancing, doubles tennis,
			or throwing a baseball or
			football?
		>10 METS	Participate in strenuous
			sports, such as swimming,
			singles tennis, football,
			basketball, or skiing?

Fig. 5-1   Assessment of METs for poor functional status.

MONITORED ANESTHESIA CARE (MAC): THE DEPTH OF SEDATION CONTINUUM

Monitored Anesthesia Care[1,10,25-28]

- A specific anesthesia service, not an anesthetic per se
- Used for diagnostic or therapeutic procedures
- Must include all aspects of anesthetic care
  - Preanesthetic evaluation
  - Intraprocedure care and monitoring
  - Postanesthetic management
- ASA standard monitors include ECG, noninvasive blood pressure (NIBP), pulse oximetry (SpO_2), end-tidal carbon dioxide ($EtCO_2$) if greater than minimal sedation; temperature available and used when indicated

Goals

- **Sedation,** as a reduction in level of consciousness
- **Analgesia,** in combinations with local, regional, or pharmacologic adjuncts
- **Anxiolysis**
- **Amnesia**
- **Stable physiologic parameters**

Medication Routes

- PO
- IV
- IM
- Transcutaneous
- Intranasal

METHODS OF ADMINISTRATION
- Intermittent IV bolus
- Continuous infusion
- Patient-controlled delivery

MEDICATIONS (Table 5-3)
- Benzodiazepines (midazolam, diazepam, lorazepam)
- Narcotics (fentanyl, alfentanil, remifentanil, sufentanil, meperidine, morphine)
- Opiate agonist-antagonists (buprenorphine, butorphanol, nalbuphine)
- Alpha-adrenergic agonists (dexmedetomidine, clonidine)
- Sedative-hypnotics (propofol, ketamine, methohexital)

Table 5-3 *Common Drugs Used for Sedation During Monitored Anesthesia Care*

Drug	Dose and Infusion Rate*
Short-Acting Opioids	
Alfentanil	5-7 µg/kg or 0.2-0.5 µg/kg/min
Fentanyl	0.3-0.7 µg/kg or 0.01-0.02 µg/kg/min
Remifentanil	0.25-0.5 µg/kg or 0.025-0.1 µg/kg/min
Sufentanil	0.05-0.15 µg/kg or 0.1-0.5 µg/kg/h
Older-Generation Opioids (slower onset, longer duration)	
Meperidine	0.2 mg/kg 10-20 mg
Morphine	0.02 mg/kg 1-2 mg
Opiate Agonist-Antagonists	
Buprenorphine	2-5 mg/kg
Butorphanol	2-7 mg/kg
Nalbuphine	0.07-0.1 mg/kg
Benzodiazepines	
Diazepam	0.05-0.1 mg/kg
Lorazepam	0.01-0.02 mg/kg
Midazolam	0.030-0.075 mg/kg
Alpha-2-Adrenergic Agonists	
Dexmedetomidine	1 µg/kg or 0.2-0.7 mg/kg/min
Alkylphenols	
Propofol	0.2-0.5 mg/kg or 10-75 µg/kg/min
Fospropofol	6.5 mg/kg
Barbiturates	
Methohexital	0.2-0.5 mg/kg
Phencyclidine	
Ketamine	0.2-0.5 mg/kg

*Based on average weight of 70 kg. Doses may vary depending on age, gender, underlying health status, and other concomitantly administered medications.

THE SEDATION CONTINUUM[26] (Table 5-4)

Table 5-4   *The Sedation Continuum*

Level of Sedation	Patient Response to Stimulation	Provider Response to Unintended Sedation Levels
Minimal	Normal response to verbal stimulation; airway, ventilation, cardiovascular function unaffected	Lighter sedation levels support preservation and maintenance of life-preserving reflexes (LPRs).[1] Patent airway Spontaneous respiration with adequate oxygenation and ventilation Swallow and gag reflex
Moderate	Purposeful response to verbal or tactile stimulation; no airway intervention; ventilation and cardiovascular function adequate	Providers of moderate sedation need ability to "rescue" should level become deeper than intended.
Deep	Purposeful response with repeated or painful stimulation; possible need for airway intervention; possible inadequate ventilation; cardiovascular function usually maintained	When ability for purposeful response is absent, *sedation* becomes "general anesthesia" regardless of need for airway instrumentation.
Transition to general anesthesia	—	When ability for purposeful response is absent, *sedation* becomes "general anesthesia" regardless of need for airway instrumentation.

Data from ASA continuum of depth of sedation: definition of general anesthesia and level of sedation/analgesia. Available at *www.asahq.org*.

- Continuum can be unpredictable, dynamic, and challenging to navigate.
- Reflex withdrawal to pain is NOT considered purposeful response.
- Deeper levels may require airway or ventilatory support (Fig. 5-2).
- Transition to general anesthesia level can include impairments, as described previously, plus cardiovascular instability.

NOTE: Providers of MAC (qualified physicians or CRNAs) should be prepared and qualified for conversion to general anesthesia.

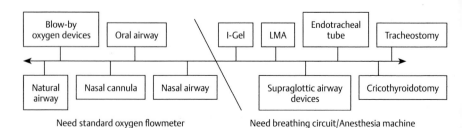

Fig. 5-2   Tools of the airway continuum.

AGENT REVERSAL

- **Benzodiazepines** are reversible with **flumazenil** (Romazicon).
  - Prepared as 0.5 mg/5 ml (0.1 mg/ml) vial
  - Initial dose of 0.2 mg IV over 15 seconds
  - May repeat 0.1-0.2 mg every 60 seconds until total dose of 1.0 mg

> **TIP:** The half-life of benzodiazepine EXCEEDS that of flumazenil; **watch for resedation.**

- **Narcotics** are reversible with **naloxone** (Narcan).
  - Prepared as 0.4 mg/1 ml vial
  - Careful titration is required, because of adverse effects of rapid opiate reversal (severe pain, seizure, pulmonary edema, hypertension, and heart failure).
  - Initial dose can be 0.1-0.2 mg.
  - Effective administration is achieved by diluting 1 vial with 10 ml normal saline solution to concentration of 0.04 mg/ml.
  - Dose is 1-2 ml (0.04 mg/ml) at a time depending on depth of respiratory depression

> **TIP:** The half-life of narcotics EXCEEDS that of naloxone; thus watch for renarcotization and recurrent respiratory depression.

GENERAL PRINCIPLES OF AIRWAY MANAGEMENT AND THE ASA DIFFICULT AIRWAY ALGORITHM

Airway choices and devices, from simple to invasive, are tailored by specific patient and surgical needs.

EVALUATION[1,29,30]

- **History** can detect factors associated with a difficult airway.
  - Previous known difficult laryngoscopy
  - Previous known difficult mask airway
  - Patient report of history of significant sore throat after anesthesia
  - Review of all available anesthetic records
  - Known medical conditions associated with difficult airway management
    - ▶ Obesity
    - ▶ OSA
    - ▶ Arthritis or ankylosing spondylitis
    - ▶ Mediastinal mass, goiter, subglottic stenosis, vocal cord paralysis
    - ▶ Acquired disease states, e.g., postradiation changes
    - ▶ Congenital syndromes, e.g., Pierre Robin sequence
- **External examination** can detect physical characteristics that might negatively affect airway management.
  - Small oral (interincisal) opening less than the desired "3 fingerbreadths"
  - Any signs of temporomandibular joint (TMJ) disorder
  - Conditions of poor dentition: Decay, loose, or missing teeth
  - Malocclusion: Overbite, underbite
  - Presence of dentures, caps, crowns, veneers, bonding, implants, braces, retainers
  - Thyromental distance less than the desired "3 fingerbreadths"
  - Thickness of neck, "bull neck"

- Limitations in cervical spine flexion and/or extension
- Inability to visualize uvula
- Narrow or high-arched palate

MANAGEMENT OF DIFFICULT AIRWAY[30]
- **Mallampati (MP) classification** (Fig. 5-3)

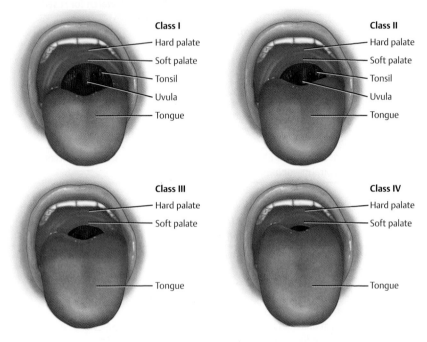

Fig. 5-3   The Mallampati score. (*Class 1,* Complete visualization of the soft palate; *class 2,* complete visualization of the uvula; *class 3,* visualization of only the base of the uvula; *class 4,* soft palate is not visible at all.)

- Used for predicting potential ease or difficulty of achieving adequate laryngoscopic view
- **MP >class 2 elevates level of concern.**
- When used alone it has poor to moderate discriminative power.
- Combination of tests (adding thyromental distance) adds incremental diagnostic value.
- ASA Practice Guidelines suggest preoperative assessment of mutiple airway features to improve predictive value of external examination.

> **NOTE:**   Avoid known "cannot ventilate–cannot intubate" patients for general anesthesia in ASC or office; consider a hospital setting.

POSITIONING[31-34]

- Shared responsibility between surgeon, anesthesiologist, and nursing staff[31]

COMPLICATIONS ASSOCIATED WITH SUBOPTIMAL PATIENT POSITIONING[32]
- **Pressure** ulcers and **muscle necrosis**
- **Alopecia (localized)**[32,33]
  - Associated with longer procedures (>6 hours), intraoperative hypotension, use of vasoconstrictors, and massive intraoperative blood loss
  - Initially focal tenderness (<24 hours) proceeds to hair loss (few days) and is usually complete by 1 month.
  - Hair regrowth begins at 3 months (most cases).
  - Case reports of permanent hair loss exist.
  - For longer procedures, gel doughnut headrests and periodic repositioning can be employed.
- **Peripheral neuropathy**[31-35]
  - Mechanisms include:
    - ▶ Stretching (traction)
    - ▶ Compression
    - ▶ Ischemia
    - ▶ Metabolic derangement
    - ▶ Surgical injury
  - ASA closed claims studies[34] have identified **nerve injuries** as **second most** frequent liability claim in anesthesia practice.
  - **Frequency of injury**
    - ▶ Ulnar ➤ brachial plexus ➤ median in frequency of injury.
    - ▶ Causes are not always easily identifiable or attributable to positioning (<10%).[31]
    - ▶ Nonpositioning-related factors include **male sex, extreme body habitus** (morbid obesity or very thin), **prolonged hospitalization.**
- **Compartment syndrome,** especially in lithotomy or lateral decubitus positions[35]
- **Thermal injuries** can occur with use of warm blankets, forced-air warming devices, and IV fluid–heating devices.
  - Recommended temperature limit for blanket warmers is **43.3° C.**
  - Forced-air warmers MUST be used with the manufacturer's blanket that disperses warm air over a wide surface area.
  - Fluid warmers can cause injury by tubing being in contact with patient's skin.
- **Corneal abrasion**[33,36]
  - **Most common injury**[33]
  - ASA closed claims database cited 41 claims settled after 1990.[36]
  - About 50% of these were associated with general anesthesia.
  - No causative event was identified in 58%.
  - 50% resulted in $12,000 median payment.
  - Incidence is decreasing over time as proportion of eye injuries in database.
  - **Prophylactic measures include:**
    - ▶ Taping or occlusive dressings to eyes
    - ▶ Sterile ophthalmic lubricant (Lacri-Lube)
    - ▶ Suturing lids closed

> ► Protective goggles
> ► Corneal protectors
>> ◆ Metal or plastic
>> ◆ Limit time of use to essential parts of procedure, because prolonged use can cause corneal ischemia.

- **Postoperative vision loss (POVL)**[33,36,37]
  - Relatively low incidence, but high debilitation
  - Mostly described in spine surgery (prone position), cardiac surgery, and head and neck surgery
  - Most closed claims (1995-2011) permanent and significant
  - One case report with prone position and protective goggles placed in addition to foam headrest, possibly compression-induced injury[38]

PATIENT-ASSOCIATED CHARACTERISTICS THAT CAN LEAD TO POSITIONING INJURIES

- Joint restrictions or cervical spine instability (rheumatoid arthritis, ankylosing spondylitis)
- H/O injuries, trauma, or inflammatory disease that affects joint mobility
- Contractures associated with chronic debilitating disease
- Fragile skin conditions of the elderly, steroid use, or autoimmune diseases
- Extremes of weight, especially if prone position is needed

MANAGEMENT OF COMPLICATIONS RELATED TO POSITIONING[33]

- **Peripheral neuropathies** are most common and enigmatic.
- Provide full disclosure and consistent information to patients.
- Avoid speculation.
- Documentation, including preexisting conditions, risk factors, limitations in positioning
- Photographic documentation of clinical findings
- Appropriate consultations, early and liberally
- Treatment dictated by findings and urgency, usually nonemergent (exception compartment syndrome)
- Involvement of risk management team
- Appropriate follow-up

PERIOPERATIVE HYPOTHERMIA[39-41] (Box 5-2)

Box 5-2   *SUMMARY OF HYPOTHERMIA PREVENTION*

- Prewarm patients for 1 hour in the preoperative area.
- Keep the OR an ambient temperature at 22.8° C.
- Monitor core temperature (esophageal or nasopharyngeal).
- Employ active warming methods.
- Employ passive covering of the exposed body surface area.
- Minimize exposure and repositioning, and resume active warming ASAP.
- Warm IV, infiltration, and irrigation fluids.
- Manage postanesthetic shivering aggressively with continuation of active-warming devices and pharmacologic intervention.

- Associated with various surgical complications and deleterious physiologic derangements[39,41]
- Patient experience and satisfaction are negatively affected.
- Normothermia averages around **37° C.**
- Range fluctuates as much as 1° C throughout the day.
- **Perioperative hypothermia is defined as <36.1° C.**
- Mild intraoperative hypothermia range is 34°-36° C.
- Plastic surgery procedures that carry a **higher risk of hypothermia** include:
  - Tumescent liposuction, especially high-volume
  - Abdominoplasty
  - Flap transfers
  - Lower body or circumferential lifts
  - Body contouring after massive weight loss

COMPLICATIONS
- Infection
- Delayed wound healing and/or dehiscence
- Seroma[39]
- Hematoma
- Coagulation disorder of decreased platelet function and impaired clot formation[41]
- Postanesthetic shivering as a source of deleterious discomfort, increased length of stay, and cost

CONTRIBUTING FACTORS
- Preoperative areas with low ambient temperatures
- Patient fasting that reduces metabolism
- Anesthesia-related inhibition of thermoregulatory defense mechanisms (neuraxial ➤ general)
- Cool intraoperative OR environments
- Body surface exposure
- Incisional heat loss from evaporation and radiation
- Use of cool irrigation, IV and infiltration fluids
- **Patient-associated risk factors** could include:
  - Increased age
  - Thin body habitus
  - Preexisting metabolic disorders, including diabetes-related autonomic dysfunction and neuropathies

ACTIVE WARMING MANEUVERS[41]
- Inadvertent hypothermia has been reported in 50%-90% of surgical patients if not preempted by active warming measures.
- Raising ambient temperature of OR to 22.8° C (73° F) is standard.
- Use of forced-air heating (e.g., Bair Hugger [Arizant Healthcare, Inc.]) has become the standard of care.
- Use of special heating blankets and mattresses, either circulating warm water or polymer-based resistive heating
- Warming irrigation fluids to 40° C in temperature-controlled warmers
- Warming IV fluids to 37° C

- Warming liposuction infiltration fluids to 37° C deemed helpful in slowing loss of body heat
- Heated, humidified anesthetic gases
- Radiant heating devices
- Investigational research methods include amino acids infusion that provokes thermogenesis.

PASSIVE WARMING MANEUVERS
- Insulating patient with standard or heated blankets and drapes
- Can only conserve, not produce, heat
- Reduces cutaneous heat loss
- *Multiple layers do not significantly increase benefit.*

> **NOTE: Heated blankets are NOT more effective than nonheated blankets, although they provide more perceptible comfort to awake patients.**

- Reflective "space caps" or wrapping the head (but not a significant source of heat loss)
- Reflective blankets

PACU RECOVERY AND RETURN TO NORMOTHERMIA
- Hypothermia on arrival to PACU may take up to **4 hours** to correct.
- Postanesthetic shivering (PAS) related to volatile anesthetics occurs in **40%-65%** of patients.
  - Related to duration of surgery and nadir of temperature
  - More common in younger patients (<60 years of age)
  - Aggravates pain
  - Increases HR, BP, release of catecholamines, oxygen consumption (200%-400%), myocardial oxygen demand—can be deleterious with preexisting cardiac disease
  - Requires aggressive active warming measures
  - Antishivering medication with meperidine 12.5-50 mg is effective but should be accompanied by other warming measures.

POSTOPERATIVE NAUSEA AND VOMITING AND POSTDISCHARGE NAUSEA AND VOMITING[8,42-45]
- Topics of *significant* patient concern and distress and affects patient satisfaction
- One of the **most frequently occurring side effects** of anesthesia
- Aesthetic surgery patients large subset of those affected
- Nausea incidence reported to be from **50%-80%**
- Vomiting incidence reported at **30%**
- Continuation or presentation of symptoms after discharge (PDNV) is 17% nausea, 8% vomiting.

CAUTION: Inadequately treated PONV can increase PACU stay or result in unplanned admission.

UNDERSTANDING MECHANISM OF EMESIS AFFECTS MANAGEMENT[42,43]

- **"Emetic zone"** located in lateral reticular formation of brainstem
- Receives afferents from the "chemoreceptor trigger zone" (CTZ) at base of fourth ventricle
- Signals to CTZ are mediated by **multiple neurotransmitters.**
  - **Serotonin (5-HT3)**
  - **Dopamine (DA)**
  - **Histamine (H-1)**
  - **Acetylcholine (Ach)**
  - **Neurokinin (NK-1)**
- Prophylaxis or therapies target blocking one or more of these receptors.

AREAS OF ATTENTION AND FOCUS[8,44,45] (Fig. 5-4; Table 5-5)

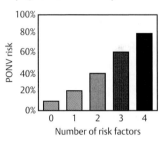

Risk Factors	Points
Female	1
Nonsmoker	1
History of PONV	1
Postoperative opioids	1
Sum =	0 ... 4

Fig. 5-4   PDNV risk factors.

Table 5-5   *Risk Factors for PONV in Adults*

Evidence	Risk Factors
Positive overall	Female sex (B1) History of PONV or motion sickness (B1) Nonsmoking (B1) Younger age (B1) General versus regional anesthesia (A1) Use of volatile anesthetics and nitrous oxide (A1) Postoperative opioids (A1) Duration of anesthesia (B1) Type of surgery (cholecystectomy, laparoscopic, gynecological) (B1)
Conflicting	ASA physical status (B1) Menstrual cycle (B1) Level of anesthetist's experience (B1) Muscle relaxant antagonists (A2)
Disproven or of limited clinical relevance	BMI (B1) Anxiety (B1) Nasogastric tube (A1) Supplemental oxygen (A1) Perioperative fasting (A2) Migraine (B1)

BMI, Body mass index; *MS,* motion sickness; *PONV,* postoperative nausea and vomiting.

- **Identify patients at risk.**
- **Tailor anesthetic plan** to reduce or mitigate baseline risk factors.
- Employ prophylaxis, pharmacologic and otherwise, based on latest evidence-based literature regarding selection, timing, risk/benefit ratio, and cost-effectiveness.[45]
- **Provide effective "rescue" therapy.**
- **Coordinate postdischarge planning** with surgeon with regard to opioid and opioid-sparing analgesia, as well as availability of PO antiemetic agents.

RISK STRATIFICATION TOOLS
- Apfel simplified risk score is tool most commonly used and validated.
- **Gan et al**[45] used meta-analysis to validate and update specific risks that include:
  - **Female sex**
  - **Nonsmoker**
  - **Younger age (<50 years)**
  - **H/O PONV or motion sickness**

ANESTHETIC-RELATED RISKS
- General versus regional anesthesia
- Volatile anesthetics, in a dose-dependent manner
- Nitrous oxide
- Postoperative opioids, in dose-dependent manner
- Duration of surgery
- Type of surgery

STRATEGIES TO REDUCE BASELINE RISK
- **Adequate hydration** allowing intake of clear liquids up to 3-4 hours before surgery
- Use of **regional anesthesia** techniques when indicated
- Preferential use of **propofol infusion** (TIVA) to avoid volatile agents
- **Minimize perioperative opioids** by:
  - Aggressive use of multimodal nonopioid analgesia
  - Liberal use of local anesthesia by surgeon
  - Use of postoperative continuous infusion pain management techniques where applicable
- **Aggressive prophylaxis** with combination or multimodal therapy based on risk stratification

COMBINATION ANTIEMETIC THERAPY (Table 5-6)
- Preferable to single drug
- **Using drugs from different classes targets multiple receptors or trigger areas in brain.**
- Effects are additive.
- *Smaller doses in different classes increases efficacy.*
- Side effects of individual drugs are decreased.
- Current literature has recommendations for doses and timing of some drugs.[45]
- Reserve at least one drug for PACU rescue administration.

Table 5-6 *Most Commonly Used Drugs (class/receptor)*

Generic Name	Trade Name
Ondansetron (5-HT3 receptor antagonist)	Zofran in IV, PO or oral dissolving (ODT)
Dexamethasone (corticosteroid)	Decadron IV
Haloperidol (butyrophenone/DA antagonist)	Haldol IV (FDA off-label use)
Meclizine (antihistamine/H-1 antagonist)	Antivert PO
Transdermal scopolamine (anticholinergic)	TransDerm Scop
Aprepitant (NK-1 antagonist)	Emend PO
Promethazine (phenothiazine/DA antagonist)	Phenergan IV, deep IM, or PO

NONPHARMACOLOGIC THERAPY

■ P6-accupressure or accupoint electrostimulation uses acupuncture principles (ReliefBand, Abbott Laboratories) and is applied to inner aspect of wrist in distribution of median nerve.
■ Recommended by several authors as effective with advantage of no additional risk.[8,45]

PACU RESCUE THERAPY

■ If prophylaxis **WAS NOT** given, can give any or combinations of:
  • Ondansetron 1.0 mg IV (dose is lower than the prophylactic dose)
  • Dexamethasone 2-4 mg IV
  • Droperidol 0.625 mg IV or haloperidol 0.5-2.0 mg
  • Promethazine 2.5-12.5 mg IV/IM
  • Propofol 20 mg IV (effect short lived)
  • Isopropyl alcohol aromatherapy (unclear efficacy but commonly used)
■ If prophylaxis **WAS** given:
  • Use drug in **different class** from those received as prophylaxis.

> **NOTE:**   Repeating any previously used drugs confers no additional benefit.

  • If >6 hours in PACU, an additional dose of ondansetron or haloperidol (not verified by clinical trials) can be given.

CAUTION: DO NOT REDOSE dexamethasone, transdermal scopolamine, or aprepitant.

MALIGNANT HYPERTHERMIA[46-49]

■ Pharmacogenetic **(autosomal dominant)** disorder triggered by:
  • Volatile anesthetic gases (desflurane, sevoflurane, isoflurane)
  • Succinylcholine
■ **Affects skeletal muscle ONLY**
■ Causes **unregulated calcium release** from sarcoplasmic reticulum
■ Can present after induction, intraoperatively, or in PACU
■ Postoperative presentation reported to be low (1.9% of cases)[49]
■ Patients have inherited MH-susceptible mutation exposed to one or both types of triggering agents.

SIGNS
- Initially can be subtle and nonspecific
  - Rigidity, with generalized muscle contraction (masseter, truncal, extremities) or whole body
  - Hypermetabolic chain reaction
  - Tachycardia
  - Increasing EtCO$_2$ *unresponsive to increased minute ventilation*
  - Increased temperature (can be late sign)
  - Hyperkalemia with ECG changes, dysrhythmias
  - Acidosis
  - Myoglobinuria
  - Cardiac arrest
  - Death
  - **Have high index of suspicion—act early**
  - **Dantrolene is the ONLY effective treatment**

MANAGEMENT
- Multiple tasks need to be executed quickly and concurrently.
- **CALL FOR HELP.**
- Halt/abort procedure, if able.
- **Call Malignant Hypothermia Association of the United States (MHAUS) Hotline: 1-800-644 -9737 or 1-800-MH-HYPER.**
  - Expert consultation is available 24/7/365.
  - They will stay on the line to guide and support crisis management.
- Get MH cart or code cart and **dantrolene.**
  - Recommend stock of 36 vials **dantrolene** (20 mg each) **OR** equivalent dose (3 vials) of new preparation **Ryanodex** (250 mg each)
  - Stop exposure to offending agent(s)
  - Hyperventilate 3-4× normal with 100% O$_2$ at HIGH FLOWS.
  - Apply activated charcoal filters (Vapor-Clean, Dynathestics) to both limbs of anesthesia circuit to accelerate reduction in concentration of anesthetic gas.
  - DO NOT take time to change machine.
  - Switch to TIVA (nontriggering anesthetic).
  - **Dantrolene ASAP!**
- **Traditional** preparations (Dantrium, Revonto)
  - Mix each 20 mg vial of powder with 60 ml sterile *nonbacteriostatic* H$_2$O.
  - **Labor intensive:** Need several people to help
  - Dose 2.5 mg/kg in repeated doses as clinically indicated up to 10 mg/kg.
  - Each 20 mg dantrolene has 3 g mannitol.
- **Newer** preparation (Ryanodex)
  - Less mixing: Use only 5 ml *nonbacteriostatic* sterile H$_2$O/250 mg vial of powder suspension.
  - **Administration is faster**
  - 1 vial Ryanodex = 12.5 vials of traditional preparation dantrolene
  - Dose 2.5 mg/kg in repeated doses as clinically indicated up to 10 mg/kg
  - Each vial has 125 mg mannitol (less than traditional preparation)
  - *Little experience with this preparation has been reported*

ADDITIONAL MANAGEMENT

- Initiate active cooling (IV fluids, surface ice packs to axilla and groin, gastric/bladder lavage).
- Place Foley catheter.
- Treat metabolic/electrolyte derangement(s).
- Provide hemodynamic support.
- **INITIATE TRANSFER PLANS TO ICU, TERTIARY CARE FACILITY.**
- Consider future testing by muscle biopsy or molecular genetics.
- Report incidence to North American Malignant Hyperthermia Registry (*http://www.mhaus.org/registry*).

> **NOTE:** MHAUS supports MH-susceptible patient as acceptable for ASCs with adequate facility resources, planning, and preparation, including transfer capabilities.

- Additional resources available at Malignant Hyperthermia Association of the United States (*MHAUS; www.mhaus.org.*)

POSTANESTHESIA RECOVERY UNIT (PACU) CARE[50-53]

PHASES OF RECOVERY
- **Phase I:** Immediate acute care
- **Phase II:** Convalescent or predischarge
- **Fast track**
  - Preferable and common in ambulatory setting
  - Expedited clinical pathway supported by appropriate anesthetic pharmacologic management with short-acting agents
  - Bypass of phase I: OR direct to phase II under direction of anesthesiologist
  - Must meet phase I criteria upon leaving OR
- **Combined phase 1 and 2**
  - Many ASCs physically merge both phases into a single unit.
  - "One stop shopping" where one nurse manages entire recovery process
  - Eliminates extra transfers and handoffs
  - Provides continuity of care
  - Provides flexibility and allows application of fast-track principles to all
- **Phase III:** Postdischarge continued recovery
  - Can last for several days
  - Continues until patient reverts to baseline preoperative status
  - Resumption of ADLs

UNPLANNED ADMISSION
- By accreditation criteria, all facilities performing aesthetic surgery must have plans in place for transfer to higher level of care.
- Reported national averages are **1%-2%**.
- Precipitated by medical conditions (cardiopulmonary, respiratory, neurologic, MH)
- Precipitated for surgical conditions (bleeding or postsurgical sequelae)
- Calls for preestablished transport protocols with a service or EMS
- Calls for preestablished agreement with receiving hospitals
- Surgeon, anesthesiologist, and/or CRNA or RN can accompany patients for continuity of care and facilitate transfer.

TOP TAKEAWAYS

➤ Regulatory agencies establish minimum standards of care in aesthetic surgery environments.

➤ ASA Standards for Basic Anesthetic Monitoring[10] (last amended 2011) must be met.

➤ Intangibles, nuances, or needs that may affect patient's satisfaction or experience in this highly specialized, consumer-driven patient population

➤ In diabetics, obtain by blood draw as preadmission testing (PAT) or by point of care testing on day of surgery

➤ The half-life of narcotics EXCEEDS that of naloxone; thus watch for renarcotization and recurrent respiratory depression.

➤ Inadvertent hypothermia has been reported in 50%-90% of surgical patients if not preempted by active warming measures

REFERENCES

1. Bennett GD. Anesthesia for aesthetic surgery. In Shiffman MA, Di Giuseppe A, eds. Cosmetic Surgery. Berlin Heidelberg: Springer, 2013.
2. Desai M. General inhalation anesthesia for cosmetic surgery. In Friedberg BL, ed. Anesthesia in Cosmetic Surgery. New York: Cambridge University Press, 2007.
3. Crowder CM, Palanca BJ, Evers AS. Mechanisms of anesthesia and consciousness. In Barash PG, Cullen BF, Stoelting RK, et al, eds. Clinical Anesthesia, ed 7. Philadelphia: Lippincott Williams & Wilkins, 2013.
4. Gertler R, Joshi GP. General anesthesia. In Twersky RS, Phillip BK, eds. Handbook of Ambulatory Anesthesia, ed 2. New York: Springer Science, 2008.
5. Raeder J, ed. Clinical Ambulatory Anesthesia. New York: Cambridge University Press, 2010.
6. Blakely KR, Klein KW, White PF, et al. A total intravenous anesthetic technique for outpatient facial laser resurfacing. Anesth Analg 87:827, 1998.
7. Friedberg BL. The dissociative effect and preemptive analgesia. In Friedberg BL, ed. Anesthesia in Cosmetic Surgery. New York: Cambridge University Press, 2007.
8. Barinholtz D. Intravenous anesthesia for cosmetic surgery. In Friedberg BL, ed. Anesthesia in Cosmetic Surgery. New York: Cambridge University Press, 2007.
9. Kataria K, Cutter TW, Apfelbaum JL. Patient selection in outpatient surgery. Clin Plast Surg 40:371, 2013.
10. ASA standards for basic anesthetic monitoring. Available at www.asahq.org.
11. ASC NSQIP Surgical Risk Calculator. Available at http://riskcalculator.facs.org/RiskCalculator/.
12. Levin N. Preanesthetic assessment of the cosmetic patient. In Friedberg BL, ed. Anesthesia in Cosmetic Surgery. New York: Cambridge University Press, 2007.
13. Ogunnaike B. Anesthesia. In Janis JE, ed. Essentials of Plastic Surgery, ed 2. New York: Thieme, 2014.
14. Committee on Standards and Practice Parameters, et al. Practice Advisory for Preanesthetic Evaluation. An updated report by the American Society of Anesthesiologists Taskforce on Preanesthesia Evaluation. Anesthesiology 116:522, 2012.
15. Mathis MR, Naughton NN, Shanks AM, et al. Patient selection for day case-eligible surgery. Anesthesiology 119:1310, 2013.
16. Choosing wisely: an initiative of the ABIM Foundation. Available at www.choosingwisely.org.

17. Cohn SL, Fleisher LA. Evaluation of cardiac risk prior to noncardiac surgery. Available at *http://www.uptodate.com/contents/evaluation-of-cardiac-risk-prior-to-noncardiac-surgery*.

18. Davenport DL, Bowe EA, Henderson WG, et al. National Surgical Quality Improvement Program (NSQIP) risk factors can be used to validate American Society of Anesthesiologists Physical Status Classification (ASA PS) levels. Ann Surg 243:636, 2006.

19. Sankar A, Johnson SR, Beattie WS, et al. Reliability of the American Society of Anesthesiologists physical status scale in clinical practice. Br J Anaesth 113:424, 2014.

20. Ansell GL, Montgomery JE. Outcome of ASA III patients undergoing day case surgery. Br J Anaesth 92:71, 2004.

21. American Society for Anesthesiologists Committee. Practice guidelines for preoperative fasting and the use of pharmacologic agents to reduce the risk of pulmonary aspiration: application to healthy patients undergoing elective procedures: an updated report by the American Society for Anesthesiologists Committee on Standards and Practice Parameters. Anesthesiology 114:495, 2011.

22. Gupta PK, Gupta H, Sundaram A, et al. Development and validation of a risk calculator for prediction of cardiac risk after surgery. Circulation 124:381, 2011.

23. Dosluoglu HH, Wang JP, Defranks-Anain L, et al. A simple subclassification of American Society of Anesthesiology III patients undergoing peripheral revascularization based on functional capacity. J Vasc Surg 47:766, 2008.

24. Visnjevac O, Davari-Farid S, Lee J, et al. The effect of adding functional classification to ASA status for predicting 30-day mortality. Anesth Analg 121:110, 2015.

25. ASA position on monitored anesthesia care. Available at *www. asahq.org*.

26. ASA continuum of depth of sedation: definition of general anesthesia and level of sedation/analgesia. Available at *www.asahq.org*.

27. Urman RD, Ehrenfeld JM, eds. Pocket Anesthesia, ed 2. Philadelphia: Lippincott Williams & Wilkins, 2013.

28. Distinguishing monitored anesthesia care ("MAC") from moderate sedation/analgesia (conscious sedation). Available at *www.asahq.org*.

29. Amadasun FE, Adudu OP, Sadiq A, et al. Effects of position and phonation on oropharyngeal view and correlation with laryngoscopic view. Niger J Clin Pract 13:417, 2010.

30. Apfelbaum JL, Hagberg CA, Caplan RA, et al. Practice guidelines for management of the difficult airway: an updated report by the American Society of Anesthesiologists Task Force on Management of the Difficult Airway. Anesthesiology 118:251, 2013.

31. Washington SJ, Smurthwaite GL. Positioning the surgical patient. Anaesth Int Care Med 10:476, 2009.

32. Dominguez E, Eslinger MR, McCord SV. Postoperative (pressure) alopecia: report of a case after elective cosmetic surgery. Anesth Analg 89:1062, 1999.

33. Hansen J, Botney R. Safe patient positioning. In Young VL, Botney R, eds. Patient Safety in Plastic Surgery. New York: Thieme Publishers, 2009.

34. Cheney FW, Domino KB, Kaplan RA, et al. Nerve injury associated with anesthesia: a closed claim analysis. Anesthesiology 90:1062, 1999.

35. Warner MA, Warner DO, Harper CM, et al. Lower extremity neuropathies associated with lithotomy positions. Anesthesiology 93:938, 2000.

36. Posner KL, Lee LA. Anesthesia malpractice claims associated with eye surgery and eye injury: highlights from the anesthesia closed claims project data request service. ASA Monitor 78:28, 2014.

37. Kara-Junior N, Espindola RF, Valverde FJ, et al. Ocular risk management in patients undergoing anesthesia: an analysis of 309,4431 surgeries. Clinics 70:541, 2015.

38. Roth S, Tung A, Ksiazek,S. Visual loss in a prone-positioned spine surgery patient with the head on a foam headrest and goggles covering the eyes: an old complication with a new mechanism. Anesth Analg 104:1185, 2007.

39. Coon D, Michaels JM V, Gusenoff JA, et al. Hypothermia and complications in post-bariatric body contouring. Plast Reconstr Surg 130:443, 2012.

40. Young VL, Watson ME. Hypothermia: prevention and consequences. In Young VL, Botney R, eds. Patient Safety in Plastic Surgery. New York: Thieme Publishers, 2009.

41. Constantine RS, Kenkle M, Hein RE, et al. The impact of perioperative hypothermia on plastic surgery outcomes: a multivariate logistic regression of 1062 cases. Aesthet Surg J 35:81, 2015.

42. Le TP, Gan TJ. Update on the management of postoperative nausea and vomiting and postdischarge nausea and vomiting in ambulatory surgery. Anesthesiol Clin 28:225, 2010.

43. Watcha MF, White PF. Postoperative nausea and vomiting. Its etiology, treatment and prevention. Anesthesiology 77:162, 1992.

44. Öbrink E, Jildenstål P, Oddby E, et al. Post-operative nausea and vomiting: update on predicting the probability and ways to minimize its occurrence, with focus on ambulatory surgery. Int J Surg 15:100, 2015.

45. Gan TJ, Diemunsch P, Habib AS, et al; Society for Ambulatory Anesthesia. Consensus guidelines for management of postoperative nausea and vomiting. Anesth Analg 118:85, 2014.

46. Young VL, Watson ME. Malignant hyperthemia. In Young VL , Botney R, eds. Patient Safety in Plastic Surgery. New York: Thieme Publishers, 2009.

47. Kim TW, Rosenberg H, Nami N. Current concepts in the understanding of malignant hyperthermia. Anesthesiology News, Feb 2014. Available at http://www.anesthesiologynews.com/download/MalignantHyperthermia_AN0214_WM.pdf.

48. MHAUS. Managing an MH crisis. Available at www.mhaus.org.

49. Litman RL, Flood CD, Kaplan RF, et al. Postoperative malignant hyperthermia: an analysis of cases from the North American Malignant Hyperthermia Registry. Anesthesiology 109:825, 2008.

50. Pregler JL, Kapur PA. Postanesthesia care recovery and management. In Twersky RS, Philip BK, eds. Handbook of Ambulatory Anesthesia. New York: Springer Science and Business Media, 2008.

51. Chung F, Lermitte J. Discharge process. In Twersky RS, Philip BK, eds. Handbook of Ambulatory Anesthesia. New York: Springer Science and Business Media, 2008.

52. Chung F, Mezei G. Factors contributing to a prolonged stay after ambulatory surgery. Anesth Analg 89:1352, 1999.

53. Apfelbaum JL, Silverstein JH, Chung FF, et al. Practice guidelines for postanesthetic care: an updated report by the American Society of Anesthesiologists Task Force on Postanesthetic Care. Anesthesiology 188:1, 2013.

RESOURCES

American Society of Anesthesiologists (ASA). Available at www.asahq.org.

American Society of Regional Anesthesia and Pain Medicine (ASRA). Available at www.asra.com.

Anesthesia Patient Safety Foundation (APSF). Available at www.apsf.org.

LipidRescue Resuscitation. Available at www.lipidrescue.org.

Malignant Hyperthermia Association of the United States (MHAUS). Available at www.MHAUS.org.

Regional Anesthesia and Pain Medicine (RAPM). Available at www.rapm.org.

Society of Ambulatory Anesthesia (SAMBA). Available at www.sambahq.org.

6. Perioperative Anesthesia Considerations for the Aesthetic Surgery Patient

Deborah Stahl Lowery

Anesthesia is an important consideration in any aesthetic procedure. Close communication between the anesthesiologist, surgeon, and patient are paramount to a safe and successful surgery. Risk stratification, proper patient selection, and optimization are needed to decrease complications.

CARDIOVASCULAR DISEASES[1-6]

HYPERTENSION
- Continue preexisting beta-blocker on day of surgery (DOS).
- Hold diuretics on DOS.
- Hold ACE inhibitors (lisinopril, ramipril, benazepril, captopril) and angiotensin-receptor blockers (ARBs) (candesartan, losartan, valsartan, irbesartan) on DOS because of exaggerated hypotension with induction of general anesthesia.

CORONARY ARTERY DISEASE

CAUTION: Defer elective surgery if diagnosed within the last 6 months.

- If history of angioplasty or stents: How many, when implanted, type, need for ongoing antiplatelet therapy or anticoagulation? **This is important!** Consult with cardiology or primary care physician (PCP).
- Cardiomyopathy
- Valvular disease
  - **Aortic stenosis is always a concern** (determine mild, moderate, severe).
- Dysrhythmias[6-8]
  - Note any cardiac implantable electronic device (CIED) such as pacemaker or automated implantable cardioverter defibrillator (AICD).

> NOTE: With bipolar electrocautery ONLY, the chance of adverse CIED interruption is minimal; safe for ambulatory surgery center office.

CONGESTIVE HEART FAILURE (CHF)
- Consider only stable, well-compensated chronic CHF for low-risk procedures.

CEREBROVASCULAR DISEASE
- Evaluate if there is a history of TIA or CVA, including presence of any residual effects.

PERIPHERAL VASCULAR DISEASE
- **Pacemakers** (elective surgery) should have device checked within **last 12 months.**
- **Defibrillators** (elective surgery) should have device checked within **last 6 months.**
- If monopolar electrocautery is necessary, consider doing these cases in hospital setting.

PULMONARY DISEASES

PULMONARY HYPERTENSION
- Patients with severe pulmonary hypertension are high risk and **should not undergo elective cosmetic surgery.**

ASTHMA[3,9,10]
- Prevalence in United States is 8.2%
- Closed claim analysis indicates incidence of intraoperative bronchospasm or laryngospasm is as low as 2%, but 90% of these type claims were for severe brain injury or death.
- Preexisting, well-controlled asthma has been associated with low increased risk of bronchospasm (1.7%).[10]
- **Most authors conclude patients with well-controlled asthma are acceptable for ambulatory surgery.**

CHRONIC OBSTRUCTIVE PULMONARY DISEASE (COPD)[3,10-12]
- Identified as **independent risk factor** for increased morbidity and mortality and unplanned intubations
- Most frequent risk factors for postoperative complications include atelectasis, pneumonia, respiratory failure, and COPD exacerbation.[3]
    - Choose a facility that allows extended PACU stay or 23-hour observation.
- Highest risk for hypoxia and hypoventilation is in the **immediate postoperative period.**

SMOKING[10,13]
- Patients who smoke >1-2 packs per day are at increased risk for perioperative respiratory complications, wound infections, flap necrosis.
- Smoking cessation *immediately* before surgery may not improve patient outcome and may actually cause **increased risk of pulmonary complications** because of increased secretions and increased airway reactivity.
- Although no definitive consensus exists in literature, Centers for Disease Control (CDC) recommends **at least 30 days of smoking cessation before and after surgery.**

POSTOPERATIVE PULMONARY COMPLICATIONS (PPCs)[10,14]
- Rate across all types of surgery is **6.8%,** according to recent systematic review.
- More prevalent in patients with known underlying disease
- **Clinically significant complications** include:
    - Atelectasis
    - Infection, bronchitis, or pneumonia
    - Respiratory failure that could result in reintubation or continued mechanical ventilation

- Exacerbation of preexisting chronic conditions
- Bronchospasm
■ **Patient-related risk factors**
  - Poor functional status
  - Poor general health status
    ▶ ASA PS class has good correlation with risk.
    ▶ ASA >II confers almost fivefold increase in risk.
  - Increasing age >50 years
  - Smoking
  - Obesity
■ **Procedure-related risk factors**
  - **Site of surgery** is single, most important factor.
    ▶ Abdominal (upper > lower) or thoracic surgery
    ▶ Abdominoplasty or massive-weight-loss procedures should promote caution.
  - Duration >3-4 hours
  - Type of anesthesia, neuraxial or regional, may confer benefit.
  - Residual neuromuscular blockade
■ PPCs are associated with increased mortality, increased length of stay, and increased cost of care.

OBSTRUCTIVE SLEEP APNEA (OSA)[15-17]

BACKGROUND
■ Rising incidence in United States
■ **Male/female** ratio **3:1**
■ Clinical correlation with **obesity**
■ High index of suspicion for difficult airway
■ Remains **largely undiagnosed** in up to **80%** of patients
■ Episodic airway obstruction results in sleep disruption/disorder and daytime hypersomnolence.
■ *Apnea* defined as **cessation** of airflow from mouth or nose for **≥10 seconds**
■ *Hypopnea* defined as **50% reduction** in airflow that causes slow respiration for **≥10 seconds**
■ Physiologic derangement includes:
  - Oxygen desaturation/hypoxia
  - Hypercarbia
  - Acidosis
  - Polycythemia
■ **Polysomnography** is the standard diagnostic test—determines apnea-hypopnea index and stratifies into *mild, moderate,* or *severe.*

PREOPERATIVE ASSESSMENT
■ American Society of Anesthesiologists (ASA) strongly recommends anesthesiologists and surgeons work together to develop protocols to evaluate patients *before* **the day of surgery** to aid in patient selection, preparation, and management.
■ **STOP-BANG questionnaire most commonly used and recommended in SAMBA (2014) Consensus Statement on OSA and Ambulatory Surgery**[17] (Fig. 6-1)

1. Do you **S**nore loudly?   Yes/No
2. Do you feel **T**ired, fatigued, or sleep during the daytime?   Yes/No
3. Has anyone **O**bserved you stop breathing during your sleep?   Yes/No
4. Have you been or are you now being treated for high blood **P**ressure?   Yes/No
5. Is your **B**ody Mass Index greater than 35 kg/m^2?   Yes/No
6. Are you over 50 years of **A**ge?   Yes/No
7. Is your **N**eck circumference greater than 40 cm?   Yes/No
8. **G**ender (male)?   Yes/No

Fig. 6-1   STOP-BANG questionnaire used for screening patients to determine the risk of OSA. Fewer than three questions positive = low risk of OSA; three or more questions positive = high risk of OSA; five to eight questions positive = high probability of moderate to severe OSA.

DECISION-MAKING AID FOR PATIENT SELECTION FOR AMBULATORY SURGERY (Fig. 6-2)

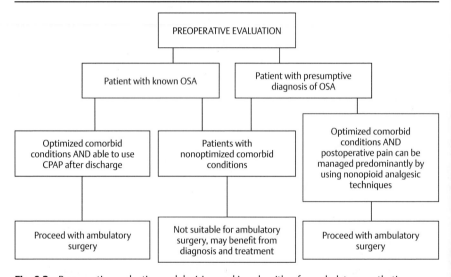

Fig. 6-2   Preoperative evaluation and decision-making algorithm for ambulatory aesthetic surgery.

GENERAL MANAGEMENT
- Minimal/judicious use of narcotics
- Use of multimodal analgesia adjuncts such as acetaminophen, gabapentin, NSAIDs or COX-2 inhibitors, ketamine, dexamethasone, centrally acting alpha-agonists
- Use of local anesthesia; peripheral, neuraxial, and other nerve blocks; home-going continuous infusion devices
- Full reversal of neuromuscular blockade
- Extubation at emergence level of fully awake
- Sedation level exceeding *minimal* should incorporate use of ventilation monitoring using capnography or other automated method. This is now an ASA standard of care.[18]

- PACU care consists of:
  - Supplemental oxygen until able to maintain baseline oxygen saturation or >90%
  - Avoidance of supine position; elevate head of bed to semiupright or lateral
  - Continued monitoring, including SPO_2, until discharge
  - Use of patient's own CPAP or other devices
  - **Discharge care** consists of:
    - ▶ Patient and caregiver education to promote vigilance regarding signs of OSA, especially with use of postoperative pain medications
    - ▶ Encouragement of patients' use of CPAP or other devices while sleeping, even during the day, using nonsupine position

DIABETES[4,19,20]

- Increasingly present in ambulatory aesthetic patient population
- **Type 2 diabetes** is not uncommon residual disease in patients having **body contouring after massive weight loss** or **large-volume liposuction** secondary to preexisting obesity.
- Recommendations by American Diabetes Association (ADA) and American Association of Clinical Endocrinologists (AACE) only target hospitalized patients, critically ill, and those undergoing major surgical stress—not always helpful for ambulatory settings.
- Consider using patient's PCP or endocrinologist for management in outpatient setting.
- Preanesthesia evaluation or preoperative clinic can also provide guidance with patient selection criteria and management.
- Ideally, glycemic control should be optimized before elective aesthetic surgery.
- **HbA1C ≤7.4** correlates with decreased infectious complications.
  - Current recommendation is to hold oral and noninsulin injectables the *day of surgery* until normal food intake is resumed.

HYPERGLYCEMIA ON DAY OF SURGERY

- **Can occur with:**
  - Preexisting inadequate or poor glycemic control
  - Inappropriate discontinuation of preoperative therapy
  - Stress response
- **Cancel or postpone surgery if evidence of:**
  - Severe dehydration
  - Ketoacidosis
  - Hyperosmolar nonketotic state
- May be acceptable to proceed if blood glucose elevated DOS but **preexisting adequate long-term control** evidenced by:
  - HbA1C ≤7.4%
  - Preprandial blood glucoses levels 70-130 mg/dl
  - Postprandial blood glucose levels <180 mg/dl
- Considerations include:
  - Coexisting comorbidities
  - Degree of end-organ impairment or autonomic dysfunction
  - Potential complications of delayed wound healing and wound infection
  - Duration of surgery: Higher levels may be acceptable in shorter procedures.
  - Invasiveness of procedure
  - Type of anesthetic technique: Symptoms of blood glucose aberrations can be masked under general anesthesia or deep sedation.
  - Expected time to resume oral intake and antidiabetic medications

---

NOTE: The optimal blood glucose level for ambulatory surgical patients is unknown.

TIP: Maintain preoperative **baseline** blood glucose levels, rather than preoperatively acutely "normalizing" them.

ADJUNCTS AND CONSIDERATIONS
■ Aggressive postoperative nausea and vomiting (PONV) prophylaxis and avoidance of emetogenic factors promote early resumption of adequate PO intake (see Chapter 5).
■ Dexamethasone dose of 4 mg IV is acceptable and provides reasonable PONV prophylaxis **without evidence of significant elevation of blood glucose or detrimental outcome.**
■ If perioperative insulin is given, discharge criteria should promote observation until likelihood of postoperative hypoglycemia has passed.
■ Discharge instructions should include plan for resuming antidiabetic therapy based on postoperative course, ability to consume adequate oral intake, and ability to self-monitor blood glucose levels.

OBESITY
■ Recent statistics (2015) indicate that adult obesity in United States is approaching **40%.**[21,22]
■ **BMI** is most commonly used to define severity of obesity (Table 6-1).

Table 6-1   *Severity of Obesity Based on BMI*

BMI (kg/m²)	Classification
25.0-29.9	Overweight
30.0-34.9	Obese class I
35.0-39.9	Obese class II
40.0-49.9	Obese class III
≥50	Supermorbid obesity

BMI, Body mass index.

■ How big is too big for safe practice in ambulatory procedures requiring anesthesia?
  • The literature is **contradictory.**
■ A 2103 study using National Surgical Quality Improvement Program (NSQIP) data found *overweight* and *obesity* to be independent risk factors for early perioperative morbidity and mortality.[23]
■ The Society for Ambulatory Anesthesia (SAMBA) Committee on Practice Guidelines performed systematic literature review (2013) in an *unsuccessful* effort to establish specific guidelines for obese patient selection.[24]
■ Literature review revealed higher incidences of clinical correlations with obesity:
  • Hypoxemia requiring supplemental oxygen
  • Need for airway maneuvers
  • Laryngospasm and bronchospasm
  • Treatment for PONV

- Based on bariatric surgery literature, morbidly obese patients **may** be candidates for ambulatory surgery with the caveat of identification and optimization of comorbidities.
- **Supermorbid obesity** (BMI ≥50 kg/m²) *did* present a higher risk; therefore these patients need thorough evaluation, optimization, and consideration before acceptance for elective ambulatory procedures.
- **Patients with BMI ≥50 kg/m² may not be suitable for freestanding ASCs or office-based practices.**
- Patients with BMI 40-50 kg/m² require careful preoperative assessments for OSA, hypoventilation syndromes, pulmonary hypertension, uncontrolled hypertension and cardiac manifestations, and diabetic control before deemed suitable for ambulatory facilities.

NOTE: There is insufficient evidence for determining an arbitrary weight limit cutoff to preclude elective ambulatory surgery.[24]

HERBAL SUPPLEMENTS[4,25-27]

- Use has become commonplace, with >50,000 dietary supplement products available[25]
- Aesthetic surgery patient profiles consistent with that of more prevalent users[26]
- Little standardization of products
- Unregulated by FDA
- No requirements for efficacy
- Various reports indicate ≥32% of U.S. population take them on a *regular* basis.
- Most patients **(>70%)** do not reveal use to health care providers.[4]
- Concern exists regarding untoward effects.[26,27]
  - Drug-drug interactions
  - Bleeding
  - Hypertension
  - Increased heart rate
  - Sedation
  - Liver failure
  - Inhibition or induction of cytochrome systems affecting drug levels
- Common herbs affecting anesthetic or surgical course include:
  - Echinacea
  - Ephedra
  - Feverfew
  - Garlic
  - Ginger
  - Ginkgo
  - Ginseng
  - Kava kava
  - St. John's wort
  - Valerian root

TIP: Ephedra is used commonly by young, overweight females.

TIP: Garlic, ginger, ginkgo, and ginseng (the four Gs) are some of the most popular supplements.

- >90 dietary supplements may affect blood clotting/increase bleeding,[25] which can affect:
  - Regional anesthesia placed for postoperative analgesia
  - Surgical homeostasis
  - Postoperative complications such as hematoma
- Prudent approach promotes careful preoperative patient inquiry to determine consumption.
- **Lack of scientific studies and comprehensive literature supports a conservative approach.**
- **ASA promotes preoperative discussions and discontinuation of herbal medications.**
  - 2- to 3-week period before elective procedure is cited most often.[1,13,28]

Top Takeaways

➤ Continue preexisting beta-blocker on day of surgery (DOS).

➤ Patients with severe pulmonary hypertension are high risk and **should not undergo elective cosmetic surgery.**

➤ Patients who smoke >1-2 packs per day are at increased risk for perioperative respiratory complications, wound infections, flap necrosis.

➤ American Society of Anesthesiologists (ASA) strongly recommends anesthesiologists and surgeons work together to develop protocols to evaluate patients *before* **the day of surgery** to aid in patient selection, preparation, and management.

➤ Patient and caregiver education to promote vigilance regarding signs of OSA, especially with use of postoperative pain medications

➤ Dexamethasone dose of 4 mg IV is acceptable and provides reasonable PONV prophylaxis **without evidence of significant elevation of blood glucose or detrimental outcome.**

References

1. Desai M. General inhalation anesthesia for cosmetic surgery. In Friedberg BL, ed. Anesthesia in Cosmetic Surgery. New York: Cambridge University Press, 2007.
2. Raeder J, ed. Clinical Ambulatory Anesthesia. New York: Cambridge University Press, 2010.
3. Kataria K, Cutter TW, Apfelbaum JL. Patient selection in outpatient surgery. Clin Plast Surg 40:371, 2013.
4. Levin N. Preanesthetic assessment of the cosmetic patient. In Friedberg BL, ed. Anesthesia in Cosmetic Surgery. New York: Cambridge University Press, 2007.
5. Cohn SL, Fleisher LA. Evaluation of cardiac risk prior to noncardiac surgery. Available at *http://www.uptodate.com/contents/evaluation-of-cardiac-risk-prior-to-noncardiac-surgery.*
6. Lau WC, Eagle KA. Managing cardiovascular risk and hypertension. In Young VL, Botney R, eds. Patient Safety in Plastic Surgery. New York: Thieme Publishers, 2009.
7. American Society of Anesthesiologists. Practice advisory for the perioperative management of patients with cardiac implantable electronic devices: pacemakers and implantable cardioverter-

defibrillators: an updated report by the american society of anesthesiologists task force on perioperative management of patients with cardiac implantable electronic devices. Anesthesiology 114:247, 2011.

8. Crossley GH, Poole JE, Rozner MA, et al. The Heart Rhythm Society (HRS)/American Society of Anesthesiologists (ASA) Expert Consensus Statement on the perioperative management of patients with implantable defibrillators, pacemakers and arrhythmia monitors: facilities and patient management this document was developed as a joint project with the American Society of Anesthesiologists (ASA), and in collaboration with the American Heart Association (AHA), and the Society of Thoracic Surgeons (STS). Heart Rhythm 8:1114, 2011.

9. Woods BD, Sladen RN. Perioperative considerations for the patient with asthma and bronchospasm. Br J Anaesth 103(Suppl 1):i57, 2009.

10. Cereda M, Neligan PJ. Managing the risk of perioperative pulmonary complications. In Young VL, Botney R, eds. Patient Safety in Plastic Surgery. New York: Thieme Publishers, 2009.

11. Alvarez MP, Samayoa-Mendez AX, Naglak MC, et al. Risk factors for postoperative unplanned intubation: analysis of a national database. Am Surg 81:820, 2015.

12. Snyder CW, Patel RD, Roberson EP, et al. Unplanned intubation after surgery: risk factors, prognosis, and medical emergency team effects. Am Surg 75:834, 2009.

13. Bennett GD. Anesthesia for aesthetic surgery. In Shiffman MA, Di Giuseppe A, eds. Cosmetic Surgery. Berlin Heidelberg: Springer, 2013.

14. Smentana GW. Evaluation of preoperative pulmonary risk. Available at www.uptodate.com.

15. Stephan PJ, Mercier D, Coleman J, et al. Obstructive sleep apnea: implications for the plastic surgeon and ambulatory surgery centers. Plast Reconstr Surg 125:652, 2009.

16. American Society of Anesthesiologists Task Force on Perioperative Management of Patients with Obstructive Sleep Apnea. Practice guidelines for the perioperative management of patients with obstructive sleep apnea: an updated report by the American Society of Anesthesiologists Task Force on Perioperative Management of patients with obstructive sleep apnea. Anesthesiology 120:268, 2014.

17. Joshi GP, Saravanan PA, Gan TJ, et al. Society of Ambulatory Anesthesia consensus statement of preoperative selection of adult patients with obstructive sleep apnea scheduled for ambulatory surgery. Anesth Analg 115:1060, 2012.

18. ASA standards for basic anesthetic monitoring. Available at www.asahq.org.

19. Braithwaite SS. Perioperative glucose control and diabetes management. In Young VL, Botney R, eds. Patient Safety in Plastic Surgery. New York: Thieme Publishers, 2009.

20. Joshi GP, Chung F, Vann MA, et al. Society for Ambulatory Anesthesia consensus statement on perioperative blood glucose management in diabetic patients undergoing ambulatory surgery. Anesth Anal 111:1378, 2010.

21. Levi J, Segal LM, Rayburn J, et al. The state of obesity: better policies for a healthier America 2015. Available at http://stateofobesity.org/files/stateofobesity2015.pdf.

22. Ogden CL, Carrol MD, Fryar CD, et al. Prevalence of obesity among adults and youth: United States, 2011-2014. NCHS Data Brief No. 219, 2015.

23. Mathis MR, Naughton NN, Shanks AM, et al. Patient selection for day case-eligible surgery. Anesthesiology 199:1310, 2013.

24. Joshi GP, Ahmad S, Riad W, et al. Selection of obese patients undergoing ambulatory surgery: a systematic review of the literature. Anesth Analg 117:1082, 2013.

25. Abe A, Kaye AD, Gritsenko K, et al. Perioperative analgesia and the effects of dietary supplements. Best Pract Res Clin Anesthesiol 28:183, 2014.

26. Broughton G, Crosby MA, Coleman J, et al. Use of herbal supplements and vitamins in plastic surgery: a practical review. Plast Reconstr Surg 119:48e, 2007.
27. Jalili J, Askeroglu U, Alleyne B, et al. Herbal products that may contribute to hypertension. Plast Reconstr Surg 131:168, 2013.
28. Gertler R, Joshi GP. General anesthesia. In Twersky RS, Phillip BK, eds. Handbook of Ambulatory Anesthesia, ed 2. New York: Springer Science, 2008.

RESOURCES

American Society of Anesthesiologists (ASA). Available at *www.asahq.org.*
American Society of Regional Anesthesia and Pain Medicine (ASRA). Available at *www.asra.com.*
Anesthesia Patient Safety Foundation (APSF). Available at *www.apsf.org.*
Regional Anesthesia and Pain Medicine (RAPM). Available at *www.rapm.org.*
Society of Ambulatory Anesthesia (SAMBA). Available at *www.sambahq.org.*

7. Procedure-Specific Anesthesia Guidelines for the Aesthetic Surgery Patient

Deborah Stahl Lowery

ANESTHESIA FOR FACIAL PLASTIC SURGICAL PROCEDURES (RHYTIDECTOMY, NECKLIFT, ETC.)[1,2]

- Patient factors
  - Usually middle-aged or older
  - May have increased burden of comorbidities, especially preexisting hypertension
  - Can have cardiac conditions for which they take antiplatelet, antithrombotic, or anticoagulant medication
  - Any disruption/resumption in blood thinners should be coordinated with primary care physician or consultant.
  - Require increased attention to positioning and padding with range of motion limitations, *including cervical spine*
- Often part of multiprocedure combination with duration ≥4 hours
  - Consider Foley catheter
  - DVT mechanical prophylaxis with sequential compression devices
  - Intermittent position checks to assess extremity and pressure point support and padding
- Multiple anesthetic techniques used successfully
  - IV sedation of varying levels
  - Total intravenous anesthesia (TIVA) (see Chapter 5)
  - Balanced technique with inhalational anesthesia
- Choice of anesthetic type frequently influenced by surgical preference

ANESTHETIC GOALS[2,3]
- Achieve optimal hemodynamic control.
  - **Hematoma** is most common complication of procedure.
  - **Preoperative systolic BP >150 mm Hg** has been identified as risk factor for hematoma.[3]
- Appreciate anxiolysis, antiemesis, and analgesia treatments as components of hemodynamic control.
- Preemptively manage changes in surgical stimuli that result in hemodynamic aberration (awareness of procedural components and their sequence).
- Be aware of placement, timing, and tolerance of compression head dressings.
- Achieve smooth emergence and extubation that prevents coughing and bucking.

PREOPERATIVE MANAGEMENT[1,4]
- Continue any home anxiolytic medications.
- Add preoperative anxiolysis with midazolam 1-2 mg IV titrated up to 0.7 mg/kg.

- Continue any home antihypertensive medications (except diuretics, angiotensin-converting enzymes [ACE-inhibitors], and angiotensin-receptor blockers [ARBs]).
- Determine baseline BP and, if known, typical ranges.
- Consider use of **clonidine:** 0.1-0.2 mg PO or 0.1-0.2 mg/d transdermal patch placed preoperatively.
- Optimize preoperative PO multimodal analgesia (celcoxib, acetaminophen, gabapentin).
- Optimize preoperative antiemesis prophylaxis (aprepitant [Emend], scopolamine patch), especially if history of PONV/PDNV.

INTRAOPERATIVE MANAGEMENT
- Ensure smooth IV induction with propofol.
- Continue **prophylactic antiemesis regimen** (with addition of promethazine, decadron, ondansetron, and/or haloperidol), as determined by Apfel score.
- Continue **opioid-sparing multimodal analgesia** regimen (ketamine, IV acetaminophen).
- Provide **neuromuscular blockade** redosing preemptively for head repositioning or injection stimulation.
- Maintain **low normotension or modest hypotension** during resection.
- Generous surgical use of **local anesthetic infiltration** and **nerve blocks**
- Bolus with shorter-acting synthetic opioids (fentanyl, sufentanil, alfentanil) to blunt:
  - Hemodynamic effects of laryngoscopy
  - Periods of intermittent stimulation during local anesthesia injection
  - Airway stimulation caused by changes in head positioning
- Total narcotic use is typically minimal and therefore lessens untoward side effects like postoperative nausea and vomiting (PONV).
- Before closing, **allow BP return to baseline range** to facilitate surgical assessment of oozing.
- **Judicious use of IV fluids** (maintenance amounts) to prevent facial edema
  - Estimated blood loss (EBL) is minimal.
  - No appreciable third space losses occur.
- **Delay emergence** until all dressings and wraps are securely in place.
- Surgeon or assistant can hold pressure to site during extubation.
- **Elevate head of bed at least 30 degrees** ASAP to minimize postprocedural edema.
- **Smooth extubation** is critical to prevent coughing or bucking that causes increased venous return and increased BP leading to hematoma.
- Use **lidocaine IV** PRN to depress airway reflexes.
- Use **esmolol IV** PRN to quickly control increases in BP.
- Timely management of any anxiety, hypertension, pain, or nausea in PACU
- In one study, hypertension in the PACU was found to be a statistically significant factor in formation of hematoma.[2]
- Rhytidectomy is unique in that these components that affect BP need to be **strictly controlled** to minimize subcutaneous bleeding and hematoma formation.

AIRWAY MANAGEMENT[1,5]
- **Endotracheal intubation** with controlled ventilation
  - Provides maximal control of airway during head position changes
  - Minimizes motion that can occur with spontaneous respiration

- Provides closed system for oxygen delivery minimizing fire risk with electrocautery
- Decrease FiO_2 to lowest level that supports adequate oxygenation.
- Secure ET tube in a way to maximize surgeon's dynamic maneuverability.
- Avoid tape by securing ET tube to incisors or canine teeth with suture or floss (inform patient of potential gum irritation, soreness, or bleeding).
- Some surgeons prefer to leave ET tube unsecured for ability to move from side to side throughout procedure.

> **TIP:**   If unsecured, mark the ET tube with an indelible marker at centimeter markings for the teeth or lip so that its position can be continually checked for initial placement depth!

- Consider preformed ET tube (oral or nasal RAE).
- Bioocclusive dressing can secure ET tube to chin to minimize tape.
- Determine level of maintenance muscle relaxation desired by surgeon to prevent unwanted facial laxity.
- **Supraglottic device** (laryngeal mask airway [LMA], I-gel)
  - Prevents facial distortion, which is less desirable for this reason
  - Assess anticipated head manipulation to prevent airway irritation or dislodgement intraoperatively.
  - Good alternative (if no contraindications) in isolated browlift, blepharoplasty, or eyelid procedures because of maintenance of neutral head positioning.
  - Facilitates smooth emergence because patients less likely to cough or buck
- **Natural airway** with spontaneous ventilation

EYE PROTECTION
- Sterile ophthalmic ointment (Lacri-Lube) ONLY

CAUTION: DO NOT confuse Lacri-Lube with Surgilube, which, if applied to the cornea, can cause severe ocular damage through probable toxic effects of chlorhexidine gluconate.[4]

- **Corneal protectors**
  - Remember to remove before emergence to avoid unpleasant patient experience and difficulty with removal when awake.

FACIAL LASER RESURFACING[1,6,7]
- Use of CO_2 laser is painful and usually requires significant analgesia both intraoperatively and immediately after procedure.
- Successful use of room air/natural airway/spontaneous ventilation techniques using TIVA have been described.
  - Need for cardiorespiratory depressants is prevented by using nonopioid analgesics in conjunction with local anesthetic nerve blocks.
  - **Supplemental oxygen and assisted ventilation are avoided**, and surgical field is freed.
  - Drawbacks[6] include eventual need for predischarge rescue opioid analgesics (>70%) and antiemetics (32%).

- Balanced technique or TIVA with use of an endotracheal tube[1,5] confers ability to:
  - Treat drug-induced respiratory depression with controlled ventilation
  - **Minimize combustion/fire risk by:**
    - ► Using closed-circuit oxygen delivery
    - ► Using laser-resistant ET tube
    - ► Decreasing FiO_2 to lowest level that supports adequate oxygenation
    - ► Communicating the level of O_2 to the surgeon before laser use in a specific laser time-out
- ET tube may need repositioning to allow surgeon to work around it, possibly unsecured.
- Eye protection with corneal protectors and saline-soaked gauzes pads are needed.
- PACU needs can include:
  - Supplemental narcotic analgesia
  - Chilled air to face
  - Application of ointment
  - Humidified face tent

RHINOPLASTY

- Well-suited for general anesthesia with controlled airway
- Alternative method is moderate-deep sedation with natural airway, although providing supplemental oxygen is more challenging.
- Position and secure ET tube over the mandible. Use of tube extenders, armored tube, or oral RAE tube facilitates surgical exposure and maneuverability and prevents crimping or compression.
- Supraglottic devices (LMA, I-gel) have also been used successfully.
- Caution is needed with osteotomies and bleeding that passively migrates to stomach causing increased incidence of PONV, risk of aspiration, and airway irritation.

> **TIP:**   If LMA is used, consider the type that allows gastric suctioning.

- Use of throat packing dampened with saline solution can decrease blood migration but can cause mucosal irritation and postprocedure sore throat.

CAUTION: Use vigilance to make sure throat packing is removed at the end of the procedure! (Add to checklist.)

- Patients should be kept anesthetized until splints are contoured and stiffened and dressings are in place.
- **Emergence entails:**
  - Being awake enough to prevent aspiration or laryngospasm, especially because mask application with positive pressure can cause injury to fresh repair
  - Being smooth enough to prevent coughing and bucking that increase bleeding
    - ► Postoperative pain is usually minimal because of local infiltration by surgeon.

ANESTHESIA FOR BREAST AND ABDOMINAL PROCEDURES

BREAST AUGMENTATION[1]

- Patients tend to be younger (most <40 years of age).
- Younger age, female sex, use of volatile agents and opioids increase Apfel PONV score; thus **PONV prophylaxis is often indicated.**

- Submuscular dissection and placement lends itself to postoperative deep muscular pain and spasm.
- Use of multimodal analgesia can include initial doses of acetaminophen, gabapentin, celecoxib or other NSAID.
  - Can add diazepam (Valium) or carisoprodol (Soma) to regimen to aid pectoralis relaxation[8]
- Position changes intraoperatively are dynamic and frequent to observe implant location and symmetry.
  - **All positioning should take into account:**
    - ▶ Pressure point padding
    - ▶ Angle of arm abduction (≤90 degrees)
    - ▶ Method of securing that allows safe transition between supine and sitting
    - ▶ Testing the bed to sitting position before prep and drape

CAUTION: Hemodynamic and vascular changes can occur with position changes.

- Coordinate timing of emergence to account for dressings, bra, elastic bandages, and if they were placed while patient was sitting or supine.
- Although general anesthesia is the mainstay for this procedure, successful use of regional techniques for sole anesthetics or postoperative pain supplements are well described, including epidural or thoracic paravertebral blocks.[9,10]
- Postoperative pain management can be augmented by local anesthesia continuous infusion pumps (On-Q, Kimberly-Clark), intercostal nerve blocks, paravertebral blocks, and/or incisional local anesthetic infiltration, including liposomal bupivacaine.
- Recommend continuation of multimodal analgesia regimen after discharge.

BREAST REDUCTION AND MASTOPEXY
- Dynamic positioning is similar to that of augmentation.
- EBL and resulting fluid balance correlate with amount of tissue resection and duration.

ABDOMINOPLASTY[1,11,12]
- Characterized as "moderate" surgical risk procedure
- Promotes thorough preoperative assessment to aid in patient and facility selection
- Concerning preoperative surgical factors are active smoking and increased HbA1C >7.4.
- **Carries increased risk of thromboembolism**
  - Increased risk can include **general anesthesia** and **operative times >140 minutes.**[10]
  - Apply sequential compression devices (SCDs) in preoperative area, ensure they are operational before anesthetic induction. (Add to checklist!)
  - Promotes attention to adequate hydration and fluid balance
  - Consider pharmacologic prophylaxis with LMW-heparin enoxaparin (Lovenox) as per risk assessment (Caprini RAM) (see Chapter 11).
  - Provide preoperative information on signs of DVT/PE, need for early ambulation.
- Warming measures include preoperative prewarming, adequate OR room temperature, active warming devices (Bair Hugger, Arizant Healthcare, Inc.), head covers, IV fluid warmers.

TIP: Preparation for procedure MUST INCLUDE testing of OR table for flexion function before patient arrives in OR.

- Preoperative multimodal analgesia can include initial doses of acetaminophen, gabapentin, and/or celecoxib.
- Preoperative **multimodal PONV/postdischarge nausea and vomiting (PDNV) prophylaxis** is indicated to prevent deleterious effects of vomiting on rectus plication (see Chapter 5).
- Keeping patient anesthetized through transition from OR table to car, maintaining flexed position for binder placement before emergence, is helpful.
- Goal is smooth emergence with avoidance of increased abdominal pressure caused by coughing and bucking.
- Provide early, aggressive pain management with adequate opioid supplementation as needed in PACU.
- Consider continuing multimodal analgesia regimen after discharge, often with the addition of a muscle relaxant, e.g., cyclobenzaprine (Flexaril).

ANESTHESIA FOR BODY CONTOURING AFTER MASSIVE WEIGHT LOSS (MWL)[13-16]

- **Increased operative duration >6** hours promotes procedural staging.
- **Body surface area (BSA) exposure** with thermoregulation challenges
- **Complex, dynamic positioning,** including prone
- **Complex, difficult, and dynamic IV access**
  - May need to change sites intraoperatively
  - May need to use lower extremity, external jugular sites, or even central venous access
- **Possible significant EBL**
- Need for extended postoperative care beyond typical PACU length of stay
- **Perioperative care can be complicated by:**
  - Possible persistent difficult intubation because of body habitus
  - Residual hypertension, diabetes mellitus, obstructive sleep apnea
  - Gastroesophageal reflux disease and/or hiatal hernia
  - Risk of aspiration, especially with gastric banding
  - Preexisting cardiac disease and/or pulmonary hypertension
  - Decreased pulmonary reserves with quicker desaturation
  - Nutritional deficiencies and anemia
  - Predisposition to infection
  - Thromboembolic risk

PHARMACOLOGIC CHALLENGES[14]

- Pharmacokinetics and pharmacodynamics can be altered as both fat and lean body weight (LBW) increase in the obese and morbidly obese.
- Dosing based on **ideal body weight (IBW)** can result in **underdosing.**
- Dosing based on **total body weight (TBW)** can result in **overdosing.**
- If patient is **not obese,** TBW, IBW, and LBW are similar, and **TBW** can be used.

POSITIONING CHALLENGES[14,16]

- May be dynamic and creative—atypical to achieve favorable surgical access
- **Requires extensive padding and securing**
- Consider allowing awake patient positioning pretest to assess for stress, compression, stretching, pinching.

- Consider allowing awake bed positioning pretest to check for safety, slippage, flexion breaks.
- Preplan for position changes.
- **Prone considerations include:**
  - Need for cart to table and back
  - Log roll supine to prone
    - ▶ With arms at sides
    - ▶ Then "sweep" arms up to head, hugging side of table.
    - ▶ Then attach arm boards, placing forearms at 90-degree angle to shoulders.
    - ▶ Reverse process at end.
  - **Prone chest rolls or frame** to relieve weight compressing/restricting chest wall and to optimize ventilation
  - **Axillary rolls** to prevent brachial plexus compression or stretching, dislocation of glenohumeral joint
  - Arm boards with adequate padding
  - Slight (15-30 degrees) dorsiflexion of wrists
  - Cervical spine kept neutral position while turning and positioning
  - Prone headrest with appropriate cut-outs for eyes, nose, and ET tube or manufactured mirrored support device (ProneView, Mizuho OSI)
  - **Avoid orbital compression** that can lead to postoperative vision loss (POVL).
  - Perform and document periodic (every 15 minutes) ocular checks.
  - **Reverse Trendelenburg 15 degrees positioning** can help to decrease intraocular pressure.
  - Check nipples, breast, abdomen, and male genitalia for compression.
- **Supine considerations include:**
  - Excess weight on chest while supine can be uncomfortable for awake patients, limiting preoxygenation.
    - ▶ Alleviate by induction with patient in semisitting position.
  - Arms abducted ≤90 degrees, padded and secured, wrists in natural position
  - Legs slightly flexed at knees
  - Heels padded

INTRAOPERATIVE CONCERNS[17]
- One study of body contouring after MWL showed lower intraoperative temperature associated with increased seroma formation, increased blood loss, and higher need for transfusion.
  - Thermoregulation: Use prewarming in preoperative area.
  - Increase room temperature (target of 21.1° C).
  - Employ active warming maneuvers, e.g., forced-warm-air blankets, warmed fluids for IV and irrigation.
  - Remember to cover areas during lengthy position changes.
  - Continue active warming into PACU.
- Foley catheter
- Antibiotics: Don't forget to redose for longer-duration surgery.
- DVT/VTE prophylaxis is imperative.

POSTOPERATIVE CONCERNS
- Anticipate longer PACU stay.
- Low threshold for 23-hour observation or overnight stay depending on complexity and duration of procedure(s)

- Need for supplemental oxygen may be prolonged.
- Extended full American Society of Anesthesiologists (ASA) monitoring with addition of nasal cannula end-tidal carbon dioxide monitor
- Continuous positive airway pressure/bilevel positive airway pressure (CPAP/biPAP) (patients to bring their own if preexisting OSA)
- Incentive spirometry (continue at home)

ANESTHESIA FOR LIPOSUCTION[18-23]

- Considered *moderately invasive* procedure
- Anticipate proposed length of procedure and plan for:
  - Positioning challenges or dynamics
  - Thermoregulation mechanisms and challenges
  - Determination of total volume of aspirate, defined as total fat + fluid removed
  - Volume/fluid management and monitoring
  - Concomitant procedures, especially those that would include additional lidocaine or other local anesthetic infiltration

CAUTION: Large-volume liposuction (>5000 cc total aspirate) should be performed in an acute care hospital or accredited facility for overnight monitoring and management.

POTENTIAL SERIOUS COMPLICATIONS

- Local anesthetic toxicity
- Fluid overload/pulmonary edema
- Thermal injury
- Pulmonary embolus
- Fat embolus
- Hypothermia
- Dilutional coagulopathy
- Metabolic/electrolyte derangement
- Viscus or vascular perforation

FLUID MANAGEMENT[18,21]

- Good communication between surgeon, anesthesiologist, and circulator is critical to track cumulative fluids, both IV and infiltrate—**this is imperative.**
- Noninvasive hemodynamic monitoring ± urinary catheter is needed to assess volume status.
- For **<5-liter** aspirate, use judicious IV fluids consisting of **maintenance.**
- For **>5-liter** aspirate, IV fluids consist of **maintenance + replacement:** Rate 0.25 ml of IV crystalloid/ml of aspirate >5 liters. (Some recommend starting this at 4-liter aspirate.)
- Most of infiltrative solution (60%-70%) is reabsorbed by patient.
- Aggressive fluid administration may increase risk of pulmonary edema.
- With aspirate <5 liters, third-space losses should be minimized by application of compression garments.
- With aspirate >5 liters, increasing amounts correlate with fluid shifts, electrolyte imbalance, need for hemoglobin assessment, attention to volume status (including use of urinary catheter), and postoperative overnight observation.

THROMBOEMBOLIC PROPHYLAXIS

- Preoperative identification/discontinuation of all herbal supplements that promote hypercoagulable state
- Preoperative identification of hypercoagulable medical conditions (e.g., Factor V Leiden deficiency), oral contraceptive use, smoking
- Use of sequential pneumatic compression devices (SCDs) with general anesthesia (place BEFORE induction) and with procedures >1-hour duration
- Consider LMW heparin prophylaxis or postoperative use.

MAINTENANCE OF CORE TEMPERATURE

- Use active-warming devices.
- Cover exposed surface areas.
- Increase OR ambient temperature.
- Warm infiltration solution.
- Warm IV fluids.
- Minimize evaporative losses from large areas of wet skin.
- Continue active warming in PACU to provide additional comfort.

ANALGESIA[1]

- Supplemental narcotics may be needed because of "feathering techniques" that may encroach into tissues where tumescent infiltration is inadequate.
  - Becomes apparent at emergence or early PACU
- Early narcotic rescue with fentanyl IV in 25 µg increments is helpful.

LIDOCAINE[18,20,22]

- An amino-amide structure
- **Most commonly used local anesthetic in wetting solutions**
- 90% undergoes hepatic metabolism, 10% is excreted unchanged in urine.
- Relative short duration of action (10-30 minutes)
- **Plasma half-life is 8 minutes.**
- **Terminal half-life is 90 minutes.**
- **Toxicity and maximal dosing limits**
  - **Subcutaneous** infiltration limits
    - ▶ **4.5 mg/kg** without epinephrine, not to exceed **300 mg**
    - ▶ **7.0 mg/kg** with epinephrine, not to exceed **500 mg**
  - **Tumescent infiltration**[19]
    - ▶ No standardized mixture; individual variations
    - ▶ **Common "recipe":**
      - ◆ 1000 ml normal saline (NS) or lactated ringers (LR) solution
      - ◆ Lidocaine 300 mg (30 ml 1% plain)
      - ◆ Epinephrine 1000 µg (1 ml 1:1000 amp)
    - ▶ **"Klein" (1987)[24] preparation**
      - ◆ 1000 ml NS
      - ◆ Lidocaine 500 mg (50 ml 1% plain)
      - ◆ Epinephrine 1000 µg (1ml 1:1000 amp)
      - ◆ Sodium bicarbonate 8.4% 12.5 ml (can eliminate if general anesthesia)
    - ▶ Calculate lidocaine dose based on total body weight.
    - ▶ Maximum dose **35.0 mg/kg** is accepted limit (ASPS Practice advisory).

▶ Maximum dose 55.0 mg/kg is a controversial megadosing in some literature.
▶ Modify preparation in obese patients or large volume; reduce concentration when necessary.

TIP: Consider omitting lidocaine when general or regional anesthesia is used.

- Peak (subtoxic) plasma concentrations can be delayed and have been reported typically as 6-14 hours (up to 23 hours)[22,23] depending on:
  - Infiltration speed
  - Patient characteristics
  - High lidocaine binding affinity to adipose tissue
  - Unequal volume of distribution in subcutaneous tissue[23]

SIGNS AND SYMPTOMS OF LIDOCAINE TOXICITY

- Dose dependent
- Typically present initially (awake patient) with **central nervous system symptoms**
- Proceeds to **cardiovascular manifestations** as plasma levels increase
- Continuum is obscured by general anesthesia.
- Pretreatment with benzodiazepines can aid by increasing the seizure threshold but also diminishes patient's ability to report early symptoms.
- Plasma levels **<3 μg/ml** are nontoxic.
- Plasma levels of **5-10 μg/ml** are more subjective and **minor** (awake patient).
  - Perioral numbness and/or facial tingling
  - Restlessness, confusion, or lethargy
  - Metallic taste
  - Vertigo
  - Slurred speech
  - Tinnitus
- Plasma levels of **10-20 μ/ml** symptoms are increasingly objective and **serious.**
  - Delirium
  - Seizures
  - Coma
- Plasma levels **>20 μg/ml** proceed to cardiac manifestations.
  - Hypotension
  - A-V block, idioventricular rhythms
  - Asystole, cardiac arrest, cardiovascular collapse
  - See the following section.

LOCAL ANESTHETIC SYSTEMIC TOXICITY (LAST)

MANAGEMENT[22,25,26]

- **Priorities consist of:**
  - Airway management
  - Circulatory support
  - Decreasing systemic effects of local anesthetics
- Can be very challenging at best, especially in an office or ambulatory surgery center (ASC)
- **CALL FOR HELP.**

- Supportive care
  - 100% FiO_2
  - Support or secure airway.
  - Hemodynamic support with IV fluids and/or vasopressors
  - Seizure suppression with IV benzodiazepines (diazepam or midazolam)
  - If no benzodiazepine available, can use small doses of propofol (caution: cardiac depression)
    - ▶ Avoid phenytoin (Dilantin).
  - Correction of acidosis with hyperventilation (avoid sodium bicarbonate as per current ACLS guidelines)

EMS AND TRANSFER PROTOCOLS
- Proceed to nearest facility with **CARDIAC BYPASS CAPABILITY.**
- Resuscitation efforts can be prolonged in this setting.
- For **refractory cardiac arrest unresponsive to standard therapy:** Consider IV fat emulsion, **Intralipid 20% (Baxter).**

INTRALIPID 20%
- Recommended dosing for 70 kg patient (lean body mass)
  - Bolus 1.5 ml/kg (about 100 ml)
  - Infusion rate 0.25 ml/kg/min (about 18 ml/min)
  - Continue BLS/ACLS chest compressions to circulate
  - Repeat bolus x 2 every 3-5 minutes circulation is restored.
  - Can double infusion rate to support circulation
  - Maximal upper dosing limit varies in literature; has been reported to be 8-10 ml/kg.

TOP TAKEAWAYS
- ➤ Patients should take their home medications the morning of surgery to maintain steady-state levels.
- ➤ Risk factors for PONV include females, nonsmokers, past history of PONV, history of motion sickness, young age, migraine history.
- ➤ Good communication between surgeon, anesthesiologist, and circulator is critical to track cumulative fluids, both IV and infiltrate—**this is imperative.**
- ➤ Preoperative identification/discontinuation of all herbal supplements that promote hypercoagulable state
- ➤ Other than procedures performed using local and mild oral tranquilization, surgery should be carried out in an accredited facility.

REFERENCES

1. Desai M. General inhalation anesthesia for cosmetic surgery. In Friedberg BL, ed. Anesthesia in Cosmetic Surgery. New York: Cambridge University Press, 2007.
2. Ramanadham SR, Costa CR, Narasimhan K, et al. Refining the anesthesia management of the face-lift patient: lesson learned from 1089 consecutive face lifts. Plast Reconstr Surg 135:723, 2015.
3. Lau WC, Eagle KA. Managing cardiovascular risk and hypertension. In Young VL, Botney R, eds. Patient Safety in Plastic Surgery. New York: Thieme Publishers, 2009.
4. Sawyer W, Burwick K, Jaworski J, et al. Corneal injury secondary to accidental Surgilube exposure. Arch Ophthalmol 129:1229, 2011.

 5. Raeder J, ed. Clinical Ambulatory Anesthesia. New York: Cambridge University Press, 2010.
 6. Blakely KR, Klein KW, White PF, et al. A total intravenous anesthetic technique for outpatient facial laser resurfacing. Anesth Analg 87:827, 1998.
 7. Friedberg BL. The dissociative effect and preemptive analgesia. In Friedberg BL, ed. Anesthesia in Cosmetic Surgery. New York: Cambridge University Press, 2007.
 8. Unger JG, Thornwell HP III, Decherd ME. Breast augmentation. In Janis JE, ed. Essentials of Plastic Surgery. New York: Thieme Publishers, 2014.
 9. Evans H, Steele SM. Regional anesthesia for cosmetic surgery. In Friedberg BL, ed. Anesthesia in Cosmetic Surgery. New York: Cambridge University Press, 2007.
10. Tahiri Y, Tran DQ, Bouteaud J, et al. General anesthesia versus thoracic paraverterbral block for breast surgery: a meta-analysis. J Plast Reconstr Aesthet Surg 64:1261, 2011.
11. Buck DW, Mustoe TA. An evidence-based approach to abdominoplasty. Plast Reconstr Surg 126:2189, 2010.
12. Rios LM, Obaid SI. Abdominoplasty. In Janis JE, ed. Essentials of Plastic Surgery. New York: Thieme Publishers, 2014.
13. Hoschander A, Strauch B, et al. Risk and safety considerations in body contouring after massive weight loss. Available at www.plasticsurgeryhyp erguide.com tutorial accessed 10/01/2014.
14. Nostro A. Anesthesia for Reconstructive Surgery After Massive Weight Loss. Available at www.plasticsurgeryhyperguide.com tutorial accessed 10/01/2014.
15. Whizar-Lugo VM, Cisneros-Corral R, Reyes-Alveleyra MA, et al. Anesthesia for plastic surgery procedures in previously morbidly obese patients. Anestesia en México 21:186, 2009.
16. Ellsworth WA, Basu CB, Iverson RE. Perioperative considerations for patient safety during cosmetic surgery-preventing complications. Can J Plast Surg 17:9, 2009.
17. Coon D, Michaels JM V, Gusenoff JA, et al. Hypothermia and complications in post-bariatric body contouring. Plast Reconstr Surg 130:443, 2012.
18. Dorin AF. Lidocaine use and toxicity in cosmetic surgery. In Friedberg BL, ed. Anesthesia in Cosmetic Surgery. New York: Cambridge University Press, 2007.
19. Constantine FC, Rios JL. Liposuction. In Janis JE, ed. Essentials of Plastic Surgery. New York: Thieme, 2014.
20. Berry MG, Davies D. Liposuction: a review of principles and techniques. J Plast Reconstr Aesthet Surg 64:985, 2011.
21. American Society of Plastic Surgeons. Practice advisory on liposuction: executive summary. Available at www.plasticsurgery.org.
22. Gonzalez-Sotomayor JA, Alshaarawi AF. Safety considerations for different anesthesia techniques. In Young VL, Botney R, eds. Patient Safety in Plastic Surgery. New York: Thieme Publishers, 2009.
23. Martinez MA, Ballesteros S, Segura LJ, et al. Reporting a fatality during tumescent liposuction. Forensic Sci Int 178:e11, 2014.
24. Klein JA. The tumescent technique for liposuction surgery. AM J Cosmetic Surg 4:1124, 1987.
25. Neal JL, Bernards CL, Butterworth JF IV, et al. ASRA practice advisory on local anesthetic systemic toxicity. Reg Anesth Pain Med 35:152, 2010.
26. Weinberg G. LipidRescue™ Resuscitation. Available at www.lipidrescue.org.

RESOURCES

American Society of Anesthesiologists (ASA). Available at www.asahq.org.
American Society of Regional Anesthesia and Pain Medicine (ASRA). Available at www.asra.com.
Anesthesia Patient Safety Foundation (APSF). Available at www.apsf.org.
LipidRescue Resuscitation. Available at www.lipidrescue.org.
Regional Anesthesia and Pain Medicine (RAPM). Available at www.rapm.org.
Society of Ambulatory Anesthesia (SAMBA). Available at www.sambahq.org.

8. Multimodal Analgesia for the Aesthetic Surgery Patient

Girish P. Joshi, Jeffrey E. Janis

UNDERSTANDING MULTIMODAL PAIN MANAGEMENT

- "Prescription drug overdose is an epidemic in the United States. All too often, in far too many communities, *the treatment is becoming the problem.*"[1]
- **80%** of patients experience acute pain after surgery.
- **75%** of U.S. patients report surgical pain rated 7 or higher (scale of 1-10).
- **59%** of patients are concerned about postoperative pain.[2]

OPIOID EPIDEMIC

- **November 2016:** U.S. Surgeon General declares epidemic of addiction—public health crisis[3]
- United States contains 4.6% of the world's total population, but consumes two thirds of the world opioid supply.
- 12.5 million people, or 4.7% of the American population, aberrantly used prescription opioids in 2015.[4]
- 1% of the U.S. population is addicted to opioids.
- **2015:** 28,647 people died in the United States due to prescription opioid overdose
- Prescription opioid use disorder is estimated to cost the American economy $53.4 billion per year.
- Resurgence of heroin
  - Cheaper
  - Inappropriate weaning strategies from prescription opioids
- Four fifths of heroin users report their initial exposure to opioids was to prescription opioids.[5]
- **2007:** Prescription opioid overdose responsible for *more deaths than heroin and cocaine combined*[6]
- **1996-2006:** Rate of prescription opioid use disorder increased by 167%[7]
  - Rates continued to rise

PRESCRIBING PATTERNS AND DEATHS
- In patients with opioid prescriptions that overdose, the mortality rate increases with escalating dose.[8]
- Increases in opioid prescription rates have not resulted in improvement in patient disability or health outcome.[9]

STATISTICS
- Accidental deaths per year in United States[10]:
  - #1: Drug poisoning
    - 40% of drug poisonings are due to opioid overdose.

- #2: Automobile accidents
- **2015:** United States—5.4% of high school seniors aberrantly used prescription opioids within the last year[11]
  - ► 40% stated that these drugs were easy to get.
- **2016:** Canada—20.6% of grade 12 high school students aberrantly used opioid medication in the last year[12]
  - ► 70% obtained the medication from their own homes.
- 44 Americans die every day of a prescription overdose.[13]
  - ► For every death there are:
    - ◆ 10 treatment admissions for abuse
    - ◆ 32 Emergency Department visits for misuse or abuse
    - ◆ 130 people who abuse or are dependent
    - ◆ 825 nonmedical users

DIVERSION

- Illicitly obtained prescription opioids are often obtained from friends or family.
- **2006-2010:** Street availability of prescription opioids increased
- **2010:** 40% of Medicaid patients with opioid prescriptions had indicators of aberrant use or diversion[14]

SURGEON'S ROLE

- Surgeons responsible for 9.8% of the total opioid prescriptions in the United States[15]
- Rates of opioid prescriptions to opioid naive patients after minor surgery increased between 2004 -2012.[16]
- *Surgeons may play a significant role in propagating the addiction crisis by exposing patients to potentially harmful and addictive opioid medications and contributing to the street supply of opioids.*
- Simple education interventions for patients to explain how to safely store and dispose of opioid medications can make a significant impact.
- Led by the surgeon and a written handout or referral to a website which explains proper opioid storage and disposal

PROPER STORAGE AND DISPOSAL

- Opioids should be stored in a locked cabinet.
- All unused medication should be returned to the pharmacy or destroyed once post-operative pain has resolved.

SURGERY AND ADDICTION

- Patients who were opioid naive before surgery shown to have a significant chance of persistent postoperative opioid use.[17]
- Many patients continue to receive opioids chronically after initially receiving them for postoperative pain control.
- Patients taking opioids chronically prior to surgery have an increased chance of still taking them 1 year later when compared with controls.

OPIOIDS AND SURGERY

- A 2016 study of elective hand surgery patients showed 13% were still taking opioids 90 days after surgery.[18]
- Another study found that 3.1% were still taking opioids at 90 days after major surgery.[19]
- Total knee arthroplasty: 1.4% chance of still taking opioids one year after surgery[20]
  - Odds ratio of 5:1 when compared to nonoperated controls
  - Another study found that older patients (>66 years old) following low-risk surgery have a 44% increased likelihood of chronic use at 1 year compared with controls.[21]

CAUTION: Surgery is a risk factor! There is a risk of persistent opioid use following exposure to opioid medications in the perioperative period, *even in opioid naive patients*.

RISK FACTORS FOR OPIOID ABUSE

- History of substance use disorder
- Comorbid psychological health conditions (i.e., anxiety, depression)
- Male sex
- Low socioeconomic status

LEFTOVERS AND DISPOSAL

- Elective hand surgery study (2012): 95% received opioids with average 30 doses[22]
- 19 doses left over after acute pain resolution
- Urology: 92% received no instructions on how to dispose of leftover opioids after surgery[23]
  - 67% had leftover opioids
  - 91% of the patients with leftovers went on to keep them in an unlocked medicine cabinet[24]
- Oral surgery and pediatric surgery: similar to above
- Thoracic and gynecological surgery: 83% had leftover opioid medication
  - ▶ 71%-73% stored the leftovers unsafely

> **SENIOR AUTHOR TIP:** Since most people with prescription opioid use disorder get them from friends and family, it is reasonable to conclude that *our postoperative analgesia prescription practices are making a significant contribution to the supply of illicit opioids.*

RECOMMENDATIONS FOR SURGEONS

- Consider the risk that an individual patient may develop persistent opioid use and proceed to an opioid use disorder.
- Consider the risk that medications prescribed postoperatively may end up diverted to nonmedical use and causing direct public health harm.
- Identify risk factors:
  - Psychiatric illness
  - History of either aberrant substance use or diagnosed substance use disorder
  - Communicate to the patient in a nonjudgmental way so that they can exercise caution in taking prescribed medications.

- Patients with an established or suspected substance use disorder should be referred to an addiction specialist *preoperatively if possible.*[25]
- Elective surgery in patients with established substance use disorders should not be performed until follow-up for substance use has been arranged.
- Efforts should be made to explain and facilitate the use of nonopioid pain control.
- Prescriptions should be limited to 20 doses of low potency, immediate release opioids unless circumstances clearly dictate otherwise.[26,27]

> **SENIOR AUTHOR TIP:**   We can make a major contribution by curbing opioid diversion in the perioperative period. We can partner with our anesthesia/pain colleagues to *identify at-risk patients* and prevent postoperative aberrant opioid use.

CAUTION: If an opioid naive patient develops an opioid use disorder after surgery, that is a surgical complication. Similarly, if members of our patient's family (i.e., children, home care workers, etc.) aberrantly use the medications we prescribe, we hold a level of responsibility for this.

PROPER PAIN MANAGEMENT

Multiple organizations have urged a shift toward nonopioid options for pain management.
- JCAHO[27]:
  - *"An individualized, multimodal treatment plan should be used to manage pain—upon assessment, the best approach may be to start with a non-narcotic"*[1]
- CDC[28]:
  - *"Health care providers should only use opioids in carefully screened and monitored patients when non-opioid treatments are insufficient to manage pain"*[2]
- ASA[29]:
  - *"A multimodal approach to pain management beginning with a local anesthetic where appropriate"*[3]

IMPACT OF INADEQUATE PAIN MANAGEMENT[30]
- Undesirable physiologic and immunologic effects
- Associated with poor surgical outcomes
- ↑ probability of hospital readmission
- ↑ cost of care
- ↓ patient satisfaction
- Postsurgical pain intensity was associated with delayed wound healing.

APPROACH TO PAIN MANAGEMENT
- Common pain management protocols are opioid based.
- Lack understanding of current literature
- Don't differentiate between acute and chronic pain
- Aren't customized to patients or surgical procedures

OPIOID-RELATED ADVERSE EVENTS[31]
- Primary component of most postoperative multimodal pain management strategies

- Associated with unwanted and severe adverse events
  - Nausea and vomiting
  - Pruritus
  - Sedation and cognitive impairment
  - Urinary depression
  - Sleep disturbances
  - Respiratory depression

ANALGESIC OPTIONS FOR MULTIMODAL ANALGESIA

- Regional analgesic techniques
  - Wound infiltration
  - Field blocks (TAP block)
  - Peripheral nerve and plexus blocks
  - Neuraxial blocks
- IV lidocaine infusion
- Acetaminophen
- NSAIDs
- COX-2 inhibitors
- Dexamethasone
- Ketamine
- Gabapentin/pregabalin
- Opioids (as rescue)

BENEFITS[32,33]

- Improve postsurgical pain control
- Permit use of lower analgesic doses
- Reduce dependence on opioids for postsurgical pain management
- Combines a variety of analgesic medication and techniques with nonpharmacological interventions[34]
  - Uses drugs with complimentary mechanisms of action
  - Targets multiple sites of the nociceptive pathway
  - Allows for lower doses of medications and potentially provides greater pain relief
- May result in fewer analgesic side effects
- May address patient differences in analgesic metabolism and pain sensitivity
- Avoid "shotgun" approach
- Type and number of analgesics should be procedure- and patient-specific
- Emphasis on function NOT pain scores

ACETAMINOPHEN, NSAIDs, AND COX-2 INHIBITORS COMBINATION

- Meta-analysis of opioid-sparing effects of acetaminophen, NSAIDs, and COX-2 inhibitors
- All analgesics resulted in lower 24-hour morphine requirement (6-10 mg).
- No clinically significant advantages shown for one group over the others
- NSAIDs associated with more bleeding
  - **NSAIDs versus Coxibs**
    - ▶ No difference in analgesic efficacy between nonselective-NSAIDs and COX-2 selective inhibitors at equipotent doses

▶ COX-2 inhibitors lack of platelet inhibition and do not influence perioperative blood loss

▶ No difference in other adverse effects (cardiovascular, renal, gastrointestinal)

PERIOPERATIVE DEXAMETHASONE AND PAIN

- Systematic review of published literature that involved 45 studies, involving 5796 patients
- **Benefits (as per systematic review):**
  - Reduced pain scores at 2 hours and 24 hours postoperatively
  - Reduced opioid requirements
  - Reduced need for rescue analgesia for intolerable pain
  - Allowed longer time to first rescue analgesic
  - Allowed shorter PACU stay
- No increase in infection or delayed wound healing
- No dose response with regards opioid sparing

GABAPENTIN/PREGABALIN FOR POSTOPERATIVE PAIN[35,36]

- Reduces postoperative pain and opioid requirements
- **Limitations:** Studies have small sample size and short duration of follow-up
- **Side effects:** Sedation, dizziness may delay discharge home
- *Selective use in surgical procedures with high incidence of persistent postoperative pain*
  - Patients with fibromyalgia, chronic pain

INTRAVENOUS KETAMINE

- Systematic review placebo-controlled, RCTs (n = 47) IV ketamine (bolus or infusion)
- Heterogeneity among studies was significant
- Reduced total opioid consumption and increase in time to first analgesic observed in all studies
- Reduced pain scores
- Reduced PONV only when pain scores decreased
- Not beneficial for surgery with mild pain (VAS <4)
- Hallucinations and nightmares significantly high when ketamine was efficacious

INFILTRATION OF LOCAL ANESTHETICS

TIMING

- Timing of the block (preincision versus postincision) does not appear to be clinically significant.
- Nerve blocks improve postoperative analgesia.
- Total dose, but not volume and concentration, of local anesthetics affects the efficiency.

SURGICAL SITE INFILTRATION: BEST CLINICAL PRACTICE[37] (Fig. 8-1)

- Use a 22-gauge, 1½-inch needle.
- Use a fanning technique ("moving needle technique").
- Needle is inserted approximately 0.5-1 cm into the tissue plane and local anesthetic solution is injected while slowly withdrawing the needle (reduces the risk of intravascular injection).

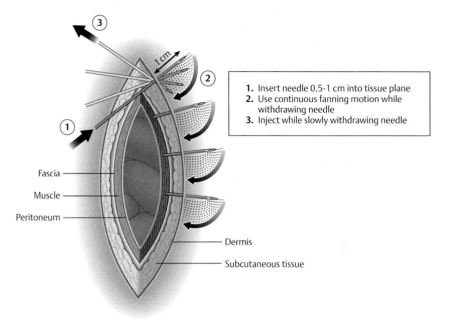

1. Insert needle 0.5-1 cm into tissue plane
2. Use continuous fanning motion while withdrawing needle
3. Inject while slowly withdrawing needle

Fascia
Muscle
Peritoneum
Dermis
Subcutaneous tissue

Fig. 8-1   Infiltration with moving needle technique to optimize distribution of the local anesthetic solution.

MULTIMODAL ANALGESIA REGIMEN

SENIOR AUTHOR TIP: The following is my own perioperative multimodal analgesia regimen for many patients (aesthetic and reconstructive), though it is tailored and individualized to the patient and specific procedure. It is intended as a demonstrative example only.

- **Night before surgery**
  - 300 mg gabapentin (Neurontin) by mouth
    - ▶ Only if no history of sleep apnea
- **Upon arrival to the surgery center or hospital**
  - 1000 mg acetaminophen by mouth liquid (2 hours prior to surgery time)
    - ▶ If no hypersensitivity, severe hepatic impairment, or severe active liver disease
  - 300 mg gabapentin by mouth (2 hours prior to surgery time)
    - ▶ Only if no history of sleep apnea
  - 400 mg celecoxib by mouth (20 minutes prior to surgery time)
    - ▶ Depends on assessment of individual patient's risks (cardiovascular morbidity, gastroduodenal ulcer history, renal and hepatic function)
  - 40 mg aprepitant (Emend), one tablet by mouth, 2 hours before surgery*
    - ▶ *(Only if history of postoperative nausea and vomiting AND ONLY preoperative, never postoperative)*

Note on NSAIDS
- Use varies depending on individual patient risks
  - Bleeding complications
  - Cardiovascular morbidity
  - Actual or recent gastroduodenal ulcer history
  - Aspirin-sensitive asthma
  - Renal function
  - Hepatic function

Intraoperative
- Multiplanar field block with 0.25% Marcaine with epinephrine
  - Or liposomal bupivacaine, if available
- Ketorolac IV (30 mg)
  - Or IV acetaminophen or IV ibuprofen
- Dexamethasone IV (8 mg)
  - Improves pain control, reduces PONV, antiinflammatory
  - No significant effect on blood glucose

Day of Surgery/POD 0
- **200 mg celecoxib** by mouth (12 hours after the morning dose)
- **1000 mg acetaminophen** tablet by mouth (every 6 hours, repeat 3 times)
- **5 mg oxycodone:** One tablet by mouth every 4 hours as needed for pain
- **100 mg docusate (Colace):** One tablet by mouth 2 times a day as needed for constipation
- **8 mg odansteron sublingual:** One dissolvable tablet every 8 hours as needed for nausea

POD 1 and After
- **200 mg celecoxib** by mouth, 3 times a day for 14 days
- **1000 mg acetaminophen** tablet by mouth every 6 hours for 14 days (with no other APAP-containing meds!)
- **5 mg oxycodone:** One tablet by mouth every 4 hours as needed for pain
- **100 mg docusate (Colace):** One tablet by mouth 2 times a day as needed for constipation for 7 days
- **8 mg odansteron sublingual:** One dissolvable tablet every 8 hours as needed for nausea

Gabapentinoids
- Beneficial when high probability of prolonged, persistent pain
- Reduce both pain and opioid requirements
- Can improve perioperative sleep and anxiety
- < 65 years old:
  - Gabapentin 300 mg by mouth 3 times a day for 7 days
- > 65 years old:
  - Gabapentin 300 mg by mouth 2 times a day for 7 days
    - ▶ Need to adjust for renal function

Alternatives
- If allergic to celecoxib or insurance won't cover, can use meloxicam 15 mg by mouth 2 times a day

- If cannot take celecoxib or meloxicam, use either ibuprofen 400 mg by mouth every 6 hours or naprosyn 440 mg by mouth every 12 hours.
  - Do not use if patient with history of peptic ulcer disease. Do not take both, only one or other.

TOP TAKEAWAYS
➤ We are in an opioid epidemic. Doctors/surgeons play a role.
➤ Be judicious in your opioid prescribing habits and be aware of overprescribing habits and diversion.
➤ Multimodal analgesia should be patient- and procedure-specific.

REFERENCES

1. US Centers for Disease Control and Prevention. Press release. Opioid painkiller prescribing varies widely among states. July 1, 2014. Available at *http://www.cdc.gov/media/releases/2014/p0701-opioid-painkiller.html*.
2. Apfelbaum JL, Chen C, Mehta SS, et al. Postoperative pain experience: results from a national survey suggest postoperative pain continues to be undermanaged. Anesth Analg 97:534, 2003.
3. Manchikanti L, Singh A. Therapeutic opioids: a ten-year perspective on the complexities and complications of the escalating use, abuse, and nonmedical use of opioids. Pain Physician 11:S63, 2008.
4. Center for Behavioral Health Statistics and Quality. (2016). 2015 national survey on drug use and health. Substance Abuse and Mental Health Services Administration, Rockville, MD.
5. Kolodny A, Courtwright DT, Hwang CS, et al. The prescription opioid and heroin crisis: a public health approach to an epidemic of addiction. Annu Rev Public Health 36:559, 2015.
6. Manchikanti L, Kaye AM, Kaye AD. Current state of opioid therapy and abuse. Curr Pain Headache Rep. May, 2016. Available from *http://link.springer.com/10.1007/s11916-016-0564-x*.
7. Dart RC, Surratt HL, Cicero TJ, et al. Trends in opioid analgesic abuse and mortality in the United States. N Engl J Med 372:241, 2015.
8. Bohnert AS, Valenstein M, Bair MJ, et al. Association between opioid prescribing patterns and opioid overdose-related deaths. JAMA 305:1315, 2011.
9. Sites BD, Beach ML, Davis MA. Increases in the use of prescription opioid analgesics and the lack of improvement in disability metrics among users. Reg Anesth Pain Med 39:6, 2014.
10. Warner M, Chen LH, Makuc DM, et al. Drug poisoning deaths in the United States, 1980-2008. [cited 2016 Nov 16]; Available from *https://stacks.cdc.gov/view/cdc/13332/cdc_13332_DS1.pdf*.
11. Johnston L, O'Malley P, Miech R, et al. Monitoring the future national survey results on drug use, 1975-2015. National Institute on Drug Abuse at the National Institutes of Health, 2016.
12. Brands B, Paglia-Boak A, Sproule BA, et al. Nonmedical use of opioid analgesics among Ontario students. Can Fam Physician Med Fam Can 56:256, 2010.
13. Centers for Disease Control and Prevention. Prescription drug overdose data. Available at *http://www.cdc.gov/drugoverdose/data/overdose.html*.
14. Mack KA, Zhang K, Paulozzi L, et al. Prescription practices involving opioid analgesics among Americans with Medicaid, 2010. J Health Care Poor Underserved 26:182, 2015.
15. Levy B, Paulozzi L, Mack KA, et al. Trends in opioid analgesic-prescribing rates by specialty, U.S., 2007–2012. Am J Prev Med 49:409, 2015.
16. Wunsch H, Wijeysundera DN, Passarella MA, et al. Opioids prescribed after low-risk surgical procedures in the United States, 2004-2012. JAMA 315:1654, 2016.

17. Mudumbai SC, Oliva EM, Lewis ET, et al. Time-to-cessation of postoperative opioids: a population-level analysis of the veterans affairs health care system. Pain Med 17:1732, 2016.

18. Johnson SP, Chung KC, Zhong L, et al. Risk of prolonged opioid use among opioid-naive patients following common hand surgery procedures. J Hand Surg 41:947, 2016.

19. Clarke H, Soneji N, Ko DT, et al. Rates and risk factors for prolonged opioid use after major surgery: population based cohort study. BMJ 348:g1251, 2014.

20. Sun EC, Darnall BD, Baker LC, et al. Incidence of and risk factors for chronic opioid use among opioid-naive patients in the postoperative period. JAMA Intern Med 176:1286, 2016.

21. Alam A, Gomes T, Zheng H, et al. Long-term analgesic use after low-risk surgery: a retrospective cohort study. Arch Intern Med 172:425, 2012.

22. Rodgers J, Cunningham K, Fitzgerald K, et al. Opioid consumption following outpatient upper extremity surgery. J Hand Surg 37:645, 2012.

23. Bates C, Laciak R, Southwick A, et al. Overprescription of postoperative narcotics: a look at postoperative pain medication delivery, consumption and disposal in urological practice. J Urol 185:551, 2011.

24. Bartels K, Mayes LM, Dingmann C, et al. Opioid use and storage patterns by patients after hospital discharge following surgery. PLoS One 11:e0147972, 2016.

25. Thorson D, Biewen P, Bonte B, et al. Acute pain assessment and opioid prescribing protocol. Inst Clin Syst Improv 2014 [cited 2016 Nov 16]; Available from http://citeseerx.ist.psu.edu/viewdoc/download?doi=10.1.1.678.4784&rep=rep1&type=pdf.

26. O'Neill DF, Thomas CW. Less is more: limiting narcotic prescription quantities for common orthopedic procedures. Phys Sportsmed 42:100, 2014.

27. The Joint Commission. Revisions to pain management standard effective January 1, 2015. http://www.jointcommission.org/assets/1/23/jconline.

28. Centers for Disease Control and Prevention. Vital signs: overdoses of prescription opioid pain relievers—United States, 1999-2010. MMWR Morb Mortal Wkly Rep 62:537, 2013.

29. American Society of Anesthesiologists Task Force on Acute Pain Management. Practice guidelines for acute pain management in the perioperative setting: an updated report. Anesthesiology 116:248, 2012.

30. Joshi GP, Beck DE, Emerson RH, et al. Defining new directions for more effective management of surgical pain in the United States: highlights of the inaugural Surgical Pain Congress. Am Surg 80:219, 2014.

31. Dasta J, Ramamoorthy S, Patou G, et al. Bupivacaine liposome injectable suspension compared with bupivacaine HCl for the reduction of opioid burden in the postsurgical setting. Curr Med Res Opin 28:1609, 2012.

32. Lovich-Sapola J, Smith CE, Brandt CP. Postoperative pain control. Surg Clin North Am 95:301, 2015.

33. Golembiewski J, Dasta J. Evolving role of local anesthetics in managing postsurgical analgesia. Clin Ther 37:1354, 2015.

34. Manworren RC. Multimodal pain management and the future of a personalized medicine approach to pain. AORN J 101:308, 2015.

35. Adam F, Menigaux C, Sessler DI, et al. A single preoperative dose of gabapentin (800 milligrams) does not augment postoperative analgesia in patients given interscalene brachial plexus blocks for arthroscopic shoulder surgery. Anesth Analg 103:1278, 2006.

36. Paech MJ, Goy R, Chua S et al. A randomized, placebo-controlled trial of preoperative oral pregabalin for postoperative pain relief after minor gynecological surgery. Anesth Analg 105:1449, 2007.

37. Joshi GP, Janis JE, Haas EM, et al. Surgical site infiltration for abdominal surgery: a novel neuroanatomical-based approach. Plast Recon Surg Glob Open 4:e1181, 2016.

PART III

Safety

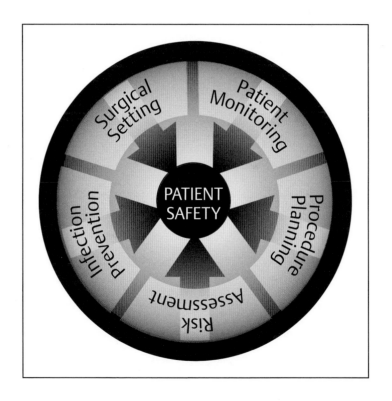

9. Safety Considerations in Aesthetic Surgery

Jeffrey E. Janis, Sumeet Sorel Teotia, J. Byers Bowen, Girish P. Joshi, Vernon Leroy Young

"The physician must . . . have two special objects in view with regard to disease, namely, to do good or to do no harm."[1]

Hippocrates

SAFETY IN OFFICE-BASED SURGERY

- Two decades ago **<20%** of surgical procedures were performed on an outpatient basis.
- Today **>80%** of all surgeries are performed in an outpatient setting.[2]
- Numerous studies have established the efficacy and safety of outpatient office-based surgical facilities.
- These studies have shown low **complication rates of 0.33%-0.7%** and extremely low **mortality rates** of approximately **0.002%**.[2-6]
- The two largest plastic surgery societies in the United States, the American Society of Plastic Surgeons (ASPS) and the American Society for Aesthetic Plastic Surgery (ASAPS), have recognized the importance of establishing a culture of safety and have accordingly established task forces that are charged with establishing guidelines for office-based surgical facilities.
- In their review of patient safety in an office-based setting, Horton, Janis, and Rohrich[7] divided this topic into four broad categories:
  1. Administrative
  2. Clinical aspects
  3. Liposuction
  4. Management of postoperative issues, in particular postoperative pain and postoperative nausea and vomiting (PONV)

ADMINISTRATIVE ISSUES[7]

- **Governance:** Policies outlining the structure of office-based surgical facilities include staff responsibilities, supervision, and a patient bill of rights.
- **Physician qualifications:** Practitioners must obtain and maintain adequate training and certification for all procedures/treatments performed in the office facility and should limit their practice to the scope of the certifying board.
- **Quality assessment:** Develop a system of quality of care with continual evaluation focused on improving patient care/safety. This includes the maintenance of the physical plant, operating room/recovery room equipment, personnel evaluations and coursework, and development and implementation of protocols and procedures.
- Accreditation and maintenance of surgical facility standards

- Protocols for management of emergency situations. This includes transfer protocols to a higher level of care (i.e., hospitals), generally, where the surgeon has admitting privileges and ideally privileges to perform the same procedures that are performed in the office-based setting.
- Informed consent process
- Maintenance of complete medical records
- Guidelines for patient discharge
- System for reporting of adverse events

CORE PRINCIPLES

- These core principles have been approved by the American College of Surgeons, the American Medical Association, and the ASPS for outpatient office-based surgery involving any level of anesthesia above local anesthesia procedures.[8]
  - **Core principle 1:** Guidelines or regulations should be developed by states for office-based surgery according to levels of anesthesia defined by the ASA Continuum of Depth of Sedation statement dated October 13, 1999, excluding local anesthesia or minimal sedation.
  - **Core principle 2:** Physicians should select patients by criteria, including the ASA Patient Selection Physical Status Classification System. This should be documented in the preoperative evaluation of the patient.
  - **Core principle 3:** Physicians who perform office-based surgery should have their facilities accredited by the Joint Commission on Accreditation of Healthcare Organizations, the Accreditation Association for Ambulatory Health Care, the American Association for Accreditation of Ambulatory Surgery Facilities, the American Osteopathic Association, or a state-recognized entity such as the Institute for Medical Quality, or the facility should be state licensed and/or Medicare certified.
  - **Core principle 4:** Physicians performing office-based surgery must have admitting privileges at a nearby hospital, or have a transfer agreement with another physician who has admitting privileges at a nearby hospital, or maintain an emergency transfer agreement with a nearby hospital.
  - **Core principle 5:** States should follow the guidelines outlined by the Federation of State Medical Boards regarding informed consent.
  - **Core principle 6:** States should consider legally privileged adverse incident reporting requirements as recommended by the Federation of State Medical Boards and accompanied by periodic peer review and a program of Continuous Quality Improvement.
  - **Core principle 7:** Physicians performing office-based surgery must obtain and maintain board certification by one of the boards recognized by the American Board of Medical Specialties, the American Osteopathic Association, or a board with equivalent standards approved by the state medical board within 5 years of

completing an approved residency training program. The procedure must be one that is generally recognized by that certifying board as falling within the scope of training and practice of the physician providing the care.

- **Core principle 8:** Physicians performing office-based surgery may show competency by maintaining core privileges at an accredited or licensed hospital or ambulatory surgical center for the procedures they perform in the office setting. Alternatively, the governing body of the office facility is responsible for a peer review process for privileging physicians based on nationally recognized credentialing standards.
- **Core principle 9:** At least one physician who is credentialed or currently recognized as having successfully completed a course in advanced resuscitative techniques (advanced trauma life support, advanced cardiac life support, or pediatric advanced life support) must be present or immediately available with age- and size-appropriate resuscitative equipment until the patient has met the criteria for discharge from the facility. In addition, other medical personnel with direct patient contact should, at a minimum, be trained in basic life support.
- **Core principle 10:** Physicians administering or supervising moderate sedation/ analgesia, deep sedation/analgesia, or general anesthesia should have appropriate education and training.

CLINICAL ISSUES RELATED TO OFFICE-BASED SURGERY

- **Preoperative evaluation:** This includes a thorough history and physical examination performed by the surgeon, with consideration for use of a standardized form to capture all information pertinent to a patient's medical history, which would allow the surgeon to adequately assess the patient's risk for surgery and optimize the outcome from the proposed procedure.
- **Anesthesia evaluation:** For any procedure that requires >simple local anesthesia (i.e., sedation or general anesthesia), anesthesia should be given by a practitioner, either a certified nurse anesthetist or anesthesiologist, in accordance with the current specific state requirements where the surgical facility exists.
- Patient selection in office-based surgery is an important concept.[9,10]
- Patients should be risk stratified based on the **American Society of Anesthesiologists (ASA) physical classification status** (Table 9-1).
  - ASA I and II patients are considered ideal candidates for all types of office-based surgery.
  - ASA III patients are considered reasonable candidates for procedures that can be performed using a local anesthetic with or without sedation (see Chapter 5).
  - ASA IV patients are candidates for only local anesthesia procedures in an office setting.
  - These are general guidelines and should be interpreted by each surgeon in consultation with the anesthesia practitioner.

Table 9-1   *American Society of Anesthesiologists Physical Status Classification*

Physical Status	Description	Example
Class 1	A normal healthy patient	Healthy, nonsmoking, no or minimal alcohol use
Class 2	A patient with mild systemic disease	Mild diseases only without substantive functional limitations. Examples include (but not limited to) current smoker, social alcohol drinker, pregnancy, obesity (BMI = 30-40), well-controlled DM/HTN, mild lung disease
Class 3	A patient with severe systemic disease	Substantive functional limitations; One or more moderate to severe diseases. Examples include (but not limited to) poorly controlled DM or HTN; COPD; morbid obesity (BMI ≥40); active hepatitis; alcohol dependence or abuse, implanted pacemaker, moderate reduction of ejection fraction; ESRD undergoing regularly scheduled dialysis; premature infant PCA <60 weeks; history (>3 months) of MI, CVA, TIA, or CAD/stents
Class 4	A patient with severe systemic disease that is a constant threat to life	Examples include (but not limited to) recent (<3 months) MI, CVA, TIA, or CAD/stents; ongoing cardiac ischemia or severe valve dysfunction; severe reduction of ejection fraction; sepsis; DIC; ARD or ESRD not undergoing regularly scheduled dialysis
Class 5	A moribund patient who is not expected to survive without the operation	Examples include (but not limited to) ruptured abdominal/thoracic aneurysm; massive trauma; intracranial bleed with mass effect; ischemic bowel in the face of significant cardiac pathology or multiple organ/system dysfunction
Class 6	A declared brain-dead patient whose organs are being removed for donor purposes	

*The addition of "E" denotes emergency surgery. An emergency is defined as existing when delay in treatment of the patient would lead to a significant increase in the threat to life or body part.

MONITORING AND MINIMIZING PHYSIOLOGIC STRESSES RELATED TO THE SURGICAL PROCEDURE

HYPOTHERMIA
- **Definition:** Core body temperature **<36° C**
- **Incidence:** 50%-90% of surgical patients if no preventative measures are used.[11]
- **Causes:**
  - Thermoregulatory mechanisms are impaired by anesthesia.
  - Core-to-peripheral heat redistribution begins soon after anesthesia.
  - Patient loses body heat to ambient temperature of OR.[12]

- **Risks:** Increased blood loss, coagulation disorders, increased risk of cardiac events, increased risk of surgical site infection, postoperative shivering, and lengthened hospital stays.
  - All of these factors secondarily contribute to increased costs.[13]
- **Prevention:** Use of cutaneous warming devices, forced-air warming blankets, and intravenous fluid warmers (see Chapter 5)
  - Actively prewarm patients for **1 hour** preoperative with forced-air heating
  - Patients not prewarmed are prone to hypothermia within 30 minutes of anesthesia induction (Fig. 9-1).[12]

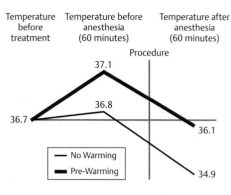

Fig. 9-1   Two-group comparison of prewarming.

- **Recommendations:** If no antihypothermia devices are available, office surgical procedures should be limited to **<2 hours' duration** and **<20% body surface area of exposure.**[9]

BLOOD LOSS
- If the anticipated blood loss is **>500 ml,** the procedure should be performed in a facility in which postoperative monitoring and blood replacement products are readily available.[9]

DURATION OF THE SURGICAL PROCEDURE
- Overall procedure length should be limited to <6 hours for office-based surgical procedures.[9]
- The safety and efficacy of outpatient office-based surgery has been established by numerous studies.[2-6]
- Some studies have correlated the length of the ambulatory surgical procedure with increased rates of postdischarge readmission to a hospital.[14]
- State regulations must be checked for details, because some states have more aggressive regulations/restrictions.

POSTOPERATIVE PAIN AND NAUSEA
- The postoperative management of office-based surgical patients affects the discharge process, the patients' overall satisfaction with the procedure and facility, and ultimately patient safety.
  - Inadequate pain control has physiologic effects on all organ systems.[15]
  - Postoperative pain is the main reason for delayed discharge and hospital readmission after ambulatory surgery.[16]
  - Inadequate pain control can also cause PONV.
  - PONV has received less attention than pain management but actually represents the **most common reason for patient dissatisfaction.** It is also a major factor in **delayed discharge** and **unplanned postoperative hospital admission.**
    - Up to 10% of patients experience PONV in the recovery room.[15,17]

- ▶ The incidence of PONV increases to 30% at 24 hours, and most patients have PONV after discharge with no access to treatment.[17]
- ▶ Long-acting narcotics and inhalational anesthetic agents should be avoided to reduce PONV.
- ▶ Propofol has been shown to have antiemetic effects.[18]
- Multimodal pain and PONV management are recommended in the preoperative, intraoperative, and postoperative phases of the office-based surgical procedure.
- Multimodal PONV involves treating all **five major** receptor systems[19,20]:
  1. Serotonin (5-HT3): These are currently the most effective and safest agents.[21]
  2. Dopamine (DA)
  3. Histamine (H-1)
  4. Acetylcholine (Ach)
  5. Neurokinin (NK-1)

For additional details, see Chapters 7 and 8.

LIPOSUCTION

- According to the 2016 American Society for Aesthetic Plastic Surgery Cosmetic Surgery National Data Bank statistics, liposuction procedures (414,335) were the most commonly performed aesthetic procedures in the United States.[22] Most of these procedures are performed in an office-based setting.

ANESTHESIA (see also Chapters 5 through 7)

- For small-volume liposuction, infiltration with a solution containing a local anesthetic may be sufficient without the need for adjunctive anesthesia, although the use of monitoring devices during the procedure is recommended.
- Bupivacaine (Marcaine) should **not** be used because of the severity of its side effects, its long half-life, and the inability to reverse toxicity.
- Lidocaine maximal dosage is **35 mg/kg.**[23]
- For larger-volume liposuction, the amount of lidocaine used should be reduced.
- Superwet (1:1) technique rather than tumescent (3:1) technique is used to reduce lidocaine dosage and infiltrate volume.
- If regional or general anesthesia is used, not using or reducing the lidocaine dose should be considered.
- **Epinephrine:** The recommended maximal dose is **0.07 mg/kg**, although up to 10 mg/kg have been used safely.[24]
- Epinephrine is avoided for patients with comorbid medical conditions that prohibit its use, including hyperthyroidism, severe hypertension, cardiac disease, peripheral vascular disease, and pheochromocytoma.
- For multiple-site liposuction procedures, infiltration is staged to decrease the epinephrine effects.[24]
- Patient selection: Liposuction is generally a safe procedure for treating localized adiposity of the abdomen, flanks, arm, trunks, and thighs. Liposuction is not a treatment for obesity. It is generally not recommended for patients with a **BMI >30.**[25]

VOLUME

- In an office-based setting, the maximal volume of lipoaspirate should be **5000 cc.**[24] Large-volume liposuction (>5000 cc) should be performed in an acute facility that

allows monitoring of fluid resuscitation requirements, and overnight observation/
hospitalization should be strongly considered.

FLUID MANAGEMENT

- Recommendations for fluid resuscitation are shown in Box 9-1.

Box 9-1 *LIPOSUCTION FLUID RESUSCITATION GUIDELINES*

Small-Volume Aspirations (<5 liters)	Large-Volume Aspirations (>5 liters)
Maintenance fluid[a]	Maintenance fluid[a]
Subcutaneous infiltrate[b]	Subcutaneous infiltrate[b]
	0.25 ml of intravenous crystalloid per millimeter of aspirate >5 liters

[a]Amount of fluid to be replaced from preoperative, NPO status.
[b]Seventy percent is presumed to be intravascular.

COMBINATION PROCEDURES

- Studies have shown a cumulative effect on the incidence of complications when multiple surgical procedures are combined in one setting.
- Studies have shown that smaller-volume liposuction can be safely and effectively combined with other plastic surgery procedures, even in office settings.
- Some states have recently restricted the combination of liposuction with any other type of surgery.
- Surgeons operating in an office-based facility must be aware of the local and state regulations.

MORTALITY

- A survey study of ASAPS members showed 95 deaths in close to 500,000 lipoplasty procedures for a mortality rate of 1 in 5224 (19.1/100,000 versus 3/100,000 for elective inguinal hernia repair)[26] (Table 9-2).
- **Pulmonary embolism (PE)** was the most common cause of death **(23%).**
- Overall lipoplasty mortality rates have been reported as 0.0021%-0.019%.[26,27]

Table 9-2 *Fatal Outcomes from Liposuction*

Cause of Death	Number of Deaths	Percentage
Fat embolism	11	8.5
Anesthesia-related complications	13	10.0
Hemorrhage	6	4.6
Thromboembolism	30	23.1
Cardiorespiratory failure	7	5.4
Gastrointestinal perforations	19	14.6
Massive infection	7	5.4
Unknown or confidential	37	28.5
Total	**130**	**~100**

COMBINATION SURGICAL PROCEDURES

- After the 2000 Florida moratorium banned the combination of abdominoplasty and liposuction, interest in evaluating the safety and efficacy of combined plastic surgical procedures has increased.[28]
- Many states have imposed arbitrary restrictions on allowable lengths of surgery for office-based surgery.
- Florida mandates that procedures lasting **>6 hours** must not be performed in the office setting, whereas Pennsylvania and Tennessee have imposed arbitrary **4-hour limits** on office-based surgery.
- Balakrishnan et al[29] reviewed the current available data and concluded: "As they [states] attempt to impose regulations on office surgery, it is evident that sufficient data do not exist to formulate immediate evidence-based policy."
- A review of the literature revealed that most studies have addressed the combination of abdominoplasty with either liposuction or gynecological procedures.[30,31]
- Unlike previous reports,[30,31] which were mainly retrospective reviews of the efficacy of combining abdominoplasty with gynecological procedures, these studies established the safety of office-based abdominoplasty and of performing concomitant aesthetic procedures with abdominoplasty.[32,33]
  - **Stevens et al (2006)[32]:** Their study showed no statistically significant difference in complication rates between a group of patients who underwent abdominoplasty with a breast procedure compared with a control group who underwent abdominoplasty alone.
  - **Melendez et al (2008)[33]:** Aside from a single episode of PE in their abdominoplasty-only group (incidence 1.03%), they reported no other major complications or mortality in either study group (i.e., abdominoplasty versus abdominoplasty with another aesthetic procedure).
  - A 2006 retrospective Canadian study[34] compared a group of 37 inpatient abdominoplasty procedures with 32 patients who underwent outpatient abdominoplasty. Most patients underwent concomitant aesthetic procedures. There was no significant difference in complications between the inpatient and outpatient groups.
- Although these studies support the safety of combining aesthetic surgical procedures, both abdominoplasty and high-volume liposuction have been established as **higher-risk surgeries for VTE,**[26,27,35] and it is prudent for surgeons to approach the combination of these two procedures with caution and maximize patient safety with appropriate VTE prophylaxis. In higher-risk patients these combination procedures should be performed in a hospital, or consideration should be given to not combining the procedures.
- **Gordon and Koch[36]** reviewed 1200 consecutive facial plastic surgeries performed in an office-based setting:
  - The duration of the procedure was >240 minutes in 1032 (86%) procedures.
  - Patients whose surgeries lasted <4 hours served as a control group for the lengthier procedures.
  - *The incidence of major morbidity was not increased in the patients undergoing procedures lasting >4 hours.*

- Clear, evidence-based criteria for the optimal duration of office-based surgery has not been established due to a paucity of objective level 1 evidence.[9,28]
- *In general, overall surgical procedure time should be* **<6 hours** *for outpatient surgery, especially in the office-based setting.*[9]

VENOUS THROMBOEMBOLISM (see also Chapter 11)

- **Incidence**
  - An ASPS study of existing data *estimated* that 18,000 cases/year of DVT may occur.[37]
  - The overall incidence of DVT in the United States is 84-1550 per 100,000 per year.[38]
  - The incidence of PE in the United States is 125,000-400,000 cases per year.[39]
  - PE is the **third most common cause of postsurgical mortality,** accounting for approximately 150,000 deaths per year.
  - The incidence of VTE varies greatly between medical and surgical specialties, as well as within a specialty, depending on the procedure performed[40] (Table 9-3).

Table 9-3   *Absolute Risk of DVT in Hospitalized Patients*

Group of Patients	DVT Occurrence (%)
Major general surgery	15-40
Major orthopedic surgery	40-60
Spinal cord injury	60-80
Multiple trauma	40-80
Neurosurgery	15-40
Stroke	20-50
Major gynecological surgery	15-40
Major urological surgery	15-40
Critical care patients	10-80
Medical patients	10-20

- McDevitt[41] found that in patients undergoing elective surgery who received no prophylactic treatment the incidence of fatal PE was 0.1%-0.8%.
- Medical comorbidities that may increase the incidence of VTE[42,43]:
  1. Chronic venous insufficiency
  2. Family history of thrombotic syndromes
  3. **Obesity**
  4. Trauma
  5. Severe infection
  6. Polycythemia
  7. Central nervous system disease
  8. Malignancy
  9. Homocystinuria
  10. History of pelvic or lower extremity radiation
  11. **Use of birth control pills**
  12. **Hormone replacement therapy (HRT)**

- **Obesity, use of birth control pills,** and **HRT** are common within our aesthetic surgery patients.
- Many body contouring surgeries are performed on patients who are trying to achieve improved appearance but may present at borderline obese BMIs or have previously been morbidly obese and underwent bariatric surgery, increasing their risk for VTE.
- Most aesthetic surgery patients are female, and although there are limited data on the incidence of use of birth control pills or HRT within these distinct aesthetic surgery populations, most patients probably use these.
  - A recent review and meta-analysis in the British Medical Journal of eight observational studies and nine randomized controlled trials showed a **twofold to threefold increased risk of VTE in women on HRT.**
    - ▶ This study also established that the risk is highest within the first year of HRT use as well as for women who are considered higher risk for VTE.
    - ▶ This review also established that transdermal HRT decreases the risk of VTE compared with the oral route of administration and appears to be safe in regard to thrombotic risk.[44]
  - Men receiving estrogen therapy for prostate cancer are also at increased risk of VTE.
  - **Smoking** compounds the VTE risk of patients who are taking oral contraceptives.
  - The prothrombotic mechanism of estrogen is related to **the decreased levels of protein S associated with elevated levels of circulating estrogen.** Smoking exacerbates this clinical scenario.
  - There are no definitive data to suggest when oral contraceptives or hormone replacement should be discontinued before surgery to minimize VTE risks, but it has been suggested that this should be done at least **2 weeks before surgery.**[42]
- Despite the recent interest in VTE prevention, evidence clearly establishing the true incidence of DVT and PE within the field of aesthetic surgery is insufficient.
  - The earliest report on the incidence of VTE in the plastic surgery literature was in 1977 when Grazer and Goldwyn[45] reported an incidence of DVT of 1.1% and PE of 0.8% in >10,000 abdominoplasty patients.
  - Hester et al[31] reported that combining abdominoplasty with another surgical procedure increased the incidence of PE.
  - Voss et al reported a 6.6% incidence of PE when abdominoplasty was combined with intraabdominal gynecological procedures.[46]

- A survey study of board-certified plastic surgeons that reviewed 496,000 liposuction procedures and PE accounted for the largest percentage **(23%)** of deaths.[26]
- DVT and PE in large-volume liposuction procedures have been reported as ranging from 0%-1.1%.[26,27,44]
- When liposuction is combined with other procedures, the incidence of mortality increases from 1 in 47,415 to 1 in 7314, an almost sevenfold increase.[27]

RISK ASSESSMENT (Fig. 9-2)

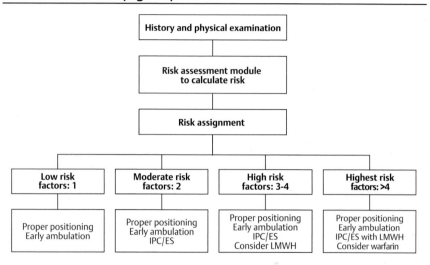

Fig. 9-2   Algorithm for venous thromboembolism prevention in plastic surgery patients. (*ES*, Elastic compression stockings; *IPC*, intermittent pneumatic compression stockings; *LMVH*, low-molecular-weight heparin.)

- Recently, a number-scoring risk assessment model was developed by Caprini and modified by Davison et al[43] to adapt it to plastic surgery patients (Table 9-4).
- Hatef et al[47] made further modifications to the Davison-Caprini risk assessment model to account for increased risk of VTE in body contouring procedures, specifically, circumferential abdominoplasty, high incidence of hormone use in plastic surgery patients, and BMI >30 (Table 9-5).

Table 9-4 *Exposing and Predisposing Risk Factors (Davison-Caprini)*

Exposing Risk Factors	Predisposing Risk Factors
1 Risk Factor (each item represents one risk score)	**1 Risk Factor**
Minor surgery	Age 40-60 Obesity >20% IBW Pregnancy or <10 month postpartum Oral contraceptive/hormone replacement therapy
2 Risk Factors (each item represents two risk scores)	**2 Risk Factors**
Major surgery Immobilization Patients confined to bed for more than 72 hours Central venous access	Age >60 Malignancy
3-4 Risk Factors (each item represents three risk scores)	**3 Risk Factors**
Previous myocardial infarction Congestive heart failure Severe sepsis Free flap	History of DVT/PE Any genetic hypercoagulable disorder Lupus anticoagulant Antiphospholipid antibodies Myeloproliferative disorders Heparin-induced thrombocytopenia Hyperviscosity Homocystinemia
>5 Risk Factors (each item represents five risk scores)	
Fracture of the hip, pelvis, or leg Stroke Multiple trauma Acute spinal cord injury	

Table 9-5 *Exposing and Predisposing Risk Factors (Hatef Modification)*

Exposing Risk Factors	Predisposing Risk Factors
1 Risk Factor	**1 Risk Factor**
Minor surgery	Age 40-60
2 Risk Factors	**2 Risk Factors**
Major surgery Immobilization Central venous access	Age >60 Current malignancy Obesity Over-the-counter progesterone (OCP) Hormone replacement therapy (HRT)
3-4 Risk Factors	**3 Risk Factors**
Previous myocardial infarction (MI) Previous congestive heart failure (CHF) Severe sepsis Free flap Circumferential abdominoplasty	History of venous thromboembolism Hypercoagulable disorder
5 Risk Factors	
Fracture of the hip, pelvis, or leg Stroke Multiple trauma	

POSTBARIATRIC SURGERY PROCEDURES AND VENOUS THROMBOEMBOLISM

- Often these procedures combine **large excisional procedures** with extensive liposuction to achieve body contouring objectives.
- Circumferential abdominoplasty procedures combine circumferential dissection/excision, increased operative time (often >6 hours), circumferential disruption of superficial veins, and increased pain, leading to difficulty with early postoperative mobilization.
  - Aly et al[48] reported an incidence of PE of 9.4% in 32 belt lipectomy procedures.
  - Hatef et al[47] studied 360 excisional body contouring procedures and stratified patients based on risk factors, BMI, type of procedure performed, and the administration of low-molecular-weight heparin for VTE prophylaxis.
    - ▶ The overall incidence of DVT in circumferential abdominoplasty patients was **7.7%**.

▶ **BMI >30** was noted to be a statistically significant factor for increased risk of DVT, and there was a nonsignificant increased trend toward PE.

▶ Patients receiving hormone replacement/birth control had a statistically significant increased rate of both DVT (8.6%) and PE (7.5%).

▶ When patients undergoing circumferential abdominoplasty were examined based on the administration of enoxaparin (Lovenox), a low-molecular-weight heparin, the incidence of DVT was 0% for those who received enoxaparin versus 20% for those who did not receive enoxaparin therapy.

▶ Enoxaparin administration demonstrated nonsignificant trends toward decreased incidence of DVT and VTE in the highest risk group of patients, as well as in those with a BMI >30.

▶ There was a statistically increased incidence of hematoma formation (7.3% versus 0.5%) and clinically significant bleeding requiring transfusion (6.6% versus 0.9%) in the enoxaparin groups.

▶ The addition of liposuction to the excisional body contouring procedure increased the incidence of VTE (6.8% versus 2.4%), which approached statistical significance ($p = 0.083$).[47]

POSTBARIATRIC BODY CONTOURING (see also Chapter 62)

■ In 2015 alone, according to American Society for Bariatric Surgery data, 196,000 Americans underwent bariatric surgery.[49]

■ Unlike many aesthetic surgery patients who are relatively healthy, most massive-weight-loss patients have preexisting medical conditions, such as diabetes mellitus or pulmonary dysfunction, as a result of their elevated BMI.

■ Even if these medical conditions have resolved after their bariatric surgery, the sequelae result in a **higher-risk patient presenting for elective surgery.**

■ These patients have a significantly different physiologic profile than that of typical plastic surgery patients.

■ To optimize aesthetic outcomes and improve safety, surgeons must address these issues during the preoperative workup and planning phase.

■ Among MWL patients, **30%-40%** showed evidence of **vitamin or mineral deficiencies** and >50% were **anemic** on routine evaluation.[50]

■ These nutritional deficiencies arise because of the malabsorptive nature of some of the gastric bypass procedures and because of the patients' altered diets in the postbariatric period during weight loss.

■ Deficiencies of both **folate,** absorbed in the duodenum and proximal jejunum, and **vitamin B$_{12}$,** which binds to intrinsic factor in the stomach and is required for vitamin B$_{12}$ to be absorbed in the terminal ileum, can lead to **anemia.**[51]

■ Observational data from body contouring surgeons showed that many of these patients are both **hypokalemic** and **hypocalcemic.**[52]

■ Hypocalcemia can increase general anesthesia risks, whereas low potassium levels are associated with persistent emesis and can lead to PONV.

■ The evaluation and treatment of anemia in these patients is important, because most of the body contouring procedures involve extensive excisional procedures associated with moderate blood loss.

■ Preoperative treatment of anemia can reduce the need for blood transfusions and their associated risks in this patient population.

■ The ASPS/ASAPS Joint Post-Bariatric Task Force recommended an extensive preoperative laboratory workup before any proposed body contouring procedures to allow assessment and preoperative treatment of any nutritional deficiencies.[52]
 • Routine preoperative laboratory test for the massive-weight-loss patient should include:[52]
  ▶ Complete blood cell count
  ▶ Complete chemistry panel
  ▶ Liver function tests
  ▶ Lipid profile
  ▶ Coagulation tests
  ▶ Iron
  ▶ Vitamin B_{12}
  ▶ Urinalysis

■ Several factors influence the sequence of surgical staging and the number of procedures performed at each stage. These factors include:
 • Patient's BMI
 • Setting of surgery (outpatient versus inpatient)
 • Size of the operating team (solo versus team surgery)
 • Surgeon's experience
 • Coverage (insurance versus fee for service)
 • Patient's goals/desires
 • The most important factor is **preoperative BMI.**
  ▶ Generally, the smaller the BMI, the fewer stages required to perform all procedures.
  ▶ Small patients are defined as **BMI <28.**
  ▶ Medium-sized patients have a **BMI of 28-32.**
  ▶ Large patients have a **BMI of >32.**
  ▶ A higher BMI has been associated with an increased risk of complications in postbariatric body contouring procedures,[53,54] in particular, risk of DVT.[55]

■ Staging of procedures can limit surgical/anesthetic times, minimize surgical blood loss, and lead to decreased surgeon fatigue, thus improving patient safety and outcomes.

■ The use of a **multiple surgeon team approach** or the use of **physician extenders** can also limit operative times and allow combination of procedures. This means fewer surgical procedures from which patients must recover.

■ Usually, staged procedures should be performed at a **minimum of 3-month intervals** to allow adequate recovery time (Table 9-6).

Table 9-6   *Surgical Planning*

Stage	Solo Approach	Team Approach
I	Abdomen	Body lift, liposuction thighs
II	Flank excision	Upper body lift
III	Breast	Thigh lift, revisions
IV	Thighs and arms	N/A
V	Arms and thighs	N/A
VI	Face	N/A

- The ASPS/ASAPS Joint Post-Bariatric Task Force provided an extensive review of body contouring after massive weight loss which details the preoperative, perioperative, and postoperative care of this unique patient population.[52]
- Consensus recommendations based on a recent review of the literature are summarized in Box 9-2.

Box 9-2 *CONSENSUS GUIDELINES*

- Weight loss is complete and stable prior to surgery.
- Preoperative smoking cessation is strongly recommended.
- Venous thromboembolism prophylaxis is initiated preoperatively and postoperatively.
- Chemoprophylaxis should be considered in addition to mechanical prophylaxis. The first dose of unfractionated or low-molecular-weight heparin should be administered within 12 hours of surgery.
- Nutritional status is assessed based on patient history and laboratory tests to detect anemia and protein malnutrition.
- Body contouring procedures should only be performed at accredited surgical facilities.
- Intraoperative hypothermia is prevented with forced-air warming blankets, warming intravenous or injectable fluid, or raised room temperature.
- Patient safety is ensured with positioning and prevention of compression injuries. When prone, the patient should be placed in 15-degree reverse Trendelenburg position to decrease intraocular pressure.

SURGICAL SITE INFECTIONS

- When proper measures are employed, up to 60% of SSIs can be prevented.[56,57]

SOURCES OF WOUND CONTAMINATION
Endogenous (i.e., the patient's own skin)[58]

- It is impossible to sterilize the skin.
- 20% skin flora resides in skin appendages: Sebaceous glands, hair follicles, sweat glands.
- The patient's own skin is direct source of contamination in only 2% of cases.
- Experiments using albumin microspheres as tracers reveal 100% of surgical wounds are contaminated with particles from sites remote to the surgical wound.

Exogenous[58]

- OR personnel (poor hand hygiene, loose surgical masks, staphylococcus carriers, poor sterile technique)
- Analysis of 655 cases revealed that **31%** of surgical gloves had a perforation by the end of the case.
- Double gloving reduces perforation of the inner glove and reduces risk of contamination.

PREVENTION OF SURGICAL SITE INFECTIONS
Sterile Technique[59]

- The introduction of computers, tablets, radios, and cell phones into the OR creates unnecessary sources of contamination. Among these devices, 44%-98% carry resistant microorganisms (gram-negative rods and *Staphylococcus aureus*).

- Do not wear scrub attire outside the OR.
- Minimize traffic in and out of the OR.
- The number of people in the OR should be limited to five or six.

PREPARATION OF THE SURGICAL TABLE[60]
- Surgical table preparation should be coordinated with draping, which is the step with the greatest risk of contamination.
- Placing the patient on the OR table, prepping, and draping results in a fourfold increase in airborne contamination.
- Containers and instruments should be covered when not in use.
- The duration of instrument tray opening correlates directly with the contamination rate (4% after 30 minutes, 15% after 1 hour, and 30% after 4 hours).

PATIENT-RELATED RISK FACTORS[61]
- Age
- Diabetes/glucose control
  - Several studies have determined that hyperglycemia before and after surgery (in diabetics and nondiabetics) is associated with a **threefold to fourfold** increase in SSI.
  - More specifically, a preoperative or postoperative serum glucose level **>125 mg/dl** produced a **4.7-fold** increased risk of SSI.
- Obesity (BMI >30)
- Smoking
- Immunosuppressive medications
- Nutrition
- Remote sites of infection
- Preoperative hospitalization

PROCEDURE-RELATED RISK FACTORS
- Preparation of patient
- Hair removal: Shaving increases the risk of infection 2.4-fold[62]
- Skin preparation
- OR staff/surgeon hand hygiene[63]
  - Rubbing hands and forearms with 75% aqueous alcohol is as effective as scrubbing with 4% povidine or 4% chlorhexidine.
- OR staff/surgeon gloving[64]
  - In an analysis of 655 operations, perforations were found in **31%** of gloves.
  - Glove perforations raises the risk of SSI **(OR = 2.0).**
  - Double gloving is associated with less perforation of the inner glove **(OR = 0.10).**
- Antimicrobial prophylaxis
- Hypothermia
- Oxygenation

ANTIBIOTIC PROPHYLAXIS
What Cases Need Prophylactic Antibiotics
- Contaminated cases
- Clean contaminated cases where the aerodigestive track is entered
- Cases that involve an implant
- Breast surgery, because the ducts contain bacteria
- For other clean cases, the evidence does not support using prophylactic antibiotics.

Timing of Prophylactic Antibiotics[65,66]

- The timing of antibiotic administration should be adjusted to maximize prophylactic efficacy.
- Therefore prophylactic antibiotics should be administered within **1 hour (30-60 minutes)** of incision.
- Prophylactic antibiotics (with the exception of vancomycin, aminoglycosides, and fluroquinolones) should be readministered during prolonged procedures or EBL of 1500 ml or greater.
- **Relationship to SSI rates revisited**
  - European data[65] (Table 9-7)
    - ▶ 3385 patients followed prospectively
    - ▶ Cefuroxime administered
    - ▶ Baseline infection rate 4.7%
  - U.S. data[66] (Table 9-8)

Table 9-7   *Relationship to SSI Rates: European Data*

Time Administered	RR	OR	p Value
<30 minutes before incision	2.0	2.0	0.02
30-59 minutes before incision	1.0	1.0	*
60-120 minutes before incision	1.8	1.7	0.05

*No p value is listed for antibiotic infusion times from 59-30 minutes before incision because that timing had the lowest risk of SSI and therefore serves as the reference or standard to which all other infusion times are compared.
OR, Odds ratio; *RR,* relative risk.

Table 9-8   *Relationship to SSI Rates: U.S. Data*

Time Administered	RR	OR (95% CI)	p Value
>120 minutes before incision or no prophylaxis	2.54	2.11 (0.68, 6.59)	0.07
61-120 minutes before incision	1.49	1.25 (0.74, 3.00)	0.26
31-60 minutes before incision	1.48	1.74 (0.98, 3.08)	0.13
1-30 minutes before incision	1.0	1.0	*
1-30 minutes after incision	2.44	1.96 (0.65, 5.95)	0.09
>31 minutes after incision	4.12	4.18 (1.37, 12.75)	0.02

*No p value is listed for antibiotic infusion times from 0-30 minutes before incision because that timing had the lowest risk of SSI and therefore serves as the reference or standard to which all other infusion times are compared.
CI, Confidence interval; *OR,* odds ratio; *RR,* relative risk.

SPECIAL CONSIDERATIONS IN SURGICAL SITE INFECTIONS

STAPHYLOCOCCUS COLONIZED PATIENTS
Potential Carriers[67]
- Athletes
- Military personnel
- Men having sex with men
- Prison inmates
- IV drug users
- Homeless persons
- Recent hospitalization
- Recent course of antibiotics

Decolonization[58,68]
- One third of the population carries staphylococcal organisms all the time; one third, part of the time; and one third, never.
- Studies examining preoperative decolonization have been inconclusive.
- Known carriers and high-risk individuals can be decolonized with mupirocin and chlorhexidine showers.

Preoperative Skin Decolonization[69,70,71]
- Showering with chlorhexidine the evening before and the morning of surgery decreases skin colonization.
- Wiping the operative area with 2% chlorhexidine-impregnated cloths is more effective than showering.
- Showering with chlorhexidine has not been shown to prevent SSI.

Dental Procedures[72]
- Patients with breast implants do not need prophylactic antibiotics for dental procedures.

Surgical Drains[73,74]
- Bacterial colonization of the drain is an independent predictor of SSI. Of patients developing an infection, 83% were of the same bacterial species documented in the drainage fluid.
- The probability of bacterial colonization of the drain rose from 33% to 80.8% between postoperative days 7 and 14.
- Despite this, drain-associated infection rates seem low and do not appear to be related to duration of use.
- *Current literature does not provide any evidence that postoperative systemic antibiotics can lower the incidence of SSI associated with drains.*
- Aggressive management of the drain insertion site with a chlorhexidine disc and irrigation of the drain bulb with Dakin solution may be more effective than systemic antibiotics for prevention of drain-associated SSI.

SENIOR AUTHOR TIP: Patient Safety Dos and Dont's for Plastic Surgeons[56]

Do:

Consider not giving prophylactic antibiotics for clean cases that do not involve an implant or the breast.

A first-generation cephalosporin (cefazolin) should be the antibiotic of first choice for prophylaxis.

For beta-lactam allergic patients clindamycin is a better choice than vancomycin for prophylaxis.

For optimum effectiveness cefazolin must be administered 30-60 minutes before the incision is made. Any other time results in a greater risk of SSI.

Cefazolin should be redosed for cases lasting longer than 3 hours or if there is an estimated blood loss 1500 ml or greater.

Use vancomycin for prophylaxis only when absolutely necessary (MRSA) carrier.

Consider not giving prophylactic antibiotics after wound closure in clean cases.

Double glove and practice good hand hygiene.

Maintain normothermia (>36° C).

Have patients stop smoking for a minimum of 4 weeks before and after surgery (confirm with a cotinine test).

Maintain tight glucose control in diabetics HbA1C <7, and glucose <200 mg/dl.

Have patients shower with chlorhexidine the morning of surgery.

Require patients to remove artificial nails before surgery.

Consider giving supplemental oxygen (FiO$_2$ of 80%)

Maintain normovolemia.

Develop and maintain a collaborative environment where staff are encouraged to voice concerns when they feel something is not right.

Stay focused: Double tasking and distractions lead to errors.

Don't:

Never use broad-spectrum antibiotics for prophylaxis.

Do not shave to remove hair at the incision site.

Have patients stop shaving for hair removal 2 weeks before and after surgery.

Drains and implants do not justify prolonged antibiotics.

Never operate on patients with infections at remote sites.

Don't give antibiotics to implant patients for dental procedures.

Don't bring unnecessary items such as brief cases and back packs into the operating room.

Top Takeaways

➤ Develop a system of quality of care with continual evaluation focused on improving patient care/safety.

➤ A first-generation Cephalosporin (Cefazolin) should be the antibiotic of first choice for prophylaxis.

➤ Consider not giving prophylactic antibiotics after wound closure.

➤ Have patients stop smoking for a minimum of 4 weeks before and after surgery.

References

1. Hippocrates, ed. Epidemics, Bk. I, (translated by WS Jones). London: William Heinemann, 1923.

2. Byrd HS, Barton FE, Orenstein HH, et al. Safety and efficacy in an accredited outpatient plastic surgery facility: a review of 5316 consecutive cases. Plast Reconstr Surg 112:636, 2003.

3. Keyes GR, Singer R, Iverson RE, et al. Analysis of outpatient surgery center safety using an internet-based quality improvement and peer review program. Plast Reconstr Surg 113:1760, 2004.

4. Hoefflin SM, Bornstein JB, Gordon M. General anesthesia in an office-based plastic surgical facility: a report on more than 23,000 consecutive office-based procedures under general anesthesia with no significant anesthetic complications. Plast Reconstr Surg 107:243, 2001.

5. Bitar GB, Mullis W, Jacobs W, et al. Safety and efficacy of office-based surgery with monitored anesthesia care/sedation in 4778 consecutive plastic surgery procedures. Plast Reconstr Surg 111:150, 2003.

6. Morello DC, Colon G, Fredricks S, et al. Patient safety in accredited office surgical facilities. Plast Reconstr Surg 99:1496, 1997.

7. Horton JB, Janis JE, Rohrich RJ. MOCS-PS CME article: patient safety in the office-based setting. Plast Reconstr Surg 122:1, 2008.

8. Rohrich RJ. Patient safety first in plastic surgery. Plast Reconstr Surg 114:201, 2004.

9. Iverson RE; ASPS Task Force on Patient Safety in Office-Based Surgery Facilities. Patient safety in office-based surgery facilities: I. Procedures in the office-based surgery setting. Plast Reconstr Surg 110:1337, 2002.

10. Iverson RE, Lynch DJ; ASPS Task Force on Patient Safety in Office-Based Surgery Facilities. Patient safety in office-based surgery facilities: II. Patient selection. Plast Reconstr Surg 110:1785, 2002.

11. Young VL, Watson ME. Prevention of postoperative hypothermia in plastic surgery. Aesthet Surg J 26:551, 2006.

12. Sessler, DI. Complications and treatment of mild hypothermia. Anesthesiology 95:531, 2001.

13. Fortier J, Chung F, Su J. Unanticipated admission after ambulatory surgery: a prospective study. Can J Anaesth 45:612, 1998.

14. Mingus ML, Bodian CA, Bradford CN, et al. Prolonged surgery increases the likelihood of admission of scheduled ambulatory surgery patients. J Clin Anesth 9:446, 1997.

15. Iverson RE, Lynch DJ. Practice advisory on pain management and prevention of postoperative nausea and vomiting. Plast Reconstr Surg 118:1060, 2006.

16. McGrath B, Elgendy H, Chung F, et al. Thirty percent of patients have moderate to severe pain 24 hr after ambulatory surgery: a survey of 5,703 patients. Can J Anaesth 51:886, 2004.

17. Watcha MF. Postoperative nausea and emesis. Anesthesiol Clin North Am 20:709, 2002.

18. Kim SI, Han TH, Kil HY, et al. Prevention of postoperative nausea and vomiting by continuous infusion of subhypnotic propofol in female patients receiving intravenous patient-controlled analgesia. Br J Anaesth 85:898, 2000.

19. Habib AS, Gan TJ. Evidence-based management of postoperative nausea and vomiting: a review. Can J Anaesth 51:326, 2004.

20. White PF, O'Hara JF, Roberson CR, et al; POST-OP Study Group. The impact of current antiemetic practices on patient outcomes: a prospective study on high-risk patients. Anesth Analg 107:452, 2008.

21. Buck DW, Mustoe TA, Kim JY. Postoperative nausea and vomiting in plastic surgery. Semin Plast Surg 20:249, 2006.

22. American Society for Aesthetic Plastic Surgery. 2016 Cosmetic surgery national data bank statistics. Available at http://www.surgery.org.

23. Fodor PB. Wetting solutions in ultrasound-assisted lipoplasty. Clin Plast Surg 26:289, 1999.

24. Iverson RE, Lynch DJ; American Society of Plastic Surgeons Committee on Patient Safety. Practice advisory on liposuction. Plast Reconstr Surg 113:1478, 2004.

25. Iverson RE, Pao VS. MOCS-PS CME article: liposuction. Plast Reconstr Surg 121:1, 2008.

26. Grazer FM, DeJong R. Fatal outcomes from liposuction: census survey of cosmetic surgeons. Plast Reconstr Surg 105:436, 2000.

27. Hughes CE III. Reduction of lipoplasty risks and mortality: an ASAPS survey. Aesthet Surg J 21:120, 2001.

28. Clayman MA, Seagle BM. Office surgery safety: the myths and truths behind the Florida Moratoria—six years of Florida data. Plast Reconstr Surg 118:777, 2006.

29. Balakrishnan R, Gill IK, Vallee JA, et al. No smoking gun: findings from a national survey of office-based cosmetic surgery adverse event reporting. Dermatol Surg 29:1093, 2003.

30. Kryger ZB, Dumanian GA, Howard MA. Safety issues in combined gynecologic and plastic surgical procedures. Int J Gynaecol Obstet 99:257, 2007.

31. Hester TR, Baird W, Bostwick J, et al. Abdominoplasty combined with other major surgical procedures: safe or sorry. Plast Reconstr Surg 86:997, 1989.

32. Stevens WG, Cohen R, Vath SD, et al. Is it safe to combine abdominoplasty with elective breast surgery? A review of 151 consecutive cases. Plast Reconstr Surg 118:207, 2006.

33. Melendez MM, Beasley M, Dagum AB, et al. Outcomes of abdominoplasty performed in an office based surgical setting. Plast Reconstr Surg 122(Suppl abstract):128, 2008.

34. Spiegelman JI, Levine RH. Abdominoplasty: a comparison of outpatient and inpatient procedures shows that it is a safe and effective procedure for outpatients in an office-based surgery clinic. Plast Reconstr Surg 118:517; discussion 523, 2006.

35. Kim J, Stevenson TR. Abdominoplasty, liposuction of the flanks, and obesity: analyzing risk factors for seroma formation. Plast Reconstr Surg 117:773; discussion 780, 2006.

36. Gordon NA, Koch ME. Duration of anesthesia as an indicator of morbidity and mortality in office-based facial plastic surgery: a review of 1200 consecutive cases. Arch Facial Plast Surg 8:47, 2006.

37. Rohrich RJ, Rios JL. Venous thromboembolism in cosmetic plastic surgery: maximizing patient safety. Plast Reconstr Surg 112:871, 2003.

38. Hirsh J, Lee AY. How we diagnose and treat deep vein thrombosis. Blood 99:3102, 2002.

39. Silverstein MD, Heit JA, Mohr DN, et al. Trends in the incidence of deep vein thrombosis and pulmonary embolism: a 25-year population-based study. Arch Intern Med 158:585, 1998.

40. Young VL, Watson ME. The need for venous thromboembolism (VTE) prophylaxis in plastic surgery. Aesthet Surg J 26:157, 2006.

41. McDevitt NB. Deep vein thrombosis prophylaxis. Plast Reconstr Surg 104:1923, 1999.

42. Seruya M, Baker SB. MOC-PS CME article: venous thromboembolism prophylaxis in plastic surgery patients. Plast Reconstr Surg 122:1, 2008.

43. Davison SP, Venturi ML, Attinger CE, et al. Prevention of venous thromboembolism in the plastic surgery patient. Plast Reconstr Surg 114:43e, 2004.

44. Canonico M, Plu-Bureau G, Lowe GD, et al. Hormone replacement therapy and risk of venous thromboembolism in postmenopausal women: systematic review and meta-analysis. BMJ 336:1227, 2008.
45. Grazer FM, Goldwyn RM. Abdominoplasty assessed by survey, with emphasis on complications. Plast Reconstr Surg 59:513, 1977.
46. Voss SC, Sharp HC, Scott JR. Abdominoplasty combined with gynecologic surgical procedures. Obstet Gynecol 67:181, 1986.
47. Hatef DA, Kenkel JM, Nguyen MQ, et al. Thromboembolic risk assessment and the efficacy of enoxaparin prophylaxis in excisional body contouring surgery. Plast Reconstr Surg 122:269, 2008.
48. Aly AS, Cram AE, Chao M, et al. Belt lipectomy for circumferential truncal excess: the University of Iowa experience. Plast Reconstr Surg 111:398, 2003.
49. American Society for Bariatric and Metabolic Surgery. Estimate of bariatric surgery numbers, 2011-2015. Available at https://asmbs.org/resources/estimate-of-bariatric-surgery-numbers.
50. Rhode BM, Maclean LD. Vitamin and mineral supplementation after gastric bypass. In Deitel M, Cowan GM Jr, eds. Update: Surgery for the Morbidly Obese Patient: The Field of Extreme Obesity Including Laparoscopy and Allied Care. Toronto, Ontario: FD Communications, 2000.
51. Brolin RE, Gorman JH, Gorman RC, et al. Are vitamin B12 and folate deficiency clinically important after roux-en-Y gastric bypass? J Gastrointest Surg 2:436, 1998.
52. Rohrich RJ. Body contouring surgery after massive weight loss. Plast Reconstr Surg 117:S1, 2006.
53. Arthurs ZM, Caudardo D, Sohn V, et al. Post-bariatric panniculectomy: pre-panniculectomy body mass index impacts the complication profile. Am J Surg 193:567, 2007.
54. Nemerofsky RB, Oliak DA, Capella JF. Body lift: an account of 200 consecutive cases in the massive weight loss patient. Plast Reconstr Surg 117:414, 2006.
55. Shermak MA, Chang D, Heller J. Factors affecting thromboembolism after bariatric body contouring surgery. Plast Reconstr Surg 119:1590, 2007.
56. Mangram AJ, Horan TC, Pearson ML, et al. Guideline for prevention of surgical site infection, 1999. Centers of Disease Control and Prevention (CDC) Hospital Control Practices Advisory Committee. Am J Infect Control 2:97; discussion 96, 1999.
57. Page CP, Bohnen JM, Fletcher JR, et al. Antimicrobial prophylaxis for surgical wounds. Guidelines for clinical care. Arch Surg 128:79, 1993.
58. Anderson DJ. Surgical site infections. Infect Dis Clin North Am 25:135, 2011.
59. Richard RD, Bowen TR. What orthopaedic operating room surfaces are contaminated with bioburden? A study using the ATP bioluminescence assay. Clin Orthop Relat Res 475:1819, 2017.
60. Dalstrom DJ, Venkatarayappa I, Manternach AL, et al. Time-dependent contamination of sterile operating-room trays. J Bone Joint Surg Am 90:1022, 2008.
61. Olsen Ma, Nepple JJ, Riew KD, et al. Risk factors for surgical site infection following orthopaedic spinal operations. J Bone Joint Surg Am 90:62, 2008.
62. Seropian R, Reynolds BM. Wound infections after preoperative depilatory versus razor preparation. Am J Surg 121:251, 1971.
63. Humphreys H. Preventing surgical site infection. Where now? J Hosp Infect 73:316, 2009.
64. Alexander JW, Solomkin JS, Edwards MJ. Updated recommendations for control of surgical site infections. Ann Surg 253:1082, 2011.
65. Weber WP, Mujagic E, Zwahlen M, et al. The timing of surgical antimicrobial prophylaxis. Ann Surg 247:918, 2008.
66. Steinberg JP, Braun BI, Hellinger WC, et al; Trial to Reduce Antimicrobial Prophylaxis Errors (TRAPE) Study Group. Timing of antimicrobial prophylaxis and the risk of surgical site infections: results from the Trial to Reduce Antimicrobial Prophylaxis Errors. Ann Surg 250:10, 2009.

67. Gould IM. Antibiotics, skin and soft tissue infection and methicillin-resistant Staphylococcus aureus: cause and effect. Int J Antimicrob Agents 34:S8, 2009.
68. Bode LG, Kluytmans JA, Wertheim HF, et al. Preventing surgical-site infections in nasal carriers of Staphylococcus aureus. N Engl J Med 362:9, 2010.
69. Webster J, Osborne S. Preoperative bathing or showering with skin antiseptics to prevent surgical site infection. Cochrane Database Syst Rev 2:CD004985, 2015.
70. Atiyeh BS, Dibo SA, Hayek SN. Wound cleansing, topical antiseptics and wound healing. Int Wound J 6:420, 2009.
71. Viega DF, Damasceno CA, Veiga-Filho J, et al. Randomized controlled trial of the effectiveness of chlorhexidine showers before elective plastic surgical procedures. Infect Control Hops Epidemiol 30:77, 2009.
72. Little JW, Falace DA, Miller CS, et al. Antibiotic prophylaxis in dentistry: an update. Gen Dent 56:20, 2008.
73. Chim JH, Borsting EA, Thaller SR. Urban myths in plastic surgery: postoperative management of surgical drains. Wounds 28:35, 2016.
74. Phillips BT, Wang ED, Mirrer J, et al. Current practice among plastic surgeons of antibiotic prophylaxis and closed-suction drains in breast reconstruction: experience, evidence, and implications for postoperative care. Ann Plast Surg 66:460, 2011.

10. Decreasing Complications in Aesthetic Surgery

Edward H. Davidson, Zoe Diana Draelos, Bridget Harrison, Ibrahim Khansa, Jeffrey E. Janis

- Successful outcomes in aesthetic surgery and nonoperative cosmetic procedures demand meticulous preparation and aftercare to ensure optimal results and minimize risk of complications.
- Preparation and aftercare regimens are commonly procedure, technique, and practitioner dependent, but general principles and considerations may be applied.
- Involving patients in their own management before and after cosmetic interventions promotes understanding, empowers them to invest in their own results, and may help to manage expectations.

PREOPERATIVE MEASURES TO REDUCE COMPLICATIONS

COMORBIDITIES
- Elective aesthetic surgery patients are usually healthy. The presence of chronic disease (including diabetes, hypertension, coronary heart disease, chronic obstructive pulmonary disease, hepatic or renal dysfunction, cancer) necessitates **preoperative medical clearance** by the patient's primary care physician or specialist.
  - **Diabetes:** Poor glycemic control places diabetic patients at increased risk of surgical site infection and delayed wound healing.[1,2]
  - **Hypertension:** Uncontrolled hypertension increases risk of bleeding and hematoma in all aesthetic procedures, and visual loss after blepharoplasty.[3]
  - **Coagulopathy:** Hematologic consultation should be considered for patients with history of coagulopathy or venous thromboembolism (VTE).
  - Most elective plastic surgery procedures performed in the United States are performed on white females. Factor V Leiden gene is found as a heterozygous mutation in **3%-7% of white females** and results in a **sixfold increase in the risk of VTE.**
  - VTE risk is increased if combined with cancer, travel, immobilization, use of oral contraceptives, hormone replacement therapy, and estrogen receptor antagonists.
- In low-risk ambulatory plastic surgery patients, preoperative laboratory testing is costly, associated with limited clinical benefit, and may be eliminated with significant cost savings.[4]
- **Mental health:** A patient's mental health should be preoperatively assessed and appropriately addressed before proceeding with any elective procedure.[5] Patients with mental health conditions—whether psychiatric disorders, such as body dysmorphic disorder or substance abuse diagnoses—who undergo outpatient aesthetic surgery seek hospital-based acute care within 30 days postoperatively **three times more often than patients without a mental health condition** (see Chapter 1).
- **Medications:** Every patient's medications must be carefully reviewed. Table 10-1, although not exhaustive, lists medications associated with postoperative complications and/or interference with some anesthesia and may require discontinuation or special precautions.

143

Table 10-1   *Medications Requiring Discontinuation or Special Precautions*

Medications That Should Not Be Taken the Day of Surgery

Acarbose	DIOVAN	Insulin (LONG	MONOPRIL
ACCUPRIL	DIURIL	ACTING–LANTUS,	Nateglinide
ACTOPLUS MET	DUETACT	LEVEMIR, insulin	NOVOLIN R
ACTOS	EDECRIN	detemir, insulin	NOVOLOG
ALDACTONE	Enalapril	glargine):	OSMITROL
ALTACE	ENDURON	Arrive at hospital	Perindopril
AMARYL	Eplerenone	before 10 AM: Hold	Pioglitazone
Amiloride	Exenatide	morning dose	Polythiazide
APIDRA	Fosinopril	Arrive at hospital	PRANDIN
ATACAND	FUROCOT	after 10 AM: Half	PRECOSE
AVANDAMET	FUROMIDE	of usual dose	PRINIVIL
AVANDARYL	Furosemide	insulin aspart,	PROBALAN
AVANDIA	Glimepiride	glulisine, lispro	Quinapril
AVAPRO	glipiZIDE	JANUMET	Ramipril
BENEMID	GLUCOPHAGE	JANUVIA	RENESE
BENICAR	GLUCOTROL	LASIX	Repaglinide
Benazepril	GLUMETZA	Lisinopril	Rosiglitazone
Bumetanide	glyBURIDE	LISPRO-PFC	Sitagliptin
BUMEX	GLYSET	Losartan	Spironolactone
BYETTA	HCTZ	LOTENSIN	STARLIX
CAPOTEN	HUMALOG	LOZOL	SYMLIN
Captopril	HUMULIN R	Mannitol	THALITONE
Chlorothiazide	Hydrocort	METAGLIP	TOLAZamide
chlorproPAMIDE	Indapamide	Methyclothiazide	TOLINASE
Chlorthalidone	INSPRA	Metformin	TOLBUTamide
COZAAR		Metolazone	Torsemide
DEMADEX		MICARDIS	Trandolapril
		MICROZIDE	Triamterene
		MIDAMOR	Valsartan
		Miglitol	VASOTEC
		Moexipril	

Medications That Should Be Stopped the Night Before Surgery

ANTARA	Fenofibrate	NIASPAN	QUESTRAN
APOKYN	FENOGLIDE	NICOMIDE-T	REQUIP
Apomorphine	Gemfibrozil	NICOTINEX	Ropinirole
Bromocriptine	LIPOFEN	OMACOR	Rotigotine
Cholestyramine	LOFIBRA	Omega-3-	Selegiline
Colesevelam	LOPID	acid ethyl esters	SLO-NIACIN
COLESTID	LOVAZA	Pergolide	TRICOR
Colestipol	NEUPRO	PERMAX	TRIGLIDE
ELDEPRYL	Niacinamide	Pramipexole	ZELAPAR
EMSAM	NIACINOL	PREVALITE	ZETIA
Ezetimibe	NIACOR		

Medications to Discuss With Doctor: Stop 1-2 Weeks Before Surgery

Abciximab	CORICIDIN	Hormone	ORGARAN
ACTRON	Cortisone	replacement	ORUDIS
ACULAR	COUMADIN	Hydrocortisone	ORUVAIL
ADVIL	Dalteparin	HUMIRA	Oxaprozin
AGGRENOX	Danaparoid	IBREN	PARNATE
ALEVE	DARVON	Ibuprofen	PLAVIX
ALKA-SELTZER	DASIN	INDOCIN	Phenelzine
AMIGESIC	DAYPRO	Indomethacin	Piroxicam
ANACIN	DECADRON	Infliximab	PONSTEL
Anakinra	Dexamethasone	INNOHEP	Prednisone
ANAPROX	Diclofenac	Isocarboxazid	PRESALIN
ANSAID	Diflunisal	JANTOVEN	PULMICORT
ANTURANE	Dipyridamole	Ketoprofen	Rasagiline
ARCALYST	DISALCID	Ketorolac	RELAFEN
ARGESIC	DOANS	KINERET	REMICADE
ARTHRA-G	DOLOBID	LANORINAL	REOPRO
ARTHROPAN	ECOTRIN	Leflunomide	RHINOCORT
ASCRIPTIN	EFFICIN	LODINE	SALATIN
ASPER-BUFF	EMPIRIN	LOVENOX	SALSALATE
ASPERCIN	ENBREL	MAGAN	Selective estrogen
ASPERGUM	ENCAPRIN	MARNAL	receptor modulators
ASPIRTAB	Enoxaparin	MARPLAN	SOLUMEDROL
ASPIR-TRIN	Ephedra	MEDROL	Sulindac
ASPROJECT	Eptifibatide	Meloxicam	TICLID
Astropan	EQUAGESIC	Methotrexate	Ticlopidine
AZILECT	Etanercept	methylPREDNISolone	Tinzaparin
BAYER	Etodolac	MIDOL	Tirofiban
Betamethasone	EXCEDRIN	MOBIC	TOLECTIN
BUFF A	FELDENE	MOMENTUM	Tolmetin
BUFFAPRIN	Fenoprofen	MOTRIN	TORADOL
BUFFERIN	FIORINAL	Nabumetone	Triamcinolone
BUFFETTS	FLECTOR	NALFON	TRIGESIC
BUFFEX	Fludrocortisones	NAPRELAN	Unfractionated
CAMA	Flurbiprofen	NAPROSYN	Heparin
CELEBREX	FRAGMIN	Naproxen	Valerian
Celecoxib	Gamma-	NARDIL	VANQUISH
Cilostazol	butyrolactone/	NASACORT	VOLTAREN
CLINORIL	gamma-	NEOPROFEN	Warfarin
Clopidogrel	hydroxybutyric acid	Oral contraceptives	ZORPRIN
COPE	(GBL/GHB)		

SUPPLEMENTS[6,7] (see Chapter 6)

- Use of herbal medicines and supplements is more prevalent in the cosmetic surgery population than in the population at large (49% versus 42%, respectively).[6]
- Nutritional supplements are not routinely recommended in lieu of a healthy, well-balanced diet.
- **60%-72%** of patients do not report use of supplements.[7]
- Many herbal medicines and supplements are cited for adverse reactions and should not be taken for 2-3 weeks before and after surgery[8] (Box 10-1), according to the American Society of Anesthesiologists.

Box 10-1 *HERBS AND SUPPLEMENTS TO AVOID TWO TO THREE WEEKS BEFORE AND AFTER SURGERY*

Bilberry	Green tea
Cayenne	Guarana
Chondroitin* (postoperative bleeding)	Hawthorne
Dong quai	Kava kava* (postoperative sedation)
Echinacea* (potentiates barbiturate and halothane toxicity, allergic reaction, immunosuppression)	Licorice root
	Ma huang
	Meadowsweet
Ephedra* (hypertension and cardiac instability)	Melatonin
	Milk thistle* (volume depletion)
Feverfew	Niacin
Fish oil	Red clover
Garlic* (perioperative bleeding)	Saw palmetto
Ginko* (postoperative sedation, perioperative bleeding)	St. John's wort
	Turmeric
Ginger	Valerian
Ginseng* (perioperative bleeding)	Vitamin E
Glucosamine* (hypoglycemia)	Yohimbe
Goldenseal* (volume depletion, postoperative sedation, photosensitization)	White willow

*Top ten herbal and supplemental medications used by cosmetic patients.[8]

Bromelain
- Pineapple extract
- Reported to reduce pain, edema, inflammation, bruising, and platelet aggregation and to potentiate antibiotics
- 500-1500 mg/day taken in divided doses 1-2 weeks preoperatively and postoperatively
- More randomized, controlled clinical trials necessary to determine its clinical potential[9]

Arnica
- Reported to reduce ecchymosis and edema postoperatively; contradictory evidence[10]
- May be equivalent to steroids in reducing postrhinoplasty edema when used postoperatively[11]

Vitamin A

■ Impairment of wound healing caused by use of corticosteroids can be reversed by the oral administration of vitamin A (retinoic acid), use 15,000 IU daily for 7 days; however, this is not common surgical practice.[12]

Vitamin B

■ Patients with true deficiencies of vitamin B_6 (pyridoxine), vitamin B_1 (thiamine), or vitamin B_2 (riboflavin) may have wound-healing problems and benefit from supplementation.[13]
■ Vitamin B–deficient patients may have other nutritional deficiencies and may be poor surgical risks.

Vitamin C

■ Vitamin C deficiency (scurvy) results in **inability to cross-link collagen fibers** and **decreased wound tensile strength,** which may be reversed by vitamin C supplementation.[14]
■ Vitamin C deficiency is extremely rare and is an indicator of otherwise poor health and poor surgical candidates.

SURGEON-PATIENT COMMUNICATION

■ Patient satisfaction is highly dependent on the initial consultation. This interaction not only affects the patient's impression of the physician, but can also influence satisfaction with surgical and overall outcomes.[15]
■ Behaviors that lead patients to not recommend surgeons to friends and family members include failure to adequately explain medical condition, failure to show interest in the patient, failure to ask if the patient has questions, and failure to answer questions.[16]

LIFESTYLE MODULATION

■ There are relative and absolute contraindications for office-based aesthetic surgery that need to be addressed with the patient before the procedure (Box 10-2).

Box 10-2 *RELATIVE AND ABSOLUTE CONTRAINDICATIONS FOR OFFICE-BASED AESTHETIC SURGERY*

Patient-Related Factors	
Poorly controlled systemic disease	History of end-stage renal failure, undergoing dialysis
Moderate to severe obstructive sleep apnea	Sickle cell disease
Morbid obesity	Myasthenia gravis
Myocardial infarction in last 6 months	Younger than 3 years old
Cerebral vascular accident in last 3 months	
Lack of an adult escort	**Procedure-Related Factors**
Implantable defibrillator or pacemaker	Liposuction >5,000 ml
Unstable psychological disease	Tumescent solution >5,000 ml
Acute substance abuse	High-volume liposuction with second procedure
History of malignant hyperthermia (if use of triggering agent planned)	Multiple procedures with abdominoplasty
	Anticipated blood loss >500 ml in adults
	Surgical duration >6 hours

Smoking
- Cigarette smoking has a well-established negative effect on the wound-healing process, resulting in tissue hypoxia and ischemia.[17]
- A common recommendation is a 4-week period of no smoking both before and after surgery.[18]
- Pharmacologic (nicotine replacement, bupropion) and nonpharmacologic (counseling, behavioral therapy, hypnosis, psychotherapy, electrical stimulation) smoking cessation strategies should be considered.
- If noncompliance is suspected, a urine cotinine (a nicotine metabolite) test is recommended preoperatively.[19,20]
- Alternatively, a blood test can measure multiple nicotine metabolites (cotinine, anabasine, nornicotine) to give a clearer picture of active smoking, passive smoke inhalation, and use of nicotine replacement therapies.

> **TIP:** A urine cotinine test is a simple and inexpensive measure to determine whether a patient has smoked within the last 4 days.

Alcohol
- Potentially alcohol-induced disorders of the liver, pancreas, and nervous system
- Heavy drinking also affects cardiac function, immune capacity, hemostasis, and metabolic stress response, and induces muscular dysfunction.
- May be associated with other nutritional deficiencies previously discussed
- Dose-response relationship between alcohol intake and an increase in postoperative morbidity
  - Complication rate is about **50% higher** in patients who drink **3-4 drinks per day** compared with 0-2 per day.[21]
- Recommend decreasing and even abstaining from alcohol 1-2 weeks preoperatively and postoperatively to decrease risk of perioperative bleeding.[22]

Diet
- The following foods may potentiate bleeding, and some physicians advise decreased intake 1-2 weeks before and after surgery (Box 10-3).

Box 10-3   *FOODS THAT MAY POTENTIATE BLEEDING*

Avocados	Fish (especially	Onions	Root beer
Apples	salmon)	Oranges	Shellfish
Apricots	Garlic	Peaches	Soybeans
Blackberries	Gooseberries	Peppers	Spicy foods
Cherries	Grapefruit	Plums	Strawberries
Cucumbers	Grapes	Potatoes	Sunflower seeds
Currants	Lemons	Prunes	Sweet potatoes
Dewberries	Melons	Raisins	Tomatoes
	Nectarines	Raspberries	Wheat germ oil

DECOLONIZATION AND SKIN ANTISEPSIS

- Surgical site infection can be a devastating complication of aesthetic surgery, especially when implanting a prosthetic material (e.g., breast augmentation).
- *Staphylococcus aureus* is the leading cause of surgical site infection, and the prevalence of methicillin-resistant *S. aureus* (MRSA) surgical site infection is increasing.
- Presurgical decolonization and skin antisepsis have been demonstrated to decrease surgical site infections drastically, particularly in cardiac and orthopedic surgery implant-based procedures, and support is emerging for similar practice in plastic surgery.[23-25]
- **Decolonization and skin antisepsis protocol:**
  - Two to 4 weeks before surgery, patients who may have an increased likelihood of MRSA infection (e.g., history of infection, health care worker, immunocompromised) are screened for *S. aureus* nasal carriage as outpatient procedures, with samples collected from both nares on a single swab. (The association with nasal carriage of *S. aureus* and subsequent infection is well established.[26,27])
  - Patients with nasal cultures positive for *S. aureus* are instructed to apply 2% mupirocin nasal ointment twice daily to both nares and to bathe with chlorhexidine (40 mg/ml Hibiscrub) daily for 5 days immediately before the scheduled surgery.
  - **Perioperative antibiotic prophylaxis:** Patients with a history of MRSA infection or type I allergy to penicillin and patients who are MRSA carriers receive vancomycin 1 g 60 minutes before surgery; all others receive cefazolin 2 g 30-59 minutes before surgery.[2]

DVT RISK ASSESSMENT (see Chapter 11)

- The **2005 Caprini Risk Assessment Model** stratifies patients by risk and guides prophylaxis decisions. Patients at **high risk (score >8)** should be considered for postoperative chemoprophylaxis.[28]
- Overall, postoperative enoxaparin does not increase rates of reoperative hematoma.[12]

INTRAOPERATIVE MEASURES TO REDUCE COMPLICATIONS

■ The World Health Organization has developed a guideline of items to prevent mortality and postoperative complications. These include three phases (sign in, time out, and sign out) (Box 10-4).

Box 10-4 *ELEMENTS OF THE SURGICAL SAFETY CHECKLIST*

Phase 1: Sign In

Before anesthesia, team members verbally note or confirm the following:
• Patient has verified his or her identity, verified the surgical site, verified the procedure, and given consent.
• Surgical site has been marked (if applicable).
• The pulse oximeter is attached to the patient and functioning.
• Team members are aware of patient allergies (if applicable).
• Airway and risk of aspiration have been assessed; appropriate equipment and assistance are available.
• Adequate access and fluids are available if blood loss is anticipated and expected to be more than 500 ml (or 7 ml/kg of body weight for children).

Phase 2: Time Out

Before incision, team members verbally note or confirm the following:
• All team members introduce themselves by name and role.
• Patient has verified his or her identity, verified the surgical site, verified the procedure, and given consent.
• A review of anticipated critical events is completed by team.
• Surgeon describes critical or nonroutine steps, expected duration of the procedure, and anticipated blood loss.
• Anesthesia team reviews patient-specific concerns.
• Nursing team confirms sterility of instrumentation, availability of equipment, and any other anticipated concerns.
• Antibiotic prophylaxis is confirmed to have been administered 60 minutes prior to incision (if applicable).
• All essential imaging results are confirmed to be present, and for the correct patient.

Phase 3: Sign Out

Before the patient leaves the operating room, team members verbally note or confirm the following:
• Nursing team reviews all of the following with the entire team:
  – Name of the procedure performed
  – Confirmation of needle, sponge, and instrument counts (as applicable)
  – Labeling of all specimen with the patient's name
  – Any equipment issues that will need to be addressed
• Surgeon, anesthesia team, and nursing team all verbally note the key concerns for the patient's recovery and care.

- *Sign in* takes place before anesthesia induction and includes confirmation of the patient, procedure, surgical site, and approval. The correct site is marked, allergies are reviewed, and anesthesia risk is identified.
- *Time out* takes place after anesthesia induction and before surgical incision. All team members must participate and introduce themselves. Patient identity, operative site, procedure, and correct positioning are confirmed. Antibiotics and their timing are identified, and availability of images is confirmed.
- *Sign out* requires confirmation of the procedure performed, documentation of surgical counts, labeling of surgical specimens, and revision of any problems in the use of devices.
- **Implementation of this checklist decreased perioperative mortality from 1.5% before checklist introduction to 0.8% afterward among patients ≥16 years of age undergoing noncardiac surgery in a diverse group of hospitals.**[29]

ANTIBIOTIC ADMINISTRATION

- The optimal time for administration of preoperative antibiotics (i.e., first-generation cephalosporins) is within **30-59 minutes** before surgical incision.
- **Fluoroquinolones** and **vancomycin** require a longer period for administration and should begin **no less than 1 hour** before incision.
- **Ancef** dosing is 2 g or 3 g for patients weighing >120 kg and should be redosed **every 4 hours**.
- **Clindamycin** dosing is 900 mg and should be redosed **every 6 hours.**
- The Surgical Care Improvement Project has emphasized limiting postoperative antibiotics; however, withholding postoperative antibiotics in prosthetic breast reconstruction is associated with an increased risk of surgical site infection.[30]
- Postoperative antibiotic prophylaxis is not routinely indicated for septorhinoplasty.[31]

SURGICAL SITE PREP

- In a review of common skin prep agents, 2% chlorhexidine gluconate (CHG) and 4% CHG (Hibiclens) demonstrated inferior antimicrobial activity to isopropyl alcohol (IPA) (70%) or 2% CHG combined with IPA (ChloraPrep).[32]
- A Cochrane analysis also suggested **4% CHG with 70% IPA has the highest probability of being effective.**[33] Alcohol-based antiseptics are probably more effective than those with an aqueous base.

CAUTION: Alcohol-based antiseptics have been associated with surgical fires and should be allowed to dry before draping.

- ChloraPrep is superior to povidone-iodine for preoperative cleansing.

PATIENT POSITIONING

- Poor patient positioning can make any procedure more challenging and lead to poor results. It can also lead to patient morbidities such as pressure sores, peripheral nerve injury, and alopecia.
- **Vertebral artery dissection** after vigorous movement of the head and neck during surgery and after prone positioning has been reported.[34]

- Prone positioning places increased pressure on the knees, chest, and pubis. Gel rolls, pillows, or foam egg crates should be used. It can also result in increased ocular pressure, and padded goggles are recommended (Fig. 10-1).[35]

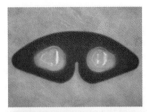

Fig. 10-1 Patient positioning.

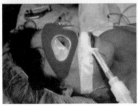
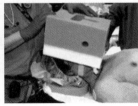

- A 1990 analysis of the American Society of Anesthesiologists Closed Claims Project database showed that 15% of claims were **for nerve injuries.** Padding and flexion of the arm and elbow to <90 degrees reduced the risk of nerve compression.[36]

STERILIZATION OF INSTRUMENTS ("FLASHING")
- Flash sterilization can be safe and effective for emergent need and immediate use of an instrument but can lead to **increased infection risks if done improperly.**
- *ANSI/AAMI ST79 Comprehensive Guide to Steam Sterilization and Sterility Assurance in Health Care Facilities*[37] asserts that immediate-use steam sterilization (flash sterilization) only be performed when instruments are properly cleaned and inspected before sterilization, delivered directly to their point of use, handled aseptically during transfer, and used immediately after flash sterilization.[38]

NORMOTHERMIA
- *Hypothermia* is defined as a core body temperature of **<36° C.**
- Anesthetic agents disrupt the body's natural thermoregulatory mechanisms and can inhibit shivering, vasoconstriction, and sweating.
- **Hypothermia** can result in **increased wound infections** by impairing immune defenses and decreasing local oxygen tension.
- Mild hypothermia may also affect coagulation, recovery time, and the rate of perioperative myocardial events.[39]
- Patient temperature can be maintained passively through blankets, surgical drapes, and humidified respiratory gasses. Active warming includes the use of radiant heat lamps, higher room temperatures, forced-air blankets, and fluid warmers (see Chapters 5 and 6).
- Standards of the Surgical Care Improvement Project require that patients have at least one documented temperature of ≥36° C within 30 minutes before or 15 minutes after the documented anesthesia end time.

SUTURE CHOICE

- Barbed sutures may expedite wound closure and decrease wound tension. The suture barbs may be unidirectional (V-Loc; Medtronic) or bidirectional (Quill; Angiotech Pharmaceuticals) (see Chapter 28).
- Barbed sutures are associated with higher rates of minor wound complications and may result in incision site erythema.[40] Foreign materials may be trapped by the suture barbs and induce an immune response. Consequently, **direct contact should be avoided with laparotomy pads or sterile drapes.**
- Despite decreased skin closure and anesthesia times with barbed sutures, current costs are six to seven times those of Vicryl or Biosyn and twice as much as Monocryl.

POSTOPERATIVE MEASURES TO DECREASE COMPLICATIONS

PAIN CONTROL

- Uncontrolled postoperative pain can delay recovery, result in unanticipated readmission, and decrease patient satisfaction.
- Liposomal bupivacaine has been used because of its prolonged analgesic benefit. It decreases postoperative pain in breast reduction and abdominoplasty, but additional product cost must be considered.
- Ketorolac is **not** associated with increased hematoma rates and is safe to use in aesthetic plastic surgery.[41]
- Single-dose oral celecoxib is effective for postoperative pain relief. It was effective in perioperative pain management after facelift surgery.[42]

VENOUS THROMBOEMBOLISM PROPHYLAXIS (see Chapter 11)

- The incidence rate of VTE in aesthetic surgery is **0.3%-1.2%.**[43]
- **Body contouring** seems to have the highest probability of VTE compared with other plastic surgery procedures, with a DVT incidence of 1.1% and pulmonary embolism (PE) incidence of 0.8 % in abdominoplasty patients.
  - **Massive-weight-loss patients** with circumferential body contouring operations are at even greater risk, with a **5.7%-9.6% incidence of VTE.**
- Every provider and institution should adopt a formal, active strategy designed to prevent VTE.
- **Primary prophylaxis** is the most useful and cost-effective strategy for reducing the risk of VTE.
- **Early ambulation** and **proper positioning** on the operating table are logical measures that should be applied to all patients undergoing surgery, regardless of their risk.
- Specific recommendations regarding mechanical and chemical prophylaxis in plastic surgery patients have not been validated to date, but Table 10-2 presents the latest recommendations.[44]

Table 10-2   *Venous Thromboembolism Prophylaxis*

Low Risk		
Healthy patients having outpatient surgery	General or regional anesthesia procedure lasting <1 hour or Sedation procedure <2 hours	Proper positioning and early ambulation
	General or regional anesthesia procedure lasting >1 hour or Sedation procedure >2 hours	Intermittent pneumatic compression or venous foot pumps
Moderate Risk		
Patients with 0-4 risk factors having surgery requiring admission and recovery in the hospital Abdominoplasty patients	Normal risk of bleeding and 3-4 risk factors	Enoxaparin 30 mg SQ daily and intermittent pneumatic compression or venous foot pumps First dose given 12 hours postoperatively
	High risk of bleeding or 0-2 risk factors*	Intermittent pneumatic compression or venous foot pumps
High Risk		
Patients with >4 risk factors having surgery requiring admission and recovery in the hospital Body contouring patients having other intraabdominal or pelvic procedures	Normal risk of bleeding	Enoxaparin 40 mg SQ daily and intermittent pneumatic compression or venous foot pumps First dose given 12 hours postoperatively
	High risk of bleeding*	Intermittent pneumatic compression or venous foot pumps

*Mechanical thromboprophylaxis should be switched to anticoagulant thromboprophylaxis when high bleeding risk decreases.

RISK FACTORS
- Major surgery
- Erythropoiesis-stimulating medications
- Venous insufficiency
- Central venous access
- Trauma
- Paroxysmal nocturnal hemoglobinuria
- Immobility of lower extremities
- Medications
- Cancer (excluding skin)
- Myeloproliferative disorders
- Cancer therapy (chemotherapy/radiotherapy)
- Obesity
- History or family history of VTE (higher in Leiden factor V carriers)
- Thrombophilia
- Age >40 years

- Nephrotic syndrome
- Pregnancy/postpartum
- Inflammatory bowel disease
- Oral contraceptives (with estrogen)
- Acute medical illness
- Hormone replacement therapy
- Selective estrogen receptor

ADJUNCTIVE THERAPIES
Postoperative Steroids[45]

- The evidence that **perioperative corticosteroids** decrease facial swelling and ecchymosis following facelift remains **anecdotal and unsubstantiated** and may be associated with increased cost and risk for complications, including exacerbation of hypertension, deterioration of glucose control, an increased rate of infection, and the potential for avascular osteonecrosis.[46-48]
- For **rhinoplasty,** perioperative corticosteroid use **decreases postoperative edema and ecchymosis**. Preoperative use is superior to postoperative use, and extended dosing is superior to singular.[11,49-51]

Lymphatic Massage

- Clears the main lymphatic collectors, favoring mobilization of edema, which can notably improve the decongestion of the face, neck, and/or extremities
  - In some instances, graduated support garments may replace or augment lymphatic massage postoperatively.
- Usually performed by trained aestheticians or physical therapists and has become particularly popular after facelifts with common protocols advocating one to three sessions spaced over postoperative days.*
- Contrary to the procedure in which drainage of the facial skin of the nonoperated face is massaged to promote drainage to the parotid, submaxillary, and occipital lymph nodes, after a facelift, the massages must be **reversed** in direction, that is, to the **medial part of the face,** and from there to the deep nodes of the neck.
- Lymphatic massage is reported to relax the parasympathetic system and tranquilize patients, reducing postoperative anxiety.[52]

SCAR MANAGEMENT[53]

- **Adhesive, microporous, hypoallergenic paper tape**
  - Applied to fresh surgical incisions and replaced every 3-7 days for up to 12 weeks is useful in low-risk patients to improve scar cosmesis and prevent hypertrophic scarring.[54-56]
- **Silicone gel sheeting and silicone gel ointments**
  - Most accepted modality in the treatment and prevention of hypertrophic scar in high-risk patients (i.e., those who have previously had abnormal scarring or are undergoing a procedure with high incidence of poor scarring such as breast surgery)
  - Should begin soon after surgical closure, when the incision has fully epithelialized, and be continued for at least 1 month

---

*References 12, 14, 20, 21, 24, 27, 28, 33, 39.

- Silicone gel sheets should be worn for a minimum of 12 hours daily, and if possible for 24 hours daily with twice-daily washing.
  - Less evidence that silicone gel ointments (e.g., Kelo-cote) are as effective in preventing scarring, but they may be more appropriate on the head and neck[27]
- Topical vitamin E, cocoa butter, onion extract cream (e.g., Mederma), allantoin-sulfomucopolysaccharide gel, glycosaminoglycan gel, and creams containing extracts from plants such as *Bulbine frutescens* and *Centella asiatica* have **not** been shown to consistently improve scar appearance as single agents.
  - Any benefits of such topical agents have been suggested to result from **massage** associated with their application; thus deep wound massage therapy is a common modality for managing scarring, but scientific evidence for its efficacy is also limited.[41,43,44]
- A new device designed to minimize tension on the scar (Embrace; Neodyne Biosciences) demonstrated a statistically significant improvement in scar appearance in a prospective, randomized multicenter clinical trial.[57,58]

TOP TAKEAWAYS

➤ Management of comorbidities must be optimized before elective aesthetic intervention.

➤ Lifestyle measures, including smoking, alcohol, and dietary habit, can affect outcomes and should be addressed.

➤ Decolonization and skin antisepsis should be considered to reduce surgical site infection, especially for prosthetic implantation.

➤ Basic skin care underpins success in achieving aesthetic rejuvenation and consists of routine exfoliating, cleansing, moisturizing, photoprotection, and antiaging treatment (i.e., topical retinoids).

➤ Risk of perioperative VTE can be reduced by following current guidelines.

➤ Adjunctive therapies such as lymphatic massage and graduated compression garments can expedite healing and enhance well-being postoperatively.

➤ Taping or silicone gel sheeting is probably the most effective and proven means to favorably modulate scar maturation.

REFERENCES

1. Guyuron B, Raszewski R. Undetected diabetes and the plastic surgeon. Plast Reconstr Surg 86:471, 1990.
2. Harrison B, Khansa I, Janis JE. Evidence-based strategies to reduce postoperative complications in plastic surgery. Plast Reconstr Surg 137:351, 2016.
3. Mejia JD, Egro FM, Nahai F. Visual loss after blepharoplasty: incidence, management, and preventive measures. Aesthet Surg J 31:21, 2011.
4. Fischer JP, Shang EK, Nelson JA, et al. Patterns of preoperative laboratory testing in patients undergoing outpatient plastic surgery procedures. Aesthet Surg J 34:133, 2014.
5. Wimalawansa SM, Fox JP, Johnson RM. The measurable cost of complications for outpatient cosmetic surgery in patients with mental health diagnoses. Aesthet Surg J 34:306, 2014.

6. Broughton G II, Crosby MA, Coleman J, et al. Use of herbal supplements and vitamins in plastic surgery: a practical review. Plast Reconstr Surg 119:48e, 2007.

7. Zwiebel SJ, Michelle L, Brendan A, et al. The incidence of vitamin, mineral, herbal, and other supplement use in facial cosmetic patients. Plast Reconstr Surg 132:78, 2013.

8. Heller J, Gabbay JS, Ghadjar K, et al. Top-10 list of herbal and supplemental medicines used by cosmetic patients: what the plastic surgeon needs to know. Plast Reconstr Surg 117:436, 2006.

9. Orsini RA. Bromelain. Plast Reconstr Surg 118:1640, 2006.

10. Lawrence WT; Plastic Surgery Educational Foundation DATA Committee. Arnica. Plast Reconstr Surg112:1164, 2003.

11. Totonchi A, Guyuron B. A randomized, controlled comparison between arnica and steroids in the management of postrhinoplasty ecchymosis and edema. Plast Reconstr Surg120:271, 2007.

12. Ehrlich HP, Tarver H, Hunt TK. Effects of vitamin A and glucocorticoids upon inflammation and collagen synthesis. Ann Surg 177:222, 1973.

13. Massé PG, Pritzker KP, Mendes MG, et al. Vitamin B6 deficiency experimentally-induced bone and joint disorder: microscopic, radiographic and biochemical evidence. Br J Nutr 71:919, 1994.

14. Alcaín FJ, Burón MI. Ascorbate on cell growth and differentiation. J Bioenerg Biomembr 26:393, 1994.

15. Ho AL, Klassen AF, Cano S, et al. Optimizing patient-centered care in breast reconstruction: the importance of preoperative information and patient-physician communication. Plast Reconstr Surg 132:212e, 2013.

16. McLafferty RB, Williams RG, Lambert AD, et al. Surgeon communication behaviors that lead patients to not recommend the surgeon to family members or friends: analysis and impact. Surgery 140:616; discussion 622, 2006.

17. Jensen JA, Goodson WH, Hopf H, et al. Cigarette smoking decreases tissue oxygen. Arch Surg 126:1131, 1991.

18. Sørensen LT. Wound healing and infection in surgery: the pathophysiological impact of smoking, smoking cessation, and nicotine replacement therapy: a systematic review. Ann Surg 255:1069, 2012.

18a. Sørensen LT. Wound healing and infection in surgery. The clinical impact of smoking and smoking cessation: a systematic review and meta-analysis. Arch Surg 147:373, 2012.

19. Krueger JK, Rohrich RJ. Clearing the smoke: the scientific rationale for tobacco abstention with plastic surgery. Plast Reconstr Surg 108:1063, 2001.

20. Rohrich RJ, Coberly DM, Krueger JK, et al. Planning elective operations on patients who smoke: survey of North American plastic surgeons. Plast Reconstr Surg 109:350, 2002.

21. Tønnesen H, Nielsen PR, Lauritzen JB, et al. Smoking and alcohol intervention before surgery: evidence for best practice. Br J Anaesth 102:297, 2009.

22. Mayo Clinic: May Medical Laboratories. Available at *www.mayomedicallaboratories.com*.

23. Chen AF, Wessel CB, Rao N. Staphylococcus aureus screening and decolonization in orthopaedic surgery and reduction of surgical site infections. Clin Orthop Relat Res 471:2383, 2013.

24. Craft RO, Damjanovic B, Colwell AS. Evidence-based protocol for infection control in immediate implant-based breast reconstruction. Ann Plast Surg 69:446, 2012.

25. Feldman EM, Kontoyiannis DP, Sharabi SE, et al. Breast implant infections: is cefazolin enough? Plast Reconstr Surg 126:779, 2010.

26. Bode LG, Kluytmans JA, Wertheim HF, et al. Preventing surgical-site infections in nasal carriers of Staphylococcus aureus. N Engl J Med 362:9, 2010.

27. Wenzel RP, Perl TM. The significance of nasal carriage of Staphylococcus aureus and the incidence of postoperative wound infection. J Hosp Infect 31:13, 1995.

28. Pannucci CJ, Dreszer G, Wachtman CF, et al. Postoperative enoxaparin prevents symptomatic venous thromboembolism in high-risk plastic surgery patients. Plast Reconstr Surg 128:1093, 2011.

29. Haynes AB, Weiser TG, Berry WR, et al. A surgical safety checklist to reduce morbidity and mortality in a global population. N Engl J Med 360:491, 2009.

30. Clayton JL, Bazakas A, Lee CN, et al. Once is not enough: withholding postoperative prophylactic antibiotics in prosthetic breast reconstruction is associated with an increased risk of infection. Plast Reconstr Surg 130:495, 2012.

31. Georgiou I, Farber N, Mendes D, et al. The role of antibiotics in rhinoplasty and septoplasty: a literature review. Rhinology 46:267, 2008.

32. Hibbard JS. Analyses comparing the antimicrobial activity and safety of current antiseptic agents: a review. J Infus Nurs 28:194, 2005.

33. Dumville JC, McFarlane E, Edwards P, et al. Preoperative skin antiseptics for preventing surgical wound infections after clean surgery. Cochrane Database Syst Rev 2015:CD003949, 2015.

34. Bund M, Heine J, Jaeger K. [Complications due to patient positioning: anaesthesiological considerations] Anasthesiol Intensivmed Notfallmed Schmerzther 40:329, 2005.

35. Shermak M, Shoo B, Deune EG. Prone positioning precautions in plastic surgery. Plast Reconstr Surg 117:1584; discussion 1589, 2006.

36. Miller RD, ed. Miller's Anesthesia, ed 8. Philadelphia: Elsevier Saunders, 2015.

37. AAMI/ANSI ST79. Comprehensive Guide to Steam Sterilization and Sterility Assurance in Health Care Facilities, ed 4. Arlington, VA: Association of Advanced Medical Instruments, 2013.

38. Carlo A. The new era of flash sterilization. AORN J 86:58, 2007.

39. Hernandez M, Cutter TW, Apfelbaum JL. Hypothermia and hyperthermia in the ambulatory surgical patient. Clin Plast Surg 40:429, 2013.

40. Cortez R, Lazcano E, Miller T, et al. Barbed sutures and wound complications in plastic surgery: an analysis of outcomes. Aesthet Surg J 35:178, 2015.

41. Stephens DM, Richards BG, Schleicher WF, et al. Is ketorolac safe to use in plastic surgery? A critical review. Aesthet Surg J 35:462, 2015.

42. Aynehchi BB, Cerrati EW, Rosenberg DB. The efficacy of oral celecoxib for acute postoperative pain in face-lift surgery. JAMA Facial Plast Surg 16:306, 2014.

43. Abboushi N, Yezhelyev M, Symbas J, et al. Facelift complications and the risk of venous thromboembolism: a single center's experience. Aesthet Surg J 32:413, 2012.

44. Venturi ML, Davison SP, Caprini JA. Prevention of venous thromboembolism in the plastic surgery patient: current guidelines and recommendations. Aesthet Surg J 29:421, 2009.

45. Pulikkottil BJ, Dauwe P, Daniali L, et al. Corticosteroid use in cosmetic plastic surgery. Plast Reconstr Surg 132:352e, 2013.

46. Echavez MI, Mangat DS. Effects of steroids on mood, edema, and ecchymosis in facial plastic surgery. Archiv Otolaryngol Head Neck Surg 120:1137, 1994.

47. Owsley JQ, Weibel TJ, Adams WA. Does steroid medication reduce facial edema following face lift surgery? A prospective, randomized study of 30 consecutive patients. Plast Reconstr Surg 98:1, 1996.

48. Rapaport DP, Bass LS, Aston SJ. Influence of steroids on postoperative swelling after facial plasty: a prospective, randomized study. Plast Reconstr Surg 96:1547, 1995.

49. Hatef DA, Ellsworth WA, Allen JN, et al. Perioperative steroids for minimizing edema and ecchymosis after rhinoplasty: a meta-analysis. Aesthet Surg J 31:648, 2011.

50. Hoffmann DF, Cook TA, Quatela VC, et al. Steroids and rhinoplasty. A double-blind study. Arch Otolaryngol Head Neck Surg 117:990, 1991.

51. Kargi E, Hoşnuter M, Babuçcu O, et al. Effect of steroids on edema, ecchymosis, and intraoperative bleeding in rhinoplasty. Ann Plast Surg 51:570, 2003.
52. Mottura AA. Face lift postoperative recovery. Aesthetic Plast Surg 26:172, 2002.
53. Khansa I, Harrison B, Janis JE. Evidence-based scar management: how to improve results with technique and technology. Plast Reconst Surg 138:1655, 2016.
54. Atkinson JA, McKenna KT, Barnett AG, et al. A randomized, controlled trial to determine the efficacy of paper tape in preventing hypertrophic scar formation in surgical incisions that traverse Langer's skin tension lines. Plast Reconstr Surg 116:1648, 2005.
55. Mustoe TA, Cooter RD, Gold MH, et al. International clinical recommendations on scar management. Plast Reconstr Surg 110:560, 2002.
56. Reiffel RS. Prevention of hypertrophic scars by long-term paper tape application. Plast Reconstr Surg 96:1715, 1995.
57. Longaker MT, Rohrich RJ, Greenberg L, et al. A randomized controlled trial of the embrace advanced scar therapy device to reduce incisional scar formation. Plast Reconstr Surg 134:536, 2014.
58. Havlik RJ. Vitamin E and wound healing. Plastic Surgery Educational Foundation DATA Committee. Plast Reconstr Surg 100:1901, 1997.

11. Venous Thromboembolism and the Aesthetic Surgery Patient

Christopher J. Pannucci, Amy Kathleen Alderman

- VTE is a life- or limb-threatening complication that can occur after surgical procedures.
- It has been designated by the CDC as the **most common cause of "preventable" hospital deaths** and has been designated by the Centers for Medicare and Medicaid Services as a "never event" for some surgical procedures.
- The annual estimate of VTE events is 500,000 cases with 100,000 deaths in the United States.
- VTE occurs in **18,000 plastic surgery patients a year,** and, although this may seem rare, it can be particularly devastating when it occurs in elective aesthetic surgery patients.
- Surgeons should consider patients' VTE risk as part of the standard aesthetic surgery workup.
- Although research in plastic surgery patients has clearly demonstrated that all VTEs are not preventable, surgeons can minimize VTE risk preoperatively, intraoperatively, and postoperatively.

WHAT DO THE GUIDELINES SAY?

- Both the American Society of Plastic Surgeons (ASPS) (2012) and American Association of Plastic Surgeons (AAPS) (2016) have published **evidence-based consensus statements** on VTE risk stratification and prophylaxis.[1,2]
- Both sets of recommendations advocate for individualized VTE risk stratification using the **2005 Caprini Risk Assessment Model (RAM).**[3]
- Both sets of recommendations recommend different VTE prevention strategies based on baseline VTE risk, characterized by Caprini score and by procedure type.
  - A "one size fits all" approach is not recommended

SUMMARY OF CURRENT GUIDELINES

- The **ASPS VTE Task Force**[1] makes recommendations for aesthetic surgery patients who have surgery under general anesthesia. Direct quotes are provided from their 2012 manuscript.
  - **Risk stratification:** *"Should consider completing a 2005 Caprini RAM . . . to stratify patients into a VTE risk category based on their individual risk factors"*
  - **For elective surgery patients with Caprini scores of ≥7:** *"Should consider utilizing risk reduction strategies such as limiting OR times, weight reduction, discontinuing hormone replacement therapy, and early postoperative mobilization"*

- **For body contouring or abdominoplasty under general anesthesia with procedure time >60 minutes:**
  - ▶ **Caprini score 3-6:** *"Should consider the option to use postoperative low-molecular-weight heparin or unfractionated heparin"*
  - ▶ **Caprini score ≥3:** *"Should consider the option to utilize mechanical prophylaxis . . . for nonambulatory patients"*
  - ▶ **Caprini score ≥7:** *"Should strongly consider the option to use extended (duration) low-molecular-weight heparin postoperative prophylaxis"*
- The **AAPS** published a systematic review/meta-analysis and consensus panel on DVT/PE prevention in 2016. Source data were largely derived from inpatient surgery, but several recommendations were applicable to the aesthetic surgery population.[2] Direct quotes are provided from their manuscript.
  - *"We recommend using nongeneral anesthesia when appropriate. When possible, consideration should be given to using monitored anesthesia care, local anesthesia with sedation, or neuraxial anesthesia instead of general anesthesia."*
  - *"We recommend using intermittent pneumatic compression to prevent perioperative VTE events in plastic surgery patients . . . intermittent pneumatic compression is superior to elastic compression stockings."*
  - *"We recommend all plastic and reconstructive surgery patients should be risk stratified for perioperative VTE risk using a 2005 Caprini score."*
  - *"We do not recommend adding chemoprophylaxis to intermittent pneumatic compression for VTE prophylaxis in the general non-risk-stratified plastic surgery population."*
  - *"We recommend that surgeons consider chemoprophylaxis on a case-by-case basis in patients with Caprini score >8."*
  - *"We do not recommend adding routine chemoprophylaxis for VTE prophylaxis in non-risk-stratified patients undergoing . . . body contouring."*

UNDERSTANDING THE CAPRINI RISK ASSESSMENT MODEL[3]

- This is a VTE risk assessment model that has been **validated in >20,000 patients,** including plastic, general/vascular/urology, gynecology oncology, and otolaryngology/head and neck.
- The Caprini RAM is a **one-page questionnaire** that is easy to complete at either the patient's initial consultation or preoperative visit (Fig. 11-1).
  - Assigns different point values for the various risk factors based on the **patient's personal medical history and family history.**
  - An aggregate risk factor score is generated and correlates with a **percentage value for postoperative VTE risk.**
  - Using this information, physicians can make a decision about chemoprophylaxis and other risk-reduction strategies.
- Current recommendations support the use of the 2005 Caprini RAM and ***not* the 2010 Caprini RAM,** which places more patients in a higher-risk category but does not increase the sensitivity of predicting VTE.[4]

Choose All That Apply

Each Risk Factor Represents 1 Point
☐ Age 41-60 years
☐ Minor surgery planned
☐ History of prior major surgery (<1 month)
☐ Varicose veins
☐ History of inflammatory bowel disease
☐ Swollen legs (current)
☐ Obesity (BMI >25)
☐ Acute myocardial infarction
☐ Congestive heart failure (<1 month)
☐ Sepsis (<1 month)
☐ Serious lung disease incl. pneumonia (<1 month)
☐ Abnormal pulmonary function (COPD)
☐ Medical patient currently at bed rest
☐ Other risk factors _____

Each Risk Factor Represents 2 Points
☐ Age 60-74 years
☐ Arthroscopic surgery
☐ Malignancy (present or previous)
☐ Major surgery (>45 minutes)
☐ Laparoscopic surgery (>45 minutes)
☐ Patient confined to bed (>72 hours)
☐ Immobilizing plaster cast (<1 month)
☐ Central venous access

Each Risk Factor Represents 5 Points
☐ Elective major lower extremity arthroplasty
☐ Hip, pelvis, or leg fracture (<1 month)
☐ Stroke (<1 month)
☐ Multiple trauma (<1 month)
☐ Acute spinal cord injury (paralysis) (<1 month)

Each Risk Factor Represents 3 Points
☐ Age over 75 years
☐ History of DVT/PE
☐ **Family history of thrombosis** *
☐ Positive Factor V Leiden
☐ Positive Prothrombin 20210A
☐ Elevated serum homocysteine
☐ Positive lupus anticoagulent
☐ Elevated anticardiolipin antibodies
☐ Heparin-induced thrombocytopenia (HIT)
☐ Other congenital or acquired thrombophilia
If yes:
Type _____
*most frequently missed risk factor

For Women Only (Each Represents 1 Point)
☐ Oral contraceptives or hormone replacement therapy
☐ Pregnancy or postpartum (<1 month)
☐ History of unexplained stillborn infant, recurrent spontaneous abortion (≥3), premature birth with toxemia or growth-restricted infant

Total Risk Factor Score ☐

Fig. 11-1   Caprini risk assessment model.

WHAT AESTHETIC SURGERY PATIENTS ARE AT HIGHEST RISK?

- Among cosmetic procedures, **abdominoplasty alone or in combination with another procedure has the highest risk of VTE.** The procedure type with the greatest risk is *circumferential abdominoplasty,* which has an associated VTE frequency of **3.40%.**[5]
- The Doctors Company has seen an increase in malpractice claims involving VTE, and a major issue is **inadequate prophylaxis in high-risk patients.**
  - In a review of 12 claims, 8 were abdominoplasty cases (6 of those 8 were combined procedures). Half of all patients had general anesthesia, the other half had IV sedation. Death occurred in 9 patients.
- Why is the risk of VTE increased with abdominoplasty?
  - **Multifactorial.** Contributing causes include length of procedure (venous pooling with general anesthesia), prone positioning for hip liposuction (increased venous pressure from hip roll), fluid shifts with liposuction, increased intraabdominal pressure from rectus plication, flexed posture and postoperative abdominal binder,[6] and decreased postoperative mobility.

WHAT CAN BE DONE BEFORE SURGERY—RISK STRATIFICATION

■ Complete a full history and physical examination and a VTE risk assessment tool such as the 2005 Caprini RAM. This tool reminds surgeons to ask about **family history of VTE** *(the most commonly missed risk factor),* genetic hypercoagulability, and current estrogen usage, among other often missed risk factors.
  • Studies among plastic surgery inpatients[7] and surgical outpatients[8] have identified an 18- to 20-fold variation in VTE risk among the overall surgical population.
  • Individualized risk stratification allows surgeons to conceptualize and quantify this risk.

NOTE: No VTE risk stratification tool has been validated for aesthetic surgery patients.

■ Data from plastic surgery inpatients not given chemoprophylaxis can be used to estimate VTE risk.[9]
  • **Caprini 3-4:** 0.32% 60-day VTE risk
  • **Caprini 5-6:** 1.22% 60-day VTE risk
  • **Caprini 7-8:** 2.55% 60-day VTE risk
  • **Caprini >8:** 8.54% 60-day VTE risk
■ If a risk stratification tool is not used, risk estimate based on procedure type can be provided and discussed during the informed consent process.[5,10,11]
  • Circumferential abdominoplasty: 3.4%
  • Abdominoplasty with intraabdominal procedure: 2.1%
  • Abdominoplasty with concomitant procedure: 0.67%
  • Abdominoplasty alone: 0.34%
  • Breast augmentation: 0.02%
  • Facelift: 0.02%
■ **Preoperative hematology consultation** can be considered if patients have family member(s) with VTE or other notable risk factors.[12]
  • Hypercoagulability testing can be affected by many drugs and clinical circumstances.
  • Hypercoagulability testing is best ordered and interpreted by a hematologist.
  • Hematologists can help to estimate level of VTE risk and can make recommendations for VTE prevention strategies in high-risk patients.
  • Aesthetic surgery is elective and can be delayed until the entire workup is complete.

WHAT CAN BE DONE BEFORE SURGERY—RISK MODIFICATION

■ **Many patient-level risk factors are potentially modifiable before surgery.**[3]
  • BMI, presence of central line or chemoport, use of estrogen-based contraceptives, among others
  • Encourage patients to lose weight, have a general surgeon remove a chemoport, wait at least 30 days between procedures, and hold estrogen products and tamoxifen for 3-4 weeks before surgery—all of these examples of risk modification will theoretically decrease VTE risk.[13]
    ▶ Help patients to understand that their safety is the principal concern.
■ Studies have associated **increased number of surgical procedures** and **increased length of surgery** with higher risk for VTE.[5,14-16] The two are related, and the driving force is unknown.

- *Limiting number of concurrent procedures, and thus operative time, is a modifiable risk factor.*
  - ▶ Aesthetic surgeons need to be aware that they often combine procedures more than any other surgical specialty for patient convenience (single recovery), expedited patient gratification, competitive market forces, and patient costs.
  - ▶ **≤6 hours should be the targeted length of aesthetic surgery.**
    - ◆ ASPS has recommended: *"Ideally, office procedures should be completed within 6 hours . . . this might involve staging multiple procedures into more than one case."*[17]
    - ◆ Surgeons should be aware of **state-based surgical time and liposuction volume limits** on office-based surgery.
- For example, compared with abdominoplasty alone, abdominoplasty plus intraabdominal procedure has **6× increased risk** (0.34% versus 2.17%), and abdominoplasty plus other procedure has **2× increased risk** (0.34% versus 0.67%).[5]
- In another example, Tracking Operations and Outcomes for Plastic Surgeons (TOPS) and CosmetAssure data suggested that among those having combined procedures, the risk of VTE increases fivefold among those having breast augmentation and 30% for those having an abdominoplasty, compared with single procedures.[10]
- ■ **Plastic surgery tourism can increase risk for VTE**
  - Screening duplex ultrasound before and after long flights in economy class showed that **4.9%** of people developed deep or superficial thrombosis during flight.
  - The clinical relevance of these asymptomatic DVTs is unclear.
  - **Below-knee elastic compression stockings** significantly decreased DVT rate from 4.5% to 0.24%.[18]
  - Systematic review of air travel and VTE showed that elastic compression stockings, but not aspirin or low-molecular-weight heparin, prevented DVT.[19]
- ■ For patients at very high risk, the decision to perform a surgical procedure is the last consideration in risk modification.
  - Surgeons may deem some patients' VTE risk as too high to safely offer an aesthetic procedure.

WHAT CAN BE DONE DURING SURGERY—RISK REDUCTION
- ■ **Type of anesthesia** is a modifiable risk factor in the intraoperative setting.
  - **General anesthesia** increases risk, compared with other anesthesia types.
  - VTE with abdominoplasty is significantly higher among patients having general versus IV sedation (OR: 0.11, CI: 0.03-0.43).[20]
    - ▶ Cause is probably **loss of calf muscle pump and resultant venous stasis,** as well as other mechanisms.
  - Nongeneral anesthetic, when feasible for surgeon and patient, is preferred and safer.
- ■ **Mechanical prophylaxis** options include elastic compression stockings and intermittent pneumatic compression.
  - Elastic compression shunts blood from the superficial to deep systems and minimizes stasis.
  - Use of stockings is more effective than nonuse in prevention of VTE.[21]
  - Intermittent pneumatic compression physically pumps blood from caudal to cranial, re-creating the action of the calf muscle pump, and activates the body's endogenous fibrinolytic mechanism.[22]

- The AAPS consensus statement recommended intermittent pneumatic compression as superior to elastic compression stockings.[2]
■ **Slight knee flexion (5 degrees)** on a pillow can promote venous egress.
■ Abdominal wall plication and bed flexion during abdominoplasty increases intraabdominal pressure.[6,23] This may cause inferior vena cava and femoral vein stasis, predisposing to DVT.
- Surgeons should plicate only when clinically necessary, and not as a matter of course.

WHAT CAN BE DONE AFTER SURGERY—RISK REDUCTION
■ **Early ambulation and adequate hydration are critical.**
■ Postoperative abdominal binders and compression garments can constrict the common femoral vein in the thigh and may require modification.[24,25]
■ Mechanical prophylaxis (intermittent pneumatic compression) can be used to mimic the calf muscle pump after surgery, at least until patients are ambulatory.
- There are no data on VTE risk reduction with postdischarge mechanical prophylaxis.
- Chemoprophylaxis, including unfractionated heparin and enoxaparin/low-molecular-weight heparin, has been studied extensively among plastic surgery inpatients.
  ▶ For inpatients, **enoxaparin** prophylaxis provided for the duration of inpatient stay reduced VTE risk among high-risk patients (Caprini scores of 7-8 and >8), but not in lower-risk patients (Caprini scores of 3-4 and 5-6).[9]
  ▶ For inpatients, postoperative enoxaparin prophylaxis **did not significantly increase bleeding risk.**[26]
  ▶ Despite the injectable delivery, enoxaparin is **well tolerated** among aesthetic surgery patients and is **affordable.**
  ▶ Preoperative or intraoperative chemoprophylaxis significantly increases bleeding risk in **body contouring**[27] and **facelift**[28] surgery.
  ▶ Providing chemoprophylaxis to all patients may have an unfavorable risk/benefit relationship.[2]
    ◆ The ASPS and AAPS recommend prophylaxis based on Caprini scores as opposed to all patients.
■ Some surgeons use oral Factor Xa inhibitors for chemoprophylaxis.
- Limited data exist, and, presently, oral Factor Xa inhibitors are not FDA approved for prophylaxis in nonorthopedic surgery patients.
- In abdominoplasty patients, oral Factor Xa inhibitors have low rates of reoperative hematoma (2.3%), but no studies on effectiveness have been published.[29]
■ Current guidelines explicitly recommend *against* aspirin as a single-agent chemoprophylaxis for VTE.[30]
■ Screening duplex ultrasound for all patients, instead of other mechanical and pharmacologic means of prophylaxis, has been recommended.[31]
- Among 200 aesthetic surgery patients, the rate of asymptomatic DVT was 0.5%.

SENIOR AUTHOR TIP: I strongly disagree with this practice of screening via duplex ultrasound when performed instead of other mechanical and pharmacologic means.

- Current American College of Chest Physicians guidelines explicitly recommend against screening duplex ultrasound, even in high-risk patients.

TOP TAKEAWAYS
➤ Risk for perioperative VTE is affected by both patient-level and procedure-level factors.
➤ Considering patients' risk based on their individual characteristics will allow surgeons to modify risk factors and implement VTE prevention strategies in the preoperative, intraoperative, and postoperative settings.
➤ Generally, outpatient aesthetic surgical procedures should be <6 hours; all patients should undergo a VTE risk assessment; appropriate measures for risk reduction should be taken; and surgeons should have a low threshold to stage cosmetic procedures.

REFERENCES

1. Murphy RX Jr, Alderman A, Gutowski K, et al. Evidence-based practices for thromboembolism prevention: summary of the ASPS Venous Thromboembolism Task Force Report. Plast Reconstr Surg 130:168e, 2012.
2. Pannucci CJ, MacDonald JK, Ariyan S, et al. Benefits and risks of prophylaxis for deep venous thrombosis and pulmonary embolus in plastic surgery: a systematic review and meta-analysis of controlled trials and consensus conference. Plast Reconstr Surg 137:709, 2016.
3. Caprini JA. Thrombosis risk assessment as a guide to quality patient care. Dis Mon 51:70, 2005.
4. Pannucci CJ, Barta RJ, Portschy PR, et al. Assessment of postoperative venous thromboembolism risk in plastic surgery patients using the 2005 and 2010 Caprini Risk score. Plast Reconstr Surg 130:343, 2012.
5. Hatef DA, Trussler AP, Kenkel JM. Procedural risk for venous thromboembolism in abdominal contouring surgery: a systematic review of the literature. Plast Reconstr Surg 125:352, 2010.
6. Huang GJ, Bajaj AK, Gupta S, et al. Increased intraabdominal pressure in abdominoplasty: delineation of risk factors. Plast Reconstr Surg 119:1319, 2007.
7. Pannucci CJ, Bailey SH, Dreszer G, et al. Validation of the Caprini risk assessment model in plastic and reconstructive surgery patients. J Am Coll Surg 212:105, 2011.
8. Pannucci CJ, Shanks A, Moote MJ, et al. Identifying patients at high risk for venous thromboembolism requiring treatment after outpatient surgery. Ann Surg 255:1093, 2012.
9. Pannucci CJ, Dreszer G, Wachtman CF, et al. Postoperative enoxaparin prevents symptomatic venous thromboembolism in high-risk plastic surgery patients. Plast Reconstr Surg 128:1093, 2011.
10. Alderman AK, Collins ED, Streu R, et al. Benchmarking outcomes in plastic surgery: national complication rates for abdominoplasty and breast augmentation. Plast Reconstr Surg 124:2127, 2009.
11. Santos DQ, Tan M, Farias CL, et al. Venous thromboembolism after facelift surgery under local anesthesia: results of a multicenter survey. Aesthetic Plast Surg 38:12, 2014.
12. Pannucci CJ, Kovach SJ, Cuker A. Microsurgery and the hypercoagulable state: a hematologist's perspective. Plast Reconstr Surg 136:545e, 2015.
13. Gupta V, Winocour J, Rodriguez-Feo C, et al. Safety of aesthetic surgery in the overweight patient: analysis of 127,961 patients. Aesthet Surg J 36:718, 2016.
14. Kim JY, Khavanin N, Rambachan A, et al. Surgical duration and risk of venous thromboembolism. JAMA Surg 150:110, 2015.
15. Howland WS, Schweizer O. Complications associated with prolonged operation and anesthesia. Clin Anesth 9:1, 1972.

16. Gravante G, Araco A, Sorge R, et al. Pulmonary embolism after combined abdominoplasty and flank liposuction: a correlation with the amount of fat removed. Ann Plast Surg 60:604, 2008.

17. Haeck PC, Swanson JA, Iverson RE, et al. Evidence-based patient safety advisory: patient selection and procedures in ambulatory surgery. Plast Reconstr Surg 124(4 Suppl):S6, 2009.

18. Belcaro G, Geroulakos G, Nicolaides AN, et al. Venous thromboembolism from air travel: the LONFLIT study. Angiology 52:369, 2001.

19. Philbrick JT, Shumate R, Siadaty MS, et al. Air travel and venous thromboembolism: a systematic review. J Gen Intern Med 22:107, 2007.

20. Hafezi F, Naghibzadeh B, Nouhi AH, et al. Epidural anesthesia as a thromboembolic prophylaxis modality in plastic surgery. Aesthet Surg J 31:821, 2011.

21. Sachdeva A, Dalton M, Amaragiri SV, et al. Elastic compression stockings for prevention of deep vein thrombosis. Cochrane Database Syst Rev 2010(7):CD001484.

22. Comerota AJ, Chouhan V, Harada RN, et al. The fibrinolytic effects of intermittent pneumatic compression: mechanism of enhanced fibrinolysis. Ann Surg 226:306; discussion 313, 1997.

23. Al-Basti HB, El-Khatib HA, Taha A, et al. Intraabdominal pressure after full abdominoplasty in obese multiparous patients. Plast Reconstr Surg 113:2145; discussion 2151, 2004.

24. Berjeaut RH, Nahas FX, Dos Santos LK, et al. Does the use of compression garments increase venous stasis in the common femoral vein? Plast Reconstr Surg 135:85e, 2015.

25. Clayburgh DR, Stott W, Cordiero T, et al. Prospective study of venous thromboembolism in patients with head and neck cancer after surgery. JAMA Otolaryngol Head Neck Surg 139:1143, 2013.

26. Pannucci CJ, Wachtman CF, Dreszer G, et al. The effect of postoperative enoxaparin on risk for reoperative hematoma. Plast Reconstr Surg 129:160, 2012.

27. Hatef DA, Kenkel JM, Nguyen MQ, et al. Thromboembolic risk assessment and the efficacy of enoxaparin prophylaxis in excisional body contouring surgery. Plast Reconstr Surg 122:269, 2008.

28. Durnig P, Jungwirth W. Low-molecular-weight heparin and postoperative bleeding in rhytidectomy. Plast Reconstr Surg 118:502; discussion 508, 2006.

29. Hunstad JP, Krochmal DJ, Flugstad NA, et al. Rivaroxaban for venous thromboembolism prophylaxis in abdominoplasty: a multicenter experience. Aesthet Surg J 36:60, 2016.

30. Gould MK, Garcia DA, Wren SM, et al; American College of Chest Physicians. Prevention of VTE in nonorthopedic surgical patients. Antithrombotic Therapy and Prevention of Thrombosis, 9th ed. American College of Chest Physicians Evidence-Based Clinical Practice Guidelines. Chest 141(2 Suppl):e227S, 2012.

31. Swanson E. Ultrasound screening for deep venous thrombosis detection: a prospective evaluation of 200 plastic surgery outpatients. Plast Reconstr Surg Glob Open 3:e332, 2015.

PART IV

Skin Care

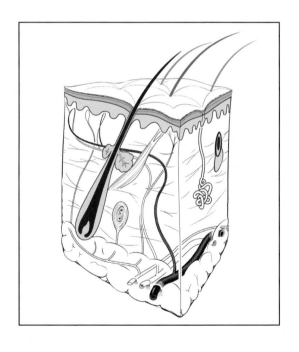

Skin Care

12. The Medi Spa and Other Practice Considerations

Rishi Jindal, Renato Saltz

PRACTICE BASICS

WHAT IS A MEDI SPA?

- Fusion of wellness spa, salon, retail store, and medical office practice with or without integrated ambulatory surgery center (ASC)
  - ASC defined by Code of Federal Regulations as "any distinct entity that operates exclusively for the purpose of providing surgical services to patients not requiring hospitalization and in which the expected duration of services would not exceed 24 hours following an admission"[1]
  - Definition varies by organization and jurisdiction, but lack of (anticipated) need for overnight admission universal
- Spa, salon, and retail services offered typically in one part of facility
- Plastic/aesthetic surgeon functions primarily on medical side in another part of facility
- Physician on site can allow more advanced "medical spa" services like deep chemical peels, laser therapies, and injectables (see Legal Considerations section).
- Retail sales of skin care products, camouflage makeup, mechanical or light-based devices (Table 12-1)

Table 12-1 *Range of Services Offered in a Comprehensive Medi Spa*

Spa, Salon, and Retail Services	Medi Spa (Noninvasive) Services	Surgical Services
Chemical peels	Deep chemical peels	Body
Facials, skin care, and cosmeceuticals	Dermal fillers	Abdominoplasty
Hand, foot, and nail care	Intense-pulsed light (IPL)	Body contouring (body lift, brachioplasty, thigh lift)
Hair care	Photorejuvenation	Hand surgery and hand rejuvenation
Laser therapies	Latisse (Allergan)	Labiaplasty
Makeup	Microdermabrasion	Liposuction
Massages	Neurotoxin injections	Scar revision
Scrubs	Postsurgical skin care	Breast (augmentation, reconstruction, reduction)
		Gynecomastia reduction
		Mastopexy
		Facelift
		Browlift
		Eyelid surgery
		Facial implants
		Hair transplant
		Otoplasty
		Rhinoplasty

> **TIP:** Medi spas can incorporate retail services, salon care, spa services, and noninvasive and surgical cosmetic procedures into one facility; it depends on the surgeon's interests, goals, and finances.

PRACTICE SETTING

- Solo practice can offer complete control over all aspects of the practice or medi spa.
- Conversely, complete responsibility of decisions and finances lies with the physician.
- Establish who will care for patients, complications, and emergencies when physician is away for personal or professional activities in solo practice.
- Group practice can offer convenience of trusted colleagues caring for patients.
- Personal goals, personality, and philosophy are important considerations when deciding to work in a solo or group practice.
- Hospital-affiliated facility versus truly private practice may affect choice for size of practice, considering "on-call" activities, overhead costs, and ease of becoming established in the specific geographic market.

OFFICE

- Consider a convenient and accessible location, while maintaining subtlety and privacy.
- Ensure adequate parking, adherence to all building and city codes, and standards of accrediting organizations.
- Provide attractive, elegant interior with efficient flow of patients, but avoid gaudy, extravagant, or ostentatious décor and atmosphere.
- Maintain separation of medical/surgical patients and consumers of retail, salon, and spa services.

STAFF

- Ensure that all staff knows the practice's philosophy and embraces it.
- Ensure the team is trustworthy, knowledgeable, intellectually curious, and dedicated.
- Hire a business manager, patient coordinator, administrative assistant; expand and focus roles as the practice and business grow.
- Schedule regular staff meetings.
- Encourage environment of working hard, generating business, and putting patient safety at the forefront of mission.
- Maintain professionalism—always lead by example!

> **TIP:** A well-trained, dedicated, trustworthy staff can be one of a physician's biggest assets in practice. Interview carefully and take the time to hire wisely!

> **SENIOR AUTHOR TIP:** Complete financial and background checks on all potential employees *before* you hire them.
>
> Embezzlement is a very common problem in medi spa and aesthetic practices. Learn how employees can embezzle and how you can prevent it from happening.
>
> I recommend staff meetings very often, at least on a monthly basis. The focus should be on patient safety, new technology, and proactive staff issues—do not allow drama!

MARKETING AND GETTING ESTABLISHED[2]
Marketing

- **Telephone** is usually the first encounter a patient has with a medi spa, so ensure someone warm and knowledgeable is answering.
- Have an attractive and informative **website;** start early, even months before the doors open, and consider a web designer familiar with medi spas.
- Communications outside the office must have a **"call to action"**—an intended response, which can be as simple as providing education and contact information to referral sources, potential patients, and community groups.
- **Internal marketing** once patients are in the door
  - Staff and physician directing communication with patients is the most effective tool.
  - **Internal branding:** Have pamphlets with services you offer, your practice name on pens and mugs, email sign-up list for offers or specials.
  - Unique aspect of medi spa is that spa and noninvasive cosmetic procedures can be direct referral into the surgical practice for patients who want to take that step.
  - Suggest complementary services, like peels for facelift patients, or offer packages that combine surgical and nonsurgical treatments.

> **TIP:** Physicians should establish a niche, identify a community's needs or what it lacks in other aesthetic surgeons, and identify why they and their medi spa are unique or novel.

- **External marketing** to get patients in the door
  - **Community outreach:** Early in their career or practice, physicians should make themselves available to as many community groups, speaking engagements, and local radio and television shows as possible.
  - Meet and engage referral sources by sending educational materials, speaking with other physicians at the local hospital, offering expertise (when it is sought), and later showing sincere gratitude for their support.

Advertising

- **Printed material:** Newspaper and magazine advertisements; direct mailings to patients, groups, or referring physicians; pamphlets in the office or handed out at events
- **Electronic material:** Email; text messages; radio and television; the website and other Internet sites (Facebook and Twitter)
- **Links from related websites**

> **SENIOR AUTHOR TIP:** I recommend having a full-time marketing director and a full-time social media manager. I also recommend a modern, attractive website that needs to be renewed every 2 to 3 years.

> **SENIOR AUTHOR TIP:** Referrals must be carefully studied at minimum every quarter.

FINANCES[3]

- Physicians should set goals for themselves and their practice for financial growth, practice expansion, patient management, and experience.
- Projections can be time consuming, and trying to calculate the cost of goals can be daunting, but goals may go unfulfilled if this is not done.
- Assets include skills and education, the staff and their knowledge, the patients, and tangibles like products, materials, equipment, and property.

- Expenses include (1) direct expenses like wages, supplies, cost of operating equipment, and (2) overhead expenses like debt, loans, taxes, monthly bills, equipment rental, and depreciation.
- Careful planning and some research will allow surgeons to project how to balance their income and assets with expenses and future goals.
- Determine when taking on partners or nonphysician providers can increase revenue, while not necessarily doubling overhead.

AMBULATORY SURGERY FACILITY CERTIFICATION AND STANDARDS

ACCREDITATION[4]

- Before 1980 there were no specific guidelines for ASCs, quality control, or patient safety standards.
- Plastic surgeons decided to create a certifying body to oversee safe, reliable patient care facilities.
- They established the American Association for Accreditation of Plastic Surgery Facilities.
- It was later extended to facilities for all surgical specialties, becoming **American Association for Accreditation of Ambulatory Surgery Facilities, Inc. (AAAASF).**
- More than 2000 facilities nationally are AAAASF certified—largest not-for-profit accrediting body of ASCs.
- In 1996 California was first to mandate AAAASF accreditation for facilities providing sedation or general anesthesia (Legislation AB595).
- Most State Departments of Health accept accreditation instead of state licensure.
- AAAASF can also provide Medicare certification.

ACCREDITATION OF AMBULATORY SURGERY FACILITY CLASSES[5] (Table 12-2)

- Accreditation requirements based on anesthesia administered in each facility
- Far fewer requirements for Class A facilities
- Similarities for other classes, with more mandates as anesthesia becomes more invasive

Table 12-2 *Accreditation of Ambulatory Surgery Facility Class Based on Anesthesia*

Class A	Class B	Class C-M	Class C
Allowed	**Allowed**	**Allowed**	**Allowed**
Topical or local anesthesia Oral medications producing minimal or moderate sedation	Class A, plus: IV and parenteral sedation Regional blocks Dissociative drugs	Class A and B, plus: IV propofol Spinal or epidural anesthesia	Class A, B, C-M, plus: Inhalational agents LMA or endotracheal intubation
Restrictions	**Restrictions**	**Restrictions**	**Restrictions**
Liposuction aspirate limited to 500 mL	Propofol Endotracheal intubation and LMA Inhalational agents	Propofol Endotracheal intubation and LMA Inhalational agents	Propofol, inhalational agents, spinal and epidural anesthetics must be administered by a CRNA, anesthesia assistant, or anesthesiologist

CRNA, Certified registered nurse anesthetist; *LMA,* laryngeal mask airway.

STANDARDS

- ASPS and ASAPS mandated in 1999 that members performing plastic surgery using more than local anesthesia or oral sedation be in a facility with:
  - State licensure
  - Medicare certification, or
  - Accreditation by an organization like AAAASF, Accreditation Association for Ambulatory Health Care (AAAHC), or Joint Commission on the Accreditation of Health Care Organizations (JCAHO)[6]
- AMA and Center for Medicare Services (CMS) have similar mandates for accreditation by these or similar agencies.[1,7]
- **Generally, physicians performing surgery must:**
  - Maintain hospital privileges for all surgical procedures performed at the ASC
  - Maintain admitting privileges or at least emergency transfer agreement with nearby hospital
  - Be a member of an American Board of Medical Specialties board
- Surgical procedures performed at the ASC should be within guidelines for that specialty's scope of practice.

> **TIP:** ASPS, ASAPS, AMA, and CMS mandate facility accreditation by one of the national accrediting organizations.

LEGAL CONSIDERATIONS

FEDERAL REGULATIONS[1]

- Code of Federal Regulations requires ASCs to participate in Medicare through CMS.
- CMS requires following all state laws for accreditation or licensure.
- Previously listed standards for hospital privileges and board certification for physicians performing surgery apply for CMS coverage.
- Limit Medicare-covered surgical procedures to those with duration generally <90 minutes and <4 hours of postsurgical recovery, and type of surgery to those that:
  - Do not generally result in extensive blood loss
  - Do not require major or prolonged invasion of body cavities
  - Do not directly involve major blood vessels
  - Are generally emergency or life-threatening in nature

STATE REGULATIONS

- These vary by state, but usually comply with federal/CMS rules.
- Many states, including California, Florida, Ohio, and Pennsylvania, have accreditation requirements.[8]
- Some such as Arizona and Kentucky require registration with state or licensure.
- Most others require credentialing for physicians without nearby hospital privileges, though some states have no ASC restrictions.
- Florida, Pennsylvania, Rhode Island, and Tennessee are the only states with surgical time limits currently (e.g., 4 hours in Pennsylvania; beyond this time, reporting violations to state department of health with an explanation is required!).
  - Longer surgeries are more likely to produce nausea, vomiting, and pain, leading to more unplanned admissions, especially procedures ending after 3 pm.[9,10]
- **Liposuction aspirate volume is limited in numerous states.**

> **TIP:** Being familiar with specific state laws is essential to avoid losing accreditation. Most are readily available online through state departments of health.

NONPHYSICIAN PROVIDERS: ADVANTAGES, GUIDELINES, AND CAUTIONS

- According to ASAPS, more than 13,000,000 cosmetic procedures were performed by board-certified doctors in the United States in 2016.[11,12]
  - Nonsurgical procedures account for 85% of total.
  - Increase of 7% in 1 year
  - $15 billion spent by Americans; injectables approximately 44% of total expenditure
  - 4.6 million botulinum toxin type A injections; 2.5 million hyaluronic acid injections
  - From 2012 data, injectable procedures increase by 20% when including those by nonphysician injectors[12]
  - Demand for nonsurgical cosmetic procedures is obviously increasing, faster than physicians alone can accommodate.
  - Productivity and revenue can multiply with surgeries, while qualified nonphysician providers perform nonsurgical cosmetic procedures.

GUIDELINES

- State laws are vague and left open to reasonable interpretation by providers.[13]
- Most imply that tasks and procedures be delegated to competent, trained, licensed nonphysician providers at the discretion of the physician.
- Medical director or physician supervisor may be required to be on site at all times, occasionally, or only available by electronic communication.
- Initial consultation and treatment plan should be created with physician.[14]
- Physician should ensure ongoing training and competency of injectors.

> **TIP:** Physicians' judgment is the underlying principle, and ultimate responsibility lies with them!

CAUTIONS

- Opinions vary regarding "losing" nonsurgical procedures to nonsurgeons as other providers become more adept with injectables—physicians need to determine the culture in their community.
- Some patients may be wary of nonphysicians providing most of their nonsurgical treatment.
- State-by-state laws and recommendations vary widely (e.g., in Ohio, physician assistant laws require physician be within 60 minutes' travel time, and one physician can supervise no more than 2 physician assistants at a time).[13,15]
- Whatever model or staff structure is chosen, it is the physician's practice and reputation.

> **TIP:** State regulations for nonphysician injectors vary widely and can be different based on the training of each provider.

PATIENT SELECTION AND PATIENT SAFETY[16-21]

PATIENT SELECTION
- Consider patient comorbidities before creating a treatment plan (see Chapters 5 through 7).

MINIMIZING PATIENT DISSATISFACTION
- Familiarize yourself with and always follow standards of care
- Informed consent: Document in detail, engage each patient in a verbal discussion before signing, and include all parts: diagnosis, proposed treatment and its benefit, risks and complications, likelihood of successful treatment, alternatives to the proposed plan, consequences of declining proposed treatment.
- Use well-lit, standardized preoperative and postoperative photography (see Chapter 3).
- Listen to patients' complaints, build rapport, and understand why they presented.
- Be warm, confident but never arrogant; do not make patients feel badly for asking questions or reciting facts they found on the internet; and make them feel comfortable from the time they walk in the door.

COMPLICATIONS AND PREVENTION
- Commit to a **culture of safety,** and ask the same of the entire staff.
- Conduct internal reviews when complications occur, and report to accrediting organization and State as mandated.
- Have a malignant hyperthermia cart with necessary supplies and dantrolene (see Chapter 5).
- Have a local anesthetic systemic toxicity cart with necessary supplies and lipid emulsion.[22]
- Common complications seen in ASCs and strategies to minimize their occurrence are discussed below.

POSTOPERATIVE PAIN, NAUSEA, AND VOMITING
- Most unplanned hospital admissions result from **nausea, vomiting, pain, and dizziness.**[16]
- **Liposuction** and **breast augmentation** cause the most pain for aesthetic surgery procedures.[23]
- Pain medication dosing postoperatively should take into account patient's BMI.
- Nausea and vomiting after discharge occur in **37%** of patients
- **Age <50 years, female gender, nonsmoking status,** and **perioperative opioid use** are risk factors.
- **Propofol, nonnarcotic analgesia** (ketorolac, IV acetaminophen), and use of **local and regional anesthesia** are known to decrease risk of postoperative nausea and vomiting.[24]

INFECTION[25]
- **14%** of all complications reported to AAAASF are infections.
- Infection rate is 0.7% overall in all cases performed.
- **Infection rate is highest in abdominoplasty (0.16%),** followed by mastopexy, breast augmentation, liposuction, and facelift.

- **Risk factors** include hypothermia, smoking, obesity, hyperglycemia, heavy alcohol use, and malnutrition but no conclusive data for patients in ASCs.
- Perioperative antibiotics, antibiotic saline irrigation, normothermia, and preoperative hair removal may help to reduce incidence.[26]

HEMATOMA[25]

- **36%** of all complications reported to AAAASF are hematomas.
- Overall hematoma rate is 0.14% in all cases performed.
- 41% of those occurred in breast surgeries (two thirds were augmentations, the rest reductions or mastopexy), followed by blepharoplasty, abdominoplasty, and liposuction.
- Remain vigilant, avoid hypotensive surgery, and evaluate patients undergoing these procedures before their discharge from PACU.

VENOUS THROMBOEMBOLISM[25]

- 1.0% of all complications reported to AAAASF are DVT, and pulmonary embolism are 1.2%.
- Deep venous thrombosis rate overall is 0.004% in all cases performed, and pulmonary embolism rate is 0.005%.

CAUTION: Odds ratio for venous thromboembolism in abdominoplasty versus all other plastic surgery procedures is 5:5!

- **Higher risk when abdominoplasty combined with other procedures** (see Chapter 11)
- Genetic factors, antiphospholipid syndrome, homocysteinemia, and contraceptive or hormone replacement therapy contribute to risk.[16]
- Consider sequential compression devices in lower-risk patients, and chemoprophylaxis preoperatively and postoperatively in higher-risk patients.[27]

MORTALITY[25]

- Rare in ambulatory surgery
- 0.0024% occurrence in all plastic surgery cases
- **PE associated with 15% mortality rate**
- Caution when considering combining abdominoplasty with any additional procedures[27]

TOP TAKEAWAYS

➤ A well-trained, dedicated, trustworthy staff can be one of a physician's biggest assets in practice. Interview carefully and take the time to hire wisely.
➤ State regulations for nonphysician injectors vary widely and can be different based on the training of each provider.
➤ State-by-state laws and recommendations vary widely.
➤ Risk factors include hypothermia, smoking, obesity, hyperglycemia, heavy alcohol use, and malnutrition.

REFERENCES

1. U.S. Government Publishing Office. Electronic Code of Federal Regulations, Title 42, Part 416. Available at *www.ecfr.gov*.
2. Nahai F, Colon GA, Lewis W, et al. The practice: models, management, and marketing. In Nahai F, ed. The Art of Aesthetic Surgery: Techniques and Principles, ed 2. New York: Thieme Publishers, 2010.
3. Kuechel MC. The practice: staffing, services, and financial planning. In Nahai F, ed. The Art of Aesthetic Surgery: Techniques and Principles, ed 2. New York: Thieme Publishers, 2010.
4. Pearcy J, Terranova T. Mandate for accreditation in plastic surgery ambulatory/outpatient clinics. Clin Plast Surg 40:489, 2013.
5. American Association for Accreditation of Ambulatory Surgery Facilities. Regular Standards and Checklist for Accreditation of Ambulatory Surgery Facilities. Available at *www.aaaasf.org*.
6. American Society of Plastic Surgeons and American Society for Aesthetic Plastic Surgery, Inc. Policy Statement on Accreditation of Office Facilities. Available at *www.plasticsurgery.org*.
7. American Medical Association. Office-based Surgery Core Principles. Available at *www.ama-assn.org*.
8. American Society of Plastic Surgeons. Office-based surgery state requirements chart. Available at *www.plasticsurgery.org*.
9. Fogarty BJ, Khan K, Ashall G, et al. Complications of long operations: a prospective study of morbidity associated with prolonged operative time (>6 h). Br J Plast Surg 52:33, 1999.
10. Fortier J, Chung F, Su J. Unanticipated admission after ambulatory surgery: a prospective study. Can J Anaesth 45:612, 1997.
11. American Society for Aesthetic Plastic Surgery. 2016 ASAPS statistics. Available at *www.surgery.org*.
12. American Society for Aesthetic Plastic Surgery. News releases: cosmetic procedures increase in 2012. Available at *www.surgery.org*.
13. American Academy of Physician Assistants. State Laws and Regulations. Available at *https://www.aapa.org*.
14. American Society of Plastic Surgeons. Guiding principles: supervision of non-physician personnel in medical spas and physician offices. Available at *http://www.plasticsurgery.org*.
15. Ohio Laws and Rules. Ohio Revised Code, Title 47, Chapter 4730. Available at *codes.ohio.gov*.
16. Iverson RE. Patient safety in office-based surgery facilities: I. Procedures in the office-based surgery setting. Plast Reconstr Surg 110:1337, 2002.
17. Kataria T, Cutter TW, Apfelbaum JL. Patient selection in outpatient surgery. Clin Plast Surg 40:371, 2013.
18. Warner MA, Shields SE, Chute CG. Major morbidity and mortality within 1 month of ambulatory surgery and anesthesia. JAMA 270:1437, 1993.
19. Davenport DL, Bowe EA, Henderson WG, et al. National Surgical Quality Improvement Program (NSQIP) risk factors can be used to validate American Society of Anesthesiologists Physical Status Classification Levels. Ann Surg 243:636, 2006.
20. Gorney M. Recognition of the patient unsuitable for aesthetic surgery. Aesthet Surg J 27:626, 2007.

21. Blackburn VF, Blackburn AV. Taking a history in aesthetic surgery: SAGA—the surgeon's tool for patient selection. J Plast Reconstr Aesthet Surg 61:723, 2008.
22. Young VL. Patient safety in aesthetic surgery. In Nahai F, ed. The Art of Aesthetic Surgery: Techniques and Principles, ed 2. New York: Thieme Publishers, 2010.
23. Chung F, Ritchie E, Su J. Postoperative pain in ambulatory surgery. Anesth Analg 85:808, 1997.
24. Keyes M. Management of postoperative nausea and vomiting in ambulatory surgery: the big little problem. Clin Plast Surg 40:447, 2013.
25. Soltani AM, Keyes GR, Singer R, et al. Outpatient surgery and sequelae: an analysis of the AAAASF internet-based quality assurance and peer review database. Clin Plast Surg 40:465, 2013.
26. Nazarian Mobin SS, Keyes GR, Singer R, et al. Infections in outpatient surgery. Clin Plast Surg 40:439, 2013.
27. Iverson RE, Gomez JL. Deep venous thrombosis: prevention and management. Clin Plast Surg 40:389, 2013.

13. Anatomy, Physiology, and Disorders of the Skin

Thornwell H. Parker III, Molly Burns Austin, Alton Jay Burns

ANATOMY[1] (Fig. 13-1)

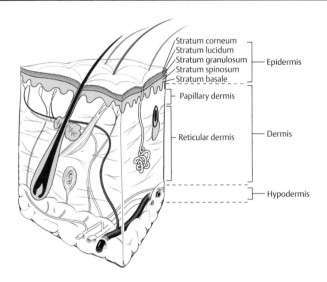

Fig. 13-1 Layers of the skin with adnexal structures.

EPIDERMIS

- The epidermis comprises the following cells:
  - *Keratinocytes:* 80% of epidermis
  - *Melanocytes:* Mostly within basal layer, pigment-producing cell, pigment provides UV protection
  - *Merkel cells:* Mostly within basal layer, mechanoreceptor, slow-adapting
  - *Langerhans cells:* Antigen-presenting/T-cell activating cells of the epidermis
- The epidermis has **five layers,** each approximately 100 µm thick:
  - *Stratum basale:* Mitotically active layer providing cells for upper layer differentiation
  - *Stratum spinosum:* Spinelike appearance of cell margins from intercellular bridging
  - *Stratum granulosum:* Intracellular granules containing materials to create skin barrier
  - *Stratum lucidum:* Clear layer of dead cells devoid of nuclei, prominent in palms/soles
  - *Stratum corneum:* Cornified layer of cells following programmed cell death of the granular layer, providing skin barrier

DERMIS
- Makes up most of skin
- Responsible for the **strength, elasticity,** and **pliability** of the skin
- Composed of primarily collagen (type I/III ratio 4:1) and elastic fibers
- Maintained by fibroblasts
- Also inhabited by macrophages and mast cells
- The dermis has **two layers:**
  - **Papillary dermis:** Superficial, similar thickness to epidermis, approximately 100 μm (thickness of all layers varies by location)
  - **Reticular dermis:** Deep, makes up most of dermis (2000-2500 μm). Collagen and elastic fibers are thicker and more organized in deeper dermis.

VASCULATURE
- Small vessels penetrate from the subcutaneous tissue and form a **horizontal vascular plexus** within the **deep reticular dermis.**
- Arterioles extend vertically from the plexus toward the epidermis, forming the subpapillary plexus at the interface of the papillary and reticular dermis.
- Individual capillary loops then extend from these end arterioles up into each papilla of the papillary dermis.

LYMPH
- Lymph vessels are important to regulating interstitial fluid balance, collecting degraded substances, and sampling for immune function

NERVES
- Nerves follow a distribution and pattern similar to those of the vasculature, with a deep reticular and subpapillary plexus.

SKIN APPENDAGES
- Hair follicles, growth cycle variable by location
  - **Anagen:** Growth phase, 2 years
  - **Catagen:** Programmed cell death, hair loss, 2 weeks
  - **Telogen:** No hair, no growth, 2 months

GLANDS
- Sebaceous glands, eccrine glands, apocrine glands
- Maintain skin hydration and assist with thermal regulation
- Provide source for epidermal regeneration—increased density on face allows resurfacing procedures, but below the jawline, reduced density delays epidermal regeneration, and can lead to scarring
- Affected by retinoids (impaired by isotretinoin, which reduces sebaceous units)

SKIN PHYSIOLOGY

NORMAL SKIN FUNCTION
- **Thermal:** Provides insulation and regulation through blood flow and eccrine secretions
- **Mechanical and chemical:** Protection against injury, infection, and water loss
- **Metabolism:** Vitamin D conversion

- **Sensation:** Sensation, temperature, pressure, and vibration
- **Aesthetics**

NORMAL SKIN AGING (Fig. 13-2)

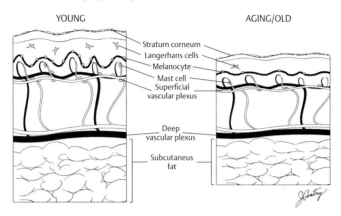

YOUNG   AGING/OLD

Stratum corneum
Langerhans cells
Melanocyte
Mast cell
Superficial
vascular plexus
Deep
vascular plexus
Subcutaneus
fat

Fig. 13-2   Histology of aging skin. Aging skin is shown on the right.

HISTOLOGY

- Thinning of epidermis
- Flattening of the rete ridges
- Thinning and degeneration of the dermis, collagen, and elastic fibers (solar elastosis)
- Atrophy of subcutaneous tissue

CLINICAL PICTURE

- Thinning skin
- Lost elasticity
- Facial laxity
- Facial rhytids
- Loss of facial volume

WOUND HEALING[2,3]

- **Inflammation (days 1 to 6)**
  - Vasoconstriction ➤ coagulation ➤ vasodilation/capillary leak ➤ chemotaxis ➤ cell migration
  - Neutrophils ➤ macrophages ➤ lymphocytes
    - ▶ **Macrophage** most important to regulate growth factors and wound healing
- **Proliferation (day 4 to week 3)**
  - Fibroblasts predominate, increased collagen synthesis, and angiogenesis
- **Maturation (week 3 to 1 year)**
  - Equilibrium between collagen deposition and breakdown
  - Increased collagen organization and stronger cross-links
  - Type I collagen replaces type III to restore 4:1 ratio
  - Healing strength begins to plateau at approximately **60 days at 80% original strength.**

- **Reepithelialization**
  - **Mobilization:** Loss of contact inhibition occurs for cells at edge of wound.
  - **Migration:** Cells migrate across wound until they meet cells from other side.
  - **Mitosis:** As edge cells migrate, cells farther back proliferate to support migration.
- **Contraction**
  - Myofibroblasts (specialized fibroblasts) appear by day 3 and are maximal by day 10 to 21, with greater numbers and contraction in full thickness/deeper wounds.

FACTORS AFFECTING WOUND HEALING

GENETIC SKIN DISORDERS
- **Cutis laxa**
  - Nonfunctioning elastase inhibitor leads to elastic fiber degeneration.
  - Skin has coarse texture, droops over all of body, and is diagnosed during neonatal or early childhood.
  - Congestive heart disease, emphysema, pneumothorax, aneurysms, and hernias may also occur.
  - It slowly worsens over time, but **surgical correction can be beneficial.**
- **Pseudoxanthoma elasticum**
  - Similarities to cutis laxa, with loose skin secondary to elastic fiber degeneration
  - **May also benefit from surgery**
- **Ehlers-Danlos**
  - Disorder of collagen cross-linking
  - Leads to fragile, hyperelastic skin, hypermobile joints, and aortic aneurysms
  - **Surgery <u>contraindicated</u> because poor wound healing**
- **Elastoderma**
  - Poorly understood cause
  - Pendulous skin over trunk and extremities, eventually entire body
  - **Surgery <u>contraindicated</u>**
- **Progeria (also known as Hutchinson-Gilford syndrome)**
  - Rapid progression and short lifespan, from childhood
  - Laxity and irregular skin contouring, craniofacial malformations, cardiac disease, ear abnormalities, and poor wound healing
  - **Surgery <u>contraindicated,</u> poor wound healing**

COMORBIDITIES
- Diabetes
- Atherosclerotic disease
- Renal failure
- Immunodeficiency

NUTRITIONAL DEFICIENCIES
- Vitamins and minerals (vitamin C, zinc, iron)
- Caloric
- Protein (check albumin, prealbumin, transferrin, and haptoglobin)

DRUGS
- **Smoking:** Vasoconstriction and decreased oxygen delivery
- **Steroids:** Impair wound healing

- **Antineoplastic agents:** Impair fibroblast proliferation and wound contraction
- **Antiinflammatory medicine:** Decreases collagen synthesis 45%
- **Lathyrogens:** Prevent collagen cross-linking

LOCAL WOUND FACTORS
- **Moisture:** Speeds epithelialization
- **Warmth:** Increased tensile strength
- **Unfavorable:** Poor oxygen delivery, infection, chronic wound, denervation, radiotherapy, free radicals

SKIN ANALYSIS[4]

SKIN QUALITY
- Skin type[5] (Table 13-1)
- Skin texture
- Thickness
- Pore size
- Sebaceous quality
- Discoloration: Hyperpigmentation, solar lentigo, rosacea, telangiectasias
- Scarring: Acne, surgery, trauma

Table 13-1   *Fitzpatrick Skin Type Classification*

Skin Type	Characteristics	Sun Exposure History
I	Pale white, freckles, blue eyes, blond or red hair	Always burns, never tans
II	Fair white, blue/green/hazel eyes, blond or red hair	Usually burns, minimally tans
III	Cream white, any hair or eye color	Sometimes burns, tans uniformly
IV	Moderate brown (Mediterranean)	Rarely burns, always tans well
V	Dark brown (Middle Eastern)	Rarely burns, tans easily
VI	Dark brown to black	Never burns, tans easily

TIP: Patients with Fitzpatrick skin types V and VI are at higher risk for hyperpigmentation, but show fewer signs of photoaging.

AGING FACE
- Laxity
- Redundancy
- Rhytids
  - **Static rhytids:** At rest, treat with resurfacing, fillers, surgery
  - **Dynamic rhytids:** Accentuated with animation, respond to neurotoxin
- Volume loss
- Volume displacement (gravity)

SKIN LESIONS
Many patients will request cosmetic nevus removal or scar revision from other procedures. Surgeons need to distinguish diagnostic features of common skin lesions and cancers to properly diagnose and treat these patients.

Common Skin Cancers
- **Basal cell cancer (BCC)**[6]
  - **No. 1 skin cancer,** accounting for 75% of all nonmelanoma skin cancers (NMSC)
  - 30% on nose[7]
  - **Risk:** Increased with fair skin, blond or red hair, blue or green eyes, UV exposure
  - **Appearance:** Translucent, rolled border, telangiectasia, central ulceration
  - **Location:** Most often head and neck
  - **Types:**
    - ▶ **Nodular:** 50% of BCC
    - ▶ **Superficial:** Appears as an erythematous, scaly, eczematous-looking patch, often on trunk
    - ▶ **Pigmented BCC:** Brown pigmentation, look-alike for melanoma
    - ▶ **Sclerotic/morpheaform:** White scarlike appearance, sometimes atrophic or depressed
- **Squamous cell cancer (SCC)**[8]
  - No. 2 skin cancer
  - Most arise from actinic keratosis (60%) or SCC in situ (Bowen disease)
  - **Location:** Favor head, neck, dorsal hands, and forearms
  - **Appearance**: Firm, flesh-colored nodule, central keratin plug, can also be erythematous and plaque
  - **Additional risk factors:** Significant increase in prevalence and aggressiveness secondary to immune suppression and radiotherapy
  - **High-risk SCC:** Merits consideration for lymph node evaluation and occasionally radiation. High-risk factors include size >2 cm, poor differentiation, recurrence, perineural or perivascular invasion, and lip and intraoral lesions.
  - **Variants**
    - ▶ **In situ:** Slowly enlarging erythematous plaque, scaly or slightly verrucous surface; if untreated, can progress to invasive SCC
    - ▶ **Keratoacanthoma:** Rapidly growing (within a few weeks) crateriform nodule, often 1-2 cm size, on sun-exposed skin, may slowly involute over a period of months. Although often known for spontaneous resolution, keratoacanthomas can metastasize on occasion and can be very destructive locally. Many consider them to be a variant of SCC.
  - *Patients with a history of one SCC are at a 50% risk of developing another NMSC*[9]
- **Melanoma**[10]
  - Third most common skin cancer, 5% of skin cancer
  - Estimated 55,000 invasive, 35,000 in situ in United States per year
  - **Men:** Upper back, upper extremities
  - **Women:** Back, lower extremities
  - **Subtypes:** Superficial spreading 50%-70%, nodular 15%-30%, lentigo maligna 4%-10% (melanoma on sun-damaged skin, commonly on the face)
  - **Prognosis: Depth** (Breslow thickness) most important to staging and prognosis, **best if <0.75 mm, worst if >4 mm;** sentinel node biopsy should be considered for anything in between.
  - **Appearance:**
    - ▶ (A)symmetry
    - ▶ (B)orders irregularity
    - ▶ (C)olor variations

- ▶ (D)iameter >6 mm
- ▶ (E)volving or changing
- **Treatment**
  - **Mohs micrographic surgery:** Treatment of choice for many skin cancers
    - ▶ Especially useful for head, neck, or hands, large, aggressive, ill-defined, or recurrent tumors[11-15]
    - ▶ Cure rate: Primary BCC >99%,[11,12,13] SCC 96%-97%,[14] MM >99%[15]
  - **Traditional surgical excision:** Standard margins typically taken based on tumor size and type
  - **Electrodessication and curettage (ED&C):** Often used on superficial BCC of the trunk or extremities, allowed to heal secondarily
  - **Cryosurgery:** Typical liquid nitrogen used to freeze actinic keratoses and precancerous lesions, causes epidermolysis and sloughing of lesion
  - **Radiotherapy:** Typically reserved for patients with combination of numerous comorbidities, limited lifespan, and number lesions requiring treatment
  - **Topical therapy:**
    - ▶ 5-FU (Carac or Efudex) used for treatment of actinic keratoses and some superficial nonmelanoma skin cancers, is approved for small superficial BCCs
    - ▶ Imiquimod (Aldara or Zyclara): Historically used for verruca, also used with some success on superficial skin cancers and actinic keratoses
  - **Photodynamic therapy (PDT):** Aminolevulinic acid (ALA) applied to skin, incubate usually 1-3 hours, then activated under blue light. For actinic keratosis, less downtime than 5-FU or imiquimod.

Premalignant Lesions
- **Actinic keratosis**
  - **Appearance:** Rough/scaly erythematous patches/plaques
  - **Location:** Sun-exposed areas, like the scalp, face (especially the forehead, cheeks, nose, rim of ear), dorsal hands/forearms
  - **Precursor to SCC:** Approximately 10% eventually progress to become SCC, and 60% of SCC arise within an actinic keratosis.[16]

Common Benign Lesions
- **Flesh colored**
  - **Sebaceous hyperplasia**
    - ▶ Small yellow or flesh-colored, finely lobulated papules, may have slight umbilicated appearance
    - ▶ May resemble BCC
    - ▶ Face, particularly forehead and cheeks
  - **Fibrous papules**
    - ▶ Small, firm, white or flesh-colored, smooth dome-shaped papule
    - ▶ Often on or around nose
    - ▶ May resemble BCC, but usually firm and white in appearance
  - **Nevi**
    - ▶ Nonpigmented nevi may resemble BCC, often more flaccid and prone to wrinkling on palpation (see Pigmented lesions)
  - **Syringomas**
    - ▶ Small, smooth, yellow or flesh-colored papules
    - ▶ On the face, particularly the lower eyelids

- **Pigmented lesions**
  - **Seborrheic keratosis**
    - ▶ Extremely common after 30 years of age, hereditary
    - ▶ Lack a true pigment network
    - ▶ Begin as sharply demarcated brown macules that evolve into elevated lesion with a warty, rough, or waxy and follicular surface, often appearing "stuck on"; color can vary from dark brown to white to flesh colored
    - ▶ Although benign and classic in appearance, patients frequently concerned about melanoma, because the lesions are "dark, ugly, growing, and raised up"
  - **Acrochordon (skin tag)**
    - ▶ Polypoid/pedunculated papule, often found on axillas, head, and neck; thought to be a variant of a seborrheic keratosis
  - **Lentigo (solar lentigo)**
    - ▶ Circumscribed, pigmented macules with "moth-eaten" border on sun-exposed skin; usually, surrounding areas have other similar macules.
    - ▶ Benign
  - **Nevi (acquired)**
    - ▶ Most grow during second and third decades of life.
    - ▶ Symmetrical with regular, sharp border, even color (white, flesh colored, red, or brown)
    - ▶ Dermal nevi and compound nevi: More often raised in appearance, with a larger population of neval cells present in the dermis; compound nevi also have neval cell activity along the dermal-epidermal junction.
    - ▶ Junctional nevi: Usually flat in appearance, neval cells mostly present along dermal-epidermal junction
    - ▶ Benign
  - **Congenital nevi**
    - ▶ Present from birth, range from small to giant size, often darker than acquired nevi
    - ▶ Increased risk for melanoma, especially with **giant congenital nevi,** up to **7%** risk; risk related to size; small congenital nevi carry relatively low risk.
    - ▶ Concern that melanoma may not be discovered until a later stage because hidden within the nevus
  - **Dysplastic nevi (atypical melanocytic nevi)**
    - ▶ Although they share some of the atypical clinical and histologic features of melanoma, these are very common and are most often considered benign.
    - ▶ Sometimes mislabeled as "premelanomas"
    - ▶ Patients with increased numbers of atypical nevi and/or a family history of melanoma are at increased risk for melanoma.
    - ▶ Not all dysplastic nevi warrant excision, but these patients require careful observation and regular screening.
  - **Dermatofibroma**
    - ▶ Often begins as a firm, erythematous papule <1 cm size, slowing involuting, and changing color to darker shades of brown
    - ▶ Benign
- **Vascular lesions**
  - **Angiomas:** Small, bright red papules, may become purple and venous
  - **Telangiectasias:** Dilated capillaries
  - **Spider angioma:** Dilated capillaries radiating from central arteriole
  - **Varicose veins:** Dilated veins
  - **Venous lake:** Venous malformation on the lip

> **SENIOR AUTHOR TIP:** Rosacea is not really a "vascular lesion" per se, but rather more of an inflammatory condition within the acne family that can result in telangiectasias on the face.

PHYSIOLOGY OF COMMON MEDICAL SKIN THERAPIES

TOPICAL RETINOID THERAPY
- DNA binding, **inhibits AP1 transcription,** decreasing metalloprotease activation
- Reverses photoaging, thins stratum corneum, thickens epidermis, reverses atypia, increases collagen and angiogenesis, and evens melanin dispersion
- Most commonly used for acne
- Daily use >4 years improves rhytids and hyperpigmentation

HYDROQUINONES
- Block conversion of dopamine to melanin by **inhibiting tyrosinase enzyme**
- Useful for preventing hyperpigmentation

KERATINOLYTIC AGENTS/CHEMICAL PEELS
- **Dissolve intercellular connections,** allowing desquamation
- Reduce fine rhytids by increased desquamation
- Melanocyte toxicity may lead to hypopigmentation, although inflammation may lead to hyperpigmentation.

5-FU (CARAC, EFUDEX)
- **Blocks DNA synthesis** as a thymine analogue
- Clinically affects sun-damaged skin, destroying actinic keratosis
- Significant irritation, erythema, pain, and pruritus often accompany a typical course of treatment. Patients may also have bleeding and crusting.

SUNSCREEN
- **Mechanical blockers**
  - Zinc and titanium products
  - Traditionally pasty white in appearance
  - Newer products contain micronized zinc and titanium, which are more translucent.
  - Provides good UVB and UVA coverage, typically with longer half-life
  - Even protective against wavelengths in the visible light range
- **Chemical blockers**
  - Historically, UVB was main concern, but increasing research showing dangers of UVA underestimated
    - ► UVA is 10× more abundant, not filtered by glass, less affected by time of day or atmosphere, and penetrates 5× deeper in skin; therefore 100× more photons reach dermis.
  - Sunscreens and sunblocks do not measure UVA blockage.
  - **SPF is UVB specific.**
  - Many sunscreens block UVB well, but block UVA poorly.
  - Block by absorption of UV
  - **Avobenzone** is most commonly used for UVA blockage, but is quickly broken down by UV in 20 minutes, limiting half-life. Helioplex by Neutrogena and Anthelios with Mexoryl by L'Oréal stabilize avobenzone and increase half-life of UV blockage.

> ## Top Takeaways
> ➤ The epidermis is composed of five layers. The two most superficial layers (stratum corneum an dstratum lucidum) are made up of nonviable keratinocytes.
> ➤ Collagen provides the tensile strength of the skin.
> ➤ Type 1 collagen replaces type III to restore a 4:1 ratio.
> ➤ Predictable physiologic and histologic skin changes occur with age.
> ➤ Patients with increased numbers of atypical nevi and/or a family history of melanoma are at increased risk for melanoma.

References

1. Chu DH, Haake AR, Holbrook K, et al. The structure and development of skin. In Freedberg IM, Eisen AZ, Wolff K, et al, eds. Fitzpatrick's Dermatology in General Medicine, ed 6. New York: McGraw-Hill, 2003.
2. Janis JE, Harrison B. Wound healing: part I. Basic science. Plast Reconst Surg 133:199e, 2014.
3. Glat P, Longaker M. Wound healing. In Aston SJ, Beasley RW, Thorne CH, et al, eds. Grabb and Smith's Plastic Surgery, ed 5. Philadelphia: Lippincott-Raven, 1997.
4. Baker TJ, Stuzin JM, Baker TM, eds. Facial Skin Resurfacing. New York: Thieme Publishers, 1998.
5. Fitzpatrick TB. The validity and practicality of sun-reactive skin types I though VI. Arch Dermatol 124:869, 1988.
6. Carucci JA, Leffell DJ. Basal cell carcinoma. In Freedberg IM, Eisen AZ, Wolff K, et al, eds. Fitzpatrick's Dermatology in General Medicine, ed 6. New York: McGraw-Hill, 2003.
7. Gloster HM Jr, Brodland DG. The epidemiology of skin cancer. Dermatol Surg 22:217, 1996.
8. Grossman D, Leffel DJ. Squamous cell carcinoma. In Freeberg IM, Eisen AZ, Wolff K, et al, eds. Fitzpatrick's Dermatology in General Medicine, ed 6. New York: McGraw-Hill, 2003.
9. Marcil I, Stern RS. Risk of developing a subsequent nonmelanoma skin cancer in patients with a history of nonmelanoma skin cancer: a critical review of the literature and meta-analysis. Arch Dermatol 136:1524, 2000.
10. Langley RG, Barnhill RL, Mihm MC Jr, et al. Neoplasms: cutaneous melanoma. In Freedberg IM, Eisen AZ, Wolff K, et al, eds. Fitzpatrick's Dermatology in General Medicine, ed 6. New York: McGraw-Hill, 2003.
11. Rowe D, Carroll R, Day C. Long-term recurrence rates in previously untreated (primary) basal cell carcinoma: implications for patient follow-up. J Dermatol Surg Oncol 15:315, 1989.
12. Cottel WI, Proper S. Mohs' surgery, fresh-tissue technique. Our technique with a review. J Dermatol Surg Oncol 8:576, 1982.
13. Mohs FE. The chemosurgical method for the microscopically controlled excision of cutaneous cancer. In Epstein E, ed. Skin Surgery. Philadelphia: Lea & Febiger, 1976.
14. Nguyen TH, Ho DQ. Nonmelanoma skin cancer. Curr Treat Options Oncol 3:193, 2002.
15. Zitelli JA, Brown C, Hanusa BH. Mohs micrographic surgery for the treatment of primary cutaneous melanoma. J Am Acad Dermatol 37:236, 1997.
16. Marks R, Rennie G, Selwood TS. Malignant transformation of solar keratoses to squamous cell carcinoma. Lancet 1:795, 1988.

14. Cosmeceuticals and Other Office Products

Sammy Sinno, Zoe Diana Draelos

Cosmeceuticals is a term combining the concepts of cosmetics and pharmaceuticals. These products are over the counter and considered active cosmetics, delivering more to the skin than simply color or scent adornment. No U.S. Food and Drug Administration–recognized category for cosmeceuticals has been established.[1,2]

> **TIP:** The primary benefit provided by cosmeceuticals is enhanced skin moisturization.

- Comprehensive treatment involves **cleansing, moisturization,** and **photoprotection.**
- Treatments are aimed at improving the appearance of dry and aging skin.
- Aging skin is induced by:[3]
  - UV exposure
  - The creation of dermal scars from reactive oxygen species
  - Chronic inflammation inducing the activation of matrix metalloproteinases (collagenase, elastase)
- Dry skin can be caused by excessive cleansing and low humidity conditions (air travel, forced-air gas heat).

CLEANSERS[4]

- Main active ingredients are **surfactants.**
- These surfactants may be formulated as bar cleansers or liquid cleansers (Table 14-1).
- Patients with **dry skin** benefit from surfactants that remove **less skin surface sebum** (i.e., cleansing cream or oil).
- High detergent surfactants may remove skin surface sebum and intercellular lipids, leading to barrier damage, inability of skin to hold water, and dry skin.
- Cleansers remove sebum, perspiration, cosmetics, dust, and microorganisms.
- Cleansers based on sodium cocoyl isethionate are low detergent and well tolerated in those with dry skin.
- Individuals with **dry skin** may benefit from using **cooler water** when washing.

Table 14-1   *Key Features of Surfactants*

Surfactant	Key Features
Superfatted soaps (bar surfactant)	Enhance mildness and lather through incomplete saponification Unreacted fatty acids/oils left in soap or added to soap during production
Transparent soap (bar surfactant)	High levels of humectants, giving a clear appearance Can cause irritation but are usually mild products
Combination bars	Combine natural soaps with milder synthetics Less likely to cause irritation
Synthetic bars	Sodium cocoyl isethionate most commonly used (adds mildness to product) Formulated in neutral pH range
Liquid surfactants	Often combined anionic (i.e., alkyl ether sulfate, alkyl sulfosuccinates) and amphoteric (i.e., cocoamphoacetate, cocamidopropyl betaine) Nonionic surfactants (i.e., acyl glycinates) increasingly more common

SENIOR AUTHOR TIP: Synthetic moisturizers, also known as *syndets,* are labeled as beauty bars and are milder because they remove less sebum.

MOISTURIZERS

Best moisturizers contain occlusives and humectants.[5,6]

PETROLATUM (OCCLUSIVE)
- Second most commonly used active ingredient (after water)
- **Very effective moisturizing agent,** reducing transepidermal water loss by **99%** (occlusive function)
- When applied to wounded skin, **enhances water retention** thus improving fibroblast migration
- Decreases fine rhytids of dehydration
- Reduces pain and itching by forming an artificial barrier
- *Often criticized by patients for being too greasy*

LANOLIN (OCCLUSIVE)
- Derived from **sheep sebaceous secretions**
- Contain **cholesterol,** which is a component of lipids in the strateum corneum
- May be a source of **allergic contact dermatitis**
- Lanolin alcohol used in some cosmetics

OILS (OCCLUSIVE)
- Important in **maintaining skin barrier**
- Include mineral oil, vegetable oils (safflower oil, sunflower oil, jojoba oil, hemp oil, grape seed oil, and olive oil), cetyl alcohol
- Oils are hydrophobic and lipophilic

DIMETHICONE (OCCLUSIVE)
- Also very common moisturizer
- Silicone derivative
- Can function as emollient, making skin smooth by **filling spaces between desquamating corneocytes**
- Does not create greasy shine in patients with oily skin

GLYCERIN (HUMECTANT)
- Draws water from dermis and epidermis into dehydrated stratum corneum
- Shown to **regulate water channels in the skin** (aquaporins), allowing passage of ions and solutes
- Thought to hydrate and improve overall appearance of skin

SENIOR AUTHOR TIP: Glycerin has a reservoir effect in the skin due to the modulation of aquaporins, which adjust skin osmotic balance.

RETINOIDS[7,8]
- **Refers to vitamin A and all of its synthetic derivatives**
- Regulate epithelial cell growth and differentiation
- Bind to specific cellular receptors
- Act as an UV filter, antimicrobial, antioxidant
- High-quality evidence to support use in prescription treatment of photoaging (tretinoin), but less effect when used in cosmeceuticals (retinol, retinyl propionate, retinaldehyde)

TIP: Retinol-based cosmeceuticals may have a beneficial effect on photoaging.

ANTIOXIDANTS[9]
Vitamin C
- L-ascorbic acid
- **Stimulates collagen synthesis,** inhibits elastase
- Photoprotective effects seen in animal studies
- Also antioxidant, regenerates vitamin E, antiinflammatory
- Many formulations unstable and cannot penetrate dermis

Vitamin E
- Tocopherols and tocotrienols
- Primary **antioxidant** preventing lipid oxidation and protecting cellular membrane from free radicals
- Shown to **enhance photoprotection** in animals

Coenzyme Q10
- **Very potent antioxidant** manufactured by the body
- **Inhibits collagenase** after UV radiation
- Considered a tertiary antioxidant

ALPHA-HYDROXY ACIDS (AHAS)
- Found in nature
- Include glycolic acid, lactic acid, malic acid, citric acid, and tartaric acid
- Glycolic and lactic acid most commonly used in cosmetic preparations
  - Glycolic acid, known as the *lunchtime peel,* used in many office treatments
  - Must be neutralized after use
  - Lactic acid used in many over-the-counter preparations
- Salicylic acid, a beta-hydroxy acid, is a chemical exfoliant used in over-the-counter preparations and in stronger concentrations for in-office peels.

- **AHAs enhance stratum corneum exfoliation.**
- Aid in treating photodamage, hyperpigmentation, and melasma
- Also used for treating dry skin, acne, rosacea

> **SENIOR AUTHOR TIP:**   Glycolic acid disrupts the ionic bonds in the skin inducing exfoliation, however it also rapidly penetrates to the dermis causing stinging and burning. It should be used with care in patients with sensitive skin.

SUNSCREENS

- Contain "filters" designed to absorb or reflect UVA and UVB radiation[3]
- **UVA** radiation is responsible for **photoaging.**
  - UVA organic filters: Benzophenones, ecamsule, anthranilates, avobenzone
- **UVB** radiation causes **sunburn.**
  - UVB organic filters: Paraaminobenzoic acid, salicylates, cinnamates

> **TIP:**   A well-formulated sunscreen should protect against both UVA and UVB radiation.

- Inorganic filters include zinc oxide and titanium dioxide.
- Inorganic filters must be used with organic filters because of the undesirable skin whitening that can occur.
- Sunscreens can prevent photoaging but cannot reverse damage.

BOTANICALS

- Primary role as **antioxidants**
- Three main categories:
  - Flavonoids (soy, silymarin)
  - Polyphenols (curcumin, green tea)
  - Carotenoids (retinol) (Table 14-2)

Table 14-2   *Common Botanicals*

Botanical	Key Features
Soy	Rich in isoflavones Estrogenic effect thought to increase collagen synthesis
Silymarin	Derived from milk thistle plant Decrease formation of pyrimidine dimers in mouse model
Curcumin	Derived from turmeric A hydrogenated form acts as moisturizer and maintains lipids in formulation[10,11]
Green tea	Decreases formation of pyrimidine dimers[12]
Retinol	Naturally occurring vitamin A Topically functions as antioxidant Cutaneously converted to retinoic acid, which is known to improve photodamaged skin
Lycopene	Found in fruits and vegetables (tomatoes, watermelon) Shown to lower oxidative stress Often found in various eye creams and moisturizers
Grape seed extract	Potent free radical scavenger

OTHER NATURAL INGREDIENTS

- **Aloe vera:** Thought to have antiinflammatory properties
  - Active constituents include salicylates, magnesium lactate, and thromboxane inhibitors
- **Ginseng:** Antiinflammatory
- **Licorice:** Antiinflammatory
- **Mushroom extract:** Antioxidant and antiinflammatory
- **Chamomile:** Thought to improve elasticity and texture of skin
  - Some patients report allergic contact dermatitis, use with caution
- **Feverfew:** Derived from a small bush with citrus leaves
  - Thought to have antiinflammatory properties
- **Turmeric:** Antiinflammatory
- **Selenium:** Protects against cellular oxidative damage

TREATMENT OF PIGMENTED SKIN

- Regimens should include a cleanser (glycolic acid) followed by tyrosinase-inhibiting serum/moisturizer (i.e., kojic acid or hydroquinone)
- Hydroquinone and kojic acid (derived from *Aspergillus, Acetobacter,* and *Penicillium* fungal species), inhibits tyrosinase
- Hydroxyquinone used in treatment of postinflammatory hyperpigmentation and melasma

---

TOP TAKEAWAYS

➤ Cosmeceuticals are cosmetics, which are not regulated by the FDA.
➤ Comprehensive treatment involves cleansing, moisturization, and UVA/UVB broad-spectrum sun protection.
➤ Petrolatum (oil based) and dimethicone (oil free) are commonly used occlusive moisturizer ingredients.
➤ Retinaldehyde is a retinol-based cosmeceutical with evidence to support an effect on photoaging.
➤ UVA radiation is responsible for photoaging, whereas UVB radiation induces sunburn.

REFERENCES

1. Aston SJ, Steinbrech DS, Walden JL. Aesthetic Plastic Surgery. Philadelphia: Saunders Elsevier, 2010.
2. Babamiri K, Nassab R. Cosmeceuticals: the evidence behind the retinoids. Aesthet Surg J 30:74, 2010.
3. Chatterjee L, Agarwal R, Mukhtar H. Ultraviolet B radiation-induced DNA lesions in mouse epidermis: an assessment using a novel 32P-postlabeling technique. Biochem Biophys Res Commun 229:590, 1996.
4. Draelos ZD. Active agents in common skin care products. Plast Reconstr Surg 125:719, 2010.
5. Friberg SE, Ma Z. Stratum corneum lipids, petrolatum and white oils. Cosmet Toilet 107:55, 1993.
6. Spencer TS. Dry skin and skin moisturizers. Clin Dermatol 6:24, 1988.

7. Duell EA, Derguini F, Kang S, et al. Extraction of human epidermis treated with retinol yields retro-retinoids in addition to free retinol and retinyl esters. J Invest Dermatol 107:178, 1996.

8. Torras H. Retinoids in aging. Clin Dermatol 14:207, 1996.

9. Sinno S, Lee DS, Khachemoune A. Vitamins and cutaneous wound healing. J Wound Care 20:287, 2011.

10. Maheux R, Naud F, Rioux M, et al. A randomized, double-blind, placebo-controlled study on the effect of conjugated estrogens on skin thickness. Am J Obstet Gynecol 170:642, 1994.

11. Menon VP, Sudheer AR. Antioxidant and anti-inflammatory properties of curcumin. Adv Exp Med Biol 595:105, 2007.

12. Katiyar SK, Perez A, Mukhtar H. Green tea polyphenol treatment to human skin prevents formation of ultraviolet light B-induced pyrimidine dimers in DNA. Clin Cancer Res 6:3864, 2000.

15. Ethnic Skin Care

Sammy Sinno, Zoe Diana Draelos

- People of color are 40% of the population in the United States.[1]
  - Hispanics and blacks are the groups growing in number most rapidly.
- Racial minorities receive approximately 20% of all cosmetic procedures.
- Unique issues to ethnic skin care can include:[2,3]
  - Restoring uniform pigmentation
  - Hair removal
  - Acne care
  - Skin hydration
- **Ethnic skin contains:**
  - More cell layers in stratum corneum (22 layers in black skin versus 17 in white skin)[4]
  - Increased lipid content
  - Increased desquamation
  - Decreased ceramide content
- Increased photoprotection with darker skin, but also robust response to epidermal/dermal injury[5]

> **TIP:** Understanding the subtleties of treating various ethnicities is essential to maximize results.

PATIENT EVALUATION

- Fitzpatrick scale was developed by Dr. Thomas Fitzpatrick, a Harvard dermatologist, in 1975 (Table 15-1).
  - Used for classifying response of different skin types to UV light[6]

Table 15-1 *Fitzpatrick Skin Type Classification*

Skin Type	Characteristics	Sun Exposure History
I	Pale white, freckles, blue eyes, blond or red hair	Always burns, never tans
II	Fair white, blue/green/hazel eyes, blond or red hair	Usually burns, minimally tans
III	Cream white, any hair or eye color	Sometimes burns, tans uniformly
IV	Moderate brown (Mediterranean)	Rarely burns, always tans well
V	Dark brown (Middle Eastern)	Rarely burns, tans easily
VI	Dark brown to black	Never burns, tans easily

> **TIP:** The number of melanocytes does not differ between skin types, but darker-skinned individuals produce more melanin.

> **SENIOR AUTHOR TIP:**   Fitzpatrick skin types are not always accurate presently as many individuals are now biracial. Persons with an African father and an Irish mother may have dark skin, but freckle with sun exposure.

- Obtain accurate patient history.
- Identify natural hydration level of skin:
  - Normal
  - Dry
  - Oily
  - Combination
- Dark-skinned people can be predisposed to oily or dry skin.[7]
  - Also can have severe reactions to treatment and poor wound healing with excessive scar formation (keloids or hypertrophic scars) and postinflammatory hyperpigmentation

HYDRATION

- Darker skin tends to dry and crack more easily and has a higher propensity to develop acne.
  - Associated with **higher transepidermal water loss** (TEWL)
- Pigmented skin scale produces ashy appearance, magnifying dry skin problems.
  - Drying over-the-counter products should be avoided.
  - Impaired barrier function can lead to inflammation, irritation, increased hyperpigmentation after treatments.

> **TIP:**   Gentle cleansers and emollient moisturizers smooth skin scale and help to optimize appearance in skin of color.

DYSCHROMIA

- **Hypopigmentation:** Melanocyte underproduction of melanin
- **Vitiligo:** A condition of skin depigmentation from absent melanin production
  - Particularly noticeable in people with darker skin, causing emotional distress
  - Possible autoimmune condition directed at melanocytes
  - Commonly associated with thyroid disorders (Hashimoto thyroiditis), pernicious anemia, diabetes
  - Diagnosis with Wood lamp (black light)
  - Some improvement can be seen with camouflage using stains, makeup, or self-tanning lotions.
  - **Treatment:** Phototherapy, immunomodulators, topical steroids
- **Hyperpigmentation:** Increased melanocyte stimulation, typically a postinflammatory response resulting in increased pigmentation
  - **Treatment:** Skin-lightening agents suppressing melanin production by inhibiting tyrosinase
  - Hydroquinone typically used in concentrations of 2% over-the-counter or 4% prescription strength
  - Irritation and contact dermatitis common complications
  - Commonly used pigmentation inhibitors listed in Table 15-2

> **SENIOR AUTHOR TIP:**   Infrared A is the source of heat from the sun, but may also induce hyperpigmentation, especially in individuals of higher Fitzpatrick skin type. Thus, persons with hyperpigmentation should also avoid heat exposure.

Table 15-2   *Commonly Used Pigmentation Inhibitors*

Inhibitor	Mechanism of Action
Hydroquinone	Inhibits tyrosinase by inhibiting DNA and RNA synthesis
Kojic acid	Chelates copper bound to tyrosinase rendering it inactive
Azelaic acid	Naturally derived from grain products and by oxygenation of oleic acid Cytotoxic to melanocytes
Lactic acid	Suppresses formation of melanocytes
Retinoids	Inhibits tyrosinase activity
Arbutin	Found naturally in cranberries Inhibits melanosome maturation Less irritating than hyroquinone

ACNE

■ Darker-skinned individuals have **thicker follicular epithelium.**[8]
  • Less likely to develop nodulocystic acne
  • More likely to keratinize and form comedones
  • Can give appearance of skin irritation
  • Commonly seen on face, back, shoulders, upper chest
  • Nodules and cysts can form, which can be complicated by keloid or hypertrophic scar formation
■ Major goal is to **prevent postinflammatory hyperpigmentation.**
  • Early intervention needed
  • Monotherapy often ineffective
  • Studies have shown combination therapy most effective: clindamycin, topical retinoid, benzoyl peroxide
■ Commonly used agents are listed in Table 15-3.

Table 15-3   *Commonly Used Agents in Treating Acne in Ethnic Skin*

Agent	Characteristics
Kojic acid	Fungal-derived antibacterial Patch test because of possibility of contact dermatitis
Lactic acid	Promotes desquamation of stratum corneum and inhibits tyrosinase Increases water content of epidermis (humectant)
Azelaic acid	Antibacterial and antiinflammatory
Retinoids	Vitamin A family Normalize follicular keratinization High risk of irritation associated with retinoic acid prevented with retinol
Licorice	Antiinflammatory Effective in preventing postinflammatory hyperpigmentation
Salicylic acid	Lipophilic Penetrates sebaceous plugs Minimal risk of topical irritation

SUNSCREEN

- Role of sunscreen in preventing skin cancers is important in skin of color.
- UVA and UVB are effectively reflected by products containing titanium dioxide and zinc dioxide, but these inorganic sunscreens can cause skin whitening in skin of color.

SENIOR AUTHOR TIP: Organic sunscreens take solar radiation and transform it to heat thereby preventing skin damage. However, heat can trigger a variety of skin conditions, including rosacea. Inorganic sunscreens are a better choice in persons with rosacea.

HAIR REMOVERS

- Use is higher in blacks because of **higher incidence of pseudofolliculitis barbae.**
- Hair removers, or chemical depilatories, cause **degradation of hair shaft disulfide bonds** and **swelling of hair shaft.**
  - *These hairs are so soft after treatment; they can be removed with rubbing.*
- Most common active ingredients are **calcium thioglycolate** and **sodium thioglycolate.**
- Blacks typically require stronger ingredients because of the coarseness of their hair; therefore the following ingredients are used:
  - Strontium sulfide
  - Barium sulfide
  - Potassium hydroxide
  - Sodium hydroxide

TIP: Chemical depilatories can be very irritating, inducing postinflammatory hyperpigmentation in skin of color.

SOFT TISSUE FILLERS

- No difference noted with injection in darker Fitzpatrick skin types compared with injection in those with lighter complexions.

TOP TAKEAWAYS
➤ Unique issues to ethnic skin care can include restoring uniform pigmentation, hair removal, acne care, and skin hydration.
➤ The Fitzpatrick scale is used to classify response of different skin types to UV light.
➤ Vitiligo is a condition of skin depigmentation from melanocyte dysfunction.
➤ Hyperpigmentation is typically a postinflammatory response.
➤ Darker-skinned people are less likely to develop nodulocystic acne, but their skin is more likely to keratinize and form comedones.
➤ For ethnic skin, combination therapy is often most effective.[9]
➤ Black patients typically require stronger ingredients for hair removal because of the coarseness of hair.

REFERENCES

1. American Society for Aesthetic Plastic Surgery. 2013 Cosmetic Surgery National Data Bank. Available at *http://www.surgery.org/sites/default/files/Stats2013_4.pdf.*
2. Berardesca E, Maibach HI. Sensitive and ethnic skin. A need for special-skin care agents? Dermatol Clin 9:89, 1991.
3. Cole PD, Hatef DA, Taylor S, et al. Skin care in ethnic populations. Semin Plast Surg 23:168, 2009.
4. Andersen KE, Maibach HI. Black and white human skin differences. J Am Acad Dermatol 1:276, 1979.
5. Reed JT, Ghadially R, Elias PM. Skin type, but neither race nor gender, influence epidermal permeability barrier function. Arch Dermatol 131:1134, 1995.
6. Odunze M, Cohn A, Few JW. Restylane and people of color. Plast Reconstr Surg 120:2011, 2007.
7. Montagna W, Prota G, Kenney JA Jr, eds. Black Skin Structure and Function. San Diego: Academic Press, 1993.
8. Weigand DA, Haygood C, Gaylor JR. Cell layers and density of Negro and Caucasian stratum corneum. J Invest Dermatol 62:563, 1974.
9. Taylor SC. Utilizing combination therapy for ethnic skin. Cutis 80(1 Suppl):15, 2007.

PART V

Noninvasive and Minimally Invasive Therapy

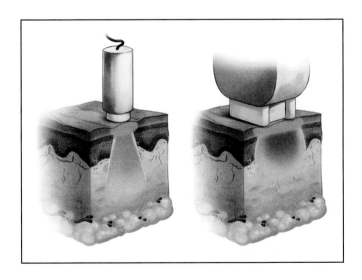

Part V

Noninvasive and Minimally Invasive Therapy

16. Basics of Laser Therapy

Darrell Wayne Freeman, Ibrahim Khansa, Molly Burns Austin, Alton Jay Burns

PHYSICS OF LASERS[1]

COMPONENTS OF LASERS
- **Excitation mechanism**
- **Medium**
  - Can be **solid** (crystal as in YAG and Ruby lasers or semiconductor as in diode laser), **liquid** (pulsed dye laser [PDL]), or **gas** (helium-neon laser)
  - Determines the wavelength of the light emitted by the laser
- **Two parallel mirrors:** One mirror 100% reflective, and the exiting mirror varies in reflectivity and how it releases energy

MECHANISM OF ACTION
- Energy is transmitted from the excitation mechanism to the medium.
- Electrons in the medium are excited to a higher-energy state.
- As the electrons fall back to their baseline state, they release a photon.
- Photons result in waves of light (energy) that can exit the medium to provide a uniform wavelength of light or that can hit an adjacent electron to further excite the medium and amplify the energy.
- The light waves are reflected back and forth between the mirrors.
- The exiting mirror can be manipulated so that only photons that hit it exactly perpendicular may exit, creating coherent waves that move in phase.

NOTE: Q-switching involves two mirrors that are 100% reflective. The exiting mirror shutters open, releasing the entire cavity at once. Q-switching creates very high powers.

PROPERTIES OF LASER LIGHT
- In phase
- Monochromatic
- Coherent

EFFECT ON TARGET
- **Reflection**
  - Off shiny surgical instruments
  - Off skin or target, which decreases energy delivered to target
  - Can cause ocular damage if wavelength-specific goggles not worn
- **Scatter**
  - Off dull objects or targets that are just off the peak of absorbent coefficients
- **Transmission**
  - The less target in the medium, the more the light will be transmitted through the medium. This varies with each laser, each with its own specific targets.

- **Absorption**
  - Laser energy absorbed by **target chromophore**
  - Energy converted to thermal energy in target chromophore *(selective photothermolysis)* or with extremely high energies and short-wavelength Q-switched lasers, which generate acoustic energy
  - Usually is the mechanism of action that provides the desired effect
  - Heat can transmit to surrounding tissues and cause a wider zone of damage if the principles of selective photothermolysis are not followed.

CHARACTERISTICS OF LASERS
- **Wavelength**
  - Each wavelength has absorption spectrum that identifies the optimal targets.
  - Within the visible light spectrum (approximately 400-750 nm), the longer the wavelength, the deeper the penetration.
- **Pulse duration**
  - Continuous: More likely to cause *nonselective tissue injury*
  - Long pulses (milliseconds)
  - Short pulses (nanoseconds), as in Q-switched laser
- **Spot size**
  - Smaller spot sizes have more scatter and may therefore not reach the dermis.
  - *Generally, the larger the spot size, the deeper the penetration.*
- **Beam shape**
  - Most lasers have a Gaussian distribution of intensity within the beam (lower intensity along the periphery).
  - Therefore some overlap between treatment zones is needed.
- **Surface cooling:** Allows protection of the epidermis while heating the deeper targets in the dermis
- **Pulse width:** Duration of time tissues are exposed to the laser
- **Fluence:** Energy delivered per surface area (J/cm^2)
- **Thermal relaxation time:** Time for tissues to lose 50% of their heat

MAJOR TYPES OF LASERS

ABLATIVE LASERS (see Chapter 17)
- Chromophore is **water.**
- Vaporize the epidermis and possibly part of the dermis
- Cause mild to significant edema and an open wound, all dependent on the depth of injury
- Have a **higher risk of scarring** and **pigmentation changes** than nonablative lasers
- Erythema longer than nonablative and is depth dependent
- Very effective for treating **moderate to severe rhytids**
- Most commonly used ablative lasers: **CO_2 laser** (10,600 nm) and the **erbium:YAG laser** (2940 nm)

NONABLATIVE LASERS
- Spare the epidermis and cause thermal damage in the **dermis**
  - Collagen is denatured when heated to 60°-70° C, stimulating **new collagen formation.**

- During the healing response, fibroblasts are activated in the papillary and midreticular dermis, increasing type I collagen and elastin deposition ➤ dermal thickening.
- Collagen reorganizes into parallel fibrils.[2]
- Skin tightens, and irregularities decrease.[3]

TIP: Although nonablative lasers allow skin rejuvenation with minimal downtime, their efficacy is significantly less than that of ablative rejuvenation methods.

FRACTIONAL LASERS
- Coagulate columns of tissue in regularly spaced arrays, while sparing intervening tissue
- Up to 3000 microscopic treatment zones (MTZs) per cm^2
- Each MTZ 70-450 μm in width, 100-1400 μm in depth
- 15%-40% of the skin area coagulated with every treatment session

NOTE: **The parameters above are highly variable between the various fractional lasers. Variation in energy delivery and safety parameters is significant; therefore surgeons should be extremely familiar with the laser system used.**

- Spare the stratum corneum[4] and epidermis if settings are appropriate

OTHER RESURFACING MODALITIES

INTENSE PULSED LIGHT
- Xenon flashlamp gives noncoherent, polychromatic intense light.
- Wavelengths range from 500-1200 nm.
  - Intense pulsed light (IPL) machines vary in energy, cooling protection, spot size, rep rate, and pulse duration. Familiarity with the system used is essential to achieve optimal results and minimize complications.

MONOPOLAR RADIOFREQUENCY
- Radiofrequency waves have a much longer wavelength than laser light.
- As the polarity of the current within the capacitive coupled electrode changes at high frequency, electrons in the tissue change direction rapidly.
- Resistance to this electron flow generates heat.
- The amount of heat generated depends on the tissue's impedance and the energy delivered.
- Collagen heated to 60°-70° C denatures, and new collagen forms over 6 months.

INDICATIONS AND CONTRAINDICATIONS

INDICATIONS
- Mild to moderate static rhytids
- Acne scars
- Immature burn scars
- Atrophic scars
- Dyschromia (solar lentigines, melasma)[5]
- Skin hypervascularity (telangiectasias, rosacea)

- Undesirable tattoo
- Undesirable hair

CONTRAINDICATIONS
- Unrealistic expectations
- Collagen vascular disease
- History of wound-healing problems
- Immunologic skin condition (such as vitiligo)
- Pregnancy (higher risk of hyperpigmentation)
- Isotretinoin use within the past 12 months[6]
- History of photosensitivity or recent use of photosensitizing drug
- Tattoo containing gunpowder
  - May catch fire and cause burns
    - ► Relative contraindications
- Skin cancer
- Fitzpatrick IV-VI skin type with laser wavelengths in the visible light spectrum
- Tattoos containing flesh-colored pigment made of iron oxides
  - Pigment may paradoxically darken with laser treatment.[7]

> NOTE: If the patient is aware of this issue and agrees to treatment, then the only way to remove the pigment is to darken it and continue to treat it; it usually fades as another tattoo once converted to a darker pigment.[8]

PREOPERATIVE EVALUATION

HISTORY
- Wound-healing problems
- Scarring problems
- Family history of wound-healing problems or excessive scarring
- Recent medication use
- Of most importance is a **history of recent tanning,** which is the most common cause of complications when treated with a laser using visible light.
- Patient expectations

> TIP: Clarification of patient expectations preoperatively is essential for patient satisfaction.

PHYSICAL EXAMINATION
- **Analyze facial skin**
  - **Fitzpatrick skin type** (Table 16-1)
    - ► Patients with darker skin have a higher risk of hypopigmentation and hyperpigmentation with laser.
    - ► Patients with lighter skin have a higher risk of prolonged postoperative erythema.

Table 16-1 *Fitzpatrick Skin Type Classification*

Skin Type	Characteristics	Sun Exposure History
I	Pale white, freckles, blue eyes, blond or red hair	Always burns, never tans
II	Fair white, blue/green/hazel eyes, blond or red hair	Usually burns, minimally tans
III	Cream white, any hair or eye color	Sometimes burns, tans uniformly
IV	Moderate brown (Mediterranean)	Rarely burns, always tans well
V	Dark brown (Middle Eastern)	Rarely burns, tans easily
VI	Dark brown to black	Never burns, tans easily

- **Static versus dynamic rhytids**
  - ▶ **Class I:** Fine wrinkles
  - ▶ **Class II:** Fine to moderately deep wrinkles, moderate number of wrinkle lines
  - ▶ **Class III:** Deep wrinkles, numerous wrinkle lines, redundant folds
- **Scarring (surgical, traumatic, burn)**
  - ▶ Assess maturity of scar
  - ▶ Assess pliability, erythema, pigmentation
- **Hypervascularity**
  - ▶ Rosacea
  - ▶ Telangiectasia
- **Dyspigmentation**
  - ▶ Solar lentigines
  - ▶ Melasma
  - ▶ Ephelides

SENIOR AUTHOR TIP: Bleaching agents like hydroquinone should not be used for patients with Fitzpatrick III and higher skin types.

Lower eyelid laxity is assessed preoperatively with a snap test to prevent ectropion with aggressive treatments.

Patients with Fitzpatrick skin types IV and higher are at increased risk of hyperpigmentation with most nonablative and ablative lasers.

PREPARATION FOR TREATMENT
- Pretreatment
  - Hydroquinone 4% and tretinoin 0.05% 4-6 weeks pretreatment
    - ▶ Stimulates faster healing and prevents posttreatment hyperpigmention
  - Discontinue oral isotretinoin (Accutane) products 6 months to 1 year before treatment because of increased risk of scarring.
- Prophylaxis
  - Antivirals 48 hours before and 7-10 days after in all patients undergoing ablative treatment, and in patients with a history if undergoing nonablative treatment

MEDICATIONS
- Herbal supplements that may increase bleeding time and should be discontinued 2-3 weeks before treatment
- Arnica, danshen, feverfew, garlic, ginger, Ginkgo biloba, kava, licorice, St. John's wort, vitamin E
  - **Anticoagulation**
    - ▶ Vitamin K antagonist stopped 5 days before the procedure unless high risk, then bridge therapy (atrial fibrillation, mechanical heart valve, venous thromboembolism)
    - ▶ Acetylsalicylic acid (ASA) stopped 7-10 days before the procedure unless moderate to high risk
    - ▶ Risk versus benefit always evaluated on a case-by-case basis

PRETREATMENT
- Antiviral therapy for herpes simplex
- Acyclovir 400 mg by mouth three times per day, famciclovir 250 mg by mouth twice per day, or valacyclovir 500 mg by mouth twice per day for 1-3 days before treatment until reepithelialization at 5-14 days

BACTERIAL INFECTIONS
- Dicloxacillin or azithromycin may be prescribed if history of bacterial infections of the face
- 1g cefazolin intraoperatively
- Chlorhexidine face scrub
- Intranasal mupirocin

ANTIFUNGAL
- One dose of fluconazole at the time of the procedure and one dose 1 week postoperatively to prevent cutaneous candidiasis
- Controversial because of the low risk of infection
- May be beneficial in patients with history of vaginal candidiasis

INFORMED CONSENT

TIP: Surgeons must understand patients' expectations before treatment is offered. Patients must understand that nonablative resurfacing methods do not have the same effectiveness as ablative resurfacing methods.

- Patients must understand that **multiple treatments are almost invariably needed** to achieve the desired effect, especially with nonablative treatments.
- **Risks of nonablative resurfacing include:**
  - Unsatisfactory result
  - Prolonged erythema
  - Prolonged edema
  - Hypopigmentation

- Hyperpigmentation
- Scarring
- Ecchymosis (with PDL)
■ Alternative procedures include:
  - Chemical resurfacing
  - Dermabrasion

TOP TAKEAWAYS

➤ Lasers are in phase, monochromatic, coherent light that can be effectively used to resurface the skin.

➤ Lasers can be ablative or nonablative, and can also be fractionated.

➤ Skin treatment, both before and after laser resurfacing is an important component to a successful result.

REFERENCES

1. Atiyeh BS, Dibo SA. Nonsurgical nonablative treatment of aging skin: radiofrequency technologies between aggressive marketing and evidence-based efficacy. Aesth Plast Surg 33:283, 2009.
2. Orringer JS, Kang S, Maier L, et al. A randomized, controlled, split-face clinical trial of 1320-nm Nd:YAG laser therapy in the treatment of acne vulgaris. J Am Acad Dermatol 56:432, 2007.
3. Friedman PM, Skover GR, Payonk G, et al. Quantitative evaluation of nonablative laser technology. Semin Cutan Med Surg 21:266, 2002.
4. Cohen SR, Henssler C, Johnston J. Fractional photothermolysis for skin rejuvenation. Plast Reconstr Surg 124:281, 2009.
5. Katz TM, Glaich AS, Goldberg LH, et al. Treatment of melasma using fractional photothermolysis: a report of eight cases with long-term follow-up. Dermatol Surg 36:1273, 2010.
6. Rubenstein R, Roenigk HH Jr, Stegman SJ, et al. Atypical keloids after dermabrasion of patients taking isotretinoin. J Am Acad Dermatol 15:280, 1986.
7. Alexiades-Armenakas M. Laser-mediated photodynamic therapy. Clin Dermatol 24:16, 2006.
8. Alster TS. Q-switched alexandrite laser treatment (755 nm) of professional and amateur tattoos. J Am Acad Dermatol 33:69, 1995.

17.   Ablative Laser Resurfacing

Darrell Wayne Freeman, Molly Burns Austin, Alton Jay Burns

Lasers were originally employed in surgery in the 1960s as a cutting instrument in lieu of a scalpel. They originally used a continuous wave CO_2 laser. As technology advanced, high-energy pulsed CO_2 lasers were developed that could selectively ablate superficial tissue with minimal residual thermal damage (RTD). This resulted in improvement of many signs of photoaging, scars, and lesions on the skin. Throughout the years, newer laser technologies have been developed to include erbium:yttrium aluminum garnet (Er:YAG) lasers and fractional lasers. The goals of all these devices are to eliminate or reduce sun-damaged collagen and encourage new collagen deposition and remodeling through a combination of tissue vaporization and collagen denaturation.

EQUIPMENT

ABLATIVE CARBON DIOXIDE (CO_2) LASER
- **10,600 nm** wavelength
- Target chromophore: **Water**
  - Absorption coefficient = 800 cm^{-1}
- Visible helium-neon laser is projected on the skin to show the targeted treatment area.
- Produces **tissue vaporization** and **thermal coagulation**[1-3]
  - Pulse duration must be <1 millisecond to prevent residual thermal damage (RTD) to surrounding tissue.
  - 5 J/cm^1 needed to produce tissue ablation (fluence)
  - ~20-30 µm of ablative tissue penetration per J/cm^1
    - ▶ **Nonlinear relationship** between the number of passes and depth of tissue ablation
    - ▶ Decreasing depth of tissue ablation with each additional pass
    - ▶ Limits ablation to ~200-300 µm deep[4]
    - ▶ Ablation limited but thermal damage is much deeper
  - 70-120 µm area of RTD
  - Surface temperatures reach 120°-200° C
- **CO_2 ablation**
  - Produces dramatic results but requires a longer healing time because of deeper RTD compared with erbium
  - Immediate postprocedure edema and erythema resolve in 1-2 weeks and final results require up to 6 months.
- **Two types**[1-3]
  - **High energy pulsed**
    - ▶ Energy delivered in 600 microseconds to 1 millisecond
    - ▶ Can produce 500 mJ of energy in <900-microseconds pulse
    - ▶ Uses a spot size of 3 mm or a computer pattern generator (CPG) supplying a pattern of up to 80 pulses with a 2.25 mm spot size

- **Scanned**
  - ▶ Energy delivered in ≤1 millisecond
  - ▶ Scan duration of 0.03-0.52 seconds with a dwell time of 300-1000 microseconds
  - ▶ Computer program scans 0.2 mm spots in a spiral design over an 8-16 mm diameter and performs the ablation.
  - ▶ No one spot is ablated more than once.

ABLATIVE ERBIUM:YTTRIUM ALUMINUM GARNET (ER:YAG)[1]

- **2940 nm** wavelength
- Chromophore: **Water**
  - Absorption coefficient 10 times greater than that of CO_2 laser (12,000 cm^{-1})
- Produces **more precise tissue vaporization** and **less thermal coagulation** than CO_2 lasers[1]
  - 1-3 µm of ablative tissue penetration per J/cm^2
  - 5-30 µm area of RTD
  - Produces 1-50 mJ/ cm^2 of energy in 300 microseconds to 10 milliseconds
  - 2-7 mm collimated or focused spot size
  - **Value:** Comprehensive and versatile. It can be the most superficial laser with quick healing times, or it can be much more aggressive and ablative than CO_2 with less RTD and an optimal efficacy safety profile (i.e., can be as aggressive or as superficial as needed).
- **Three types**
  - **Single pulse**
    - ▶ Pulse duration of 250-350 microseconds
  - **Variable pulse**
    - ▶ Pulse duration of 10-50 milliseconds (longer duration causes more RTD with more secondary collagen deposition); however, the RTD never reaches that of CO_2
  - **Dual ablation/coagulation** mode (tunable erbium)
- **Er:YAG ablation**[5]
  - Most versatile ablative laser
  - Can produce superficial wounds from 10 µm that can give quick recovery times and usually require repeat treatments
  - Can produce the deepest of all wounds because of the extremely high ablation threshold of 5 J/cm^2
  - Excellent results possible with even the deepest rhytids
  - Less residual thermal damage, so faster healing than with CO_2, even for the same depths (5-20 nm residual thermal damage [RTD], compared with 70-120 µm RTD for CO_2)

ABLATIVE FRACTIONAL LASERS[6-9]

- CO_2, Er:YAG, and yttrium scandium gallium garnet (YSGG) models available
- Wide variety of models and handpieces provides different fluence and penetration depths.
- Produces **microthermal zones (MTZ) of ablation injury** with surrounding layer of denatured collagen heated to 55°-62° C for optimal long-term collagen deposition/ remodeling
  - MTZ/cm^2 can be manually set. (Both depth of injury and density of MTZ can be set.)
  - Ablation depth up to 1.6 mm (varies based on fluence, wavelength, and spot size)

- Settings relate to laser used and desired target (dyschromia, pores, rhytids).
- The deeper the ablation depth, the greater zone of coagulation and denatured collagen.
- Decreased postprocedure erythema and complications
- Complete healing and reepithelialization by 1 week[9]
- For more aggressive treatments, erythema may last up to 6-8 weeks.
- **Fractionated lasers**
  - Multiple treatments are needed, because only a fraction of the skin is treated per session.
  - Open wounds last 3-4 days, with erythema lasting 2-8 weeks for aggressive treatment protocols.
  - Laser of choice for lower eyelids, acne, and large pore size[5]

TECHNIQUE

SAFETY (LASER INSTITUTE, OCCUPATIONAL SAFETY)

- American National Standards Institute (ANSI)[10] provides policies for laser safety.
- Occupational Safety and Health Administration (OSHA)[11] provides oversight.
- Proper documentation of safety training is required for all perioperative personnel.
- Laser Safety Officer (LSO) provides control over administrative, procedural, and engineering controls.
- Each treatment area must define the nominal hazard zone (NHZ), have proper signage for eyewear, and have limited access by trained personnel.
- Windows must be covered with appropriate opaque material.
- Laser must be test fired before the procedure.
- Antiflammable precautions, including saline-soaked clothes, irrigation solution, and fire extinguishers
- Smoke evacuation to remove laser plume
- Laser kept in standby mode when not actively in use

MARKINGS

- Each aesthetic unit to be treated is outlined.
- Light blending between aesthetic units provides a smooth transition.
- Full-face treatment gives best blend but is not always indicated.

ANESTHESIA

- *Ablative lasers cause more pain than nonablative treatments;* therefore, when treating areas not easily blocked by local anesthesia, general anesthesia may be indicated for more aggressive settings. Patient preference for comfort is also a consideration.
- For very superficial laser resurfacing, topical anesthesia may suffice for limited areas.
  - Lidocaine cream (LMX) or lidocaine and prilocaine cream (EMLA) 30-90 minutes before procedure
  - 15 g BLT triple anesthetic cream (20% **b**enzocaine, 6% **l**idocaine, and 4% **t**etracaine) applied 20 minutes before procedure and again after first laser pass[12]
  - Cold-air cooling

NOTE: Use of topical agents should be limited after deepithelialization because of potential lidocaine toxicity. Topical use is limited to one or two areas; lidocaine toxicity is a known issue when large areas are treated.

Local Anesthesia[1,13]

- **Central face,** including central forehead, cheek, nose, upper and lower lips
  - 1%-2% lidocaine with 1:100,000 or 1:200,000 epinephrine
- **Lateral face**
  - 2% lidocaine with 1:100,000 epinephrine, 0.5% bupivacaine, 1:10 8.4% $NaHCO_3$, and 75 U hyaluronidase
  - Or, equal parts of 1% lidocaine with 1:100,000 epinephrine and 0.5% marcaine with 1 ml hyaluronidase for every 9 ml local anesthesia
- **Nerve blocks:** 4% articaine hydrochloride
  - Supraoribital nerve
  - Supratrochlear nerve
  - Infraorbital nerve
  - Maxillary nerve
  - Mandibular nerve
  - Mental nerve
- **Orbital anesthesia**
  - Three drops of 0.5% proparacaine ophthalmic solution to each eye before application of lubricated eye shields
- **Tumescent local anesthesia**
  - Kessels et al[14] reported using 0.11% solution of 500 ml lactated Ringer solution, 20 ml 1% ropivacaine, 20 ml 2% xylocaine, and 0.5 ml epinephrine
  - Minimum of 6 ml/kg

CAUTION: Tumescent anesthesia introduces water into the tissue which decreases the depth of penetration which may not be desired.

Systemic Analgesia/Anesthesia[1,13] (see Chapters 5 through 7)

- **Oral**
  - 10 mg diazepam 30 minutes before procedure
- **Intramuscular**
  - 100 mg meperidine 30 minutes before procedure
  - 25 mg hydroxyzine 30 minutes before procedure
- **Inhalation**
- **Intravenous**[4]
  - Propofol 1-2 mg/kg loading dose, 4-8 mg/kg/hr continuous infusion
  - Midazolam 0.05-0.1 mg/kg
  - Fentanyl 50-100 µg
  - Ketamine 10-20 mg (must administer glycopyrrolate 0.2 mg, propofol, and midazolam first)
  - Laryngeal mask adaptor (LMA) necessary with heavy sedation

---

TIP: Adding $NaHCO_3$ to the local anesthesia to the lateral face neutralizes the pH, whereas the hyaluronidase increases tissue diffusion.

TIP: A wetting solution of 0.1% lidocaine and 1:1,000,000 epinephrine anesthetizes the cheeks.

TIP: All procedure rooms need adequate ventilation systems, smoke evacuators, and laser protective masks to control toxic gases from the laser plumes.

> **TIP:**   Surrounding the treatment area with saline-soaked towels helps to prevent an accidental fire.

> **TIP:**   Safety glasses do not protect against direct laser exposure.

CARBON DIOXIDE (CO$_2$) LASER TECHNIQUE[1,15]

- Resurfacing begins by ablating tissue in the treatment area in a **nonoverlapping** manner and only once.
    - ▶ Debris is removed with a normal saline–soaked gauze.
    - ▶ The skin is completely dried.
    - ▶ The treatment area will have **a pink color** as the papillary dermis is exposed.
- A second pass is performed in a **nonoverlapping** manner.
    - ▶ The debris is removed with a normal saline–soaked gauze, and the skin is completely dried.
    - ▶ The treatment area will transition to **a yellow color,** and the dermis will contract.
    - ▶ Most treatment areas will only need **two or three passes** to achieve optimal results.
    - ▶ **Endpoint for adequate treatment**
        - ◆ Yellow-brown discoloration
        - ◆ No further skin contraction
        - ◆ Disappearance of the photodamaged area or rhytid
- Additional laser treatment may be applied to deep rhytids to soften transition zones.
    - ▶ Excessive laser exposure should be avoided: *Brown coloration signifies thermal necrosis and charring of the skin.*

CAUTION: This treatment should NOT be carried out unless a clear understanding of the endpoint is appreciated. The procedure requires training and experience and a great appreciation of the endpoint before it is incorporated into practice.

> **TIP:**   Water remaining on the skin surface during laser treatment may block dermal penetration.

> **TIP:**   Applying a single pass of Er:YAG at the conclusion of CO$_2$ treatment removes debris and decreases reepithelialization time.

ER:YAG LASER TECHNIQUE[1]

- ▪ Resurfacing begins by ablating tissue in the treatment area in an **overlapping** manner by free hand or a scanner.

> **NOTE:**   **Understanding the laser in detail is essential, because the amount of overlap depends on the energy distribution profile for each laser. As much as 50% overlap should be used on the most popular erbium laser system, but this overlap does not apply to other systems.**

- A common misconception is that erbium is a more superficial laser. *This is unequivocally false.* The erbium laser can penetrate deeply if an adequately powered system is used.

- Erbium's affinity for water is **11 times that of CO_2**; therefore it ablates dermis much more readily than CO_2.
- If no coagulation is used, then the endpoint is the bleeding pattern common with debriding burn wounds; i.e., fine fibrillar bleeding is from papillary dermis, and larger bleeding spots that are less dense imply reticular bleeding.
- The proper endpoint is **eradication of the rhytid or penetration to the midreticular dermis.**

CAUTION: Understanding endpoints is critical to using this device. Users should be very comfortable with these endpoints before employing the procedure in practice.

- ▶ Skin contraction is usually **not** visible when a short-pulsed laser is used but may be seen with a variable-pulsed laser, which increases dwell time and coagulation with increased pulse widths.
- ■ Removing debris during passes is unnecessary because of high water affinity.
  - ▶ Debris is wiped off after final pass to cleanse wound, and an occlusive moist dressing like Flexzan is applied.

POSTOPERATIVE CARE

- **Metal eye shields** are removed and eyes are flushed with normal saline solution.
- **Dressing**
  - CO_2/aggressive erbium
    - ▶ **Biooclusive dressing**[4,15-19]
      - ◆ Common examples include composite foam Flexzan (Dow Hickam Pharmaceuticals), hydrogel 2nd Skin (Bionet), plastic mesh N-Terface (Winfield Laboratories), and polymer film Silon-TSR (Bio Med Sciences).
        - – Exudate buildup through perforations is removed with normal saline solution.
        - – Meticulous wound care with frequent dressing changes minimizes increased risk of infection with occlusion.
        - – Placing and keeping it on may be difficult.
        - – More expensive than open wound care
        - – Improved patient comfort
      - ◆ Applied for 24-72 hours
        - – Longer use may predispose to *Pseudomonas* infection
      - ◆ Ice water or 2% acetic acid solution soaks
        - – Starting when final dressing removed on day 2-5 depending on protocol, soaking for 20-30 minutes every 2-3 hours while awake
        - – Frequency of soaks decreased to every 3-4 hours while patient is awake, and a petroleum-based ointment is applied after soaks until reepithelialization
        - – After reepithelialization, transition from soaks to gentle cleansing and application of a mosturizer and sunscreen
    - ▶ **Open wound care**
      - ◆ Ice water, normal saline solution, or 0.25% acetic acid soaks beginning postoperatively for 20-30 minutes every 2-3 hours
        - – Removes exudate buildup
        - – Minimizes edema
      - ◆ Petroleum-based healing ointment applied after each soak

- ◆ Decreased frequency of soaks as the skin reepithelializes
- ◆ Less expensive than a closed dressing
- ◆ Risk that patient may not properly apply ointment and inadvertantly damage their face by allowing certain areas to dry out, or may abrade wound
- ◆ Increased pain and patient dissatisfaction
- • **Superficial Er:YAG aggressive fractional ablative**[20]
  - ▶ Petroleum-based ointment until reepithelialization in 7-10 days
  - ▶ Diluted peroxide or diluted vinegar washes 3-4 times daily
  - ▶ Ice packs to minimize edema
  - ▶ Mosturizer and sunscreen after reepithelialization
- ■ Continuation of antiviral therapy
- ■ Dicloxacillin or azithromycin if the patient has a history of bacterial infections
- ■ Pain control: Acetaminophen or oxycodone
- ■ **Preventing hyperpigmentation**
  - • Application of a bleaching mixture containing 2% hydroquinone and 15% glycolic acid; or Klingman regimen consisting of 5% hydroquinone, 0.1% tretinoin, and 1% dexamethasone[21]; or Lytera (SkinMedica), which has been shown to be equally effective as 4% hydroquinone, with no risk of ochronosis and no prescription required, but more expensive
  - • Sunscreen
    - ▶ At least SPF 30 should be used until erythema resolves, starting a few days after reepithelialization.
    - ▶ Wanitphakdeedecha et al[22] suggested sunscreen containing licochalcone-A and glycyrrhetinate starting on day 1, which reduces the risk of postinflammatory inflammation associated with early sunscreen use.
  - • Avoidance of sunlight

> **TIP:** Avoiding antibiotic ointments such as mupirocin, bacitracin, and bacitracin-polymyxin B helps to prevent dermatitis.

COMPLICATIONS

CO_2[4,17,19,23-26]
- ■ **Major**
  - • **Infection**
    - ▶ Herpes simplex 2%-7.4%
    - ▶ Candida <1%
    - ▶ Gram-positive and gram-negative 3%-47%
    - ▶ All patients treated with antivirals for herpes preoperatively and postoperatively
    - ▶ Antifungals and antibiotics reserved for active infections

> **SENIOR AUTHOR TIP:** Usual signs of infection are not present without epithelium; therefore a multimodality approach is often initially indicated with post-laser/pre-epithelium infections.

  - • **Hypopigmentation (16%-57%[1,27,28])**
    - ▶ **Immediate**
      - ◆ Resurfaced skin appears hypopigmented compared to untreated, photodamaged skin

- ◆ Can also perform a chemical peel or fractional resurfacing on the photodamaged skin to soften the transition between the treated and untreated areas
  - ▶ **Delayed (16%[1])**
    - ◆ Appears 6-12 months after resurfacing
    - ◆ Usually permanent but sunlight, UV light therapy, and glycolic acid peels can be attempted
    - ◆ Can blend edges with fractional laser treatment
    - ◆ Hypopigmentation much less with erbium
- **Postinflammatory hyperpigmentation (5%-83%)**
  - ▶ Increasing risk with increasing Fitzpatrick number
  - ▶ Treated with 4% hydroquinone, a retinoid, and sunlight avoidance[29,30] or Lytera
- **Scarring (0.1%-1%)**
  - ▶ Most common sites[23]
    - ◆ Upper lip
    - ◆ Mandible
    - ◆ Malar region
    - ◆ Periorbital region
    - ◆ Neck
    - ◆ Minimizing laser passes, energy, and RTD lowers risk
    - ◆ Treated with topical and intralesional steroids injections, silicone gel sheets, and IPL treatments

SENIOR AUTHOR TIP: Care is needed when treating areas that have decreased skin appendages that are usually helpful in reepithelialization (e.g., extensive and comprehensive laser hair removal, electrolysis, and Accutane).

- **Ectropion (2%[31])**
  - ▶ Rare
  - ▶ May have a history of blepharoplasty or rhytidectomy or senile laxity
  - ▶ Treated with tape and massage
  - ▶ May require surgical correction with a lateral canthal suspension
- ▪ **Minor**
  - **Prolonged erythema (30%[4])**
    - ▶ Typically lasts 1-4 months
    - ▶ Much less erythema in intensity and longevity with erbium compared with CO_2
    - ▶ Up to 1 year
  - **Treatment**
    - ▶ Camouflage makeup
    - ▶ Topical steroids: 1% hydrocortisone 2-3 times daily for 2 weeks after reepithelialization[14]
    - ▶ Intense pulsed light (IPL) lasers
    - ▶ LED therapy
  - **Edema**
    - ▶ Most severe postoperative days 1-3
    - ▶ Ice packs
    - ▶ Head of bed elevated at night
    - ▶ Corticosteroids, if severe

- **Pruritus (2.3%)**
  - ▶ Usually noticed in the first month and may last 3 months
  - ▶ Antihistamines

SENIOR AUTHOR TIP: Patients who itch significantly should always be evaluated, because this may be a sign of a complication such as infection or deeper injury.

- **Acne and milia (1%-30%[2,31])**
  - ▶ May be worsened by occlusive dressings
  - ▶ Seen more frequently in patients with a history of acne
  - ▶ Respond to typical antiacne treatments such as tretinoin
  - ▶ Isotretinoin may worsen postoperative scarring and should not be used.
- **Contact dermatitis (10%-65%[23])**
  - ▶ Usually from topical antibiotics and home remedies that patients take

ER:YAG[21,32]
- ■ **Major**
  - • Hypopigmentation[33]
- ■ **Minor**
  - • Prolonged erythema
    - ▶ Typically lasts 1 month
  - • Edema
  - • Hyperpigmentation
    - ▶ Transient directly postoperatively

FRACTIONAL ABLATIVE LASER[28,34]
- ■ Erythema
  - • Short-term 100%
  - • >3 months 7%
- ■ Xerosis 87%
- ■ Edema 82%-100%
- ■ Flaking 60%
- ■ Superficial scratches 47%
- ■ Pruritus 37%
- ■ Postinflammatory hyperpigmentation 20%-27%

OCULAR DAMAGE AND BLINDNESS
- ■ Protective eyewear with appropriate optical density (OD) for everyone present in the treatment area
- ■ Protective eye shields for patients

FIRE
- ■ Drapes, cloth, and other flammable materials can easily catch fire.
- ■ All makeup should be removed.
- ■ Alcohol prep and skin cleansing solutions are allowed to completely dry.
- ■ Laser must not be used near sources of oxygen.

TOP TAKEAWAYS

➤ Resistance to transition from using CO_2 to erbium laser resurfacing is common because many more CO_2 systems are in place and, if used properly, produce a fine cosmetic result with an adequate safety profile. There is also a misconception that erbium laser is only effective for superficial treatments. Erbium is a highly versatile laser with the ability to treat superficially or deeply a vast array of skin targets. The safety profile is far superior to that of CO_2. This paradigm shift is the major shift in ablative lasers over the last 5-10 years.

➤ Fractional lasers vary greatly in efficacy, safety, and ease of use. Users should be aware of manipulated "knockoff" fractional devices, because their safety and efficacy profiles can be dangerous in inexperienced hands.

➤ Adding $NaHCO_3$ to the local anesthesia to the lateral face neutralizes the pH, whereas the hyaluronidase increases tissue diffusion.

REFERENCES

1. Alexiades-Armenakas MR, Dover JS, Arndt KA. The spectrum of laser skin resurfacing: nonablative, fractional, and ablative laser resurfacing. J Am Acad Dermatol 58:719, 2008.
2. Brightman LA, Brauer JA, Anolik R, et al. Ablative and fractional ablative lasers. Dermatol Clin 27:479, 2009.
3. Walsh JT Jr, Flotte TJ, Anderson RR, et al. Pulsed CO2 laser tissue ablation: effect of tissue type and pulse duration on thermal damage. Lasers Surg Med 8:108, 1988.
4. Fitzpatrick RE, Williams B, Goldman MP. Preoperative anesthesia and postoperative considerations in laser resurfacing. Semin Cutan Med Surg 15:170, 1996.
5. Burns JL. Lasers in plastic surgery. Sel Read Plast Surg 10:23, 2008.
6. Cartee TV, Wasserman DI. Commentary: Ablative fractionated CO2 laser treatment of photoaging: a clinical and histologic study. Dermatol Surg 38:1790, 2012.
7. Hantash BM, Bedi VP, Kapadia B, et al. In vivo histological evaluation of a novel ablative fractional resurfacing device. Lasers Surg Med 39:96, 2007.
8. Tierney EP, Hanke CW, Petersen J. Ablative fractionated CO2 laser treatment of photoaging: a clinical and histologic study. Dermatol Surg 38:1777, 2012.
9. Rahman Z, MacFalls H, Jiang K, et al. Fractional deep dermal ablation induces tissue tightening. Lasers Surg Med 41:78, 2009.
10. Laser Institute of America. ANSI Z136 standards. Available at http://www.lia.org/publications/ansi.
11. U.S. Department of Labor. Occupational Safety & Health Administration. Laser hazards. Available at https://www.osha.gov/SLTC/laserhazards/.
12. Oni G, Rasko Y, Kenkel J. Topical lidocaine enhanced by laser pretreatment: a safe and effective method of analgesia for facial rejuvenation. Aesthet Surg J 33:854, 2013.
13. Saedi N, Hamilton HK, Arndt KA, et al. How to prepare patients for ablative laser procedures. J Am Acad Dermatol 69:e49, 2013.
14. Kessels JP, Ostertag JU. The use of tumescent local anaesthesia in ablative laser treatments. J Eur Acad Dermatol Venereol 26:1456, 2012.
15. Batra RS, Ort RJ, Jacob C, et al. Evaluation of a silicone occlusive dressing after laser skin resurfacing. Arch Dermatol 137:1317, 2001.
16. Batra RS. Ablative laser resurfacing—postoperative care. Skin Therapy Lett 9:6, 2004.

17. Manuskiatti W, Fitzpatrick RE, Goldman MP, et al. Prophylactic antibiotics in patients undergoing laser resurfacing of the skin. J Am Acad Dermatol 40:77, 1999.
18. Goldman MP, Roberts TL III, Skover G, et al. Optimizing wound healing in the face after laser abrasion. J Am Acad Dermatol 46:399, 2002.
19. Manuskiatti W, Fitzpatrick RE, Goldman MP. Long-term effectiveness and side effects of carbon dioxide laser resurfacing for phyotoaged facial skin. J Am Acad Dermatol 40:401, 1999.
20. DiBernardo BE, Pozner JN, Codner MA, eds. Techniques in Aesthetic Plastic Surgery Series: Lasers and Non-Surgical Rejuvenation. Philadelphia: Saunders Elsevier, 2009.
21. Papadavid E, Katsambas A. Lasers for facial rejuvenation: a review. Int J Dermatol 42:480, 2003.
22. Wanitphakdeedecha R, Phuardchantuk R, Manuskiatti W. The use of sunscreen starting on the first day after ablative fractional skin resurfacing. J Eur Acad Dermatol Venereol 28:1522, 2014.
23. Ratner D, Tse Y, Marchell N, et al. Cutaneous laser resurfacing. J Am Acad Dermatol 41:365, 1999.
24. Nanni CA, Alster TS, Complications of carbon dioxide laser resurfacing. An evaluation of 500 patients. Dermatol Surg 24:315, 1998.
25. Nanni CA, Alster TS. Complications of cutaneous laser surgery. A review. Dermatol Surg 24:209, 1998.
26. Sriprachya-Anunt S, Fitzpatrick RE, Goldman MP, et al. Infections complicating pulsed carbon dioxide laser resurfacing for photoaged facial skin. Dermatol Surg 23:527, 1997.
27. Bolognia JL, Jorizzo JL, Schaffer JV, eds. Dermatology, ed 3. Philadelphia: Elsevier, 2012.
28. Dijkema SJ, van der Lei B. Long-term results of upper lips treated for rhytides with carbon dioxide laser. Plast Reconstr Surg 115:1731, 2005.
29. Fabi S, Massaki N, Goldman MP. Efficacy and tolerability of two commercial hyperpigmentation kits in the treatment of facial hyperpigmentation and photo-aging. J Drugs Dermatol 11:964, 2012.
30. Sriprachya-Anunt S, Marchell NL, Fitzpatrick RE, et al. Facial resurfacing in patients with Fitzpatrick skin type IV. Lasers Surg Med 30:86, 2002.
31. Ward PD, Baker SR. Long-term results of carbon dioxide laser resurfacing of the face. Arch Facial Plast Surg 10:238, 2008.
32. Rostan EF, Fitzpatrick RE, Goldman MP. Laser resurfacing with a long pulse erbium:YAG laser compared to the 950 ms pulsed CO(2) laser. Lasers Surg Med 29:136, 2001.
33. Wheeland RG, Bailin PL, Ratz JL. Combined carbon dioxide laser excision and vaporization in the treatment of rhinophyma. J Dermatol Surg Oncol 13:172, 1987.
34. Fisher GH, Geronemus RG. Short-term side effects of fractional photothermolysis. Dermatol Surg 31:1245, 2005. International Electrotechnical Commission. Safety of Laser Products—Part 1: Equipment Classification and Requirements, ed 2. Geneva, Switzerland: International Electrotechnical Commission, 2007.

18.   Nonablative Laser Resurfacing

Ibrahim Khansa, Molly Burns Austin, Alton Jay Burns

EQUIPMENT

Two types of nonablative lasers, and two additional modalities, are commonly used in nonablative resurfacing.

MIDINFRARED LASERS

- Longer wavelength allows **deeper penetration into the dermis** and **partially spares melanin.**
- Target **dermis** without a specific chromophore
- **Not** very effective for epidermal signs of photoaging, such as dyschromia

ND:YAG LASER

- **1320 nm, long pulses**
- One of the earliest lasers used for nonablative resurfacing
  - Early applications did not include a cooling device, and this resulted in a high rate of scarring, hyperpigmentation, and pain.
- Newer models include a cryogenic cooling spray, which keeps the epidermis temperature around 40°-48° C, while the dermis is heated to 60°-70° C.[1,2]
- Effective in resurfacing **atrophic acne scars**[3,4]

Q-SWITCHED ND:YAG LASER

- **1064 nm, very short pulses**
- Coupled with a cryogenic cooling device
- Very effective at **treating tatoos**[5]

> **SENIOR AUTHOR TIP:**   This laser does not see "brown pigment" well so it is an excellent choice for treating tattoos in darker skin types.

DIODE LASER

- **1450 nm**
- Has not demonstrated a significant effect on rhytids[6]
- Effective in resurfacing **atrophic acne scars**[7]

ERBIUM-DOPED FRACTIONAL LASER

- Fraxel (Solta Medical)
- **1550 nm**
- The **most frequently used nonablative laser** and has **multiple applications,** such as dyschromia,[8,9] fine rhytids,[8,9] acne scars,[10] burn scars,[8,9,11] striae distensae[12]
- **Treatment of dyschromia:** Same effectiveness as nonablative, nonfractionated lasers[13,14]

- **Treatment of rhytids:** More effective than nonfractionated, nonablative lasers, but less effective than ablative fractional or fully ablative lasers[13,14]
- Requires three to six treatments, spaced at 2- to 4-week minimum intervals
- Other fractional lasers include the Lux 1540 fractional laser (1540 nm, Cynosure) and the Affirm laser (1320 nm + 1440 nm, Cynosure).[15]

> **SENIOR AUTHOR TIP:**   Currently our most frequently used laser is actually a dual hybrid laser 1440 nm/2970 nm firing simultaneously in the same spot. The 1440 nm is less painful yet equally effective to the 1550 nm fractional laser and the 2970 nm adds quicker healing time and greater dermal change.

VISIBLE LIGHT LASERS
- **Pulsed dye laser**
  - **585-595 nm**
  - Of limited use in dark skin types because of high affinity for melanin
    - ▶ Risk of hypopigmentation and hyperpigmentation
  - Shown to increase the quantity of collagen and elastin in the dermis[16]
  - *Photodynamic therapy:* Effect can be potentiated by topical application of a photosensitizer, such **as 5-aminolevulinic acid.**[17]
  - For aging treatment, fluencies used are below those typically used for the treatment of vascular lesions, and pulse width durations are longer than those used to treat port-wine stains to minimize purpura.
  - Best used for signs of **hypervascularity** and **dyschromia**
  - Most effective laser for **port-wine stain treatment**

INTENSE PULSED LIGHT
- **Not a laser.** Intense polychromatic light including **multiple wavelengths** from 500-1200 nm.[18]
- Filters can be added to allow only certain wavelengths, thus targeting specific chromophores.
- Of limited use in dark skin types (IV-VI) because of affinity for melanin
- Excellent in the treatment of **hypervascularity,** such as **rosacea** and **telangiectasia**[19]
  - Very good in the treatment of dyspigmentation, such as solar lentigines[13]
  - **Broadband light (BBL)** is a form of IPL and has proven to be effective in genetic transcription to a more youthful genomic expression with multiple frequent treatments at least three times per year for several years[20]
- *Photodynamic therapy:* Effect can be potentiated by topical application of a photosensitizer, such as 5-aminolevulinic acid.[21]

RADIOFREQUENCY
- ThermaCool (Solta Medical)
  - Radiofrequency waves cause collagen denaturation when heated to 55°-62° C, and the amount of collagen in the skin increases over time.[22]
  - Amount of tissue heating and the placement of that heating zone can be controlled by modifying the fluence of the radiofrequency waves and the intensity of the cryogenic cooling spray.
  - Heat is delivered at high fluence (70-150 J/cm^2) for short pulses (<2.3 seconds) (*flash heating*).

- Because radiofrequency does not target melanin, it **can be used safely in patients of all skin phenotypes.**
- Used in patients with **mild skin laxity**
- Does not address underlying structural ptosis
- Several studies analyzing the efficacy of monopolar radiofrequency showed measurable improvement in skin laxity.
  - ▶ However, most studies were not blinded, randomized, or comparative.[12,23]
  - ▶ Overall, results were modest and inconsistent.[24,25]
- Can be painful to the patient
- Low risk of complications, although multiple reports have described fat atrophy from heat damage to adipose tissue early in the treatment's evolution.[26] Current treatment protocols greatly minimize or eliminate this risk.

TECHNIQUE

ANESTHESIA
- Nonablative lasers are **not as painful** as ablative lasers in general, but can vary depending on the depth; i.e., a deep, nonablative laser treatment could possibly cause more pain than a superficial ablative laser treatment.
- Topical anesthesia, typically with EMLA (2.5% prilocaine/2.5% lidocaine) or LMX (4% or 5% lidocaine), is usually sufficient.
- It must be applied at least 1 hour before treatment, covered with an occlusive dressing, and wiped off just before treatment.

SAFETY
- Medical lasers are all class **IV devices**.
  - They are hazardous to view directly, under reflection or under scatter.
  - Therefore all persons in the room must wear wavelength-specific safety goggles.
  - A warning sign must be placed on each entrance, with extra goggles hanging outside the door.
- Corneal eye shields are placed, with ophthalmic ointment lubrication.
- If patient is under general anesthesia, a laser-safe ET tube must be used if treating around the mouth, and the lowest possible FiO_2 should be given.
  - Wet towels should be applied around the treatment area to absorb heat energy.
- If treating viral warts, live viral particles can be transmitted into personnel's airway.
  - Therefore appropriate masks and ventilation systems must be in place.

TECHNIQUE
- During the first treatment, inexperienced users can start with a test area to find the optimal fluence for the patient's skin; however, the use of test spots is very unusual beyond a novice level of experience.
  - Clinical endpoints for nonablative lasers are usually based on guidelines determined by experts and depend on the treatment goal. There is usually no visual endpoint for nonablative lasers used for the treatment of rhytids.
    - ▶ Hypervascularity: Mild purpura
    - ▶ Tattoo removal: Skin whitening
- In subsequent treatments, the choice of fluence can be made based on the effect observed with prior treatments.
- Multiple passes may be needed before the clinical endpoint is observed.

- Most authors recommend a **10%-20% overlap** between treatment zones because of the Gaussian distribution of intensity within each treatment zone if using a PDL.

APPLICATIONS
Rhytids
- Near-infrared nonablative lasers are variably and mildly effective at reducing fine rhytids.
- Perioral rhytids are difficult to improve and may require fully ablative lasers and/or soft tissue fillers.[27]

Scars
- Nonablative and fractional lasers are effective at improving burn scars, traumatic scars, and unfavorable, hypertrophic surgical scars, but require multiple treatments.
- Multiple modalities may be combined to treat different aspects of the scar:
  - **Fractional laser** for scar pliability, texture[28]
  - **PDL** for erythema and irritation of immature scar[29,30,31,32]
  - **IPL** for chronic folliculitis, scar dyschromia[33]

> **SENIOR AUTHOR TIP:**   In difficult scar cases we rub 5-fluorouracil or steroids over the fractionally treated scar to enhance results.

Dyschromia
- Lentigines respond to lasers that target melanin, such as the 510 nm PDL, 532 nm KTP laser, and IPL devices.
- Of these, IPL devices show the most dramatic effects with the shortest downtime and greatest safety profile.

Hypervascularity
- Best response is usually obtained with **PDL** and **IPL** devices; the difference is that PDL is prone to greater efficacy in one treatment if pushed to produce purpura.
- IPL devices more often require repeat treatments but cause no purpura if treated within normal guidelines.

Tattoo Removal
- Pigment is embedded in the dermis as large particles.
  - The goal of laser therapy is to **break up the large particles into smaller particles** that can be phagocytized by macrophages by a photoacoustic effect from the laser.
- Ideal laser **depends on the tattoo color,** but **Q-switched lasers** are ideal tattoo removal devices.
  - **Black-blue** absorbs a wide range of lasers: 694 nm Q-switched ruby, Q-switched 1064 nm Nd:YAG, Q-switched alexandrite
  - **Green:** Q-switched alexandrite[34]
- Up to 10-15 treatments may be needed.[34]

Hair Reduction
- Chromophore is **melanin.**
- Laser needs to reach the **dermal papilla** to destroy the follicle.

- Typical lasers used are the 810 nm diode, 755 nm alexandrite, 1064 nm ND:YAG, and 694 nm ruby.
- Wavelengths in the visible light spectrum have a higher risk of complications with darker skin types.
- The ruby laser has the highest incidence of hyperpigmentation, hypopigmentation, and blistering in darker skin types and tanned individuals.[35]
- Up to 6-8 treatments may be needed.

> **TIP:** Laser hair reduction is most effective in people with dark hair and fair skin.

POSTOPERATIVE CARE

- Because nonablative modalities do not leave an open wound, **no dressing is usually needed.**
- If blistering occurs, triple antibiotic ointment is applied until the area heals.
- Sun avoidance and the use of sunscreen with SPF 30+ are extremely important.
- Ice packs as needed for swelling.
- Patients must finish course of antivirals and antibiotics as prescribed.

COMPLICATIONS

- **Unsatisfactory result**
- Nonablative techniques are not as effective as ablative techniques at removing moderate to severe rhytids.

> **TIP:** Up to eight treatments may be needed to achieve the desired clinical result.

- **Hypopigmentation (10%-20%)[36]**
  - Thought to be caused by melanocyte destruction by heat energy
  - Usually transient and self-limiting
  - Rarely, delayed hypopigmentation can develop 6-12 months after treatment.
  - Skin type is not a predictor.

> **SENIOR AUTHOR TIP:**   This complication is extremely rare in nonablative treatments and is more common in aggressive CO_2 resurfacing.

- **Blistering**
  - Usually mild and self-limiting
  - Petrolatum ointment used until healed
- **Scarring**—very rare
- **Subdermal fat atrophy**
  - Reported with the monopolar radiofrequency device
  - Frequency unclear

SIDE EFFECTS

> **NOTE:**   Side effects differ from complications. Side effects occur predictably, and must be included as common occurrences patients must accept after laser treatment.

- **Erythema occurs very commonly (60%).**[13]
  - Usually lasts for 24-48 hours
  - Self-limiting
- **Swelling occurs commonly (15%-20%).**[13]
  - Usually lasts 24-48 hours
  - Self-limiting
  - Ice pack used as needed
- **Hyperpigmentation**
  - Thought to be caused by **melanocyte stimulation by heat energy**
  - Patients with **dark skin types** are at much higher risk.
    - ▶ General incidence 0.7%
    - ▶ 0.3% in Fitzpatrick skin type I, 33% in Fitzpatrick skin type V[37]
  - Risk is higher with low-wavelength lasers and IPL (have high affinity for melanin) and/or lasers with longer pulse durations.
  - Risk is higher if sun avoidance and sunscreen use are not practiced, i.e., tan is present.
  - Pretreatment and posttreatment with hydroquinone and tretinoin recommended[5]
  - At the first sign of hyperpigmentation, **bleaching cream** is started: Hydroquinone/ Lytera and tretinoin.
  - When treating solar lentigines, lesions typically darken for 1 week before improving.
  - Self-limiting
- **Purpura**
  - Very common when treating hypervascularity with the PDL
  - Lasts 1-2 weeks and is self-limiting
- **Herpes simplex virus outbreak (2%-7%)**[37]
  - Most common in patients with a prior history of herpes simplex virus outbreak

SENIOR AUTHOR TIP: I am often asked, "If you could only buy one machine, which one would you buy?" This is impossible to answer, because it depends on the patient population and practice characteristics, but my most common answer is an IPL/BBL device. (NOTE: Currently, many platform options allow physicians to purchase one device and add to it as their knowledge and practice grow. This is a very reasonable approach to building a laser- and light-based practice.

TOP TAKEAWAYS

➤ When treating with visible-light wavelengths, patients with unrecognized tans have the highest rate of complications.

➤ Patients treated with nonablative lasers should be informed that their result is directly related to the response of their immune system and genetic factors beyond their control or the surgeon's control. They are paying for minimal downtime but accepting the risk of variability of result. The time spent explaining this openly and honestly will benefit the patient and prevent liability issues if it is documented well.

➤ IPL/BBL treatment several times per year over several years is probably the most effective nonablative light treatment from a cost-effective standpoint. More youthful skin is the rule.

REFERENCES

1. Kelly KM, Nelson JS, Lask GP, et al. Cryogen spray cooling in combination with nonablative laser treatment of facial rhytides. Arch Dermatol 135:691, 1999.
2. Kono T, Kikuchi Y, Groff WF, et al. Split-face comparison study of cryogen spray cooling versus pneumatic skin flattening in skin tightening treatments using a long-pulsed Nd:YAG laser. J Cosmet Laser Ther 12:87, 2010.
3. Bellew SG, Lee C, Weiss MA, et al. Improvement of atrophic acne scars with a 1,320 nm Nd:YAG laser: retrospective study. Dermatol Surg 31:1218, 2005.
4. Rogachefsky AS, Hussain M, Goldberg DJ. Atrophic and a mixed pattern of acne scars improved with a 1320-nm Nd:YAG laser. Dermatol Surg 29:904, 2003.
5. Goldberg DJ, Cutler KB. Nonablative treatment of rhytids with intense pulsed light. Lasers Surg Med 26:196, 2000.
6. Hohenleutner S, Koellner K, Lorenz S, et al. Results of nonablative wrinkle reduction with a 1,450-nm diode laser: difficulties in the assessment of "subtle changes." Lasers Surg Med 37:14, 2005.
7. Tanzi EL, Alster TS. Comparison of a 1450-nm diode laser and a 1320-nm Nd:YAG laser in the treatment of atrophic facial scars: a prospective clinical and histologic study. Dermatol Surg 30:152, 2004.
8. Cohen JL, Ross EV. Combined fractional ablative and nonablative laser resurfacing treatment: a split-face comparative study. J Drugs Dermatol 12:175, 2013.
9. Collawn SS. Fraxel skin resurfacing. Ann Plast Surg 58:237, 2007.
10. Ong MW, Bashir SJ. Fractional laser resurfacing for acne scars: a review. Br J Dermatol 166:1160, 2012.
11. Glaich AS, Rahman Z, Goldberg LH, et al. Fractional resurfacing for the treatment of hypopigmented scars: a pilot study. Dermatol Surg 33:289, 2007.
12. Guimarães P, Hadad A, Sabino Neto M, et al. Striae distensae after breast augmentation: treatment using the nonablative fractionated 1550-nm erbium glass laser. Plast Reconst Surg 131:636, 2013.
13. Fodor L, Peled IJ, Ullmann Y, et al. Using intense pulsed light for cosmetic purposes: our experience. Plast Reconstr Surg 113:1789, 2004.
14. Lupton JR, Williams CM, Alster TS. Nonablative laser skin resurfacing using a 1540 nm erbium glass laser: a clinical and histologic analysis. Dermatol Surg 28:833, 2002.
15. Weiss RA, Gold M, Bene N, et al. Prospective clinical evaluation of 1440-nm laser delivered by microarray for treatment of photoaging and scars. J Drugs Dermatol 5:740, 2006.
16. Zelickson BD, Kilmer SL, Bernstein E, et al. Pulsed dye laser therapy for sun damaged skin. Lasers Surg Med 25:229, 1999.
17. Alexiades-Armenakas MR. Laser-mediated photodynamic therapy. Clin Dermatol 24:16, 2006.
18. Bitter PH. Noninvasive rejuvenation of photodamaged skin using serial, full-face intense pulsed light treatments. Dermatol Surg 26:835, 2000.
19. Sadick NS, Schecter AK. A preliminary study of utilization of the 1320-nm Nd:YAG laser for the treatment of acne scarring. Dermatol Surg 30:995, 2004.
20. Chang AL, Bitter PH Jr, Qu K, et al. Rejuvenation of gene expression pattern of aged human skin by broadband light treatment: a pilot study. J Invest Dermatol 133:394, 2013.
21. Dover JS, Bhatia AC, Stewart B, et al. Topical 5-aminolevulinic acid combined with intense pulsed light in the treatment of photoaging. Arch Dermatol 141:1247, 2005.
22. Low DW. Lasers in plastic surgery. In Thorne CH, Bartlett SP, Beasley RW, et al, eds. Grabb and Smith's Plastic Surgery, ed 6. Philadelphia: Lippincott Williams & Wilkins, 2007.

23. Fitzpatrick R, Geronemus R, Goldberg D, et al. Multicenter study of noninvasive radiofrequency for periorbital tissue tightening. Lasers Surg Med 33:232, 2003.
24. Hruza G, Taub AF, Collier SL, et al. Skin rejuvenation and wrinkle reduction using a fractional radiofrequency system. J Drugs Dermatol 8:259, 2009.
25. Hsu TS, Kaminer MS. The use of nonablative radiofrequency technology to tighten the lower face and neck. Semin Cutan Med Surg 22:115, 2003.
26. Youn A. Nonsurgical face lift. Plast Reconstr Surg 119:1951, 2007.
27. Cohen SR, Henssler C, Johnston J. Fractional photothermolysis for skin rejuvenation. Plast Reconstr Surg 124:281, 2009.
28. Haedersdal M, Moreau KE, Beyer DM, et al. Fractional nonablative 1540 nm laser resurfacing for thermal burn scars: a randomized controlled trial. Lasers Surg Med 41:189, 2009.
29. Parrett BM, Donelan MB. Pulsed dye laser in burn scars: current concepts and future directions. Burns 36:443, 2010.
30. Allison KP, Kiernan MN, Water RA, et al. Pulsed dye laser treatment of burn scars. Alleviation or irritation? Burns 29:207, 2003.
31. Donelan MB, Parrett BM, Sheridan RL. Pulsed dye laser therapy and z-plasty for facial burn scars: the alternative to excision. Ann Plast Surg 60:480, 2008.
32. Hultman CS, Edkins RE, Wu C, et al. Prospective, before-after cohort study to assess the efficacy of laser therapy on hypertrophic burn scars. Ann Plast Surg 70:521, 2013.
33. Erol OO, Gurlek A, Agaoglu G, et al. Treatment of hypertrophic scars and keloids using intense pulsed light (IPL). Aesth Plast Surg 32:902, 2008.
34. Alster TS. Q-switched alexandrite laser treatment (755nm) of professional and amateur tattoos. J Am Acad Dermatol 33:69, 1995.
35. Lanigan SW. Incidence of side effects after laser hair removal. J Am Acad Dermatol 49:882, 2003.
36. Handley JM. Adverse events associated with nonablative cutaneous visible and infrared laser treatment. J Am Acad Dermatol 55:482, 2006.
37. Graber EM, Tanzi EL, Alster TS. Side effects and complications of fractional laser photothermolysis: experience with 961 treatments. Dermatol Surg 34:301, 2008.

19. Chemical Peels

George Broughton II, Ahmed M. Hashem, Christopher Chase Surek,
James E. Zins

PREOPERATIVE EVALUATION

- Consultation with the patient to establish realistic goals and expectations
- Does the patient have an indication for chemical resurfacing?
    - Superficial or deep rhytids/photoaging
    - Preneoplastic or neoplastic lesions such as actinic keratoses and lentigines
    - Underlying skin disease such as acne
    - Pigmentary dyschromias
    - Demarcation lines secondary to other resurfacing procedures
- Any contraindications (Box 19-1)?

Box 19-1 *CONTRAINDICATIONS FOR CHEMICAL PEELS*

Absolute
- Poor physician-patient relationship
- Lack of psychological stability and mental preparedness
- Unrealistic expectations
- Poor general health and nutritional status
- Isotretinoin therapy within the last 6 months*
- Complete absence of intact pilosebaceous units on the face
- Active infection or open wounds (such as herpes, excoriations, or open acne cysts)

Relative
- Medium-depth or deep resurfacing procedure within the last 3-12 months*
- Recent facial surgery involving extensive undermining, such as a facelift*
- History of abnormal scar formation or delayed wound healing
- History of therapeutic radiation exposure
- History of particular skin diseases (such as rosacea, seborrheic dermatitis, atopic dermatitis, psoriasis, and vitiligo) or active retinoid dermatitis
- Fitzpatrick skin types IV, V, and VI*

---

*These contraindications are for medium- and deep-depth peels and do not apply to touchups.

- Comprehensive medical and surgical history and physical examination
    - Bleeding complications/risks from prescription and herbal medicine
- Is the patient taking isotretinoin, birth control pills, or immunosuppressants?
    - Is the patient pregnant?
    - Patients having a history of cold sores require herpes simplex prophylaxis.
    - **All patients should receive antiviral prophylaxis regardless of history.**
    - Does the patient have a history of hypertrophic or keloid scars?

- Does the patient have a history or risk of hepatitis or HIV?
- Does the patient have certain cutaneous diseases in the operative site?

TIP: Patients with rosacea, seborrheic dermatitis, atopic dermatitis, psoriasis, or vitiligo may be at increased risk for postoperative complications, including disease exacerbation, prolonged erythema, contact hypersensitivity, or delayed healing. Patients with rosacea have a vasomotor instability and may develop an exaggerated inflammatory response.

- What skin regimens have been used and what were the results?
- If patient has history of skin rejuvenation, what type of rejuvenation was done, what were results, and did problems occur?
- Identify dyschromias and determine the best depth of peel (Box 19-2).
- Determine depth of pigmentation using a Wood lamp.
  - ▶ View patient in darkest room possible.
  - ▶ Hold lamp 8-12 inches from patient's face and rotate wrist to change angles.
  - ▶ Under a Wood lamp, epidermal hyperpigmentation is bright and accentuated. Deep dermal hyperpigmentation is not seen or is less pronounced.

TIP: The worse the patient looks under a Wood lamp, the more superficial the pigmentation.

Box 19-2   *PEEL RESULTS FOR DIFFERENT DYSCHROMIAS*

Superficial Peel	Medium-Depth Peel
Excellent Results	***Excellent Results***
Ephelides	Ephelides
Epidermal hyperpigmentation	Epidermal melasma
Epidermal melasma	Epidermal postinflammatory hyperpigmentation
	Lentigines simplex
	Senile lentigines
Variable Results	***Variable Results***
Lentigines simplex	Dermal and mixed melasma
Mixed (epidermal and dermal) melasma	Dermal and mixed postinflammatory hyperpigmentation
Mixed postinflammatory hyperpigmentation	Seborrheic keratoses
Senile lentigines	
Poor Results	***Poor Results***
Dermal melasma	Nevi
Dermal postinflammatory hyperpigmentation	Some exophytic seborrheic keratoses
Junctional nevi	
Seborrheic keratoses	

- Determine and document patient's skin type (using the Fitzpatrick skin type classification)[1] and photoaging grouping (Tables 19-1 and 19-2), degree of actinic damage, sebaceous gland density, dyschromias, suspicious lesions, and scarring.
- Point out any skin excess and gravitational changes that will **not** be corrected by chemical peels.

- Standard preoperative photographs for surgical planning (see Chapter 3)
- Presurgical arrangement and understanding about financial responsibilities for revisions
- Analysis and operative planning based on patient's desires, clinical examination, and photographs.

Table 19-1 *Fitzpatrick Skin Type Classification*

Skin Type	Characteristics	Sun Exposure History
I	Pale white, freckles, blue eyes, blond or red hair	Always burns, never tans
II	Fair white, blue/green/hazel eyes, blond or red hair	Usually burns, minimally tans
III	Cream white, any hair or eye color	Sometimes burns, tans uniformly
IV	Moderate brown (Mediterranean)	Rarely burns, always tans well
V	Dark brown (Middle Eastern)	Rarely burns, tans easily
VI	Dark brown to black	Never burns, tans easily

Table 19-2 *Glogau Photoaging Scale*

Type	Description	Features
I (mild)	Wrinkles not present or minimal	Early photoaging No keratoses, pigmentary changes Patient generally wears minimal or no makeup Typical age range: 20s-30s
II (moderate)	Wrinkles present only when skin is in motion	Early to moderate photoaging Early actinic keratoses Sallow color Smile lines begin Patient generally wears some makeup Typical age range: Late 30s-40s
III (advanced)	Wrinkles present when skin is at rest	Advanced photoaging Dyschromias, telangiectasias Actinic keratoses Persistent wrinkling Patient always wears makeup Typical age range: 50s or older
IV (severe)	Only wrinkles	Severe photoaging Yellow-gray skin Dynamic/gravitational wrinkling throughout Actinic keratoses ± skin malignancies No normal skin Patient wears makeup, but coverage is poor (it cakes or cracks) Typical age range: 60s or older

NONFACIAL PEELING

INDICATIONS

- **Back**
  - To remove sunburn freckles across the shoulders and upper back
  - To improve acne scars
  - To improve postinflammatory hyperpigmentation from acne
- **Chest**
  - To improve hyperpigmented macules, usually lentigines or flat seborrheic keratoses and sunburn freckles
  - To improve acne scars, especially in areas of hypopigmented scars and hyperpigmented actinic damage
  - To improve postinflammatory hyperpigmentation from acne
  - To improve fine wrinkling (usually vertical lines over the sternum)
- **Hands and forearms**
  - To improve hyperpigmented macules (age spots)
  - To improve superficial wrinkling
  - To improve rough texture

SOME KEY POINTS[2]

- It usually takes **nonfacial** areas **50%-100% longer** to heal than the face. Patients need to be sure they have time to undergo this type of therapy before having it done.
- Dermal peels on the arms, hands, neck, and chest are more prone to scarring or abnormal textural changes. It is safer to perform **epidermal peels** in these areas. Dermal hyperpigmentation and most types of scars on nonfacial areas should not be treated with chemical peeling, because they will not improve significantly.
- Most nonfacial peels are done to improve fine wrinkling and blotchy discoloration (including age spots). One intraepidermal peel is usually not sufficient to give these patients their best results. Nonfacial peels are usually repeated several times to achieve the best response.
- Most nonfacial peels are performed on large areas of skin (a larger surface area than the face). If a peeling agent with potential toxicity is used, there is a greater risk of developing a systemic reaction.
- The larger the area treated and subsequently wounded, the more difficult it is for patients to care for it, and the greater the chance of a complication, particularly premature peeling or infections.

INFORMED CONSENT[3]

Recommended items to be included in the informed consent:

- No warranties, guarantees, or special contracts about the success and longevity of the procedure
- Review of the healing process and how the patient will look and for how long
- Possible need for additional surgeries/procedures
- Complications, especially pigment changes (hyperpigmentation and hypopigmentation), scarring (including keloids, hypertrophic scarring), fever blisters (herpes simplex) activation, infection, milia, and "pink areas" (erythema)
- Review (with the patient) the things chemical peels can and cannot do (Box 19-3).

Box 19-3 *THINGS CHEMICAL PEELS CAN AND CANNOT DO*

Things Chemical Peels CAN Do	Things Chemical Peels CANNOT Do
Correct sun damage (actinic degeneration)	Decrease pore size—chemical peels might increase pore size
Flatten mild scarring	Improve skin laxity
Remove rhytids	Improve deep scarring
Improve irregular hyperpigmentation	Totally remove hyperpigmentation in dark-skinned whites, Asians, and blacks
	Remove vascular lesions

PEEL PREPARATION

- Chemical peels may be classified as:
  - **Superficial** (epidermal injury)
  - **Medium-depth** (superficial dermal injury to the papillary dermis)
  - **Deep** (mid-dermal injury to the reticular dermis).
- **Degree of injury** is dependent on:
  - Chemical agent used
  - Concentration
  - Time of application before neutralization
  - Number of coats and the amount of peeling agent placed with each application (i.e., degree of wetness of the applicator)

Fig. 19-1 is a review of skin anatomy. The different chemical peel formulations commonly used are summarized in the section Common Chemical Peel Agents.

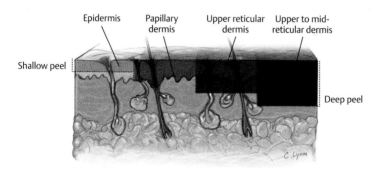

Fig. 19-1   Skin anatomy and chemical peel depth.

COMMON CHEMICAL PEEL AGENTS

GLYCOLIC ACID[4]
- **The product**
  - Not light sensitive: Does not need to be stored in a dark bottle
  - Very stable (>2 years)
  - Deliquescent (absorbs moisture): Must be kept in a tightly capped bottle

- ■ **Features**
  - Most practitioners use 30%-70% glycolic acid and neutralize the skin with a bicarbonate solution or rinse with water at the onset of erythema.
  - Caution must be used, because uneven peeling and dermal wounding can occur.
  - White, scattered frosting indicates epidermal necrosis and dermal inflammation.
  - Moy et al[5] found a protocol of 10%-15% glycolic acid applied twice daily and 50%-70% glycolic peels given weekly for 4 weeks effective in the treatment of fine wrinkles and superficial lesions. Van Scott and Yu,[6] using a similar protocol for 10 months, reduced wrinkles in 21 of 27 patients.
  - Glycolic peels are less effective for solar keratoses and solar lentigos.
  - Piacquadio[7] concluded that retinoids, light TCA peels, and glycolic lotion represent a better consumer value than glycolic acid peels.

> **TIP:**   Glycolic acid is an alpha-hydroxy acid (AHA) made from sugar cane. Other AHAs include lactic acid (from sour milk), malic acid (from apples), citric acid (various fruits) and tartaric (from grape wine).

JESSNER SOLUTION[4]

Formulated by Dr. Max Jessner. The combination allows decreasing the concentration and toxicity of each ingredient.

- ■ **The product**
  - Contains **resorcinol, salicylic acid, lactic acid,** and **ethanol**
  - Retains strength for up to 2 years if container is opened for only 5 minutes per month
  - *Light and air sensitive!* May develop a salmon-colored tone on exposure to light and air—store in a dark amber bottle with a tight cap
- ■ **Features**
  - It creates a uniform-depth peel that results in an excellent exfoliation.
  - It is useful in treating hyperpigmentation by increasing epidermal turnover and yielding a decrease in the number of melanin-containing keratinocytes.
  - Complications are rare because of the limited penetration.
  - Use is limited to the face because of the potential for salicylate (tinnitus, headache, nausea) or resorcinol (methemoglobinemia and hypothyroidism with prolonged use) toxicity.
  - It is thought to break the intracellular bridges between keratinocytes and has the capacity to remove the epidermis.
  - Used alone, it causes superficial epidermal peel.
  - Depth is controlled by **number of applications.**
  - No neutralization is needed.
  - It can be combined with TCA for a medium peel.
  - Application first causes a faint erythema followed by a more pronounced erythema on second application. After further applications, a frost begins to form. Significant exfoliation is seen for 8-10 days when a frost is achieved; however, no weeping or crusting is seen, because it remains an intraepidermal peel.

TRICHLOROACETIC ACID (TCA)
- **The product**
  - **Not** light sensitive
  - Refrigeration **not** needed
  - Stable for at least 23 weeks in an opened container
  - 20%-100% TCA stored in an unopened TCA-resistant clear plastic container for 2 years—TCA concentration within 3% of the labeled strength
  - Colorless and clear
  - Free of precipitate
- **Features**
  - **TCA** is commonly used in **30%-35%** concentration for medium-depth peeling penetrating into the upper reticular dermis.
  - The concentration, skin preparation, pretreatment skin type, and method of application contribute to the peel depth obtained.
  - An intraepidermal, epidermal, or papillary dermal peel can be successfully obtained with 20% TCA. Superficial papillary dermal necrosis was shown histologically in a porcine model at 24 hours using 20% TCA; however, no change in the number of fibroblasts or elastic fibers was detected at 28 weeks after the peel.[8]
  - Dolezal[9] suggested four levels of superficial and intermediate TCA peels.
    - **Level 0:** Has no frost, and the skin looks slick and shiny, which represents removal of the stratum corneum.
    - **Level 1:** Has an irregular, light frost with some erythema; this is an intraepidermal peel that creates 2-4 days of light flaking.
    - **Level 2:** Has a pink-white frost, which suggests a full-thickness epidermal peel, and heals in about 5 days.
    - **Level 3:** Has a solid white frost and is thought to extend into the superficial retinacular dermis. Johnson et al[10] described an additional sign of "epidermal sliding" for a papillary dermal peel.

CROTON OIL PEEL
- **The product**
  - Initially utilized by "lay peelers." The formula was obtained by Tom Baker in the early 1960s. The original Baker Gordon formula utilized high concentrations of phenol and croton oil (50% phenol, 2.1%-2.4% croton oil). Although excellent results could be obtained, long-term hypopigmentation became a problem and croton oil peeling fell into disfavor.
  - Phenol-croton oil peeling regained popularity in the early 2000s due to the work of Hetter[11-14] and later Stone and colleagues.[15-16] Hetter refuted a number of the concepts espoused by Baker (phenol-croton oil peeling is an "all or none phenomenon," and decreasing concentrations of phenol led to deeper injury). But most importantly both Hetter and Stone demonstrated by reducing the concentration of phenol and croton oil, complications could be significantly reduced while the results could be maintained.
- **Features**
  - Stone suggested that the depth of peeling is dependent on the concentration of both the phenol and croton oil, whereas Hetter suggested that croton oil is the critical agent determining peel depth.
  - Ozturk et al[17] stated that a concentration of 33% phenol and 1.1% croton oil is associated with acceptable side effects in Fitzpatrick I and II skin types, especially in the perioral area.

- Gatti et al[18] stated that treatment of the lower lids with phenol 22% and 1.1% croton oil is effective in treating hyperpigmentation and fine lines.
  - ► Standard concentration 88%
  - ► Used alone causes medium-depth peel
  - ► Causes keratin protein coagulation
  - ► Rapidly absorbed through skin, metabolized in the liver, excreted renally
  - ► Can lead to renal failure, hepatotoxicity, directly irritates myocardium causing **arrhythmias**
  - ► Requires **cardiac monitoring** and testing of kidney, liver, cardiac function
  - ► Hypopigmentation and scarring significantly minimized by reducing concentrations of phenol and croton oil.
  - ► Peel in subunits, allowing 15-20 minutes per site between units.

PHENOL-CROTON OIL AND TCA PEELS

- Although traditionally TCA was considered a medium-depth peeling agent and phenol-croton oil a deep peeling agent, this has clearly been disproven by Hetter and Stone. Using modern peeling understanding, both agents can peel in subunits to superficial (epidermal), intermediate (papillary dermal), or deep (mid-reticular dermal) levels depending on:
  1. Concentration of agents used
  2. Number of applications
  3. Wetness of the applicator
- Most critical to the level of the peel is the **degree and nature of the frost obtained.**
  - *Pink-white* frost suggests injury to the papillary dermis; *dense white* frost suggests superficial reticular dermal injury, and *gray-white* suggests mid-reticular dermal injury.
- Therefore, TCA and croton oil peels should not be thought of as intermediate or deep peeling agents only, but as agents that can peel to any depth desired. This significantly increases their respective versatility.

SALICYLIC ACID

- **The product**
  - Made into a paste and spread over the skin using a tongue depressor
  - Formula: Salicylic acid powder USP, 50%; methyl salicylate, 16 drops; Aquaphor, 112 g
- **Features**
  - The incidence of significant complications is low, and it is easy to use.
  - Deep penetration is difficult.
  - It is effective for the treatment of hyperpigmented age spots on the hands and arms. Patients will need to have their hands/arms wrapped in plastic wrap and gauze for 48 hours.
  - In concentrations of 3%-5% it is keratolytic and enhances topical penetration of other agents.
  - It has mild potency as a fungicide.
  - Symptoms of salicylate toxicity include ringing in the ears, muffled hearing, dizziness, and/or headache several hours after the peel. Increased water intake and removal of the bandage may improve mild salicylism.

- Application of salicylic acid will cause mild stinging for 1-3 minutes followed by superficial anesthesia to light touch. After 5 minutes of air drying, the face should be washed with water.
- Peeling starts around days 3-5 and continues until day 10.

BETA-LIPOHYDROXY ACID[19]
- **The product**
  - Eight-carbon fatty chain linked to a benzene ring (derivative of salicylic acid)
  - Available in formulations of 5% and 10%
- **Features**
  - The safety profile is good with less skin irritation, compared with glycolic acid, and neutralization is not required.
  - It reduces melanosome clustering and epidermal pigmentation and is used for treatment of photoaged skin and acne.
  - It increases the skin's resistance of UV-induced damage.
  - It has antibacterial and antifungal effects.
  - The corneosome-corneocyte interface is targeted to cleanly detach individual corneosomes, preventing desquamation in clumps and resulting in skin smoothness.

KEY POINTS FOR ETHNIC SKIN
- Ethnic skin may respond unpredictably to chemical peels regardless of phenotype.
  - Latino and Hispanic patients are prone to an increased incidence of *melasma* and *postinflammatory hyperpigmentation,* and chemical peels should only be approached with caution in this patient population. Prolonged pretreatment suppression with 4% hydroquinone is critical.
- Consider modifying the peel technique: Spot treat lesions instead of treating the entire face.
- Indications
  - Dyschromia
  - Acne
  - Scarring
  - Postinflammatory hyperpigmentation
  - Melasma
  - Pseudofolliculitis barbae
- Chemical peel formulations considered safe to use in ethnic skin include:
  - Beta-lipohydroxy acid: 5%-10%
  - TCA: 10%-20%
  - Glycolic acid: 20%-70%
  - Salicylic acid: 20%-30%
  - Lactic acid
  - Jessner solution

PRECONDITIONING THE SKIN: "PRIMING"
- Preparation of patients may include oral antibiotics and antivirals, facial cleansing, and some preprocedure skin creams. Light peels that only injure the stratum corneum often require no preprocedure prophylaxis, whereas deeper peels may place susceptible patients at higher risk of herpetic outbreaks and should be covered with an appropriate antiviral agent. Skin preparation may include vigorous cleansing with an exfoliant to remove oils and debris.

■ **For medium to deep peels:** Patients should be instructed to start a vitamin A (retinoic acid 0.1% cream daily for a minimum of 2 weeks before the peel) and glycolic acid skin conditioning program for 6 to 8 weeks before the procedure. Preconditioning the skin causes treated skin to heal faster by 3-4 days by increasing its metabolism—from accelerated cellular division and new collagen formation.[20-22]

> **TIP:** All-*trans*-retinoic acid (tretinoin) will speed epidermal healing and enhance the effect of the peel.[22]

■ **Patients with dyschromias:** Patients undergoing a peel to improve hyperpigmentation (any depth) need to use **tretinoin in combination with a bleaching agent** before the peel. This is also true for patients at risk for developing a postinflammatory hyperpigmentation (determined by history—does the patient's scar turn dark?). In addition to tretinoin, two other products are available, hydroquinone and kojic acid, in the following preparations: [23-24]
  • 4% Hydroquinone preparation
  • 2% Hydroquinone with 10% glycolic acid gel
  • 2% Hydroquinone with 2% kojic acid and 6% AHA gel base

> **TIP:** 4% Hydroquinone is prescription strength, and 2% is not. However, 2% hydroquinone combined with 10% glycolic acid is equally effective. Kojic acid is an alternative bleaching agent that can be used on patients who do not tolerate hydroquinone.

TECHNIQUES

SAFETY CHECK BEFORE PEELING
■ Always check the label on the bottle of any chemical to be applied to a patient's skin. Accidental application of the wrong acid can create serious problems.
■ Never pass an open container of acid (or an applicator wet with acid) over a patient's face. Acid could accidentally spill onto the skin.
■ Never perform a peel with a patient lying completely flat. Always elevate the patient's head at least 30-45 degrees. Failure to elevate the head increases the chances of acid collecting around the eye.
■ Always have water nearby to flush the eyes in case acid gets into them.
■ Watch for tears with all peels. A tear running down the cheek onto the neck can create an area of peeling on the neck.
■ When using a different brand of peeling agent (or if a different pharmacist makes the solution), always know whether the preparation is made by the same weight-to-volume measurement. With glycolic acid, note whether the pH of the new solution is the same as the pH of the previous one.
■ Before peels, always ask patients whether they:
  • Recently had a facial waxing
  • Recently used a facial depilatory
  • Recently had electrolysis
  • Recently had head or neck surgery

- Have taken isotretinoin (13-*cis*-retinoic acid [Accutane]) within the past 1-2 years
- Are currently using retinoic acid (Retin A) or AHAs
  - ▶ Patients who answer "yes" to any of these questions may react more strongly to a peel.
    - ◆ All patients undergoing any peel type should take oral acyclovir or valcyclovir starting 2 days before and until healing is complete.
    - ◆ All patients undergoing any type of treatment for photodamage must use a broad-spectrum sunscreen daily.

ANESTHESIA: OFFICE-BASED[1,2]

- **Superficial peels**: Anesthesia is generally not needed. Explain to patients they will feel a warm stinging-burning discomfort that will last for 15-30 minutes. If there are no contraindications, patients can take over-the-counter NSAIDs before the procedure to help with discomfort.
- **Medium-depth peels**: These peels are more uncomfortable than superficial peels. The pain is intense and lasts for 2-3 minutes. Strategies to address the pain include:
  - Patients can take NSAIDs an hour before the procedure.
  - Use a fan to cool patients during the peel.
  - Perform the peel in anatomic units to allow one section to cool before performing the next.
  - Narcotics: Intramuscular meperidine and hydroxyzine, or intravenous midazolam or fentanyl, or oral diazepam is given before the procedure.
  - Nerve blocks: The entire face can be adequately anesthetized with 12 injections (Fig. 19-2). Patients must decide if 12 injections is a fair trade for 3 minutes of burning pain.
  - Topical anesthetics (EMLA): Topical anesthetics vasoconstrict and can increase the depth of a TCA peel.

> **SENIOR AUTHOR TIP:**   With topical anesthetics, apply a lower strength of TCA than originally planned, because unrecognized vasoconstriction will lead to a deeper peel.

Fig. 19-2   Location of injection sites for central face nerve block and mapping of nerve distribution. The entire face can be mapped with 12 injections (five on each side and two centrally). Usually, only 1 ml of lidocaine is needed at each site. The infraorbital nerve *(IO)* can be blocked by intraoral needle placed cephalad between the bicuspid teeth above the periosteum in the midpupillary line. Alternatively, an injection can be performed just cephalad and lateral to the nasolabial fold. The mental nerve *(M)* is reached by inserting the needle between the first and second molars caudally to the halfway point down the mandible. The remaining sites are anesthetized with a direct, transcutaneous approach. *(AE,* External branch of the anterior ethmoidal nerve; *IT,* infratrochlear nerve [V2]; *SO,* supraorbital nerve [V1]; *ST,* supratrochlear nerve [V1].)

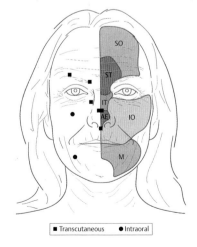

■ Transcutaneous   ● Intraoral

DEGREASING THE SKIN
- Before a chemical peel, the skin must be adequately prepared with a degreasing agent to remove debris and allow a uniform penetration. *Proper degreasing allows deeper penetration of the agent.*
  - **Office-based**
    - ▶ The patient removes all makeup, washes the face with an antiseptic skin cleanser (povidone-iodine or chlorhexidine) and then self-scrubs with acetone on gauze for 3 to 5 minutes. Patients will almost always underscrub themselves. The physician or nurse should wipe the skin again with isopropyl alcohol and then vigorously scrub it with acetone for 2 minutes to strip the stratum corneum. A handheld fan can be used to disperse acetone fumes.
  - **In the operating room**
    - ▶ Wipe the face off with isopropyl alcohol and then scrub the face with acetone for 2 minutes.
- **Acetone** is a very effective degreasing agent. Rubbing alcohol and Hibiclens have also been used and have been shown to be equally effective as acetone.[23] Acetone has the disadvantage of being highly flammable and therefore not available in hospitals or ambulatory surgery centers. Rubbing alcohol is a mixture of isopropyl alcohol, acetone, methyl isobutyl ketone, and water. Hibiclens is a detergent and surfactant, nontoxic, and has a pH of 5-6.5. It has the disadvantage of the additional step of rinsing the skin thoroughly and drying it to eliminate surface residue.

CHOICE OF APPLICATOR AND MODE OF APPLICATION
- Pouring the wounding agent into a glass cup before application will eliminate contamination of the master bottle, prevent cotton-tipped applicator disintegration, and conserve product.
- **Cotton balls**: Cotton balls are a reservoir for product and are best used for quickly applying a lotion of glycolic acid.
- **Cotton-tipped applicators:** One moist cotton-tipped applicator rubbed on the surface with moderate pressure will deliver more solution than a single, lightly applied, slightly damp applicator. Rubbing the surface with two cotton-tipped applicators with hard pressure will deliver more product than a single applicator.
- **4- by 4-inch gauze sponge:** A 4 × 4 gauze sponge wrung out, damp or wet, can deliver more wounding agent to a larger area.
- **Sable brush:** A 1-inch sable brush used with Jessner solution delivers more agent than a 4 × 4 gauze sponge.
- **Proctology swabs:** A large cotton-tipped applicator is a reservoir for the agent and can deliver product over a large area. The large surface area prevents streaking with uneven application, but it will waste a lot of product. *These swabs should not be used with phenol solutions because it will deliver too much phenol to skin.*

TIP: Sable brushes are available in art supply stores and can be cleaned with povidone-iodine solutions.

DILUTION
- Once frosting appears, penetration of the agent has already occurred—*adding water to an aqueous wounding agent on the skin before frosting dilutes the agent and will affect the concentration and reproducibility of the peel.*

- TCA peels do not need to be "neutralized" or diluted.
- AHAs (i.e., glycolic acid) do not frost in the same manner as TCA peels and are dependent on **contact time** with the skin. Washing them from the skin after a given time is important. A 10% sodium bicarbonate solution can also be used.

OCCLUSION

- Taping after phenol-croton oil peeling is thought to increase the depth of injury.[24]
- A mechanical tape barrier is more effective than an immediate application of an occlusive ointment for absorption and penetration of phenol.
- Tape can applied to selected problem areas, and taping the entire face is not imperative.
- Clinically, the results can be the same with or without taping.

SUGGESTED ORDER OF AREAS TO BE PEELED (SUPERFICIAL AND MEDIUM-DEPTH)

- Begin with the most sensitive area first (periorbital) so the patient is alert, cooperative, and still (before the inevitable squirming that will occur once frosting starts).
- **Areas and order to be peeled:** Lower eyelash area ➤ upper eyelid ➤ nose ➤ cheeks ➤ perioral area ➤ forehead

PERIORBITAL PEELING TECHNIQUE (Fig. 19-3)

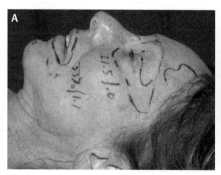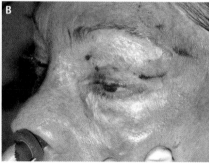

Fig. 19-3   A, Photograph demonstrating preprocedure markings and planned phenol/croton oil chemical peel concentrations specific to each aesthetic subunit. High concentrations of phenol and croton oil will peel deeper than lower concentrations, given similar application process (i.e., number of swipes). For this patient an upper lip and cheek peel with phenol 33%/croton oil 1.1% and periorbital peel with phenol 27%/croton oil 0.105%. **B,** Photograph immediately following phenol 27%/croton oil 0.105% peel. Note the *pink-white frost* indicative of controlled injury at the depth of the papillary dermis.

- The cotton-tipped applicator should be **wrung out** and **semidry** to prevent dripping of product into the eyes.
- Generally, except for the crow's-feet area, the entire periorbital complex is thin skinned, and one applicator should be used for better control.
- The applicator must not be passed over the eye. A syringe or bulb of saline solution should be available to flush the eyes in case product is introduced into them.

■ **Steps in periorbital peel:**
1. The head is elevated to 30-45 degrees.
2. Tears are wiped away during the peeling process with a cotton-tipped applicator at the medial and lateral canthus while the eye is held open to prevent capillary action from wicking product into it.
3. For the lower eyelid, the eye is opened and the patient looking up. Product is applied within millimeters of the eyelash margin by moving from the lateral crow's-feet to the medial canthal area.
4. For the upper eyelid, the eye is closed. Application proceeds from the lateral to inner canthal area. Product is not applied below the superior tarsal plate to prevent edema. However, if sun damage is severe enough to warrant peeling within millimeters of the upper eyelashes, a superficial peeling agent no stronger than 35% TCA is used.
5. Ice pack application over the eye will help with postpeeling swelling—5-10 minutes for TCA peel and 6 to 8 hours after phenol application.
■ If performing periorbital peel only: Always peel to the orbital rims to prevent a line of demarcation. A superficial agent beyond these areas will never hurt and will help in blending the demarcated areas.

TIP: Some physicians advocate using protective ophthalmic ointment petrolatum. The ointment may promote excessive tearing and blinking and is unnecessary if the cotton-tipped applicator is well wrung out.

PERIORAL PEELING TECHNIQUE
■ Peeling agent should be applied 3 mm onto the vermilion border.
■ Manually stretching the skin will allow deeper and more even penetration.
■ The wooden end of a cotton-tipped applicator can be used to apply agent to an individual rhytid, especially on a repeat peel.
■ For especially deep, severely damaged actinic skin damage, aggressive pre-peel defatting of the area with heavy application of the agent seems to work well. Another method is to use selective occlusion.
■ If peeling the perioral area only, agent is applied to at least immediately beyond the nasolabial fold and the rest of the face is feathered with superficial peeling agent to prevent lines of demarcation.

TECHNICAL TIPS

GLYCOLIC ACID
■ The skin is cleaned with a gentle wipe of acetone or alcohol. Excessive defatting before a 70% glycolic acid peel may cause undesirable erythema or pigmentation.
■ The agent is applied rapidly, covering the entire face within 20 seconds. Glycolic acid comes as a liquid or lotion. A large cotton applicator or cotton balls are used to apply the product. To create an even peel, the product must have the same contact time throughout the face. See Table 19-3 for recommended glycolic acid concentrations and lengths of time the product is left on for different clinical scenarios.
■ After the desired time has passed or severe erythema occurs, the agent is wiped off with water-soaked gauze, or the patient can go to the sink and splash water over the face. *Ensuring the entire product is diluted is critical.*

TIP: Marketed purified water or commercial neutralizers with sodium bicarbonate have NO advantage over tap water. Ensuring that water-soaked gauzes or a 10% sodium bicarbonate solution is available *before* applying the agent is essential.

Table 19-3   *Suggested Glycolic Acid Concentrations and Duration for Different Indications*

Indication	Glycolic Acid (%) (pH ≤2.5)	Contact Time (minutes)
Acne	50-70	1-3
Melasma	50-70	2-4
Actinic keratoses	70	5-7
Fine wrinkles	70	4-8
Solar lentigines	70	4-6
Back or chest—any indication	70	5-10

TIP: Glycolic acid can create dermal wounds. Never tell patients it is a "risk-free" peel.

Glycolic acid peels usually need to be repeated several times for best results.

Some patients will have amazing results from glycolic acid peels and others will not. Stress to the patient that results **do vary.**

Glycolic acid peels **always need to be diluted to terminate their action.** The longer the peel is left on the skin, the deeper it will penetrate.

Glycolic acid peels can induce postinflammatory hyperpigmentation and create significant inflammation.

JESSNER SOLUTION

■ Jessner solution is excellent for use in acne patients, because resorcinol is a well-known treatment for acne. To prevent systemic absorption and the combined effects of resorcinol and salicylic acid, *it should not be used over large surface areas of the body.*
  • Clean skin with a gentle wipe of acetone or alcohol.
  • Apply Jessner solution in a uniform layer. Any of the applicators mentioned previously can be used. Most advocate using a sable brush.
    ▶ Rubbing the solution in with 2 × 2 gauze will enhance penetration and should be the method used for patients with thick, sebaceous skin.
    ▶ Patients with thin, sensitive skin should have the solution applied with a softer applicator: sable brush, cotton-tipped applicators, or cotton balls.
  • Observe for skin changes based on the level of peel. Each deeper level requires additional coats of Jessner solution, and each coat takes 4-6 minutes for the full skin reaction to occur.
    ▶ **Level 1**: Requires one coat of Jessner solution. Very superficial peel—faint erythema and light, powdery-looking whitening on the face (not to be confused with frost). The white powder can be wiped off the face with a finger or cotton ball.
    ▶ **Level II:** Requires two or three coats. With deeper penetration, erythema becomes more pronounced, turning bright red. Some smaller areas of white frost may appear. (This cannot be wiped off.) Patients may feel some light burning and

stinging for 15-30 minutes. The next 1-3 days will develop persistent, mild red-brown coloration. For 2-3 days, patients may feel like cellophane is on their face, and for the next 2-4 days their face exfoliates (appearing windburned instead of actually peeling).

➤ **Level III:** Requires three or four coats. Looks similar to a level II peel except exfoliation may take as long as 8-10 days. Some actual peeling may occur.

• Dilution or neutralization is **not** needed.

TRICHLOROACETIC ACID
Key Points About the Application of TCA

■ The head should be elevated 45 degrees—patients are more comfortable and there is less chance of acid pooling around the eyes.

■ The head should be stabilized with one hand so the other hand can press fairly hard with a gauze applicator as the acid is applied.

■ When applying the TCA below the eyes and in the crow's-feet area, the surrounding skin is pulled tight so that the acid gets to the bottom of the wrinkles and prevents acid from wicking into the eye along the wrinkle.

■ Overlapping coats of TCA will increase the depth of the peel. When using low strengths (<25% TCA), this is not much of a problem, but with higher concentrations, an area of accidental overlap can be a problem. This is prevented by always following the same pattern of application. *It may be helpful to count the number of strokes applied to each area to ensure a similar amount of acid is applied to all areas.*

■ TCA is a chemical cauterant, which coagulates proteins in the skin. This is the basis for the formation of the white frost seen when TCA is applied to the skin. The deeper the peel performed with TCA, the more intensely white the frost. Again, the nature and density of the frosting is the critical factor determining the depth of injury as espoused by Obagi.[10,25]

Application of TCA

■ The patient is seated at 45 degrees.

■ TCA is applied with folded 2 × 2 gauze sponges to allow the TCA to be rubbed into the skin. The sponge should be wet enough to allow a few drops to escape if squeezed.

■ TCA is applied in a systematic fashion (Fig. 19-4).

• Left forehead ➤ left upper eyelid ➤ Right forehead ➤ right upper eyelid ➤ nose ➤ PAUSE

• Left lower eyelid ➤ left cheek ➤ perioral area (left to right) ➤ PAUSE

• Right lower eyelid ➤ right cheek

➤ The pause will allow patient to cool and recover from the burn before proceeding.

➤ Pausing also allows for observation of the depth of the peel

• An alternative application procedure has the advantage of applying TCA to the sensitive areas first.

➤ Lower eyelash area ➤ upper eyelid ➤ nose ➤ cheeks ➤ perioral area ➤ forehead

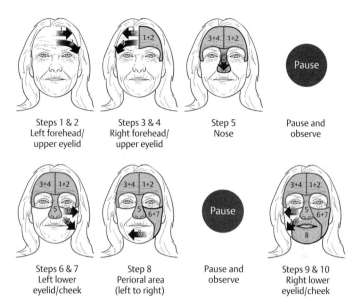

Fig. 19-4 Sequence for a TCA peel. After step 5, the physician pauses to observe the results and to allow the patient's skin to cool. After step 8, the physician pauses again to observe results of steps 6 through 8.

TIP: Levels of frosting: pink-white (papillary dermal), dense white (superficial reticular dermal), gray-white (mid-reticular dermal).

Maneuvers to Increase Depth of Peel

■ A second coat of acid is applied over the area that has already frosted. (It is safest to decrease the strength of TCA in the second coat by 5%-10% to prevent too deep a peel.)
■ When applying the TCA to the next (previously untreated) area on the face:
  • A gauze sponge that is wetter is used. It will allow application of a greater quantity of acid, which will create a deeper peel.
  • The acid-soaked gauze is rubbed more aggressively into the skin, in an attempt to overlap areas of application.
■ Once the appropriate frost has been achieved, rinsing the patient's face with room temperature water to wash off any excess acid that may remain on the skin is optional.
■ Some physicians advocate applying ice packs to the skin after the peel to cool the skin and to decrease residual burning. Many patients are hypersensitive immediately after the peel, and ice packs may be too uncomfortable for them.

TIP: If water or ice compresses are applied to the skin after a TCA peel, the stratum corneum will be hydrated and more TCA cannot be reapplied, because the acid will be rapidly diluted by the water trapped in the stratum corneum.

COMBINATION PEELS

Combination peels allow deeper penetration at lower concentrations. The following are common combinations.

JESSNER SOLUTION AND TRICHLOROACETIC ACID[26]

- Skin is cleaned in the normal fashion.
- One to four layers of Jessner solution is applied to the face with the endpoint of fairly uniform erythema with areas of little frost. Wait 5 minutes between applications.
- TCA 35% is applied in the usual manner. This penetrates more rapidly and uniformly than when it is applied to untreated skin.
- In patients with thick, sebaceous skin, several coats of Jessner solution may be needed. Patients with thin or dry skin generally do not need this combination treatment.

> **TIP:** If TCA concentrations of >35% are used with Jessner solution, a deep peel can be created. Jessner solution stings and burns—after it is applied, patients will be more sensitive and uncomfortable when TCA is applied. Applying coats of Jessner solution will add an additional 15-30 minutes to the procedure.

GLYCOLIC ACID AND TRICHLOROACETIC ACID[27]

- Patients are primed as usual, but the skin is not cleaned.
- Glycolic acid 70% is applied to the face for 2 minutes and then washed off with water.
- TCA 35% is applied in the normal fashion.

Things to Consider

- *Glycolic acid peels are uneven—it is counterintuitive to use a caustic peel on top of an uneven one.*
- Applying water to dilute a glycolic acid peel will hydrate the stratum corneum and may dilute TCA when applied.
- Dots are placed along the mandibular ramus as a reminder **not** to use the peel caudal to this line.
- An IV line is placed and LR started. Patients who have been fasting are given a bolus of 500 ml. Phenol is detoxified in the liver and excreted by the kidneys.
- Cardiac monitoring equipment is placed, a pulse oximeter and blood pressure monitor.
- Sedation and analgesia are given. A facial nerve block is performed, longer-acting anesthetics—bupivacaine, ropivacaine, or etidocaine may be used.
- The face should have been thoroughly washed the night before and morning of surgery. Patients should have NO makeup on.
- The skin is cleaned using Septisol (hexachlorophene with alcohol) or acetone. **Adequate degreasing is imperative for good results.**

- The phenol wounding agent should be applied with moist but not very wet cotton-tipped applicators or 2 × 2. Deep rhytids can be individually addressed before the rest of the cosmetic unit.
- The wound agent should be applied to each cosmetic unit in this order:
  • Forehead
  • Left cheek
  • Right cheek
  • Perioral area
  • Nose
  • Periorbital area
- Phenol does not affect hair growth and should be feathered into the hair-bearing areas.
- To minimize the risk of renal and cardiac toxicity, 10-15 minutes should elapse between applications to cosmetic units before a new coat is applied. Thus the peel is completed in 60-120 minutes.

TIP: Applicators and wound agent SHOULD NEVER PASS OVER A PATIENT'S EYES.

TAPING (INCREASES DEPTH OF INJURY) OR PETROLATUM (ALLOWS WOUND OBSERVATION)

- Tape is applied to each segment as the peel progresses or, if using the croton oil peel, after the peel is completed.
- Tape is precut into 1.5-4 cm strips.
- The tape is applied along the inferior border of the mandible in a sawtooth pattern. This pattern will produce an irregular line that is less noticeable. Tape placement is expanded out from there by applying the tape 1-2 cm parallel to the inferior border of the mandible.
- Stuzin et al[24] found that application of petrolatum (Vaseline) immediately after the peel is an alternative to taping. It will provide a vapor barrier to prevent phenol evaporation and increased maceration and penetration.

SENIOR AUTHOR TIP: Petrolatum (Vaseline) should be applied as a thick layer immediately after a region of the face has been treated with the wounding agent. THE WOUND SHOULD NOT BE ALLOWED TO DESICCATE. Taping increases the depth of the injury of the peel.

- Tape removal
  • The mask is removed in 48 hours when the exudate has lifted the tape. The mask should be removed as a single unit, not as individual strips of tape.

TIP: Repeat peeling can be performed in 12-18 months if necessary. Individual rhytids or spot areas can be retouched in 6 months.

POSTPEEL CARE AND INSTRUCTIONS TO PATIENTS

ALPHA-HYDROXY ACID PEELS (GLYCOLIC ACID)[25]

- Do not expect to really "peel." Most patients have a little redness for 12-24 hours. Occasionally, mild flaking may occur in a few localized areas for 1 or 2 days. Rarely, an area of crusting may develop. If this occurs, apply an antibiotic ointment to the area and notify the office if it fails to improve within 24 hours.
- Apply a bland moisturizer to the skin as often as needed. Do not apply any medications or glycolic acid products during this time—it will irritate the skin.
- Do not expect to see much reaction to this peel. Most patients look normal the day after a glycolic acid peel. The maximum benefit of this procedure is not really apparent until about 2-3 weeks after the peel.

JESSNER PEELS

- The face may appear slightly redder than usual for 7 days. In general, the peeled area will appear mildly or moderately sunburned.
- Peeling usually occurs from day 2-5 after treatment. The skin will become very dry, and small cracks may develop.
- Skin should be cleaned with a nondrying cleanser such as Dove, Neutrogena, or Cetaphil, and proper moisturizer such as Complex 15, Lubriderm, Nutraderm, or Aquaphor should be applied.
- Makeup may be applied as usual.
- Light peel treatments may be spaced at 2- to 4-week intervals.
- Topical medications such as retinoic acid (Retin A) and glycolic acid should not be applied for several days after the peel.

TRICHLOROACETIC ACID PEELS[25,28]

- Blistering, crusting, and peeling skin can occur for about a week.
- Treated skin should not be picked or rubbed.
- When washing hair, the head is tilted backward in the shower or in the sink. Too much water will cause premature peeling and leave red, sore areas that may lead to scarring or the need to be treated again.
- Large pieces of hanging, peeling skin may be carefully cut off with a pair of blunt-nose scissors.
- Avoid the sauna, Jacuzzi or strenuous exercise. Sweating will sting and cause premature peeling.
- Minimize facial expressions for a week after the peel. Excessive facial movements will cause the skin to crack prematurely.
- The face should be washed gently for 20-30 seconds twice a day using a mild, quality liquid soap (Dove, Neutrogena, or Cetaphil). The soap is lathered in the hands and gently patted onto the face. Rinse with a splash of lukewarm water. Dry by patting gently with a clean towel.
- A petrolatum-containing ointment (Aquaphor, Vaseline) or Preparation H should be used after washing. A tube is more sterile than a jar.
- Do not let the skin dry out. Ointment can be applied 10 times a day to prevent the skin from drying. A well-moisturized face will reduce tightness and will enhance comfort.
- **Avoid sunlight.** Exercise by walking in the early morning or late evening when the sun is barely out.

- Swelling may occur during the first 2-3 days after the peel. In extreme cases, the eyes may swell almost closed during the first two mornings. This is a normal response and will resolve on its own. Sleeping with an extra pillow to elevate the head may help to decrease swelling.
- Ice packs or cold compresses should **NOT** be applied to the face to decrease the swelling. The moisture from these may cause the skin to peel prematurely.
- Sleep on the back to prevent rubbing the peeling skin against the pillow. This could create an area of prematurely peeled skin.
- Sunscreen must always be worn when outside.
- Makeup may be worn 1-2 days after peeling is complete.

CAUTION: If unexpected irritation, a cold sore, or possible infection develops, instruct the patient to contact the office immediately.

CROTON OIL PEEL[28]

- Clear liquids sipped through a straw or soft foods should be taken for the first 48 hours until the bandages are removed (if present). Cool ice packs may be applied to the outside of the bandages.
- If no bandages are in place, those areas should be kept moist consistently with ointment.
- Swelling will be considerable, and drainage may appear underneath the tape after the first 12 hours until the tape is removed.
- Sleep with the head elevated on several pillows.
- Minimize talking or biting/chewing after peeling; sipping liquids through a straw is helpful.
- After the tape is removed, wash in the shower with a mixture of Betadine Skin Cleanser and white, unscented Dove liquid soap by using a splashing action and fingers only. Do not use a washcloth or other exfoliating aides. After each washing, a moisturizing ointment should be applied as a thick coat. If no tape is present, wash in the shower after 48 hours.
- Swelling begins to subside after day 5, and the peel is usually healed by day 14.
- DO NOT PICK AT THE CRUST.
- Avoid prolonged constrictive use of caps, shower caps, eyeglasses, or visors in peeled areas until the skin has healed over.
- If pain or fever blisters develop anytime during the peel process, have the patient call the office immediately for evaluation.
- Itching 7-14 days after healing is common. Excessive redness and itching may be caused by allergy to the ointment. If this happens, switching to Vaseline or Crisco is appropriate.
- Most patients can return to work as soon as day 14. Makeup and sunscreen can be applied on any area that has healed.
- Working out and jogging should be avoided for 30 days, because increased blood flow may result in microhemorrhages and red blotching.
- A retouch of specific areas or re-peeling 6 months after peeling may be required for selected deep wrinkles.
- Complete avoidance of the sun is critical. Exposure to sunlight, getting pregnant, or taking birth control pills before the redness has disappeared may cause blotchiness or postinflammatory hyperpigmentation.

- The redness from deep peeling is usually resolved 90-180 days after peeling. Occasionally, localized areas may persist as long as 18 months.
- In lighter-skinned individuals (Fitzpatrick I), redness is more persistent and may last for months.

SIMULTANEOUS FACELIFT AND CHEMICAL PEEL

- Originally, we thought that the skin flap from a facelift cannot be safely resurfaced simultaneously with a chemical peel.[29-31]
- Fulton[31] has shown that a Jessner/TCA peel can be safely used on the skin flap from a facelift.
- A deep, full-face phenol peel should NOT be done simultaneously over undermined facelift flaps to prevent injury to the subdermal plexus and compromised wound healing. However, croton oil peeling can be performed at the same time as a facelift in areas not undermined. Therefore, perioral and periorbital peeling at the time of facelifting is safe.[17]
- All preoperative considerations for a face peel should be followed for the facelift.
- Patients can expect the skin to begin peeling around day 3 or 4 after the peel. The duration of exfoliation is directly related to the depth of the peeling.
- Skin hydration with a petrolatum-based moisturizer is paramount.

EXPECTED RESULTS (Figs. 19-5 through 19-8)

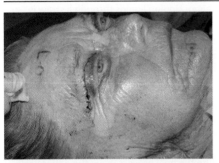

Fig. 19-5 Photograph during chemical peel of the face. In the region of the cheek note the abating dense white frost in the cheek. The concentration in the cheek was phenol 33%/croton oil 1.1%.

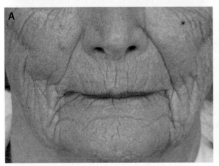
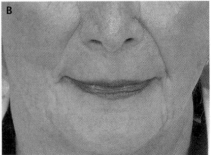

Fig. 19-6 **A,** Preprocedure photograph. **B,** Postprocedure photograph 3 years after full-face phenol 33%/croton oil 1.1% peel and upper blepharoplasty. Note the significant improvement of perioral rhytids with minimal hypopigmentation of the skin.

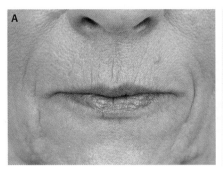 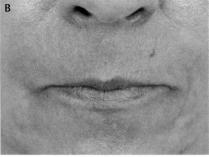

Fig. 19-7 A, Preprocedure photograph. **B,** Postprocedure photograph 3 years after facelift, fat injection to nasolabial folds, and perioral phenol 33%/croton oil 1.1% peel. Note the significant improvement of perioral rhytids with minimal hypopigmentation of the skin.

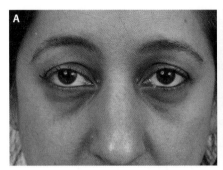 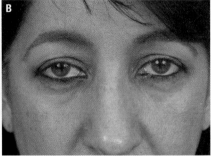

Fig. 19-8 A, Preprocedure photograph demonstrating periorbital hyperpigmentation. **B,** Postprocedure photograph 5 years after periocular phenol 27%/croton oil 0.105% peel. Note the significant improvement in hyperpigmentation.

COMPLICATIONS[32]

- Complications can be divided into three categories: during procedure, early postprocedure, and late postprocedure.

DURING PROCEDURE COMPLICATIONS
- Usually a result of errors in technique
- **Tears dripping onto the neck**
  - Tears can drip down the cheek and dilute the acid. This will result in a strip of skin where the peel is more superficial than on the rest of the face.
  - Tears can drip down the cheek and neck, bringing acid with them. The path of an acidic tear can burn the skin, easily scarring the neck (especially if the acid concentration is high).

> **SENIOR AUTHOR TIP:** Someone should watch the patient and blot any tears immediately with cotton-tipped applicators. If a tear should reach the neck, the area should be washed with water to dilute the acid.

- **"Streaky" or "blotchy" results**
  - This is usually caused by inadequate degreasing with acetone.
  - This can also be caused by overlapping of peeled areas.
    - ▶ Reapplication of TCA or phenol and croton oil produces a deeper wound.
- **Cardiac arrhythmias**
  - May occur with phenol-based peels
  - Usually premature atrial and ventricular contractions
  - Cardiac monitoring necessary with phenol-based peels
  - Most arrhythmias reversed with hydration, supplemental oxygen, and stopping the peel. Whether phenol-croton oil peel is causative with regard to arrhythmias is, however, debatable.

EARLY POSTPROCEDURE COMPLICATIONS
- **Infection**
  - *Staphylococcus* and *Streptococcus* species are the most common.
  - Less common causes are *Pseudomonas* species, mycobacteria, and fungi.
  - Bacterial and fungal infections are rare in the absence of prolonged occlusive taping methods.
- **Reactivation of dormant herpetic infections**
  - Early detection and aggressive treatment can prevent long-term and disastrous sequelae.

> **TIP:** In the face of prophylactic antiviral therapy, significant herpes infections are rare and generally mild. Sudden deterioration of the peeled area is suggestive of infection and requires an immediate office visit.

- **Premature peeling:** The necrotic skin created by the peel functions as a protective biologic dressing. When it is picked off prematurely, it can lead to infection, postinflammatory hyperpigmentation, persistent erythema, and scarring. The following are common signs of premature peeling:
  - A sharply demarcated area of bright erythema
  - A peel that is completed within 1-2 days of the expected halfway point of the peel.
  - No evidence of old peeling skin can be found. (Usually compliant patients will have small areas of peeling skin in the hairline.)

> **TIP:** Patients with signs or symptoms of premature peeling should be confronted about the possibility of them picking at the scab. This should be documented in the medical record and the patient counseled about the possible complications.

LATE POSTPROCEDURE COMPLICATIONS

■ **Milia:** A common benign condition of keratin-filled cysts that appear as small white bumps
- Usually occurs 3 weeks after procedure
- Found most often around the periorbital area
- Responds well to topical vitamin A derivatives, which prevents future outbreaks with continued use
- Can also be physically extracted

■ **Acneiform" eruptions:** Tender erythematous follicular papules. Caused by follicular occlusion from emollients or ointments.
- Treatment: Topical antibiotic therapy with clindamycin or erythromycin or systemic therapy with tetracycline and erythromycin
- Typically clear in 5-10 days

■ **Hypopigmentation and hyperpigmentation**
- Can occur as early as 10-14 days, but most cases occur 4 weeks postoperatively.
  - ▶ Hypopigmentation
    - ◆ Observe for 3-6 months while inflammation resolves.
    - ◆ Hypopigmentation that persists after 3-6 months is unlikely to resolve spontaneously.
    - ◆ There is no good treatment for hypopigmentation—patients will need to camouflage the affected areas with makeup.
  - ▶ Hyperpigmentation
    - ◆ Early treatment with topical bleaching agents (4% hydroquinone ointment) can resolve the problem completely
    - ◆ If a strong inflammatory component is also present, topical steroids can be added.
    - ◆ Patients who do not respond to medical therapy may need nonablative laser treatment to diminish pigment.

■ **Prolonged erythema** (pink areas)
- This is almost completely self-limiting within 6 months (most within 3 months)
- Patient will need reassurance.
- Topical steroid treatment will resolve the erythema for very anxious patients.

■ **Scarring**
- This results from excessively deep penetration.
- It can also occur from exaggerated inflammatory response (as in keloid formation).
- Treatment of the scar with serial intralesional triamcinolone injections often resolves the problem.
- Resistant scars may need dermabrasion or laser resurfacing followed by silicone sheet therapy.

TOP TAKEAWAYS

➤ Chemical peeling is a time-tested, safe, and effective modality to treat the skin.

➤ The goal of chemical peeling is to produce a controlled partial-thickness skin injury, mitigating pigmentary disorders, solar damage, and aging.

➤ Pretreatment (priming) with Retin-A and hydroquinone is helpful to minimize posttreatment hyperpigmentation, especially in darker-skinned patients.

➤ Pretreatment with Retin-A and AHAs can smooth skin texture, optimizing the peeling outcome. Moisturizers and sun-blocking agents further enhance the result.

➤ The propensity for complications and untoward reactions is directly related to the depth of peeling.

➤ Categorizing peels as superficial intermediate and deep is an antiquated concept. Phenol-croton oil and trichloroacetic acid (TCA), formerly considered deep and intermediate peeling agents respectively, can instead be used as superficial, intermediate or deep peeling agents. This is readily accomplished by reducing the concentration of agents used, reducing the number of applications, or the wetness of the applicator.

➤ Critical to predicting the depth of injury is assessing the nature and intensity of frosting: pink-white suggests injury to the level of the papillary dermis; dense white, the superficial reticular dermis; and gray-white, the mid-reticular dermis.

➤ Any peel can induce untoward effects if used with excessive frequency, in inappropriate concentrations, or even with aggressive skin preparation.

➤ Secondary alteration of skin pigmentation is the most common complication.

➤ Damage to the melanocytes at the epidermal-dermal junction leads to hypopigmentation. This is more common in fair-skinned patients, and especially after phenol peeling.

➤ Hyperpigmentation usually results from peeling induced inflammation, with melanocyte overstimulation. Darker-skinned patients are more prone to this complication, especially with premature sun exposure.

➤ Scarring, the most serious, although rare, complication, is usually secondary to extension of damage to the deep reticular dermis. It is most often encountered in the perioral and mandibular areas. Heralded by persistent erythema, it usually begins as an area of induration. It should be aggressively treated with dilute Kenalog injection (3 mg/ml) on a weekly (not monthly) basis until it is resolved. Surgical revision may be required.

➤ Treatment of the lower lids with dilute phenol and croton oil is effective in treating hyperpigmentation and fine lines.

REFERENCES

1. Fitzpatrick TB. The validity and practicality of sun-reactive skin types I through VI. Arch Dermatol 124:869, 1988.
2. Collins PS. Trichloroacetic acid peels revisited. J Dermatol Surg Oncol 15:933, 1989.
3. Duffy DM. Informed consent for chemical peels and dermabrasion. Dermatol Clin 7:183, 1989.
4. Clark CP III. Office-based skin care and superficial peels: the scientific rationale. Plast Reconstr Surg 104:854, discussion 865, 1999.
5. Moy LS, Murad H, Moy RL. Glycolic acid peels for the treatment of wrinkles and photoaging. J Dermatol Surg Oncol 19:243, 1993.
6. Van Scott EJ, Yu RJ. Alpha hydroxy acids: procedures for use in clinical practice. Cutis 43:222, 1989.
7. Piacquadio D, Dobry M, Hunt S, et al. Short contact 70% glycolic acid peels as a treatment for photodamaged skin. A pilot study. Dermatol Surg 22:449, 1996.
8. Roenigk RK, Brodland DG. A primer of facial chemical peel. Dermatol Clin 11:349, 1993.
9. Dolezal J. Trichloroacetic acid solutions and basic pharmacy. In Rubin MG, ed. Manual of Chemical Peels: Superficial and Medium Depth. Philadelphia: Lippincott Williams & Wilkins, 1995.
10. Johnson JB, Ichinose H, Obagi ZE, et al. Obagi's modified trichloroacetic acid (TCA)-controlled variable-depth peel: a study of clinical signs correlating with histological findings. Ann Plast Surg 36:225, 1996.
11. Hetter GP. An examination of the phenol-croton oil peel: Part IV. Face peel results with different concentrations of phenol and croton oil. Plast Reconstr Surg 105:1061; discussion 1084, 2000.
12. Hetter GP. An examination of the phenol-croton oil peel: Part III. The plastic surgeons' role. Plast Reconstr Surg 105:752, 2000.
13. Hetter GP. An examination of the phenol-croton oil peel: Part II. The lay peelers and their croton oil formulas. Plast Reconstr Surg 105:240; discussion 249, 2000.
14. Hetter GP. An examination of the phenol-croton oil peel: Part I. Dissecting the formula. Plast Reconstr Surg 105:227; discussion 249, 2000.
15. Stone PA. The use of modified phenol for chemical face peeling. Clin Plast Surg 25:21, 1998.
16. Stone PA, Lefer LG. Modified phenol chemical face peels: recognizing the role of application technique. Clin Plast Surg 9:351, 2001.
17. Ozturk CN, Huettner F, Ozturk C, Bartz-Kurycki MA, Zins JE. Outcomes assessment of combination face lift and perioral phenol-croton oil peel. Plast Reconstr Surg 132:743e, 2013.
18. Gatti JE. Eyelid phenol peel: an important adjunct to blepharoplasty. Ann Plast Surg 60:14, 2008.
19. Kornhauser A, Coelho SG, Hearing VJ. Applications of hydroxy acids: classification, mechanisms, and photoactivity. Clin Cosmet Investig Dermatol 3:135, 2010.
20. Hevia O, Nemeth AJ, Taylor JR. Tretinoin accelerates healing after trichloroacetic acid chemical peel. Arch Dermatol 127:678, 1991.

21. Nemeth AJ, Eaglstein WH, Falanga V, et al. Methods to speed healing after skin biopsy or trichloroacetic acid chemical peel. Prog Clin Biol Res 365:267, 1991.
22. Mandy SH. Tretinoin in the preoperative and postoperative management of dermabrasion. J Am Acad Dermatol 15:878, 1986.
23. Peikert JM, Krywonis NA, Rest EB, et al. The efficacy of various degreasing agents used in trichloroacetic acid peels. J Dermatol Surg Oncol 20:724, 1994.
24. Stuzin JM, Baker TJ, Gordon HL. Chemical peel: a change in the routine. Ann Plast Surg 23:166, 1989.
25. Rubin MG, ed. Manual of Chemical Peels: Superficial and Medium Depth. Philadelphia: Lippincott Williams & Wilkins, 1995.
26. Monheit GD. The Jessner's-trichloroacetic acid peel. An enhanced medium-depth chemical peel. Dermatol Clin 13:277, 1995.
27. Coleman WP III, Futrell JM. The glycolic acid trichloroacetic acid peel. J Dermatol Surg Oncol 20:76, 1994.
28. Brody HJ. Chemical Peeling and Resurfacing, ed 2. St Louis: Mosby–Year Book, 1997.
29. Baker TJ. Chemical face peeling and rhytidectomy. A combined approach for facial rejuvenation. Plast Reconstr Surg Transplant Bull 29:199e, 1962.
30. Litton C. Chemical face lifting. Plast Reconstr Surg Transplant Bull 29:371, 1962.
31. Fulton JE. Simultaneous face lifting and skin resurfacing. Plast Reconstr Surg 102:2480, 1998.
32. Roy D. Ablative facial resurfacing. Dermatol Clin 23:549, 2005.

20. Dermabrasion

George Broughton II, James L. Baker, Jr.

PREOPERATIVE EVALUATION[1-4]

- Consultation with the patient to establish **realistic goals and expectations** (see Chapter 4)
- Comprehensive medical and surgical history and physical examination. Some medical conditions are contraindications to dermabrasion (see Box 20-2).
  - Bleeding complications/risks from prescription and herbal medicine
    - ▶ Is the patient taking isotretinoin, birth control pills, or immunosuppressants?
  - Is the patient pregnant?
  - History of cold sores requires herpes simplex prophylaxis
  - History of hypertrophic or keloid scars?
  - History or risk of hepatitis or HIV?

> **TIP:** Dermabrasion results in aerosolization of tissue and blood. Physicians and their assistants (including the anesthesiologist) must take appropriate measures to protect themselves. This involves wearing a gown, face shield, face mask, and gloves.

- History of connective tissue disorders, cold intolerance, or Raynaud phenomenon? (These patients may not be candidates if a refrigerant is used.)
- Current and past skin regimens and their results?
- Prior history of skin rejuvenation? When and what kind? Results/problems from those treatments?
- Tanning history: Does the patient have hyperpigmentation or hypopigmentation?
- Documentation of patient's skin type (Fitzpatrick skin type classification) (Table 20-1) and photoaging grouping (Table 20-2), degree of actinic damage, sebaceous gland density, dyschromias, suspicious lesions, and scarring.
- Skin excess and gravitational changes that will **not** be corrected by dermabrasion are pointed out.

Table 20-1 *Fitzpatrick Skin Type Classification*

Skin Type	Characteristics	Sun Exposure History
I	Pale white, freckles, blue eyes, blond or red hair	Always burns, never tans
II	Fair white, blue/green/hazel eyes, blond or red hair	Usually burns, minimally tans
III	Cream white, any hair or eye color	Sometimes burns, tans uniformly
IV	Moderate brown (Mediterranean)	Rarely burns, always tans well
V	Dark brown (Middle Eastern)	Rarely burns, tans easily
VI	Dark brown to black	Never burns, tans easily

> **SENIOR AUTHOR TIP:** Skin types I through III will have a uniform blended skin color postoperatively. Types IV proceed with caution and best to not dermabrade types V and VI due to hyperpigmentation postoperatively.

■ Standard preoperative photographs for surgical planning
  • Patients evaluated for facial rejuvenation or scar improvement are asked to provide photographs of themselves (in repose) when they were younger.
  • Preoperative and postoperative photographs are helpful for those who had prior surgery on their face.
■ Preoperative arrangement and discussion of financial responsibilities for revisions
■ Analysis and operative planning based on patient desires, clinical examination, and photographs
■ Patients are given an antibacterial cleanser to wash and shampoo with the night before and the morning of surgery and prescriptions for cephalexin 500 mg twice per day for 5-7 days, acyclovir 1 g once per day (twice per day for patients with history of oral herpes, start the day before the procedure) for 5-7 days, diazepam (or similar relaxant), and narcotic pain medication.
■ Test spot close to the area to be treated should be considered. This allows the patient to experience the procedure in a limited fashion and provides some information about expected results. Usually a 1 cm area is abraded with the patient under local anesthesia.

TIP: The test spot should be placed close to the area to be treated but in an obscured area that can be easily camouflaged or hidden if further treatment is not performed. For example, for patients who will have facial or neck dermabrasion, the spot can be made behind the ear. Stressing that the test spot is *not* predictive of the overall outcome is critical.

Table 20-2   *Glogau Photoaging Scale*

Type	Description	Features
I (mild)	Wrinkles not present or minimal	Early photoaging No keratoses, pigmentary changes Patient generally wears minimal or no makeup Typical age range: 20s-30s
II (moderate)	Wrinkles present only when skin is in motion	Early to moderate photoaging Early actinic keratoses Sallow color Smile lines begin Patient generally wears some makeup Typical age range: Late 30s-40s
III (advanced)	Wrinkles present when skin is at rest	Advanced photoaging Dyschromias, telangiectasias Actinic keratoses Persistent wrinkling Patient always wears makeup Typical age range: 50s or older
IV (severe)	Only wrinkles	Severe photoaging Yellow-gray skin Dynamic/gravitational wrinkling throughout Actinic keratoses ± skin malignancies No normal skin Patient wears makeup, but coverage is poor (it cakes or cracks) Typical age range: 60s or older

INDICATIONS AND CONTRAINDICATIONS (Boxes 20-1 and 20-2)

Box 20-1   *CONDITIONS TREATABLE WITH DERMABRASION*

Acne rosacea	Lichenified dermatoses
Actinically damaged skin	Linear epidermeral nevus
Active acne	Discoid lupus erythematosus
Adenoma sebaceum	Mibelli porokeratosis
Angiofibromas of tuberous sclerosis	Multiple pigmented nevi
Basal cell carcinoma (superficial type)	Multiple seborrheic keratoses
Blast tattoos (gunpowder)	Multiple trichoepitheliomas
Chloasma	Neurotic excoriations
Chronic radiation dermatitis (mild)	Postacne scars
Congenital pigmented nevi	Pseudofolliculitis barbae
Darier's disease	Rhinophyma
Dermatisis papillaris capillitii	Scleromyxedema
Early operative scars	Smallpox or chickenpox scars
Facial rhytids	Striae distensae
Favre-Racouchot syndrome	Syringomas
Fox-Fordyce disease	Syringocystadenoma papilliferum
Freckles	Tattoos (decorative and traumatic)
Hair transplantation (elevated recipient sites)	Telangiectasias
	Traumatic scars
Hemangiomas	Verrucous nevus
Hypertrophic scars	Vitiligo
Keratoacanthomas	Xanthelasma
Lentigines	Xeroderma pigmentosum
Lichen amyloidosis	

Box 20-2   *CONTRAINDICATIONS TO DERMABRASION*

Absolute	Relative
Isotretinoin therapy within the last 6-12 months*	History of hypertrophic scars
	History of keloids
Congenital ectodermal defects	Burns—deep thermal or chemical
Radiodermatitis (only if severe)	Fitzpatrick skin types IV, V, VI (test patch should be tried first)
Pyoderma	
Psychosis	History of hepatitis or HIV†
Active herpes labialis	

*Seven patients with atrophic acne scars on the face taking oral isotretinoin to treat facial acne had manual dermabrasion on an area approximately 1 cm.[2] At the 6-month follow-up, all patients had normal cicatrization, and the atrophic acne scar revision was deemed excellent.[5] In another study, 10 patients treated with oral isotretinoin for acne had a medium-depth chemical peel applied to the entire face and manual sandpaper dermabrasion (until the appearance of a blood dew) 1-3 months after the isotretinoin therapy was concluded. At the 6-month follow-up, all patients had normal cicatrization, and no hypertrophic scars or keloids were observed. Depressed acne scar revision was satisfactory.[6]
†Personal decision of the surgeon.

PHYSICAL EXAMINATION[1,3,7]

- Thorough inspection of the type or condition to be treated. Dermabrasion has been used for numerous traumatic and medical conditions. (Box 20-1 contains a partial list.)
- Characterization of the scar. Deep, wide, or ice-pick scars may not be appreciably helped by dermabrasion and may require multiple procedures.
- Evaluation of the patient's scar for potential of dyspigmentation

INFORMED CONSENT[1,2]

Recommended items to be included in the informed consent:
- Location of the area(s) to be treated
- A statement that reads, "Dr.___ has placed markings on my face and/or body. I have examined these markings completely with Dr.__, and I understand that they represent the location where dermabrasion will be done."
- No warranties, guarantees, or special contracts about the success and longevity of the procedure
- The possible need for additional surgeries/procedures
- **Complications:** Scarring, catastrophic intraoperative disaster (avulsion of soft tissue such as lips and eyelids), dyspigmentation, and failure of the procedure to adequately improve the treated area
- A complete understanding from the patient that some skin conditions have malignant potential, and that any recurrence or new growth at the treated areas requires immediate evaluation

EQUIPMENT AND PREPARATION[1,3]

Standard equipment includes personal protective gear for everyone in the operating room, a dermabrader, a standard surgical tray, a cryogenic spray or local anesthetic, and a choice of planing tips—diamond fraises, serrated wheels, and wire brushes.
- Dermabraders can be electrical or gas powered. The choice of dermabrader is dependent on the physician's level of comfort with the device's rotational speed and torque.
  - Compressed-gas–powered units generate greater torque and higher rotational speed.
  - Electrical-powered dermabraders are more convenient but have slower rotational speeds and torque. Some units have foot pedal control and can achieve a variable speed ranging from 400-40,000 rpm.

> **TIP:**   The rotations per minute of devices with high torque will not decrease in response to friction caused by the downward pressure of the planing tip onto the skin.

- Abrading tips are available in a wide range of sizes (width, length, and coarseness), with three basic types:
  - **Diamond fraise.** Stainless steel wheels with industrial-grade diamonds bonded to them. They are graded according to barrel width, shape, and coarseness. The coarser the diamond surface and the faster the cutting speed, the greater penetration into the tissue.

TIP: For novice surgeons, a wide-barrel fraise with fine-grade diamonds offers the greatest margin of safety.

- **Wire brush**. Stainless steel bristles are tightly fixed to a wheel and may be angulated or straight. Great care is required with this planing device, because it can easily cause horrific tissue damage. Most experienced surgeons think a wire brush is more effective than a fraise tip.

TIP: Wire brush tips tend to cause significant dissemination of particulate matter, blood, and tissue.

- **Serrated wheel**. A circular wheel with small surface spikes. The spikes are widely spaced on a barrel-type tip and can easily cause tissue gouging. This tip is not used much and should be employed by experienced surgeons because of its greater potential to cause tissue damage.
- **Manual spot dermabrasion.**[8] Manual spot dermabrasion involves abrading devices for dermabrasion, including wire brush, diamond fraise, sandpaper, Bovie scratch pads, abrasive cloth, and drywall or plaster sanding screen. These instruments are used manually in a back-and-forth or circular motion.

SENIOR AUTHOR TIP: Wrapping a sheet of sanding screen paper around the barrel of a 3 ml syringe provides a controlled and easy-to-use method of spot dermabrasion.

- **Microdermabrasion.** A variety of microdermabraders are available on the market. Common to all systems is a pump that generates a high-pressure stream of aluminum oxide or salt crystals, a connecting tube that delivers the crystals to the handpiece, a handpiece, and a vacuum to remove the crystals and exfoliated skin. The crystals are discarded and cannot be recycled. Handpieces can be reusable or disposable. The reusable handpieces must be resterilized after each use.

TECHNIQUES

DERMABRASION[1,3]
Treatment Areas
The most commonly treated area is the face; however, dermabrasion can be used on any body part to treat scars or traumatic tattoos.

Preprocedure Details
- Antibiotics are started the day before the procedure if taken orally or just before the procedure if given intravenously. Oral postoperative antibiotics should be continued for a week after the procedure, or until complete reepithelialization.
- Patients with a history of cold sores are treated with antiviral agent (acyclovir or valacyclovir) on the day before the procedure, the morning of the procedure, and for approximately 7 days after the procedure.
- The skin is cleaned with antibacterial soap. Patients should not apply makeup on the day of the procedure, and all of it should be removed before arriving for the procedure.
- Anesthesia is required. A general anesthetic or sedation with a nerve block is used.
- The surgeon and everyone else in the room MUST wear protective eyeglasses to shield against airborne tissue flung by the dermabrader.

■ The valley of deep rhytids and acne pits should be marked with a surgical marker to help determine the depth of treatment.

> **TIP:**   Deep rhytids are marked with a fine-tipped marker. Marking the pit of acne scars with an outline around the area of maximum scarring will help to identify the depth and extent of dermabrasion needed.

Performance Details

■ When working around tissues with free edges, the rotation should always be toward the leading edge, and the dermabrasion drum should always be moved toward the direction of rotation (Fig. 20-1).

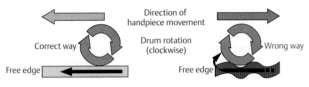

Fig. 20-1   Correct way to move the handpiece of a dermabrader. When the handpiece is moved in the direction of rotation (correct way), the tissue is swept away from the rotating drum. When the handpiece is moved in the direction opposite the drum's rotation, the abrasive tip will clutch the tissue; the rotating drum, in combination with the moving handpiece, will "dig into" the tissue and cause the upcoming tissue to be forcefully and rapidly pulled toward the rotating drum. A free edge would be dragged up and over the drum. This can forcefully avulse tissues with free edges (lips and eyelids).

■ For treatment around the lips, the **rotational speed should be decreased,** and the drum should be swept over the vermilion-cutaneous border to prevent lip avulsion. For treatment of nasolabial lines and crow's-feet, the movement of the handpiece and the direction of rotation should be AWAY from the nose and AWAY from the eye, respectively.
■ *Care is needed when holding a gauze around the dermabrader.* If it is caught, it will be ripped from the physician's hand and whipped around, possibly injuring the eye or soft tissue.
■ The abraded surface needs to be wiped frequently with a gauze to observe the bleeding pattern. **Uniformly spaced, punctate bleeding is the goal.**
■ The fraise or brush is held **parallel to the skin.** If the drum is angulated, the leading edge will cut into the skin.
■ After dermabrasion treatment, the skin is cleaned using a saline solution rinse and a soft bristle brush or rough gauze to remove excess skin debris.

> **TIP:**   Laying a nonadherent dressing soaked in epinephrine solution (1:1,000,000) over the open wounds can decrease bleeding.

Dressing

- Treated areas can be left uncovered, and the patient can apply antibacterial or white petrolatum ointment.
- Ointment can be generously applied and nonadherent dressings or petrolatum gauze placed on the treated areas.

Postoperative Care

- Patients are reminded to complete their full course of oral antibiotic and antiviral therapy.
- The importance of wearing sunblock EVERY day—regardless of the season and whether the patient works inside or outside—must be stressed.
- Persistent redness can be treated with topical steroid cream (Temovate [clobetasol propionate] 0.05%) applied twice per day for 2 weeks. This regimen is repeated until normal skin color returns. Patients are counseled against using it continuously and not on the eyelids (unless specifically instructed to do).

TIP: A green-base makeup applied to the red skin will neutralize the color, and a light layer of natural makeup can be applied over it.

MICRODERMABRASION[7]

Microdermabrasion works by blasting aluminum oxide crystals at high speeds toward the skin surface, creating a "sandblaster effect" that produces a superficial ablation, primarily in the epidermis. A vacuum is used to remove the abrasive crystals, sloughed skin, and debris.

Microdermabrasion has several advantages that make it a popular office-based procedure (Box 20-3). Because it only affects the epidermis, the procedure is ineffective for deeper wrinkles and scars. Indications for performing microdermabrasion include treatment for minor degrees of sun damage, fine wrinkling, acne/superficial scarring, and blending of treatment boundaries. In select patients, microdermabrasion can be an effective treatment with minimal risk and rapid recovery.

Treatment Areas

- The most commonly treated area is the face; however, the neck, hands, and chest can be treated.
- The depth of the treatment depends on:
  - The strength of flow of the crystals
  - The rate of movement of the handpiece against the skin
  - The number of passes over the treatment area
- Longer contact of the abrasive crystals with the skin by slowly moving the handpiece and performing more passes will result in a deeper abrasion. Two passes will exfoliate to a depth of 15-25 μm.

Box 20-3   *ADVANTAGES AND DISADVANTAGES OF MICRODERMABRASION*

Advantages	Disadvantages
Does not require anesthesia	Multiple treatments needed
Painless	Good effectiveness only in very select
Can be repeated within short intervals	patients
Simple and quick to perform	
Less operator-dependent than dermabrasion	
Consistent depth of tissue loss (adjustable)	
Less blood exposure than with dermabrasion	
Risks of hyperpigmentation/ hypopigmentation and scarring low	
Rapid recovery—erythema resolves after 24 hours	
Can be performed by a physician, nurse, or licensed aesthetician	

Preprocedure Details
- Premedication is usually not necessary.
- Skin is cleaned of all makeup and oil.
- Topical or local anesthetic is usually not necessary.
- Contact lenses must be removed, and eye protection is worn to prevent injury from stray crystals.

Performance Details
- The **key technical maneuver** for successful microdermabrasion is to **create an effective vacuum** by placing the skin under tension. This is achieved by stretching the treatment area with the nondominant hand and using the dominant hand to guide the handpiece. When the neck is treated, it is placed in extension to ensure the most skin tension.
- Treatment sessions generally last 30-40 minutes for the face and 20 minutes for the neck.

TIP: The key aspect of successful microdermabrasion is an effective vacuum seal. The skin is tensed with the nondominant hand while using the dominant hand to control the handpiece.

Controlling the Handpiece
- The handpiece is moved over the treatment area in a single, smooth stroke.
- A foot pedal controls the pressure of the crystal stream. Pressure is decreased when treating the thinner skin of the lower eyelids and upper cheek.
- Thicker skin, such as that on the forehead, chin, and nose, can be treated aggressively.
- All strokes are vertically oriented for treating the neck.

- The second treatment path is perpendicular to the first for treatment of the face.
- Between treatments, the face is cleaned of residual crystals.
- Two treatments per session are sufficient for the face.
- The endpoint is **erythema.**
- Specific areas, such as acne scars or age spots, can be more aggressively and individually treated with additional passes.

Postprocedure Details
- The treated area is cleaned with a wet cloth to remove any residual crystals.
- A moisturizer or ointment is applied. The use of a moisturizer or ointment is continued postoperatively until the erythema resolves, because exfoliation may occur.
- Patients may have a mild sunburnlike sensation for a couple of days.
- Sunscreen should be used liberally.

SENIOR AUTHOR TIP: Patients must avoid direct sun exposure, even with sunblock, for at least 3 months. Avoid sitting near a swimming pool or on a boat as sun reflects off the water and can affect the facial skin even when a broad brim hat is worn.

Follow-Up Care
- Usually **5-12 treatments** are needed, although more may be warranted in heavily scarred/damaged areas.
- The first several treatments are performed weekly or biweekly, and maintenance treatments are performed monthly to biannually.

COMPLICATIONS[1,3]

HYPERPIGMENTATION AND HYPOPIGMENTATION
- **Proper patient selection** is the best treatment of these complications.
- **Hypopigmentation** occurs from dermabrasion that is too deep. Time will usually correct this problem.
- **Hyperpigmentation** occurs most commonly in patients with type III or IV skin and in those who have not used sunblock. Hyperpigmentation can be minimized with 2 g of ascorbic acid (vitamin C) daily. Pigmentation is usually limited to the superficial epidermis and treatable with topical applications of Retin-A, hydroquinone, and glycolic acids. If pigmentation persists after several months of adequate skin care treatment, a medium-depth trichloracetic acid chemical peel will usually be necessary.

MILIA
- Milia are small white cysts over the surface of the treated area. One third of patients will develop them.
- They typically appear within 2-4 weeks after treatment and will clear spontaneously in most patients.
- These small cysts can be unroofed with a buff puff or a mildly abrasive skin cleaner.

RESIDUAL RHYTIDS AND SCARS
BEFORE the procedure, physicians should emphasize that deep rhytids and all scars will not be completely removed. Multiple treatments and soft tissue fillers may be needed to achieve the aesthetic goal.

SCARRING

- **Linear scars** are usually caused by gouging from an inadvertent angling of the dermabrasion drum. If recognized at the time of the procedure, the defect should be closed with fine suture.
- Dermabrasion that was too deep and postprocedure infection can cause hypertrophic scarring. Early steroid injection helps to minimize it.

INFECTION

- Infection after dermabrasion should be rare. Occlusive dressings can hide an infection and should be used with caution.
- Patients with an oral herpes history are pretreated with an antiviral agent. If a lesion appears, it should be very aggressively treated.

> **SENIOR AUTHOR TIP:** It is a good practice to place all dermabrasion patients on an antiviral drug as prophylaxis.

TOP TAKEAWAYS

➤ The dermabrasion drum should always be moved toward the leading edge of soft tissue.

➤ The drum should always be positioned parallel to the skin to prevent gouging that can occur if it is angled.

➤ Antibiotic and antiviral coverage is required (in patients with a history of oral herpes and/or fever blisters).

➤ Postprocedure sun protection is essential.

➤ Patients with deep rhytids and/or acne scars should be counseled about the probable need for multiple treatments.

REFERENCES

1. Baker JL. Dermabrasion. In Nahai F, ed. The Art of Aesthetic Surgery: Principles & Techniques. New York: Thieme Publishers, 2005.
2. Duffy DM. Informed consent for chemical peels and dermabrasion. Dermatol Clin 7:183, 1989.
3. Hruza GJ. Dermabrasion. Facial Plast Surg Clin North Am 9:267, 2001.
4. Coleman S, ed. Structural Fat Grafting. New York: Thieme Publishers, 2004.
5. Bagatin E, dos Santos Guadanhim LR, Yarak S, et al. Dermabrasion for acne scars during treatment with oral isotretinoin. Dermatol Surg 36:483, 2010.
6. Picosse FR, Yarak S, Cabral NC, et al. Early chemabrasion for acne scars after treatment with oral isotretinoin. Dermatol Surg 38:1521, 2012.
7. Holck DE, Ng JD. Facial skin rejuvenation. Curr Opin Ophthalmol 14:246, 2003.
8. Dubina M, Tung R. Management of complications of microdermabrasion and dermabrasion. In Tosti A, Beer K, De Padova MP, eds. Management of Complications of Cosmetic Procedures: Handling Problems and More Uncommon Problems. Berlin, Heidelberg: Springer, 2012.

21. Botulinum Toxin

Joshua Lemmon, Smita R. Ramanadham, Miles Graivier

DEFINITION

Botulinum toxin is a neurotoxin that is produced by *Clostridium botulinum,* a gram-positive anaerobic bacterium.

HISTORY AND PHYSIOLOGY[1,2]

BOTULISM

- The toxin was identified as the cause of a symmetrical, neuroparalytic illness.
- Foodborne botulism occurs from the ingestion of the neurotoxin and rarely occurs in the modern era, except in home-canned goods or rare instances.
- **Wound botulism** occurs when the bacteria colonize a wound and produce the toxin, causing progressive weakness.
- **Infant botulism**—the most common in the United States (100 infants/year)—results from the ingestion of clostridial spores, colonization of the gut with the bacteria, and production of toxin.

TOXINS[3]

- *Clostridium botulinum* produces eight toxins, of which seven have paralytic properties: serotypes A through G.
  - Antigenetically distinct with different sites of action[4]
- **Mechanism of action**
  - The neurotoxin acts at presynaptic nerve terminals to **inhibit the release of acetylcholine,** producing a chemodenervation.
  - The protein consists of a heavy and light chain. The heavy chain irreversibly binds to the nerve terminal, and the toxin is internalized through endocytosis, where it renders the nerve terminal nonfunctional and blocks the release of acetylcholine into the neuromuscular junction.[4]
  - It targets the **SNAP/SNARE docking protein complex and the vesicle-associated membrane protein (VAMP)** (type B toxin).
  - Recovery is through **two phases:**
    - Phase 1: Accessory terminals sprout from the affected axon to stimulate the postsynaptic target.
    - Phase 2: After 28 days, the main axon teminal begins slow recovery of its acetylcholine release ability. At appromately **90 days** recovery is complete.[4]
- Type A was purified in crystalline form in 1946.
  - In the 1970s type A was first used clinically in treating **strabismus** and then **facial dystonias.**
  - Carruthers and Carruthers[5] then described the first aesthetic use of toxin for the treatment of glabellar frown lines in 1992.

- **Types A and B are FDA approved** for clinical use.
  - **Type A** is approved for multiple clinical uses, including the cosmetic improvement of glabellar rhytids and crow's-feet in patients 65 years or younger.
    - ▶ Expanded to include hyperhidrosis, blepharoptosis, and cervical dystonia.
  - **Type B** is approved for cervical dystonia.
- Three preparations of type A are available for facial cosmetic use (Table 21-1).

Table 21-1 *Preparations of Type A Botulinum Toxin*

	Botox: OnabotulinumtoxinA (Allergan)[6]	Dysport: AbobotulinumtoxinA (Medicis Aesthetics)	Xeomin: IncobotulinumtoxinA (Merz Pharmaceuticals)
FDA approval granted	2002 for treatment of glabellar rhytids 2013 for the treatment of crow's-feet	2009 for treatment of glabellar rhytids and cervical dystonia	2010 for treatment of cervical dystonia and blepharoptosis 2011 for glabellar rhytids[7]
Availability	50 and 100 U vials	300 U vials	50 and 100 U vials
Preparation	Vacuum-dried	Freeze-dried	Lyophilized powder
Dilution	Typically, final concentration of 2.5-4 U/0.1 ml	Typically, diluted to a final concentration of 10-30 U/0.1 ml[8-10]	Typically, diluted to a final concentration of 2.5-4 U/0.1 ml
Dosing		**1:2 or 1:2.5 dosing ratio between Botox and Dysport** **Ratio may be up to 1:4 or 1:5 in some data**[11-12]	**1:1 dosing ratio between Botox and Xeomin in consensus study**[8-10] In study comparing 1:1 dosage between Botox and Xeomin, Botox found to be stronger[7]
Other characteristics		Larger area of action with greater diffusion and spread compared with Botox[12]	Does **NOT** require refrigeration

INDICATIONS AND CONTRAINDICATIONS[2,13]

INDICATIONS
- Despite limited FDA approval, widely used off-label to improve *dynamic* facial rhytids

CONTRAINDICATIONS
- **Active infection** at the proposed injection site
- Known **hypersensitivity** to any ingredient in the formulation, including albumin

PRECAUTIONS
- **Botulinum toxin is used cautiously in:**
  - Patients with **neuromuscular disorders** including ALS, myasthenia gravis, and Lambert-Eaton syndrome, because they may have significant side effects
  - Coadministration with **aminioglycoside antibiotics** or other agents that interfere with neuromuscular transmission, which can potentiate the effect of type A toxin

- **Pregnant women** (category C): Adverse effects shown in animal pregnancy studies, but inadvertent use has not resulted in problems in humans
- **Lactating patients,** as it is unknown whether the toxin is excreted in human milk
- **Inflammatory skin conditions** are the site of planned injection

PATIENT EVALUATION

HISTORY
- Age
- Gender
- Medical comorbidities
- History of prior treatments and preferences
- NSAID use and other medications (may increase bruising)

ANALYSIS
- Evaluate static and dynamic rhytids in the upper and lower face.
- Identify platsymal bands.
- Assess brow symmetry and aperture width.
- Identify any preexisting brow or upper lid ptosis.

OTHER CONSIDERATIONS
- Skin quality: More toxin is generally required for thicker skin.
- Muscle mass: Male patients tend to have larger facial muscles and require more toxin.

PHOTOGRAPHS
- Static and dynamic (animated) preprocedure photographs are helpful, especially for patients not previously treated.

PATIENT EXPECTATIONS
- Patients have varying desires for treatments. Some request near-complete denervation, whereas others prefer a more limited treatment.
- Static lines frequently soften, but they are rarely eliminated. Treatment improves *dynamic* rhytids.
- Longevity is approximately **3 months** on average, but varies by dose, muscle bulk, and injection site.

> **TIP:** In patients who have had prior treatments, a history including results and preferences is especially important.

INFORMED CONSENT

The risks, benefits, and alternatives to the procedure need to be presented. The planned injection sites may not be FDA-approved indications and are considered off-label use.
- Recommended items to be included in the informed consent:
    - A general description of the procedure and location of injections
    - A sufficient description of potential risks
        - ▶ Pain at injection site
        - ▶ Bleeding

- ▶ Bruising
- ▶ Eyelid or brow ptosis
- ▶ Headache
- ▶ Allergic reaction
- ▶ Nausea
- ▶ Facial asymmetry
- ▶ Dysphagia
- ▶ Respiratory compromise

PREPARATION AND EQUIPMENT[2,13]

RECONSTITUTION
- The powder is usually reconstituted gently with 0.9% sterile saline solution.
- When reconstituted, the solution should be clear, colorless, and free from particulate matter.

> **SENIOR AUTHOR TIP:**   Studies have shown that injection site discomfort is less when using *preserved* saline.[14,15]

STORAGE
- Before reconstitution, unopened vials should be stored at **2°-8° C.**
  - **Xeomin** can be stored on the shelf at **room temperature.**
- The manufacturer recommends using the toxin within 4 hours of reconstitution and storing it at 2°-8° C.
- Literature indicates efficacy is maintained for up to 6 weeks with proper storage.

SYRINGE AND NEEDLES
- **1 ml syringes** allow injection of a precise volume of solution.
  - Tuberculin or insulin syringes are most frequently used.
- **30-gauge** or **32-gauge** needles
  - Ultrafine needles limit injection site pain and allow tactile perception of muscular penetration.

> **SENIOR AUTHOR TIP:**   When performing multiple injections, changing needles after each syringe use is recommended. The fine tips dull quickly.

ANESTHESIA
- Use of ice or cold packs, topical local anesthetic combinations, and other modalities can limit procedural discomfort.
- This is not required, and use varies by physician and patient.

IMMUNOGENICITY[11]

- Neurotoxins are macromolecular protein complexes with molecular weights of 300-900 kDa comprising a 150 kDa neurotoxin protein and varying amounts of nontoxin proteins.

- The immune system may recognize any component of the protein complex and initiate an immune reaction, decreasing the effect of botulinum toxin over time.
- Xeomin lacks a 900 kDa complexing protein. It has been postulated that this may result in a less immunosuppressant response compared with Botox and Dysport.

TECHNIQUE[13]

- Treatment must be individualized based on muscle strength, skin thickness, degree of rhytids, choice of neurotoxin, and previous treatments.
- Recommended doses are based on administration of Botox and Xeomin. Recommended ratio of 1:2 or 1:2.5 pertains to Dysport.

GLABELLAR COMPLEX
Vertical frown lines are the result of contraction of the muscles within the glabellar complex.

Anatomy
- The **corrugator supercilii, procerus,** and **depressor supercilii** (medial orbicularis oculi) are the muscles responsible for brow depression.
  - **Corrugator supercilii muscles** are composed of a **transverse** (larger) and an **oblique** head.
    - ▶ **Origin:** Frontal bone at the superomedial orbital rim
    - ▶ **Insertion:** Dermis at the middle third of the eyebrow, interdigitating with orbicularis occuli and frontalis muscle fibers
    - ▶ **Action:** Depresses and adducts the eyebrows
    - ▶ **Dynamic rhytids:** Vertical glabellar lines
  - The **procerus** muscle is a flat, pyramidal muscle present on the bridge of the nose.
    - ▶ **Origin:** Inferior aspect of the nasal bone and upper lateral nasal cartilages
    - ▶ **Insertion:** Dermis overlying the nasal root
    - ▶ **Action:** Depresses the medial brow
    - ▶ **Dynamic rhytids:** Transverse lines on the nasal dorsum
  - The **depressor supercilii** muscle is a portion of the medial orbicularis oculi, just inferior to the medial brow.
    - ▶ Vertically oriented and just superficial to the corrugators at the superomedial orbital rim
    - ▶ **Action:** Brow depression
    - ▶ **Dynamic rhytids:** Contributes to both vertical and transverse glabellar lines and a lower static medial brow position

Injection
- Five to seven injection sites are recommended (Fig. 21-1).
- Starting doses are approximately 20-30 U for women and 30-40 U for men.
- Midline injection should be at the nasal root to treat the procerus muscle.
- Injection of the depressor supercilii can raise the static position of the medial brow if desired.

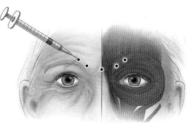

Fig. 21-1   Injection points for glabellar complex and vertical forehead lines.

> **TIP:**   The corrugators lie immediately superficial to the periosteum medially.

> **SENIOR AUTHOR TIP:**   Injection only above the orbital rim to prevent diffusion resulting in eyelid ptosis requires caution.

NASAL REGION
Bunny lines are downward-radiating lines along the nasal sidewalls.

Anatomy
- The transverse portion of the nasalis muscle arises from the maxilla and expands into a thin aponeurosis over the nasal dorsum and interdigitates with the caudal edge of the procerus.
- Contraction compresses the nasal bridge, depresses the nasal tip, and elevates the lateral alae.
- Bunny lines result from **nasalis** contraction.

Injection
- Small doses are usually sufficient: 4-6 U.
- Three injections sites are usually chosen (Fig. 21-2).
- Injections should be relatively superficial.

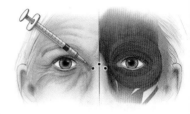

Fig. 21-2   Injection points for bunny lines.

FOREHEAD
Dynamic transverse forehead lines result from contraction of the **frontalis muscle.**

Anatomy
- The frontalis is a large, paired muscle that is the continuation of the galea aponeurotica inferior to the coronal suture.
- Variable decussation and interdigitation of the muscle in the midline are responsible for the diversity of shape of transverse forehead rhytids.
- Laterally, the frontalis terminates in the conjoined tendon at the temporal ridge.
  - **Origin:** Galea aponeurosis
  - **Insertion:** Dermis at the level of the supraorbital rim
  - **Action:** Brow elevation
  - **Dynamic rhytids:** Transverse forehead lines

Injection
- Injection varies depending on gender.
  - Men generally require large doses because they have thicker muscles.
  - The **female** brow is **arched,** whereas the **male** brow is usually more **horizontal.**
    - ▶ Injection patterns should be tailored with this in mind.
- Complete paralysis should be prevented because it leads to brow ptosis and significantly limits facial expression.
  - This is best prevented by injecting **2 cm above the eyebrow.**
  - Lateral injections should be high (especially in women) to prevent drooping of the lateral brow.
- Starting doses are approximately 10-20 U for women and 20-30 U for men.

TIP: Brow asymmetry and lateral elevation can be improved with injection of the superior lateral orbicularis oculi immediately below the eyebrow—sometimes called a *chemical browlift.*

LATERAL PERIORBITAL REGION

Crow's-feet are radial, lateral periorbital rhytids that result from orbicularis oculi contraction and photoaging.

Anatomy
- The **orbicularis oculi** muscle is a thin, sphincterlike muscle that encircles the eyes.
  - Composed of **palpebral** and **orbital** portions
  - Functions to close the eyelids, but also acts as a brow depressor and weak elevator of the malar region
  - Muscle is very superficial, **immediately beneath the thin skin** in this region
- Redundant skin laterally bunches over the contracting muscle, leading to lateral rhytids

Injection
- Injections are given near the lateral orbital rim with the needle pointing away from the globe.
- **Superficial,** subcutaneous injections are given.
- Two to five injection points are chosen, and starting doses are 8-16 U per side (Fig. 21-3).
- In patients with lower lid laxity

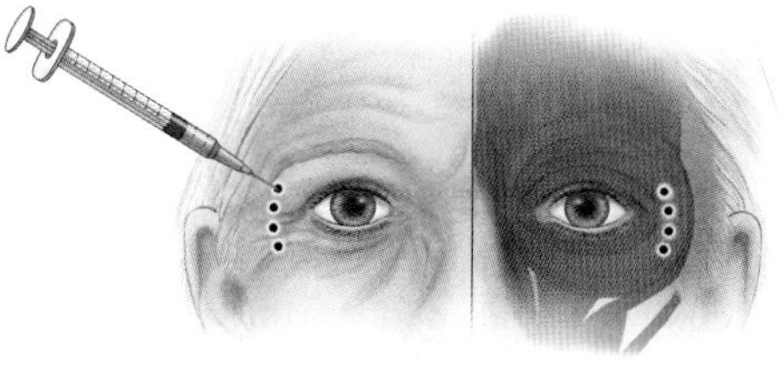

Fig. 21-3   Injection points for crow's-feet.

or laxity of the lateral canthal tendon, caution is necessary in this area to prevent postinjection scleral show and lower lid retraction.

TIP: To prevent injection of the zygomaticus major muscle, injections should not be given below the zygomatic arch.

TIP: Undertreatment is common, and patients frequently benefit from reassessment and additonal injection 2 weeks after the initial procedure.

PERIORAL REGION

Vertical perioral rhytids result from contraction of the **orbicularis oris muscle.**

Anatomy
- The orbicularis oris is a layered sphincter muscle that encircles the mouth.
  - Functions to close the mouth and pucker the lips

Injection
- Injections are **superficial** and **within 5 mm** of the vermilion border (Fig. 21-4).

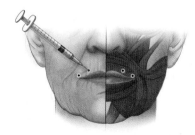

Fig. 21-4   Injection points for perioral rhytids.

- Injection sites should be symmetrical, and inexperienced injectors should avoid the lower lip.
- Low doses should be used initially, with starting doses of 4-10 U, evenly divided by injection sites.

CAUTION: Overtreatment can result in significant impairment and must be avoided.

SENIOR AUTHOR TIP: Injections in patients who use their lips for their professions, such as musicians or public speakers, are not recommended.

- Perioral region is often **more sensitive,** and topical anesthesia is often beneficial in this location.

TIP: Low-dose botulinum toxin injection is an excellent accompaniment to dermal fillers in the lips.

CHIN
A dimpled chin results from loss of subcutaneous fat and contraction of the **mentalis muscles.**

Anatomy
- The mentalis muscles are paired muscles that originate from the mandible, course downward, and insert into the skin of the chin.
  - Functions to raise the chin and protrude the lower lip

Injection
- Low doses are usually adequate: 2-6 U.
- It can be given as a midline injection just inferior to the tip of the chin or as paired lateral injections.
- Needle should be angled superiorly, as the muscle originates cephalad to its site of insertion.

NECK
The cause of plastymal banding is multifactorial and is historically most frequently treated surgically. Botulinum toxin is an alternative treatment in selected patients.

Anatomy[14]
- The **plastyma** is a sheetlike, quadrangular muscle enveloped by the superficial and deep layers of the superficial fascia in the neck.[16]
- Fibrous bands anchor the dermis to superficial fascia and therefore can result in skin "banding" with muscular contraction.
  - **Origin:** Pectoralis major muscle fascia
  - **Insertion:** Contralateral plastyma, mandible, risorius muscle
  - **Action:** Depresses the jaw, lower lip, oral commissures

Injection
- Treatment with botulinum toxin is indicated in patients with preserved skin elasticity and a paucity of submental fat.

- Band should be grasped with the nondominant hand and injected in three to six sites along its length.
- Starting doses are variable and usually are within a range of **10-20 U per band.**
- Low doses should be used initially, starting with doses 4-10 U, evenly divided by injection sites.

> **TIP:**   Can also be used in postrhytidectomy patients with residual bands.

MASSETER[17]

Masseter hypertrophy can lead to a wide contour of the lower face. In 1994 Moore and Wood[18] first used botulinum toxin for functional reasons. Rijsdijk et al[19] later used the toxin for aesthetic wrinkle reduction.

Anatomy
- **Three layer** skeletal muscle consisting of superficial, middle, deep layers.
- The myofibers within these layers are arranged in different directions.
  - **Superficial layer** arises from the anterior zygomatic arch and passes posteriorly and inferiorly, inserting onto the masseter tuberosity.
  - The thinner, **middle layer** arises from the posterior arch and travels downward to the front and inserts into the masseter tuberosity.
  - The **deep layer** arises from the posterior arch as well and passes back and downward to insert on the masseter tuberosity.
  - These three layers fuse together in the lower third of the muscle.

Injection
- Bulging characteristics of masseter vary on clenching. Five different bulging types:
  - **Type I:** Minimal bulging, no obvious bulge
  - **Type II:** Mono, local single longitudinal bulge
  - **Type III:** Double, two separate longitudinal bulges
  - **Type IV:** Triple, three longitudinal bulges
  - **Type V:** Excessive, massive single bulge
- **Most prominent point of muscle bulge is injected.** Injection is adapted to static thickness, because thickness correlates with force of muscle.
- 20 U is the effective minimal dosage and is increased depending on strength of muscle.
- Results have shown a decrease in masseter thickness and improved contour of the lower face.

POSTOPERATIVE CARE
- Postinjection instructions vary widely by physician and are frequently unwarranted.
- Generally, patients are instructed not to massage the injection sites and to briefly limit activity.
  - Refraining from strenuous activity may be beneficial by limiting ecchymosis and edema.
- Onset is generally within 3-4 days and plateaus at 14 days after injection.
- At 14 days, results are assessed and touchups performed if needed.
- Treatment is repeated every 3-6 months.

COMPLICATIONS

- ■ **Hypersensitivity reactions**
  - • Very rare; possible allergic reaction to human albumin, which is also present within the vial
- ■ **Dysphagia**
  - • Also uncommon, and very unlikely after cosmetic use
  - • Seen rarely after treatment for cervical dystonia
- ■ **Transient eyelid ptosis**
  - • *The most commonly reported adverse effect (5%)*
  - • Prevented by following previously mentioned suggestions
- ■ Headache, nausea, malaise, vasovagal response, bruising, pain at injection site are probably related to the injection itself rather than the toxin.

TOP TAKEAWAYS

➤ There are three FDA-approved neurotoxins generally used for treatment of dynamic facial rhytids.

➤ The toxin works by preventing acetylcholine release at the neuromuscular junction.

➤ Intramuscular injection is facilitated by knowledge of anatomic location and depth.

➤ Effects are seen after several days and plateau 2 weeks after injection.

➤ Complete paralysis is avoided, and attention is given instead to aesthetic facial shaping and softening of dynamic rhytids.

REFERENCES

1. Bartlett JG. Clostridial infections. In Goldman L, Ausiello DA, Arend W, et al, eds. Cecil Medicine, ed 23. Philadelphia: Saunders Elsevier, 2008.
2. Botox® Cosmetic Package Insert. Allergan, Inc., Irvine, CA. Available at *http://www.allergan.com/assets/pdf/botox_cosmetic_pi.pdf.*
3. Rohrich RJ, Janis JE, Fagien S, et al. The cosmetic use of botulinum toxin. Plast Reconstr Surg 112(5 Suppl):S117, 2003.
4. Kim EJ, Ramirez AL, Reeck JB, et al. The role of botulinum toxin type B (Myobloc) in the treatment of hyperkinetic facial lines. Plast Reconstr Surg 112(5 Suppl):S88, 2003.
5. Carruthers JD, Carruthers JA. Treatment of glabellar frown lines with C. botulinum-A exotoxin. J Dermatol Surg Oncol 18:17, 1992.
6. Lorenc ZP, Kenkel JM, Fagien S, et al. A review of onabotulinumtoxinA (Botox). Aesthet Surg J 33(1 Suppl):S9, 2013.
7. Yielding RH, Fezza JP. A prospective, split-face, randomized, double-blind study comparing OnabotulinumtoxinA to IncobotulinumtoxinA for upper face wrinkles. Plast Reconstr Surg 135:1328, 2015.
8. Lorenc ZP, Kenkel JM, Fagien S, et al. A review of abobotulinumtoxinA (Dysport). Aesthet Surg J 33(1 Suppl):S13, 2013.
9. Matarasso A, Shafer D. Botulinum toxin neurotoxin type A-ABO (Dysport): clinical indications and practice guide. Aesthet Surg J 29(6 Suppl):S72, 2009.

10. Maas C, Kane MA, Bucay VW, et al. Current aesethic use of abobotulinumtoxin a in clinical practice: an evidence-based consensus review. Aesthet Surg J 32(1 Suppl):S8, 2009.
11. Klein AW, Carruthers A, Fagien S, et al. Comparisons among botulinum toxins: an evidence-based review. Plast Reconstr Surg 121:413e, 2008.
12. Nguyen AT, Ahmad J, Fagien S, et al. Cosmetic medicine: facial resurfacing and injectables. Plast Reconstr Surg 129:142e, 2012.
13. Carruthers J, Fagien S, Matarasso SL; Botox Consensus Group. Consensus recommendations on the use of botulinum toxin type a in facial aesthetics. Plast Reconstr Surg 114(Suppl 6):S1, 2004.
14. Kwiat DM, Bersani TA, Bersani A. Increased patient comfort utilizing botulinum toxin type a reconstituted with preserved versus nonpreserved saline. Ophthal Plast Reconstr Surg 20:186, 2004.
15. Alam M, Dover JS, Arndt KA. Pain associated with injection of botulinum A exotoxin reconstituted using isotonic sodium chloride with and without preservative: a double-blind, randomized controlled trial. Arch Dermatol 138:510, 2002.
16. Vistnes LM, Souther SG. The platysma muscle: anatomic considerations for aesthetic surgery of the anterior neck. Clin Plast Surg 10:441, 1983.
17. Xie Y, Zhou J, Li H, et al. Classification of masseter hypertrophy for tailored botulinum toxin type a treatment. Plast Reconstr Surg 134:209e, 2014.
18. Moore AP, Wood GD. The medical management of masseteric hypertrophy with botulinum toxin type A. Br J Oral Maxillofac Surg 32:26, 1994.
19. Rijsdijk BA, van Es RJ, Zonneveld FW, et al. Botulinum toxin type A treatment of cosmetically disturbing masseteric hypertrophy. Ned Tijdschr Geneeskd 142:529, 1998.

22. Soft Tissue Fillers

Ashkan Ghavami, Miles Graivier

RELEVANT ANATOMY AND GENERAL CONCEPTS[1,2]

> NOTE: This chapter is meant to discuss all current filler applications. We will concentrate on FDA-approved fillers and their most common clinical indications. Use in some anatomic locations may not be approved by the FDA or specifically advocated by the filler manufacturers.

FOREHEAD
- Indications for fillers are mostly for filling lines.
- Lines and deep furrows, particularly in glabellar region, may not be fully correctable with muscle chemodenervation alone.
- Deep transverse lines may require fillers as adjuncts to botulinum toxin.
- Volume is as much an issue here as in other areas.

PERIORBITA
Upper
- Deep upper sulcus, either congenital or from aggressive fat removal through blepharoplasty, may require soft tissue filling.
- Lateral "tail" of brow can be lifted slightly with soft tissue fillers, in addition to chemodenervation of lateral orbicularis.

Lower
- **Tear trough deformity:** Medial groove from region of medial canthus to orbital rim
  - Multifactorial in severity, relates to: Position of orbital rim, thickness of skin, pigment of skin, amount of medial fat in lower lid, characteristic of orbicularis retaining ligament (ORL), variation in orbicularis muscle insertion (tarsal, septal, and orbital portions), and insertion of orbital septum
  - Good indication for soft tissue filling with **small-molecule hyaluronic acid (HA)**
- Lower lid–cheek junction
  - Severity varies.
  - Depth of presentation varies from the tear trough/nasojugal fold toward the lateral orbital thickening.
  - It is not necessarily related to position of ORL, orbicularis, or arcus marginalis.
  - Position is relatively stable throughout facial aging.[3]
  - **Small-particle fillers** can be very beneficial in rejuvenation.

MIDFACE
Malar Shape and Projection
- Fullness in malar region from lateral zygomaticomaxilllary junction to the nasomaxillary region below the tear trough is very important in overall facial rejuvenation.

■ Fat compartments in this region are deep and superficial.
  • Various depths require **multilevel filling.**
■ Cheek fold, when present, should be corrected for balance.
■ This is an excellent indication for **large-molecule HA fillers and/or hydroxyapatite.**

Nasolabial Fold
■ Cause not fully known: Severity may be related to dermal insertions of deeper fascial attachments and position of mobile lateral soft tissue against more fixed medial upper lip region.[4]
■ Depth and location vary.
  • **Multilevel filling** can be useful.
■ Some upper-segment depth is natural and desired.
■ *Overcorrection should be avoided.*

LOWER FACE
Lateral Perioral Lines
■ Formed mostly during animation
■ When present on repose, good indication for filling
■ Usually lateral to lowest point of nasolabial fold
■ May require **multilevel filling**

Upper Lip Lines
■ Superficial lines extend radial (perpendicular) to vermilion border.
■ Skin resurfacing (laser versus peeling) and botulinum toxin, along with volume restoration and filling of each specific line, gives most optimal correction when lines are severe.
■ Vermilion-cutaneous junction and upper lip augmentation are usually required.

Lips (Fig. 22-1)
■ Youthful characteristics
  • Upper lip/lower lip height ratio should be ⅓:⅔.
  • Cupid's bow is sharp and well-defined.
  • Full philtral columns
  • Gentle concave sloping from nasal base and labiomental groove
  • Oral commissures slightly upward in orientation
  • Full medial tubercle
  • Sharp white rolls (vermilion-cutaneous junction)

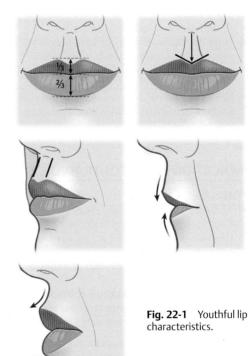

Fig. 22-1   Youthful lip characteristics.

Labiomental Groove
- Depth should be harmonious relative to nose-lip-chin projection.
- Deep crease with cracked appearance would benefit from filling.

Chin Dimpling
- Botulinum toxin along with filling can correct
- Often only botulinum toxin required, however

Perimental Hollows ("Prejowl Sulcus")
- Good indication for deep-level filling with large-particle HA or hydroxyapatite

OTHER LOCATIONS
Nasal Contouring
- Cephalad and/or caudal to a dorsal hump to blend and balance overall nasal appearance
- Postrhinoplasty correction
  - Nostril and alar imbalances

Scar Filling
- Acne, posttraumatic, chicken pox

Crow's-Feet
- **Chemodenervation** is best treatment.
- Once the skin is severely aged or thinned and separated from the underlying orbicularis muscle, then botulinum toxin is less helpful. Fillers are only rarely effective in this area when skin is thick and well adherent to the underlying orbicularis.

> **TIP:** Consider the facial fat compartments[5] and recognize/perform other complementary procedures that will blend facial zones and create overall facial youth and harmony through proper volume restoration.

INDICATIONS AND CONTRAINDICATIONS

FOLDS AND CREASES
- As discussed previously, any crease, furrow, or line can be filled.
- Caution should be used in filling lines in the forehead, because superficial placement is usually required, which can lead to vascular complications, ulcerations, and visible product.
- Evaluate if botulinum toxin may be a substitute or if botulinum toxin–filler combination would be optimal.
- **Thickness of overlying skin/soft tissues** is important.
  - Lower lid–cheek junction and tear trough have thin skin that requires deep, conservative placement with a small-particle hydroxyapatite.

CAUTION: Calcium hydroxyapatite should *NOT* be injected in the lower lid–cheek junction and tear trough area.

  - Nasolabial fold has thicker skin and multilevel injection technique with mutiple types of fillers may be used

VOLUME RESTORATION

- Recent literature has helped our understanding of facial aging with respect to volume and position of soft tissue compartments.
- Thorough knowledge of the fat compartments of the face and proper balance between fullness of these facial zones is essential.
- *Example*: Malar fullness with submalar hollowing is a desirable aesthetic relation and a strong visual indication of youth.
- Overcorrection can lead to an awkward "overdone" appearance.

ENHANCEMENT
Lips
- An unnatural appearance should be avoided.
- Adherance to the desired aesthetic proportions is vital.

> **NOTE: Some patients may demand overcorrection. Extreme caution should be used, as overcorrection should be avoided.**

> **TIP:**   The lips are a vital and central portion of the face. It is a primary location that is subconsciously and consciously evaluated during social interactions. The lips evoke emotion, sensuality, youth, and vitality. Overcorrection in this region is commonly seen and makes many wary of soft tissue fillers. An incremental approach should always be used, with reevaluation from multiple views during injection.

CHIN PROJECTION
- The appearance of minimal chin projection and fullness at the pogonion can be achieved with hydroxyapatite-based fillers.

PREINJECTION EVALUATION

HISTORY
- Presence of a collagen-vascular disease process may interfere with healing at the injection site and compromise skin blood supply.
- Any active skin or soft tissue inflammatory or infectious process should completely subside before injections.
- Smoking may delay or interfere with healing and longevity of the product, especially if a collagen response is necessary for results.
- Any immunocompromise indicates the need for extra caution.
- Skin testing: Most fillers today do not require a skin test, however bovine collagen-based products can be used. (See the discussion on collagen-based fillers.)

AESTHETIC EVALUATION
Lips
- Proper proportions should be understood, and all portions relating to improving lip aesthetics should be treated to optimize results.
- Philtral columns, downturned oral commissures, and vermilion-cutaneous junction should not be ignored.
- Volume and contour require treatment.

Lower Lid/Tear Trough
- Evaluate depth and skin type.
- Evaluate height of lower lid.
- Evaluate requirement for multilevel filling.
- Often, malar augmentation is also necessary.

Midface-Malar
- Facial fat compartment locations should be assessed and understood.
- Asymmetry should be documented. (One side is always wider than other.)
- Middle cheek fold can be filled to blend the fat compartments.
- This region is complementary with lower lid injections.
- Multiple syringes are often required.

Lines/Furrows/Creases
- The contribution of dynamic muscle motion, if any, is determined.
- The best treatment is selected: chemodenervation, fillers, or a combination of both modalities.
- Small static lines (periorbital and perioral) are a good indication for small-particle collagen.

INFORMED CONSENT

Should include, but not be limited, to the following:
- **Edema:** Patients need to know timeline, because returning to their work and other activities is always important. Some fillers and locations produce more edema than others.

> **SENIOR AUTHOR TIP:**   Radiesse (Merz Aesthetics) injections deep in the malar region may allow return to work the same day whereas injections in the nasolabial fold may produce edema and erythema. Lips usually become edematous from the high vascularity.

- **Ecchymosis:** Patients should not take aspirin, NSAIDs, and other blood-thinning medication for at least 1 week before injection.
- **Cosmetic outcome:** As with any cosmetic procedure, the possibility of a poor cosmetic outcome or asymmetry should be discussed with patients.
  - Lumpiness, in particular, should be discussed with patients.
  - Contour irregularity
  - Overcorrection or undercorrection
- **Allergic reaction/hypersensitivity:** Rare hypersensitivity has been reported with all filler materials. However, bovine collagen–based products can produce a localized hypersensitivity and 1%-5% of negative skin test patients can produce an allergic reaction to facial injection.[6] Previous hypersensitivity to a specific filler is a contraindication to repeat treatment.
  - Cystic and granulomatous reactions are possible.
  - Cystic abscesses have been reported.

- **Skin necrosis/ulcerations:** Rare, but should be mentioned; more likely in poorly selected patients (e.g., cocaine abusers and those with autoimmune disease or collagen-vascular disorders); upper third of nasolabial fold near base of nose, and locations with watershed vascularity or thin overlying skin where superficial placement increases risk (e.g., glabella).
- **Pain/discomfort:** Very temporary and easily minimized with proper technique; reduced by anesthetic block and icing. Prolonged discomfort or reaction at injection site may require corticosteroid treatment (injection or oral).
- Recent laser or chemical peel treatment may increase the risk of **inflammatory complications.**
- **Infection:** Rare. Risk is increased if active inflammatory or infectious skin process coexists at injection site(s). Delaying treatment may be needed.
    - *Herpetic reactivation*
        - ▶ Patients with a history of facial herpetic outbreaks should be pretreated for several days with oral antiviral therapy.
- **Tyndall effect or Rayleigh scattering**: If injection is too superficial with any HA, a *bluish discoloration* will result (particulate bolus scattering shorter wavelength blue light).

EQUIPMENT

NECESSARY MATERIALS
Needles
- Often provided in packaging
- A 1¼-inch 27-gauge needle helpful for long, linear threading and for large areas such as the malar and nasolabial fold.
- Otherwise, a ½-inch 27-gauge needle often used
- 30-gauge needles good for superficial injections

Topical Anesthetic
- Custom-compounded triple-anesthetic combinations can be special ordered from most pharmacies.
- Requires application 15 minutes before procedure
- Useful adjunct that should be placed before or at same time as local anesthetic blocking techniques

Local Anesthetic Block[7]
- Agent: 1% lidocaine with or without epinephrine versus Septocaine

> **SENIOR AUTHOR TIP:**   Septocaine causes less discomfort.

- **Nerve block**
    - Posterior superior alveolar nerve (PSA)
    - Infraorbital nerve (ION)
    - Mental nerve
    - Inferior alveolar nerve (IAN)
    - Superior alveolar nerve branches
    - Buccal branches (intraoral/mucosal)

Ice
- Useful before and during injection
  - Apply with pressure immediately before needle entry and between injections to prevent or minimize bruising and swelling.
- May use ready-made iced rollers
- Icing with pressure if bruise noted can minimize ecchymotic progression.

IDEAL SOFT TISSUE FILLER CHARACTERISTICS[1]
- FDA approved
- Biocompatible
- Nonantigenic
- Nontoxic
  - Proven safety profile
- Easy to use (i.e., filler material flows smoothly, needle and other equipment durable and does not fail easily)
  - Long-lasting

> **NOTE: Permanence is not necessarily desirable. For example, some patients may not want their lips to be full for the rest of their life. As soft tissue and skin ages, delfates, and atrophies, permanent fillers will remain and look awkward.**

  - Predictable outcome ("What you see is what you get.")
  - Potentially reversible
  - Nonpalpable and soft where necessary
  - Readily available
  - Minimal downtime
  - No migration
  - Reproducible
  - Durable

HYALURONIC ACID FILLERS[8-12]

NONANIMAL STABILIZED HYALURONIC ACID (NASHA) BACKGROUND
- Not animal based
- NASHA products such as Restylane (Galderma) and Perlane (Galderma) are manufactured with blocks of gel passing through sizing screens (sieving) and dispersed within a lubricant. This creates a less homogeneous particle size, which is the characteristic of the Hylacross HAs such as Juvéderm products (Allergan).
- Normal component of ground substance of many tissues (skin, cartilage, bone, and synovial fluid)
  - ▶ Amounts decrease with age.
- Glycosaminoglycan biopolymer of repeating disaccharide units of N-acetylglucosamine and glucuronic acid
- **NO skin test required, NO immunologic activity**
- Hydrophilic (accounts for initial swollen/overcorrected appearance)
- Degree of cross-linking and molecular weight differs between products.

NASHA AND OTHER HA PRODUCTS THAT ARE FDA APPROVED

- **Restylane**: First FDA-approved NASHA (December 2003)
- **Perlane** is a larger-particle HA indicated for deeper folds and used often for malar augmentation.
- **Other versions**
  - **Restylane Silk:** A very-low-molecular-weight HA
  - **Restylane-L:** Restylane with lidocaine
  - **Perlane-L:** Perlane with lidocaine
- **Juvéderm Ultra , Juvéderm Ultra Plus, and Juvéderm Voluma**
  - All *above* also available in "XC" form (Voluma available only as XC form), which denotes lidocaine in the product.
  - Particle size increases from Ultra to Ultra Plus and Voluma
    - ► Most commonly used: Juvéderm Ultra (smaller-particle HA) and Juvéderm Ultra Plus (larger-particle HA)
    - ► **Juvéderm Voluma XC:** Highest viscosity and particle size; indicated for deep folds and malar augmentation
- **Belotero Balance (Merz Aesthetics)**
  - Considered a cohesive polydensified matrix (CPM) HA
  - Longevity comparable to other HA fillers: 12 months
  - **No Tyndall effect or Rayleigh scattering**
    - ► Possibly because product has a more homogeneous intradermal distribution pattern. An absence of specific boluses prevents blue light scattering.
    - ► Transient skin blanching can be seen with more superficial injection.
  - Various Belotero products from Merz Aesthetics available in United States include:
    - ► **Belotero Soft:** Superficial rhytids, crow's-feet, forehead lines
    - ► **Belotero Balance:** Moderate perioral lines, nasolabial fine lines, glabellar folds, marionette lines, oral commissures
    - ► **Belotero Intense:** Deeper areas such as nasolabial folds and lines, lips
    - ► **Belotero Volume:** Malar and other areas requiring volume
    - ► **Belotero Hydro:** Contains glycerol, which the company indicates helps firm volume restoration of face, hands, neck

INDICATIONS AND TECHNIQUE FOR HYALURONIC ACID FILLERS[9]

> **NOTE:** The FDA has approved specific indications, but most practitioners use these products for various indications that are considered off-label.

> **NOTE:** Juvéderm is less viscous than Restylane, requiring a different injection technique, speed, and feel to product placement.

- Injection is performed with an even flow to prevent lumpiness and irregularities. If lumpiness is seen or felt, then massage immediately to smooth the product.
- Different locations are best served with different injection techniques. For example, the white roll of the vermilion necessitates linear threading, whereas commissures may be best treated with cross-radial injections (Fig. 22-2).

> **TIP:**   Avoid injecting a large-particle filler in a thin-skinned area or superficially. If volume restoration and overlying wrinkle correction are required, then consider a multiproduct and multilevel injection technique. Customize the HA filler type and size to preference and "feel" for a particular filler for a specific area. Evaluate the skin thickness, and look for veins and scar tissue, which can cause bruising or unexpected tissue resistance. Much of the success with fillers depends on injecting the proper amount and type and appreciating the "feel" of the product, which comes with time and experience.

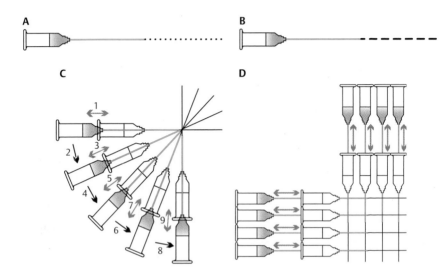

Fig. 22-2   A, Serial puncture. **B,** Linear threading. **C,** Fanning technique. **D,** Cross-radial technique or cross-hatching.

- Inject to a final desired volume.
  - Overcorrection is not required with HAs, in general

CALCIUM HYDROXYAPATITE FILLER[13,14]

RADIESSE (MERZ AESTHETICS)
- FDA-approved
- Composed of synthetic **calcium hydroxyapatite** microspheres (30%) suspended in an aqueous carrier gel (70%)
  - Microspheres: 25-45 μm
  - Similar to mineral portion of bone and teeth
- Packaged as 1.3 cc or 0.6 cc syringes
- Biocompatible, nontoxic, nonirritating, and nonantigenic[13]
- When placed into soft tissue, immediate correction noted
  - Over time: Carrier gel absorbed and a collagen response surrounds microspheres
  - Dermal matrix integration without granuloma, ossification, or foreign body reaction noted at 1 and 6 months[13]

Longevity
- Over time: Broken down into calcium and phosphate ions
- Maximum volume effect seen at *4-6 weeks*
- Results clinically seen up to **9-12 months**
- Varies by location
  - As with any filler, increased muscle motion and patient factors influence longevity.

Indications and Technique
- Ideal sites are generally in regions with overlying thicker skin.
  - Nasolabial folds
  - Malar augmentation
  - Submalar augmentation
  - Oral commissures
  - Marionette lines
  - Labiomental crease
  - Jawline
    - ▶ Prejowl/premental depression
  - Chin augmentation

NOTE: Significant augmentation should not be expected, but some minimal improvement in overall lower third facial balance can be achieved.

TIP: Radiesse is an excellent filler for malar and nasolabial fold augmentation. Injection technique is less forgiving than with HA fillers. Because of longevity, not injecting where product should not be injected is critical (e.g., superficial dermis/epidermis). Massage of product is not as effective as with softer, more malleable HA fillers.

Specific Technical Considerations
- As with most fillers, a nerve block technique of choice should be used (intraoral or extraoral).
- Radiesse is ideally injected with a 27-gauge needle, most commonly one with 1¼-inch length.
- Injection should be in *deep dermis or superficial subcutaneous level.*
- The needle is preloaded with product.
- Deposition of product is best performed **during needle withdrawal.**
  - *Mindfulness of skin entry and exit sites is essential, because product may be inadvertently deposited superficially.*
- **Fanning technique** is most useful, because product is placed during needle withdrawal.
- Postinjection massage
  - Handheld vibration is also useful to evenly distribute product.

NOTE: Meticulous product placement is most critical.

Nasolabial Folds (Fig. 22-3)
- Fanning technique useful
- Multiple injection points along fold
- Can use cross-radial technique for certain, stubborn locations along fold

Malar Augmentation (see Fig. 22-3)
- A very effective treatment for this region
  - Requires as many syringes as needed for desired shape
    - ► Commonly one or two syringes (1.3 cc each) per malar side
- Can start deep in subcutaneous or preperiosteal level and layer
- Fanning technique from lateral submalar point and/or medially at upper nasolabial fold
  - Cross-hatching and overlapping passes important to prevent linear-appearing deposition of product
- Augment entire malar region.
- Can extend inferiorly along medial zygoma
- Malar augmentation is important and complementary to lower lid–tear trough treatments with HA agents.
  - Allows comprehensive and natural blending of the periorbital with malar subcutaneous compartments
- DO NOT inject in region of lower eyelid.
  - One finger held at infraorbital rim to block inadvertent needle passes
- Very effective for HIV-associated lipoatrophy of malar region

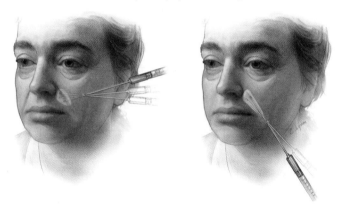

Fig. 22-3   Injection technique. Injection of the nasolabial folds and malar mounds with Radiesse.

Other Lower-Third Facial Locations
- **Prejowl sulcus**
  - Important to stay deep
  - Start from lateral to medial and use fanning.
- **Marionette lines**
  - As with HA filler technique
  - Fanning and/or cross-hatching technique
- **Oral commissures**
  - Fanning/cross-hatching
  - Do not overcorrect.
- **Chin augmentation**
  - Fanning with cross-hatching and deep serial threading is most useful.
  - Approach chin bilaterally with a central entry site when necessary.

- **Nasal contouring**
  - Has received recent attention as a dorsal augmentation filler in "nonsurgical rhinoplasty"
  - Injected cephalad to a dorsal hump and sometimes caudal to it to balance the sagittal appearance of the nose

POLY-L-LACTIC ACID (PLLA)[1,15-17]

SCULPTRA (GALDERMA)
- **FDA approved** for HIV lipoatrophy of the face
- Injectable poly-L-lactic acid (PLLA)
  - PLLA has been used in dissolvable sutures for more than two decades.
- Synthetic polymer
  - Biodegradable, biocompatible, immunologically inert
  - No skin test required
- Delivered as microparticles that are broken down by nonenzymatic hydrolysis into lactic acid monomers
  - Lactic acid polymers are then broken down to CO_2 or glucose.
- Initial effect results from an inflammatory process between the soft tissue and PLLA.
  - Macrophages and fibroblasts form a capsule around the microspheres.
  - PLLA is eventually all degraded and **replaced with collagen.**

NOTE: The initial, robust appearance of the product is from edema and inflammation, and patients can expect this result.

- Patients should be informed that the results will diminish and return at approximately 8-12 weeks as collagen replacement is under way.

Longevity
- May last up to **2 years**[15-17]
- May require **three to six treatments**

Indications and Technique
- Approved for **facial lipoatrophy associated with HIV infection**
- Typically, this involves the malar and submalar areas and parts of the zygomatic process and arch.
- Has been used for temporal wasting as well
- Must be injected in deepest dermis and/or subcutaneous tissue
  - Can also be multilayered starting with preperiosteal deposition
- **Technical considerations**
  - **Must be *reconstituted* 2 hours before injection** with 3-5 ml of sterile water
    - ▶ More water will allow easier injection, because viscosity is lowered.
  - After reconstitution, can be stored at room temperature for **72 hours**
  - Vial must be agitated or rolled (preferred).
  - Local block(s) of choice

- **Requires a larger-bore needle** (26-gauge is the smallest possible)
  ▶ Some use a 25- or 23-gauge, which is easiest.
- Multiple injection entries with cross-radial and/or fanning overlaps allow smooth product placement.
  ▶ Injection at preperiosteal level
    ♦ Small "parcels" are injected, the product is spread over bone with finger manipulation.
- Sometimes mutiple sessions are more effective than correcting to 100% at one session.
  - Average is three to six treatment sessions

POLYMETHYLMETHACRYLATE (PMMA)[18,19]

- Bovine collagen–coated PMMA beads
  - Collagen serves only as a transport vehicle and is absorbed over 4-6 weeks.
- Synthetic and biologically active
- **Skin test required**
- Volume of soft tissue augmented is from connective tissue increase around beads.
- Considered a *PERMANENT* **filler**
  - However, more filler may be required at 1½ years.
  - Initial results may not be seen for 6-8 weeks.

INDICATIONS

- Useful for deep acne scars and lines
  - Nasolabial fold and deep marionette lines
  - Can be used in malar augmentation
- Permanency makes product very unforgiving.

> **TIP:** As soft tissue and skin atrophies with age, the product will become more visible with time. It should be placed very carefully and conservatively. It is NOT safe for superficial rhytids or locations prone to skin ulceration/atrophy.

TECHNICAL CONSIDERATIONS

- High viscosity makes Artefill a very technique-dependent filler; it has a higher resistance to injection compared with other fillers.
- Use a 26-gauge needle.
- Product is injected during withdrawal.
- Injection is in deepest dermis in ONLY areas with thick overlying skin.
- Massage is needed to make sure no lumpiness is present.
- For depressed scars
  - Release scar first (18-gauge or "pickle fork" instrument/subcision).
  - Scar is filled gradually using serial injection over several weeks to months.
- Postinjection irregularities should be treated with dilute doses of Kenalog (0.2 mg/ml).
  - In refractory cases, direct incision may be required.
  - Granulomas have been reported.[19,20]

POSTINJECTION CARE

> **TIP:** Injectables are known as *minimal* or *no downtime* treatments by the lay public, which is a misperception. Ask patients about their plans for the next several days to weeks after treatment. Some may be planning to attend a wedding in 24 hours and expect to have no bruising or swelling!

- **Tissue manipulation**
  - Most beneficial if performed by the injecting physician during or immediately after injection.
  - Massaging at home is only rarely helpful and may be detrimental if done incorrectly.
  - Filler volume and shape should be optimal before the patient leaves the office.
  - *There should, therefore, be no need for at-home manipulation or "shaping" of product when injected properly.*
- **Cooling/icing**
  - Initial ice application may help to reduce facial edema.
  - Cooling can be applied for 20 minutes on and 20 minutes off during first 12-24 hours
- **Position/activity**
  - Patients are instructed to limit activity that increases heart rate for 3-7 days.
  - Head of bed is up (45 degrees) for 3-5 days if possible.
    - ► Only recommended if multiple fillers injected throughout face to prevent excess/additive edema
- **Prophylactic antibiotics**
  - Usually not needed if no active infection and proper skin preparation with alcohol or chlorhexidine
  - Continued orally for 3-5 days every 8 hours
- **Steroids**
  - Oral steroids
    - ► Very rarely indicated. If a lot of fillers are injected at one time (e.g., malar augmentation, nasolabial fold, lips, and tear trough) then a 5- or 6-day oral steroid regimen may be useful.
  - Injectable diluted Kenalog (Kenalog 10)
    - ► Helpful for granulomas or resistant, persistent lumpiness
    - ► Less helpful for HA agents

> **NOTE:** Persistent lumps are refractory to steroid injection, and overcorrection can be treated with hyaluronidase injections.

- **Diet**
  - Patients can resume previous diet as tolerated.
  - As with any cosmetic procedure, limiting salt intake may to help decrease edema slightly.

- **Herbs, other postinjection medication**
  - "Hypersensitive/atopic-type" patients may benefit from an oral antihistamine before and/or after injection for several days.
  - *Arnica montana* oral dosing for 2-5 days after injection may be beneficial.
  - Bromelain, a high-dose pineapple extract helpful for ecchymosis and edema, can be started before injection for most efficacy, if surgeon prefers.

COMPLICATIONS[1,20,21]

> **SENIOR AUTHOR TIP:**   Use light source and possibly loupes to see small- to medium-sized veins. This is useful in areas such as the lateral periorbita.

- **Edema**
  - Initial edema may last up to 3-5 days.
  - Bruising can last as long as 1-2 weeks and depends on individual.
    - ▶ If a medium-sized vein is punctured, this can cause up to 3 weeks of discoloration.
- **Lumpiness**
  - More likely with less malleable products or semipermanent to fully permanent products
  - Related to improper technique, fast injection, wrong level (too superficial), and placement of disproportionate filler material in one spot
  - **Should be treated immediately** when seen, with massage to smooth out
    - ▶ May place adjacent product to balance out the area
  - HA fillers can be dissolved using **hyaluronidase**—Vitrase (Bausch & Lomb) or Hylenex (Halozyme Therapeutics)—ovine 200 USP units/ml
    - ▶ Amount of injection varies according to size of area and amount of filler requiring dissolution.
    - ▶ Excess injection volumes when overcorrected can affect native HA.
- **Overcorrection**
  - Inject more adjacent to site to help balance area out; e.g., if upper lip is too full, consider injecting more to lower lip to achieve proper lip balance.
  - Excess HA can be treated with hyaluronidase in extreme cases.
  - Reassurance is sometimes best, because appearance will improve in most cases in several weeks.
  - Injection of appropriate volume of hyaluronidase is essential.
- **Asymmetry**
  - Most commonly seen with lips
  - Vital to be aware of preinjection lip anatomy and inherent asymmetries

> **NOTE: Everyone has a fuller-lip side or a unilaterally more-pronounced vermilion-cutaneous border.**

- Corrected by touchup injection, immediately or at subsequent session
- Initial asymmetry may be from first side injection (which may appear fuller at the end of injection session) or from a bruise or internal venous puncture on only one side.

- **Ecchymosis/hematoma**
  - Usually venous, from rupture of a medium- to large-sized vein
  - Treat immediately with pressure and cooling to minimize progression.
  - Prevent with careful attention to venous architecture during injection.
  - May be more common at vascular crosspoints (lateral orbit, oral commissure, base of nose/upper nasolabial fold, mid–lid-cheek junction)
  - A true hematoma is rare.
- **Hypersensitivity**
  - Rare
    - ▶ May occur if improper skin testing done before injecting an animal-based product
  - Can treat with oral antihistamine
  - Light topical steroid
  - Self-limiting over several weeks
- **Granulomas/nodules**
  - Very rare but can occur with any filler
  - May be more common with more permanent fillers such as Artefill or discontinued fillers such as Hydrelle
  - Treat with steroid injection or surgical excision if refractory.

TOP TAKEAWAYS
➤ Calcium hydroxyapatite should *NOT* be injected in the lower lid–cheek junction and tear trough area.
➤ The appearance of minimal chin projection and fullness at the pogonion can be achieved with hydroxyapatite-based fillers.
➤ Presence of a collagen-vascular disease process may interfere with healing at the injection site and compromise skin blood supply.
➤ Different locations are best served with different injection techniques. For example, the white roll of the vermilion necessitates linear threading, whereas commissures may be best treated with cross-radial injections.

REFERENCES
1. Born TM. Soft tissue fillers in aesthetic facial surgery. In Nahai F, ed. The Art of Aesthetic Surgery: Principles & Techniques. New York: Thieme Publishers, 2007.
2. Fagien S, Klein AW. A brief overview and history of temporary fillers: evolution, advantages, and limitations. Plast Reconstr Surg 120(6 Suppl):S8, 2007.
3. Lambros V. Observations on periorbital and midface aging. Plast Reconstr Surg 120:1367, 2007.
4. Yousif NJ, Gosain A, Sanger JR, et al. The nasolabial fold: a photogrammetric analysis. Plast Reconstr Surg 36:239, 1994
5. Rohrich RJ, Pessa J. The fat compartments of the face: anatomy and clinical implications for cosmetic surgery. Plast Reconstr Surg 119:2219, 2007.
6. Somerville P, Wray RC Jr. Asymmetrical hypersensitivity to bovine collagen. Ann Plast Surg 30:449, 1993.
7. Zide BM, Swift T. How to block and tackle the face. Plast Reconstr Surg 10:840, 1998.

8. Carruthers A, Carruthers J. Non-animal-based hyaluronic acid fillers: scientific and technical considerations. Plast Reconstr Surg 120(6 Suppl):S33, 2007.

9. Rohrich RJ, Ghavami A, Crosby MA. The role of hyaluronic acid fillers (Restylane) in facial cosmetic surgery: review and technical considerations. Plast Reconstr Surg 120(6 Suppl):S41, 2007.

10. Sundaram H, Cassuto D. Biophysical characteristics of hylauronic acid soft-tissue fillers and their relevance to aesthetic applications. Plast Reconstr Surg 132(4 Suppl):S5, 2013.

11. Lorenc ZP, Fagien S, Flynn TC, et al. Review of key Belotero balance safety and efficacy trials. Plast Reconstr Surg 132(4 Suppl):S33, 2013.

12. Flynn TC, Thompson DH, Hyun SH. Molecular weight analysis and enzymatic degradation profiles of the soft-tissue fillers Belotero Balance, Restylane, and Juvéderm Ultra. Plast Reconstr Surg 132(4 Suppl):S22, 2013.

13. Marmur ES, Phelps R, Goldberg DJ. Clinical, histologic, and electron microscopic findings after injection of a calcium hydroxylapatite filler. J Cosmet Laser Ther 6:223, 2004.

14. Graivier MH, Bass, Lawrence S, et al. Calcium hydroxylapatite (Radiesse) for correction of the mid- and lower face: consensus recommendations. Plast Reconstr Surg 120(6 Suppl):S55, 2007.

15. Woerle B, Hanke CW, Sattler G. Poly-L-lactic acid: a temporary filler for soft tissue augmentation. J Drugs Dermatol 3:385, 2004.

16. Sterling JB, Hanke CW. Poly-L-lactic acid as a facial filler. Skin Therapy Lett 10:9, 2005.

17. Borelli C, Kunte C, Weisenseel P, et al. Deep subcutaneous application of poly-L-lactic acid as a filler for facial lipoatrophy in HIV-infected patients. Skin Pharmacol Physiol 18:273, 2005.

18. Lemperle G, Romano JJ, Busso M. Soft tissue augmentation with Artecoll: 10-year history, indications, techniques, and complications. Dermatol Surg 29:573, 2003.

19. Alcalay J, Alkalay R, Gat A, et al. Late-onset granulomatous reaction to Artecoll. Dermatol Surg 29:859, 2003.

20. Lombardi T, Samson J, Plantier F, et al. Orofacial granulomas after injection of cosmetic fillers. Histopathological and clinical study of 11 cases. J Oral Pathol Med 33:115, 2004.

21. Alam M, Dover JS. Management of complications and sequelae with temporary injectable fillers. Plast Reconstr Surg 120(6 Suppl):S98, 2007.

23. Fat Grafting

George Broughton II, Sydney R. Coleman

PREOPERATIVE EVALUATION[1]

- Consultation with the patient to establish realistic goals and expectations (see Chapter 4)
- Comprehensive medical and surgical history and physical examination
  - Surgical implants are at risk for rupture or puncture with fat grafting techniques.
  - Bleeding complications/risks are possible from prescription and herbal medicine.
  - History of cold sores requires herpes simplex prophylaxis.
  - Patients planning weight loss should wait until weight goal is achieved.
- Standard preoperative photographs for surgical planning (see Chapter 3)
  - Patients being evaluated for facial rejuvenation are asked to provide photographs of their younger selves in repose.
  - Preoperative and postoperative photographs are helpful for patients who had prior surgery on their face.
- Presurgical arrangement and understanding financial responsibilities for revisions
- Analysis and operative planning based on patient desires, clinical examination, and photographs

INFORMED CONSENT[1]

RECOMMENDED ITEMS TO BE INCLUDED IN THE INFORMED CONSENT

- Locations where fat will be harvested and placed
- A statement that reads, *"Dr.___ has placed markings on my face and/or body. I have examined these markings completely with Dr.___, and I understand they represent the location for placement and/or removal of fat and planned incisions."*
- No warranties, guarantees, or special contracts about the success and longevity of the procedure
- Possible need for additional surgeries/procedures
- Complications (including donor site complications)

EQUIPMENT AND PREPARATION[1-3]

CHOICE OF HARVEST SITE

- There is **no difference** on grafted fat longevity based on donor site.
- Fat should be harvested from sites that will enhance body contour and are easily accessible in the supine position.
- Most common sites used are the **abdomen** and **medial thigh.** Other sites include the knees, and lateral and anterior thigh.
- Incisions should be placed in creases, previous scars, stretch marks, and hirsute areas. The pubic region is the most useful site—it allows access to the abdomen, medial thigh, and anterior thigh.

- Incisions are closed with a single stitch of nylon or plain gut.
- Recommended incision sites are shown in Fig. 23-1.

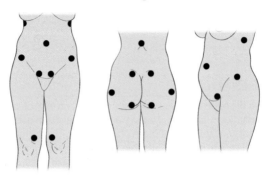

Fig. 23-1   Recommended incision sites for fat harvest.

HARVEST CANNULAS

- A two-holed cannula with a blunt tip and dull distal openings at the end is used for harvesting (Fig. 23-2). Cannula lengths are 23 and 15 cm. The advantageous greater reach of the 23 cm cannula can be offset by the frustration of broken syringe tips, resulting from the greater torque generated by the longer cannula.
- A 10 cc Luer-Lok syringe is used.

NINE-HOLE HARVESTING CANNULAS

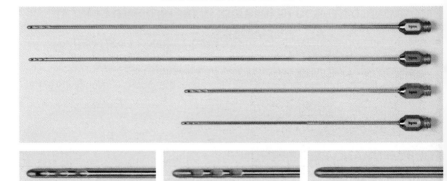

Right oblique view   Left oblique view   Back view

Fig. 23-2   Harvest cannulas.

TECHNIQUE

- The harvest areas are surgically prepared.
- A solution of 0.5% lidocaine with 1:200,000 epinephrine is infiltrated at the incision site using a 25-gauge needle.
- A stab incision is made with a No. 11 blade just large enough for the harvesting cannula (2-3 mm).
- A Lamis infiltrator can be used to infiltrate lidocaine at a volume of 1 ml of lidocaine for every cubic centimeter of fat harvested. For larger volumes or multiple sites, a solution of lactated Ringer with a 1:400,000 epinephrine is used instead. Wait 7 minutes before harvesting.

SENIOR AUTHOR TIP: Superwet or tumescent techniques are not used during the harvesting phase, because the large volumes of fluid may break up the parcels of fatty tissue into smaller components of tissues and cells. This will decrease the survival of the injected fat. The extra volume of liquid aspirated with the harvested fat will decrease the yield of fat for each syringe and increase operative time.

- The plunger is manipulated on a 10 cc syringe to generate 1 to 2 cc of negative pressure space.

TIP: If excessive fluid is in the syringe, set it on the back table with the plunger side down to allow the fat and liquid to separate. Express the excess liquid out of the syringe and continue to use it to collect more fat.

TIP: The oil separated from the fat can be used to lubricate the cannula to minimize the risk of superficial burns.

- After the syringe is filled, the cannula is removed and a dual-function Luer-Lok plug is used to cap the syringe (Fig. 23-3). With the syringe tightly capped, the plunger is removed and the syringe placed in a centrifuge for **3 minutes at 3000 rpm.**

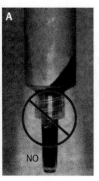 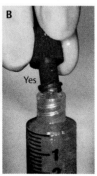

Fig. 23-3   Separating the fat. **A,** The plugs that accompany the syringe should not be used, because they frequently allow the aqueous portion of the contents to leak. **B,** The preferred plug is a dual-function Luer-Lok plug, which is twisted on to create a seal that will prevent spillage during the centrifuging process.

SEPARATION OF COMPONENTS

After centrifugation, the harvested fat will separate into **three layers** (Fig. 23-4).

- The dual-function Luer-Lok plug SHOULD NOT be removed. First, pour the upper oil layer into a medicine cup and save it for lubricating the cannulas.
- After the oil is decanted, the syringe is kept upright (Luer-Lok–side down) and the Luer-Lok plug removed. The lower aqueous layer will run out. If a tissue plug prevents the aqueous layer from draining, the syringe should be gently tapped or pulled out.
- The syringe is placed with the middle viable fat cells in a test tube rack (Luer-Lok–side down) and a Codman neuropad is placed into the syringe to wick the fat. The wick should be replaced every 4 minutes, and this should be done at least twice (Fig. 23-5, *A*).

NOTE: Fat sticking to the Codman neuropad is an indication that the fat has been exposed to the air too long and should be discarded (Fig. 23-5, *B*).

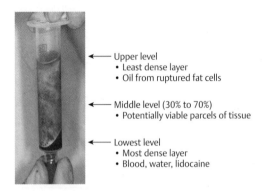

Upper level
- Least dense layer
- Oil from ruptured fat cells

Middle level (30% to 70%)
- Potentially viable parcels of tissue

Lowest level
- Most dense layer
- Blood, water, lidocaine

Fig. 23-4   Three different layers of harvested fat after centrifugation.

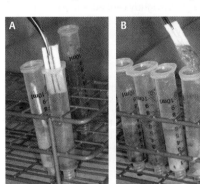

Fig. 23-5   Wicking. **A,** The wick should be replaced every 4 minutes, and this should be done at least twice. **B,** Fat is seen sticking to the Codman neuropad. This is an indication that the fat has been exposed to the air too long. This syringe of fat should be discarded.

- The plunger is replaced and the excess air carefully expressed out of the syringe.
- The fat is transferred into a 1 cc Luer-Lok syringe by inserting the Luer-Lok tip of the 10 cc syringe into the back of the plungerless 1 cc syringe. (The syringes must be vertical and nothing should block the tip of the 1 cc syringe, to allow air to escape). The plunger to the 1 cc syringe is replaced once it is filled (Fig. 23-6).
- Alternatively, a double-sided female connector can be used to join both syringes together (and their plungers), and fat from the 10 cc syringe is passed into the 1 cc syringe. (The plunger on the 1 cc syringe should be fully mobile before the transfer so it can slide to accommodate the transferred fat).

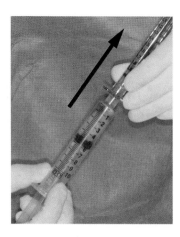

Fig. 23-6   Transfer of fat into a 1 cc Luer-Lok syringe.

FAT PLACEMENT[1,3,4]

- The recipient site is surgically prepped and draped.
- The recipient site is infiltrated with a dilute solution of epinephrine (1:400,000 in lactated Ringer solution) to minimize bruising, hematoma, and the possibility of arterial embolization.
- Incisions should be placed in wrinkle lines, folds, or hair-bearing areas.
- **The level of fat placement is dictated by the goal:**
  - To strengthen soft tissue projection over bony prominences, fat should be injected deep against bone or cartilage.
  - To support skin for an aesthetic appearance, fat should be layered immediately under the skin.
  - To fill, plump, or restore fullness, fat is placed in the intermediate layers between skin and the appropriate underlying tissue.
- The volume of fat to be infused is a difficult decision. The recipient site will be distorted by accumulating volumes of blood and infiltration solution. The volume of fat to be injected will be diluted with blood, lidocaine, and oil. It will be displaced by postoperative muscle contraction and lost to necrosis/absorption.
- Fat is infiltrated into the desired sites with a blunt cannula or a V-dissector (pickle fork). There are three types of blunt cannulas, and the recipient site determines which one is best.

- **Cannula types** (Fig. 23-7)
  - The **V-dissector** is used for correction of scars.
  - **Type I:** Completely capped on the tip, it minimizes injury to nerves, vessels, glands. It lays out the most stable placement of fat.
  - **Type II:** Similar to type I, but not completely capped at the tip
  - **Type III:** Flat on the end, it allows dissection through tissue. Useful for scars or fibrous tissue and for placing fat in intermediate subcutaneous tissue such as lower eyelid or the white roll of the lip.

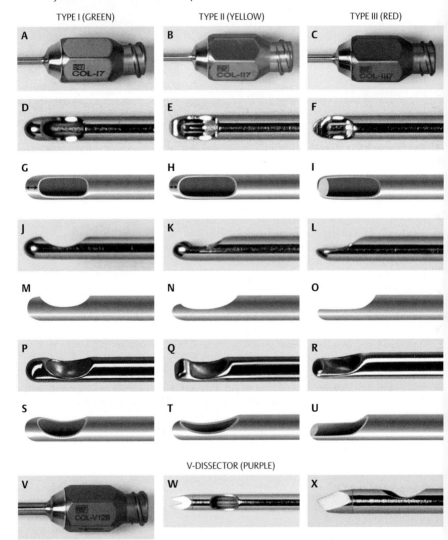

Fig. 23-7   Cannula types.

POSTOPERATIVE CARE[1]

EDEMA
- **Postoperative edema** is the most common problem.
- Patients are informed PREOPERATIVELY about what to expect.

SENIOR AUTHOR TIP: The following is a timetable "of what to expect":

Week 1, "Monster": Patients are not recognizably human—swelling at worst on day 3.

Week 2, "Human": Patients begin to look like a younger, "beat-up version" of themselves. The bruising is resolving but swelling remains.

Week 3, "Recognizable": Patients begin to recognize themselves.

Weeks 3-5, "Acceptance": Patients begin to understand and like their new look.

Up to 16 weeks: Some swelling is present in varying degrees.

TREATMENT AND PREVENTION OF EDEMA[1]
- Elevation and cold therapy should be used immediately for up to 48 hours postoperatively.
- Microfoam tape is placed immediately over the treated areas and left in place for 3 to 4 days. The tape helps to keep the transplanted fat in place and minimizes edema.
- Patients are counseled against placing any pressure on their treated areas, especially while they sleep.
- Patients are encouraged to massage their donor site as soon as tenderness in the area will permit. **The recipient site should not be massaged until 2 weeks after the procedure.**

CAUTION: Fat placed in folds or grooves should not be massaged.

TREATMENT OF SELECTED AREAS

NASOLABIAL FOLDS AND MARIONETTE GROOVES (Fig. 23-8)[1,2]

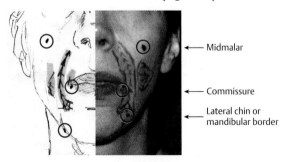

← Midmalar

← Commissure

← Lateral chin or mandibular border

Fig. 23-8   Preoperative markings of nasolabial folds and marionette grooves for location to transfer fat (^) and location of stab wounds *(red circles)* to introduce the fat grafting cannulas.

- **Anesthesia**
  - 0.5% lidocaine with 1:200,000 epinephrine
- **Incision placement**
  - A lower midmalar incision is used for perpendicular placement of fat to the nasolabial fold, and a lateral chin or mandibular border for parallel placement. An access incision at the commissure is sometimes used for different angle of placement. An alternative location is an incision at the most cephalad portion of the nasolabial fold, just lateral to the alar groove.
- **Recommended infiltrating cannula**
  - A Coleman type II is most commonly used for the nasolabial fold. A Coleman type III or V-dissector cannula may be used in areas of very fibrous adhesions.
- **Level of infiltration**
  - The primary level is at the **subdermal plane.**
- **Volume range**
  - For the nasolabial fold, 2-11 cc is needed depending on the depth. For marionette grooves, usually 1-3 cc is needed.
- **Most likely technical mistake**
  - Fat is placed into the deepest part of the fold without feathering into the surrounding area. This can lead to reformation of wrinkles in the areas adjacent to the infiltrated fatty tissue.
- **Postoperative care**
  - **Dressing:** 1-inch Microfoam tape
  - **Massage:** Massaging the nasolabial area IS NOT recommended.
  - **Recovery:** Quick. Bruising is minimal, and patients look acceptable within a few days.
- **Problems**
  - Folds medial or distal to the older folds recur, because fat was not feathered around the fold.

SENIOR AUTHOR TIP: If multiple sites are addressed on the face, the nasolabial folds and marionette grooves should be approached before the cheek or lower eyelid.

Placement of structural fat into the nasolabial fold and marionette grooves requires a complex matrix for support. At least two layers should be placed in different directions.

Feathering should always be done, except in fuller areas.

Signs of vertical folds on the upper lip medial to the nasolabial fold should be identified and feathered over at least to that area.

Surgeons should not create too much of a mound lateral to the fold, because it can accentuate an already existing fold.

Perforation of the mucosa should be carefully avoided; this is a primary cause of infection.

Fat grafted to the subcutaneous planes does not have the same effect as intradermal injections of collagen, hyaluronic acid, and other materials.

TIP: To minimize the risk of postoperative infection, patients should be instructed to gargle with Peridex a few days preoperatively.

LIPS (Fig. 23-9)[1,2]

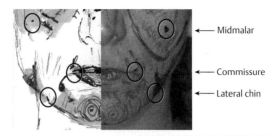

←— Midmalar

←— Commissure

←— Lateral chin

Fig. 23-9   Preoperative marking of lips and chin for location to transfer fat and location of stab wounds *(red circles)* to introduce the fat grafting cannulas.

- **Anesthesia**
  - 1% lidocaine with 1:100,000 epinephrine is used for an infraorbital and mental block. A solution of 0.5% lidocaine with 1:200,000 epinephrine is used in the dermis around the incision sites and in the superficial muscle and submucosal planes of the lip. (A Coleman type III cannula is recommended.)
- **Incision placement**
  - Incisions are placed at the commissures; occasionally, an incision is made in a wrinkle radiating from the lip or a midmalar incision is used to approach the cutaneous lip.
- **Recommended infiltrating cannula**
  - Coleman type III infiltration cannula
- **Level of infiltration**
  - Fat needs to be placed with precise accuracy in the plane immediately deep to the mucosa or vermilion. Placement within the muscle only creates a fat lip (Fig. 23-10).
- **Volume range**
  - 0.75-1.25 cc to restructure the white roll and the same volume for the lower lip rim. In the body of the upper lip, volumes range from 0.75-4 cc; the volume used for the body of the lower lip is twice that used for the upper lip.

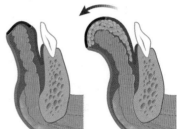

Correct superficial fat placement

Fig. 23-10   Fat used for lip augmentation should be placed with precise accuracy in the plane immediately deep to the mucosa or vermilion and should not be infiltrated into the muscle.

- **Most likely technical mistake**
  - Placing fat under the skin above the white roll (and not directly under it) or placing fat under the skin of the upper and lower lip, creating a "cutaneous lip."
- **Postoperative care**
  - **Dressing:** None. To prevent chapping, tell patients to keep their lips moist with lip balms or ointments.
  - **Massage:** Gentle massage of the lips after 1 or 2 weeks on the skin but not on the mucosa. Patients are encouraged to "work" their orbicularis oris the first week to encourage lymphatic drainage.

- **Recovery:** Slow. Patients will have significant swelling for 1 to 2 weeks; by 4 weeks the swelling is usually resolved. Cold therapy helps to decrease the swelling time. Some patients report still being able to feel changes in texture and size of their lips for up to 8 months.
■ **Problems**
  - Splitting of the lip. Splitting of the lower lip has been seen when the volume infiltrated is too much. Lacerations should be closed with simple interrupted chromic sutures.

SENIOR AUTHOR TIP: If multiple sites are addressed on the face, the lip should be treated last to prevent contaminating the other areas of the face or body.

To augment the lip with increased vermilion show, fat should not be placed deep to the cutaneous portion of the lip. This can expand the lip and actually decrease the amount of vermilion show.

Small lumps are amazingly well tolerated in the lip; large lumps are not.

Flipping the lip outward can shorten the upper lip in two ways:
  - By shortening the distance from the columellar base to the height of the Cupid's bow—the action of turning up the lip.
  - By increasing the amount of vermilion visible—the relative proportion of the cutaneous lip to the vermilion lip is adjusted.

Maxillary incisor show will be influenced by lip augmentation. With eversion of the upper lip, it is possible to obtain a significant increase in maxillary incisor show. In some patients, maxillary incisor show may be less because of a slight descent of the upper lip.

Mandibular incisor show can also be changed during lip augmentation. The aging lip descends to increase visibility of the lower incisors; raise the entire lip slightly, by placing more fat into the submucosal plane of the lower lip and sometimes into the orbicularis oris muscle itself.

The philtrum is approached in one of two ways:
  - By simply running a type III cannula up into the philtral columns while placing fat below the white roll. Although the 90-degree angle may appear sharp, it is usually easy to navigate.
  - By making a central incision in the vermilion about half a centimeter inferior to the Cupid's bow and passing a type III cannula up through the base of the philtral column to the columella. This begins by placing the fat deep using 5-8 passes to deposit less than 1/30 cc each time.

Augmentation of the muscle will initially evert the lip vermilion and mucosa from edema overlying the muscle. As the swelling subsides, so does the eversion of the vermilion and the apparent augmentation.

TROUBLESHOOTING[1]: PATIENTS WHO HAVE HAD PERMANENT FILLERS PLACED IN THEIR LIPS

- **Nonintegrated, permanent soft tissue fillers**
  - Some of the most difficult patients in whom to achieve a natural correction are those who have had nonintegrated, permanent soft tissue fillers placed, such as Gore-Tex, solid silicone, dermal fat grafts, or fascia grafts. If these substances can be removed from the lip, they should be removed.

> **SENIOR AUTHOR TIP:** In patients in whom the substance was left in place, the lip retained an unnatural feel.

- **Integrated, permanent fillers**
  - Patients whose lips have been injected with permanent fillers such as silicone, Artecoll, DermaLive, and polyacrylamide gel present a difficult challenge. Because it is impossible to remove these substances, surgeons who choose to operate on these patients must devise a careful plan that will NOT make the lips worse.

TEAR TROUGH AND CHEEK (Fig. 23-11)[1,2]

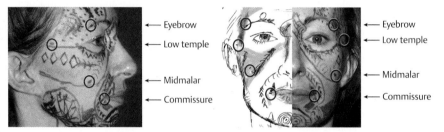

— Eyebrow
— Low temple
— Midmalar
— Commissure

— Eyebrow
— Low temple
— Midmalar
— Commissure

Fig. 23-11 Preoperative markings of tear trough and cheek for locations to transfer fat and location of stab wounds *(red circles)* to introduce the fat grafting cannulas.

- **Anesthesia**
  - A solution of 0.5% lidocaine with 1:200,000 epinephrine using a blunt cannula (type I) to prevent injuring infraorbital nerve
- **Incision placement**
  - Four primary incisions are used on each side: The lateral eyebrow, lateral inferior temple at the level of the zygomatic arch, lower midmalar region, and the lateral lip.
- **Recommended infiltrating cannula**
  - For placement against the periosteum of the anterior and lateral malar region: Type I cannula
  - Deep soft tissue: Type II cannula (A curved cannula is used to follow the curvature of the maxilla and zygoma.)
  - Superficial placement around the lower eyelids: Type III cannula

- **Level of infiltration**
  - Immediate subdermal plane: This provides structural support to the skin that eliminates wrinkles, reduces pore size, and can lighten the eyelid skin.
  - Anterior malar fold: Fat is placed at every level from the periosteum to the skin (Fig. 23-12). This pattern is used over the entire malar region. In the midmalar and lateral malar cheeks, stay deep to provide structural support.
  - Lower eyelids superior to the infraorbital rim: Stay superficial. Fat is placed in the immediate subdermal plane or in the orbicularis oculi muscle.
  - Buccal cheek: Superficial infiltration to help with skin texture and decrease risk of neurovascular injury.
- **Volume range (Table 23-1)**

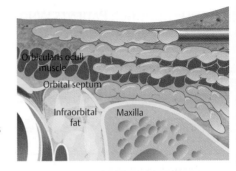

Fig. 23-12 For the anterior malar fold, fat is placed at every level from the periosteum to the skin over the entire malar region. In the midmalar and lateral malar cheeks, stay deep to provide structural support.

Table 23-1 *Volume Ranges of Fat Infiltration*

Location	Volume (cc)
Superficial anterior malar fold	1-3
Between the anterior malar fold and nose	0.25-1
Infraorbital rim lateral to the anterior malar fold	1-5
Lateral eyelid	0.25-1.5
Anterior malar region	1-5
Midmalar cheek	1-7
Lateral malar cheek	1-8
Buccal cheek	1-10

- **Most likely technical mistakes**
  - Not feathering over to the nose and leaving an area of depression between the nose and anterior malar cheek
  - Infraorbital irregularities if fat is infiltrated in volumes larger than 1/10 cc in the lower eyelid or if molding the fat into shape
  - Overcorrection, especially in the anterior malar fold

- **Postoperative care**
  - **Dressing:** Microfoam tape on the lower eyelids from below the ciliary margin beyond the limits of fat placement. A layer of Microfoam tape is placed over the malar and buccal cheeks (Fig. 23-13). Dressings are removed between days 3 and 5, and patients are instructed to start massaging the treated areas. Ice compresses can be used, but cautiously if the fat grafting was difficult, because the compression may cause contour irregularities.

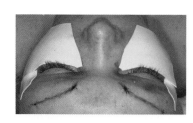

Fig. 23-13 Recommended dressing following malar fat grafting consists of using Microfoam tape on the lower eyelids from below the ciliary margin beyond the limits of fat placement.

  - **Massage:** After dressings are removed, patients should start massaging the treated areas. They should start gentle downward rolling massage to encourage lymphatic drainage four to six times a day for 1 minute on each lower eyelid.
  - **Recovery:** Quick. Swelling is usually minimal. Patients may have black and blue discoloration for a few weeks.
- **Problems**
  - Contour irregularities from fat deposited in lumps. The problem is corrected by aspirating the excess fat using a type I cannula or open removal. Some patients may have prolonged infraorbital hyperpigmentation (probably from hemosiderin deposits from resolving hematoma).

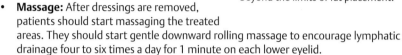

SENIOR AUTHOR TIP: Note the aperture direction and removal of grafted fat. Although the direction of the aperture is not usually a concern, keeping the cannula facing upward toward the skin and maneuvering the cannula so that the fat is between the cannula and the skin will allow aspiration of unwanted fat easier.

Special care should be taken during fat grafting in the lower eyelid. Only miniscule amounts are placed with each withdrawal of the cannula. If a visible lump is noted after infiltration, immediate measures are taken to remove the lump (it will not get better postoperatively). Digital pressure and smoothing the fat can be attempted, but if it is not flattened, then it is removed by suctioning with a type I cannula.

During infiltration of the lower eyelids, the thumb is used as a guide and to protect the globe (Fig. 23-14). The thumb can also be used to detect the correct level for placement and to guide the cannula to that level, whether deep or superficial. This added sensory input can be helpful, particularly along the entire infraorbital rim, from the medial commissure to the lateral commissure.

As the placement moves to a more superficial plane, placing traction on the skin to detect the position of the cannula more accurately is sometimes helpful. This can be accomplished by pulling the skin with the fingers of the nondominant hand.

Continued

When infiltrating the lower eyelid, traction on the upper eyelid can provide better visualization of the skin of the lower eyelid.

The prominence of the cheek is identified preoperatively and maintained at that proposed height. The attractive malar prominence is usually most protuberant along a line running from the alar base to the base of the auricular helix. This line is marked with the patient standing and participating. (I use diamonds to mark this line so there is no confusion with other marks.) These marks will keep surgeons oriented when placing infiltrate in the malar prominence. If the markings are not visible when the malar prominence is determined, careful attention should be paid to these landmarks to ensure the prominence will be maintained in an attractive direction and level.

A type I cannula is used near veins and arteries. At times, it is difficult to remain in the proper plane with a type I or the tissues are too fibrous for placement with a type I. In such situations, surgeons can try to force a plane in the tissue with a type I or II cannula. After a plane is somewhat established, a type III cannula is used for fat placement. This does not always work, but I have found it helpful many times.

The use of a V-dissector in the periorbital region is not recommended.

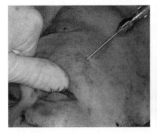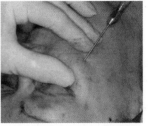

Fig. 23-14   During infiltration of the lower eyelids, the thumb is used as a guide and to protect the globe. The thumb can also be used to detect the correct level for placement and to guide the cannula to that level, whether deep or superficial. This added sensory input can be helpful.

COMPLICATIONS[1-5]

- Inaccurate volume causing undercorrection or overcorrection
- Poor preoperative planning, fat necrosis, poor viability of fat caused by excessive negative pressure during fat harvest, exposure to air, mechanical trauma during harvesting, or placement

FATE OF TRANSPLANTED ADIPOCYTES[6]

- In vitro studies showed that transplanted adipocytes are susceptible to an ischemic death, whereas adipose-derived stromal cells can remain viable for 3 days.
- Most adipocytes died on day 1, with only some survivors.
- Seven days after grafting, there was an increase in viable adipocytes, suggesting that repair and regeneration of dead adipocytes was under way.
- There are **three zones** of transplanted fat:
  1. A surviving area (adipocytes survived)
  2. A regeneration area (adipocytes died and adipose-derived stromal cells survived to replace dead adipocytes)
  3. A necrotic area (where both adipocytes and adipose-derived stromal cells died)
- **Irregular contour: Dips, lumps, and bumps**
  - Large globule of fat undergoes central necrosis, collapses, and causes depression.
  - Large globule of fat is aggressively molded intraoperatively or postoperatively and results in central necrosis and depression.
  - Fat placement is isolated, without feathering or intradermal placement.
- **Fat migration**
  - Muscle motion causes intrinsic pressure and displacement, which occurs most often around the glabella.
  - External pressure can displace recently transplanted fat. Patients should not manipulate treated areas or wear objects that can cause pressure such as glasses and hats.
- **Infection**
  - Proper surgical scrub at the donor and recipient sites
  - Perioperative antibiotics
  - Antiviral prophylaxis in patients with history of fever sores if fat is grafted around mouth
  - Avoid introducing foreign bodies with the fat. The most likely source is cotton fibers from sponges or Telfa used to wick fatty oils.

> **TIP:** Use Codman neuropad to prevent this complication.

- **Nerve injury**
  - Almost always temporary
  - Most likely to occur if sharp needle is used to inject fat; preventable when blunt cannulas are used
- **Muscle injury** caused by needles or cannulas and is most noticeable in the face
- **Parotid gland injury** caused by needles or cannulas and may result in parotitis
- **Cutaneous injury** at harvest/recipient sites causing prolonged erythema and inflammation. Friction caused by the cannula can cause thermal injury to the skin.

> **TIP:** Using a patient's own residual oil left over from the fat harvest can lubricate the cannula and minimize this problem.

- Hematoma from infiltration of the local anesthetic. If a hematoma is encountered on the face, the opposite side is treated first. The volume to be grafted on the hematoma side is based on the volume used on the nonaffected side and preoperative plan.
- **Arterial occlusion**
    - Intraarterial injection of fat will result in excruciating pain followed by skin loss.
    - Central arterial injection can cause blindness, stroke, and soft tissue necrosis. This complication can result from introduction of fat (filler) around the supratrochlear and supraorbital arteries.

SENIOR AUTHOR TIP: There are ways to prevent complications caused by intraarterial injections.[1]

Do not use sharp cannulas or needles; instead, use larger, blunt cannulas.

Use epinephrine—a vasoconstricted vessel is much harder to cannulate than a dilated one.

Inject small volumes (1/10 cc) around danger areas.

Use small syringes—controlling the injected volume is much easier using a 1 cc Luer-Lok syringe than a 10 or 20 cc syringe.

Do not use mechanical assistance devices for injecting fat that can generate high and destructive pressures in soft tissues.

TOP TAKEAWAYS
➤ There is **no** difference in grafted fat longevity based on donor site.
➤ Fat sticking to the Codman neuropad is an indication that the fat has been exposed to the air too long and should be discarded.
➤ Incisions should be placed in wrinkle lines, folds, or hair-bearing areas.
➤ Postoperative edema is the most common problem.

REFERENCES
1. Coleman SR. Structural Fat Grafting. New York: Thieme Publishers, 2004.
2. Coleman SR. Facial recontouring with lipostructure. Clin Plast Surg 24:347, 1997.
3. Coleman SR. Long-term survival of fat transplants: controlled demonstrations. Aesthetic Plast Surg 19:421, 1995.
4. Coleman SR. Structural fat grafts: the ideal filler? Clin Plast Surg 28:111, 2001.
5. Coleman SR. Hand rejuvenation with structural fat grafting. Plast Reconstr Surg 110:1731; discussion 1745, 2002.
6. Eto H, Kato H, Suga H, et al. The fate of adipocytes after nonvascularized fat grafting: evidence of early death and replacement of adipocytes. Plast Reconstr Surg 129:1081, 2012.

24. Treatment of Prominent Veins

Edward J. Ruane, Girish S. Munavalli

PROMINENT VEINS[1]

- Can occur in the presence or absence of either symptoms or an underlying functional venous disorder[2]
- Present in up to **50%** of individuals
- **Risk factors** include:
  - Advancing age
  - Family history
  - Ligamentous laxity
  - Prolonged standing
  - Increased BMI
  - Smoking
  - Sedentary lifestyle
  - History of trauma
  - History of venous thrombosis
  - Arteriovenous shunting
  - High estrogen states, including pregnancy in women
- **Telangiectasias,** often referred to as *spider veins,* are most common.
- **Varicose veins** are dilated, elongated, tortuous, subcutaneous veins ≥3 mm.[3]
- **Goals of treatment**
  - Improvement of symptoms (including pain or aching, heaviness, swelling, dry and/or irritated skin, and tightness)
  - Improvement of appearance

TREATMENT OPTIONS

CONSERVATIVE MANAGEMENT
- Extremity elevation
- Exercise
- Compression therapy

SCLEROTHERAPY
Indications
- Treatment of choice for most superficial leg veins
- Appropriate for the treatment of telangiectasias, reticular veins, and small varicose veins[4]

Contraindications
- Acute venous thrombosis or phlebitis
- Pregnancy
- Diabetes mellitus (relative)

- Moderate to severe peripheral artery disease (relative)
- Patent foramen ovale (relative)[5]

Preoperative Evaluation

- For patients who are **asymptomatic** but find the cosmetic appearance of their veins distressing, sclerotherapy can be performed after physical examination without further diagnostic studies, because these patients are unlikely to have underlying venous reflux.
- **Symptomatic** patients should undergo further evaluation with venous duplex imaging to identify the presence of **superficial or deep venous insufficiency.**

Informed Consent

- Veins will lighten and become less noticeable but may not completely disappear.
- **Multiple treatments** are typically required to achieve the desired effect.
- **Hyperpigmentation** is a relatively common complication.

TIP: Veins are documented photographically before each treatment and reviewed with the patient periodically.

Equipment[6-7] (Table 24-1)

Table 24-1   *Common Sclerosing Agents for the Treatment of Prominent Veins*

Agent	Vessel Size (mm)	Concentration (%)	Volume (ml)	Maximum Dose	Advantages	Disadvantages
Sodium tetradecyl sulfate	0.3-1 1-3 3-5 >5	0.1-0.25 0.25-0.5 0.5-1 1-3	0.25 0.5 0.5-1 1-2	10 ml of 3%	Less telangiectatic matting	Allergy Hyperpigmentation at high concentrations Ulceration/necrosis
Polidocanol	<0.5 0.5-1 1-3	0.25 0.5 1	0.1-0.3 0.1-0.3 0.1-0.3	2 mg/kg	Painless Nontoxic Rare ulceration No necrosis	Allergy Telangiectatic matting Hyperpigmentation
Hypertonic saline	<0.5 0.5-1 1-3	11.7 11.7 23.4	0.25 0.5 0.5-1	None	No allergy	Pain Muscle cramping Ulceration/necrosis Hyperpigmentation
Glycerin[8]	<1	25-72	0.25	10 ml of 72%	No matting No ulceration No necrosis	Contact sensitivity Urethral colic Hematuria (rare) Off-label, not FDA approved

Technique

- Sclerosants may be used in their liquid form or mixed with room air as a foam, to increase their surface area for the treatment of larger veins.
- **Tessari method** involves using a three-way stopcock and two syringes, mixing air with liquid to create a foam.[9]
- After the sclerosant liquid or foam (with or without lidocaine) is mixed into a syringe at the appropriate concentration, attach the syringe to a 27- or 30-gauge needle.
- Place the patient in **Trendelenburg position** to discourage refilling of injected veins.
- Apply alcohol to clean the area, introduce the needle into the vein, **aspirate to ensure intraluminal position,** and inject using a low pressure, a fixed amount of the sclerosant.
- Withdraw the needle, apply compression, and massage the treated area to prevent refilling of the injected vein.
- Secure a compressive dressing in place with tape while advancing to other treatment areas.

SENIOR AUTHOR TIP: The use of 2-way Baxa connectors are an easier, more rapid way to generate foam.

TIP: Larger underlying reticular veins should be obliterated before more superficial telangiectasias are treated.

Postoperative Care

- Compressive stockings should be worn continuously for at least 24 hours and then daily for 2-3 weeks.[10]
- Avoid strenuous exercise and sun exposure for 2-4 weeks.
- Repeat injections are not performed for at least 4-6 weeks.
- Clearance of **60%-80%** of treated telangiectasias, reticular veins, and small varicose veins can be expected.[11]

SENIOR AUTHOR TIP: In the sclerotherapy consultation, inform patients that new spider veins will occur over time and annual maintenance treatments are encouraged.

Complications[12]

- **Minor**
  - **Pain**
  - **Ulceration**
    - Reported incidence: 1%-5% of patients treated
    - Usually small and heal with local wound care in 4-6 weeks
  - **Telangiectatic matting**
    - Consists of multiple, fine dilated vessels in the area of the injection site
    - Relatively common, occurring in 15%-24% of patients
    - Usually resolves **within 3-12 months**[13]

- ▶ Check for the presence of local feeding vessels
- ▶ Consider treating using sclerotherapy with 72% glycerin
- ▶ Minimize incidence by using the minimum strength concentration of sclerosant to achieve effective treatment
- **Hyperpigmentation**
  - ▶ Caused by deposition of hemosiderin in the skin
  - ▶ Occurs in up to 30% of patients
  - ▶ Resolves spontaneously in 80% of patients within 2 years

SENIOR AUTHOR TIP: Minimize incidence of matting and hyperpigmentation by using the minimum strength concentration of sclerosant to achieve effective treatment.

- **Major (rare)**
  - **Superficial thrombophlebitis**
  - **Deep venous thrombosis**
  - **Microembolic** events
    - ▶ Occur in <1% of patients
    - ▶ Symptoms include visual disturbance (scotoma), migraine-like headache, and neurologic deficits.
  - **Anaphylaxis**

LASER THERAPY
Indications[14]
- Patients who do not tolerate or fail sclerotherapy
- Superficial vessels that are too small to cannulate with a sclerotherapy needle
- Needle phobia on the part of the patient

Contraindications
- Acute venous thrombosis or phlebitis
- Pregnancy
- Diabetes mellitus (relative)
- Moderate to severe peripheral artery disease (relative)
- Fitzpatrick skin types III-VI (relative)

TIP: A test spot should be performed before proceeding with laser therapy on patients with Fitzpatrick skin types III-VI out of concern for either hyperpigmentation or hypopigmentation.

Preoperative Evaluation
- In the absence of signs of venous reflux, laser and light therapy can be performed after a physical examination.

Informed Consent
- Multiple treatments are typically required.
- Alterations in skin pigmentation can occur.

Equipment[15] (Table 24-2)

Table 24-2 *Common Laser and Light Sources for the Treatment of Prominent Veins*

Source	Wavelength (nm)	Vessel Size (mm)	Skin Type (Fitzpatrick)	Advantages	Disadvantages
Alexandrite	755	>0.4	I/II/III	High penetration depth Less painful	Purpura Telangiectatic matting
Diode	800, 810, 940, 980	<4	I/II/III/IV	Treats larger veins	Unpredictable results
KTP	532	0.5-1.5	I-III	Less painful	Pigmentary changes
Nd:YAG	1064	0.3-3.0	I-IV	High clearance rate Less pigmentary changes	Pain
PDL	585-595	<1.5	I-III	Less pigmentary changes	Purpura
IPL	585+	<1 (red)	I-III	Large spot size Less purpura	Limited evidence

IPL, Intense pulsed light; *KTP,* potassium titanyl phosphate; *Nd:YAG,* neodymium:yttrium-aluminum-garnet; *PDL,* pulsed dye laser.

Technique
- The U.S. Occupational Safety and Health Administration (OSHA) requires that protective eyewear be worn when operating class 4 lasers.
- Enter the selected treatment parameters into the laser/light control panel.
- First, cool the skin, and then activate the laser/light over the target vessel or vessels.
- A visible clearing of the vein should be seen, but, if not, the vessel can be treated again and/or the laser parameters can be adjusted.

CAUTION: To prevent burns, no more than three attempts should be made over the same area.

Postoperative Care
- No dressings are needed.
- Patients may return to their normal daily activities immediately.
- Avoidance of sun exposure to the treated areas is critical.
- Repeat therapy may be performed within 4-8 weeks.

Complications
- **Minor**
  - **Pain**
    - Usually lasts only seconds to minutes after treatment
    - Application of topical anesthetic for 30-60 minutes prior may lessen pain[16]
  - **Bruising**

- **Pigmentation changes**
    - ▶ Common in patients with skin types III-VI
    - ▶ Usually develop within 3 weeks after treatment
    - ▶ Hyperpigmentation—usually temporary
    - ▶ Hypopigmentation—may be permanent
- Telangiectatic matting
- **Major**
    - **Superficial thrombophlebitis**
        - ▶ May take up to 6 weeks to resolve
        - ▶ Rarely has sequelae

ENDOVENOUS LASER ABLATION (EVLA)

- Percutaneous technique using **laser energy** to ablate incompetent superficial veins
- **Axial veins** (i.e., great, small, or accessory saphenous veins) are the primary target for this therapy.
- Varicose vein recurrence reported to occur in 7%-14% of patients in the long-term[17]

Contraindications

- Venous thrombosis or phlebitis
- Pregnancy
- Moderate to severe peripheral artery disease
- Severe tortuosity, which may limit passage of the device
- Superficial veins (<1 cm deep), in which skin burns may result
- Aneurysmal veins (>2.5 cm diameter), in which the risk of failure may be greater

Complications

- Bruising/hematoma
- Skin burns
- Superficial thrombophlebitis
- Deep venous thrombosis (DVT)
- Cutaneous nerve injury[18]

RADIOFREQUENCY ABLATION (RFA)

- Percutaneous technique that uses **thermal energy** to ablate incompetent veins
- **Axial veins** (i.e., great, small, or accessory saphenous veins) are the primary target, but intersaphenous veins or perforator veins can also be treated with specialized probes

Contraindications

- Venous thrombosis or phlebitis
- Pregnancy
- Diabetes mellitus
- Moderate to severe peripheral artery disease
- Veins <5 mm or >15 mm in diameter[19]

Complications

- Superficial thrombophlebitis
- DVT
- Cutaneous nerve injury

NONENDOTHERMAL ENDOVENOUS ABLATION
- Percutaneous access, with direct injection into saphenous veins
- 1% Polidocanol microfoam-injected directly into the saphenous veins. FDA approved for treatment of the great saphenous vein and tributaries
- Cyanoacrylate glue: Injected directly into the saphenous veins. FDA approved for treatment of the great saphenous vein and tibuaries

SURGERY
- Largely supplanted by less invasive methods
- Remains the standard to which other techniques are compared
- Most commonly used to manage **large varicose veins** (>1.5 cm diameter) and **complications of varicose veins** (e.g., varicose vein hemorrhage, recurrent phlebitis)
- Surgical techniques involve ligation and/or removal of veins through multiple incisions.
- Specific techniques include:
  - Saphenous vein inversion and removal
  - High ligation of the saphenous vein
  - Ambulatory phlebectomy
  - Transilluminated phlebectomy
  - Conservative venous ligation (CHIVA)
  - Perforator ligation
- Surgical techniques are associated with 20%-28% varicose vein recurrence rates.[20]

Contraindications
- Venous thrombosis or phlebitis
- Diabetes mellitus
- Moderate to severe peripheral artery disease
- Significant cardiopulmonary comorbidities, increasing the risk of anesthesia

Complications
- Bruising/hematoma
- Infection
- Superficial thrombophlebitis
- DVT
- Cutaneous nerve injury
- Lymphatic leakage

TOP TAKEAWAYS
➤ Sclerosants may be used in their liquid form or as a foam to increase their surface area for the treatment of larger veins.
➤ Clearance of 60%-80% of treated telangiectasias, reticular veins, and small varicose veins can be expected.
➤ To prevent burns, no more than three attempts should be made over the same area.
➤ Never double pulse veins with diode or 1064 Nd:YAG laser.
➤ A test spot should be performed before proceeding with laser therapy on patients with Fitzpatrick skin types III-VI.
➤ The U.S. Occupational Safety and Health Administration (OSHA) requires that protective eyewear be worn when operating class 4 lasers.

References

1. Callam MJ. Epidemiology of varicose veins. Br J Surg 81:167, 1994.
2. Chiesa R, Marone EM, Limoni C, et al. Chronic venous disorders: correlation between visible signs, symptoms, and presence of functional disease. J Vasc Surg 46:322, 2007.
3. Chang CJ, Chua JJ. Endovenous laser photocoagulation (EVLP) for varicose veins. Lasers Surg Med 31:257, 2002.
4. Langer RD, Ho E, Denenberg JO, et al. Relationships between symptoms and venous disease: the San Diego population study. Arch Intern Med 165:1420, 2005.
5. Davis LT, Duffy DM. Determination of incidence and risk factors for postsclerotherapy telangiectatic matting of the lower extremity: a retrospective analysis. J Dermatol Surg Oncol 16:327, 1990.
6. Schwartz L, Maxwell H. Sclerotherapy for lower limb telangiectasias. Cochrane Database Syst Rev 18:CD008826, 2011.
7. Tisi PV, Beverley C, Rees A. Injection sclerotherapy for varicose veins. Cochrane Database Syst Rev CD001732, 2006.
8. Leach BC, Goldman MP. Comparative trial between sodium tetradecyl sulfate and glycerin in the treatment of telangiectatic leg veins. Dermatol Surg 29:612; discussion 615, 2003.
9. Tessari L, Cavezzi A, Frullini A. Preliminary experience with a new sclerosing foam in the treatment of varicose veins. Dermatol Surg 27:58, 2011.
10. Weiss RA, Sadick NS, Goldman MP, et al. Post-sclerotherapy compression: controlled comparative study of duration of compression and its effects on clinical outcome. Dermatol Surg 25:105, 1999.
11. Hamahata A, Yamaki T, Sakurai H. Outcomes of ultrasound-guided foam sclerotherapy for varicose veins of the lower extremities: a single center experience. Dermatol Surg 37:804, 2001.
12. Munavalli GS, Weiss RA. Complications of sclerotherapy. Semin Cutan Med Surg 26:22, 2007.
13. Gillet JL, Guedes JM, Guex JJ, et al. Side-effects and complications of foam sclerotherapy of the great and small saphenous veins: a controlled multicentre prospective study including 1,025 patients. Phlebology 24:131, 2009.
14. McCoppin HH, Hovenic WW, Wheeland RG. Laser treatment of superficial leg veins: a review. Dermatol Surg 37:729, 2011.
15. Eremia S, Li C, Umar SH. A side-by-side comparative study of 1064 nm Nd:YAG, 810 nm diode and 755 nm alexandrite lasers for treatment of 0.3-3 mm leg veins. Dermatol Surg 28:224, 2002.
16. Chen JZ, Alexiades-Armenakas MR, Bernstein LJ, et al. Two randomized, double-blind, placebo-controlled studies evaluating the S-Caine Peel for induction of local anesthesia before long-pulsed Nd:YAG laser therapy for leg veins. Dermatol Surg 29:1012, 2003.
17. Ravi R, Trayler EA, Barrett DA, et al. Endovenous thermal ablation of superficial venous insufficiency of the lower extremity: single-center experience with 3000 limbs treated in a 7-year period. J Endovasc Ther 16:500, 2009.
18. Desmyttère J, Grard C, Wassmer B, et al. Endovenous 980-nm laser treatment of saphenous veins in a series of 500 patients. J Vasc Surg 46:1242, 2007.
19. Merchant RF, Pichot O; Closure Study Group. Long-term outcomes of endovenous radiofrequency obliteration of saphenous reflux as a treatment for superficial venous insufficiency. J Vasc Surg 42:502; discussion 509, 2005.
20. Michaels JA, Campbell WB, Brazier JE, et al. Randomised clinical trial, observational study and assessment of cost-effectiveness of the treatment of varicose veins (REACTIV trial). Health Technol Assess 10:1, 2006.

PART VI

Adjuncts to Aesthetic Surgery

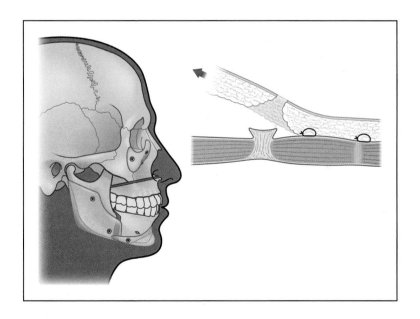

PART VI

Adjuncts in Aesthetic Surgery

25. Tissue Glues

Joseph Meyerson, Renato Saltz

PRINCIPLES OF THE PERFECT TISSUE ADHESIVE

- High bonding strength
- Ease of operative applications
- Reproducible outcomes
- Nontoxic to tissue
- Affordable cost

FIBRIN SEALANT

HISTORY

- Fibrin powder used as hemostat and sealant by Bergel[1] in 1909
- Described as an adhesive for skin grafts in 1940s[2,3]
- Approved by FDA in 1998 for use as a hemostatic agent and as a tissue sealant in liquid form; fibrin sealant patch approved in 2010[4]
  - Artiss (Baxter) is the only fibrin sealant approved specifically for autologous skin grafting and flap adherence in rhytidectomy.
- Fibrin sealant approved by the FDA as a **hemostat, adhesive, and sealant**

MECHANISM OF ACTION[5]

- **Fibrin clot** forms from a polymerized fibrin compound resulting from the reaction of fibrinogen and thrombin.
  - Thrombin cleaves larger subunits of fibrinogen, creating fibrin subunits, which in turn polymerize.
  - Factor XIII and calcium cause cross-linking and formation of a stable fibrin clot.
- Fibrin clot will degrade in approximately **10-14 days.**

DELIVERY SYSTEM[6,7,8]

- Delivery systems consist of **two separate components of fibrin and thrombin** that combine on exiting the device through a double-barrel syringe with a Y-connector.
  - May be applied locally or aerosolized for larger surfaces
- Commercially available products contain components from varied sources.
  - Fibrinogen from human pooled plasma or a patient's own plasma
  - Thrombin of human or bovine origin
  - Aprotinin (antifibrinolytic protein)
  - Factor XIII and calcium (catalysts)
  - Equine collagen and cellulose matrix available for fibrin patch design

PRICING[9]
- Liquid form approximately $50/ml of fibrin sealant
- Fibrin sealant patches range $600-$800/patch

NOTE: **Prices for these products may vary based on contracting.**

COMPLICATIONS[10]
- Commercial preparations of fibrin sealants have risk of **bloodborne pathogens** (viral, prions).
- Products with **bovine** components can cause **disseminated coagulopathy.**
- **Aprotinin-containing** products can cause **anaphylaxis, rash.**
- **Air emboli** can occur with **pressurized applications.**
- Thick layers of fibrin allowed to polymerize before tissue apposition can **inhibit wound healing** and act as an **antiadhesive.**

APPLICATIONS
- Conflicting studies exist for the outcomes of fibrin sealant used in cosmetic procedures.
- Lower levels of thrombin (5 units/ml) allow the sealant to set at a slower rate, resulting in extended time for flap manipulation.
- **Rhytidectomy**[11,12,13]
  - Multiple studies show statistically significant decrease in drain output with fibrin sealant versus control.
  - Varied reports in decreasing hematoma, edema, and ecchymosis formation.
  - Randomized controlled, blinded trial compared one side of the face without fibrin sealant and the addition of fibrin sealant on the other. The fibrin sealant side reduced average drainage volumes (20 ml without fibrin glue versus 7.7 ml with fibrin glue, p <0.0001) without increasing the incidence of hematoma or seroma.
  - Prospective, double-blind, randomized, controlled trial on the use of fibrin sealant in 20 consecutive patients undergoing facelifts by the same surgeon. Each patient was randomized for the use of fibrin sealant on either the right or the left side of the face with the contralateral side acting as the control. Total drainage was recorded on each side for 24 hours before drains were removed. The side treated with fibrin glue had a median drainage of 10 ml and the control side 30 ml (p <0.002).
  - Prospective, nonblinded, randomized, controlled trial in 30 patients undergoing facelifts. Patients were their own controls and were randomized to having glue on one side of their face. Drainage on glued side was 7.5 ml less than unglued in 24 hour output, but not thought to be clinically significant (p <0.05).

SENIOR AUTHOR TIP: I have used tissue glues in all my facial rejuvenation procedures since 1991. They help to "seal" the space after SMAS treatment is completed. They appear to reduce swelling, bruising, and small seromas/hematomas.

- **Abdominoplasty**[14]
  - Fibrin sealants have been shown to lower rates of seroma postoperatively.
  - One prospective study demonstrated fibrin sealant may be inferior to surgical drains or quilting.
    - Forty-three patients were randomly placed into three groups during abdominoplasty and evaluated with ultrasound for evidence of seroma

postoperatively. Group one, abdominoplasty with suction drains alone. Group two, abdominoplasty with quilting suture, and group three, abdominoplasty with fibrin sealant. Seroma formation was significantly lower in drain (13.9 ml) and quilting (16.1 ml) groups compared with the fibrin sealant (53.6 ml) group (p <0.05).

- **Blepharoplasty**[15]
  - Shown to be an acceptable alternative or adjunct to sutures for closure in upper blepharoplasty.
  - When compared with standard suture techniques, the incidence of minor problems such as milia formation was lower, with the only complication of glue only technique was one wound separation in 16 patients. Endorses using fibrin glue and a minimal number of sutures for blepharoplasty patients.
- **Browlift**[16]
  - A retrospective study of endoscopic browlifts found that fixation with only fibrin sealant resulted in loss of brow elevation 3 months postoperatively.
  - In 538 patients two different fixation methods were compared.
    - ▶ Group one had fibrin glue and group two had polydioxanone sutures used as fixation.
    - ▶ At 1 month postoperatively, each fixation technique remained equivocal and stable in regards to brow elevation.
    - ▶ At 3 months postoperatively, there was a significant difference in brow elevation with a higher number of relapses in ptosis in the patients treated with only fibrin glue (p <0.01).

SENIOR AUTHOR TIP: The use of tissue glues after endoscopic midface suspension has decreased the postoperative swelling from 4 to 2 weeks, as well as the bruising and pain involved.

CYANOACRYLATES

HISTORY
- Originally synthesized in 1949
- Coover et al[17] reported on adhesive properties in 1959.[17]
- New forms of cyanoacrylates (N-butyl-2-cyanoacrylate and octyl-2-cyanoacrylate) demonstrate less tissue toxicity than earlier compounds.[18]
- Approved by FDA in 1998 for **topical wound closure**

MECHANISM OF ACTION[19]
- Reaction of cyanoacrylate monomer with hydroxyl groups of water creates exothermic reaction and polymerizes in 30-60 seconds, generating adhesive film.
- Commercial preparations are often paired with purple dye to assist with application (D&C Violet 2) and with a plasticizer for more flexible, less brittle product.

DELIVERY SYSTEM
- Various tip applicators are available from different manufacturers allowing exact drop application or blunt-tip application.
- New polyester mesh adhesive tape and cyanoacrylate adhesive combinations have been designed to perform tissue approximation for larger surgical incisions (Prineo, Ethicon).[20,21]

COMPLICATIONS

- **Not for internal use:** Cyanoacrylates have been associated with foreign body reactions and carcinogenicity and tissue necrosis.[22]
- Wound dehiscence is more common in areas of skin tension.
- Wound healing is impeded if polymerization occurs between wound edges.
- Contact with eyes may cause corneal abrasion; use of petroleum-based antibiotic ointment assists with removal of cyanoacrylate glue.

APPLICATIONS

- Cyanoacrylates should be applied on clean, well-approximated, and tension-free wounds.
- Prospective randomized trials of cyanoacrylates in plastic surgery procedures have shown equivalent rates of wound infections, wound dehiscence, and cosmesis as conventional closure methods, but with the added benefit of decreased operating time, eliminating need for suture removal or secondary dressings.[23,24,25,26]
- Study of 133 patients undergoing breast surgery were randomly placed into two groups, monofilament skin closure and cyanoacrylate only skin closure, with 1 year follow-up.
  • No difference in cosmetic score or complications.
  • Patient satisfaction significantly higher when closed with cyanoacrylate versus standard suture ($p <0.0001$).
  • Application of the tissue adhesive was significantly faster than that for standard suture ($p <0.001$).
  • Total costs were less in the tissue adhesive group, mainly due to lower postoperative costs of physician and assistant services ($p <0.001$).[23]
- A retrospective review of 670 consecutive bilateral reduction mammaplasties comparing cyanoacrylate and suture closure, demonstrated decreased operative times by 25 minutes or 20% less surgical time ($p <0.05$).[24]
- Prospective, randomized, blinded study comparing cosmetic and functional outcome in blepharoplasty closure with cyanoacrylate versus conventional suturing in same patient. There was no statistical difference in wound complications, duration of healing, inflammation, time for closure or final incision appearance.[25]

> **SENIOR AUTHOR TIP:**   I have used skin glues without significant complications in all my areolar incisions, eliminating layers of closure, suture removal, and expediting recovery time.

TOP TAKEAWAYS

➤ Commercial preparations of fibrin sealants have risk of bloodborne pathogens (viral, prions).

➤ Cyanoacrylates have been associated with foreign body reactions and carcinogenicity and tissue necrosis (not for internal use).

➤ Prospective randomized trials of cyanoacrylates in plastic surgery procedures have shown equivalent rates of wound infections, wound dehiscence, and cosmesis as conventional closure methods, but with the added benefit of decreased operating time, eliminating need for suture removal or secondary dressings.

REFERENCES

1. Bergel S. Uber Wirkungen des Fibrins. Dtsch Med Wochenschr 135:663, 1909.
2. Cronkite EP, Lozner EL, Deaver JM. Use of thrombin and fibrinogen in skin grafting. JAMA 124:976, 1944.
3. Tidrick RT, Warner ED. Fibrin fixation of skin transplants. Surgery 15:90, 1944.
4. Spotnitz WD. Fibrin sealant: past, present, and future: a brief review. World J Surg 34:632, 2010.
5. Buchta C, Hedrich HC, Macher M, et al. Biochemical characterization of autologous fibrin sealants produced by CryoSeal and Vivostat in comparison to the homologous fibrin sealant product Tissucol/Tisseel. Biomaterials 26:6233, 2005.
6. Package insert. Tissel. Baxter, 2014.
7. Package insert. Artiss. Baxter, 2014.
8. Package insert. Evicel. Baxter, 2014.
9. Spotnitz WD. Fibrin sealant: the only approved hemostat, sealant, and adhesive—a laboratory and clinical perspective. ISRN Surg 2014:203943, 2014.
10. O'Grady KM, Agrawal A, Bhattacharyya TK, et al. An evaluation of fibrin tissue adhesive concentration and application thickness on skin graft survival. Laryngoscope 110:1931, 2000.
11. Hester TR Jr, Shire JR, Nguyen DB, et al. Randomized, controlled, phase 3 study to evaluate the safety and efficacy of fibrin sealant VH S/D 4 s-apr (Artiss) to improve tissue adherence in subjects undergoing rhytidectomy. Aesthet Surg J 33:487, 2013.
12. Oliver DW, Hamilton SA, Figle AA, et al. A prospective, randomized, double-blind trial of the use of fibrin sealant for face lifts. Plast Reconstr Surg 108:2101, 2001.
13. Marchac D, Greensmith AL. Early postoperative efficacy of fibrin glue in face lifts: a prospective randomized trial. Plast Reconstr Surg 115:911, 2005.
14. Bercial ME, Sabino Neto M, Calil JA, et al. Suction drains, quilting sutures, and fibrin sealant in the prevention of seroma formation in abdominoplasty: which is the best strategy? Aesthetic Plast Surg 36:370, 2012.
15. Mandel MA. Minimal suture blepharoplasty: closure of incisions with autologous fibrin glue. Aesthetic Plast Surg 16:269, 1992.
16. Jones BM, Grover R. Endoscopic brow lift: a personal review of 538 patients and comparison of fixation techniques. Plast Reconstr Surg 113:1242, 2004.
17. Coover HW Jr, Joyner FB, Shearer NH, et al. Chemistry and performance of cyanoacrylate adhesives. Soc Plast Eng J 15:413, 1959.
18. Leonard F, Kulkarni RK, Brandes G, et al. Synthesis and degradation of poly(alkyl α-cyanoacrylates). J Appl Polymer Sci 10:259, 1966.
19. Package insert. Dermabond. Ethicon, 2014.
20. Richter D, Stoff A, Ramakrishnan V, et al. A comparison of a new skin closure device and intradermal sutures in the closure of full-thickness surgical incisions. Plast Reconstr Surg 130:843, 2012.
21. Blondeel PN, Richter D, Stoff A, et al. Evaluation of a new skin closure device in surgical incisions associated with breast procedures. Ann Plast Surg 73:631, 2014.
22. Toriumi DM, Raslan WF, Friedman M, Tardy ME. Histotoxicity of cyanoacrylate tissue adhesives. A comparative study. Arch Otolaryngol Head Neck Surg 116:546, 1990.
23. Gennari R, Rotmensz N, Ballardini B, et al. A prospective, randomized, controlled clinical trial of tissue adhesive (2-octylcyanoacrylate) versus standard wound closure in breast surgery. Surgery 136:593, 2004.
24. Scott GR, Carson CL, Borah GL. Dermabond skin closures for bilateral reduction mammaplasties: a review of 255 consecutive cases. Plast Reconstr Surg 120:1460, 2007.

25. Greene D, Koch RJ, Goode, RL. Efficacy of octyl-2-cyanoacrylate tissue glue in blepharoplasty. A prospective controlled study of wound-healing characteristics. Arch Facial Plast Surg 1:292, 1999.
26. Nipshagen MD, Hage JJ, Beckman WH. Use of 2-octyl-cyanoacrylate skin adhesive (Dermabond) for wound closure following reduction mammaplasty: a prospective, randomized intervention study. Plast Reconstr Surg 122:10, 2008.

26. Fixation Devices

Brian H. Gander, Renato Saltz

BACKGROUND

- Multiple devices have been described for fixation during browlift, midface lift, and neck rejuvenation.
  - Plates and screws[1]: Screws can be removed during follow-up
  - K-wires[2]: Can be either temporary or permanent
  - Bolsters[3]
  - Fibrin glue[4]
  - Absorbable tack[5]
  - Direct needle suture fixation
- More recent methods of fixation use bioabsorbable devices that anchor soft tissues; however, permanent implantable devices are still in plastic surgeons' armamentaria.
- Barbed suture is a useful adjunct for rhytidectomy, body contouring, and breast surgery.

FIXATION FOR BROWLIFTS, MIDFACE LIFTS, AND NECKLIFTS

DIRECT NEEDLE SUTURE FIXATION

- Uses permanent or absorbable suture depending on the surgeon's preference

ENDOTINE TACK (COAPT SYSTEMS)[6,7]

- Made of 82:18 ratio of polylactic acid/polyglycolic acid
- Triangular tack 0.5 mm thick
- Five tines up to 3.5 mm thick and a bone bolt 3.75 mm thick
- To secure the tack, the Endotine drill bit is used to drill through the outer cortex of the calvarium. Octyl-2-cyanoacrylate (ISO-DENT, Ellman International) cement is used to fix device into the calvarium.
- Soft tissues are secured to the tack using digital pressure.
- Bioabsorbable
  - Degrades through hydrolysis and enzymatic activity.
  - The polyglycolic component goes through hydrolysis quicker than the polylactic acid component.
  - The tack is completely absorbed in **12 months.**
- **Advantages**
  - Speedy, direct fixation
  - Bioabsorbs in 12 months
  - Can be used in conjunction with an endoscope
  - Low learning curve
- **Disadvantages**
  - Possibility of palpability until device absorbs
  - Postoperative tenderness over the device
  - Difficult to address temporal laxity and severe brow ptosis with the Endotine device
  - Added cost to surgical procedure for the device

ULTRATINE TACK (COAPT SYSTEMS)[8-10]

- The FDA approved the device in 2006.
- Composed of polylactic acid and polyglycolic acid
  - Ratio is unknown at this time given proprietary nature.
- Undergoes hydrolysis at a **faster rate** than Endotine
  - **50%** of the device is absorbed in **4 months,** and **70%** is absorbed in **10 months.**
- Fixated to calvarium and soft tissues in same method as Endotine
- **Advantages**
  - Absorbs more rapidly than Endotine
  - In one study with 12 patients who underwent coronal browlift, with one side fixated with Endotine and the other with Ultratine, decreased palpability and increased satisfaction noted on the Ultratine fixated side.[10]
- **Disadvantages**
  - Potential loss of fixation from quickened absorption
  - Reports of inflammatory retention cysts that histologically demonstrated chronic granulomatous inflammation that has necessitated surgical correction[8]
  - Added cost to the surgical procedure for the device

ENDOTINE RIBBON (COAPT SYSTEMS)[11,12]

- Used for ptosis of cheeks, jowls, and neck
- A 16 cm long ribbon 0.5 mm thick and 5 mm wide
- Seventeen rows of double tines that are 2.5 mm tall, with holes between the tines. The proximal third of the device has no tines and is used as a "leash" and area for fixation.
- Fixated to fascia with absorbable or permanent sutures
- Same components and composition as Endotine tack
- Bioabsorbable. This device loses its mass at 3 months and is absorbed in **12 months.**
- **Advantages**
  - Useful adjunct for correction of ptosis at the cervicomental junction
  - Can address temporal laxity[12]
  - Same composition as Endotine tack and is absorbed in **12 months**
- **Disadvantages**
  - Does not address anterior cervical banding
  - Potential for palpability of the ribbon in patients with thin soft tissue
  - Possible early loss of fixation when absorbable suture is used for fixation of the device
  - Added cost to the surgical procedure for the device

MITEK ANCHOR (ETHICON)[13]

- Can be used for medial and/or lateral canthoplasty
- Allows fixation of soft tissues to bone
- Three different sizes, with **Mini-Mitek** anchor most appropriate for facial aesthetic surgery
  - The anchor portion is 1.8 mm in diameter, 5.4 mm in length. It is composed of a titanium alloy and has two barbs that are 180 degrees apart and angled retrograde for fixation against the cortical bone.
- For fixation, a hole is drilled into the desired bone, and the anchor is inserted into the drilled hole.
- Attached to the anchor is a double-armed suture of 3-0 Ethibond Excel (Ethicon) suture for fixation of soft tissues (braided polyester).

- **Advantage**
  - Ability to secure soft tissues to bone with relative ease
- **Disadvantages**
  - Potential for device to be palpable in area of thin soft tissue
  - Permanent device
  - Added cost to the surgical procedure

V-Loc Barbed Suture (Covidien)[14]

- Used in closure of skin and subcutaneous tissues in body contouring and breast surgery
- Composed of both bioabsorbable (polyglyconate) and permanent material of variable length (6, 12, 18, and 23 inches)
- It is **unidirectional barbed suture** with a cutting or tapered needle at one end and a loop at other end for fixation.
- The V-Loc suture is run in a subcutaneous or dermal plane in a **single direction.** To complete suturing, the V-Loc can be brought out through the skin at the edge of the wound, or, once the end of the wound has been reached, it can be run in the reverse direction for a number of passes and brought out through the skin.
- Absorbable sutures have variable lengths of time for absorption (Table 26-1).

Table 26-1   *V-Loc Suture Tensile Strength and Absorption Time*

Suture Material	Days Implanted	Tensile Strength (%)	Time to Absorption (days)
V-Loc 90	7	90	90-110
(polyglyconate)	14	75	90
V-Loc 180	7	80	180
(polyglyconate)	14	75	180
	21	65	180

- **Advantages**
  - Shortens operative time during the closure of wounds
  - Lessens the number of buried knots in the subcutaneous and dermal planes thus decreasing the risk of suture extrusion during wound healing
  - Evenly distributes tension along the wound
  - Potential to shorten scars through the "accordian effect" of barbed suture
  - Possible decreased surgical cost because of decreased operative time while closing and the use of fewer surgical packs
- **Disadvantage**
  - Reported risk of suture extrusion

Quill Suture (Angiotech Pharmaceuticals)[15,16]

- Also used in the closure of subcutaneous tissues in body contouring and breast surgery
- Composed of both bioabsorbable (polydioxanone or monoderm) and permanent material
- **Bidirectional barbed suture** of variable length with a tapered needle at both ends
- Suture is run in a subcutaneous plane starting in midportion of the created wound and run **in both directions.** To complete the suture, the Quill is run to the end of the desired point and either run back toward the midline of the wound or cut at the end of the desired endpoint.
- The absorbable products have variable lengths of time for absorption (Table 26-2).

Table 26-2   *Quill Suture Tensile Strength*

Suture Material	Days Implanted	Tensile Strength (%)
Polydioxanone	42	47-79
Monoderm	7	64-76
Monoderm	14	40

ADVANTAGES AND DISADVANTAGES OF VARIOUS FIXATION DEVICES (Table 26-3)

Table 26-3   *Advantages and Disadvantages of Various Fixation Devices*

Device(s)	Advantages	Disadvantages
Plates and screws	Well-established fixation device Possibility of using bioabsorbable plates and screws	Opportunity of palpation Potential risk of extrusion Requires secondary procedure for removal of nonabsorbable hardware
K-wires	A well-established means of fixation Speed of fixation Possibility for permanent or temporary placement of K-wires	Potential for extrusion May require secondary procedure for removal
Bolsters	Ease of fixation	Unsightly appearance while in place If removed prematurely, potential loss of fixation
Fibrin glue	Ease of fixation Decreased ecchymosis[17,18,19] Decreased serous drainage thereby reducing postoperative sweeping and recovery time[17,18,19]	Subjective application can lead to possible loss of fixation Low but possible risk of allergic reaction

> **TIP:** The use of fibrin glue during rhytidectomy has been associated with decreased ecchymosis postoperatively.

OUTCOMES

- Endotine and Ultratine Tack: Servat and Black (2012)[8]
  - A retrospective chart review of 138 patients comparing Endotine to Ultratine demonstrated a statistically significant higher rate of cyst formation and late loss of fixation (after 31 days postoperatively) in the Ultratine cohort.
- Endotine Ribbon: Cervelli (2009)[12]
  - A retrospective review of 30 patients undergoing browlift surgery showed symmetric lateral eyebrows and correction of temporal laxity without complication. Authors state this is an effective, safe and easy fixation method with high patient satisfaction
- Mitek Anchor: Bartsich et al (2012)[13]
  - Retrospectively assessed 12 patients who underwent revision canthoplasty following trauma or cosmetic surgery. With a mean 2-year follow-up, all patients

had proper position of the anchor and were satisfied with eyelid shape and function with no postoperative infections or implant extrusion.

- V-Loc barbed suture: Grigoryants and Baroni (2013)[20]
  - A prospective review of 30 patients followed for at least 12 months who underwent lipoabdominoplasty with one side closed in a traditional three-layer closer and the experimental side with a two-layer V-Loc closure. The experimental side was closed significantly faster than the control side and wound-healing complications were more common in the control side while both sides had similar Vancouver Scar Scale scores.
- Fibrin glue/tissue sealants: Por et al (2009)[17]
  - A meta-analysis of prospective randomized control trials where patients undergoing facelifts acted as their own control. There was no statistical significance between the two sides but there was a strong trend in reduction in posteroperative drainage 24 hours after surgery and decreased ecchymosis on the treatment side.

COMPLICATIONS

- Palpability of an implant is always possible.
- Postoperative retention cysts with bioabsorbable fixation devices which may be higher with Ultratine[8]
- Visible skin dimpling may occur with direct needle fixation.
- Suture or device extrusion can be more likely with products that have a longer duration of absorbability or that are permanent and also in patients with thin soft tissues.

> **SENIOR AUTHOR TIP:**   In my experience since 2002, Endotine is the most reliable fixation for endoscopic browlift.
>
> I have used fibrin glue in facelifts since 1991 and have shown it reduces swelling, bruising, and recovery time by decreasing the lymphatic drainage, dead space (gluing tissues to each other), and bleeding.

TOP TAKEAWAYS
- ➤ There are multiple means of fixation for browlift, midface lift, and necklifts, but not all address all areas that may need to be corrected.
- ➤ Ultratine has higher patient satisfaction and less palpability compared to Endotine but is associated with retention cysts.[8]
- ➤ Palpability is possible with all devices, especially in patients with thin soft tissue.

REFERENCES

1. Bähr W. Pretapped and self-tapping screws in the human midface: torque measurements and bone screw interface. Int J Oral Maxillofac Surg 19:51, 1990.
2. Kim SK. Endoscopic forehead-scalp flap fixation with K-wire. Aesthetic Plast Surg 20:217, 1996.
3. Smith DS. A simple method for forehead fixation following endoscopy. Plast Reconstr Surg 98:1117, 1994.
4. Marchac D, Ascherman J, Arnaud E. Fibrin glue fixation in forehead endoscopy: evaluation of our experience with 206 cases. Plast Reconstr Surg 100:704, 1996.

 5. Landecker A, Buck JB, Grotting JC. A new resorbable tack fixation technique for endoscopic brow lifts. Plast Reconstr Surg 111:380, 2002.
 6. Saltz R, Ohana B. Thirteen years of experience with the endoscopic midface lift. Aesthet Surg J 32:927, 2012.
 7. Holzapfel AM, Mangat DS. Endoscopic forehead-lift using a bioabsorbable fixation device. Arch Facial Plast Surg 6:389, 2004.
 8. Servat JJ, Black EH. A comparison of surgical outcomes with the use of 2 different biodegradable multipoint fixation devices for endoscopic forehead rejuvenation. Ophthal Plast Reconstr Surg 28:401, 2012.
 9. Savar A, Shore J. Ultratine retention: report of a case. Ophthal Plast Reconstr Surg 25:501, 2009.
10. Apfelberg DB, Newman J, Graivier M, et al. Multispecialty contralateral study of clinical experience with the Ultratine forehead fixation device: evolution of the original Endotine device. Arch Facial Plast Surg 10:280, 2008.
11. Knott PD, Newman J, Keller GS, et al. A novel bioabsorbable device for facial suspension and rejuvenation. Arch Facial Plast Surg 11:129, 2009.
12. Cervelli V. An original application of the Endotine Ribbon device for brow lift. Plast Reconstr Surg 124:1652, 2009.
13. Bartsich S, Swartz KA, Spinelli HM. Lateral canthoplasty using the Mitek Anchor system. Aesthetic Plast Surg 36:3, 2012.
14. Nguyen AT, Ritz M. Body contouring surgery with the V-loc suture. Plast Reconstr Surg 128:332, 2011.
15. Hurwitz DJ, Reuben B. Quill barbed sutures in body contouring surgery: a 6-year comparison with running absorbable braided sutures. Aesthet Surg J 33(3 Suppl):S44, 2013.
16. Moya AP. Barbed sutures in body surgery. Aesthet Surg J 33(3 Suppl):S57, 2013.
17. Por YC, Shi L, Samuel M, et al. Use of tissue sealants in face-lifts: a metaanalysis. Aesthetic Plast Surg 33:336, 2009.
18. Guyron B. An evidence-based approach to face lift. Plast Reconstr Surg 126:2230, 2010.
19. Marchac D, Greensmith AL. Early postoperative efficacy of fibrin glue in face lifts: a prospective randomized trial. Plast Reconstr Surg 115:911; discussion 917, 2005.
20. Grigoryants V, Baroni A. Effectiveness of wound closure with V-Loc 90 sutures in lipoabdominoplasty patients. Aesthet Surg J 33:97, 2013.

27. Implants and Alloplasts (Nonbreast)

Jason K. Potter, Edward O. Terino

- *Biomaterials* are naturally occurring and synthetic materials used to replace, reconstruct, or augment tissues in the human body.
- Biomaterials are frequently used in aesthetic surgery for **volume or contour augmentation.**
- Factors to consider when choosing a biomaterial are shown in Box 27-1.

Box 27-1 *IDEAL PROPERTIES FOR GENERIC BIOMATERIAL*

Chemically inert	Sterilizable
Biocompatible	Easy to handle
Nonallergenic	Radiopaque
Noncarcinogenic	Ability to stabilize
Cost-effective	

- The most important clinical aspect of an implanted material is its permanence.
  - The long-term biocompatibility of a material is a function of the dynamic relationship between the host and implant.
  - Permanence is therefore achieved with harmony between host and chemical and mechanical factors.
- Frequently, the interaction between host and implant is not ideal, and various biologic reactions may be observed (Box 27-2).

Box 27-2 *BIOLOGIC REACTION TO FOREIGN BODY*

Immediate inflammation with early rejection	Incomplete encapsulation with ongoing cellular reaction
Delayed rejection	Slow resorption
Fibrous encapsulation	Incorporation

- **Definitions**
  - **Autografts:** Living tissue derived from the host
  - **Allografts:** Nonliving tissue derived from same species donor (i.e., cadaver)
  - **Xenografts:** Nonliving tissue derived from different species donor (i.e., bovine)
  - **Alloplasts:** Synthetic material

AUTOGRAFTS

ADVANTAGE
- Benchmark because of their tolerance and biologic integration into the host

DISADVANTAGES
- Requires a second operative site, increasing patient morbidity
- Requires increased operative time to harvest
- Limited in quantity
- Plagued by variable amounts of resorption over time

BONE
General Characteristics
- All free bone grafts undergo some degree of resorption and remodeling.
- The degree to which each type of graft is affected is unclear.
- **Cortical grafts** maintain their volume significantly better than cancellous grafts regardless of embryologic origin.[1]
- **Fixation** reduces graft resorption when they are placed under mobile tissues.[2]
- Sources include calvarium, iliac crest, rib, tibia, radius, and mandible.

Advantages
- Relative resistance to infection
- Incorporation by the host into new bone
- Lack of host response against the graft

Disadvantages
- Donor site morbidity
- Variable graft resorption
- Limited ability to contour some types of bone

CARTILAGE
General Characteristics
- Infection and resorption are rare.[3]
- Histologic studies have shown the survival of chondrocytes within normal matrix and a general absence of fibrous ingrowth and resorption of the graft.[2,4-7]
- Postulated that cartilage grafts will calcify with time[8]
- Main sources: Cartilaginous nasal septum, conchal cartilage, rib
- Frequently used for soft tissue augmentation, nasal and ear reconstruction

Advantages
- Ease of harvest
- Flexibility
- Limited donor site morbidity

Disadvantages
- Donor site morbidity given the need for separate incision to obtain
- Inherent memory, and can be difficult to mold[9]
- Tendency to warp[4,10,11]

ALLOGENEIC MATERIALS

GENERAL CHARACTERISTICS

- Allogeneic materials (allografts, homografts) and xenografts **contain no living cells.**
- May possess **osteoinductive** and/or **osteoconductive** properties
- Become incorporated into host tissues by providing a **structural framework or scaffolding** for ingrowth of host tissues
- Do not require a second operative site
  - Require less operative time
  - Abundant in supply
- Both xenograft and allogeneic materials are processed by various methods to reduce antigenicity.
- **Xenografts** have more antigenic potential than **homografts.**
  - Used less frequently
- Before placement of xenografts, surgeons should inquire about previous use of xenografts in the patient, because delayed hypersensitivity reactions have been reported.[12]
- Despite meticulous and careful sterilization techniques, the risk of transmission of infectious disease is the most worrisome disadvantage of allogeneic materials.
- Variable resorption is common.

LYOPHILIZED FASCIA

- Sources
  - Lyophilized dura
  - Lyophilized tensor fascia lata
- Resorption rates reported to be up to 10% of the original graft volume.[13]
- Carries the risk of transmitting infectious disease
  - Creutzfeld-Jakob disease was reported with a case of lyophilized dura implantation.[14]

HOMOLOGOUS BONE

- Provides a scaffold for new bone formation and has the same working properties of autogenous bone
- Slower to become incorporated and revascularized than autogenous bone[15]
- Associated with few complications when used for reconstructing the maxillofacial skeleton[16]
- Supplied in many forms, including whole bone cribs

HOMOLOGOUS CARTILAGE

- Undergoes ossification and calcification with time[4,17]
- Greater tendency for homologous cartilage to undergo resorption and replacement with fibrous tissue than with autogenous cartilage[3-6]
- Preserved cartilage has significantly greater amounts of resorption and increased rates of infection.[3]

SENIOR AUTHOR TIP: Despite the report of Vuyk and Adamson,[3] in my more than 20 years of experience using irradiated homologous nasal cartilage in more than 500 rhinoplasties, little significant absorption and no infections have occurred. This work, however, was never published.

HOMOLOGOUS DERMIS (ALLODERM, LIFECELL; FLEXHD, ETHICON)[18,19]
- Cadaveric human dermis processed to remove all cellular elements, leaving only the extracellular matrix scaffolding.
- Host response minimal, because no antigenic cells remain
- Incorporates into the host tissue
- Resorption varies.
- Applications include fascial replacement, soft tissue volume augmentation, and breast implant coverage.

BILAMINATE NEODERMAL MATRIX (INTEGRA, INTEGRA LIFESCIENCES)
General Characteristics
- Bilayered dermal regenerate template used for skin replacement
  - The top layer is **silicone.**
    - ► Provides temporary epidermal coverage
    - ► Controls fluid loss
    - ► Imparts strength and mechanical protection to the matrix
  - The bottom layer is a collagen/glycosaminoglycan matrix.
    - ► Promotes cellular ingrowth to create a dermal regenerate
    - ► Silicone layer is removed after approximately 21 days, and the dermal regenerate is covered with a thin, split-thickness skin graft.

Advantages
- The greatest advantage is **creation of a new dermis** that allows reconstruction of pliable skin.
- Reconstruction of large defects
- Can place over exposed tendon without paratenon, exposed cartilage without perichondrium, exposed bone without periosteum
- Can be particularly effective when soft tissue coverage is needed with limited donor sites (exposed tendon or bone).[20]

Disadvantages
- Very expensive
- Limited application in aesthetic surgery
- Easily infected

ALLOPLASTIC MATERIALS
ADVANTAGES
- Off-the-shelf availability
- Lack of donor site morbidity
- All elicit some degree of host reaction to the material, because they are seen as foreign bodies.
- Cost

NONRESORBABLE ALLOPLASTS
Metals
- **General characteristics**
  - Types
    - ► Stainless steel
    - ► Vitallium alloy

- ▶ Titanium alloys
  - ▶ Titanium alloys have become the most commonly used material
- **Advantages**
  - Titanium is approximately 10 times stronger than bone.
  - Easy to bend
  - Extremely well tolerated by the host.
- **Disadvantages**
  - Titanium has a low fatigue tolerance.
  - Failure may develop from cyclic loading of the implant.
  - Available in plates, screws, mesh, and custom implants

High-Density Porous Polyethylene (HDPE) (Medpor, Stryker)

- Pure polyethylene implant
- Processed specifically to include and control pore size
  - Pore size is engineered to range in size: 100-200 μm, >50% are larger than 150 μm.[21]
  - Pore size directly influences the rate and amount of bony and fibrovascular ingrowth into the implant.[18]
- Available in many different shapes
- Should be soaked in an **antibiotic solution** before placement
- Easily and reliably stabilized with screws[22]
- **Advantages**
  - Highly biocompatible
  - Insoluble in tissue fluids
  - Does not resorb or degenerate
  - Incites minimal surrounding soft tissue reaction
  - High tensile strength
  - Excellent tissue ingrowth[23]
  - Versatile, with complication rate <10% in craniofacial reconstruction[24]
- **Disadvantages**
  - Is not radiodense so its position cannot be easily visualized on immediate postoperative CT scans
  - Cost

Hydroxyapatite

- **General characteristics**
  - $[Ca_{10}(PO4)_6(OH)_2]$: Calcium phosphate salt that is a major constituent of bone
  - Several forms are available for reconstruction of the facial skeleton.
    - ▶ **Dense hydroxyapatite (HA):** Produced synthetically through high-pressure compaction of calcium phosphate crystals, which are then sintered (fused) into a solid form.
    - ▶ **Porous HA** can be produced synthetically or naturally. Various pore sizes may be engineered into the synthetically produced material.
    - ▶ A **"natural" HA** can be produced by heating marine coral at elevated pressures in the presence of aqueous phosphate solutions. This causes a chemical substitution of calcium phosphate for calcium carbonate in the preexisting porous skeleton of the coral.
- **Advantages**
  - Highly biocompatible
  - Minimal inflammatory reaction in the surrounding tissues
  - Produces a strong mechanical bond with host bone

- Allows ingrowth of host tissue, providing a scaffold for bone repair
- Demonstrates limited resorption[25]
- Off the shelf
- HA (all types) has a favorable infection rate of 2.7% for craniofacial reconstruction.[20]

▪ **Disadvantages**
- Brittle
- Difficult to shape/carve intraoperatively
- Very difficult to remove totally from soft tissues or bone when removal in aesthetic procedures is necessary or desired
  - ▶ Can possibly endanger the mental nerve or infraorbital nerve resulting in excessive or additional bleeding, and/or seromas, hematomas, and undesirable scar tissue

Silicone
▪ **General characteristics**
- *Silicone* refers to a group of polymers based on the element *silicon*.
- Sand (silicon dioxide [SiO_2]) is one of the most abundant compounds on earth.
- The polymer used medically is polydimethylsiloxane (PDMS).
- *Medical-grade* refers to material that is pure and consistent in composition.
- Classified as a medical device, meaning silicone does not achieve its primary intended purpose by chemical action or through its metabolism
- FDA approved the use of silicone breast implants in 2006, citing no health risks directly linked to the implants.[26]

▪ **Advantages**
- Thermal and oxidative stability
- Chemical and biological inertness
- Hydrophobic nature
- Sterilization capability
- Implant infections with smooth silicone rubber when placed in faces on bone can often be eliminated without removal.

SENIOR AUTHOR TIP: The trick is to start antibiotic therapy immediately when any swelling or color change (usually pinkish and blanching on pressure) occurs, sometimes with mild discomfort. If resolution does not begin within 48 hours, IV antibiotic is started and continued for at least 10 days. Needle aspiration of possible fluids in the implant pocket, or even the surrounding soft tissues, should be obtained and sent for cultures before antibiotics have been started.

- When indicated and necessary, small drains (suction if possible) are used percutaneously rather than intraorally.
- Implants can be made in various sizes, shapes, and consistencies such as for facial implants.[27]

SENIOR AUTHOR TIP: Encapsulation is an advantage, because it rapidly secures the silicone implant firmly onto the bone, causing permanent immobility but facilitating easy removal or exchangeability when medically necessary or desired.

- Experience using facial implants helps surgeons learn subtle variables of facial contours with individual faces, which they can apply to modifying silicone rubber implants quite easily during surgery and outside the patient. Because of its extreme flexibility in and out, trial introduction into the dissected pocket can be done with ease.
- **Disadvantages**
  - Becomes encapsulated not incorporated
  - Unsubstantiated concerns for silicone-linked illnesses
  - Very difficult to remove totally from soft tissues or bone when removal in aesthetic procedures is necessary or desired
    - ▶ May possibly endanger the mental or infraorbital nerve, resulting in excessive or additional bleeding, and/or seromas, hematomas, and undesirable scar tissue

Expanded Polytetrafluoroethylene (ePTFE) (Gore-Tex, SoftForm and UltraSoft [Tissue Technologies, Inc.], and Advanta [Atrium Medical Corp.])

- **Advantages**
  - Available in sheets, tube form, or strands
  - Nonresorbable
  - Porosities allow some degree of tissue ingrowth.
  - Various applications include soft tissue augmentation and fascial replacement.
- **Disadvantages**
  - Soft tissue augmentation: Palpability, extrusion, altered lip movement
  - Fascial replacement: Modest tissue ingrowth results in weak adherence between ePTFE and abdominal wall.

> **SENIOR AUTHOR TIP:**   The use of ePTFE has a moderate incidence of infections in the lips and malar region.

RESORBABLE ALLOPLASTS
Polylactide (PLLA) Derivatives

- **Advantages**
  - Advocates think these systems perform comparably to metal fixation systems.
  - Complete resorption, preventing growth interference or late complication
  - No long-term or lifelong risk of complications characteristic of nonresorbable alloplasts
- **Disadvantages**
  - Less precise conformation to osseous structures versus metal alloys
  - Instrumentation: Requires tapping screw hole
  - Lactosorb (Zimmer Biomet) is a biodegradable copolymer of polylactic and polyglycolic acids that has been in use clinically for >10 years.
  - Studies have demonstrated that this copolymer formulation has a more rapid rate of degradation (9-15 months) compared with PLLA and therefore might be better suited for use as an orbital implant.[21]
  - Clinical studies have demonstrated good results with Lactosorb throughout the craniofacial skeleton.[28-31]

Polyglactin 910
- Most commonly known as the suture material *Vicryl,* a resorbable, synthetic material composed of lactide and glycolide acids
- Both film and mesh forms are available.

Polydioxanone
- Resorbable aliphatic polyester polymer
- Undergoes hydrolysis in 10-12 weeks
- Can fragment leading to significant soft tissue fibrous reaction
- Because of this, it is not approved for orbital reconstruction in the United States.[9]

Gelatin Film
- **General characteristics**
  - Bioabsorbable sheeting material manufactured from denatured collagen
  - Clear, nonporous, 0.075 mm thick, brittle when dry but pliable when wet
  - Suggested for the repair of small orbital floor defects (<5 mm) or as an interpositional material between the periorbital tissues and reconstructive plates or mesh[24]
- **Advantage**
  - Reportedly entirely absorbed within 2-3 months[24]
- **Disadvantages**
  - Brittle
  - Poor mechanical properties to reconstruct true orbital defects

---

TOP TAKEAWAYS
➤ *Biomaterials* are naturally occurring and synthetic materials used to replace, reconstruct, or augment tissues in the human body.
➤ All free bone grafts undergo some degree of resorption and remodeling.
➤ Despite meticulous and careful sterilization techniques, the risk of transmission of infectious disease is the most worrisome disadvantage of allogeneic materials.
➤ Implant infections with smooth silicone rubber when placed in faces on bone can often be eliminated without removal.

REFERENCES
1. Ozaki W, Buchman SR. Volume maintenance of onlay grafts in the craniofacial skeleton: microarchitecture versus embryologic origin. Plast Reconstr Surg 102:291, 1998.
2. Lin KY, Bartlett SP, Yaremchuck MJ, et al. The effect of rigid fixation on the survival of onlay bone grafts: an experimental study. Plast Reconstr Surg 86:449, 1990.
3. Vuyk HD, Adamson PA. Biomaterials in rhinoplasty. Clin Otolaryngol 23:209, 1998.
4. Peer LA. Diced cartilage grafts. Arch Otolaryngol 38:156, 1943.
5. Peer LA. Cartilage grafting. Br J Plast Surg 7:250, 1954.
6. Ballantyne DL, Rees TD, Seidman I. Silicone fluid: response to massive subcutaneous injections of dimethylpolysiloxane fluid in animals. Plast Reconstr Surg 36:330, 1965.
7. Werther JR. Not seeing eye to eye about septal grafts for orbital fractures. J Oral Maxillofac Surg 56:906, 1998.

8. Converse JM, Smith B. Reconstruction of the floor of the orbit by bone grafts. Arch Ophthalmol 44:1, 1950.

9. Potter JK, Malmquist M, Ellis E III. Biomaterials for reconstruction of the internal orbit. Oral Maxillofac Surg Clin North Am 24:609, 2012.

10. Antonyshyn O, Gruss JS, Galbraith DJ, et al. Complex orbital fractures: a critical analysis of immediate bone graft reconstruction. Ann Plast Surg 22:220, 1989.

11. Waite PD, Clantons JT. Orbital floor reconstruction with lyophilized dura. J Oral Maxillofac Surg 46:727, 1988.

12. Celikov B, Duman H, Selmanpakoglu N. Reconstruction of the orbital floor with lyophilized tensor fascia lata. J Oral Maxillofac Surg 55:240, 1998.

13. Prichard J, Thadani V, Kalb R, et al. Rapidly progressive dementia in a patient who received a cadaveric dura mater graft. JAMA 257:1036, 1987.

14. Ellis E. Biology of bone grafting: an overview. Sel Read Oral Maxillofac Surg 2:1, 1991.

15. Ellis E III, Sinn DP. Use of homologous bone in maxillofacial surgery. J Oral Maxillofac Surg 51:1181, 1993.

16. Chen JM, Zingg M, Laedrach K, et al. Early surgical intervention for orbital floor fractures. A clinical evaluation of lyophilized dura and cartilage reconstruction. J Oral Maxillofac Surg 50:935, 1992.

17. Romano JJ, Iliff NT, Manson PN. Use of medpore porous polyethylene implants in 140 patients with facial fractures. J Craniofac Surg 4:142, 1993.

18. Liu DZ, Mathes DW, Neligan PC, et al. Comparison of outcomes using AlloDerm versus FlexHD for implant-based breast reconstruction. Ann Plast Surg 72:503, 2014.

19. Ho G, Nguyen DJ, Shahabi A, et al. A systematic review and meta-analysis of complications associated with acellular dermal matrix-assisted breast reconstruction. Ann Plast Surg 68:346, 2012.

20. Yeong EK, Chen SH, Tang YB. The treatment of bone exposure in burns by using artificial dermis. Ann Plast Surg 69:607, 2012.

21. Haug RH, Kimberly D, Bradick JP. A comparison of microscrew and suture fixation of porous high density polyethylene orbital floor implants. J Oral Maxillofac Surg 51:1217, 1993.

22. Holmes R, Hagler H. Porous hydroxyapatite as a bone graft substitute on cranial reconstruction: a histometric study. Plast Reconstr Surg 81:662, 1988.

23. Rai A, Datarkar A, Arora A, et al. Utility of high density porous polyethylene implants in maxillofacial surgery. J Maxillofac Oral Surg 13:42, 2014.

24. Ridwan-Pramana A, Wolff J, Raziei A, et al. Porous polyethylene implants in facial reconstruction: outcome and complications. J Craniomaxillofac Surg 43:1330, 2015.

25. Rubin PJ, Yaremchuck MJ. Complications and toxicities of implantable biomaterials used in facial reconstructive and aesthetic surgery: a comprehensive review of the literature. Plast Reconstr Surg 100:1336, 1997.

26. Rohrich RJ. Silicone breast implants: outcomes and safety update. Plast Reconstr Surg 120:S1, 2007.

27. Terino EO, Flowers RS, eds. The Art of Alloplastic Facial Contouring. St Louis: Mosby–Year Book, 2000.

28. Enislidis G, Pichornes S, Kainberger F, et al. Lactosorb panel and screws for repair of large orbital floor defects. J Craniomaxillofac Surg 25:316, 1997.

29. Ahu DK, Sims CD, Randolph MA, et al. Craniofacial skeletal fixation using biodegradable plates and cyanoacrylate glue. Plast Reconstr Surg 99:1508, 1997.

30. Epply BL, Sadove AM, Havlik RJ. Resorbable plate fixation in pediatric craniofacial surgery. Plast Reconstr Surg 100:1, 1997.

31. Mermer RW, Orban RE. Repair of orbital floor fractures with absorbable gelatin film. J Craniomaxillofac Trauma 1:30, 1995.

28. Progressive Tension Sutures

Terri A. Zomerlei, Todd A. Pollock, Harlan Pollock

DEFINITION: PROGRESSIVE TENSION SUTURES

- Progressive tension sutures (PTSs) securely anchor flaps over multiple points of fixation in an advanced position.

MECHANISM OF ACTION[1,2]

- **Reduces or eliminates dead space**
  - Compartmentalize space to smaller-volume areas more easily absorbed
  - Eliminate the need for postoperative drains
- **Prevents repeated disruption of weak, early healing from body motion**
  - Tissues covered by overlying flaps in a highly mobile part of the body (e.g., abdomen, latissimus donor site) may shift with repeated movement.
  - Repeated disruption of early healing leads to inflammation.
  - Andrades and Prado's analysis of seroma fluid[2] showed inflammatory exudate consistent with this mechanism.
- **Minimizes tension on the flap closure**
  - Splinting healing wounds improves scar quality.
  - Reduces scar migration from flap tension
  - Distributes tension over multiple points of fixation, improving circulation to the distal flap and preventing complications such as necrosis/dehiscence
  - Secures a skin element in a new position (e.g., secures the brow in a browlift)

INDICATIONS AND CONTRAINDICATIONS

> **SENIOR AUTHOR TIP:** PTSs are based on a simple surgical concept that can be applied to any procedure involving an advancement flap. Therefore they have no *specific* indications or contraindications.

INDICATIONS

- **Abdominoplasty:** Large area of dead space and skin excised and advanced in a highly mobile region of the body. PTS advancement and fixation:
  - Eliminates disruptive shearing forces on the healing flap
  - Reduces dead space
  - Actively advances the flap

- Internally splints the healing skin flap and distal incision
- Allows in-continuity umbilical inset: Sutures placed from deep surface of flap, facilitating a natural, inverted umbilicus
- **Facelift**[3]
  - Reduces dead space
  - Allows a controlled redraping of the skin after subcutaneous dissection
- **Subcutaneous browlift**[4]
  - Provides an accurate and secure positioning and shaping of the brows
  - Advances the flap
  - Reduces dead space
  - Allows skin closure under minimal tension
  - Eliminates the need for drains or lifting devices
- **Reconstructive advancement flaps**[5]
  - Reduces dead space
  - Actively and securely advances the flap
  - Prevents shearing forces on the healing flap

CONTRAINDICATIONS

- Progressive tension suturing is an adjunctive technique that can be applied to most conventional skin flap procedures. No unique contraindications are related to the addition of fixation sutures.

PREOPERATIVE EVALUATION

- PTSs require no unique steps in preoperative evaluation or preparation.

INFORMED CONSENT[1,6,7]

TIP: The addition of PTSs has been shown to reduce complications without adding significant risk; informed consent discussions should include the relative safety, effectiveness, and ease of recovery, compared with those of standard procedures.

- In addition to the overall risks of surgery, plastic surgeons should discuss:
  - Seroma: Use of PTSs significantly reduces the risk but does not eliminate it.
  - Skin dimpling
    - ▶ Although this is a frequent concern, dimpling is uncommon and almost always temporary.
    - ▶ Some applications are more predisposed to dimpling. In browlifts and facelifts, PTSs are applied directly to the skin, increasing the possibility of dimpling, although it is typically temporary. In abdominoplasty, proper PTS placement between superficial fascia and deep fascia makes permanent dimpling highly unlikely.

SENIOR AUTHOR TIP: If PTSs are properly placed, all tension is on the fascia—not on the skin—and permanent dimples are unlikely.

■ Revisions: No greater than with traditional techniques

> **TIP:**   The internal splinting effect of PTSs allows early ambulation in an upright posture without restrictions. The obvious benefit is patient comfort, but by eliminating a flexed posture, venous circulation is improved and VTE reduced.[7]

EQUIPMENT
■ Absorbable suture
  • **Interrupted:** Polyglactin suture: #0 or #00 sutures for PTSs
  • **Continuous:** Barbed polydioxanone suture
    ▸ Quill (Angiotech Pharmaceuticals) is a bidirectional barbed suture secured and started in the middle of the incision area.
    ▸ V-Loc (Medtronic) is a unidirectional barbed suture.

> **SENIOR AUTHOR TIP:**   Surgeons choose the type or size of suture material and the exact placement or number of sutures to obtain a secure fixation of the skin flap in an advanced position.

TECHNIQUE[7,8]

TECHNIQUE FOR PROGRESSIVE TENSION SUTURES
■ **Interrupted sutures** (Fig. 28-1)

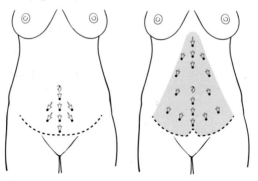

Fig. 28-1   Progressive tension sutures.

  • Incision for an abdominoplasty depends on the surgeon's preference. (See Chapter 57 for detailed variations.)

- Undermining is performed at the level of the deep fascia, wide enough to allow adequate flap advancement.
  - ► The lower abdominal dissection is full width of the abdomen, whereas the epigastric dissection is more limited. The width of dissection should be wide enough to repair the diastasis rectus without causing fullness.
  - ► Midline rectus plication is performed with #0 suture in the standard fashion.
  - ► Patient is placed in moderate flexion.
  - ► The surgeon controls the flap with the nondominant hand while placing the PTS through the superficial fascia, maximally advances the flap to determine the location of the level of the fixation to the deep fascia, and places the suture (Fig. 28-2).
  - ► The surgeon ties the suture while an assistant flap holds the flap in the advanced position. Once the suture is tied, minimal dimpling will be noticeable on the skin surface because of the tension of the advancement in that location.
    - ◆ Excessive or obvious dimpling once the next suture is tied may result from:
      - – Too superficial suture placement
      - – Excessive advancement of the flap
      - – Placement of the sutures in the wrong direction

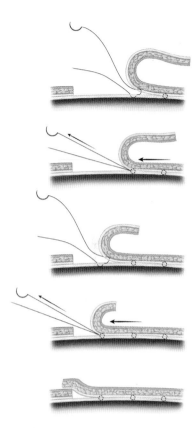

Fig. 28-2   Progressive tension suture.

SENIOR AUTHOR TIP: Placement of the midline PTS results in a midline depression that mimics a natural aesthetic contour.

  - ► This technique is repeated in the upper midline to the level of the umbilicus. The umbilicus is inset in continuity by placing sutures from the deep surface of umbilical stalk to the deep fascia (Fig. 28-3).

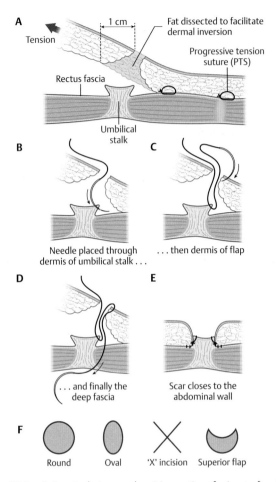

Fig. 28-3 Suture technique and excision options for inset of umbilicus.

▶ Several additional PTSs are placed in the lower midline and laterally as required to accomplish the fixation and advancement of the flap.
▶ The excess skin is removed, and three point sutures are placed to approximate superficial fascia anchored to the deep fascia.
▶ Skin is closed with buried interrupted dermal and continuous subcuticular sutures.

- **Continuous sutures**[4,9,10]
  - A smooth, running absorbable suture or a barbed suture may be used.
    - ▶ An assistant or the surgeon maintains tension and flap position while the sutures are placed and secured (Fig. 28-4).

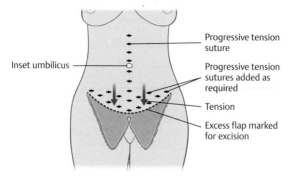

Fig. 28-4   Progressive tension sutures.

- ▶ The sutures are spaced at approximately 1-2 cm intervals in both the vertical and horizontal plane (Fig. 28-5).
- ▶ Several patterns for placement of continuous PTSs have been described that anchor the flap in an advanced position. It is based on surgeon's preference.
- ▶ Barbed PTSs maintain the tension of the advancement once suture is placed and engaged. Smooth sutures are also effective and less expensive.

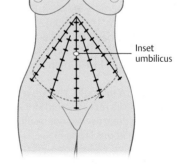

Fig. 28-5   Continuous sutures.

TIP: A midline mark on the underside of an abdominal flap will ensure that the surgeon does not skew the flap to one side when placing PTSs.

POSTOPERATIVE CARE[7,8]

- Dressing is changed in 24 hours if patient is hospitalized overnight.
- A semi-Fowler position in bed is most comfortable, but patient comfort determines exact bed elevation.

- Once patient is adequately awake, ambulation in a comfortable upright position with assistance is encouraged. Most patients are able to comfortably stand erect immediately, but patient determines a comfortable position.
- Compression garments are used for patient comfort. Patient and caregivers, including nursing staff, should understand the reason for the garment and be instructed to loosen, reposition, or remove it as necessary.
  - Abdominal binder
  - Postsurgical shapewear and girdles

> **SENIOR AUTHOR TIP:** The patient's position in bed, standing posture, and pressure garments are guided by patient comfort.

- Sutures are removed at approximately 1 week, and patients are instructed to gradually resume normal activities, avoiding strenuous activity for approximately 6 weeks. Comfort should be the guide.

OUTCOMES

SEROMA
Several longitudinal studies have demonstrated that seroma formation is reduced with the use of PTSs.

Antonetti and Antonetti (2010)[6]
- Retrospective review of 517 consecutive abdominoplasties with patients being allocated to one of five groups based on postoperative care and use of drain and PTSs. PTSs placed according to Pollock and Pollock description[1]
  - Group A were inpatients (surgery performed between 1981-1990), Group B were kept overnight (surgery between 1991-1994), and Group C were patients who had outpatient surgery (1995-2005).
  - Group D patients had PTSs and drains (2006-2007) and Group E included patients with PTSs and no drains (2006-2008).
  - Seroma rates were 9.6% (Group A), 24% (Group B and C), 4.5% (Group D), and 1.7% (Group E).
  - Earlier groups (A through C) underwent extensive undermining which may account for some of the increased seroma incidence.
  - Discontinuing drain use did not result in an increased rate of seroma when PTSs were utilized (Groups D and E).

Pollock and Pollock (2012)[7]
- Retrospective chart review of 597 consecutive abdominoplasties with PTSs and no drains
- One patient developed a seroma that was treated with aspirations.

Macias et al (2016)[11]
- Retrospective review of 453 abdominoplasties over 7 years with 324 traditional with use of drains and 127 with no drains and PTSs
  - Seroma rate with traditional abdominoplasty was 9%.
  - Seroma rate with PTSs only was 2%.

Isaac et al (2017)[12]

- 502 patients underwent a drainless abdominoplasty with use of barbed PTSs
- 4% of patients developed a seroma. All were treated successfully with percutaneous aspiration.
- While growing evidence indicates that the rate of seroma is much less in those with PTSs, there is no well-powered level I evidence to support this claim.

GENERAL COMPLICATIONS

- Forgoing drains with the use of PTSs in abdominoplasties is safe and reliable with no statistically significant increased incidence of complications[6,11,12]
  - Antonetti and Antonetti[6]: Hematoma rate 1.7% in Group D (PTSs + drains) and E (PTSs alone)
  - Pollock and Pollock[8]: One patient with a hematoma and local wound complications of 4.2%
  - Macias et al[11]: Hematoma in no patients in the PTS group and in three patients (1%) of those with traditional abdominoplasty. Wound-healing complications were 12% in the drain group and 15% in the PTS group.
  - Isaac et al[12]: Hematoma in one patient (0.2%) and infection in four patients (0.8%)
- Any skin dimpling is temporary and resolves with time
- Anecdotally, high levels of patient satisfaction are noted when drains are not used with abdominoplasties. Patients may find drain care daunting and cumbersome[6,11]

TOP TAKEAWAYS

➤ For trained surgeons, no special skills are required to perform this simple technique, and the learning curve is short.

➤ PTSs are a simple concept and technique—fixation and advancement sutures—that can be incorporated into multiple procedures that involve a basic advancement flap.

➤ The primary challenges for surgeon are to control the flap while placing the suture and to secure the suture in coordination with an assistant.

➤ Once surgeon-assistant coordination is achieved, placement of the sutures takes 20-30 minutes, including the in-continuity inset of the umbilicus.

➤ Compared with the time, patient anxiety, expense, and inconvenience of managing a complication, the surgical time added is insignificant.

➤ When PTSs are used, there is virtually no restriction on extent or location of liposuction if it is limited to the deep fat (beneath the Scarpa fascia).

➤ If a PTS is properly placed, dimpling is noted once tension is released from the flap, but it resolves after placement of the next PTS. If the depression persists, the suture may be too superficial or misdirected and can be removed and replaced. A slight, temporary depression or dimple may appear early postoperatively because of tissue edema.

➤ Overwhelming data prove that drains are unnecessary and that patients are delighted to avoid them; however, the use of drains is the surgeon's prerogative.

REFERENCES

1. Pollock H, Pollock T. Progressive tensions sutures: a technique to reduce local complications in abdominoplasty. Plast Reconstr Surg 105:2583, 2000.
2. Andrades P, Prado A. Composition of postabdominoplasty seromas. Aesthetic Plast Surg 31:514, 2007.
3. Pollock H, Pollock T. Management of face lifts with progressive tension sutures. Aesthet Surg J 23:28, 2003.
4. Pollock H, Pollock T. Subcutaneous brow lift with progresssive tension suture fixation and advancement. Aesthet Surg J 27:388, 2007.
5. Rios JL, Pollock T, Adams WP. Progressive tension sutures to prevent seroma formation after latissimus dorsi harvest. Plast Reconstr Surg 112:1779, 2003.
6. Antonetti JW, Antonetti AR. Reducing seroma in outpatient abdominoplasty: analysis of 516 consecutive cases. Aesthet Surg J 30:418, 2010.
7. Pollock H , Pollock T. Progressive tension sutures in abdominoplasty: a review of 597 consecutive cases. Aesthet Surg J 32:729, 2012.
8. Pollock H, Pollock T. No-drain abdominoplasty with progressive tension sutures. Clin Plast Surg 37:515, 2010.
9. Gutowski KA, Warner JP. Incorporating barbed sutures in abdominoplasty. Aesthet Surg J 33(3 Suppl):S76, 2013.
10. Warner jP, Gutowski KA. Abdominoplasty with progressive tension closure using a barbed suture technique. Aesthet Surg J 29:221, 2009.
11. Macias LH, Kwon E, Gould DJ, et al. Decrease in seroma rate after adopting progressive tension sutures without drains: a single surgery center experience of 451 abdominoplasties over 7 years. Aesthet Surg J 36:1029, 2016.
12. Isaac KV, Lista F, McIsaac MP, et al. Drainless abdominoplasty using barbed progressive tension sutures. Aesthet Surg J 37:428, 2017.

PART VII

Facial Surgery

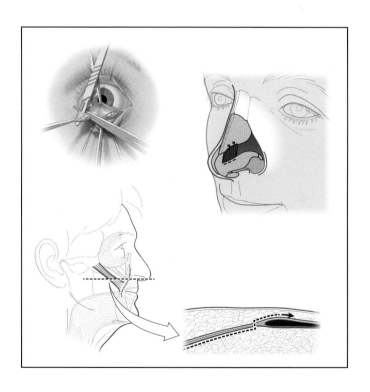

Facial Surgery

29. Periorbital Anatomy

Jason K. Potter, Grant Gilliland

SKELETAL AND SURFACE ANATOMY[1]

KEY SKELETAL LANDMARKS OF THE PERIORBITAL REGION (Fig. 29-1)

- **Superior orbital rim:** Fixed landmark to assess brow position
- **Inferior orbital rim:** Position relative to anterior surface of globe; important in determining positive versus negative vector of orbit
- **Temporal ridge:** Delineates lateral border of forehead from temporal fossa
- **Supraorbital notch:** Delineates location of supraorbital neurovascular bundle

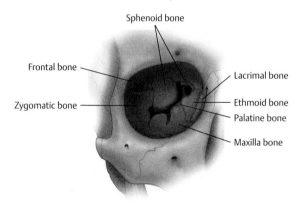

Sphenoid bone

Frontal bone

Zygomatic bone

Lacrimal bone

Ethmoid bone

Palatine bone

Maxilla bone

Fig. 29-1   Bony anatomy of the orbit.

EYEBROW SURFACE ANATOMY

UPPER FOREHEAD ARRANGED IN WELL-DEFINED LAYERS

- Skin
- Subcutaneous tissue
- Galea aponeurosis
- Loose areolar tissue
- Periosteum
  - At origin of frontalis muscle, the **galea** splits into a **superficial** and **deep** layer to encase the muscle.
  - The deep layer splits again at the midforehead level to surround the galeal fat pad, and again caudal to the fat pad to form the **glide plane space** of the brow.
  - The subgaleal space, deep layer of the galea, and periosteum fuse in the lower forehead and are firmly attached to the frontal bone.

- Movement of the brow is produced through the action of brow elevators and depressors and is enhanced by the presence of the galeal fat pad, glide plane space, and subgaleal space.
- The periosteum of the frontal bones is reflected at the arcus marginalis to become the periorbita of the periorbital bones. The arcus marginalis is a thick condensation of periorbita as it enters the orbit.

EYELID SURFACE ANATOMY[1,2] (Fig. 29-2)

- Protects the eye from injury and excessive light and prevents desiccation of the cornea.
- Provides nutrients to the avascular cornea, distributes oil throughout the tear film, debrides the ocular surface of foreign matter, and secretes antiinflammatory substances onto the cornea
- Promotes drainage from the lacrimal system
- Consists of **two lamellae:**
  1. Skin/orbicularis oculi
  2. Tarsoconjunctival layer

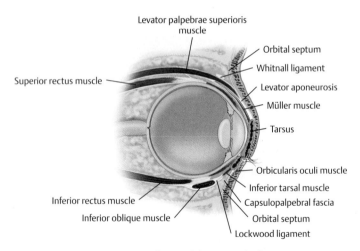

Fig. 29-2 Sagittal view of the periocular layers.

- Palpebral fissure: Aperture between upper and lower eyelids (Fig. 29-3)
  - 8-12 mm vertically, 28-30 mm horizontally
- Upper lid margin rests 0.5-1.0 mm below the upper limbus.
- Lower lid margin lies at the level of the lower limbus.

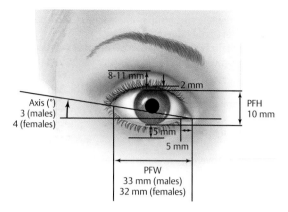

Fig. 29-3 Typical topographical measurements of the periorbita. (*PFH*, Palpebral fissure height; *PFW*, palpebral fissure width.)

SKIN
■ Eyelid skin is the **thinnest on the body.**
  • Minimal subcutaneous fat
■ Adjacent brow and malar skin are notably thicker.
■ Surgical incisions within the skin of the eyelid generally heal with almost imperceptible scarring.
■ Age-related changes in the skin include decreased type I collagen and increased dermal collagenase activity.

MUSCLES
■ **Frontalis**
  • Originates from the galea aponeurosis and inserts into the dermis of the lower forehead
  • Interdigitates with procerus and orbicularis at its insertion
  • **Elevates brow,** produces transverse forehead rhytids
■ **Corrugator supercilii** (Fig. 29-4)
  • Corrugators start 3 mm lateral to midline and end about 85% of distance to lateral orbital rim.[3]
  • **Oblique head:** Originates from the supero-medial orbit and inserts into the dermis of the medial brow

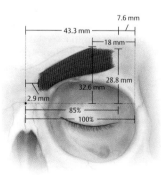

Fig. 29-4 Comprehensive corruga-tor supercilii muscle dimensions.

- **Transverse head:** Originates from superomedial orbit and inserts into dermis superior to the medial third of the medial brow
  - **Depresses and medializes the medial brow,** produces vertical glabellar rhytids
  - Lies deep to frontalis muscle
- **Depressor supercilii**
  - Originates from superomedial orbit and inserts into the dermis of the medial brow, medial to the insertion of the orbicularis
  - Lies superficial to the corrugator
  - **Depresses the medial brow**
- **Procerus muscle**
  - Originates from fascia covering lower part of nasal bone
  - Inserts onto glabellar dermis
  - **Depresses the glabella**
- **Orbicularis oculi** (Fig. 29-5)
  - Encircles the periorbital region
  - Primary **constrictor of the lids**
  - Innervated by the facial nerve (CN VII)
    - ▶ Runs on the deep surface of the muscle
  - *Pretarsal fibers* lie over the region of the tarsal plate.
    - ▶ Responsible for involuntary blink
  - *Preseptal fibers* overlie the orbital septum.
    - ▶ Assist with blink
      - ◆ Both voluntary and involuntary fibers
  - *Orbital fibers* overlie the orbital rims.
    - ▶ Produce voluntary, forceful closure

NOTE: Age-related changes in the orbicularis oculi are secondary to muscle relaxation and increasing ptosis.

NOTE: Changes result in visibility of the inferior muscle border with formation of a malar crescent[4]

- **Muscle of Riolan:** Portion of the pretarsal orbicularis comprising the "gray line" in the eyelid margin. Promotes secretion from the meibomian glands.
- **Horner tensor tarsi muscle:** Portion of the pretarsal orbicularis attaching to the posterior lacrimal crest. Encircles the canaliculi and promotes lacrimal drainage.
- **Jones muscle:** Posterior preseptal orbicularis muscle fibers that insert on the posterior lacrimal crest and promote tear drainage.

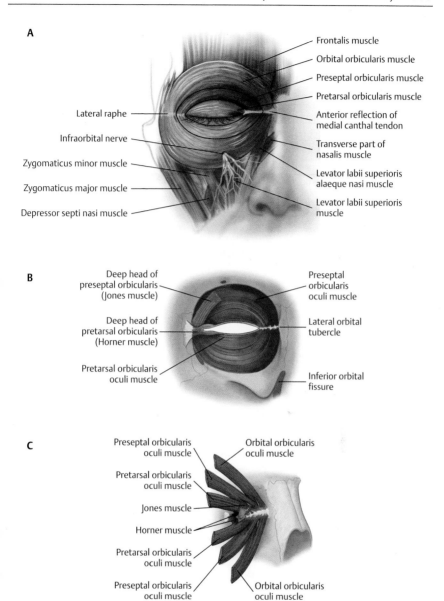

A,

Frontalis muscle

Orbital orbicularis muscle

Preseptal orbicularis muscle

Pretarsal orbicularis muscle

Anterior reflection of medial canthal tendon

Transverse part of nasalis muscle

Levator labii superioris alaeque nasi muscle

Levator labii superioris muscle

Lateral raphe

Infraorbital nerve

Zygomaticus minor muscle

Zygomaticus major muscle

Depressor septi nasi muscle

B,

Deep head of preseptal orbicularis (Jones muscle)

Deep head of pretarsal orbicularis (Horner muscle)

Pretarsal orbicularis oculi muscle

Preseptal orbicularis oculi muscle

Lateral orbital tubercle

Inferior orbital fissure

C,

Preseptal orbicularis oculi muscle

Pretarsal orbicularis oculi muscle

Jones muscle

Horner muscle

Pretarsal orbicularis oculi muscle

Preseptal orbicularis oculi muscle

Orbital orbicularis oculi muscle

Orbital orbicularis oculi muscle

Fig. 29-5 Muscular anatomy of the periorbital region. **A,** View from outside the orbit. **B,** View from inside the orbit. **C,** Complex insertion of the orbicularis muscle at the medial canthus.

- **Eyelid retractors**
    - **Upper lid** (Fig. 29-6)
        - ▶ **Levator muscle**
            - ◆ Origin at the posterior orbit on the annulus of Zinn
            - ◆ Insertion onto the superior tarsal border
            - ◆ Insertion through the orbicularis onto the subdermal skin at the lid crease (in whites, lower insertion or none at all onto subdermal pretarsal skin in Asians)

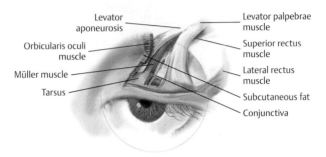

Fig. 29-6   Levator muscle and Müller muscle relationship.

- ▶ **Müller muscle** (Fig. 29-7)
    - ◆ Innervated by the sympathetic nervous system
    - ◆ Arises from the inferior surface of the levator approximately 10-12 mm above the upper border of the tarsal plate and inserts onto the superior edge of the tarsus
    - ◆ Loss of function results in 2-3 mm of ptosis.

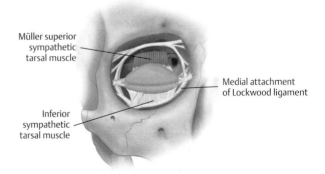

Fig. 29-7   Müller muscle after the levator muscle is cut away.

- ▶ **Levator palpebrae superioris**
    - ◆ Innervated by the superior division of CN III
    - ◆ Originates from the lesser wing of the sphenoid above the optic foramen at the annulus of Zinn and extends forward to insert onto the superior edge of

the tarsus; also, attaches to the posterior lacrimal crest through the medial horn of the levator tendon, the lateral orbital tubercle, and the pretarsal skin forming the eyelid crease

- **Lower lid**
  - ▶ **Inferior tarsal muscle** is analogous to Müller muscle in the upper eyelid (Fig. 29-8).
    - ◆ Innervated sympathetically and may result in 1 mm of lower eyelid retraction when sympathetic defects are present
    - ◆ Arises from posterior border of capsulopalpebral fascia and inserts onto the inferior border of the lower eyelid tarsal plate

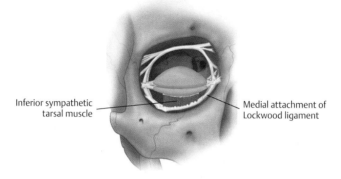

Inferior sympathetic tarsal muscle

Medial attachment of Lockwood ligament

Fig. 29-8   Inferior tarsal sympathetic muscle.

LIGAMENTOUS FRAMEWORK OF THE PERIORBITA (Fig. 29-9)
- **Upper lid**
  - **Whitnall ligament** serves as a fulcrum and suspensory ligament to redirect the vector of pull from a horizontal to a superior direction to effect lid retraction. Upward gaze is limited when the orbital septum is pulled against Whitnall ligament.
  - **Intermuscular transverse ligament** lies below Whitnall ligament and acts as a sleeve for the fulcrum of the levator muscle.

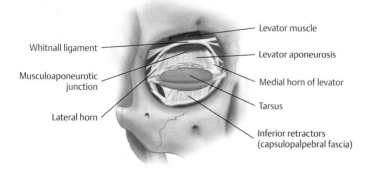

Whitnall ligament

Musculoaponeurotic junction

Lateral horn

Levator muscle

Levator aponeurosis

Medial horn of levator

Tarsus

Inferior retractors (capsulopalpebral fascia)

Fig. 29-9   Ligamentous framework of the periorbita.

- **Lockwood ligament** is analogous to Whitnall ligament in the upper eyelid. Serves as a fulcrum for change in direction of force of the capsulopalpebral fascia in the lower eyelid.
- **Lower lid**
  - **Capsulopalpebral fascia** is a condensation of fibroelastic tissue anterior to Lockwood ligament that joins with the inferior tarsus (Fig. 29-10).

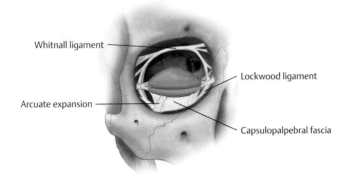

Fig. 29-10   Capsulopalpebral fascia.

  ▶ Arises from a condensation of the inferior rectus muscle sheath and envelopes the inferior oblique muscle
  ▶ Attaches to the inferior fornix of the conjunctiva and to the inferior tarsus
  ▶ Serves as the lower lid retractor
  ▶ Smooth muscle fibers in this condensation are known as the inferior tarsal muscle.
- Lateral canthal tendon (Fig. 29-11)

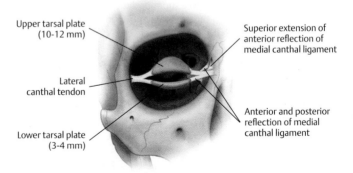

Fig. 29-11   Medial and lateral canthal tendon origins and insertions.

- Connects lateral tarsal plate with Whitnall tubercle—3 mm inside lateral orbital rim
- 2-3 mm higher than medial canthal tendon
- Deep and superficial head

- Composed of contributions from preseptal and pretarsal orbicularis, Lockwood ligament, lateral horn of levator aponeurosis, and the check ligaments of the lateral rectus muscle.[5,6]
- **The inferior ligament of Schwalbe**
  - The condensation of the lateral horn of the levator below the lacrimal gland as it attaches to Whitnall tubercle, located approximately 1-2 mm inside the lateral orbital rim.
- **Medial canthal tendon**

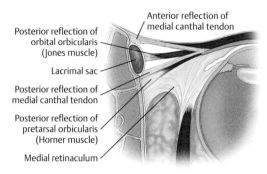

Fig. 29-12   Axial view of the lacrimal sac and enveloping medial canthal tendon.

- Connects medial tarsal plate with lacrimal crest
- Anterior thicker limb lies anterior to lacrimal sac.
- Posterior thinner limb inserts on posterior lacrimal crest.
- Superior limb inserts above lacrimal sac (Fig. 29-12).
- Composed of contributions from preseptal orbicularis (Jones muscle) and pretarsal orbicularis (Horner muscle), orbital septum, medial end of Lockwood ligament, medial horn of levator aponeurosis, check ligaments of medial rectus muscle, and Whitnall ligament[7,8]
- Arcuate expansion (Fig. 29-13)
  - Fibrous postseptal ligament that connects lateroinferior orbital rim to medial canthal tendon
  - Limits excursion of inferior oblique muscle
  - **Lateral orbital thickening:** Triangular condensation of superficial and deep fascia attaching the deep surface of the orbicularis oculi to the lateral aspect of the lateral orbital rim and deep temporal fascia[9]

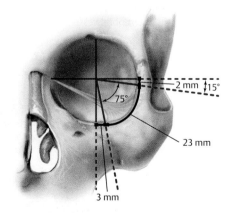

Fig. 29-13   Arcuate expansion.

- **Orbital retaining ligament** (Fig. 29-14)
  - Bilaminar membrane consisting of reflection of the orbital septum and a continuation of the membrane covering the preperiosteal fat over the zygoma[9]
  - Directly continuous with the lateral orbital thickening at the inferolateral orbital rim
  - The orbital retaining ligament, lateral orbital thickening, and lateral palpebral raphe form an anatomic unit connected to the deep head of the lateral canthal tendon by the orbicularis muscle fascia.

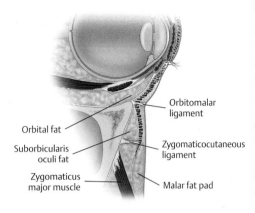

Fig. 29-14   Sagittal view of the orbitomalar ligament (orbital retaining ligament).

  - Release of the orbital retaining ligament and the lateral orbital thickening from the periosteum therefore allows movement of this complex as a single unit.
- **Soemmering ligaments**
  - Small check ligaments suspending the lacrimal gland within the superolateral orbital rim depression–lacrimal fossa.

BLOOD SUPPLY OF THE FOREHEAD
- **Internal carotid system**
  - Supraorbital vessels: 1.5 cm from midline; 10% can exit through foramen instead of supraorbital notch
  - Supratrochlear vessels: 2.7 cm from midline
- **External carotid system**
  - Superficial temporal vessels

BLOOD SUPPLY TO EYELIDS (Fig. 29-15)

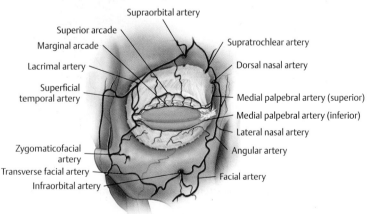

Fig. 29-15   Periorbital arterial supply.

- **Arteries**
  - The **marginal** and **peripheral arcades** provide the primary blood supply to the lids.
    - ► Located approximately 2-3 mm from lid margin and at the superior and inferior border of the tarsal plates in the upper and lower eyelid, respectively
  - Contributions are made from both the **external** and **internal carotid** systems.
  - The **upper lid** is primarily supplied by branches of the **ophthalmic** artery.
  - The **lower lid** is primarily supplied by branches of the **facial** artery.
- **Venous drainage** (Fig. 29-16)
  - Through the external jugular and the internal jugular system
  - Venous arcade of the eyelids drains into the facial vein and ultimately the external jugular system

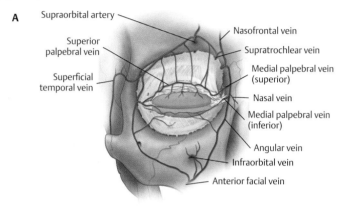

A

Supraorbital artery

Superior palpebral vein

Superficial temporal vein

Nasofrontal vein

Supratrochlear vein

Medial palpebral vein (superior)

Nasal vein

Medial palpebral vein (inferior)

Angular vein

Infraorbital vein

Anterior facial vein

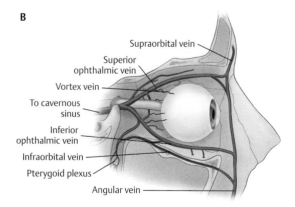

B

Supraorbital vein

Superior ophthalmic vein

Vortex vein

To cavernous sinus

Inferior ophthalmic vein

Infraorbital vein

Pterygoid plexus

Angular vein

Fig. 29-16   Venous drainage. **A,** Periorbital. **B,** Orbital.

- ► The posterior eyelids and orbit drain into the superior and inferior ophthalmic veins which ultimately drain into the internal jugular system.

INNERVATION OF BROW
- **Supraorbital nerve (V$_1$)**
  - Emerges with corresponding vessels
  - Exits orbit and divides into **superficial** and **deep** branches
    - ▶ Superficial branch enters frontalis muscle and transitions to superficial plane to supply forehead.
    - ▶ Deep branch passes deep to glide plane space, superficial to periosteum, traveling superiorly through the galeal fat pad. It exits fat pad and travels along deep galeal plane passing parallel and approximately 0.5-1 cm medial to the superior temporal line.

CAUTION: The deep branch location renders it susceptible to injury during browlifting procedures.

- **Supratrochlear nerve (V$_1$)**
  - Emerges with corresponding vessels
  - Pierces corrugator to supply central forehead

INNERVATION OF EYELID
- **Sensory innervation** is provided by the **trigeminal nerve** (Fig. 29-17).
  - The **upper** lid is supplied by the **first division (V$_1$).**
  - The **lower** lid is supplied by the **second division (V$_2$).**

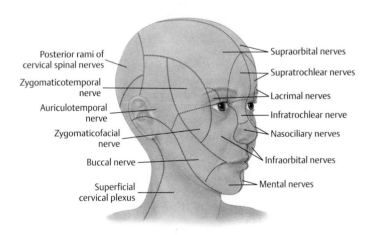

Fig. 29-17   Sensory innervation to the head and neck.

- **Motor innervation** (Fig. 29-18)
  - Provided by the facial nerve
  - The frontal, zygomatic, and buccal branches supply motor innervation to the periorbital tissue.
  - Laterally the zygomatic branch enters the orbicularis muscle from its undersurface at a right angle and courses 2.5 cm from the lateral canthus.
  - The buccal branch innervates the procerus and corrugator which is also innervated by the frontal branch of the facial nerve.

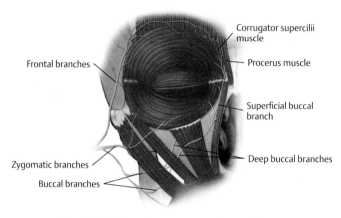

Fig. 29-18   Motor innervation to the periorbita.

LYMPHATICS

- The lymphatics drain laterally to the preauricular node (Fig. 29-19).
- Medially the lymphatics drain to the submandibular nodes
- Lymphoscintigraphy has demonstrated 72% drainage to preauricular nodes regardless of the location of the injection of the tracer[10]

ORBITAL SEPTUM

- Consists of a dense fibrous membrane attached to the periosteum of the orbital rim and extending through the lid to join the tarsus

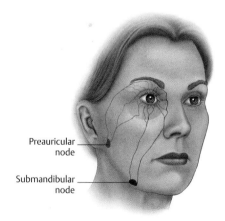

Fig. 29-19   Lymphatic drainage of the periorbita.

- Separates the orbital contents from the periorbital soft tissues
- *Arcus marginalis* is the fusion of the orbital septum with the periosteum of the orbital rim.
- Upper lid: Septum inserts onto the levator aponeurosis 2-5 mm above the tarsus.
- Lower lid: Septum inserts onto the inferior border of the tarsus.
- **Key anatomic relationships of the orbital septum**[8] (Fig. 29-20)
  - Laterally, the septum lies superficial to lateral canthal tendon.
  - Superomedially, the arcus marginalis forms the inferior portion of the superior orbital groove.
  - Medially, the septum passes superficial to the superior oblique trochlear pulley and then lies deep to the deep heads of the orbicularis oculi muscle and inserts onto the posterior lacrimal crest—above the level of the medial canthal tendon.
  - Inferomedially, the septum attaches to the anterior lacrimal crest and the inferior orbital rim.
  - Inferolaterally, the septum attaches just inferior to the inferior orbital rim creating the recess of Eisler and the interposed Eisler fat pocket.
- Attenuates posterior to the lacrimal sac, which is why a dacryocystitis may spread into the orbit readily

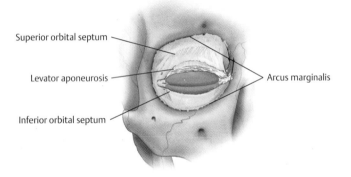

Fig. 29-20   Orbital septum.

TARSUS (Fig. 29-21)
- Located adjacent to the lid margin
- Approximately 1-2 mm thick
- Laterally, tarsi become fibrous condensations that join to form the canthal tendons.
- Composed of fibrocollagenous tissue and not cartilage
  - **Upper lid**
    - ▶ Approximately 10-14 mm cephalocaudal
    - ▶ Superior margin is the site of attachment for Müller muscle and the levator aponeurosis.

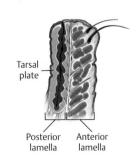

Fig. 29-21   Sagittal view of the tarsal plate.

- **Lower lid**
  - ► Approximately 6 mm cephalocaudal
  - ► Inferior margin is continuous with the capsulopalpebral fascia (analogous structure to the levator aponeurosis in the upper eyelid).
- **Eyelid margin:** Location of eyelashes and multiple apocrine and holocrine glands
  - ► **Eyelashes:** Approximately **75-180 lashes** are present in the **upper** eyelid and **60-80** are present in the **lower** eyelid.
- **Meibomian glands (holocrine):** Oil-secreting glands with an orifice located on the lid margin posterior to the eyelashes. Inspissation of oil results in formation of chalazion. Other glands include (Fig. 29-22):
  - ► Moll (apocrine)
  - ► Zeis (holocrine)
  - ► Krause (eccrine)
  - ► Wolfring (eccrine)

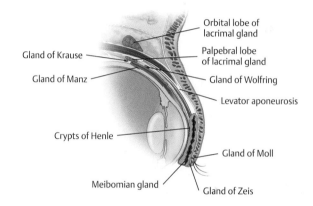

Fig. 29-22   Accessory lacrimal glands.

CONJUNCTIVA
■ Mucosal layer adjacent to the surface of the eye
  - **Palpebral portion** lines the inner surface of eyelid.
  - **Bulbar portion** lines the sclera and attaches at the limbus.
  - **Glands of Krause and Wolfring** are primary secretors of the aqueous tear film and are located in the superior conjunctival fornix.

FAT (Fig. 29-23)

- **Postseptal (intraorbital) fat**
  - **Upper lid:** Two compartments separated by superior oblique muscle
    - ► Nasal: Lighter in color, firmer
    - ► Middle
  - **Lower lid:** Three compartments
    - ► Nasal
    - ► Middle
    - ► Lateral

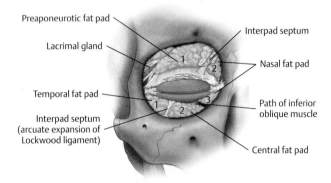

Fig. 29-23   Periorbital fat pads.

- **Preseptal (extraorbital) fat** (Fig. 29-24)
  - **Upper lid:** Retroorbicularis oculi fat (ROOF) fibrocollagenous fatty tissue
    - ► Lies deep to orbicularis overlying the lateral orbital rim
  - **Lower lid:** Suborbicularis oculi fat (SOOF)
    - ► Lies deep to orbicularis. Ptosis may contribute to formation of malar bags.

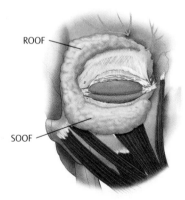

Fig. 29-24   Retroorbicularis oculi (ROOF) and suborbicularis oculi (SOOF) fat pads.

REFERENCES
1. Knize DM. The forehead and temporal fossa, anatomy and technique. Ann Plast Surg 47:585, 2001.
2. DiFrancesco LM, Codner MA, McCord CD. Upper eyelid reconstruction. Plast Reconstr Surg 114:98e, 2004.
3. Janis JE, Ghavami A, Lemmon JA, et al. The anatomy of the corrugator supercilii muscle: part II. Supraorbital nerve branching patterns. Plast Reconstr Surg 121:233, 2008.
4. Hamra ST. The zygorbicular dissection in composite rhytidectomy: an ideal midface plane. Plast Reconstr Surg 102:1646, 1998.
5. Ousterhout DK, Weil RB. The role of the lateral canthal tendon in lower eyelid laxity. Plast Reconstr Surg 69:620, 1982.
6. Jelks GW, Jelks EB. The influence of orbital and eyelid anatomy on the plapebral aperture. Clin Plast Surg 18:183, 1991.
7. McCord C Jr, Codner MA, Hester TR Jr, eds. Eyelid Surgery: Principles and Techniques. Philadelphia: Lippincott-Raven, 1995.
8. Zide BM, Jelks GW, eds. Surgical Anatomy of the Orbit. New York: Raven Press, 1985.
9. Muzaffar AR, Mendelson BC, Adams WP Jr. Surgical anatomy of the ligamentous attachments of the lower lid and lateral canthus. Plast Reconstr Surg 110:873; discussion 897, 2002.
10. Nijhawan N, Marriott C, Harvey JT. Lymphatic drainage patterns of the human eyelid: assessed by lymphoscintigraphy. Ophthal Plast Reconstr Surg 26:281, 2010.

30. Face and Neck Anatomy

John H. Hulsen, Jeffrey E. Janis

FACE AND NECK ANATOMY

- Mastery of the three-dimensional anatomy of the face and neck is essential for safe and effective aesthetic surgery.
- Anatomic variation is the rule, not the exception.

SOFT TISSUE LAYERS OF THE FACE[1-3]

- The face is anatomically arranged in related concentric layers to create a balanced structure that produces facial movement.
  - Skin
  - Superficial fat
  - Superficial fascia (or superficial musculoaponeurotic system [SMAS])
  - Mimetic muscles
  - Deep fat and anatomic spaces (buccal space)
  - Deep facial fascia (parotidomasseteric fascia)
  - Deepest plane
- **Skin**[1,2]
  - The epidermis is composed of keratinocytes, melanocytes, and antigen-presenting Langerhans cells.
  - The dermis is rich in fibroblasts and type I collagen.
  - Dermal thickness is variable throughout the face and neck and is related to its function.
    - ▶ **Thickness is usually inversely proportional to its mobility.**
    - ▶ Eyelid dermis is the thinnest, whereas forehead and nasal tip dermis is the thickest.
  - Thinner dermis is more susceptible to deterioration and signs of aging.
- **Subcutaneous tissue**[1,2,4,5]
  - Comprises two components
    - ▶ **Subcutaneous fat:** Provides facial volume
    - ▶ **Fibrous retinacular cutis:** Binds dermis to the underlying musculoaponeurotic system
    - ▶ **Retinacular cutis** is the name given to the portion of a retaining ligament as it passes through the subcutaneous layer.
  - The proportion and orientation of these components are variable in different regions of the face.
    - ▶ Compact subcutaneous fat is present in specialized areas as in the lip and eyelid.
    - ▶ Regions of thick subcutaneous tissue have longer retinacular cutis fibers that are predisposed to weakening with age.

- **Subcutaneous fat compartments**[1,2,6-10] (Fig. 30-1)
  - Subcutaneous fat in the face is partitioned into distinct anatomic compartments and may not age as a confluent mass.
  - A youthful face has smooth transitions between compartments, whereas aging can lead to abrupt contour changes.
  - Shearing between adjacent compartments may contribute to soft tissue malpositioning.

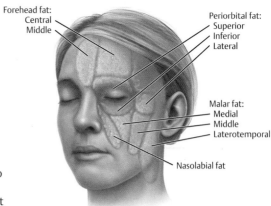

Forehead fat:
  Central
  Middle

Periorbital fat:
  Superior
  Inferior
  Lateral

Malar fat:
  Medial
  Middle
  Laterotemporal

Nasolabial fat

Fig. 30-1   Superficial facial fat compartments.

  - **Forehead**
    - ▶ **Central:** Located in the midline region of the forehead. Bordered on sides by middle temporal compartment and inferiorly by the nasal dorsum
      - ◆ Perforating vessels from the supratrochlear artery travel through the septum that borders this compartment.
    - ▶ **Middle temporal:** On either side of central forehead fat. Inferior border is orbicularis retaining ligament, lateral border is superior temporal septum.
    - ▶ **Laterotemporal:** Connects lateral forehead fat to lateral cheek and cervical fat
  - **Orbit**
    - ▶ **Superior:** Bounded by the orbicularis retaining ligament as it courses around the superior orbit
    - ▶ **Inferior:** Thin subcutaneous layer immediately below the inferior lid tarsus
    - ▶ **Lateral:** Superior border is the inferior temporal septum, inferior border is the superior cheek septum.
  - **Cheek**
    - ▶ **Superficial cheek compartment**
      - ◆ **Medial:** Lateral to the nasolabial compartment. Superior border is orbicularis retaining ligament and the lateral orbital compartment.
        - – Perforating vessels from the facial and infraorbital arteries are found within the medial limiting septum.
        - – Facial vein is found on the deep surface of the medial cheek fat.
      - ◆ **Middle:** Anterior and superficial to the parotid gland
        - – Perforating vessels of the transverse facial artery course within the middle cheek septum.
        - – The plane between the middle and lateral cheek compartments can easily lead to into the deepest plane and buccal fat pad with associated neurovascular structures.

◆ **Laterotemporal cheek:** Immediately superficial to the parotid gland, connects temporal fat the cervical subcutaneous fat
– The lateral cheek septum is anterior to the laterotemporal compartment and contains perforating vessels from the superficial temporal artery.
▶ **Deep medial cheek compartment**
◆ Found deep to the medial and middle superficial cheek compartment and inferior to orbicularis oculi muscle
◆ Orbicularis retaining ligament is superior boundary, SOOF is inferior boundary.

TIP: Potential space for fat transfer exists between the periosteum and the deep medial fat (Ristow space).

• **Nasolabial**
▶ Found anterior to the medial cheek fat overlapping jowl fat
▶ Most medial of the facial compartments
◆ Perforating vessels from the angular artery course within the nasolabial septum.
◆ The volume of the nasolabial fat is preserved.

TIP: One reason for a prominent nasolabial fold with aging is a pseudoptosis of the nasolabial fat secondary to loss of volume of the deep medial fat compartment and subsequent decreased midface projection of the deep and superficial cheek fat.

• **Jowls**
▶ Separate from the nasolabial fat
▶ Adherent to the depressor anguli oris muscle
▶ Bound medially by the lip depressor muscle and inferiorly by membranous fusion of platysma muscle
■ **Superficial fascia (SMAS)**[1-3,11-14]
• This is an upward extension of the superficial cervical fascia.
• The superficial fascial form is continuous throughout the face and neck.
• This layer is variably named according to the region and superficial muscles that it invests.
▶ In the scalp: **Galea**
▶ In the temple: **Temporoparietal fascia** (also called *superficial temporal fascia*)
▶ In the periorbital area: **Orbicularis fascia**
• The SMAS is divided into **fixed** and **mobile** portions.
▶ **Fixed:** Firmly adherent, relatively immobile, found in the lateral face over the parotid gland
▶ **Mobile:** Nonadherent to underlying structures, found directly over mimetic muscles and parotid duct and anterior to parotid gland
■ **Mimetic muscles**[2,15]
• Mimetic muscles are responsible for the coordinated movement of the midface and lips and control the size and shape of the mouth. These muscles commonly overlap and are described in **four anatomic layers** arranged from superficial to deep.
1. Depressor anguli oris, superficial portion of zygomaticus minor, orbicularis oculi
2. Platysma, risorius, zygomaticus major, deeper portion of zygomaticus minor, levator labii superioris alaeque nasi
3. Levator labii superioris and orbicularis oris
4. Mentalis, levator anguli oris, buccinator

- Muscles of the **first three layers** are innervated by the facial nerve on their **deep** surfaces, whereas muscles of the **fourth** are innervated by the facial nerve on their **superficial** surfaces.

SENIOR AUTHOR TIP: This is a common test question.

- **Deep facial fascia (parotidomasseteric fascia)**[2,3,16]
  - In the neck the deep cervical fascia is found along the superficial surface of the strap muscles.
  - The deep facial fascia is a continuation of the superficial layer of the deep cervical fascia from the neck onto the face.
  - Branches of the facial nerve within the cheek, as well as the parotid duct, are deep to the deep facial fascia.
  - As with the superficial fascia, this layer is variably named according to the specific region of the face.
    - ► Over the parotid: **Parotid capsule,** or investing fascia of the parotid
    - ► Over the masseter: **Masseteric fascia**
    - ► Superior to the zygomatic arch: **Deep temporal fascia**
  - The relationship of the superficial and deep facial fascia:
    - ► These layers may either be separated by an areolar plane or firmly adherent to each other.
      - ◆ In the temporal region the frontal branch of the facial nerve and the superficial temporal artery can initially be found in the areolar plane on the undersurface of the temporoparietal fascia (superficial facial fascia). Deep to this plane is the deep temporal fascia (deep facial fascia).

TIP: The frontal branch becomes invested by temporoparietal fascia.

      - ◆ The superficial and deep facial fascia are firmly attached along the zygomatic arch, overlying the parotid gland, and along the anterior border of the masseter.
- **Deepest plane**[2,3,15]
  - Found deep to the deep facial fascia (parotidomasseteric fascia)
  - As the facial nerve branches continue peripherally, they pierce the parotidomasseteric fascia to innervate the mimetic musculature.
  - The buccal fat pad, parotid duct, facial artery/facial vein, and zygomatic and buccal branches of the facial nerve are found within this plane.
    - ► Buccal fat pad[15,17]
      - ◆ Contributes to cheek and facial contour
      - ◆ Consists of a central body with temporal, pterygoid, and buccal extensions
      - ◆ Zygomatic and buccal branches of the facial nerve course superficial to the buccal extension.
      - ◆ The parotid duct separates the buccal extension from the central body.
- **Fascia of the neck**[18]
  - **Superficial fascia**
    - ► The deep thoracic fascia covering the pectoralis major and deltoid muscles gives rise upward to the superficial fascia of the neck.
      - ◆ This is contiguous with the superficial facial fascia (or SMAS) above the jawline.
      - ◆ Laterally, the superficial fascia fuses with the investing deep fascia of the sternocleidomastoid and trapezius muscles.

- **Deep fascia**
  - ▶ The investing deep fascia is the most superficial deep fascial layer.
    - ◆ The investing deep fascia is also called the *superficial layer of the deep cervical fascia.*
    - ◆ It acts as a visual and mechanical barrier during platysma dissection.
      - – No vital midline structures are present in the subplatysmal space while superficial to the investing deep fascia.

SENIOR AUTHOR TIP: Preservation of the cervical investing fascia is essential to addressing and placating the platysmal bands. To achieve a longer-lasting result without dehiscence, obtain suture bites of both and anterior AND posterior investing fascia (since the attenuated anterior fascia that led to the bands in the first place is insufficiently strong to hold in the long term).

- **Fascia of the infrahyoid muscles**
  - ▶ Formerly known as the middle fascia
  - ▶ Superficial layer: Invests the sternohyoid and omohyoid muscles
  - ▶ Deep layer: Invests the sternothyroid and thyrohyoid muscles
- **Visceral fascia**
  - ▶ Pretracheal fascia: Covers larynx and trachea and splits to invest the thyroid cartilage
  - ▶ Buccopharyngeal fascia: Invests the buccinator muscle and dorsal esophagus
- **Prevertebral fascia**
  - ▶ Encases the vertebral column and its associated muscles and forms the floor of the posterior triangle of the neck

NERVES[2,18]

SENSORY INNERVATION

- Sensation to the scalp, face, and neck is supplied by divisions of the trigeminal nerve (CN V_1, V_2, V_3) and cervical spinal nerves (dorsal and ventral rami), and the auditory canal is given by the vestibulocochlear (CN VIII) and vagus (CN X).
  - **Ophthalmic division** (CN V_1)
    - ▶ The frontal nerve enters through superior orbital fissure above muscles and divides into **supratrochlear** and **supraorbital** branches.
      - ◆ Supratrochlear branch exits orbit medially and courses upward along with the supratrochlear artery to innervate the central forehead.[19,20]
      - ◆ Supraorbital branch passes through a supraorbital notch or foramen along with the supraorbital artery to supply the remaining forehead and scalp.
      - ◆ The lateral branch of the supraorbital nerve is the major sensory nerve of the scalp and runs along or medial to the temporal crest.

SENIOR AUTHOR TIP: The supraorbital nerve and supratrochlear nerve can exit through a true bony foramen (40% and 18%, respectively) or through a notch, which always has a ligamentous floor.

- **Maxillary division** (CN V$_2$)
  - ▶ Sensation to the midface is provided by the zygomaticotemporal, zygomaticofacial, and infraorbital branches of the maxillary division of the trigeminal nerve.
- **Mandibular division** (CN V$_3$)
  - ▶ The auriculotemporal, mental, and buccal nerve branches are part of the mandibular division of the trigeminal nerve.
    - ◆ **Auriculotemporal nerve:** Travels with the superficial temporal artery and supplies sensation to the temple superior to the ear
    - ◆ **Buccal branch:** Communicates with the buccal branches of the facial nerve and supplies sensation to the skin of the cheek over the buccinator
    - ◆ **Mental nerve:** Supplies sensation to the chin and lower lip
- **Cervical spinal nerves** (Fig. 30-2)

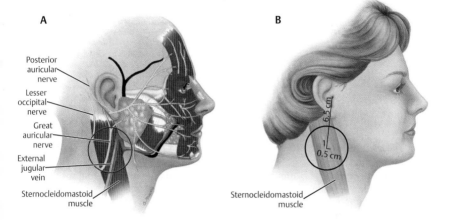

A

Posterior auricular nerve

Lesser occipital nerve

Great auricular nerve

External jugular vein

Sternocleidomastoid muscle

B

6.5 cm

1
0.5 cm

Sternocleidomastoid muscle

Fig. 30-2 A, Anatomy of the great auricular nerve. **B,** Danger zone for the great auricular nerve.

- ▶ Supply sensation to the entire neck, lower ear, lower posterior face, and posterior scalp
- ▶ **Lesser occipital nerve (C2):** Provides sensation over the postauricular mastoid area[21]

SENIOR AUTHOR TIP: The lesser occipital nerve arises behind the posterior edge of the sternocleidomastoid muscle, cephalad to the great auricular nerve, and approximately 5.3 cm below the lowest part of the external auditory canal and 6.5 cm from the posterior midline.

- ▶ The **greater occipital nerve** is a medial branch of the dorsal ramus of C2 that runs up to supply the posterior scalp to the vertex.[22]
- ▶ The **great auricular nerve** arises from the dorsal rami of C2-3.

TIP: The great auricular nerve is found at McKinney point: 6.5 cm below the external auditory canal at the midtransverse belly of the sternocleidomastoid.

▶ **Anterior branch:** Supplies the skin of the face over the parotid
▶ **Posterior branch:** Supplies the medial and lateral surfaces of the ear, including the concha and lobule

MOTOR INNERVATION: FACIAL NERVE[2,11] (Fig. 30-3)

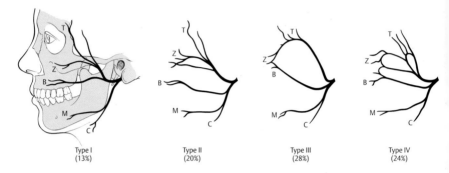

Fig. 30-3   Variations in the branching pattern of the facial nerve. (*B*, Buccal branch; *C*, cervical branch; *M*, mandibular branch; *T*, temporal branch; *Z*, zygomatic branch.)

▪ The facial nerve exits the stylomastoid foramen and is protected as it pierces the parotid gland.
▪ The nerve divides into an upper and lower portion and then into **five major branches** within the parotid gland.
  1. Temporal (or frontal)
  2. Zygomatic
  3. Buccal
  4. Marginal mandibular
  5. Cervical
▪ The branches emerge medially from the gland and course on the superficial surface of the masseter. This is deep to the deep facial fascia.
▪ Anterior to the masseter the facial nerve branches are found over the buccal fat pad at the same depth as the parotid duct and facial vessels in the so-called deepest plane.
▪ Branches proceed to innervate the most superficial three layers of mimetic muscles on their deep surface and the fourth and deepest layer (mentalis, levator anguli oris, and buccinator) on their superficial surface.

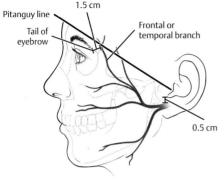

Pitanguy line
1.5 cm
Tail of eyebrow
Frontal or temporal branch

Fig. 30-4   Frontal branch course.

0.5 cm

- **Frontal branch**[11] (Fig. 30-4)
  - Follows a superficial course once it has crossed the zygomatic arch. It crosses the arch at approximately the midpoint of a line drawn from the tragus to the lateral canthus.
  - Courses superficially within the areolar plane between the temporoparietal fascia (superficial facial fascia, SMAS) and the deep temporal fascia (deep facial fascia). It eventually becomes invested by the temporoparietal fascia.
- **Zygomatic and buccal branches**
  - Injuries to the buccal and zygomatic branches of the facial nerve are rare, or rarely noticed, because of their location (deep to SMAS and deep facial fascia) and multiple redundant interconnections between these branches.
- **Marginal mandibular branch**[23,24]
  - Extends anteriorly and inferiorly within parotid
  - After exiting parotid, it is protected by thick SMAS-platysma layer and is found at or below the mandibular border.
    - ▶ Found 1-1.2 cm below the border of the mandible in 19%-53% of people
    - ▶ Once the nerve crosses the facial vessel, it may continue to run below the mandible for 1.5 cm before turning upward to cross the inferior border. However, it usually runs above the border of the mandible at the landmark of the facial vessels.
- **Cervical branch**
  - Located roughly half the distance from the mentum to the mastoid and approximately 1 cm below this line at the level of the angle of the mandible.[25]
  - Exits the inferior portion of the parotid slightly anterior to the angle of the mandible.
  - Immediately perforates the deep cervical fascia and then runs in the fibroareolar tissue that attaches to the platysma at its superolateral border
  - Platysma should be dissected at this superolateral border from the deep fascia bluntly to prevent injury.
  - Injury to the cervical branch leads to "pseudoparalysis of the mandibular branch," with an asymmetrical full denture smile. This is distinguished from marginal mandibular nerve injury by the ability to evert and purse the lower lip.[26,27]
  - Cervical branch injury is generally associated with complete recovery within 3-4 weeks on average.[27]

TIP: To prevent injury to the marginal mandibular branch, begin dissection at least 2 cm below the mandibular angle.

FACIAL DANGER ZONES[16] (Fig. 30-5)

■ Seven areas where motor and sensory nerves are at significant risk during facial surgery

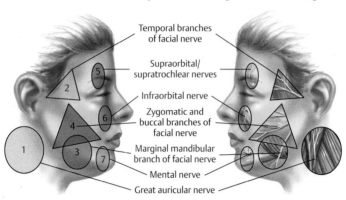

Facial Danger Zone	Location	Nerve	Relationship to SMAS	Sign of Zonal Injury
1	6.5 cm below external auditory canal	Great auricular	Posterior to	Numbness of inferior two thirds of ear, adjacent cheek and neck
2	Below a line drawn from 0.5 cm below tragus to 2 cm above lateral eyebrow and above zygoma	Temporal branch of facial	Beneath	Paralysis of the forehead
3	Midmandible 2 cm posterior to oral commissure	Marginal mandibular branch of facial	Beneath	Paralysis of the lower lip
4	Triangle formed by connecting dots on malar eminence, posterior border of mandibular angle, and oral commissure	Zygomatic and buccal branches of facial	Beneath	Paralysis of the upper lip and cheek
5	Superior orbital rim above midpupil	Supraorbital and supratrochlear	Anterior to	Numbness of forehead, upper eyelid, nasal dorsum, scalp
6	1 cm below inferior orbital rim below midpupil	Infraorbital	Anterior to	Numbness of side of upper nose, cheek, upper lip, lower eyelid
7	Midmandible below second premolar	Mental	Anterior to	Numbness of half of lower lip and chin

SMAS, Superficial musculoaponeurotic system.

Fig. 30-5   Facial danger zones: motor and sensory nerves.

VASCULAR SUPPLY[2,28]

ARTERIAL SYSTEM

- The blood supply to the face, scalp, and neck is robust and is based on the carotid system.
- Branches from the **external carotid artery** are the main vascular supply.
    - Superior thyroid
    - Ascending pharyngeal
    - Lingual
    - Facial
    - Occipital
    - Posterior auricular
    - Maxillary
    - Superficial temporal
- Maxillary and superficial temporal arteries are terminal branches of the external carotid.
- The **internal carotid** contributes a small portion to the vascular territory by supplying **supratrochlear** and **supraorbital branches** of the ophthalmic artery.
- **Vascular territories of the face:**
    - **Anterior facial arterial supply:** Facial, superior labial, inferior labial, supratrochlear, supraorbital
    - **Lateral facial arterial supply:** Transverse facial, submental, zygomaticoorbital, anterior auricular
    - **Scalp and forehead arterial supply:** Superficial temporal—frontal and parietal branches, posterior auricular, occipital
- The **anterior** face is supplied by a large network of **musculocutaneous** perforators.
- The **lateral** face, scalp, and forehead are supplied by **fasciocutaneous** perforators.
- The transition between the anterior skin supplied by musculocutaneous perforators and the lateral region supplied by fasciocutaneous perforators consistently occurs immediately lateral to the nasolabial fold.

> **TIP:** Undermining skin during a facelift will divide the lateral fasciocutaneous perforators, thus basing the facial skin flap on the medial musculocutaneous perforators.

VENOUS SYSTEM[2,18] (Fig. 30-6)

- The venous drainage of the face and neck is divided into a **superficial** and **deep system.**
- Typically, concerns of aesthetic surgery are limited to the superficial system.
- *Sentinel vein:* The larger (and more medial) of the paired zygomaticotemporal veins, located above the zygoma and lateral to the orbital rim
    - Anatomic landmark for identifying the frontal (temporal) branch of the facial nerve

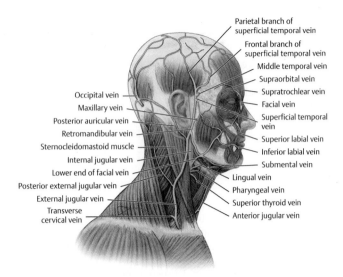

Fig. 30-6   Venous anatomy.

TIP: The frontal nerve often will course 1 cm above the sentinel vein.

■ *Facial vein:* Supratrochlear and supraorbital veins drain forehead and join to form the facial vein. It eventually crosses the inferior border of the mandible, runs over the submandibular gland and posterior belly of digastric muscle, and joins the internal jugular vein at the level of the hyoid bone.
   • Communicates with cavernous sinus through its tributaries
   • Contains no valves

TIP: Because of the lack of valves and anatomic connection, any infection involving the facial vein may extend into the intracranial system.

■ **External jugular vein:** Originates at the level of the mandibular angle, courses down the neck to the midclavicle, and enters subclavian posterior to the clavicle. It is covered by platysma over most of its course.
   • Great auricular nerve (C2-C3) ascends, along with vein, toward the head.
■ **Anterior jugular veins:** Course along mylohyoid and sternohyoid musculature descending toward the sternal notch

---

TIP: Both external jugular and anterior jugular veins are at risk during subplatysmal dissection and may cause substantial bleeding if not respected.

FACIAL BONES[2]

FRONTAL
- Forms the forehead
- Articulates with the zygoma anterolaterally, and with the nasal bones, maxilla, and lacrimal bone centrally
- Above the orbits are paired supraciliary arches that are more prominent in males. The smooth area between these arches is the glabella.
- The supraorbital neurovascular structures run through the supraorbital notch or foramen located at the junction of the medial third and lateral two thirds of the supraorbital rim.
- Half of all patients will have a frontal notch or foramen 1 cm medial to the supraorbital foramen through which pass the supratrochlear neurovascular structures.

ZYGOMA
- Forms the cheek and contributes to the lateral wall of the orbit
- The lateral canthal ligament inserts into Whitnall tubercle located behind and within the orbital margin approximately 1 cm below the zygomaticofrontal suture.
- One or two foramina are located on the lateral surface of the bone near the orbital border through which pass the zygomaticofacial neurovascular structures.

NASAL BONES
- Nasal bones are paired, oblong, thin, and variable in size and shape.
- The bones are covered by the nasalis and procerus muscles.

MAXILLA
- Forms the upper jaw, roof of the mouth, and the floor of the orbit and nose
- Connects to the zygoma, frontal, and nasal bones
- The **infraorbital foramen** is located approximately **1 cm below the infraorbital rim.**
- Vertical height undergoes substantial loss with age and tooth loss.

MANDIBLE
- Forms the lower jaw, the largest and strongest of the facial bones
- Body is arch shaped with two vertical rami.
- Midline symphysis marks the line of fusion during fetal development.
- The **mental foramen,** through which pass the mental neurovascular structures, is located approximately **1 cm below the first and second premolars.**
- The mandible is reduced in size with age and the alveolar portion is resorbed after tooth loss.
- The angle between the mandibular body and rami becomes more obtuse with age.

RETAINING LIGAMENTS OF THE FACE AND NECK[2,11,29]

- **Retaining ligaments** are strong fibrous attachments that take origin from the periosteum or deep facial fascia and travel perpendicularly through fascial layers to insert onto dermis.
- Ligaments "arborize" like limbs of a tree and function as anchor points that retain and stabilize the skin and superficial fascia (SMAS) to the underlying deep fascia and facial skeleton in predictable anatomic locations.

TEMPORAL AREA[12] (Fig. 30-7)

- Currently, there is no consensus on the accurate nomenclature of the retaining ligaments of the temporal area.
- The lateral third of the brow above the orbit is held in position by the **temporal ligamentous adhesion** or orbital ligament.
- Extending posteriorly along the temporal crest is the **superior temporal septum** (or zone of adhesion/fixation).
- Coursing medially along the supraorbital rim is the **supraorbital ligamentous adhesion.** This is where the deepest layer of the deep galea is adherent to the periosteum.[29-31]

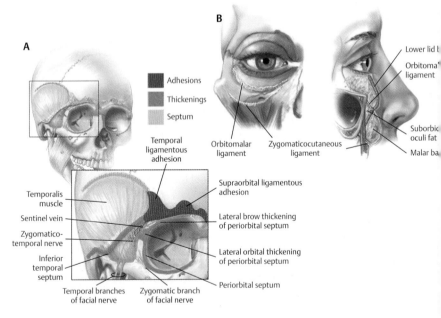

Fig. 30-7   Retaining ligaments of the temporal and orbital regions.

TIP: This descriptive confusion should not detract from the importance of the role of the retaining ligaments in mobilization for surgical facial rejuvenation.

PERIORBITAL AREA[2,24,30-33] (see Fig. 30-7)

- The **orbicularis retaining ligament (ORL)** (or orbitomalar ligament [OML]) is an osteocutaneous ligament that originates from the perisoteum of the orbital rim.
  - It passes through the orbicularis oculi and inserts into the skin of the lid-cheek junction. The ORL extends along the superior orbital rim and reaches the lateral orbit where it terminates as the **lateral orbital thickening.**
    - ▶ The *lateral orbital thickening* is known as the **superficial lateral canthal tendon,** which connects the ORL to the lateral canthal tendon through the orbicularis deep fascia (septum orbitale) and the tarsal plate. This forms a single anatomic unit.
- A **tear tough ligament** has been described along the adherent medial origin of the orbicularis oculi. This becomes continuous with the ORL.[24]

CHEEK AND MANDIBLE[1-3,14,34] (Fig. 30-8)

- **Two types** of retaining ligaments are often described:
  - **True osteocutaneous ligaments:** *True ligaments* because of their direct connection from the periosteum to the dermis
    - ▶ **Zygomatic osteocutaneous ligament**
      - ◆ Fibers originate at the inferior border of the zygomatic arch and course anteriorly to the junction with the zygoma through the malar fat pad extending to dermis.
    - ▶ **Mandibular osteocutaneous ligament**
      - ◆ Originates in the anterior third of mandible 1 cm above inferior border and inserts directly onto dermis
  - **Fasciocutaneous:** Coalescence of superficial and deep facial fascia that fixes fascial layers to overlying dermis
    - ▶ **Masseteric cutaneous and parotidocutaneous ligaments**
      - ◆ Located along the anterior border of masseter muscle and along the parotid, respectively, where superficial and deep facial fascia are intimately adherent
      - ◆ A series of fibrous bands anchor dermis to fascia.

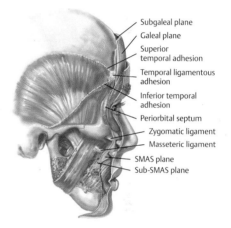

Subgaleal plane
Galeal plane
Superior temporal adhesion
Temporal ligamentous adhesion
Inferior temporal adhesion
Periorbital septum
Zygomatic ligament
Masseteric ligament
SMAS plane
Sub-SMAS plane

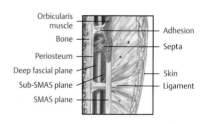

Orbicularis muscle
Bone
Periosteum
Deep fascial plane
Sub-SMAS plane
SMAS plane
Adhesion
Septa
Skin
Ligament

Fig. 30-8 Retaining ligaments of the cheek and mandible regions.

> **TIP:**   From the original description, the exact structure McGregor[35] described as a "patch" is not clear. Conventionally, this term is used as a descriptor for part of the zygomatic ligament. McGregor described the association of a buccal branch of the facial nerve with an arterial perforator at this location, and bleeding at this point should be attended to with caution.

NECK[18] (Fig. 30-9)

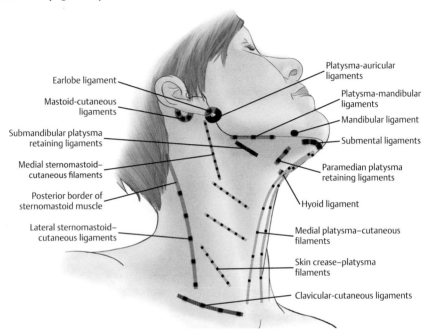

Fig. 30-9   Retaining ligaments and filaments of the neck.

■ The retaining structures that anchor the neck skin in position comprise six ligaments and three filaments:

Ligaments	Filaments
Mandibular	Medial platysma–cutaneous
Submental	Medial sternomastoid–cutaneous
Mastoid cutaneous	Skin crease–platysma
Platysma-auricular	
Lateral sternomastoid– cutaneous	
Clavicular-cutaneous ligaments	

■ Three retaining ligaments anchor the platysma to deeper tissue: Hyoid ligament, paramedian platysma retaining ligament, and submandibular platysma retaining ligament

- To understand the functional significance of these ligaments and their relationship to the facial structures is to understand, at least in part, the anatomic basis for the stigmata of the aging face.[2]
- The retaining ligaments can weaken and relax with age, causing facial soft tissue, particularly fad pads, to pivot around them.
  - Weakened **zygomatic ligaments** lead to **malar soft tissue descent.**
  - Weakened **masseteric ligaments** lead to migration of cheek tissue below the mandibular border, with resultant **jowling** as the tissue is tethered by the mandibular ligament.

ANTERIOR TRIANGLE OF THE NECK[2,18]

- Bound by the sternocleidomastoid, the median line of the neck, and the lower border of the mandible
  - **Digastric muscles**
    - ► Each muscle consists of two muscles joined by a tendon.
      - ◆ The longer posterior muscle is innervated by CN VII.
      - ◆ The shorter anterior muscle courses near the symphysis and is innervated by CN V.
  - **Submental triangle**
    - ► The region between the anterior bellies of the digastric muscles and the body of the hyoid bone
    - ► The subplatysmal fat resides deep to the platysma within this triangle.
  - **Submandibular triangle**
    - ► Contains submandibular gland, facial vessels, lingual nerve, and marginal mandibular branch of the facial nerve
      - ◆ Submandibular gland has large superficial lobe and smaller deep lobe, the bulk of which is under the body of the mandible.
      - ◆ The facial vessels cross the posterior and superior aspect of the gland.
  - **Subplatysmal fat**[9]
    - ► Located above the mylohyoid muscle
    - ► Found in discrete compartments: Central, medial, and lateral
    - ► The fascia separating supraplatysmal from subplatysmal fat is very thin.
      - ◆ Overaggressive removal of central subplatysmal fat can lead to a distorted contour.

TOP TAKEAWAYS

➤ Subcutaneous fat in the face is partitioned into distinct anatomic compartments and does not age as a confluent mass.

➤ The superficial facial fascia is an upward extension of the superficial cervical fascia and is variably named according to the region and superficial muscles that it invests.

➤ Superficial mimetic muscles are innervated by the facial nerve on their deep surfaces, whereas only the mentalis, levator anguli oris, and the buccinator are innervated on the superficial surface.

➤ The inconsistent nomenclature of the retaining ligaments should not detract from the importance of their role in mobilization for surgical facial rejuvenation.

Continued

- Anatomic variation is the rule, not the exception.
- The face is anatomically arranged in related concentric layers to create a balanced structure that produces facial movement.
- The epidermis is composed of keratinocytes, melanocytes, and antigen-presenting Langerhans cells.
- Potential space for fat transfer exists between the periosteum and the deep medial fat (Ristow space).
- The lesser occipital nerve arises behind the posterior edge of the sterno-cleidomastoid muscle cephalad to the great auricular nerve approximately 5.3 cm below the lowest part of the external auditory canal and 6.5 cm from the posterior midline.
- To prevent injury to the marginal mandibular branch, begin dissection at least 2 cm below the mandibular angle.

REFERENCES

1. Mendelson BC, Wong CH. Anatomy of the aging face. In Neligan PC, ed. Plastic Surgery, vol 2, ed 3. Aesthetic. New York: Elsevier, 2013.
2. Nahai F, Mejia JD, Nahai FR. Applied anatomy of the face and neck. In Nahai F, ed. The Art of Aesthetic Surgery: Principles and Techniques, ed 2. New York: Thieme Publishers, 2010.
3. Stuzin JM, Baker TJ, Gordon HL. The relationship of the superficial and deep facial fascias: relevance to rhytidectomy and aging. Plast Reconstr Surg 89:441, 1992.
4. Song R, Ma H, Pan F. The "levator septi nasi muscle" and its clinical significance. Plast Reconstr Surg 109:1707, 2002.
5. Chopra K, Calva D, Sosin M, et al. A comprehensive examination of topographic thickness of skin in the human face. Aesthet Surg J 35:1007, 2015.
6. Rohrich RJ, Pessa JE, Ristow B. The youthful cheek and deep medial fat compartment. Plast Reconstr Surg 121:2107, 2008.
7. Rohrich RJ, Pessa JE. The fat compartments of the face: anatomy and clinical implications for cosmetic surgery. Plast Reconstr Surg 119:2219, 2007.
8. Rohrich RJ, Pessa JE. The retaining system of the face: histologic evaluation of the septal boundaries of the subcutaneous fat compartments. Plast Reconstr Surg 121:1804, 2008.
9. Rohrich RJ, Pessa JE. The subplatysmal supramylohyoid fat. Plast Reconstr Surg 126:589, 2010.
10. Schaverien MV, Rohrich RJ, Pessa JE. Vascularized membranes determine the anatomical boundaries of the subcutaneous fat compartments. Plast Reconstr Surg 123:695, 2009.
11. Barton FE. Aesthetic surgery of the face and neck. Aesthet Surg J 29:449, 2009.
12. Mendelson BC. Extended sub-SMAS: dissection and cheek elevation. Clin Plast Surg 22:325, 1995.
13. Mitz V, Peyronie M. The superfical musculo-aponeurotic system (SMAS) in the parotid and cheek area. Plast Reconstr Surg 58:80, 1976.
14. Stuzin JM, Baker TJ, Gordon HL, et al. Extended SMAS dissection as an approach to midface rejuvenation. Clin Plast Surg 22:295, 1995.
15. Freilinger G, Gruber H, Happal W, et al. Surgical anatomy of the mimic muscle system and the facial nerve: importance for reconstructive and aesthetic surgery. Plast Reconstr Surg 80:686, 1987.

16. Seckle BR. Facial Danger Zones: Avoiding Nerve Injury in Facial Plastic Surgery. New York: Thieme Publishers, 1994.
17. Dubin B, Jackson IT, Hahm A, et al. Anatomy of the buccal fat pad and its clinical significance. Plast Reconstr Surg 83:257, 1989.
18. Feldman JJ. Surgical anatomy of the neck. In Feldman JJ, ed. Neck Lift. New York: Thieme Publishers, 2006.
19. Janis JE, Hatef DA, Hagan R, et al. Anatomy of the supratrochlear nerve: implications for the surgical treatment of migraine headaches. Plast Reconstr Surg 3131:743, 2013.
20. Janis JE, Ghavami A, Lemmon JA, et al. The anatomy of the corrugator supercilii muscle: part II. Supraorbital nerve branching patterns. Plast Reconstr Surg 121:233, 2008.
21. Dash KS, Janis JE, Guyuron B. The lesser and third occipital nerves and migraine headaches. Plast Reconstr Surg 115:1752, 2005.
22. Mosser SW, Guyuron B, Janis JE, et al. The anatomy of the greater occipital nerve: implications for the etiology of migraine headaches. Plast Reconstr Surg 113:693, 2004.
23. Dingman RO, Grabb WC. Surgical anatomy of the mandibular ramus of the facial nerve based on the dissection of 100 facial halves. Plast Reconstr Surg 29:266, 1962.
24. Wong CH, Hsieh MKH, Mendelson B. The tear trough ligament: anatomical basis for the tear trough deformity. Plast Reconstr Surg 129:1392, 2012.
25. Chowdhry S, Yoder EM, Cooperman RD, et al. Locating the cervical motor branch of the facial nerve: anatomy and clinical application. Plast Reconstr Surg 126:875, 2010.
26. Ellenbogen R. Pseudo-paralysis of the mandibular branch of the facial nerve after platysmal face-lift operation. Plast Reconstr Surg 63:364, 1979.
27. Daane SP, Owsley JQ. Incidence of cervical branch injury with "marginal mandibular nerve pseudo-paralysis" in patients undergoing face lift. Plast Reconstr Surg 111:2414, 2003.
28. Whetzel TP, Mathes SJ. Arterial anatomy of the face: an analysis of vascular territories and perforating cutaneous vessels. Plast Reconstr Surg 89:591, 1992.
29. Alghoul M, Codner MA. Retaining ligaments of the face: review of anatomy and clinical applications. Aesthet Surg J 33:769, 2013.
30. Knize DM. Anatomic concepts for brow lift procedures. Plast Reconstr Surg 124:2118, 2009.
31. Knize DM. The superficial lateral canthal tendon: anatomic study and clinical application to lateral canthopexy. Plast Reconstr Surg 109:1149, 2002.
32. Ghavami A, Pessa JE, Janis J, et al. The orbicularis retaining ligament of the medial orbit: closing the circle. Plast Reconstr Surg 121:994, 2008.
33. Muzaffar AR, Mendelson BC, Adams WP Jr. Surgical anatomy of the ligamentous attachments of the lower lid and lateral canthus. Plast Reconstr Surg 110:873, 2002.
34. Furnas DW. The retaining ligaments of the cheek. Plast Reconstr Surg 83:11, 1989.
35. McGregor M. Face Lift Techniques. Presented to the Annual Meeting of the California Society of Plastic Surgeons. Yosemite, California, 1959.

31. Facial Analysis

Janae L. Kittinger, Raman C. Mahabir

SKIN QUALITY[1,2]

- **Skin type and complexion**
  - **Fitzpatrick classification:** Ranks the skin's tendency to tan or burn after actinic exposure (Table 31-1)
- **Skin texture and thickness**
  - Total dermal thickness decreases approximately 6% per decade.
  - Actinic exposure and smoking increase the rate of dermal deterioration.
- **Photoaging**
  - **Glogau classification**: Ranks the degree of skin wrinkling and severity of photoaging (Table 31-2)
- **Severity of facial rhytids**
  - **Classification of rhytids**
    - ► Grade I: No rhytids at rest or on animation
    - ► Grade II: Superficial rhytids on animation only
    - ► Grade III: Deep rhytids on animation only
    - ► Grade IV: Superficial rhytids at rest, deep on animation
    - ► Grade V: Deep rhytids at rest, deeper on animation

Table 31-1 *Fitzpatrick Skin Type Classification*

Skin Type	Sun Exposure History/Skin Color
I	Never tans; burns easily and severely; extremely fair skin
II	Usually burns; tans minimally
III	Burns moderately; tans moderately
IV	Tans moderately and easily; burns minimally
V	Rarely burns; dark brown skin
VI	Never burns; dark brown or black skin

Table 31-2 *Glogau Classification*

Photoaging Group	Degree of Skin Wrinkling and Photoaging
I Mild (age 28-35)	Little wrinkling or scarring; no keratosis; requires little or no makeup
II Moderate (age 35-50)	Early wrinkling, mild scarring; sallow color with early actinic keratosis; requires little makeup
III Advanced (age 50-65)	Persistent wrinkling; discoloration with telangiectasias and actinic keratosis; wears makeup always
IV Severe (age 60-75)	Wrinkling; photoaging: gravitational, dynamic; actinic keratosis with or without skin cancer; wears makeup with poor coverage

FACIAL CANONS OF DIVINE PROPORTION[3]

Classical Greek canons of proportion were formulated and documented by the Renaissance artists. These neoclassical canons are as follows (Fig. 31-1):

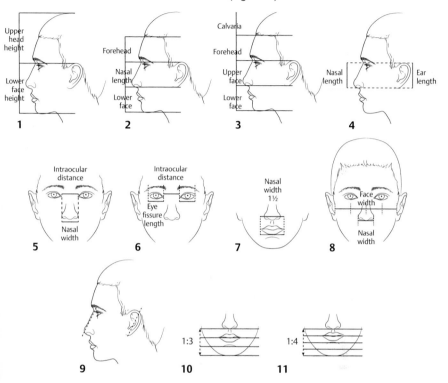

Fig. 31-1   Neoclassical canons. **1,** The head can be divided into equal halves at a horizontal line through the eyes. **2,** The face can be divided into equal thirds, with the nose occupying the middle third. **3,** The head can be divided into equal quarters, with the middle quarters being the forehead and nose. **4,** The length of the ear is equal to the length of the nose. **5,** The distance between the eyes is equal to the width of the nose. **6,** The distance between the eyes is equal to the width of each eye (the face width can be divided into equal fifths). **7,** The width of the mouth is 1½ times the width of the nose. **8,** The width of the nose is one fourth the width of the face. **9,** The nasal bridge inclination is the same as the ear inclination. **10,** The lower face can be divided into equal thirds. **11,** The lower face can be divided into equal quarters.

- The head can be divided into equal halves by a horizontal line through the eyes.
- The face can be divided into equal thirds, with the nose occupying the middle third.
- The head can be divided into equal quarters, with the middle quarters being the forehead and nose.
- The length of the ear is equal to the length of the nose.
- The distance between the eyes is equal to the width of the nose.

- The distance between the eyes is equal to the width of each eye. (The face width can be divided into equal fifths.)
- The width of the mouth is 1½ times the width of the nose.
- The width of the nose is a fourth the width of the face.
- The nasal bridge inclination is the same as the ear inclination.
- The lower face can be divided into equal thirds.
- The lower face can be divided into equal quarters.

> **TIP:**   The golden ratio of Fibonacci (1:1.618) is a common theme seen throughout facial aesthetics.

FRONTAL VIEW[4]
- Vertical fifths: Lines drawn adjacent to the most lateral projection of the head, the lateral canthi, and the medial canthi (Fig. 31-2, *A*)
- Horizontal thirds: Lines drawn adjacent to the menton, nasal base, brows at the supraorbital notch level, and hairline
  - The lower third can be divided into an upper third and lower two thirds by a line drawn through the oral commissures (Fig. 31-2, *B*).
  - The lower third can be divided into halves by a horizontal line adjacent to the lowest point of the lower lip vermilion (Fig. 31-2, *C*).
- Horizontal line through the labiomental groove divides the stomion-to-menton distance into a 1:2 ratio (Fig. 31-2, *D*).
- Width of the mouth and the stomion-to-menton distance are equal (Fig. 31-2, *E*).
- Width of the mouth approximates the distance between the medial limbi of the corneas (Fig. 31-2, *F*).
- The width of the face at the malar level is equal to the distance from the brows to the menton (Fig. 31-2, *G*).
- The distance from the infraorbital rim to the base of the nose equals the nasal base length, which is equal to half of the length of the middle third of the face (Fig. 31-2, *H*).

LATERAL VIEW[4]
- The face profile can be divided into horizontal thirds.
  - The lower third can be divided into an upper third and lower two thirds by a line drawn through the oral commissure (Fig. 31-3, *A*).
- The distance from the mandibular angle to the menton is half the distance from the hairline to the menton (Fig. 31-3, *B*).
- The desired lip-chin complex relationship is an upper lip that projects ~2 mm more than the lower lip (Fig. 31-3, *C*).
  - In women the chin lies slightly posterior to the lower lip.
  - In men the chin is slightly stronger.

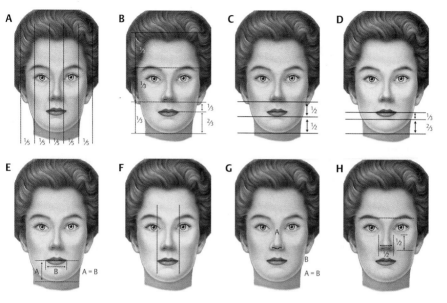

Fig. 31-2 **A,** Vertical fifths. **B,** Horizontal thirds. **C,** Division of the lower third. **D,** 1:2 ratio of the lower third. **E,** Stomion to menton *(A)* and the width of the mouth *(B)* are equidistant. **F,** Distance between the medial limbi approximates the width of the mouth. **G,** Width of the face at the malar level *(A)* is equal to the distance from the brow to the menton *(B).* **H,** Infraorbital rim to base of nose length is equal to the nasal base length, which is equal to half the length of the middle third of the face.

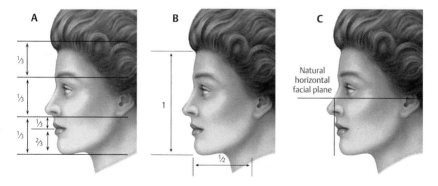

Fig. 31-3 **A,** Horizontal thirds. **B,** Distance from the mandibular angle to menton is half the distance from the hairline to the menton. **C,** Desired lip-chin complex relationship.

REGION-SPECIFIC ANALYSIS

Analysis of the region starts with the upper third, then goes to the middle third, then finally the lower third.

UPPER THIRD
Forehead[1]

- Assess for proportion and contour.
- Forehead height: Measure from hairline to midpupil (fixed point rather than hairline to brow).
- Assess for both active and passive frontalis (transverse) forehead rhytids.
- Assess for both active and passive corrugator (vertical) and procerus (horizontal) rhytids at the glabella.
- Brow position
  - Assess for compensated brow ptosis. (The brow is ptotic but compensated for by frontalis hyperactivity.)
  - Assess the medial and lateral brow position and the relationship of the brow to the upper lid.
    - ▶ With lid closed, the brow should be 2-2.5 cm above the upper lid margin.
    - ▶ At midpupil, the ratio of the aperture of the eye (1) to the distance from brow to lash line (1.618) is consistent with the golden ratio.
    - ▶ Highest portion should be at (or just lateral to) the lateral third point, corresponding to lateral edge of the limbus in straight gaze.
    - ▶ The medial portion of the brow should be caudal to the lateral portion.
    - ▶ Greatest degree of brow descent often occurs at the lateral orbit (lateral brow hooding).

Upper Eyelid[1]

- Assess for redundant skin, skin quality, fat herniation, and soft tissue excess (subcutaneous fat, preseptal fat, lacrimal gland ptosis).
- Intercanthal distance is 31-33 mm; however, 33-36 mm can be considered attractive.
- Intercanthal axis is normally tilted slightly upward from medial to lateral. (Lateral canthus is 2 degrees higher.)
- Vertical opening is ~10 mm.
- Lid position
  - Upper lid extends down at least 1.5 mm below the upper limbus but no more than 3 mm.
  - Pretarsal skin is visualized on relaxed forward gaze: 3-6 mm (varies with ethnicity).
  - The distance from the lower edge of the eyebrow to the open lid center margin should never be less than three times the measurement of the visualized pretarsal skin.

- Supratarsal fold
  - 7-11 mm from lash line
  - Indicator of levator dehiscence: Elevation of supratarsal fold; accentuated supratarsal hollow[5] (Fig. 31-4)

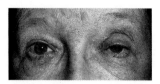

Fig. 31-4 This woman shows classic signs of left levator dehiscence with ptosis, a high lid crease, and thinning of the lid above the tarsal plate.

Lower Eyelid

- Assess for redundant skin, skin quality, rhytids (crow's-feet), tarsal laxity, skin pigmentation (blepharomelasma), festoons, fat herniation, tear trough deformity, and scleral show.
- The lower lid ideally covers 0.5 mm of the lower limbus but no more than 1.5 mm.

> **TIP:** The lid-cheek junction must also be assessed and factored into the analysis, because it is one of the more complex areas of the face.

Globe

- Determine whether positive, neutral, or negative vector relationship exists.
- Assess for globe prominence/proptosis, enophthalmos/exophthalmos, dystopia, visual acuity, and Bell palsy.

MIDDLE THIRD
Nose[4,6]

- First, evaluate skin type and texture.
  - Thick and sebaceous skin does not drape as well, and edema takes longer to subside.
  - Thin skin may drape too well and can show small deformities underneath the skin.
- Evaluate for deviation: A line drawn from midglabella to menton should bisect the nasal bridge, nasal tip, and Cupid's bow (Fig. 31-5, *A*).
- The width of the body of the nose at the nasal-cheek junction should equal 80% of the alar base width (Fig. 31-5, *B*).
- The alar base width should be about the same as the intercanthal distance, which should be the same as the width of an eye (Fig. 31-5, *C*).
  - If interalar width is wider than intercanthal width, determine whether it is caused by increased interalar width or alar flaring.
  - Normal alar flaring in white females is 2 mm wider than alar base; if it is greater than this, alar base resection should be considered.
  - If interalar width is increased, then nostril resection may be indicated.

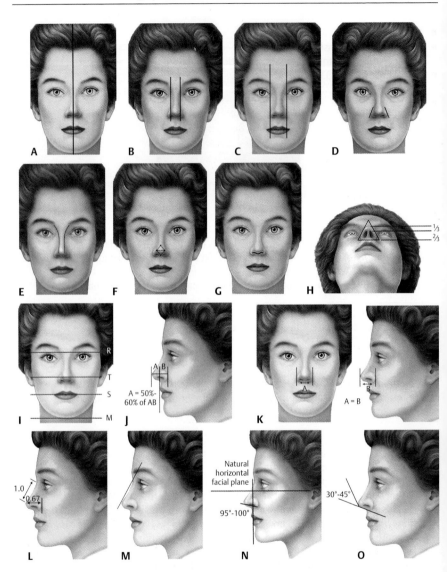

Fig. 31-5   A, Deviation of the nose is evaluated by drawing a line from the midglabella to the menton. **B,** The body of the nose at the nasal-cheek junction should equal 80% of the alar base width. **C,** Alar base width should equal the intercanthal distance. **D,** Alar rims flare slightly outward inferiorly. **E,** Slightly curved divergent lines should extend from the medial supraciliary ridges to the tip-defining points on the dorsum. **F,** The tip-defining points bilaterally, the supratip break above, and the columellar-lobular angle below should form two equilateral triangles. **G,** Gull-wing appearance of the columella. **H,** Basal view. **I,** Nasal length evaluation; RT = 1.6 × TS. **J,** Evaluation of the nasal tip projection. **K,** Alar base width *(A)* equals tip projection *(B)*. **L,** Tip projection equals 0.67 RT (nasal length). **M,** Nasal dorsum evaluation. **N,** Nasolabial angle. **O,** Columellar-lobular angle. (*M, Menton; R, radix, S, stomion; T, tip.*)

- The alar rims should flare slightly outward in an inferior direction (Fig. 31-5, *D*).
- Two slightly curved divergent lines should extend from the medial supraciliary ridges to the tip-defining points on the dorsum (Fig. 31-5, *E*).
- Nasal tip evaluation: Locate the tip-defining points bilaterally, supratip break above, and the columellar-lobular angle below; these should form two equilateral triangles (Fig. 31-5, *F*).
- Columella evaluation: Should hang just inferior to the alar rims, giving a gentle gull-wing appearance (Fig. 31-5, *G*).
- Basal view: An equilateral triangle is visualized with a 2:1 ratio of columella to lobular portion; the nostrils should be teardrop shaped (Fig. 31-5, *H*).
- Nasal length evaluation
  - Ideal nasal length (RT) should equal the distance from the stomion to menton (SM), which equals 1.6 × distance from tip to stomion (TS) (Fig. 31-5, *I*).
  - Nasal length should be approximately two thirds of midfacial (middle third) height.
- Nasal tip projection evaluation
  - A line drawn from the alar-cheek junction to the tip of the nose, when bisected by a vertical line drawn adjacent to the most projecting portion of the upper lip, should have 50%-60% of the horizontal line anterior to the vertical line (Fig. 31-5, *J*).
    - ▶ If >60% of the tip is anterior to the vertical line, the tip is overprojected and should be reduced.
    - ▶ If <50% of the line lies anterior to it, projection is inadequate and should be augmented.

TIP: This relationship only holds true if the upper lip projection is normal.

  - Tip projection equals the alar base width (Fig. 31-5, *K*).
  - Tip projection should be approximately 0.67 RT (Fig. 31-5, *L*).

TIP: This relationship only holds true if the nasal length is correct.

- Nasal dorsum evaluation
  - In women it lies 2 mm behind and parallel to a line connecting the nasofrontal angle with the desired tip projection; a slight supratip break is preferred (Fig. 31-5, *M*).
  - In men it lies slightly more anteriorly.
  - If it is too far posterior to this line, augmentation will be required.
  - If it is too far anterior to this line, reduction is indicated.
- Tip rotation
  - This is determined by the degree of the nasolabial angle.
  - Draw a straight line through the most anterior and posterior points of the nostrils on lateral view. Where this bisects with a perpendicular line to the natural horizontal facial plane is the nasolabial angle (Fig. 31-5, *N*).
    - ▶ In women 95- to 100-degree angle is preferred.
    - ▶ In men 90- to 95-degree angle is preferred.

> **TIP:**   A nose with a high dorsum without a supratip break will appear less rotated than one with a low dorsum and supratip break, even though the degree of rotation is the same.

■ Columellar-lobular angle: Formed by the junction of the columella with the infratip lobule (Fig. 31-5, O)
  • It is usually 30-45 degrees.
  • Increased fullness in this area (usually caused by prominent caudal septum) will give the appearance of increased tip rotation even though the angle of rotation (nasolabial angle) is within normal limits.
■ Intranasal examination
  • Inspect airways, nasal valve, septum, and turbinates.
■ Ethnic variations in nasal structure
  • Compared with nasal ideals for whites, the nose of black patients and those of Middle Eastern descent have the following characteristics.
    ▶ Blacks (Fig. 31-6)
      ◆ Wide, low nasal dorsum
      ◆ Decreased nasal length and tip projection
      ◆ Poor nasal tip definition
      ◆ Acute columellar-labial angle
      ◆ Alar flaring

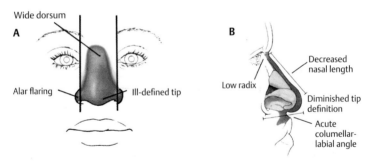

Fig. 31-6   Typical characteristics of the noses of black patients.

    ▶ Middle Eastern (Fig. 31-7)
      ◆ Wide nasal bones
      ◆ Thick, sebaceous skin
      ◆ Ill-defined bulbous tip

- ◆ High dorsum and overprojecting radix
- ◆ Acute columellar-labial angle
- ◆ Slight alar flaring

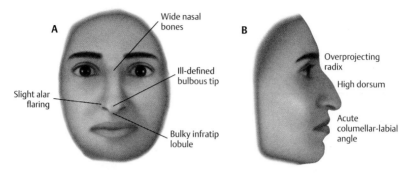

Fig. 31-7   Typical characteristics of the noses of patients of Middle Eastern descent.

Cheek
- ■ Assess rhytids, lid-cheek junction, volume of facial fat, descent of the malar fat pad, and skeletal proportions.
- ■ A youthful face has high cheekbones with concavity in the buccal area.

Ears[7,8] (Fig. 31-8)
- ■ Normal ear aesthetics
  - • The ear is positioned approximately one ear length posterior to the lateral orbital rim and centered in the middle third horizontal plane.
  - • Long axis inclines posteriorly ~20 degrees from the vertical plane.
  - • Width is ~55%-60% of height.
  - • Anterolateral aspect of helix protrudes 21-30 degrees (1.5-2 cm) from scalp.
  - • Helix should project 2-5 mm more laterally than antihelix in frontal view.

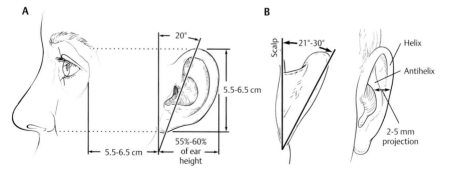

Fig. 31-8   Normal ear aesthetics.

LOWER THIRD
Mouth
- Assess dental occlusion.
- Lips
  - Examine key landmarks, including vermilion-cutaneous junction, Cupid's bow, and philtral columns.
  - Assess for presence of perioral rhytids.
  - Assess for volume loss.
  - Assess lateral angles of the mouth; aging lowers this, causing downward slant.
  - Upper lip length: At rest with the lips slightly separated, the upper lip should expose approximately one half of the incisor teeth.
- Nasolabial grooves and marionette lines (lines from the corner of the mouth to the mandibular border): Assess depth at rest and during animation.

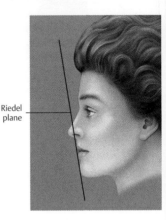

Riedel plane

Chin
- Assess projection in relation to other facial proportions; pogonion should be 3 mm posterior to the nose-lip-chin plane.
- Nasal length (RT) = Vertical chin length (SM).
- Riedel plane: Line touching projected lips should touch pogonion (Fig. 31-9).
- Assess labiomental groove definition, which should be approximately 4 mm deep.

Fig. 31-9   Riedel plane.

Neck[9]
- Assess skin for quality, tone, excess, and rhytids.
- Evaluate for subcutaneous and preplatysmal fat.
- Assess for static or dynamic platysmal banding.
- Look for submandibular gland ptosis.
- Mandibulocutaneous ligament: Tethering of the descending facial tissues at this ligament produces the appearance of jowls.
- Qualities of a youthful neck
  - Distinct inferior mandibular border
  - Subhyoid depression
  - Visible thyroid cartilage bulge
  - Visible anterior border of the sternocleidomastoid
  - Cervicomental angle of 105-120 degrees

TOP TAKEAWAYS
➤ Skin quality will dramatically affect the results.
➤ Consider facial relationships both from a static and dynamic standpoint.
➤ It is equally important to look at both the individual parts of the face as well as the face as a whole.
➤ Preoperative counseling is imperative. Areas that will not be addressed should be pointed out to patients so that they can recognize them and accept that they will be present postoperatively.
➤ These are only guidelines. Many aesthetically pleasing faces do not have these proportions. These assessments are useful in determining factors that are responsible for individual appearances.
➤ Ensure that what a patient wants is congruent with what you, the surgeon, can do. It is acceptable to say NO.

REFERENCES

1. Barton FE Jr, ed. Facial Rejuvenation. New York: Thieme Publishers, 2008.
2. Nahai F, ed. The Art of Aesthetic Surgery: Principles & Techniques. New York: Thieme Publishers, 2005.
3. Bashour M. History and current concepts in the analysis of facial attractiveness. Plast Reconstr Surg 118:741, 2006.
4. Gunter JP, Rohrich RJ, Adams WP Jr, eds. Dallas Rhinoplasty: Nasal Surgery by the Masters. New York: Thieme Publishers, 2002.
5. McCord CD Jr, Codner MA, eds. Eyelid & Periorbital Surgery. New York: Thieme Publishers, 2008.
6. Byrd HS, Hobar PC. Rhinoplasty: a practical guide for surgical planning. Plast Reconstr Surg 91:642; discussion 655, 1993.
7. Janis JE, Rohrich RJ, Gutowski KA. Otoplasty. Plast Reconstr Surg 115:60e, 2005.
8. Ha RY, Trovato MJ. Plastic surgery of the ear. Sel Read Plast Surg 11:1, 2011.
9. Ellenbogen R, Karlin JV. Visual criteria for success in restoring the youthful neck. Plast Reconstr Surg 66:826, 1980.

32. Hair Transplantation

Michelle Coriddi, Jeffrey E. Janis, Alfonso Barrera

There are many patients that can benefit from hair transplantation, not only men (male pattern baldness) but also females with androgenic alopecia and iatrogenic alopecia, i.e., postrhytidectomy hair loss.

Additionally, there are many examples of reconstructive situations that may benefit from hair transplantation, including eyebrows, eyelashes, moustache and beard, after burns, and after accidents or tumor removal.

With the latest technology in hair transplantation we have today, we cannot make new hair, but rather we can only redistribute the patient's own hair roots. Suitable candidates have a favorable ratio of supply and density of the donor area as it compares to the size of the area that needs to be transplanted (the "supply and demand" factor).

DEFINITION OF PROBLEM

- **Alopecia:** Hair loss resulting from a diminution of visible hair[1,2]
- **Three phases** of hair growth: Anagen, catagen, and telogen (Fig. 32-1)
    - **Anagen:** Active growth
    - **Catagen:** Degradation phase
    - **Telogen:** Resting phase
- Thinning and baldness develop when anagen phase shortens and telogen phase is prolonged.[2]

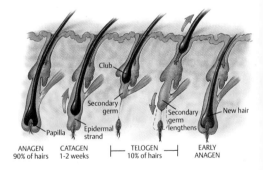

Fig. 32-1 Three phases of hair growth.

GOALS OF TREATMENT[2]

PROVIDE A NATURAL LOOK
- Hair growing in a natural and consistent direction with a natural appearance
    - In adult males a natural and mature hairline, with some degree of frontotemporal recession, and the absence of this recession on the female patient
- Absence of detectable scarring

INDICATIONS[1,2]

- Androgenic alopecia in males and females
- Secondary scarring alopecia (postsurgical, burns, radiotherapy-induced, traumatic injuries, postfungal infection scarring)
- Congenital hair loss

CONTRAINDICATIONS

- Chronic lupus erythematosus, lichen planopilaris, frontal fibrosing alopecia, classic pseudopelade of Brocq, folliculitis decalvans, central centrifugal cicatricial alopecia

PREOPERATIVE EVALUATION

NORWOOD CLASSIFICATION SYSTEM FOR MALE PATTERN BALDNESS[3,4]
(Fig. 32-2)

- **Type I:** Minimal or no hairline recession at the frontotemporal areas
- **Type II:** Symmetrical triangular frontotemporal recessions extend posteriorly no more than 2 cm anterior to the coronal plane drawn between the external auditory canals
- **Type III:** Symmetrical triangular frontotemporal recessions extend posteriorly more than 2 cm
- **Type III vertex:** Primarily vertex hair loss; may be accompanied by frontotemporal recession that conforms to type III guidelines
- **Type IV:** Sparse or absent vertex hair with more severe frontotemporal recession; areas separated by a band of moderately dense hair that extends across the top of the head
- **Type V:** Same as type IV, but more severe hair loss; band of hair narrower and more sparse
- **Type VI:** Absent band, and two areas interconnect
- **Type VII:** Most severe form; only a narrow horseshoe-shaped band of fine, sparse hair
- **Type a variants:** Applies to 3% of cases in which baldness starts at the anterior hairline without a peninsula of hair and advances in a posterior direction

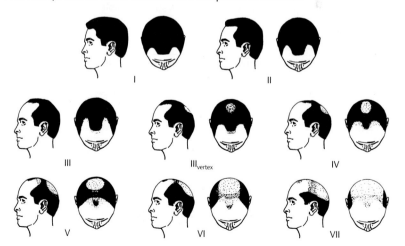

Fig. 32-2   Norwood classification of male alopecia.

LUDWIG CLASSIFICATION SYSTEM FOR FEMALE PATTERN BALDNESS[5] (Fig. 32-3)

- **Grade I:** Mild hair loss
- **Grade II:** Moderate hair loss
- **Grade III:** Severe hair loss

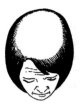

Grade I   Grade II   Grade III

OTHER CONSIDERATIONS

- **Hair density**[1,2,6,7]
  - Normal hair density: 140-220 hairs/cm^2
  - Need only **70-110 hairs/cm^2** for normal-appearing density

Fig. 32-3   Ludwig classification of female alopecia.

> **SENIOR AUTHOR TIP:**   This can usually be accomplished in two sessions (sometimes three, depending on the thickness and type of hair).

- **Male pattern baldness**[1,2,8]
  - When we do 2500 grafts, each graft having one, two, three, or four hairs per graft, this equates to somewhere about 5000-6000 hairs in a single session, so double that in two sessions or about 10,000-12,000 hairs in two sessions (see Fig. 32-5).[1,2]
- **Donor site dominance**
  - Concept that hair will retain growth characteristics of donor site
  - Best donor sites are **occipital** and **temporal**
- **Straight versus curly hair**[1]
  - Natural results are easier to obtain using curly hair in a single session.
- **Hair color**[1]
  - Dark hair on light skin tone may require more sessions to mask the contrast and create the optimal appearance of hair fullness.
- **Age**[1]
  - For patients <23 years of age, a trial of medical treatment (e.g., minoxidil [Rogaine] or finasteride [Propecia]) is recommended because of incipient baldness.

PREOPERATIVE CARE[1,2]

- Patients need to stop medications that may cause excessive bleeding (NSAIDs, acetyl salicylic acid).
- Patients are assessed for allergies.

INFORMED CONSENT[1]

- Patients must have realistic expectations and understand that the procedure redistributes existing hair; therefore hair density is limited.
- Currently no method to create new hair exists.
- The final result will not be seen until 1 year after transplantation.
- Several sessions may be necessary.

EQUIPMENT[1]

- Basic surgical equipment
- No. 10 Bard-Parker blades
- No. 11 feather blades
- No. 22.5 and 15-degree Sharpoint blades
- 3-0 polypropylene
- Mantis microscope (10×)
- Magnifying loupes (3.5×)
- Background lighting for graft dissection
- Chilled Petri dishes for graft preservation
- Aftercare: Adaptic, Polysporin ointment, Kerlix, 3-inch Ace bandage

TECHNIQUE[1]

ANESTHESIA

- Intravenous sedation with midazolam and fentanyl
- Supraorbital, supratrochlear, occipital nerve blocks
- Field blocking of the recipient site and the caudal margin of the donor area
- Tumescence infiltration: To minimize bleeding, produces temporary thickness to facilitate easier implantation of the FUs, completes anesthesia.
  - Solution of 120 ml normal saline solution, 20 ml 2% lidocaine, 1 ml epinephrine 1:1000, 40 mg triamcinolone (Kenalog) injected intradermally and subcutaneously, not subgaleally into of the recipient scalp 5-10 minutes before micrografting

DONOR SITE HARVESTING (Fig. 32-4)

- A long, narrow donor ellipse is planned in the occipital area.
- Ellipses are limited by scalp elasticity and pliability.
- Strip sizes can vary from 1 by 10 cm to 1.5 by 30-32 cm depending on FUs needed and donor site hair density.

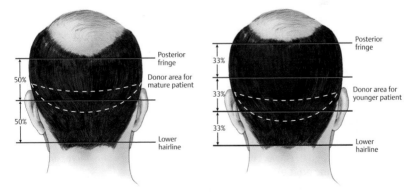

Fig. 32-4   The donor strip is harvested from the area with the thickest healthier, most durable hair, generally halfway between the upper border of baldness (or thinning) and the lower neck hairline.

> **SENIOR AUTHOR TIP:**   Generally 1 cm in width and as long as needed depending on the number of grafts planned. When planning on 2000, I make an ellipse 1cm in width and about 20-22 cm in length.

- Hair is harvested in the deep subcutaneous plane.
- Donor ellipses are harvested segmentally, allowing graft preparation to begin while the rest of the donor ellipse is harvested.
- Donor ellipses are closed primarily and without tension, undermining when necessary, with running nonabsorbable suture.

GRAFT DISSECTION
- Dissection team processes donor ellipse under magnification into 1.5-2 mm thick slices, **parallel to hair shafts.**
- Natural grouping patterns of hair follicles are preserved (Fig. 32-5).
  - **Micrografts** contain one or two hairs per graft.
  - **Minigrafts** contain three or four hairs per graft.

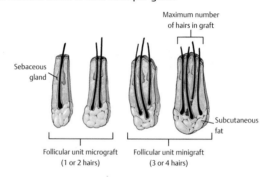

Fig. 32-5   Minigrafts and micrografts.

GRAFT INSERTION
- Recipient area is infiltrated with tumescent solution.
- Stick and place technique: Blade is inserted then tilted to open the entrance of the slit for graft insertion. Graft is inserted, and the blade holds the graft in place as forceps are withdrawn (Fig. 32-6).
- No. 22.5 Sharpoint blade is used for front 2 cm of the hairline, No. 11 feather blade for posterior and crown.

CAUTION: Hair bulb must not be gripped.

- Initially, placed 4-5 mm apart, returning to graft spaces in between after 20 minutes.
  - Allows fibrinogen to convert to fibrin, holding graft in place and decreasing the likelihood of the graft extrusion.
  - Repeated as needed until grafts are **1-2 mm apart.**

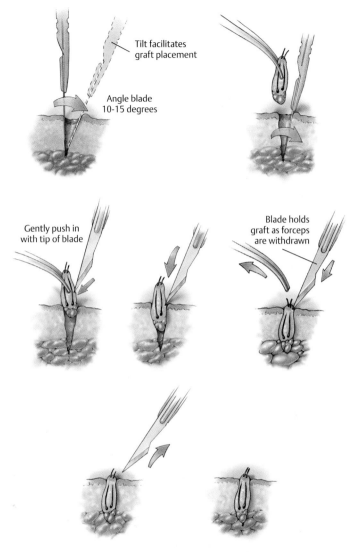

Fig. 32-6 Graft insertion: stick and place technique.

■ Epidermis of the graft should be slightly superficial to scalp epidermis to prevent cysts and ingrown hairs
■ **Inserted at proper angles**
  • **Frontal hairline:** 45-60 degrees
  • **Posterior to hairline:** 75-80 degrees
  • **Crown/vertex:** 90 degrees, whorl pattern
  • **Posterior to crown:** 45-60 degrees downward
  • **Lateral fringes:** Following direction of existing hair

- Inserted in random patterns
- **Uneven** frontal hair design
  - 8 cm from eyebrow in males
  - 5-8 cm from eyebrow in females
- 1 FU micrografts inserted in the first 1 cm of hairline
  - Can use 2 FU micrografts and minigrafts posterior to this

FOLLICULAR UNIT EXTRACTION
- Method of single FU harvest from donor area
- Limited by donor area hair density
- Prevents linear scar in donor area
- Can extract body hairs (submental beard, chest)
- Can be used to thin minigrafts or plugs
- Sharp and dull punch systems as well as robotic Artas system (Restoration Robotics) available
- Size of punches range from 0.8-1 mm.
- Major challenge is identifying subcutaneous course of the follicles.

COMBINED FOLLICULAR UNIT EXTRACTION AND TRANSPLANTATION
- Untouched strip technique for cases of more advanced baldness (Norwood types V, Va, VI, occasionally IV and VII) (Fig. 32-7)
- Second procedure using untouched strip performed at 1 year as needed

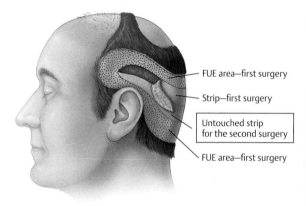

FUE area—first surgery

Strip—first surgery

Untouched strip for the second surgery

FUE area—first surgery

Fig. 32-7   Strip technique extraction and transplantation.

SENIOR AUTHOR TIP: When planning to do as many grafts as possible you may combine the strip technique with FUE (Follicular Unit Extraction). This way you may do an extra 700-800 grafts in a single session. That is you may end up with about 3500-4000 grafts as shown here.

POSTOPERATIVE CARE[1,2]
- Donor grafts are covered with nonstick dressings (Adaptic) and wrapped in Kerlix and Ace bandage.
- Patients are instructed to rest for first 72 hours and to keep head elevated at 45 degrees.

- Eyelids and forehead can swell from normal saline solution and local anesthetic and usually resolves by postoperative day 7.
- After the postoperative bandage is removed on postoperative day 2, the patient should wash hair daily with warm water and mild shampoo under low pressure.
- Patients should wear a hat for protection.
- Optional: 5% minoxidil applied twice daily for 6 months to speed the growth of newly transplanted hair
- Patients should not smoke or perform strenuous exercise for 2 weeks and should avoid sun and excessive heat for 3 weeks.
- Stitches will be removed on postoperative day 10.
- Patients are counseled that their hair initially will grow for 10 days and then shed as grafts shift into telogen phase.
  - New hair growth can be seen at 3-4 months with **visible difference at 5-6 months.**
  - Final results are not evident until **1 year postoperatively.**

COMPLICATIONS

- Overall complication rate approximately 4.7%[9]

GENERAL[1,2]

- Hemorrhage
- Lidocaine toxicity
- Hiccups
  - Can affect procedure
  - Treat with sedation and possibly chlorpromazine
- Herpes zoster
  - Rare but can manifest on postoperative day 4 or 5
  - Treated with acyclovir or valcyclovir
- Seborrheic dermatitis
  - More common in patients with oily scalp
  - Treatment involves shampoo containing selenium sulfide or coal tar.
  - Mineral or vegetable oil helps to remove scales.
  - Serious cases may require keratolytics.

DONOR SITE[1]

- Bleeding
  - Hematoma drained, and drain removed
- Wound dehiscence
  - Can rarely occur after suture removal
- Telogen effluvium
  - Temporary, usually from excessive tension and ischemia at closure site
  - Treated with local massage
- Scar widening or hypertrophic scarring
  - Prevented by limiting tension on closure
  - Treated by resecting the scar, undermining borders, and closing in two layers
  - May require tissue expanders in extreme cases.
- Hyperesthesia
  - Rare but can be caused by neuroma

- Hypoesthesia
  - More frequent and can last for 3-12 months
  - Treated with local massage

RECIPIENT SITE[1]
- Milia
  - Rare but can occur after postoperative week 2
  - Treated by rupturing the pustules with fine forceps and expressing their contents
  - Apply antiseptic solution
  - Keep scalp open
  - Wash daily with antiseptic soap
- Cysts and granulomas
  - Can appear after postoperative month 3
  - Treated with incision and extrusion of necrotic material
- Poor hair growth
  - Rare and usually caused by a donor area with poor hair quality and low density
  - Treated with minoxidil
- Swelling
  - By postoperative day 2-4, 10% of patients develop forehead and eyelid edema.
  - Usually resolves without problems

TOP TAKEAWAYS
➤ For patients <23 years of age, a trial of medical treatment (e.g., minoxidil [Rogaine] or finasteride [Propecia]) is recommended because of incipient baldness.
➤ Patients must have realistic expectations and understand that the procedure redistributes existing hair; therefore hair density is limited.
➤ Smoking and strenuous exercise should be avoided for 2 weeks and sun and excessive heat for 3 weeks.
➤ Hair will initially grow for 10 days and then shed as grafts shift into telogen phase.

REFERENCES
1. Barrera A, Oscar Uebel C. Hair Transplantation: The Art of Follicular Unit Micrografting and Minigrafting, ed 2. New York: Thieme Publishers, 2014.
2. Janis JE, ed. Essentials of Plastic Surgery, ed 2. New York: Thieme Publishers, 2014.
3. Norwood OT. Male pattern baldness: classification and incidence. South Med J 68:1359, 1975.
4. Norwood OT, Shiell RC, eds. Hair Transplant Surgery, ed 2. Springfield, IL: Charles C Thomas, 1984.
5. Ludwig E. Classification of the types of androgenic alopecia (common baldness) occurring in the female sex. Br J Dermatol 97:247, 1977.
6. Limmer B. The density issue in hair transplantation. Dermatol Surg 23:747, 1997.
7. Marritt E. The death of the density debate. Dermatol Surg 25:654, 1999.
8. Bernstein RM, Rassman W. The aesthetics of follicular transplantation. Dermatol Surg 23:785, 1997.
9. Salanitri S, Gonçalves AJ, Helene A Jr, et al. Surgical complications in hair transplantation: a series of 533 procedures. Aesthet Surg J 29:72, 2009.

33. Browlift

Joshua Lemmon, Michael R. Lee, David M. Knize

IDEAL FACIAL AESTHETICS[1-3]

FOREHEAD
- The forehead, including the eyebrows, comprises the upper third of an aesthetically proportioned face.
- The anterior hairline is typically 5-6 cm superior to the eyebrow level.
- Transverse, vertical, oblique, and glabellar forehead skin lines should be subtle and soft and rarely present without facial animation.
- *Dynamic rhytids* are skin lines present with facial animation. These rhytids are amenable to chemodenervation with botulinum toxin.
- *Static rhytids* are skin lines present without facial animation but with sustained facial muscle hypertonicity. Treatment of deep static rhytids may require surgical treatment with redraping of the involved skin.

IDEAL EYEBROW SHAPE AND POSITION WILL VARY BY GENDER
- **Female** (Fig. 33-1)
  - The eyebrow forms a gentle arch that peaks at the junction of the middle and lateral thirds just above the lateral limbus of the eye.
  - Eyebrow level is typically 3-5 mm above the supraorbital rim.
  - Medially, the eyebrow begins at the level of a perpendicular line extending from the medial canthus through the outer edge of the ipsilateral nasal ala.
  - The lateral end of the eyebrow is positioned slightly higher than the medial end and extends laterally to the level of an oblique line that passes through the outer edge of the ipsilateral nasal ala and the lateral canthus.
  - The medial end of the eyebrow is club shaped, whereas the lateral end is tapered.

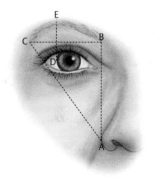

Fig. 33-1 Spatial relationships of the ideal eyebrow. (*A,* Nasal ala; *B,* medial bow; *C,* lateral tail of brow; *D,* lateral limbus; *E,* brow apex.)

- **Male**
  - Eyebrow level is at or near the level of the supraorbital rim.
  - The shape is relatively horizontal with minimal arching or peaking.
- **Effects of change in position of the eyebrow segments for males and females**
  - The medial eyebrow segment projects an angry appearance when this segment is depressed and a surprised appearance when it is elevated.
  - The lateral eyebrow segment projects a sad and tired appearance when this segment is depressed and a quizzical appearance when it is elevated.

ANATOMY[3-8]

SOFT TISSUE LAYERS OF THE FOREHEAD
- Skin
- Subcutaneous tissue
- Superficial plane of the galea aponeurosis
- Frontalis muscle
- Deep plane of the galea aponeurosis
- Loose areolar tissue
- Periosteum

GALEA APONEUROSIS
- At the origin of the frontalis muscle from the galea aponeurosis at approximately the level of the frontal hairline, the galea aponeurosis splits into a **superficial** and a **deep** layer, and these layers **encase the frontalis muscle.**
  - In the midforehead region, the deep galeal plane splits again to envelop the galeal fat pad, which extends down over the lower forehead to the eyebrow level.
- Deep to the lower third of the galea fat pad in the lower forehead region, the deep galeal plane splits again to form the *glide plane space,* located under the transverse head of the corrugator muscle as this muscle passes through the galeal fat pad area.
- The deepest layer of the deep galeal plane extends inferiorly to the supraorbital rims and bonds with the periosteum over a 2 cm wide horizontal strip just cephalad to the supraorbital rims.

BONY ANATOMY, ZONES OF FIXATION, AND RETAINING STRUCTURES
- The **supraorbital rim** is palpable above the upper eyelid and serves as a fixed position from which to assess eyebrow ptosis.
- The **temporal ridge** along the lateral margin of the frontal bone is produced by the temporal fusion line of the skull. The temporal ridge delineates the forehead area from the temporal fossa area.
- The soft tissues of the forehead are fused to the underlying bony skeleton in specific areas, and these areas must be adequately released from bone to effectively reposition the soft tissues.
- Just medial to the temporal ridge, the layers of the deep galeal plane of the forehead and scalp bond with the underlying periosteum and fuse to bone within a 5-6 mm wide zone of fixation (Fig. 33-2).
- The *orbital ligament* is a fibrous band that secures the superficial temporal fascia to the superolateral orbital rim near the lateral end of the eyebrow (see Fig. 33-6).
- Over the lower 2 cm of the frontal bone just above the supraorbital rims, the deep galeal plane and periosteum are fused together and fixed to bone, as described previously. Otherwise, the overlying skin, subcutaneous tissue, and frontalis muscle move freely over the orbital rim without direct attachment to bone.
- The **medial eyebrow segment is less mobile** than the lateral segment because of the anchoring effect produced by the supraorbital and supratrochlear nerves that exit bone and pass through the overlying medial frontalis muscle.

SENIOR AUTHOR TIP: Some authors have described a brow-retaining ligament[7] under the medial end of the eyebrow, but I think no ligaments are present between bone and dermis under the medial end of the eyebrow that restrict movement of the medial eyebrow.

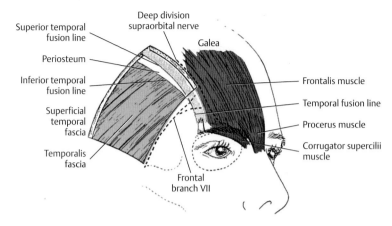

Fig. 33-2   The temporal fossa and forehead structures. Both the confluence of the superficial temporal fascia with the galea aponeurotica and the confluence of the temporalis fascia with the frontal bone periosteum are located within the zone of fixation *(stippled area)*. These planes are bonded together, and their deeper layers are fixed to bone over the 5-6 mm wide zone of fixation just medial to the temporal fusion line and the superior temporal line. The lateral margin of the frontalis muscle either terminates or abruptly attenuates over this zone. The inferior temporal line of the skull forms the perimeter of the temporalis fascia. The plane of the frontal branch of the facial nerve within the superficial temporal fascia is shown.

MUSCLES OF THE FOREHEAD (Fig. 33-3)

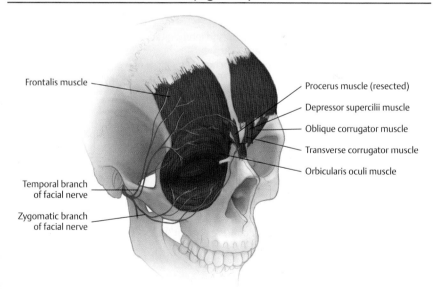

Fig. 33-3   Periorbital motor nerves and the muscles they activate. Corrugator supercilii muscle; depressor supercilii muscle; frontalis muscle; procerus muscle; temporal branch of facial nerve; zygomatic branch of the facial nerve; zygomaticus major muscle.

FRONTALIS
- **Origin:** Galea aponeurosis (at approximately the level of the typical frontal hairline)
- **Insertion:** Primarily interdigitates with the orbicularis oculi and procerus muscles, which insert into the dermis under the eyebrows
- **Innervation:** Frontal (temporal) branch of facial nerve (CN VII)
- **Action:** Eyebrow elevation primarily produced by suspending the superior orbicularis oculi muscle. Muscle contraction produces transverse forehead skin lines.

CORRUGATOR SUPERCILII
- **Origin:** Superomedial orbital rim
- **Insertion:**
  - *Oblique head* inserts into dermis under the medial head of the eyebrow.
  - *Transverse head* inserts into dermis under the middle third of the eyebrow.

> **NOTE:**   Clinically, the two heads of the muscle are often not clearly delineated, because the fibers sometime rapidly coalesce into a singular corrugator muscle mass.

- **Innervation:**
  - *Oblique head*
    - ▶ Zygomatic branches of the facial nerve
  - *Transverse head*
    - ▶ Frontal branch
- **Action:** Movement of the medial eyebrow medially and downward, which produces vertical and oblique lines in the glabellar skin

PROCERUS
- **Origin:** Dorsal surface of the nasal bones
- **Insertion:** Dermis in the glabellar region and interdigitation with the inferior medial fibers of the frontalis muscle on each side
- **Innervation:** Frontal and zygomatic branches of the facial nerve
- **Action:** Medial eyebrow depression, which produces transverse rhytids at the nasal root

ORBICULARIS OCULI
- **Origin:** Various structures in the medial canthal region
- **Insertion:** Dermis under the medial brow and the lateral palpebral raphe
- **Innervation:** Zygomatic branch of the facial nerve
- **Action:** Flat, circumferential sphincter muscle of the eyelids that primarily provides eyelid closure
  - The medial orbital portion depresses the medial brow and contributes to oblique skin line formation in the glabellar area.
  - The lateral orbital portion depresses the lateral brow and creates radial, lateral periorbital rhytids with contraction ("crow's-feet").

DEPRESSOR SUPERCILII
- **Origin:** Superomedial orbital rim, where it is often described as a portion of the medial orbicularis oculi muscle
- **Insertion:** Dermis of the medial eyebrow (medial to the dermal insertion of the fibers from the orbicularis oculi muscle and anterior to the dermal insertion of the oblique head of the corrugator supercilii muscle)
- **Innervation:** Zygomatic branch of the facial nerve
- **Action:** Medial brow depression

VASCULAR SUPPLY TO THE FOREHEAD
- Supply is from branches of both the internal and external carotid arteries
- Centrally, **supraorbital** and **supratrochlear** arteries arise off the **internal carotid** artery from the ophthalmic artery.
- Laterally, frontal branches of the **superficial temporal** artery arise from the **external carotid** artery.
- Vast communications exist between these vessels of the forehead and those of the posterior scalp, providing rich vascularity.

SENSORY INNERVATION

SUPRATROCHLEAR NERVE[9]
- A branch of the ophthalmic division of the trigeminal nerve (V_1)
- Emerges from its bony foramen within the medial orbit along with the supratrochlear artery
- Pierces the medial end of the corrugator muscle and supplies sensation for the medial forehead skin on each side

SUPRAORBITAL NERVE[10]
- A branch of the **ophthalmic division of the trigeminal nerve (V_1).** The supraorbital nerve trunk emerges from its bony exit point, the supraorbital notch (or foramen), along with the supraorbital artery.
- The supraorbital nerve trunk divides into a **superficial** and **deep** division.
- **Superficial division**
  - Pierces the frontalis muscle after dividing from the supraorbital trunk and travels cephalad, first within the frontalis muscle and later in the subcutaneous plane to the frontal scalp level
  - Supplies sensation to the dermis of the forehead skin and anterior scalp on each side
- **Deep division**
  - After dividing from the supraorbital trunk, the deep division initially runs superolaterally over the surface of the periosteum.
  - When the deep branch is almost at the temporal ridge, it turns cephalad and runs parallel with the temporal ridge to the scalp, remaining within 0.5-1.5 cm medial to the ridge.
    - ▸ Along this course, this branch progressively passes up through the plane of the deep galea to terminate in the dermis of the frontoparietal scalp.
    - ▸ The deep division passes across the forehead and provides only a few tiny branches to periosteum in this part of its course.

NOTE: Coronal incisions made through the galeal plane always transect the deep branch at the level of the incision.

CAUTION: The deep division can also be injured over the lower forehead during dissection in the subgaleal plane, because this nerve moves from the surface of periosteum into the deep galea plane at a level approximately 2-3 cm above the orbital rim.

TIP: In about 10% of patients, the deep division of the supraorbital nerve exits the frontal bone from a foramen lateral to the supraorbital notch. This foramen is usually just medial to the temporal ridge and just superior to the laterosupraorbital rim. Surgeons must be prepared for the presence of the aberrant course of the deep division and prevent inadvertent transection, which would produce dysesthesia or anesthesia of the ipsilateral frontoparietal scalp.

PATIENT EVALUATION

HISTORY SHOULD INCLUDE
- Age
- Gender
- Bleeding tendency in the past
- Medications, including herbal medicines
- Other medical comorbities
- Patient's expectations for skin smoothness and eyebrow shape and position

ANALYSIS OF THE FOREHEAD SHOULD INCLUDE
- Eyebrow position, shape, and symmetry
- Presence of dynamic and/or static rhytids
- Presence of upper lid ptosis or dermatochalasis

HAIRLINE[11]
- **See the Surgical Techniques section for descriptions of techniques mentioned here.**
- **High hairline** typically describes a brow-to-hairline distance of >5 cm in women and >6 cm in men. In these cases, an **anterior hairline technique** to prevent further elevation of the hairline should be considered.
- **Low hairline** typically describes a brow-to-hairline distance of <5 cm in women and <6 cm in men. For these cases, a **coronal incision** should be considered to allow elevation of the hairline.
- **Atypical hairline** patients are often challenging, with thin or balding hair. Often, small incisions for **endoscopic-assisted procedures or custom incisions** are made for these patients (Fig. 33-4). For males who have residual hair in the temporal scalp area, the limited incision procedure is often appropriate.
- Guyuron and Lee[12] have published a treatment algorithm based on forehead elongation, forehead lines, and brow ptosis (Fig. 33-5).

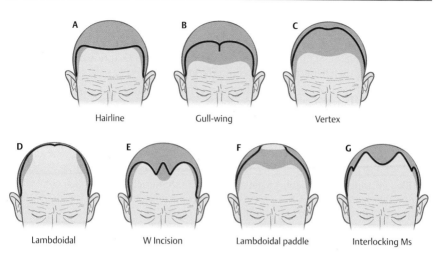

Fig. 33-4 Several types of coronal incisions used in browlift surgery. The indications for each are discussed in the text.

	Forehead Elongation Minimal	Forehead Elongation Moderate	Forehead Elongation Severe
Lines None or Minimal	Endoscopic forehead lift	Pretrichial incision Lateral brow suspension	Pretrichial incision Posterior scalp advancement
Lines Moderate	Endoscopic forehead lift Glabellar muscle resection or Limited incision and transpalpebral corrugator resection	Pretrichial incision Glabellar muscle resection Lateral brow suspension	Pretrichial incision Glabellar muscle resection Posterior scalp advancement Lateral brow suspension
Lines Severe	Incision 1-1.5 cm behind the hairline Subcutaneous dissection Glabellar musculature resection	Pretrichial incision Subcutaneous dissection Glabellar musculature resection Lateral brow suspension	Pretrichial incision Subcutaneous dissection Glabellar muscle resection Posterior scalp advancement Lateral brow suspension
	Minimal Brow Ptosis	**Moderate Brow Ptosis**	**Severe Brow Ptosis**

Fig. 33-5 Treatment algorithm for a senescent forehead.

OTHER CONSIDERATIONS
- Skin quality issues, such as the presence of actinic damage and/or dyschromia
- Adjunctive treatment methods to help restore skin tone and texture and to improve skin appearance (chemical peels, laser resurfacing, etc.)

PHOTOGRAPHS (see Chapter 3)
- Photos should include the AP, lateral, and oblique views of the entire face and a separate series of views of the forehead and periorbita.
- Dynamic photos are also useful for planning surgical treatment of frontalis and corrugator muscles.

> **TIP:** Postoperative patients sometimes question the surgical benefit they obtained from their surgical procedure. A review of the preoperative photographs will often help these patients to more fully appreciate their surgical result.

SURGICAL TECHNIQUES

PREOPERATIVE PLANNING
- These surgical techniques should be tailored to each patient, based on thorough analysis followed by thoughtful preoperative planning.
- This planning should include selection of the appropriate skin incision, the plane of dissection, options for muscle resection or alteration, and flap fixation method.
- Understanding the relationship between surgical goals and underlying anatomy is essential to delivering reliable aesthetic outcomes[13] (Boxes 33-1 and 33-2).

Box 33-1   *GOALS OF ANY FOREHEADPLASTY PROCEDURE*

Smoother glabellar skin lines
Smoother transverse nasal skin lines
Resuspend ptotic eyebrows
Resuspended pseudoexcess upper eyelid skin
Smoother transverse forehead skin lines

Box 33-2   *STRUCTURES THAT MUST BE RELEASED WITH ANY FOREHEADPLASTY PROCEDURE*

Zone of fixation
Orthical ligament
Periosteum/galea plan attachments to the superior orbital rim

INCISION OPTIONS
- **Direct forehead skin excision**
  - **Design**
    - ▶ Transverse elliptical excisions of forehead skin superior to the eyebrows at the superciliary or midforehead level are used to elevate the eyebrow.
    - ▶ The incisions are made within **deep transverse rhytids**, when possible, or along the **superior margin of the eyebrow** in an attempt to minimize scar visibility.

- **Advantages**
  - ▶ Simplicity
  - ▶ The proximity of the skin excision to the eyebrow provides for predictable, stable eyebrow elevation
  - ▶ Allows easy correction of eyebrow asymmetry
  - ▶ Excellent option in men with baldness and transverse forehead rhytids, when coronal, temporal, and endoscopic incision scars cannot be hidden
- **Disadvantages**
  - ▶ Visible scarring is present in some cases.
  - ▶ Forehead and anterior scalp hypesthesia can be permanent.
- ■ **Transblepharoplasty**
  - • **Design**
    - ▶ The suborbicularis oculi fascia under the lateral eyebrow is sutured to periosteum through an upper blepharoplasty incision.
    - ▶ The eyebrow is modestly elevated.
  - • **Advantages**
    - ▶ A simultaneous blepharoplasty can be performed, if indicated.
    - ▶ Incisional scars are limited and minimally visible.
    - ▶ Sensory innervation of the forehead and scalp can be preserved.
    - ▶ Resection of the corrugator supercilii muscle and transection of the procerus muscle can be accomplished while using this approach.[9,14]
  - • **Disadvantages**
    - ▶ Although corrugator supercilii muscle resection and procerus muscle transection can be done under direct vision in conjunction with this technique, these muscle modifications require a working understanding of the local anatomy.
    - ▶ Elevation of the eyebrow is often limited.

SENIOR AUTHOR TIP: It is always more efficient to suspend tissues rather than attempt to "push them up" to elevate the tissues. When the transblepharoplasty approach is used to elevate the eyebrow, the eyebrow tissue must be "pushed up," and this limited elevation is maintained with sutures placed into the periosteum. The range of elevation of the eyebrow is far more limited than with the use of any one of the other eyebrow suspension procedures. However, it is often the "last resort" procedure for totally bald males who will not accept more visible scarring than is produced with a blepharoplasty. In my (D.K.) experience, the transblepharoplasty approach provides excellent access to treat the corrugator supercilii, depressor supercilii, medial orbicularis oculi, and procerus muscles that produce glabellar skin lines.

- ■ **Coronal**
  - • **Design**
    - ▶ A coronal incision (see Fig. 33-4) is made in the hair-bearing scalp with the angle of the scalpel blade positioned to be **parallel to the hair follicles** when the incision is made.
    - ▶ With the incision placed approximately 5 cm posterior to the frontal hairline, a 2-3 cm wide strip of scalp along the anterior edge of the incision can be excised and the forehead flap advanced to leave the final position of the postoperative scar at least 2 cm posterior to the frontal hairline.
    - ▶ The dissection plane for elevation of the forehead flap is usually at the **subgaleal level**.

> **TIP:** For every 1 mm of eyebrow elevation desired, the frontal hairline must be elevated about 1.5 cm with cephalad transposition of the forehead flap.

- **Advantages**
  - ▶ Direct access to the entire surface of the frontal bone periosteum is possible, with direct visualization of all of the muscles whose actions produce glabellar skin rhytids.
  - ▶ Because this technique elevates the frontal hairline, it can be useful for patients presenting with a low frontal hairline.
  - ▶ Surgical scar is in hair-bearing scalp.
- **Disadvantages**
  - ▶ Risk of postsurgical alopecia
  - ▶ Expected scalp paresthesias posterior to the incision
  - ▶ Should not be performed in patients with a high frontal hairline (unless the incision is placed in the anterior hairline position, as described below).
- **Anterior hairline**
  - **Design**
    - ▶ The incision is typically made along the anterior hairline and carried into the hair-bearing temporal scalp on each side.
    - ▶ The beveled incision **perpendicular to the hair follicles** transects the hair follicles at the hairline, as shown in Fig. 33-6, with the goal that these transected hair follicles will regrow through the scar[15] and hide it.

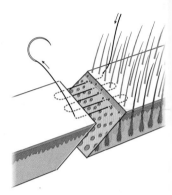

Fig. 33-6 An anterior hairline incision is beveled perpendicular to the hair follicles so that hair can grow into and anterior to the scar.

> **TIP:** Sometimes it may be beneficial to create a wavy, rather than straight, incision so as to camouflage a straight-line scar.

- **Advantages**
  - ▶ Can maintain the preoperative hairline level, or it can lower the anterior hairline for patients who present with a high hairline requesting a lower anterior hairline.
- **Disadvantages**
  - ▶ Depending on hairstyle, the incision can be relatively visible.
  - ▶ The same issues described for the coronal procedure (sensation changes, incisional alopecia, etc.).
- **Limited incision[16]**
  - **Design**
    - ▶ Historically, was used to address lateral brow ptosis, but was only marginally effective because of inadequate soft tissue release from bone. Current design incorporates wide soft tissue release from bone through bilateral 4.5 cm long temporal scalp incisions to allow effective forehead flap transposition and eyebrow elevation.
    - ▶ After incisions are made in the hair-bearing temporal scalp bilaterally, the zone of fixation along the temporal ridge is released before subperiosteal dissection of

the forehead flap. This protects the deep division of the supraorbital nerve (Fig. 33-7), which runs superficial to periosteum en route to the anteroparietal scalp.
► The temporal fossa area is dissected between the superficial temporal and deep temporal fascial planes.
► The advanced forehead flap is fixated by suturing the superficial temporal fascia lining the flap to the stable deep temporal fascia.

TIP: If medial eyebrow elevation is indicated, this can be accomplished by weakening the medial eyebrow depressor muscles in the glabellar muscle complex using the transblepharoplasty approach. This will allow unopposed frontalis muscle tone to modestly elevate the medial eyebrow segment.

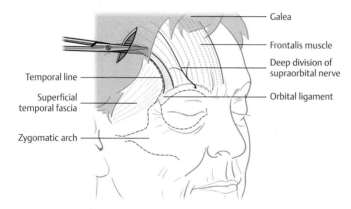

Fig. 33-7 Eyebrow elevation through a limited incision in the temporal scalp. A forehead flap is raised at the subperiosteal level. Here, the orbital ligament is transected for maximum upward movement of the superficial temporal fascia.

• **Advantages**
  ► Sensory innervation of the forehead is spared, especially the sensory innervation of the anteroparietal scalp.
  ► The lateral and middle eyebrow segments are effectively elevated.
  ► The short incision scars are in hair-bearing scalp.
• **Disadvantages**
  ► Closing the scalp incisions under tension risks alopecia.
  ► Limited exposure to the corrugator muscle group and the procerus muscle requires additional techniques. This browlift procedure is usually combined with a transblepharoplasty approach to the glabellar area to resect/modify these muscles.
  ► The technique does not elevate the medial end of the eyebrow without additional techniques. The medial eyebrow depressor muscles (procerus, depressor supercilii, and oblique head of the corrugator supercilii muscles and the medial fibers of the orbicularis oculi muscle) are treated with the addition of the transblepharoplasty approach to the glabellar area.
  ► The ability to address deep transverse forehead rhytids is limited with techniques that require access to the deep surface of the frontalis muscle.

> **TIP:** The scalp wound-closure tension should be borne by the superficial temporal fascia lining the forehead flap and not by the skin level of the flap. Tension-free reapproximation of the scalp skin wound edges will minimize local ischemia, which will preserve hair follicles and result in less scalp scarring.

- **Endoscopic-assisted**
  - **Design**
    - ▶ Developed to minimize long scars, scalp paresthesias, and scalp alopecia
    - ▶ Typically include a central incision and small, bilateral temporal incisions to elevate the forehead flap, usually at the subperiosteal level
    - ▶ Critics argue that these techniques are less powerful, because they simply reposition redundant skin rather than excise it, but no studies have demonstrated a superiority of specific techniques.
    - ▶ The zone of fixation and the periorbital attachments of periosteum/galea are released, and the eyebrows are elevated with the advanced forehead flap, which is fixated in its new position using a variety of fixation methods (see Methods of Fixation section).
  - **Advantages**
    - ▶ Small (1.5 cm) scalp incisions
    - ▶ Preservation of sensation
    - ▶ Excellent visualization of glabellar muscles for resection/modification
  - **Disadvantages**
    - ▶ Steep learning curve
    - ▶ Additional expensive endoscopic equipment is required.
    - ▶ Limited ability to address deep transverse forehead rhytids

DISSECTION PLANES FOR ELEVATION OF A FOREHEAD FLAP

SUBCUTANEOUS
- **Concept**
  - Less invasive plane of dissection, and the elevated skin flap allows direct elevation of the eyebrow
  - Used relatively infrequently today
- **Advantages**
  - Simple anatomic dissection
  - Preserves scalp sensation because deep division of the supraorbital nerve is deep to the level of dissection
  - No requirement to release soft tissues from bone because transposed skin plane elevates the eyebrows
  - Treatment of deep transverse forehead rhytids is facilitated with skin redraping.
  - Hairline position can be lowered or raised.

■ **Disadvantages**
  • **Forehead flap vascularity is decreased**, which may increase risks of skin slough and scalp alopecia.
  • Sensibility of the central forehead can be decreased by trauma to branches of the supratrochlear nerve and the superficial division of the supraorbital nerve that run in the subcutaneous plane. This sensory loss is usually only temporary, however.
  • Transition to a deeper plane is required to treat the corrugator and procerus muscles.

SUBGALEAL
■ **Concept**
  • Historically, this "natural cleft" in the forehead soft tissues invites its use for dissection.
■ **Advantages**
  • Relatively avascular dissection plane
  • Allows excellent exposure of the deep surface of the frontalis muscle for scoring and excision, in the infrequent cases where frontalis muscle modification is indicated
  • Allows rapid dissection for forehead flap elevation
  • Can facilitate dissection of the forehead flap through dissection from the subgaleal plane into the "glide plane" space

---

TIP: The *glide plane space* exists within the layers of the deep galeal plane over the lower forehead. This space is filled with only areolar tissue, and it provides gliding surfaces for the movement of the overlying transverse head of the corrugator supercilii muscle.

■ **Disadvantages**
  • Will place the deep division of the supraorbital nerve at risk of transection (see Sensory Innervation section).

SUBPERIOSTEAL
■ **Concept**
  • Developed as an alternative to the subgaleal plane
  • Most frequently used in endoscopic-assisted and limited-incision techniques
■ **Advantages**
  • Plane relatively avascular
  • Avoids deep division of the supraorbital nerve
  • All vascularized tissues of the forehead are elevated into the forehead flap.
  • Some authors argue that the inelasticity of the periosteum allows a more sustained forehead flap elevation.
■ **Disadvantages**
  • Periosteal and galeal attachments along the superior and lateroorbital rims must be released to allow forehead flap transposition.
  • Periosteum must be penetrated to treat the muscles that act on glabellar skin.

METHODS OF FIXATION[17]

- ▪ **Concept**
  - Once the forehead flap has been transposed to the desired position, stable fixation of flap position is performed to maintain the surgical result at the eyebrow level. Some authors question the need for fixation,[18] whereas others suggest the need to secure at multiple locations.[19]

> **TIP:**   According to the "elastic band principle," the effectiveness of any fixation method to suspend a forehead flap decreases as the suspension point is placed farther from the eyebrow level. However, the decision where to place a fixation point involves the "trade off" between this advantage of proximity to the eyebrow and the undesirable cosmetic effects that the method of fixation produces.

- ▪ **Skin excision**
  - When skin is excised immediately superior to the eyebrow using the "direct" technique, the amount of eyebrow elevation is usually **equal to the width of the elliptical skin excision at a 1:1 ratio**, and the tension of the wound closure is usually sufficient to maintain long-term fixed eyebrow position.
  - After scalp is excised from the leading edge of the forehead flap with the coronal technique, closure of the resultant scalp wound similarly becomes the fixation method. In contrast to the "direct" technique, however, the scalp tissue must be advanced approximately **1.5 cm** to obtain **1 mm** of eyebrow elevation because of the greater distance of the fixation point from the eyebrow. In this and any method of skin excision fixation, wound-closure tension requires care to prevent local ischemia and secondary wound-healing issues, including scalp alopecia.
- ▪ **Fascial suspension**
  - The eyebrow can be elevated when the galeal plane superior to the eyelid is vertically shortened using a plication suture technique and produces a stable fixation effect.
  - Suturing the galea to periosteum can elevate the eyebrow with long-term effectiveness.
  - A screw placed into the skull or a short tunnel made in the outer cortex of the skull can serve as an anchor point for a suture to suspend the galea plane to elevate and fix the eyebrow level.
- ▪ **Novel devices** (see Chapter 26)
  - Absorbable anchoring devices are emerging to facilitate stable fixation of soft tissue to bone.
  - Technical difficulty is decreased.

SURGICAL MODIFICATION OF MUSCLE

■ **Concept**
  • Skin lines and grooves occur in a perpendicular orientation to the direction of contraction of the underlying muscles. Resection or modification of the underlying muscle can be expected to make the rhytid less deep and make the skin smoother. Although chemodenervation of muscle with botulinum toxin yields excellent, but temporary, control of motor function, surgical treatment offers permanent control.

■ **Frontalis**
  • This muscle can be "scored" (incised) either horizontally, vertically, or both to denervate the muscle; however, this technique is infrequently used today.
  • A strip of the muscle can be excised to weaken its capacity to contract.
  • When these techniques are used, care must be taken to preserve the inferior 2 cm of frontalis muscle to maintain enough residual function to move the eyebrows.

SENIOR AUTHOR TIP: These techniques often produce a forehead with a "frozen'" appearance and are uncommonly done today. The transverse forehead line formation can often be remarkably improved, while retaining normal frontalis muscle function, simply by removing excess upper eyelid skin with a blepharoplasty. The presence of excess upper eyelid skin stimulates reflex hypertonicity of the frontalis muscle to elevate the eyebrow and lift the irritating skin off of the eyelid at the expense of transverse forehead line formation. After removal of the excess skin producing the reflex, the forehead skin becomes smoother. However, eliminating this reflex will also result in a lower eyebrow level in the absence of the induced frontalis muscle tone that had suspended them. Performing an upper blepharoplasty without also planning for management of eyebrow position can result in the cosmetic problem of undesirably low positioned eyebrows. This issue should always be considered when planning to do only an upper blepharoplasty procedure on a patient. In my (D.K.) experience, it is often unwise to do an upper blepharoplasty without also performing some form of browlift procedure.

■ **Muscles that act on glabellar skin**
  • Resection of the corrugator supercilii muscle group
  • Transection of the procerus muscle
  • Myotomy of the medial fibers of the orbicularis oculi muscle

SENIOR AUTHOR TIP: In my experience, complete rather than partial excision of the corrugator supercilii muscle group is advisable. When the corrugator muscle is only partially excised, the remaining muscle fibers will continue to contract, and this often produces the appearance of small "horns" in the glabellar area. In contrast, simple transection of the procerus muscle has proved adequate treatment to weaken this muscle's function with its production of transverse lines across the root of the nose. The function of the medial fibers of the orbicularis oculi muscle to produce oblique glabellar skin lines can be controlled with a 1 x 1 cm myotomy directly under the medial head of the eyebrow.

- To prevent excessive brow widening, the medial retaining structures must not be overly released.[20]

> **SENIOR AUTHOR TIP:**   The existence of medial retaining ligaments is not agreed on in the literature. Ligamentous structures adherent to the medial supraorbital rim bind with the overlying deep galeal plane. However, there is no anatomic evidence that these structures extend more superficially into the plane of the frontalis muscle or orbicularis oculi muscle, much less into the dermis under the medial end of the eyebrow. To "retain" the medial eyebrows from bone, any retaining ligament would have to pass through the frontalis muscle to the overlying dermis. Widening of the medial ends of the eyebrows has been observed after browlift procedures that include modification or resection of the transverse head of the corrugator supercilii muscle, whose contraction causes the medial ends of the eyebrows to move closer together. When this muscle is excised, the medial eyebrows would be expected to move apart, perhaps to the level that they were before hypertonicity of the corrugator supercilii muscle developed over time.

POSTOPERATIVE CARE

FOCUSED ON LIMITING EDEMA AND PROTECTING THE EYES
- Elevate head above the level of the heart.
- Apply continuous cool compresses over the eyes.
- Saline eye drops and protective ointments are important when blepharoplasty is performed concurrently with a browlift procedure, because temporary lagophthalmos is frequently present. Often, a temporary lateral tarsorrhaphy is effective.
- Drains are often placed and are usually removed in 24 hours.
  - Sutures in the eyelids are removed in 5-7 days, and surgical staples or sutures in the scalp are removed in 7-14 days.

COMPLICATIONS

- **Scalp paresthesias**
  - Dissection with the limited incision, endoscopic-assisted, and subcutaneous browlift technique can protect the deep division of the supraorbital nerve from permanent injury, although temporary paresthesias of the forehead skin and/or scalp occur often.
  - With **anterior hairline** or **coronal** incisions, the deep division of the supraorbital nerve is usually transected, producing **permanent dyesthesias** posterior to the level of the incision.
  - Injury to the deep division of the supraorbital nerve is more common with subgaleal dissection.
  - When this outcome is expected, it should be explained to patients as part of appropriate informed consent.
  - Byun et al[21] conducted a systematic review and reported technique-associated complications:
    - **Anterior hairline incision with subcutaneous dissection**: Alopecia (8.5%), paresthesia (5.4%), scar revision (2.1%), skin necrosis (1.8%)
    - **Coronal incision with subperiosteal dissection:** Nerve injury (6.4%), scar revision (2.5%), hematoma (1.0%)

▶ **Endoscopic techniques with subperiosteal dissection** had the highest number of complications overall: Asymmetry (3.6%), lagophthalmos (2.7%), recurrence (2.4%).

■ **Postsurgical alopecia of the scalp**
  • Thinning or loss of scalp hair can result from excessively tight wound closure, which can produce local ischemia.
  • Thermal injury from superficial use of monopolar cautery can destroy hair follicles. Use of bipolar cautery might limit the zone of thermal injury.

■ **Facial nerve injury**
  • The frontal (temporal) branch of the facial nerve is vulnerable to injury from excessive traction or transection during dissection in the temporal fossa area.
  • A working knowledge of the anatomy of this nerve is essential for browlift procedures.

■ **Overelevation of the medial eyebrow segment**
  • Excessive elevation of the eyebrow produces a "surprised" appearance, and this problem is very difficult to correct.

TIP: Although the lateral eyebrow segment must always be elevated, elevation of the medial segment is rarely indicated.

■ **Contour deformities**
  • Skin surface deformities can result from aggressive scoring or excision of the frontalis muscle.
  • A skin depression across the root of the nose at the level of transection of the procerus muscle can occur. A small graft of fascia placed across the transected procerus muscle has been effective.
  • Resection of the corrugator supercilii rarely leaves a skin depression or deformity. Some surgeons have placed soft tissue grafts, such as fat, in the area of the resected corrugator muscle, but this is usually unnecessary.

TOP TAKEAWAYS

➤ Surgeons who become students of forehead and temporal fossa anatomy will benefit from having more confidence in performing any browlift procedure, and patients will benefit by undergoing the procedure with less risk of a preventable complication.

➤ Surgeons should know the advantages and limitations of each browlift procedure and apply the appropriate procedure to each patient based on the unique presenting physical findings.

➤ Each patient should be carefully evaluated for appropriate indications for undergoing a surgical procedure and provided with appropriate informed consent to proceed with the surgical procedure.

➤ Every browlift procedure (except direct excision) requires adequate release of the soft tissues from their deep attachments before the tissues can be transposed cephalad.

➤ Reliable fixation of the transposed position is essential for reliable long-term stability of the surgical result.

➤ There is no clear evidence showing the superiority of either the open or endoscopic browlift technique.[22,23]

REFERENCES

1. Gunter JP, Antrobus SD. Aesthetic analysis of the eyebrows. Plast Reconstr Surg 99:1807, 1997.
2. Fruend RM, Nolan WB. Correlation between brow lift outcomes and aesthetic ideals for eyebrow height and shape in females. Plast Reconstr Surg 97:1343, 1996.
3. Codner MA, Kikkawa DO, Korn BS, et al. Blepharoplasty and brow lift. Plast Reconstr Surg 126:1e, 2010.
4. Knize DM, ed. The Forehead and Temporal Fossa: Anatomy and Technique. Philadelphia: Lippincott Williams & Wilkins, 2001.
5. Knize DM. Reassessment of the coronal incision and subgaleal dissection for foreheadplasty. Plast Reconstr Surg 102:478, 1998.
6. Knize DM. An anatomically based study of the mechanism of eyebrow ptosis. Plast Reconst Surg 97:1321, 1996.
7. Byrd HS, Burt JD. Achieving aesthetic balance in the brow, eyelids, and midface. Plast Reconstr Surg 110:926, 2002.
8. Janis JE, Ghavami A, Lemmon JA, et al. Anatomy of the corrugator supercilii muscle: part I. Corrugator topography. Plast Reconstr Surg 120:1647, 2007.
9. Janis JE, Hatef DA, Hagan R, et al. Anatomy of the supratrochlear nerve: implications for the surgical treatment of migraine headaches. Plast Reconstr Surg 131:743, 2013.
10. Janis JE, Ghavami A, Lemmon JA, et al. The anatomy of the corrugator supercilii muscle: part II. Supraorbital nerve branching patterns. Plast Reconstr Surg 121:233, 2008.
11. Janis JE, Potter JK, Rohrich RJ. Brow lift techniques. In Fagien S, ed. Putterman's Cosmetic Oculoplastic Surgery, ed 4. Philadelphia: Elsevier, 2007.
12. Guyuron B, Lee M. A reappraisal of surgical techniques and efficacy in forehead rejuvenation. Plast Reconstr Surg 134:426, 2014.
13. Knize DM. Anatomic concepts for brow lift procedures. Plast Reconstr Surg 124:2118, 2009.
14. Knize DM. Transpalpebral approach to the corrugator supercilii and procerus muscles. Plast Reconstr Surg 95:52; discussion 61, 1995.
15. Guyuron B. Corrugator supercilii resection through blepharoplasty incision. Plast Reconstr Surg 107:606, 2001.
16. Camirand A, Doucet J. A comparison between parallel hairline incisions and perpendicular incision when performing a facelift. Plast Reconstr Surg 99:10, 1997.
17. Knize DM. Limited-incision forehead lift for eyebrow elevation to enhance upper blepharoplasty. Plast Reconstr Surg 97:1334, 1996.
18. Rohrich RJ, Beran SJ. Evolving fixation methods in endoscopically assisted forehead rejuvenation: controversies and rationale. Plast Reconstr Surg 100:1575, 1997.
19. Troilius C. Subperiosteal brow lifts without fixation. Plast Reconstr Surg 114:1597, 2004.
20. Drolet BC, Phillips BZ, Hoy EA, et al. Finesse in forehead and brow rejuvenation: modern concepts, including endoscopic methods. Plast Reconstr Surg 134:1141, 2014.
21. Byun S, Mukovozov I, Farrokhyar F, et al. Complications in brow lift techniques: a systematic review. Plast Reconstr Surg 130(5S-1):S90, 2012.
22. Sullivan PK, Saloman JA, Woo AS, et al. The importance of the retaining ligamentous attachments of the forehead for selective eyebrow reshaping and forehead rejuvenation. Plast Reconstr Surg 117:95, 2006.
23. Graham DW, Heller J, Kurkjian TJ, et al. Brow lift in facial rejuvenation: a systematic literature review of open versus endoscopic techniques. Plast Reconstr Surg 128:335e, 2011.

34. Upper Blepharoplasty

Ashkan Ghavami, Foad Nahai

RELEVANT ANATOMY[1-3] (Fig. 34-1)

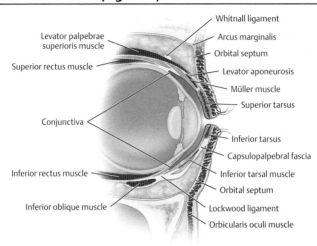

Fig. 34-1 Cross section of the upper and lower eyelids.

Upper Eyelid Layers

- **Anterior lamella:** Skin, subcutaneous tissue (retroorbicularis oculi fat [ROOF] and suborbicularis oculi fat [SOOF]), and orbicularis oculi muscle (OOM)
- **Middle lamella:** Orbital septum

> **NOTE:** Problems in this layer most commonly lead to the continuum of cicatricial contraction (more common in the lower lid).

- **Posterior lamella:** Tarsus and conjunctiva

ORBICULARIS OCULI MUSCLE

- **Innervation** (Fig. 34-2)
  - Frontal, zygomatic, and buccal contributions from facial nerve (CN VII)
  - Medial and lateral innervation points

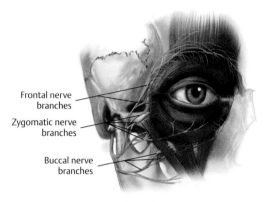

Frontal nerve
branches

Zygomatic nerve
branches

Buccal nerve
branches

Fig. 34-2   Medial and lateral innervation points warrant consideration of orbicularis oculi muscle nerve preservation (particularly the pretarsal portion) to avoid postoperative adverse effects.

- **Three portions** (Fig. 34-3)

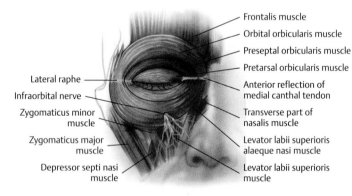

Frontalis muscle

Orbital orbicularis muscle

Preseptal orbicularis muscle

Pretarsal orbicularis muscle

Lateral raphe

Infraorbital nerve

Zygomaticus minor
muscle

Zygomaticus major
muscle

Depressor septi nasi
muscle

Anterior reflection of
medial canthal tendon

Transverse part of
nasalis muscle

Levator labii superioris
alaeque nasi muscle

Levator labii superioris
muscle

Fig. 34-3   Muscular anatomy of the periorbital region.

TIP: Considering the OOM as a sphincter muscle with three segments facilitates understanding the consequences of eyelid surgery, botulinum toxin administration, ligament release, and preservation of muscle innervation.

- **Orbital**
  - ▶ Outermost portion
    - ◆ Superficial to corrugator supercilii muscle (CSM) and procerus muscles
      - – Interdigitates laterally and medially with CSM under dermis and with frontalis muscle fibers
  - ▶ Voluntary action
  - ▶ Functions as **tight closure of eye**
- **Preseptal**
  - ▶ Directly overlies septum
  - ▶ Voluntary and involuntary components
  - ▶ Assists with **blinking mechanism**
- **Pretarsal**
  - ▶ Tightly adherent to tarsal plate
  - ▶ Involuntary
  - ▶ Responsible for **blink mechanism**
  - ▶ Innervation from zygomatic branch of facial nerve
  - ▶ Most involved in **proper tear movement**

TIP: The preseptal orbicularis is adherent to the septum, and careful dissection in the proper submuscular plane is required. No pinkish hue or transverse fibers should be left on the septum, which would indicate retained orbicularis fibers and an improper plane. At least a **6 mm** strip of pretarsal orbicularis must be preserved for proper eyelid "sphincter" function.

TARSOLIGAMENTOUS COMPLEX

- **Upper tarsus**
  - • 7-11 mm wide
  - • Müller muscle inserts onto superior border of tarsal plate.
  - • Anterior levator aponeuorosis fibers insert onto superior tarsal border.
- **Fascial insertions on the upper border of the tarsus1-4:**
  - • Help to form shape, position, and magnitude of upper eyelid crease
  - • Levator aponeurosis
  - • Orbital septum
- **Orbicularis fascia:** Firmly attached at posterior surface of orbicularis "sphincter"; fuses with levator aponeurosis at level of lid fold; offers mechanical and nutritional (possibly lymphatic) support[4]
  - • Fuses with orbicularis retaining ligament (ORL)[5-9]
- **Conjoined fascia:** Present between the eyelid fold and lash line (deep to orbicularis and superficial to tarsal plate). This is an extension or fusion of the orbicularis fascia with the levator aponeurosis at a variable location superior to the tarsus.
- **Lateral raphe**
  - • Lateral extension of the OOM along the lateral orbital rim and zygomatic complex
  - • Deep and superficial components of orbicularis insertion form lateral canthal tendon and lateral raphe.
  - • Contributes to *"lateral orbital thickening"* against the lateral orbital rim, where the ORL fuses[5-7]
  - • Acts as lateral anchor (fulcrum) for eyelids

- **Lateral canthal tendon (anterior and posterior limbs)** (Fig. 34-4)
  - Formed by:
    - ► Lateral horn of levator palpebrae superioris
    - ► Lockwood ligament
    - ► Check ligament of the lateral rectus muscle
    - ► Deep preseptal and pretarsal orbicularis muscle

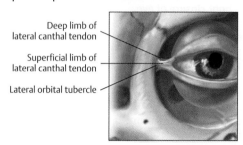

Deep limb of
lateral canthal tendon

Superficial limb of
lateral canthal tendon

Lateral orbital tubercle

Fig. 34-4   The lateral canthal tendon has posterior and anterior limbs.

MEDIAL CANTHAL TENDON
- Tripartite structure (anterior horizontal, posterior horizontal, and vertical components)
- Formed by:
  - Deep head of pretarsal orbicularis
  - Medial Lockwood ligament
  - Check ligament of medial rectus muscle
  - Whitnall ligament

ORBICULARIS RETAINING LIGAMENT[6-9] (Fig. 34-5)
- Also known as *orbitomalar ligament*[8] or *malar septum*[9] in lower periorbita
- "Near-circumferential" retaining structure encircling upper and lower orbit[7]
- Lax and longer laterally; more taut (short) medially
  - Lateral laxity may partially explain lateral hooding.
  - Medial tightness may be the reason for lack of medial hooding and tear trough phenomenon (medial depression/line at inferomedial periorbita).
- Extends from OOM to the periosteum
- True retaining ligament
- May have lymphatic properties
- Protects ocular contents: Semipermeable membrane

TIP: Blunt or sharp transection/disruption of ORL helps to smooth the tear trough and blend the lid-cheek junction. Release in the upper periorbita is required for effective browlifting. Medial preservation in the corrugator region may minimize medial brow splaying.

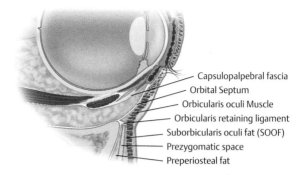

Fig. 34-5   Orbicularis retaining ligament (*ORL*). Orbicularis oculi muscle (*OOM*).

PRESEPTAL FAT
- Between orbital septum and orbicularis muscle
- Can contribute to upper eyelid lateral hooding
- **Upper lid:** ROOF
- **Lower lid:** SOOF

ORBITAL SEPTUM
- Protective function
- Extension of orbital periosteum
  - Fuses with periosteum to form the *arcus marginalis* in upper and lower periorbita
- **Upper septum:** Extends from superior orbital rim to insertion on levator aponeurosis at varying levels (10-15 mm above superior tarsal border)
- **Lower septum:** Extends from inferior orbital rim to the capsulopalpebral fascia (5 mm below lower tarsal border)
- Can have attachments with the ORL

LEVATOR PALPEBRAE MUSCLE
- **Muscle origin:** Lesser wing of sphenoid
- **Insertion:** Superior edge of tarsus (conjoined fascia)
- **Innervation:** CN III
- **Action:** 10-15 mm upper lid excursion and sustained lid elevation from contractile tone

NOTE: The amount of excursion and function is helpful in selecting an eyelid ptosis procedure.

- **Whitnall ligament:** Fascial condensation 14-20 mm from superior edge of tarsus. translates posterior vector of pull into a superior direction

TIP: The main cause of postoperative upper eyelid ptosis is "unrecognized" preoperative ptosis. Examination for upper eyelid ptosis preoperatively is essential.

Müller Muscle
- Posterior lamella of levator palpebrae muscle
- **Origin:** Levator muscle
- **Insertion:** Superior edge of tarsus
- **Innervation:** Sympathetic system
- **Action:** 2-3 mm of upper lid lift

> **TIP:**   If inadvertent lid ptosis is caused by diffusion of botulinum toxin as a result of improper technique (i.e., violation of the ORL), then the use of pharmacologic eyedrops that stimulate the Müller muscle can help until full levator function returns.

Orbital Fat Pads
- **Distinct compartments** (Fig. 34-6)
    - **Two** compartments in **upper** lid (medial and middle)
        - ▶ Medial is more pale, vascular, and fibrous.
        - ▶ Trochlea of superior oblique muscle separates the medial and middle compartments.
        - ▶ Minor lateral fat pad (Eisler fat pad) is present in some.
    - **Three** in **lower** lid (medial, central, and lateral)
        - ▶ Inferior oblique muscle separates medial and central compartments.

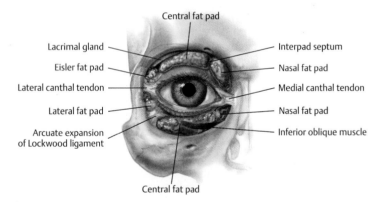

Central fat pad

Lacrimal gland —   — Interpad septum

Eisler fat pad —   — Nasal fat pad

Lateral canthal tendon —   — Medial canthal tendon

Lateral fat pad —   — Nasal fat pad

Arcuate expansion of Lockwood ligament —   — Inferior oblique muscle

Central fat pad

Fig. 34-6   Controversy exists regarding the true distinction of separate fat compartments; however, preservation of fat volume during blepharoplasty is a hallmark of the modern surgical approach.

Lacrimal Apparatus
- Palpebral and orbital segments separated by levator aponeurosis
- Located posterior to lateral portion of superior orbital rim
    - **Lacrimal drainage system**
        - ▶ Punctum drains to canaliculus, which drains to lacrimal sac, which drains to nasolacrimal duct.

  ▶ **Active pump mechanism**
    ◆ Blinking creates negative pressure in lacrimal sac, allowing tears to pass through the punctum and canaliculus into the sac.
    ◆ Eye opening increases sac pressure and passes tears into the nasolacrimal duct.

TEARS
- **Function**
  - Lubrication for lid excursion
  - Antibacterial properties
  - Oxygenation of corneal epithelium
  - Smooth, refractive globe surface
- **Three layers**
  - **Lipid layer:** Superficial and thin; reduces evaporative loss; secreted by meibomian glands and accessory sebaceous glands of Zeiss and Moll
  - **Aqueous:** Thicker, secreted from lacrimal gland and accessory glands of Wolfring and Krause
  - **Mucoid:** Maintains lid contact with globe; produced by mucin goblet cells
- **Basic secretion**
  - Accessory lacrimal glands of Wolfring and Krause, mucin goblet cells, and meibomian glands
- **Reflex secretion**
  - Main lacrimal gland, parasympathetic

INDICATIONS AND CONTRAINDICATIONS

CLASSIC INDICATIONS (UPPER EYELID)
- Excess upper eyelid skin
- Upper eyelid fold excess
- Lack of upper eyelid fold
  - Asian ethnicity with indistinct lid crease (see Chapter 34)

> **NOTE:** The fold may be present but masked by excess fat and poorly formed or positioned conjoined fascia.

- Fine periorbital or eyelid rhytids

> **TIP:** A brow evaluation is critical in all patients (see Chapter 33). Often, a browlift unmasks a poorly defined or visible upper lid crease.

EYELID PATHOLOGY AND DEFORMITIES
- **Dermatochalasis:** True excess of upper eyelid skin
- **Steatoblepharon:** Excess fat protruding through septum

- **Blepharochalasis**
  - Thin upper and lower lid skin allows presentation of cyclical lid edema (with or without erythema).
  - IgE and histamine are released.
  - In 80% of patients, onset is before 20 years of age.
  - Edema is refractory to antihistamines and steroids.
- **Blepharoptosis**
  - Drooping of upper eyelid
  - Measured by distance to light reflex of pupil (marginal reflex distance [MRD])
  - See Chapter 39 for further details.
- **Pseudoblepharoptosis**
  - Eyelid margin is in normal position; however, excess upper lid and/or brow weight is ptotic (MRD is within normal limits).
  - This may indicate blepharoplasty in conjunction with a browlift procedure.
- **Ptosis adipose:** Excess attenuation of canthus and septum

> **TIP:**   Blepharoptosis is not a contraindication to blepharoplasty, but it must be fully evaluated, informed, discussed, and treated.

> **SENIOR AUTHOR TIP:**   Eyelid ptosis should be corrected during blepharoplasty.

PREOPERATIVE EVALUATION

HISTORY
- Patient expectations
  - Functional versus aesthetic
  - Detailed discussion is needed to inform patients of the cause of the problem (with the aid of a handheld mirror) and what can be done to correct it.
  - Unrealistic expectations are unmasked and discussed.
  - Video imaging has been most helpful in discussing patients' expectations and whether they are realistic.

> **SENIOR AUTHOR TIP:**   With the Internet and media as a prevailing "pseudoeducational" force, patients may come in telling the doctor what procedure they need or want, as if ordering at a restaurant (e.g., "I don't want a browlift or anything fancy, just a little of this excess skin removed.") Patient education is more and more critical in today's practice environment. Surgeons should always recommend and do what they think is correct. Our job is to inform patients, make the recommendations that we think are best, and discuss the procedure or procedures, risks, and expected outcomes, including the quality of the result and the expected recovery. With this information, patients can make a truly informed decision.

PERTINENT MEDICAL CONDITIONS
- Eyelid inflammatory conditions (Reiter syndrome)
- Grave disease
- Benign essential blepharospasm

- Dry eye syndrome
  - Ask about eyedrop use and probe for details about dry eye symptomalogy.
  - Contact lens use
  - Bell phenomenon test
  - Consider Schirmer test

TIP: A history of dry eyes with decreased tear production (frequent use of eye lubricants), combined with postblepharoplasty tear film loss from lagophthalmos, can lead to corneal exposure (keratoconjunctivitis or ulceration). An abnormal Bell phenomenon increases the risk of corneal complications. A more conservative blepharoplasty with possible temporary tarsorrhaphy may be best versus no surgery at all for this group of patients.

- History of LASIK surgery
  - Best to **wait 12 months after LASIK surgery** to allow corneal incision time to heal

---

SENIOR AUTHOR TIP: Some ophthalmologists even recommend allowing 24 months to heal following LASIK surgery.

- Epiphora: Excess tearing
  - History of Bell palsy (crocodile tearing)
  - Gustatory epiphora
- Blepharoptosis
  - Discussed previously and in Chapter 39.
- General medical conditions
  - Coagulopathies
    - ▶ Anticoagulant/antiplatelet therapy or medication

CAUTION: Postoperative bleeding/hematoma after blepharoplasty is a serious complication that can lead to blindness. Early recognition is critical.

  - Severe "periorbital" allergic symptomatology
  - Thyroid dysfunction
  - Hypertension
  - Renal or cardiac abnormalities
  - Neurologic
    - ▶ Myasthenia gravis
    - ▶ Horner syndrome

OCULAR EXAMINATION

- The best **visual acuity** for each eye is recorded.
  - May require a more accurate assessment by an ophthalmologist (especially with insurance-related cases)
    - ▶ Patient referred to ophthalmologist if any abnormalities noted
- **Bell phenomenon:** If lids are forcibly held open while patient attempts to close them, then globe should rotate upward.
  - Built-in protective mechanism
  - When not present, patient more susceptible to dry eye exacerbation with even minimal postoperative lagophthalmos

LACRIMAL FUNCTION TEST
- Most important in elderly and patients with a history of dry eyes
  - May consider ophthalmologic referral preoperatively
- **Schirmer test I:** Basic and reflexive secretions
  - Whatman filter paper (Whatman, Inc.): 5 by 35 mm, distal 5 mm folded; fold placed on lateral sclera
  - More than 10 mm wetting after 5 minutes is normal.
- **Schirmer test II:** Basic secretion
  - Performed after topical anesthesia applied (eliminates reflex component)
  - Usually <40% of Schirmer test I
- More advanced tests: Tear film breakup, rose bengal staining, tear lysozyme electrophoresis

AESTHETIC EVALUATION (Fig. 34-7)

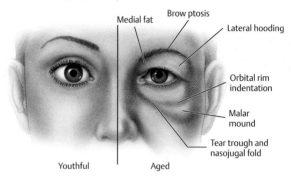

Medial fat
Brow ptosis
Lateral hooding
Orbital rim indentation
Malar mound
Tear trough and nasojugal fold
Youthful   Aged

Fig. 34-7   Characteristics of the aging periorbital region.

- **Forehead and brow**
  - **Brow asymmetry**
    - ▶ Compensated brow ptosis
      - ◆ Definition: Brow is ptotic but frontalis hyperactivity compensates.
      - ◆ With patient's eyes closed and brow fully relaxed (may require massage and major effort by surgeon during examination), frontalis is immobilized with gentle to moderate pressure/massage. Patient is then asked to open both eyes.
      - ◆ If brow position is lower than when the patient is looking straight forward, **compensated brow ptosis** is diagnosed.

> **NOTE:** If this test is not done, falsely positioned brows may lead to skin overresection, and upper blepharoplasty alone may exacerbate brow ptosis postoperatively.

- **Frontalis crease(s):** Indicate excessive frontalis hyperactivity
    - ▶ May require concomitant browlift with treatment of frontalis creases' relief of frontalis muscle activity
- **Glabellar lines**
    - ▶ Evaluate for CSM muscle hyperactivity.
    - ▶ Evaluate with patient in repose and in various positions of animation.

▶ Failure to treat overactive corrugators or moderate to severe glabellar lines and muscle bulging will produce imbalanced periorbital rejuvenation.
- **Supraorbital rim-to-globe relation**
  ▶ Often overlooked
  ▶ Distance and position of supraorbital rim relative to the superior globe margin will influence aesthetics.
  ▶ A deep sulcus or large distance may indicate less fat removal and possible fat injection.
  ▶ A shallow sulcus (short distance) may require more ROOF removal and more detailed sculpting of the sulcus.
  ▶ Prominence of orbital rim:
    ◆ Can exacerbate lateral lid-to-brow distance after blepharoplasty, resulting in an awkward appearance.
  ▶ General proptosis, enophthalmos, negative vector (for lower lid-to-malar tissue relation)
    ◆ Hertel exophthalmometer allows a more detailed evaluation.
    ◆ Normal globe prominence is **16-18 mm** from lateral orbital rim.

TIP: Transpalpebral corrugator muscle resection is a powerful adjunct to upper blepharoplasty when a full browlift is not indicated or desired by the patient. Recent anatomic details on the corrugator may assist in a more thorough and accurate resection.[10,11]

■ **Upper eyelid**
- **Measurements** (Fig. 34-8)
  ▶ **Palpebral fissure:** 12-14 mm vertically, 28-30 mm horizontally
  ▶ **Upper lid margin:** At level of upper limbus (may be slightly below; can be attractive in certain faces). Highest point is just medial to pupil.
  ▶ **Visible pretarsal skin:** 3-6 mm (may be cultural). Makeup preferences influence amount of show.
  ▶ **Lash line to supratarsal crease:** 7-8 mm in women and slightly more in men
  ▶ **Lateral canthus:** 1-2 mm above medial canthus (aesthetic canthal tilt)
    ◆ Look for excess scleral show if <1-2 mm, which may require concomitant canthoplasty.
  ▶ **Midpupillary line measurements:**
    ◆ Anterior hairline to brow: 5-6 cm
    ◆ Brow to orbital rim: 1 cm laterally at junction of first and second third
    ◆ Brow to supratarsal crease: 16 mm, minimum 12 mm
    ◆ Brow to midpupil: 2.5 cm

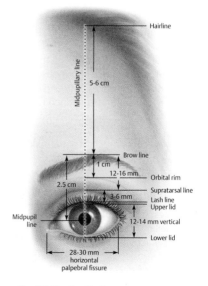

Fig. 34-8   Aesthetic measurements.

> **TIP:**   As with any aesthetic evaluation, sensitivity to ethnic and specific patient morphology is critical. For example, some patients may look better with their lid margin slightly below the upper limbus or a brow tail that is low.

- **Redundant skin**
  - Location of excess
  - Lateral hooding
  - Pseudoptosis
- **Position of supratarsal fold**
  - Examine this with patient in downward gaze.
  - High supratarsal fold indicates disassociation in conjoined fascia and possible levator malposition or dehiscence.
    - ▶ This should provide a clue about the possibility of ptosis.
- **Amount and location of excess orbital fat**[12]
  - "Pseudoherniation" of fat contents (weak septum)
  - Excess ROOF
  - Excess subcutaneous fat
  - Preaponeurotic fat (supralevator fat)
    - ▶ Lacrimal gland prolapse or ptosis
    - ▶ Fold asymmetry

> **NOTE:**   All asymmetries and findings should be pointed out to patients and documented in their chart.

ASIAN EYELID (see Chapter 36)
- **Anatomy: Smaller features, including orbits, narrower tarsal plates, smaller eyelid folds**
  - All layers infiltrated with more fat than in white eyelids
  - Small fold present but obscured by fatty infiltration
  - **KEY differences** between Asian and white eyelid morphology:
    - ▶ Absence of conjoined fascia[13]
    - ▶ Lack of fibrous extensions to pretarsal orbicularis and tarsus allows a "prolapse" of fatty lid tissue.
    - ▶ Therefore levator excursion and power are not effectively transmitted to soft tissues.

INFORMED CONSENT
Includes, but is not limited to, the following:
- Swelling: Patients need to know timeline for this to estimate returning to work and other activities.
- Ecchymosis: Often more profound in lower lid
  - Some darker-pigmented ethnic patient subgroups can show long-term "staining" of thin eyelid tissues.
- Chemosis, lagophthalmos (normal amount should be discussed)
- Infection: Abscess, preseptal and postseptal cellulitis
- Hematoma (retrobulbar): Include treatment and severity (i.e., blindness).

- Dry eyes: Exacerbation
- Epiphora
- Worsened or uncorrected asymmetries
- Temporary versus permanent injury of innervation to orbicularis, frontalis, and other muscles
- Injury to extraocular muscles
- Postblepharoplasty ptosis (temporary versus permanent)
  - Some patients with excess dissection and handling in preaponeurotic fat layer may have mild temporary ptosis from levator muscle edema and/or ecchymosis.
- Lid malposition, scleral show
- Entropion, ectropion
- Vision loss (extremely rare)

> **TIP:** Preoperative asymmetries (brow, lid position) should be pointed out to the patient, and no guarantees should be made about their correction.

> **TIP:** Even an excellent aesthetic outcome can be thwarted by lack of informed consent if the usual spectrum of swelling, bruising, and convalescence is not fully discussed.

EQUIPMENT

STANDARD BLEPHAROPLASTY TRAY
- Blepharoplasty hooks, tenotomy and iris scissors, mosquito hemostats, cotton-tipped applicators, cotton pledgets, fine needle holders

IMPORTANT SPECIAL EQUIPMENT
- Coated, thermoresistant instruments: Desmarres, malleable, and Ragnell
- Corneal protectors
- Loupes (≥2.5×) if transpalpebral CSM muscle resection
- Cautery with Colorado needle
- 1% lidocaine with 1:100,000 epinephrine with 27-gauge needle

SURGICAL TECHNIQUE: UPPER BLEPHAROPLASTY (Fig. 34-9)

PATIENT PREPARATION
- Critical to avoid NSAIDs, acetylsalicylic acid (ASA), vitamin E
- All makeup removed, including creams
- Antihypertensive medication taken the morning of surgery
- Helpful to position patient in reverse Trendelenburg position during the procedure

MARKINGS
- Use of sharp-cut edge of wooden cotton-tipped applicator dipped in methylene blue is more precise than marking pen.
  - **Lower line**
    - ► Preliminary marking of upper eyelids should be made in holding area.

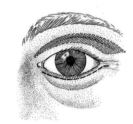

Fig. 34-9 Blepharoplasty markings.

- ▶ Skin pincher and calipers will help to determine amount of true skin excess with brows in a normal position (not compensated or falsely high) (NOTE: Green forceps are very useful for this and not uncomfortable to patient.)
- ▶ Mark lower line with patient in upright position while applying gentle upward traction on upper lid to reveal pretarsal line.
- ▶ **General guidelines**
    - ◆ Start at midpupil and taper to follow arc of crease.
    - ◆ DO NOT extend nasal to caruncle.
    - ◆ Males: 7-8 mm above lash line
    - ◆ Females: 8-9 mm
    - ◆ Asian eyelids: Sometimes <7 mm

> **TIP:** Evaluate the entire periorbita, upper sulcus, aperture, brow position, and makeup preferences, and determine what position would look best. Many Asian women may require a low crease position, but some want a higher crease to facilitate makeup application. A hollow upper lid sulcus may allow a higher crease. The measurements provided previously are a guideline.

- • **Upper line**
    - ▶ This is more dependent on amount of skin excess.
    - ▶ A planned concomitant browlift needs to be considered.
    - ▶ Extend the lateral incision by canting upward from lower line to upper line medially, and then extend beyond lower line, laterally as needed.
        - ◆ Follow crow's-feet or natural rhytid.
        - ◆ Generally, 5-6 mm above lash line at lateral canthus
        - ◆ Extent beyond lateral canthus tends to vary with age: 5 mm (young), 10 mm (middle age), 15 mm (older).
        - ◆ Males: Do not extend incision beyond lateral orbital rim (sometimes not concealable without makeup).
        - ◆ Preserve approximately **10 mm** of skin between lateral brow and incision.

> **TIP:**   Recognizing and showing patients the fold and brow asymmetries is essential. Make as symmetrical and precise a crease as possible. Perform asymmetrical skin resection when necessary. Although measurement and predetermined templates are useful, surgeons should always individualize the markings based on each patient's morphology and quality and amount of excess skin.

UPPER LID BLEPHAROPLASTY
- ■ **Anesthesia**
    - • Upper lid surgery can be done with the patient under straight local, local with conscious sedation, or general anesthesia.
    - • The choice depends on surgeon's preference and concomitant procedures.
- ■ **Technique**
    - • Caveats
        - ▶ Maintain hemostasis throughout procedure on low settings to prevent tissue staining.

- ▶ When injecting local anesthesia, stay in only the planes to be dissected to prevent unnecessary ecchymosis.
- Make lower incision first with a No. 15 blade and countertraction, then upper incision to meet lower incision.
- Excise skin ONLY, starting lateral to medial using a No. 15 blade or tenotomy scissors. Preserve orbicularis at this point.
- Excise orbicularis oculi strip (if needed) with scissors.
  - ▶ Maintain pretarsal OOM.
  - ▶ **Advantage:** Can help with postoperative adherence and create sharper supratarsal crease with closure; necessary in Asian eyelids to allow creation of conjoined fascia
  - ▶ **Disadvantage:** May distract from a desired more youthful/natural upper lid fullness in some patients[14,15]
- Incise orbital septum.
  - ▶ A more superior incision is safest to prevent levator palpebrae injury (which dives deeply in superior orbit).
  - ▶ Use separate, small incisions (versus opening widely) for each fat pad.
- ROOF or "prelevator" fatty tissue can be removed through OOM incision before completing orbital septal incisions.
- Excise excess intraorbital fat.
  - ▶ Preserve enough fat to allow a natural, youthful fullness.
  - ▶ Use a hemostat and cautery of fat on top of hemostat for a more even excision.
  - ▶ Medial fat is more dense, paler, and more vascular.
  - ▶ Preserve some fat between the nasal and central fat lobules to prevent an "A-frame" deformity.[1]
- Assess lacrimal gland. Consider pexy if it is prolapsed.
- Close skin.
  - ▶ Take very small bites with 5-0 or 6-0 running subcuticular monofilament suture (usually polypropylene or nylon).
  - ▶ Use intermittent 6-0 fast-absorbing plain gut to equalize irregular areas and for added safety.
  - ▶ Remove sutures within 4 to 6 days.

SENIOR AUTHOR TIP: Although the traditional techniques for upper lid blepharoplasty always included removal of muscle and fat, the current trend is toward fat and volume preservation, and more commonly volume is added. I rarely resect fat beyond the nasal pocket.

CREATION OF SUPRATARSAL CREASE OR LID FOLD
- **Indications**
  - Asian eyelids
  - Preoperative lid fold <4-6 mm that looks awkward
  - Secondary blepharoplasty
  - Males with brow ptosis
  - Asymmetrical supratarsal crease

- **Multiple techniques described**
  - Fernandez[16]: "Lid invagination technique." Major contribution to Asian eyelid surgery.
  - Siegel[17]: Creation of a new "conjoined fascia" position at a predetermined location, which becomes the future lid fold location.
    - ▶ Dissect levator aponeurosis edge inferiorly, release it, and suture it to desired lid location to dermis (three or four sutures only).
  - Flowers[18]: "Anchor blepharoplasty." Permanent sutures used to suture dermis to tarsus and levator.
  - Sheen[19]: Suture pretarsal orbicularis to levator.

TRANSCONJUNCTIVAL UPPER LID BLEPHAROPLASTY[1,20]
- **Indications**
  - Minimal to no excess upper lid skin, i.e., revision or secondary cases
  - Excess fat limited to medial pocket
  - In primary cases, can be combined with browlift or skin resurfacing, which may address minimal skin redundancy
- **Procedure**
  - Incision made in bare area of conjunctiva below medial horn of levator aponeurosis
  - Incision medial and opened only to obtain bulging medial fat
  - No need to close incision

> **SENIOR AUTHOR TIP:**   The procedure is best for patients whose only problem is excess nasal fat.

ADJUNCTIVE OPERATIONS
- **Direct browpexy**
  - Can be done through same upper eyelid incision
  - Technique uses Endotine device (Coapt Systems) or sutures (see Chapter 33)
  - Technique
    - ▶ Selective release of ORL where elevation desired, along with release of arcus marginalis of upper periorbita
    - ▶ Fixation of deep galea to periosteum or deep temporal fascia
    - ▶ Prevent pleating of brow skin.
    - ▶ Elevation limited with this technique

> **SENIOR AUTHOR TIP:**   This is a very useful technique for subtle brow elevation. I always place a suture rather than a device. I also almost always add this to the male upper lid blepharoplasty.

- **Transpalpebral corrugator supercilii resection[10,11]** (Fig. 34-10)
  - CSM topography is now well defined.[10]
    - ► Can mark dimensions on skin preoperatively
  - Use loupes.
  - Prevent nerve injury.
  - Resect muscle fibers as completely as possible.
    - ► Asymmetrical or incomplete resection or simple transection will likely result in unpredictable return in CSM activity and irregularities on animation.[21]
  - Use same incision.

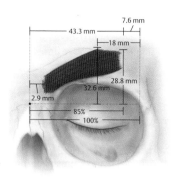

Fig. 34-10   Comprehensive corrugators supercilii muscle dimensions.

   - ► Incise preseptal and orbital OOM up high along medial supraorbital rim.
   - ► Use cephalad retraction to tent CSM fibers, which travel obliquely from nasal side.
   - ► CSM is located deep on galeal aponeurosis and periosteum medially and laterally.
   - ► Avoid frontalis resection.
   - ► Minimal medial OOM resection may be helpful, because this is a brow depressor.
   - ► Procerus muscle can be accessed and resected or transected for elimination of transverse dynamic rhytids.

SENIOR AUTHOR TIP: This is now my preferred method to modify the corrugator and procerus muscles. No special equipment is needed, just loupes. If a large amount of muscle is removed, I advise placing a small piece of fat, usually fat resected from the nasal pocket, into the defect left in the muscle to prevent a depression.

POSTOPERATIVE CARE

TIP: If the patient is a "cougher," smokes, or has Valsalva maneuvers during awakening from anesthesia, placing cold, soaked eye pads on orbits and applying steady pressure to prevent immediate bleeding complications are helpful.

SUTURES AND DRESSING
- Subcuticular suture removed on postoperative day 4-6
- Cold compress:
  - Swiss Therapy eye mask (Invotec) (excellent)
  - Ice-cold, soaked gauze pads in recovery
  - Cool compress (pack of frozen peas or corn) or eye mask gel therapy every 4 hours (20 minutes at a time) for the next 24 hours

ACTIVITY AND POSITION
- Instructed to limit activity that increases heart rate for 5-7 days
- Head of bed elevated (45 degrees) for 3-5 days

PROPHYLACTIC ANTIBIOTICS
- One dose of first-generation cephalosporin given before incision
- Single perioperative dose usually sufficient for "clean" case (CDC classification)

STEROIDS
- Short (5-6 day) steroid taper (Medrol Dosepak)
  - Recommended to decrease edema
- IV dose (Decadron 8 mg) should be given perioperatively.

EYE LUBRICATION
- Artificial tears (Refresh Plus during day and Lacri-Lube or Refresh PM at night)
  - Only needed until normal tearing function returns
  - Can do as often as needed
- Have a low threshold to treat infection or chemosis early.
  - Give a combination steroid and ophthalmologic suspension such as tobramycin (TobraDex).
  - Protect eye.
  - Irrigate with artificial tears.

DIET
- Patient can resume previous diet as tolerated.
- Salt intake is limited to help decrease edema.
- Edema, if prolonged, is more common with:
  - Disruption of ORL (especially when combined with lower lid surgery)
  - Browlift procedures
  - Supralevator (ROOF) fat resection

HERBS AND OTHER POSTOPERATIVE MEDICATIONS (see Chapter 13)
- *Arnica montana* oral dosing for 3-5 days postoperatively may be beneficial.
- Bromelain (high-dose pineapple extract) may be helpful for ecchymosis and edema.
- Management of blood pressure, pain, and nausea in the immediate postoperative period, as with all facial procedures, will decrease the risk of bleeding and reduce postoperative swelling and bruising.

COMPLICATIONS[15,22-26]

ASYMMETRY
- **Most common complication**
- May be revised in office with patient under local anesthesia

RETROBULBAR HEMATOMA
- See algorithm in Fig. 34-11.
- Results most often from bleeding vessel during orbital fat excision
  - **Signs/symptoms**
    - ▶ Pain (first sign)
    - ▶ Proptosis
    - ▶ Lid ecchymosis (more than usual and with turgor)

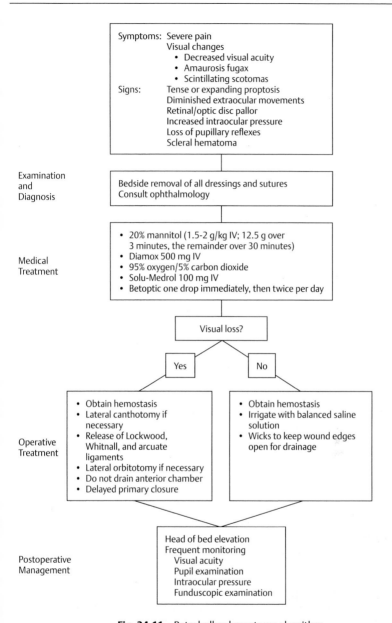

Examination and Diagnosis

Symptoms: Severe pain
Visual changes
- Decreased visual acuity
- Amaurosis fugax
- Scintillating scotomas

Signs: Tense or expanding proptosis
Diminished extraocular movements
Retinal/optic disc pallor
Increased intraocular pressure
Loss of pupillary reflexes
Scleral hematoma

Bedside removal of all dressings and sutures
Consult ophthalmology

Medical Treatment

- 20% mannitol (1.5-2 g/kg IV; 12.5 g over 3 minutes, the remainder over 30 minutes)
- Diamox 500 mg IV
- 95% oxygen/5% carbon dioxide
- Solu-Medrol 100 mg IV
- Betoptic one drop immediately, then twice per day

Visual loss?

Yes / No

Operative Treatment

Yes:
- Obtain hemostasis
- Lateral canthotomy if necessary
- Release of Lockwood, Whitnall, and arcuate ligaments
- Lateral orbitotomy if necessary
- Do not drain anterior chamber
- Delayed primary closure

No:
- Obtain hemostasis
- Irrigate with balanced saline solution
- Wicks to keep wound edges open for drainage

Postoperative Management

Head of bed elevation
Frequent monitoring
Visual acuity
Pupil examination
Intraocular pressure
Funduscopic examination

Fig. 34-11   Retrobulbar hematoma algorithm.

- ► Decrease in vision and extraocular muscle activity
- ► Dilated pupils
- ► Scotomas
- ► Increased intraocular pressure
- • **Treatment**
  - ► Elevate head of bed.
  - ► Release surgical incision.
    - ◆ Entire length of incision does not require release.
  - ► Mannitol (12.5 g IV bolus over 3-5 minutes)
  - ► Acetazolamide (Diamox): 500 mg IV bolus
  - ► Steroids (Solu-Medrol): 100 mg IV
  - ► Have patient rebreathe in bag or mask to elevate CO_2.
  - ► Topical beta blocker (Betoptic)
  - ► **Emergent ophthalmologic consultation**
  - ► Reoperation
    - ◆ May require another visit to operating room with ophthalmologist
  - ► If signs/symptoms are not relieved from above treatment and hematoma is still suspected, **perform lateral cantholysis.**
    - ◆ Place 1% lidocaine with epinephrine-soaked cottonoids on incision.
  - ► Admit patient to hospital for observation.

> **TIP:** Check on the patient and vision in recovery once he or she is alert. Recognizing early signs of retrobulbar hematoma is critical.

BLINDNESS
- 0.04% incidence
- Most common cause is a bleeding complication that is untreated or recognized too late.
- Pathophysiology:
  - • Retrobulbar hematoma causes central artery occlusion or optic nerve ischemia from pressure.
  - • **After 100 minutes: Considered irreversible!**

LAGOPHTHALMOS
- 2-3 mm of lagophthalmos is acceptable immediately intraoperatively, and even desired.
- Greater degrees may improve over time.
- If not improving, need to treat:
  - • Taping at night
  - • Lubrication is vital (lubricant before sleep); artificial tears throughout the day
  - • If these measures do not help, then consider skin grafting.

> **TIP:** The risk of lagophthalmos is decreased if measurement and a pinch test are performed preoperatively while the patient is sitting. Surgeons must consider the effects of a concomitant browlift and trust their preoperative markings.

CORNEAL INJURY
- This may occur during surgery or when removing corneal shields.
- Confirm injury with fluorescein testing.

- Consider ophthalmologic consultation.
- Treatment:
  - Superficial injury: Topical antibiotic ointment, topical anesthetic (briefly), and eye patching
  - Should resolve within 24-72 hours

DIPLOPIA
- Most often from lower lid surgery
- If from upper lid: Likely from **superior oblique muscle injury**
- Commonly resolves spontaneously
- May require corrective muscle surgery by an ophthalmologist

PTOSIS
- Most common cause of postoperative ptosis is unrecognized preoperative ptosis.
- May occur from direct injury to levator muscle or aponeurosis
- Most often a temporary occurrence from manipulation, edema, or ecchymosis of levator apparatus
  - Be cognizant of levator location at all times.
  - Minimize levator handling, if at all.

DRY EYE SYNDROME
- Keratoconjunctivitis sicca
- More common in patients with preoperative signs/symptoms
- **Imperative to inquire about eyedrop use and history of dry eyes preoperatively**
  - If positive findings, be ultraconservative during lid surgery
- May be more common in lower lid when patient is "morphologically prone"[22]
  - *Negative vector* lower lid–cheek relation
  - Proptosis or native exophthalmic globe position
- May consider Schirmer testing preoperatively

AESTHETIC RESULTS
- Prevent "A-frame" deformity medially from overresection of soft tissue between nasal and central fat pads.
- Address brow symmetry to improve results.
- Some Asian patients can be very critical of even the slightest asymmetry.
  - Creating a symmetrical lid fold position is critical.

TOP TAKEAWAYS
➤ The preseptal orbicularis is adherent to the septum, and careful dissection in the proper submuscular plane is required.
➤ Blunt or sharp transection/disruption of ORL helps to smooth the tear trough and blend the lid-cheek junction.
➤ Video imaging has been most helpful in discussing patients' expectations and whether they are realistic.
➤ The risk of lagophthalmos is decreased if measurement and a pinch test are performed preoperatively while the patient is sitting. Surgeons must consider the effects of a concomitant browlift and trust their preoperative markings.

REFERENCES

1. Nahai F. Aesthetic plastic surgery. In Nahai F, ed. The Art of Aesthetic Surgery: Principles and Techniques, ed 2. New York: Thieme Publishers, 2007.
2. Zide B, Jelks GW, eds. Surgical Anatomy Around the Orbit. New York: Lippincott Williams & Wilkins, 2007.
3. Siegel RJ. Surgical anatomy of the upper eyelid fascia. Ann Plast Surg 13:263, 1984.
4. Siegel RJ. Personal communication, 2008.
5. Moss CJ, Mendelson BC, Taylor GI. Surgical anatomy of the ligamentous attachments in the temple and periorbital regions. Plast Reconstr Surg 105:1475, 2000.
6. Muzaffar A, Mendelson BC, Adams WP. Surgical anatomy of the ligamentous attachments of the lower lid and lateral canthus. Plast Reconstr Surg 110:873, 2002.
7. Ghavami A, Pessa JE, Janis JE, et al. The orbicularis retaining ligament of the medial orbit: closing the circle. Plast Reconstr Surg 121:994, 2008.
8. Kikkawa DO, Lemke BN, Dortzbach RK. Relations of the superficial musculoaponeurotic system and characterization of the orbitomalar ligament. Ophthal Plast Reconstr Surg 12:77, 1996.
9. Pessa JE. The malar septum, the anatomical basis of malar mounds. Presented at the Annual Meeting of the American Society for Aesthetic Plastic Surgery, Dallas, TX, April 1994.
10. Janis JE, Ghavami A, Lemmon JA, et al. Anatomy of the corrugator supercilii muscle: part I. Corrugator topography. Plast Reconstr Surg 120:1647, 2007.
11. Guyuron B, Michelow BJ, Thomas T. Corrugator supercilii muscle resection through blepharoplasty incision. Plast Reconstr Surg 95:691, 1995.
12. Castanares S. Blepharoplasty for herniated intraorbital fat: anatomical basis for a new approach. Plast Reconstr Surg 8:46, 1951.
13. Siegel RJ. Advanced upper lid blepharoplasty. Clin Plast Surg 19:319, 1992.
14. Fagien S. Advanced rejuvenative upper blepharoplasty: enhancing aesthetics of the upper periorbita. Plast Reconstr Surg 110:278, 2002.
15. Rohrich RJ, Coberly DM, Fagien S, et al. Current concepts in aesthetic upper blepharoplasty. Plast Reconstr Surg 113:32e, 2004.
16. Fernandez LR. Double eyelid operation in the Oriental in Hawaii. Plast Reconstr Surg 25:257, 1960.
17. Siegel RJ. Asian "double eyelid" blepharoplasty: the contribution of L. Fernandez. Plast Reconstr Surg 116:1808, 2005.
18. Flowers RS. The art of eyelid and orbital aesthetics: multiracial surgical considerations. Clin Plast Surg 14:703, 1987.
19. Sheen JH. Change in the technique of supratarsal fixation in upper blepharoplasty. Plast Reconstr Surg 59:831, 1977.
20. Nahai F. Transconjunctival upper lid blepharoplasty. Aesthet Surg J 25:292, 2005.
21. Guyuron B. Endoscopic forehead rejuvenation: limitations, flaws, and rewards. Plast Reconstr Surg 117:1121, 2006.
22. Rees TD, LaTrenta GS. The role of the Schirmer's test and orbital morphology in predicting dry-eye syndrome after blepharoplasty. Plast Reconstr Surg 82:619, 1988.
23. Rees TD, Jelks GW. Blepharoplasty and the dry eye syndrome: guidelines for surgery? Plast Reconstr Surg 68:249, 1981.
24. Lisman RD, Hyde K, Smith B. Complications of blepharoplasty. Clin Plast Surg 15:309, 1988.
25. Fagien S. Reducing the incidence of dry eye symptoms after blepharoplasty. Aesthet Surg J 24:464, 2004.
26. Jelks GW, McCord CD Jr. Dry eye syndrome and other tear film abnormalities. Clin Plast Surg 8:803, 1981.

35. Lower Blepharoplasty

Jason K. Potter, Ted H. Wojno

ANATOMY (Fig. 35-1)

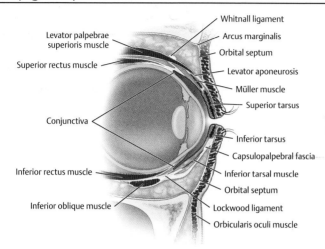

Fig. 35-1 Cross section of the upper and lower eyelids.

TERMINOLOGY

- **Dermatochalasis:** Excess eyelid skin
- **Blepharochalasis:** Thin, excessive eyelid skin secondary to recurrent bouts of painless lid edema
  - 80% may have onset prior to age 20.
- **Blepharoptosis:** Drooping or ptosis of the upper eyelid
- **Ectropion:** An outward turning of the eyelid margin
  - Senile: Results from age-related laxity of lower lid
  - Cicatricial: Results from scar-induced retraction of lower lid
- **Entropion:** Rolling of eyelid margin inward toward the sclera
  - May result in irritation of the cornea or sclera by lashes

- **Retraction:** A downward displacement of the lid margin resulting in inferior scleral show
- **Steatoblepharon:** Excess or protruding fat through a lax septum

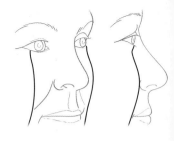

AESTHETIC EVALUATION OF THE LOWER LID[1,2]

- **Lid position:** Lower lid should rest at level of limbus without scleral show between the limbus and lid margin.
- **Pretarsal bulge:** Pretarsal orbicularis oculi hypertrophy considered by many to be aesthetic component of the youthful lower lid.
  - Often present in attractive eyes
  - Results from pretarsal orbicularis muscle fullness
- **Lid-cheek junction:** Smooth, convex, essentially imperceptible transition from lid to cheek in youthful patients (Fig. 35-2)
  - Stigmata of aging include:
    - ▶ Excess skin, pseudoherniation of intraorbital fat, malar pad descent, nasojugal groove, visible inferior orbital rim
    - ▶ Hollowed appearance from paucity of intraorbital fat

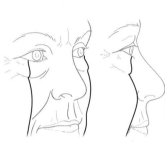

Fig. 35-2   Comparison of lid-cheek junction appearance in youth versus aged.

CHARACTERISTICS OF THE AGING LOWER LID (Fig. 35-3)

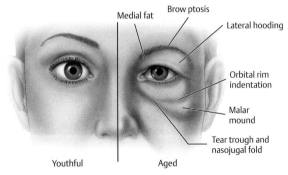

Fig. 35-3   Characteristics of aging periorbital region.

- **Skin quality**
  - Redundant with excessively thin and crêpey qualities
  - Rhytids, fine and deep (crow's-feet)
  - Residual lines or wrinkles inevitable postoperatively

- **Skin pigmentation** (blepharomelasma)
  - Hyperpigmentation of the skin
- **Orbit vector:** Position of globe relative to the inferior orbital rim
  - Useful for predicting postoperative tendencies of lid position
  - **Negative vector orbits** have poor lower lid suspension and are at risk for postoperative ectropion and retraction.
- **Lid laxity:** Horizontal lid laxity has significant risk for postoperative lid malposition.
  - **Snap-back test:** is delayed return of the lid margin to native position when retracted downward with finger traction.
  - **Pull-away test:** is abnormal when the examiner grasps the lid margin between the index finger and thumb and pulls it away from the globe more than 10 mm.
  - Best corrected with supplemental canthal anchoring procedures (see Chapter 38)
- **Redundant, ptotic orbicularis oculi muscle** *(festoon)*
  - **Squint (or squinch) test:** Forced closure of eyelids improves festoon if secondary to ptotic orbicularis oculi muscle
  - **Malar bag:** Shelving of orbicularis oculi muscle over orbital retaining ligament with excess intraorbital fat
    - ▶ Correction involves improving lid-cheek junction (Loeb procedure, septal reset, midface lift).
- **Bulging orbital fat:** Weakening of the orbital septum may result in herniation of orbital fat pads creating visible deformity of the lower lid.
  - This may be corrected by fat removal, repair of septum without fat removal, and fat relocation.
  - Current techniques emphasize *fat preservation.*
- **Tear trough** (see Chapter 29)
  - According to Barton et al,[3] created by herniation of orbital fat, tight attachment of the orbicularis along the arcus marginalis, and malar retrusion
  - According to Codner et al,[4] created by herniation of fat over the orbitomalar ligament, which arises from periosteum and attaches to skin
    - ▶ According to this definition, the tear trough arises over a triangular space defined by the orbitomalar ligament, levator labii superioris, and levator alaeque nasi.

NOTE: The terms orbitomalar ligament, orbital retaining ligment, orbicularis retaining ligament refer to the same anatomic structure.

  - Pronounced tear trough deformity may not be corrected with traditional blepharoplasty techniques alone.
- **Visible palpebromalar and nasojugal grooves**
- **Lacrimal function:** All patients should be questioned about dry eye symptoms.
  - Blepharoplasty may contribute to or worsen dry eye symptoms in susceptible patients.
  - Ophthalmologic consultation may be warranted.
- **Scleral show**
  - Lower lid should be at or within 2 mm of inferior limbus.
  - Tarsal laxity, negative vector orbit, exophthalmos, or middle lamellar contracture of lower lid can be present.

SURGICAL TECHNIQUES

> **NOTE:**   Numerous lower lid blepharoplasty techniques have been reported. The following lists include the most commonly performed techniques.

SKIN RESURFACING
Patients with isolated fine lines may be treated with skin resurfacing techniques alone such as chemical peel or laser resurfacing (see Chapters 16 through 18).

SKIN-ONLY BLEPHAROPLASTY (PINCH BLEPHAROPLASTY)
- **Indications**
  - Patients with minimal redundant skin or fullness, usually isolated to the pretarsal region, and not associated with more significant age-related periorbital changes such as fat herniation, lid laxity or orbicularis ptosis
- **Technique**[5]
  - Forceps are used to gently pinch the redundant skin over the pretarsal orbicularis oculi to determine the width of skin to be resected.
  - Appropriate width of skin to be resected is that which does not induce changes in the position of the lower lid.
  - Skin to be excised is marked with a fine-tipped marker.
  - Incision is performed with a No. 15 blade and excision of skin-only is performed with cautery.
  - No undermining or elevation of a skin flap

> **NOTE:**   If pretarsal orbicularis hypertrophy is present and contributing to excessive fullness, a strip of pretarsal muscle may be excised as well.

> **NOTE:**   The pinch technique for skin excision may be combined with other blepharoplasty maneuvers such as transconjunctival fat removal in appropriate patients.

TRANSCONJUNCTIVAL FAT REMOVAL (Fig. 35-4)

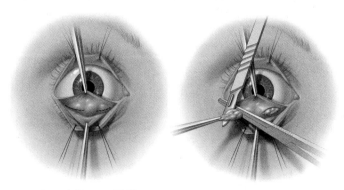

Fig. 35-4   Transconjunctival fat removal.

- **Indications**
  - Young patients with excessive fat and no excess skin or orbicularis ptosis
- **Technique**
  - Incision made through conjunctiva to expose postseptal fat compartments
  - Usually two separate incisions for access to three fat compartments
  - Skin resurfacing may be performed as needed.

NOTE: Skin excision may be added to transconjunctival fat removal when mild skin excess is present without noticeable orbicularis oculi muscle ptosis.

EXTERNAL LOWER BLEPHAROPLASTY AND ORBICULARIS SUSPENSION (Fig. 35-5)

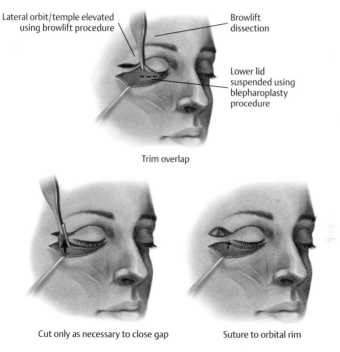

Lateral orbit/temple elevated using browlift procedure

Browlift dissection

Lower lid suspended using blepharoplasty procedure

Trim overlap

Cut only as necessary to close gap

Suture to orbital rim

Fig. 35-5   Orbicularis suspension.

- **Indications**
  - Skin excess and orbicularis ptosis
- **Technique**
  - Subciliary skin incision
  - Elevation of pretarsal and preseptal skin flap
  - Elevation of preseptal orbicularis oculi muscle flap
  - Release of orbital retaining ligament and lateral orbital thickening
  - Irrigation with Kenalog solution (2.5 mg in 0.5 ml saline solution)

- Suspension of orbicularis oculi to lateral orbital rim with a pennant flap
- Canthal anchoring
- Redundant skin trimmed and incision closed

TIP: External skin–only techniques do not adequately address orbicularis ptosis and in most cases do not adequately correct the lower lid deformity.

SENIOR AUTHOR TIP: A major consideration in lower eyelid blepharoplasty is when to perform canthal anchoring and, if so, whether to do canthopexy or canthoplasty. The decision to perform canthal anchoring is based upon the amount of horizontal laxity (based on the "snap-back test" and the "pull-away test"), the prominence of the globe (positive or negative vector), the amount of skin or skin/muscle resection planned and other ancillary procedures performed (facial rhytidectomy, laser facial resurfacing, chemical peel, etc.). In general, canthopexy, of which there are a multiplicity of variations, is quicker and easier to perform and less likely to lead to postoperative problems. It is therefore the treatment of choice for surgeons who may feel less than completely comfortable in this region. It can correct mild degrees of lid laxity and functions well as a "just in case" addition to the procedure.

When there is more significant lid laxity, canthopexy will not suffice and canthoplasty must be performed. Canthoplasty is more complex and time-consuming and more prone to postoperative problems such as dehiscence, conjunctival chemosis, and lid asymmetry. Again, there are several variations on the theme but all can be conceptualized as either resection of a redundant block of tarsal plate, formation of a strip of tarsus from the redundant lid, or anchoring the tarsus via a drill hole in the lateral orbital rim. Canthoplasty gives a greater degree of horizontal shortening with increased stability of the lid margin.

Another consideration is when to add a spacer graft to the lower eyelid retractors to counter the downward forces in a negative vector eye. Again, there are no hard and fast rules but it should be considered when the exophthalmometry readings exceed 15 mm and obviously rises as this figure increases. This is tempered by the amount of skin or skin/muscle resection planned by the surgeon. If the surgeon wishes to avoid supporting grafts in the posterior lamella, one can purposely undercorrect the amount of anterior lamella resected to compensate in a negative vector eye.

EXTERNAL LOWER BLEPHAROPLASTY WITH ORBICULARIS SUSPENSION AND SEPTAL RESET (Fig. 35-6)

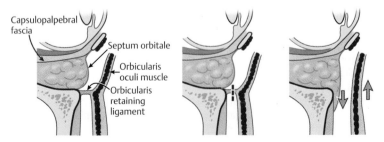

Fig. 35-6   Septal reset procedure.

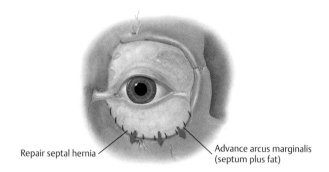

Repair septal hernia

Advance arcus marginalis
(septum plus fat)

Fig. 35-6, cont'd

- **Indications**
  - Skin excess and orbicularis oculi ptosis
  - Visible nasojugal groove and fat herniation
  - Tear trough triad
- **Technique**
  - Subciliary skin incision
  - Elevation of pretarsal and preseptal skin flap
  - Elevation of preseptal orbicularis oculi muscle flap
  - Release of orbital retaining ligament and lateral orbital thickening
  - Release of arcus marginalis and extrusion of lower lid fat
  - Suture reset of septum and orbital fat to anterior orbital rim periosteum
  - Irrigation with Kenalog solution (2.5 mg in 0.5 ml saline solution)
  - Suspension of orbicularis to lateral orbital rim with pennant flap
  - Canthal anchoring
  - Redundant skin trimmed and incision closed

TIP: Septal reset procedures should be performed with the lower lid under tension (by temporary Frost suture) to prevent excessive tightening of the septum and predisposing patients to ectropion.

SENIOR AUTHOR TIP: I do not place a temporary tarsorrhaphy suture while performing septal reset procedure as recommended here but completely agree that a degree of caution is needed to reduce the risk of inducing postoperative lower lid retraction. In general, if the orbital septum is widely opened and the orbital fat prolapsed out and transposed over the inferior rim then the risk is relatively low. If the actual septum itself is transposed then the risk is greater. This is because the septum is stiffer than the orbital fat and more closely attached to the tarsal plate. Therefore, the same degree of transposition of the septum risks lid retraction more so than the transposition of the orbital fat. When performing either procedure, I always look at the tarsal plate to see if there is any inferior movement when suturing the transposed tissue. I also feel the tension along the inferior border of the tarsal plate by pulling superiorly with a forceps before and after suturing the tissue to be certain that the tension is not excessive.

OTHER CONSIDERATIONS

ORBICULARIS INCISION AND PARALYTIC ECTROPION

- Whether orbicularis oculi muscle incision leads to paralytic ectropion after blepharoplasty is controversial.
- Pretarsal innervation is usually maintained through medial branches if the incision is made only in the lateral portion of the muscle.
- With any muscle splitting technique, proper preoperative risk assessment and **routine lateral canthal anchoring procedures** are requisite to a successful outcome.

POSTOPERATIVE CARE

- All patients are advised to expect swelling, ecchymosis, and some restriction with upward gaze.
- Generally, most patients can expect to look "presentable" at 2-3 weeks.
- Some use postoperative compressive bandages.
- Cool compresses can be used intermittently for the first 24-36 hours to improve postoperative edema.
- Moisturizing eyedrops and/or ophthalmic lubricating ointment should be provided to prevent dry eye symptoms and desiccation of the sclera.
- If no canthopexy is performed, a Frost suture should be placed to prevent lid retraction.
- Patients should be counseled to refrain from using contact lenses in the postoperative phase.

COMPLICATIONS

PERIBULBAR HEMATOMA

- Usually results from bleeding of the orbicularis oculi muscle
- Vision is usually not threatened.
- If seen intraoperatively, they should be evacuated.
- Small hematomas seen in the postoperative phase can be watched.
- Larger hematomas can be evacuated at 7-10 days after they have undergone liquefaction.
- Prevention is aimed at meticulous perioperative blood pressure control; postoperative ice packs and elevation of the head are essential.[6]

RETROBULBAR HEMATOMA

- Rare but serious complication (0.04% incidence)[7]
- Can compress neurovascular structures and cause retinal ischemia and optic nerve compression
- Symptoms include severe pain, visual changes, proptosis, and ecchymosis.

CAUTION: This constitutes a surgical emergency and should prompt reexploration immediately.

- Medical treatment of retrobulbar hematomas includes mannitol, acetazolamide, and systemic and topical steroids.

DRY EYE SYNDROME

- Symptoms include itching, foreign body sensation, burning, secretions, and frequent blinking.
- Documented dry eyes, history of dry eyes, and abnormal orbital and periorbital anatomy such as lower lid laxity are predictors of postoperative dry eye complications.
- Blepharoplasty should be delayed for **at least 6 months** in patients who previously have undergone laser in situ keratomileusis (LASIK).
- Prevention is largely related to proper patient screening.
- Patients who wear contact lenses without difficulty have adequate tear production to proceed with blepharoplasty.[8]
- Treatment includes lubricating drops and ointment.
- Eye patch or Frost suture can also be used if lubricating measures do not improve symptoms.
- In prolonged cases (>3 months), cyclosporine ophthalmic can be used to increase tear production.[8]

SENIOR AUTHOR TIP: Dry eye syndrome in the postoperative period can also be treated by temporary or permanent punctal plugs which partially block the lacrimal outflow apparatus. This increases the volume of tears available to the ocular surface. Also keep in mind that ocular rosacea can mimic all of the symptoms of dry eye. This can activate in the eyelids in individuals so predisposed after eyelid surgery. A history compatible with rosacea may suggest that a trial of low-dose tetracycline is in order.

CHEMOSIS[9]

- Can be caused by manipulation of the conjunctiva or prolonged scleral exposure leading to desiccation
- Frequent moisturizing with wetting drops, ophthalmic lubricating ointments, and intermittent forced lid closure prevents exposure-related desiccation.
- Most cases will resolve spontaneously.
- Treatment involves artificial tears and ointment.
- Steroid drops can be used under careful surveillance in refractory cases.[10]
- Physicians can also give 2.5% Neo-Synephrine eyedrops, because they suppress inflammation and constrict conjunctival blood vessels.

SENIOR AUTHOR TIP: The treatment of conjunctival chemosis has probably generated more arcane solutions than anything else that I can imagine. I have seen cases where the edema persisted over 6 months from the time of the surgery. The conjunctiva is well supplied with lymphatic vessels that drain into the preauricular node (from the upper eyelid) and to the submandibular node (from the lower eyelid). Surgical procedures on the lids disrupt the normal lymphatic drainage. This seems to be especially true when a canthotomy and cantholysis is performed in the lower eyelid. In time, the lymphatic channels recanalize and the chemosis resolves. In addition to the treatments suggested here are massage, hypertonic saline drops and ointments, diuretics, and pressure patches. I have on occasion actually cut into the swollen conjunctiva with sharp scissors and found immediate and permanent resolution of the problem. I have also found instances in which cutting into the conjunctiva was not at all helpful. My feeling is that we tend to believe that whatever treatment we rendered immediately before the spontaneous resolution of the problem is what worked.

INFECTION
- Rare complication of blepharoplasty
- Dry eye is a predisposing factor.
- Can be treated with **topical antibiotics**

LOWER LID MALPOSITION
- The **most common complication** after lower lid blepharoplasty
- May range from mild inferior scleral show to severe ectropion
- Can be caused by cicatricial and/or gravitational forces overcoming the support mechanisms of the lower eyelid[11]
- Laxity of the tarsoligamentous sling causes a loss of normal upward tensile strength and dynamic elasticity of the lower lid.[9]
- Preoperative identification of patients at risk for lid retraction is critical and includes patients with proptosis, malar hypoplasia, and high myopia.
- Mild lid malposition can be managed with eyelid massage.
- If needed, operative intervention is delayed until the late postoperative period.

LAGOPHTHALMOS
- Occurs from lid edema, excessive skin resection trauma to the orbicularis oculi, and iatrogenic orbital septal shortening
- Typically resolves as muscles relax and edema subsides
- Treatment includes light massage and nocturnal lubrication.
- If conservative measures fail, surgery may be necessary.

TOP TAKEAWAYS
➤ Accurate, individualized assessment of each patient's orbital morphology and lid deformity is central to the proper approach to lower lid blepharoplasty.
➤ A graduated treatment plan is developed for each patient depending on the presence of skin laxity, orbicularis oculi ptosis, fat herniation, and tear trough deformities.
➤ Canthal anchoring techniques should be considered a routine aspect of lower lid blepharoplasty.

REFERENCES
1. Flowers RS, DuVal C. Blepharoplasty and periorbital aesthetic surgery. In Aston SJ, Beasley RW, Thorne HM, et al, eds. Grabb and Smith's Plastic Surgery, ed 6. Philadelphia: Lippincott Williams & Wilkins, 2007.
2. Guyuron B. Blepharoplasty and ancillary procedures. In Achauer BH, Eriksson E, Guyuron B, et al, eds. Plastic Surgery: Indications, Operations, and Outcomes. St Louis: Mosby–Year Book, 2000.
3. Barton FE, Ha R, Awada M. Fat extrusion and septal reset in patients with the tear trough triad: a critical appraisal. Plast Reconstr Surg 13:2115, 2004.
4. Codner MA, Kikkawa DO, Korn BS, et al. Blepharoplasty and brow lift. Plast Reconstr Surg 126:1e, 2010.

5. Kim, EM, Bucky LP. Power of the pinch: pinch lower lid blepharoplasty. Ann Plast Surg 60:532, 2008.
6. Trussler AP, Rohrich RJ. MOC-PSSM CME article: blepharoplasty. Plast Reconstr Surg 121 (1 Suppl):S1, 2008.
7. Wolfort FG, Vaughan TE, Wolfort SF, et al. Retrobulbar hematoma and blepharoplasty. Plast Reconstr Surg 104:2154, 1999.
8. Pacella SJ, Codner MA. Minor complications after blepharoplasty: dry eyes, chemosis, granulomas, ptosis, and scleral show. Plast Reconstr Surg 125:709, 2010.
9. Lelli GJ Jr, Lisman RD. Blepharoplasty complications. Plast Reconstr Surg 125:1007, 2010.
10. Weinfeld AB, Burke R, Codner MA. The comprehensive management of chemosis following cosmetic lower blepharoplasty. Plast Reconstr Surg 122:579, 2008.
11. McCord CD Jr. The correction of lower lid malposition following lower lid blepharoplasty. Plast Reconstr Surg 103:1036, 1999.

36. Asian Blepharoplasty

Jerome H. Liu, Richard Y. Ha, Lily Daniali, William Pai-Dei Chen

BACKGROUND

- Mikamo performed first reported double-eyelid operation in 1896.[1]
  - Nonincision method using three sutures of silk thread removed postoperatively
- Sayoc,[2] Millard,[3] and Fernandez[4] first reported on it in Western literature in 1950s.
- Operation gained popularity in Asia after World War II following the influx of whites.
  - Upper lid blepharoplasty is now the most common plastic surgery procedure in Asia.
- Approximately 30%-50% of Asians have a natural supratarsal crease.[5]
- Not a "Westernizing" of the eyelid
  - Patients typically request a natural look that opens the eye, while respecting their Asian identity.[6]

DIFFERENCES BETWEEN WHITE AND ASIAN EYELIDS[7]

- **Characteristics of "single fold" eyelid** (Fig. 36-1)
  - Absent or short superior palpebral crease
  - Preseptal fibroadipose tissue or orbicularis muscle thickening
  - Diffuse, poorly defined and variable insertion of septum into levator aponeurosis
    - ▶ Can insert as low as 2 mm below superior tarsal border
  - Inferior descent of preaponeurotic (prelevator) fat
  - Short tarsal height (Asians 6.5 ± 8.0 mm; whites 11.3 ± 1.7 mm)[8]
  - Medial epicanthal fold

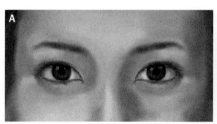 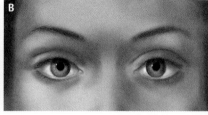

Fig. 36-1   Corresponding cross sectional fascial anatomy of **A,** an Asian eyelid and **B,** a white eyelid.

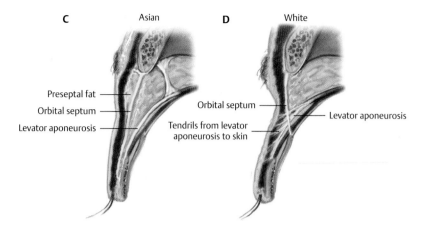

Fig. 36-1, cont'd Note the low fusion of the septum and levator in the **C,** Asian eyelid versus the high fusion in the **D,** white eyelid. Also note the presence of abundant preseptal fat and the lack of fascial attachments from the levator to the orbicularis and skin.

- ■ **Two theories of superior palpebral crease formation**
  - • **Levator-dermal expansion**[2,9-13]
    - ▶ Traditional theory describes fibrous extensions of the levator inserting into dermis to create the palpebral crease in whites.
    - ▶ Expansions from levator aponeurosis pierce orbicularis and insert into dermis or subcutaneous tissue of pretarsal skin.
    - ▶ Anchoring produces characteristic fold in upper eyelid.
    - ▶ **Asians lack a palpebral fold,** because the levator does not penetrate the septum. Therefore there are no fibrous extensions of the levator into the skin or subcutaneous tissue.

> **SENIOR AUTHOR TIP:**   I support the view of **levator-dermal extension.** Since Collins' paper in the 1980s, electron microscopy (EM) studies have confirmed the presence of microtubules (microfibrils) that extend to the undersurface of skin, in addition to wraparound intermuscular fascia of the orbicularis oculi.

- • **Levator-septal variable union**[13-17]
    - ▶ There are no clearly defined dermal expansions from the levator; there are expansions from the levator to the orbicularis muscle.[14]
    - ▶ The formation of the crease is based on the level of union between the levator aponeurosis and orbital septum, creating a *conjoined fascia.*
    - ▶ Crease formation is a result of the fusion of the levator and septum with adherence of the orbicularis muscle and the overlying skin.

▶ Whites have a high union between the levator and the orbital septum at or above the superior border of the tarsal plate, allowing a well-defined palpebral crease.

▶ Asians have a low or variable union between the levator and orbital septum below the superior border of the tarsal plate.

▶ The low attachment allows descent of preaponeurotic orbital fat between the levator and the septum to extend inferiorly.

▶ Abundance of preseptal fat creates a glide plane and prevents adherence between levator-septal complex and orbicularis muscle.

▶ Primary insertion of levator aponeurosis into orbicularis muscle occurs closer to the eyelid margin.

■ **Soft tissue differences between Asian and white eyelids**[7,13,18]
  • Asian skin has **thicker dermis** with higher collagen content.
  • Asian upper lid has more prominent **preseptal fibroadipose tissue.**
    ▶ Submuscular fibroadipose layer is directly continuous with eyebrow fat pad.
    ▶ Brow fat can inferiorly extend to lash line.
    ▶ Preseptal fat adds thickness and fullness to upper lid.
    ▶ Can be continuous or intimately associated with retroorbicularis oculi fat (ROOF).
  • Asians have **thicker pretarsal subcutaneous tissue.**
    ▶ Presence of pretarsal fibroadipose tissue
  • Asians have **thicker and bulkier orbicularis oculi muscle.**
  • Abundance of bulky soft tissue contributes to poorly defined palpebral crease.
■ **Epicanthal fold**
  • Appears as a skin web that overlies portion of the medial canthus and obscures the lacrimal caruncle, and possibly the medial portion of the sclera.

SENIOR AUTHOR TIP: The term *epicanthal fold* has been overapplied even to normal Asian individuals who do not have clinically significant epicanthal folds (as seen in patients with congenital syndromes like Down syndrome and blepharophimosis syndrome). The treatment, epicanthoplasty, has been overprescribed as a surgical solution when the finding is merely a medial upper lid fold (a term which I prefer), in which half of the exposed caruncle is easily seen. Because the finding of medial upper lid fold is common and easily corrected as part of tissue removal in a double-eyelid crease procedure through incisional approach, the myriad methods of epicanthoplasty all seem to work since the findings are quite mild and often not pathological enough to be called a *true epicanthal fold.*[19]

  • Johnson[20] first described the four types of epicanthus (Fig. 36-2). At the time they were described as pathological entities, although the epicanthus tarsalis in its mildest form seems to overlap with what one should consider a normal finding in Asians who have no upper lid crease, or even in those who are born with a natural crease.

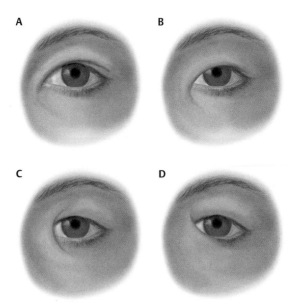

Fig. 36-2   Types of epicanthus. **A,** Tarsalis. **B,** Superciliaris. **C,** Palpebralis. **D,** Inversus.

▶ *Type 1. Epicanthus tarsalis:* Fold is seen along medial upper eyelid, and covers part of the medial pretarsal region. May block view of the dermal portion of the caruncle, which is normally seen as opposed to the deeper conjunctival portion at its base.

SENIOR AUTHOR TIP: Many Asians have a medial upper lid fold without it blocking any of the medial portion of the pretarsal region, and the caruncle can still be seen. I do not consider these patients as having epicanthus tarsalis.

▶ *Type 2. Epicanthus superciliaris:* Fold originates from the brow and follows down to the lacrimal sac in an inferonasal oblique fashion, may block portion of the superonasal iris, and covers caruncle from view.
▶ *Type 3. Epicanthus palpebralis:* Bridges both upper and lower eyelids; covers the caruncle from view.
▶ *Type 4. Epicanthus inversus:* Main portion of this fold sits along medial portion of lower eyelid, and arches up superonasally to cover medial canthal angle as well as caruncle view.
• Epicanthal folds, especially the last three types, are usually seen associated with rare conditions like blepharophimosis, congenital ptosis, Down syndrome, or as an isolated finding.

SENIOR AUTHOR TIP: In patients being considered for Asian upper blepharoplasty (with construction of upper lid crease), the reduction or excision of any medial upper lid fold should be considered as part of the upper blepharoplasty, rather than labeled as a mild form of pathological epicanthus tarsalis necessitating the creation of a special "epicanthoplasty" to be added to the surgical procedure.

AESTHETICS

- ■ **Skin evaluation**
  - • Thickness
  - • Fitzpatrick classification
- ■ **Brow relationship**
  - • Need accurate evaluation of brow position
    - ▶ Asian skin can camouflage frontalis function or activation.
    - ▶ Asian blepharoplasty can be followed by "brow drop," especially in those with borderline brow position or reflex frontalis activation.
  - • Evaluation of crease/brow ratio
- ■ **Classification of crease**
  - • **Taper:** Crease and pretarsal show tapers from lateral to medial.
    - ▶ Nasal crease tapers to or into fold medially.
  - • **Parallel:** Crease is parallel to the lid margin along its entire course; no tapering occurs down into an epicanthal fold.
- ■ **Determine pretarsal show**
  - • Pretarsal show is different between whites and Asians.
  - • Patient decision
  - • Based on aesthetics
  - • Ideally, approximately **1-4 mm** of pretarsal show[13,21,22]
- ■ **Evaluate for aging eyelid and senile changes**
  - • Upper eyelid margin is normally 1-1.5 mm below superior corneal limbus.
  - • Distance from central upper eyelid margin to pupillary light reflex is margin-reflex distance (MRD).
  - • Ptosis is present when MRD <3 mm.
  - • Asymmetry is present with MRD difference of ≥0.5 mm between the two upper eyelids.
- ■ **Evaluate for crease symmetry and presence of multiple folds/creases.**

PREOPERATIVE EVALUATION AND SURGICAL PLANNING

STANDARD HISTORY AND PHYSICAL EXAMINATION
- ■ Blepharoplasty workup
- ■ History of dry eyes

MARKINGS (Fig. 36-3)
- ■ Determine level of palpebral crease fixation.
- ■ Determine degree of pretarsal show and thus amount of skin resection (if needed).
- ■ Determine need for debulking of preaponeurotic fat.

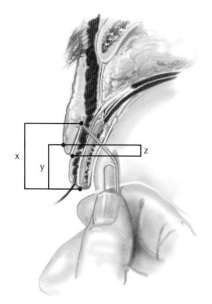

Fig. 36-3   Measure how much skin overhang to remove *(z)* to obtain the desired amount of visible pretarsal skin *(y)*. Double the length of *z*, and add 1.5 mm for the caudal bend, depending on skin thickness, to calculate the amount of skin to be removed at that point on the lid. This exercise may be repeated at two or more points along the lid. Pretarsal height is shown *(x)*. If a frontal lift will be performed, assess the skin in this same way, but with the measured lid's corresponding eyebrow held at the level of "best guess" estimate of where the "postlift" brow will reside in 6 months.

Browlift Options
- Endobrow
- Temporal brow
- Coronal brow

Incisional Versus Nonincisional
- **Nonincisional technique (also known as *suture, minimal incision*, or *closed*)**
  - Higher incidence of relapse
  - Best reserved for eyelids requiring **minimal change**
  - **Relative indications**
    - ▶ Patient is young with thin upper lids.
    - ▶ Patient has no redundant upper lid skin or requirements for debulking.
    - ▶ Patient does not want a visible scar.
  - **Relative contraindications**
    - ▶ Excessive amount or thickness of subcutaneous fat
    - ▶ Dermatochalasis or excess fat and skin
- **Incisional technique**
  - More common technique
  - Lower incidence of relapse
  - **Relative indications**
    - ▶ Need concomitant removal of skin or fat
    - ▶ Thick eyelids that require debulking
  - **Relative contraindications**
    - ▶ Patient does not want a visible scar.

SENIOR AUTHOR TIP: The buried suture methods were the first to be used in the early twentieth century when understanding of anatomy was rudimentary. During the period from 1930-1960 there was greater integration of awareness of anatomy of the face and eyelids with advances in techniques that are selectively targeted. External incision methods and suture methods became more common. The great rivalry between the proponents of the two schools of Asian eyelid crease surgery fueled greater evolution of simple and complex methods in each school.

Eventually, every practitioner needs a greater understanding of the physiology and biodynamic of the complex layers of the upper lid, as well as techniques that suit his or her technical capability. It would be simplistic and foolhardy to think that the upper lid is a homogeneous layer of flesh 1.5-4.0 mm thick that can withstand indiscriminate incision and excision in external incision methods, along with multiple needle passes in buried suture methods in which permanent sutures are placed at various distances *above* the superior tarsal border without affecting the excursion, contractility, and function of the levator muscle and Müller muscle.

Patients are often surprised to find that after "nonincisional" methods, permanent nondissolvable suture material was placed within their upper eyelid layers, or that opening or closing their eyelids does not occur quite as naturally. They often describe a strained feeling or tightness.

EPICANTHOPLASTY
- **Clinical evaluation of epicanthal fold severity**
  - **Mild:** Fold is present without local distortion.
  - **Moderate:** Fold extends to level of lower limbus.
  - **Severe:** Fold extends (a) >1 mm below level of lower limbus and creates appearance of telecanthus or internal strabismus or (b) to lower lid and reflects laterally *(epicanthus inversus)*.
  - Epicanthoplasty is considered for moderate or severe epicanthal folds.
- **Indications for epicanthoplasty**[21]
  - Patient preference
    - ▶ If patient desires a parallel crease, epicanthal fold will need to be addressed.
  - Prominent folds that give appearance of telecanthus or strabismus
  - Epicanthus inversus with fold turning laterally onto lower eyelid
  - Lid crease diving beneath the epicanthal canopy

TECHNIQUE

INCISIONAL TECHNIQUES WITH LEVATOR-DERMAL FIXATION
- Many authors have described the levator release technique.[2,17,23-25]
- **Basic concept**
  - Supratarsal incision with excision of a strip of orbicularis muscle

- Removal of excessive fat and soft tissue
- Anchoring of muscle/skin flap to the levator aponeurosis at the upper tarsal edge
■ **Technique**
  - Skin incision marked with fine-tipped pen (Fig. 36-4, *A* through *D*)
    ▶ Lower incision is typically 6-9 mm above the ciliary margin.
    ▶ Skin excision markings are conservative and vary with technique.

A   B

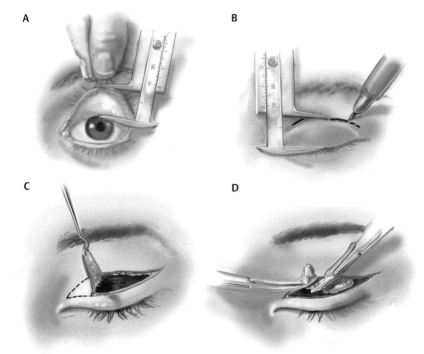

C   D

Fig. 36-4   **A,** In the operating room, the lid is turned over and the tarsus measured. **B,** With the skin under uniform traction, the incision or the lower margin of the skin excision is marked with a Jameson caliper 8-9 mm above the lashes for a 4 mm tall pretarsal segment, 8 mm for a 2.5-3 mm segment, and 7 mm for a 1.5-2 mm pretarsal segment. The 2 mm added by including the lashes and lid margin compensate for the tightly stretched skin and the inward curvature necessary to reach the anterior tarsus. The skin excision rarely extends beyond the orbital rim and the actual lid creasing. **C** and **D,** A sliver of orbicularis bordering the pretarsal skin flap is removed. Never tent this during excision to prevent transecting aponeurosis.

- Skin and muscle resection
  ▶ Incise and remove skin.
  ▶ Trim underlying preseptal muscle in thin strips.
  ▶ Remove preseptal muscle and underlying orbicularis fascia to match skin excision.
  ▶ Remove small strip of muscle along upper edge of tarsus.
- Remove sliver of conjoined fascia (Fig. 36-5, *A* and *B*).
  ▶ Conjoined fascia is superficial to tarsal plate.

- ▶ Fascia is fairly adherent.
- ▶ As the levator and orbital septum retract upward, the upper tarsus is exposed.

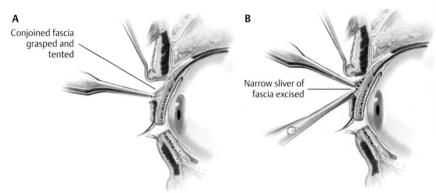

A, Conjoined fascia grasped and tented

B, Narrow sliver of fascia excised

Fig. 36-5   A, The conjoined fascia is superficial to the tarsal plate. Delicate forceps grasp the fairly adherent conjoined fascia. **B,** A narrow sliver of conjoined fascia is resected.

- • Incise remainder of the septal levator junction.
  - ▶ Opens the preaponeurotic fat space
  - ▶ Releases the septum from the levator aponeurosis
  - ▶ Conservative fat removal if indicated
- • Smooth and redrape pretarsal tissues.
- • Reattach levator (Fig. 36-6, *A* and *B*).
  - ▶ Advance free edge of levator to pretarsal tissue.
  - ▶ Suture aponeurosis to anterior tarsus and dermal margin of lower incision.
  - ▶ Skin closure

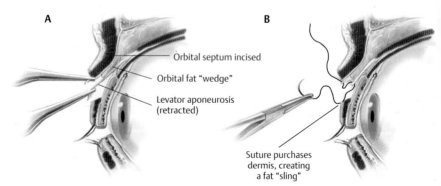

A,
Orbital septum incised
Orbital fat "wedge"
Levator aponeurosis (retracted)

B,
Suture purchases dermis, creating a fat "sling"

Fig. 36-6   A, The forceps hold the two components of the fat sling. The upper forceps is on the edge of the orbital septum, while the lower places have the medial free edge of the levator aponeurosis on tension, pulling down and revealing the fibers of the levator muscle. A small, highly vascularized fat wedge separates the two layers. **B,** After the pretarsal tissues are smoothed and advanced nasally, sutures approximate the free edge of the levator aponeurosis to the pretarsal tissue. In this case, the aponeurosis is sutured to both the anterior tarsus and the dermis at the margin of the lower incision.

SENIOR AUTHOR TIP: The notion that levator aponeurosis should be surgically detached (or euphemistically "released" in the construction of an upper lid crease) seems heavy-handed and unnecessary to me. Why the early writers mention this as a *necessary* step puzzles me, when the goal to construct an eyelid crease that indents along the superior tarsal border should require preserving all the contractile strength available, gently guiding the correct amount at the right location to generate a natural, dynamic crease. Too high a placement of crease-fixation sutures can risk fixing the deeper-located elevating muscles (levator aponeurosis and Müller muscles) to the surrounding tissues at a more proximal point, up along its contractile axis, impairing the range of excursion and causing a Faden-like decrease in overall contractility (strength, force).[26] This often results in a mild secondary ptosis even if the levator has not been "released" before being reattached. (This phenomenon is often observed but not mentioned enough in conjunction with buried suture methods or nonincisional techniques.)

INCISIONAL TECHNIQUES WITHOUT LEVATOR RELEASE
- **Basic concept**
  - Promote adherence of tarsal plate to pretarsal skin
  - Adjust amount of excess tissue and fat with graded debulking
    - ▶ Periincisional tissue
    - ▶ Pretarsal tissue
    - ▶ Orbital fat
    - ▶ Preseptal fat
    - ▶ Orbicularis muscle
  - No need to interfere with tarsal-levator junction
- **Technique**
  - Supratarsal incision with planned periincisional tissue excision
  - Pretarsal tissue debulking
  - Preseptal excision
  - Orbital fat excision if necessary
  - Suture fixation of skin to anterior surface of tarsus at desired level of the crease
  - Skin closure

TRAPEZOIDAL DEBULKING OF PREAPONEUROTIC TISSUES IN ASIAN BLEPHAROPLASTY

SENIOR AUTHOR TIP: Trapezoidal debulking of preaponeurotic tissues allows precise, physiologic, and on-plane debulking and requires the fewest steps of all upper blepharoplasty techniques.

- This technique allows selective removal of layers of tissues in a beveled approach,[27,28] coupled with construction of a dynamic, natural-appearing lid crease.
  - Beveled approach allows selective removal of tissues that may be impeding crease construction; optimally aligns the wound for closure

- Depending on the limited amount of skin that needs to be removed, the excision of soft tissues can be performed in an elegant, trapezoidal block.[25-27]
  - ▶ This preserves more of the orbicularis oculi than traditional excision and allows clearing of a greater surface of the aponeurosis.
  - ▶ In most cases, a small amount of skin is necessarily removed to reduce the lid fold.
  - ▶ These tissues need not be removed layer by layer, which risks nonuniform treatment through the tissue planes.
  - ▶ Rarely, when skin is not removed, only a single lid crease mark is incised; after a beveled passage through the orbicularis oculi allows a triangular cross segment of orbicularis oculi and some septal to be cleared.
- Crease **height** is primarily based on the central upper tarsal height.
- **Shape** chosen is included in the design.
- After the crease incision (lower incision line) and upper incision have been made through the skin using a surgical blade, the next step is a superiorly-beveled traverse through the upper incision's orbicularis oculi and orbital septum to the preaponeurotic space (Fig. 36-7).

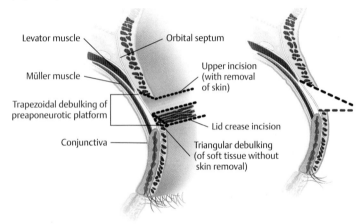

Fig. 36-7   The concept of trapezoidal and triangular debulking of eyelid tissues as applied in Asian upper blepharoplasty.[26,27]

- The strip of myocutaneous tissues backed by the orbital septum (in most cases) is then rotated forward and trimmed along the superior tarsal border toward the lid crease incision, using light application of monopolar cautery on cutting mode with good control of vascular oozing.
- Small strands of redundant fibroadipose tissues may be selectively thinned along the crease incision and superior tarsal border.
- The wound-injury involvement of the layers is staggered and distributed.

> **SENIOR AUTHOR TIP:**   With this beveled approach, access through the skin, orbicularis oculi, and orbital septum allows en bloc removal, preventing the need to excise each individual layer, as well as allowing graded handling of the preaponeurotic fat, depending on the clinical finding.

- The tissue planes are reset appropriately through release of any constraining surgical drapes.
- The upper edge of the incision wound will fall in place naturally without exaggerated wound tension over the aponeurotic tissue along the superior tarsal border; the crease invagination is easily observed intraoperatively even before closing the wound edges.
- Five to six crease-enhancing 6-0 sutures are applied from the skin to the superficial strands of the levator aponeurosis, and back to skin as interrupted sutures.
- The wound is further approximated with a running 7-0 suture.

> **NOTE:**   The orbicularis oculi muscle, orbital septum, and preaponeurotic fat pad are intentionally not embedded in the crease wound, further reducing the incidence of malformation of the crease and suboptimal results. In this technique, buried sutures are not used, and all sutures are removed at 1 week.

> **SENIOR AUTHOR TIP:**   The elegance of the beveled approach is that instead of removing a square or rectangular cross sectional block (preaponeurotic skin, orbicularis oculi, and possibly fat), a beveled approach through orbicularis removes a smaller amount of these tissue layers. Fat excision is minimal to prevent a sunken sulcus. This preserves more of the orbicularis oculi than traditional excision and allows clearing of a greater surface of the aponeurosis. In most cases, a small amount of skin is necessarily removed to reduce the lid fold.

- This technique has the following **advantages:**
  - Spreads the wound injury among the eyelid layers in different depths and locations
  - Allows a tension-free closure
  - Preserves most of the preaponeurotic fat (as a glide zone buffer)[13]
  - It provides flexibility and access to all layers of the upper lid.
  - Aims to preserve and even enhance the biodynamics of tissue layers
    - ▶ The biodynamics of the upper lid relies on a glide plane[13] (consisting of preaponeurotic fat, fourth layer) to exist between the anterior and posterior lamella.
    - ▶ This permits the formation of a dynamically pulled-in crease between the interphase of activated levator–Müller muscle with a relaxed skin-orbicularis oculi (lid fold).
    - ▶ The anterior lamellar components of skin-orbicularis-orbital septum acts as a functional unit, innervated by the facial nerve branches.
    - ▶ The posterior lamella components are much more dynamic among its layers; there are movements at the boundary between the levator muscle and the preaponeurotic fat pad in front, as well as co-contraction of the Müller muscle.
- This technique relies on the spatial optimization of the different tissue layers relative to each other.

- Rather than rely on suture compression or ligation of upper lid tissues with permanent sutures, it creates a more favorable anatomic environment for a crease to form naturally.
- It avoids encircling sutures (temporary or permanent) on any muscles by using strategic attachment of only fractional strands of the distal levator aponeurotic fibers, redirecting it toward the skin along the superior tarsal border, and dissolvable suture materials are not used.
- All sutures are removed at 1 week. The concept and technique are equally applicable to revisions.[28]

NONINCISIONAL TECHNIQUES
Basic Concept
- Creates transtarsodermal fixation of eyelid skin to superficial portion of tarsal plate
- Combines suture apposition and scarring to create the palpebral crease

Technique
- Determine the fold height
  - Position relative to the epicanthal fold
  - Desires of the patient
  - Personal aesthetics
- Eversion of lid and measurement of tarsal height with calipers
- Mark desired fold (usually at or slightly inferior to the superior margin of the tarsal plate), following natural curve of upper eyelid
- Mark incision/suture line
  - Width of marking should be at or slightly less than tarsal width for younger patients.
  - Width of marking should be slightly wider than tarsal width for older patients.
- Single or multiple buried suture technique
  - Single suture[29] (Fig. 36-8)

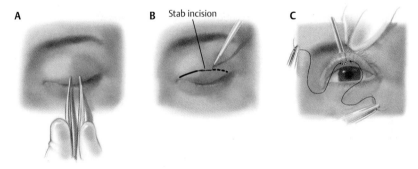

Fig. 36-8   Design of the position and conjunctival passage of the suture. **A,** The two points of entry are determined by marking the desired fold using a fine forceps. **B,** The points of entry of the suture are marked with methylene blue. **C,** The lid is everted and a double-armed 6-0 Prolene suture is inserted through the conjunctiva.

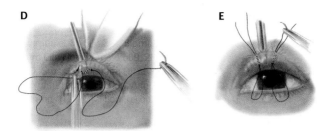

Fig. 36-8, cont'd   D, One end of the double-armed suture is passed back through the lid, entering through the same needle hole on the conjunctival surface and exiting through the stab incisions in the skin. **E,** The other end of the suture is passed back to the skin.

- Small stab incisions performed at identified points of entry along new superior palpebral crease with the steps of stabbed incisions. Technically one is no longer in a nonincisional technique, as these stab incisions are closed also with 6-0 nylon/ polypropylene.
- Suture inserted through conjunctiva, entering and exiting through same hole
- Passes through full thickness of lid
- Enter and exit through same skin incision so needles come through stab incision together
- Knot tied and released to bury it subcutaneously
- Essentially is a buried, full-thickness, horizontal mattress suture
- Alternatively, can do multiple through-and-through mattress sutures[21] (Fig. 36-9)

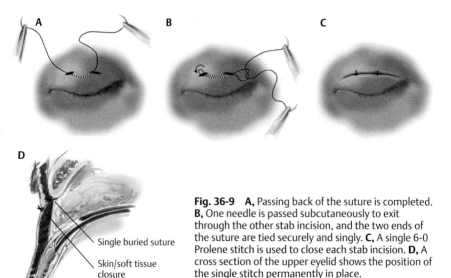

Fig. 36-9   A, Passing back of the suture is completed. **B,** One needle is passed subcutaneously to exit through the other stab incision, and the two ends of the suture are tied securely and singly. **C,** A single 6-0 Prolene stitch is used to close each stab incision. **D,** A cross section of the upper eyelid shows the position of the single stitch permanently in place.

Single buried suture

Skin/soft tissue closure

- Continuous buried tarsal suture[21,30,31] (Fig. 36-10)

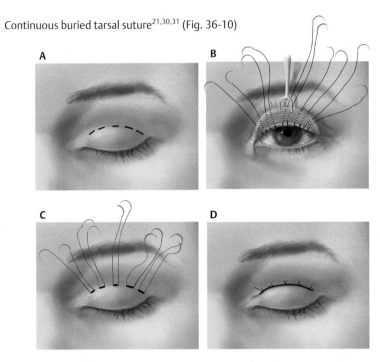

Fig. 36-10   The closed technique is commonly used in Asia for lid surgery in those without fat excess or significant skin redundancy and heavy eyelid skin and tissues. **A,** The top of the tarsus is located and defined and the cephalad margin of tarsus on the skin is delineated. **B,** Tiny incisions will allow knots to bury deep beneath skin. **C,** Nonabsorbable sutures, placed through the lid, run subconjunctivally on the deep side of the upper tarsus and exit and travel subdermally to create a nice lid fold. Large external incisions are not necessary. **D,** Sutures securely tied and cut. This technique is especially useful when combined with frontal lifting.

- Equidistant incisional dots are marked along marked fold.
  - ▶ At each point, 2-3 mm skin incision is made with No. 11 blade deep to orbicularis oculi muscle.
  - ▶ Double-armed 6-0 monofilament polypropylene suture is used. One arm enters and traverses medial stab incision with deep bite through superior tarsus, exiting and reentering the next lateral stab incision.
  - ▶ This pattern of tarsal fixation suturing continues at every other point to the lateral end.
  - ▶ Conjunctiva is inspected after each deep intratarsal bite to ensure no suture exposure through conjunctiva.
  - ▶ Using the second arm of the suture, alternating tarsal fixation sutures are placed until both ends exit laterally.
  - ▶ Needles are cut off, sutures tied to one another, and the knot buried.
  - ▶ Essentially, the technique is a **continuous buried horizontal mattress suture** (Fig. 36-11).

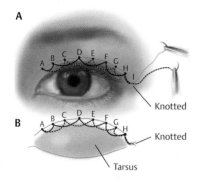

A

B

Knotted

Knotted

Tarsus

Fig. 36-11   A, Modified continuous buried tarsal stitch technique. Incisional dots are marked at points *A* through *H;* both threads reenter at lateral ends *(I),* and the knot is tied. **B,** Cross section of a continuous buried tarsal stitch.

SENIOR AUTHOR TIP: The frequent association of secondary consecutive ptosis when the crease fixation was performed excessively high (aggressive) will often generate pressure on the surgeon to prophylactically perform a mild ptosis correction. Conjointly this is achieved either by tucking the levator aponeurosis in incisional methods, or by passing one to three buried suture sets even higher above the superior tarsal border (by several millimeters) to create a skewed, posteriorly directed and upwardly beveled passage across the thickness of the upper lid, causing a plication or tucking of the levator aponeurosis and Müller muscle.

NOTE: **Fig. 36-12 shows typical placement of buried sutures in nonincisional methods. In the short term, it gives the appearance of a lift in the upper lid margin but is often associated with a longer-term graded weakening of the levator muscle, with minimal to mild consecutive ptosis. This is akin to a Faden-like effect of sutures used ophthalmologically in strabismus repair. Fig. 36-13 illustrates the mechanism involved in Faden-like weakening of the contractility of levator aponeurosis with long-term placement of nondissolvable sutures fixating the Müller, levator, and orbicularis muscles.**

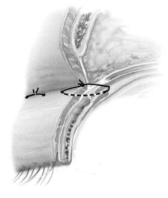

Fig. 36-12   Cross section showing placement of a buried suture that encircles the orbicularis oculi, levator aponeurosis, and underlying Müller muscle. It is a *suture loop* of 7-0 nylon or polypropylene. Often, a small fragment of preaponeurotic fat pad and orbital septum may be inadvertently included in the ligature.

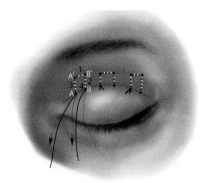

Fig. 36-13 In buried suture methods, three double-armed 6-0 or 7-0 nylon are typically used. This left upper eyelid shows the typical passages for the medial set of buried suture. The first passage *(1)* involves everting the upper lid margin and passing it subconjunctivally for 3-4 mm at a level typically several millimeters *above* the superior tarsal border *(A'-B')*. The second passage is trans-lid *(2)* and directs one needle toward the skin side along the path of *B'-B*, aiming just over the upper border of the tarsus. Similarly, for the other arm of the suture, the third passage *(3)* goes from *A'* to *A*. If each suture thread is tied on the skin at this moment, it will be a full-thickness compression ligature encompassing (plicating) the Müller muscle, the levator aponeurosis, and orbicularis oculi muscle in a posterosuperiorly biased fashion along the axis of the levator muscle's contractility. It also inadvertently creates a Faden-like effect at each of the two locations of *B'-B* and *A'-A*. Essentially, the second needle exiting the skin at *A* is repassed *(4)* subcutaneously to join *B*, exiting at a ministab skin opening there. The nylon ends are "firmly" tied and the knot sunken into the small surgical opening. In addition to the Faden-like effect, this results in a horizontal contraction in the width of levator aponeurosis at the two locations of *A'-B'* and *A-B*. Traditionally, the suture methods use three sets of these sutures, one each at the medial third, central third, and lateral third. With three sets of sutures, the restrictive effect is tripled.

SENIOR AUTHOR TIP: Three sets of these buried sutures means that three encircling loops are placed around the levator/Müller muscle layers from the subcutaneous plane from the front skin surface. Patients who have these procedures often have an exaggerated stare or an elevated upper lid margin; in essence, a prophylactic correction has been included. It may also be marketed as a form of ptosis repair. This is a classic example of an overdiagnosed condition (ptosis) with overprescribed countermeasures, sometimes in an overcomplicated fashion.

EPICANTHOPLASTY
- **Basic concept**
  - Local flaps to rearrange tissue and expose the caruncle
  - Flaps designed to pull skin medially
  - Requires exercising caution, because it may produce hypertrophic or unsightly scarring
- **Multiple designs have been reported (e.g., W-plasty, Z-plasty)** (Fig. 36-14)

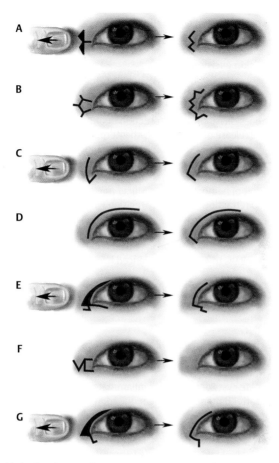

Fig. 36-14   Published techniques for correcting Asian epicanthal folds. **A,** The modified Uchida method. **B,** Matsunaga's modified "M-plasty" method. **C,** Fuente's transpositional flap. **D,** Jordan's "deep tissue approach" flap. **E,** Yoon's "one-armed jumping man" method. **F,** Wu's square-flap method. **G,** Park's "Z-plasty" method.

COMPLICATIONS

ASYMMETRY
- Common source of dissatisfaction in 13%-35%[20]
- Minimized by consistent and meticulous technique
- Hyaluronic acid filler injection into superior sulcus can lower a surgically created eyelid crease and may be alternative to reoperation for patients with asymmetrical creases.[32]
- **Causes**
  - **Swelling**
    - ▶ 6 weeks minimum
    - ▶ Can last up to 3-6 months

- **Resolution of compensatory frontalis activation**
  - ▶ May require browlift to achieve brow symmetry
  - ▶ May require revision blepharoplasty
- **Discrepancy in skin excision**
  - ▶ May require revision blepharoplasty to improve symmetry

MULTIPLE UPPER EYELID FOLDS
- From scar tissue adhesions and/or overresection of underlying tissues
- May require surgical release of adhesions with interposition of tissue (orbital fat, orbicularis oculi)[33]

PTOSIS OR LID RETRACTION
- Ptosis may be a result of hemorrhage into Müller muscle.
- Definite ptosis or lid retraction needs early revision within 1-2 weeks.

RELAPSE
- More common in suture techniques and in bulkier lids
  - Rates range from 2.9% to 4.5% in experienced hands and with good patient selection.[29,30]
- **Early relapse:** Consider repair within first 2-3 weeks
- **Late relapse:** Allow 3-6 months to pass

SCARRING/DIMPLING
- Scarring is usually more of a problem with epicanthoplasty than with blepharoplasty.
  - Epicanthoplasty scarring is extremely difficult to revise.
- Dimpling results from subdermal suture.
  - Sutures may create cysts or other local inflammatory reaction.
  - Suture removal after 3 months may be required.

TOP TAKEAWAYS
➤ Asians lack a palpebral fold, because the levator does not penetrate the septum and it appears that there are no fibrous extensions of the levator into the skin or subcutaneous tissue.
➤ Trapezoidal debulking of preaponeurotic tissues allows precise, physiologic, and on-plane debulking and requires the fewest steps of all upper blepharoplasty techniques.

REFERENCES
1. Shirakabe Y, Kinugasa T, Kawata M, et al. The double-eyelid operation in Japan: its evolution as related to cultural changes. Ann Plast Surg 15:224, 1985.
2. Sayoc BT. Plastic construction of the superior palpebral fold. Am J Ophthalmol 38:556, 1954.
3. Millard DR Jr. Oriental peregrinations. Plast Reconstr Surg (1946) 16:319, 1955.
4. Fernandez LR. Double eyelid operation in the Oriental in Hawaii. Plast Reconstr Surg Transplant Bull 25:257, 1960.
5. Cho M, Glavas IP. Anatomic properties of the upper eyelid in Asian Americans. Dermatol Surg 35:1736, 2009.

6. Lee CK, Ahn ST, Kim M. Asian upper lid blepharoplasty surgery. Clin Plast Surg 40:167, 2013.

7. Seiff SR, Seiff BD. Anatomy of the Asian eyelid. Facial Plast Surg Clin North Am 15:309, 2007.

8. Kakisaki H, Goold LA, Casson RJ, et al. Tarsal height. Ophthamology 116:1831, 2009.

9. Cheng J, Xu FZ. Anatomic microstructure of the upper eyelid in the Oriental double eyelid. Plast Reconstr Surg 107:1665, 2001.

10. Sayoc BT. Absence of superior palpebral fold in slit eyes; an anatomic and physiologic explanation. Am J Ophthalmol 42:298, 1956.

11. Zubiri JS. Correction of the Oriental eyelid. Clin Plast Surg 8:725, 1981.

12. Morikawa K, Yamamoto H, Uchinuma E, et al. Scanning electron microscopic study on double and single eyelids in Orientals. Aesthetic Plast Surg 25:20, 2001.

13. Chen WP. The concept of a glide zone as it relates to upper lid crease, lid fold, and application in upper blepharoplasty. Plast Reconstr Surg 119:379, 2007.

14. Collin JR, Beard C, Wood I. Experimental and clinical data on the insertion of the levator palpebrae superioris muscle. Am J Ophthalmol 85:792, 1978.

15. Doxanas MT, Anderson RL. Oriental eyelids. An anatomic study. Arch Ophthalmol 102:1232, 1984.

16. Jeong S, Lemke BN, Dortzbach RK, et al. The Asian upper eyelid: an anatomical study with comparison to the Caucasian eyelid. Arch Ophthalmol 117:907, 1999.

17. Siegel R. Surgical anatomy of the upper eyelid fascia. Ann Plast Surg 13:263, 1984.

18. Kim DW, Bhatki AM. Upper blepharoplasty in the Asian eyelid. Facial Plast Surg Clin North Am 15:327, 2007.

19. Chen WP. Asian blepharoplasty. Update on anatomy and techniques. Ophthal Plast Reconstr Surg 3:135, 1987.

20. Johnson CC. Epicanthus and epiblepharon. Arch Ophthalmol 96:1030, 1978.

21. Flowers RS. Asian blepharoplasty. Aesthet Surg J 22:558, 2002.

22. Yoon KC, Park S. Systematic approach and selective tissue removal in blepharoplasty for young Asians. Plast Reconstr Surg 102:502, 1998.

23. Fernandez LR. The East Asian eyelid-open technique. Clin Plast Surg 20:247, 1993.

24. Flowers RS. Upper blepharoplasty by eyelid invagination. Anchor blepharoplasty. Clin Plast Surg 20:193, 1993.

25. Siegel RJ. Contemporary upper lid blepharoplasty—tissue invagination. Clin Plast Surg 20:239; discussion 245, 1993.

26. Chen WP, ed. Asian Blepharoplasty and the Eyelid Crease, ed 3. Philadelphia: Elsevier Sciences, 2016.

27. Chen WP. Concept of triangular, trapezoidal, and rectangular debulking of eyelid tissues: application in Asian blepharoplasty. Plast Reconstr Surg 97:212, 1996.

28. Chen WP. Beveled approach for revisional surgery in Asian blepharoplasty. Plast Reconstr Surg 120:545; discussion 553, 2007.

29. Baek SM, Kim SS, Tokunaga S, et al. Oriental blepharoplasty: single-stitch, nonincision technique. Plast Reconstr Surg 83:236, 1989.

30. Wong JK. A method in creation of the superior palpebral fold in Asians using a continuous buried tarsal stitch (CBTS). Facial Plast Surg Clin North Am 15:337, 2007.

31. Wong JK, Zhou X, Ai T, et al. A simple, minimally invasive method for creation of the superior palpebral fold in Asians with the modified continuous buried tarsal stitch. Arch Facial Plast Surg 12:269, 2010.

32. Choi HS, Whipple KM, Oh SR, et al. Modifying the upper eyelid crease in Asian patients with hyaluronic acid fillers. Plast Reconstr Surg 127:844, 2011.

33. Lew DH, Kang JH, Cho IC. Surgical correction of multiple upper eyelid folds in east Asians. Plast Reconstr Surg 127:1323, 2011.

37. Correction of the Tear Trough Deformity

Jason K. Potter, Grant Gilliland

- Soft tissue depressions at the lid-cheek junction represent some of the most challenging, and difficult to correct, age-related deformities of the periorbital region.
- The term **"tear trough deformity"** was first coined by Flowers and refers to the development of **visible depression along the medial third of the lower lid.**[1]
- Contemporary use of the term *tear trough deformity* refers to a variable spectrum of soft tissue deformities across the lid-cheek junction that are a direct result of the interplay of complex, age-related changes that occur in the lower lid and midcheek.
  - Correction of these deformities may therefore include procedures directed at rejuvenating both the lower lid and midcheek areas depending on their severity.

TERMINOLOGY[2]

- **Nasojugal groove:** Natural sulcus directly overlying the medial one third of the inferior orbital rim.
  - "Tear trough deformity" refers to a prominent nasojugal groove.
- **Palpebromalar groove:** Prominent depression at lid-cheek junction inferolateral to nasojugal groove.
  - It is confluent with nasojugal groove.
- **Midcheek:** Region of cheek medial to a line extending from the frontal process of the zygoma to the oral commissure and from the lower lid to the nasolabial fold.
  - Prezygomatic part: Overlies the skeleton of the midcheek.
  - Infrazygomatic part: Covers the vestibule of the oral cavity.
- **Tear trough triad:** Association of several anatomic characteristics giving rise to a prominent tear trough (Fig. 37-1).
  - Herniation of orbital fat
  - Tight attachment of the orbicularis retaining ligament along the arcus marginalis
  - Malar retrusion

GRADING SYSTEM (Table 37-1)

- An objective system for grading the severity of deformity has been proposed by Barton et al.[3]
  - More severe deformities are characterized by changes not limited to the nasojugal groove.

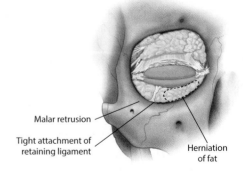

Malar retrusion

Tight attachment of retaining ligament

Herniation of fat

Fig. 37-1   Tear trough triad.

Table 37-1   *Grading System for Tear Trough Deformity*

Deformity	Grade
No medial or lateral lines indicating the arcus marginalis or the orbital rim Contour is smooth and youthful; no transition at the orbit-cheek junction	0
Medial line or shadow is mild or subtle Lid-cheek junction has a smooth lateral transition	I
Lid-cheek junction shows a moderate prominence, extending from medial to lateral	II
Orbit-cheek junction shows a severe prominence, with an obvious step between orbit and cheek	III

CLASSIFICATION OF MIDFACE MORPHOLOGY (Fig. 37-2)

■ Classification system incorporating the global changes occurring at the eyelid-cheek junction and midface.[4]

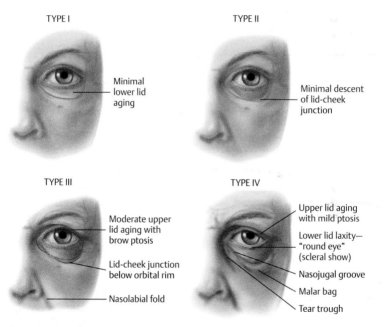

TYPE I — Minimal lower lid aging

TYPE II — Minimal descent of lid-cheek junction

TYPE III — Moderate upper lid aging with brow ptosis / Lid-cheek junction below orbital rim / Nasolabial fold

TYPE IV — Upper lid aging with mild ptosis / Lower lid laxity—"round eye" (scleral show) / Nasojugal groove / Malar bag / Tear trough

Fig. 37-2   Classification of midfacial morphology involving lid and cheek.

ANATOMIC CONSIDERATIONS CONTRIBUTING TO DEFORMITIES AT THE LID-CHEEK JUNCTION[5-7]

Periorbital and midcheek anatomy has been reviewed in detail in Chapter 22.

MEDIAL FAT PAD

■ Bulge extends anteriorly in a position superior to the inferiomedial orbital rim.
   • Visually, this creates an apparent increase in the depth of the nasojugal groove.

- Inferior descent is limited by the tight, direct attachment of the orbicularis to the medial orbital rim.

> **SENIOR AUTHOR TIP:**   The medial fat pad can be quite vascular and care must be taken in the dissection of this fat pad to prevent vascular injury that retracts into the orbit, which can result in a retrobulbar hematoma.

CENTRAL FAT PAD

- Inferior descent over the central orbital rim is not restricted and therefore occurs progressively.
- Inferior descent distends the orbicularis retaining ligament (ORL) inferiorly several millimeters.
- Inferior descent and distention of the ORL creates an apparent increase in the depth as well as the length of the nasojugal groove.
- With increasing magnitude of descent, a sulcus develops lateral and inferior to the central fat bulge—the *palpebromalar groove.*
  - Palpebromalar groove creates a visible demarcation of the lid-cheek junction laterally.

> **SENIOR AUTHOR TIP:**   The medial and lateral fat pads are separated by the "arcuate expanse." This is a fibrous extension from the arcus marginalis inferolaterally extending medially to the medial canthal tendon. It is a retroseptal structure which functions to prevent overaction of the inferior oblique muscle.

FESTOONS

- Can be multifactorial
- Skin and skin/muscle festoons can be addressed by redraping the skin and/or skin/muscle in a more anatomic position.
- Dermal festoons are more difficult to treat and are related to the interdigitation of the orbitomalar retaining ligament with the subdermal collagen as the direction of the collagen fibers change from circumocular in the eyelid to more vertical in the cheek.

> **SENIOR AUTHOR TIP:**   It is very important to identify festoons and their etiology prior to surgery so that they can be addressed and patient expectations for swelling in this area can be properly addressed.

INDICATIONS AND CONTRAINDICATIONS

- Main indication is the presence of enough deformity so that surgery may make a difference.[8]
- Patients who would clearly benefit from surgery are those with **orbital fat herniation** and **significant skin laxity**.[4]
  - Patients who have these characteristics should be discouraged from injectables alone, as they are highly likely to have an undesirable result.

■ Nonsurgical management with injectables is a good option for **mild** to **moderate** tear trough deformities, but patient selection is paramount.[9]

NONSURGICAL AND SURGICAL TREATMENT OPTIONS

PREOPERATIVE EVALUATION FOR NONSURGICAL AND SURGICAL TREATMENT

■ Consideration of perorbital form and function, along with anatomy and patient expectation, must be balanced with protecting lid function.[10]
■ **Evaluation of the lower eyelid should include:**
  • The distance from the pupil to the lower eyelid margin (MRD-2)
  • The distance from the pupil to the tear trough
  • The width of the tear trough
  • The intercanthal angle
■ These quantitative measurements can allow for objective preoperative and postoperative assessment and allow for more predictable results.[11]

> **SENIOR AUTHOR TIP:**   Assessment of lower eyelid laxity via the snap test is important in assessing whether lower eyelid tightening, and/or shortening, should be performed at the time of blepharoplasty surgery.

INFORMED CONSENT FOR NONSURGICAL AND SURGICAL TREATMENT

■ Managing patient expectations cannot be overstated.
■ All risks and benefits of the procedure should be clearly laid out.
■ Correction, not elimination of the defect, should be properly emphasized.
■ If injectables are selected, a discussion about embolization should be included in the consent.[12]

NONSURGICAL TREATMENT
Hyaluronic Acid Filler Injections[13]

> **NOTE:**   **Hyaluronic acid products are FDA approved for filling moderate to severe facial wrinkles and folds around the nose and mouth. Use in treatment of tear trough deformities is an off-label use of the product.**

■ **Indications**
  • Visible, mild to moderate tear trough deformity
  • Good skin tone without significant wrinkling
■ **Advantages**
  • Minimal downtime
  • Cost
  • Minimally invasive
  • Small particle hyaluronic acid fillers have been found to offer correction for up to 6-9 months.[14]
■ **Disadvantages**
  • Temporary[8]
  • Does not address skin pigmentation, wrinkles, or redundancy
  • Very small but serious risk of vision loss[15]

- **Technique**
  - With patient in upright position, mark area to be injected and provide local anesthesia.
  - Injection of material deep to dermis either in the orbicularis or at the **supraperiosteal level** using parallel feathering technique to treat the area of deformity
  - To prevent bumps, injection should only be performed *when the needle is being withdrawn* and never when stationary.
  - Injection should cease before retracting the needle from the dermis.

> **TIP:**   Superficial injection in the dermis may result in noticeable lumps that persist for long periods of time (1 year) if untreated. It may also lead to persistent discoloration of the lower lid.

  - ► The material is massaged to produce a smooth result.
- **Complications**
  - Bruising
  - Irregularities
  - Bluish discoloration from superficial injection (Tyndall effect with Rayleigh scattering)

> **TIP:**   Irregularities may be corrected with massage. Overfill may be corrected with injection of hyaluronidase (75 units in 3 cc of local anesthetic).

NONVASCULARIZED FAT GRAFTING
- Injection of fat grafts has been reported and is extremely technique sensitive.
- Irregularities may be permanent.
- Gain in graft volume leading to disfigurement has been reported with generalized weight gain.

SURGICAL TREATMENT
- Historically the deformity was treated by excision of herniating fat.
- Improved understanding of the deformity and the effects of volume loss and soft tissue displacement have altered treatment philosophies.
  - **Fat preservation and repositioning** is preferred over fat excision in younger patients.
  - **Excision of fat** may be necessary in older patients or those with an increased volume of orbital fat.
- Loeb first reported redraping of the orbital fat for management of the deformity.[16]
- Hamra refined the technique into what is now referred to the **septal reset procedure.**[17,18]
  - Barton has substantiated the role of the septal reset in management of tear trough deformities.[19]
  - Care must be exercised to prevent lower eyelid malposition which is a well-known sequelae of the **septal reset procedure.**

> **TIP:**   When performing the septal reset procedure, it is helpful to have the lower eyelid on stretch during the suturing of the orbital septum to its new position to prevent excessive shortening of the middle lamella and **thereby** minimize risk of lid malposition.

External Lower Blepharoplasty and Orbicularis Suspension[20] (Fig. 37-3)

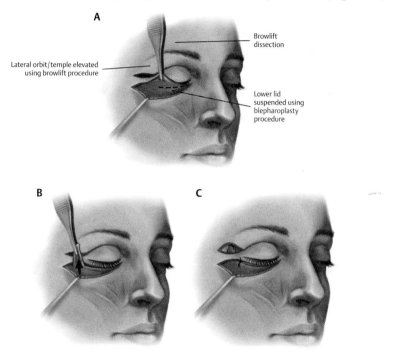

Fig. 37-3   Lower lid blepharoplasty with orbicularis suspension. **A,** Trim overlap. **B,** Cut only as necessary to close gap. **C,** Suture to orbit rim.

■ For mild deformity with vector positive or vector neutral orbits
■ Visible depression over the arcus marginalis can be improved approximately 50% by release of the orbicularis retaining ligaments and orbicularis redraping.

External Lower Blepharoplasty With Orbicularis Suspension and Septal Reset[20] (Fig. 37-4)
■ Moderate to severe deformity: Vector negative orbits with tear trough triad

- **S**ub **O**rbicularis **O**culi **F**at (SOOF) pad suspension from the arcus marginalis in conjunction with septal reset, or by itself, can improve the lid-cheek junction.
  - Provides removal of redundant skin, redraping of the orbicularis, and redraping of intraobital fat across the orbital rim for correction of the deformity.

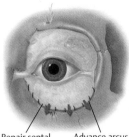

Transblepharoplasty Midface Lift[21]

- Comprehensive technique to address changes at the eyelid-cheek junction as well as repositioning ptotic midface soft tissues.
- Slightly higher incidence of complications (lateral orbital skin excess, deformities of the lateral canthus, and lower lid malposition) than traditional lower blepharoplasty techniques.
- Careful attention to lower lid laxity, orbit vector status, and lower lid supporting techniques (canthopexy) are critical to successful outcome.

Repair septal
hernia

Advance arcus
marginalis
(septum plus fat)

Fig. 37-4   Septal reset.

Tear Trough Grafts

- Initially described by Flowers,[1] due to the thin tissue qualities, grafts in the tear trough may be palpable and create visible irregularities.

TOP TAKEAWAYS

➤ Management of tear trough deformities requires an intimate knowledge of the local anatomy, recognition of the patient's characteristics and extent of deformity, and limitations of specific techniques in order to best discuss treatment options with the patient.

➤ Patients should be educated that improvement in the contours and not complete elimination is the goal.

➤ Patients should be informed that pigmentation characteristics of the skin may not be changed but improving the contours will improve shadowing that can dramatically affect the perception of pigmentation.

REFERENCES

1. Flowers RS. Tear trough implants for correction of tear trough deformity. Clin Plast Surg 20:403, 1993.
2. Mendelson BC, Muzaffar AR, Adams WP. Surgical anatomy of the midcheek and malar mounds. Plast Reconstr Surg 110:885, 2002.
3. Barton FE, Ha R, Awada M. Fat extrusion and septal reset in patients with the tear trough triad: a critical appraisal. Plast Reconstr Surg 113:2115, 2004.

4. Hester TR Jr, Codner MA, McCord CD, et al. Evolution of technique of the direct transblepharoplasty approach for the correction of lower lid and midfacial aging: maximizing results and minimizing complications in a 5-year experience. Plast Reconstr Surg 105:393; discussion 407, 2000.

5. Haddock NT, Saadeh PB, Boutros S, et al. The tear trough and lid/cheek junction: anatomy and implications for surgical correction. Plast Reconstr Surg 123:1332, 2009.

6. Pessa JE. An algorithm of facial aging: verification of Lambros's theory by three-dimensional stereolithography, with reference to the pathogenesis of midfacial aging, scleral show, and the lateral suborbital trough deformity. Plast Reconstr Surg 106:479; discussion 467, 2000.

7. Mendelson BC. Discussion: Fat extrusion and septal reset in patients with the tear trough triad: a critical appraisal. Plast Reconstr Surg 113:2122, 2004.

8. Lambros VS. Hyaluronic acid injections for correction of the tear trough deformity. Plast Reconst Surg 120(6 Suppl):74S, 2007.

9. Hirmand H. Anatomy and nonsurgical correction of the tear trough deformity. Plast Reconstr Surg 125:699, 2010.

10. Jindal K, Sarcia M, Codner MA. Functional considerations in aesthetic eyelid surgery. Plast Reconst Surg 134:1154, 2014.

11. Rohrich RJ, Ghavami A, Mojallal A. The five-step lower blepharoplasty: blending the eyelid-cheek junction. Plast Reconstr Surg 128:775, 2011.

12. Bailey SH, Fagien S, Rohrich RJ. Changing role of hyaluronidase in plastic surgery. Plast Reconstr Surg 133:127e, 2014.

13. Lambrose VS. Hyaluronic acid injections for correction of the tear trough deformity. Plast Reconstr Surg 120(6 Suppl):74S, 2007.

14. Donath AS, Glasgold RA, Meier J, et al. Quantitative evaluation of volume augmentation in the tear trough with a hyaluronic acid-based filler: a three-dimensional analysis. Plast Reconstr Surg 125:1515, 2010.

15. Beleznay K, Carruthers JD, Humphrey S, et al. Avoiding and treating blindness from fillers: a review of the world literature. Dermatol Surg 41:1097, 2015.

16. Loeb R. Fat pad sliding and fat grafting for leveling lid depressions. Clin Plast Surg 8:757, 1981.

17. Hamra ST. Arcus marginalis release and orbital fat preservation in midface rejuvenation. Plast Reconstr Surg 96:354, 1995.

18. Hamra ST. The role of septal reset in creating a youthful eyelid-cheek complex in facial rejuvenation. Plast Reconstr Surg 113:2124, 2004.

19. Barton FE, Ha R, Awada M. Fat extrusion and septal reset in patients with the tear trough triad: a critical appraisal. Plast Reconstr Surg 113:2115, 2004.

20. Barton FE. Eyelids. In Facial Rejuvenation. New York: Thieme Publishers, 2008.

21. Hester RT, Codner MA, McCord CD, et al. Evolution of technique of the direct transblepharoplasty approach for the correction of lower lid and midfacial aging: Maximizing results and minimizing complications in a 5 year experience. Plast Reconstr Surg 105:393, 2000.

38. Lateral Canthopexy

Jason K. Potter, Steve Fagien

- Lateral canthopexy is an important adjunctive procedure to plastic surgeons performing blepharoplasty surgery.
- Classically, lateral canthopexy was reserved for **lax lower eyelids** or with **correction of lower eyelid deformities.**
- **Distortion of the lower lid** is the most common complication of lower lid blepharoplasty.[1]
  - Malposition results from the interaction of the patient's anatomy, the effects of mechanical distraction secondary to cicatricial and gravitational forces, and attenuation of lid supporting structures.
  - Secondary forces result from eyelid edema, hematoma, chemosis, and disruption of orbicularis innervations.
- Lateral canthopexy should be considered as a routine component of lower blepharoplasty in the appropriate patient.[2,3]
- Contemporary blepharoplasty techniques aim to correct more than merely skin laxity and therefore have the potential for increased distracting forces on the lower lid.
  - These techniques should be used in conjunction with the consideration of routine lateral canthopexy.[4]

TERMINOLOGY (Fig. 38-1)

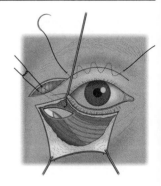

Fig. 38-1 Lateral retinacular suspension. Performed most often through the existing upper and lower blepharoplasty incision. The release allows for disinsertion of the superficial component of the lateral canthal tendon from the orbicularis muscle. A double-armed suture is placed from the lower blepharoplasty incision and passes superolateral to the internal orbital rim periosteum above Whitnall tubercle and exits the lateral upper eyelid incision. This direction can be vectored according to the patient's unique presentation and orbital morphology.

- **Lateral canthopexy:** Tightening of the lateral canthus while *maintaining the lateral attachment* of the canthus to the orbital rim
- **Lateral canthoplasty:** Tightening or repositioning the lateral canthus using transection or resection and *repositioning of the lateral canthal attachment* to the orbital rim

TIP: These terms are sometimes used interchangeably and a canthopexy, as originally described by Flowers et al,[5] was a simple suture canthal suspension without any release. A canthoplasty was used to indicate surgical division of the lateral commissure in preparation for a horizontal shortening procedure such as the lateral tarsal strip (LTS) procedure. The LTS or surgical cantholysis of the lateral commissure is rarely necessary in primary cosmetic lower blepharoplasty.

ABSOLUTE INDICATIONS FOR LATERAL CANTHOPEXY

- **Lower lid deformity:** Any procedure attempting to correct a preexisting lower lid deformity, even in a situation of primary blepharoplasty without prior surgery, should incorporate a lateral canthopexy.
  - Scleral show between the lower lid margin and inferior limbus may indicate lower lid deformity.
  - Canthal dystopia where the lateral canthal position is caudal to the lid margin and/or medial canthus.
- **Lower lid laxity:** Lower lid laxity is an indication for lateral canthopexy and is critical in preventing lid deformities from blepharoplasty when any significant tension is created, either with a skin or skin/muscle flap or skin resurfacing.
  - **Distraction (pull-away) test:** Manual anterior distraction of the lid from the globe >10 mm indicates significant lid laxity.
  - **Snap-back test:** Lid is pulled inferiorly and released to assess the speed of return to its normal position. Delayed return or persistent eversion indicates lid laxity.

RELATIVE INDICATIONS FOR LATERAL CANTHOPEXY

- Any blepharoplasty procedure involving more than isolated transconjunctival fat removal or isolated minimal skin excision

PREOPERATIVE EVALUATION

- Seven key examination findings in preoperative preparation[6]
  1. Vector analysis
  2. Tarsoligamentous integrity
  3. Scleral show
  4. Canthal tilt
  5. Distance from lateral canthus to orbital rim soft tissue
  6. Midface projection and position
  7. Vertical restriction

CHARACTERIZATION OF LOWER LID DEFORMITY

- Understanding the cause of a lower lid deformity is essential in selecting a lateral canthopexy technique.
  - **Senile ectropion:** Results from acquired laxity of the normal lower lid support mechanism
    - ▶ Manual elevation of the lid **to or beyond the superior limbus**
    - ▶ Traditional canthopexy techniques will provide sufficient augmentation of lower lid support to prevent deformity postoperatively.

- **Cicatricial ectropion:** Results from contractile forces of the scarring process; may occur secondary to prior surgery, injury, or inflammatory process
  - ▶ Manual elevation of the lid displays **minimal superior excursion** of the lid from its retracted position.
  - ▶ Correction of cicatricial ectropion benefits from powerful canthopexy techniques (transosseous) to counteract the forces of scarring and prevent recurrent deformity.

TECHNIQUES

SUPERFICIAL RETINACULAR LATERAL CANTHOPEXY
- Involves tightening lateral retinaculum to superomedial aspect of lateral orbital rim[6] (Fig. 38-2)

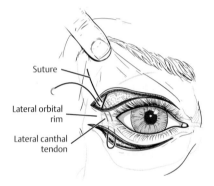

Suture

Lateral orbital rim

Lateral canthal tendon

Fig. 38-2   Lateral retinacular suspension.

- Does not disinsert lateral canthus
- May raise position of lateral canthus

SENIOR AUTHOR TIP: I originally described this form of lateral retinacular (canthal) suspension (LRS) to stabilize the lower eyelid in conjunction with a variety of lower eyelid surgical procedures utilizing, in most situations, existing upper and lower eyelid incisions with release of the superficial head of the lateral canthal tendon as well as the retinacular orbicularis muscle, to allow mobilization of a portion of the tendon rather than a simple suture canthopexy without release that was typically temporary at best. The release allows for further mobilization as well as the ability to suspend the orbicularis muscle separately and more securely with separate vectoring. This provides both canthal suspension and stabilization that allows for the appropriate orbicularis suspension that improves lower eyelid/cheek junction deformities and also provides additional lower eyelid support allowing for appropriate skin resection while avoiding lower eyelid malposition.

Unlike what has been a concern regarding lateral canthal procedures when one considers them all "the same," they certainly are not and suspension procedures like the LRS only temporarily cause an exaggerated canthal tilt that allows for lower eyelid stabilization during the healing phase of blepharoplasty and the eyelid position and canthal tilt more commonly return to the preoperative state in a matter of weeks.

In-Line Canthopexy

■ Involves tightening lateral canthus directly to Whitnall tubercle[2] (Fig. 38-3)

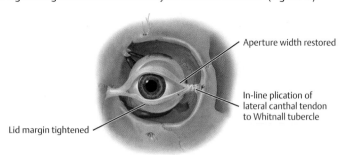

Aperture width restored

In-line plication of lateral canthal tendon to Whitnall tubercle

Lid margin tightened

Fig. 38-3   In-line lateral canthopexy.

• Does not alter position of lateral canthus

> **TIP:**   Similar to the LRS, this provides temporary lid stabilization without exaggerated canthal tilt. It may be more effective if other forms of lower eyelid stabilization (i.e., orbicularis suspension) or release are performed simultaneously.

Transcantho-Canthopexy[7]

■ Similar to in-line canthopexy, this is a temporary lid stabilization technique (Fig. 38-4).

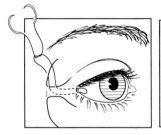
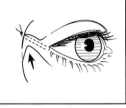

Fig. 38-4   Transcantho-canthopexy.

Orbicularis Suspension

■ Although not truly a canthopexy, this maneuver, in addition to redraping the ptotic orbicularis oculi, aids in offsetting deleterious forces on the lower lid resulting from composite facelifting and midface lifting techniques[8] (Fig. 38-5).

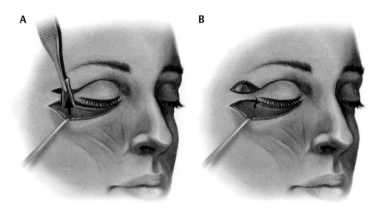

Fig. 38-5   A, An orbicularis pennant flap is created consisting of laterally based strip of pretarsal orbicularis. **B,** The pennant flap is then used to provide upward mobilization of the ptotic orbicularis, tunneled deep to the lateral canthus and then anchored with permanent suture to the superomedial aspect of the lateral orbital rim periosteum.

> **SENIOR AUTHOR TIP:**   Orbicularis suspension should be considered as an integral component of comprehensive lower blepharoplasty as it accomplishes a combination of benefits including additional lower eyelid support as well as repositioning ptotic orbicularis muscle and more effectively blends the lower eyelid-cheek junction.

TRANSOSSEOUS CANTHOPEXY
- Provides a significantly powerful canthopexy useful in situations such as cicatricial ectropion
  - Canthal anchoring suture is passed through a burr hole in the lateral orbital rim and secured to the deep temporal fascia[7] (Fig. 38-6).

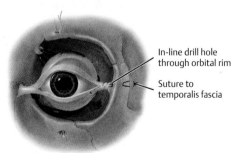

In-line drill hole through orbital rim

Suture to temporalis fascia

Fig. 38-6   Transosseous canthopexy is reserved mostly for constructive/secondary lower blepharoplasty (usually in the presence of a cicatrix) when secure fixation and lower lid repositioning cannot be achieved with standard canthoplasty or canthopexy.

> **SENIOR AUTHOR TIP:**   Originally popularized by Flowers, "drill hole" canthopexy was pioneered with the assumption that additional support and more permanent fixation to the "bone" was required where a greater canthal deformity existed. This, however, did not consider that lack of long-term fixation/canthal suspension in complicated situations also required that a point of fixation at the commissure oftentimes led to regression and failure.

HORIZONTAL LOWER LID SHORTENING
■ Effective in patients with significant horizontal lid laxity[9] (Fig. 38-7)

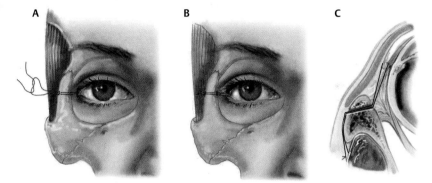

Fig. 38-7   Horizontal lid shortening.

TARSAL STRIP RELEASE
■ The tarsal strip anchors the tarsus to the periosteum of the inferolateral orbit.
■ It is located inferoposterior to the lateral canthal tendon.
■ This tethering effect can limit effectiveness of lateral canthoplasty.
■ Release of the tarsal strip improves effectiveness of canthopexy.[2]

> **SENIOR AUTHOR TIP:**   This maneuver is more often required in scarred and cicatrized situations where release is necessary for mobilization of the lower eyelid. However, it can also be helpful when significant movement is required to correct canthal dystopia in primary blepharoplasty.

CANTHOPLASTY CONSIDERATIONS
■ Periorbital anatomic factors can influence the successful performance of canthoplasty procedures.[10]
  • **Deep-set eyes:** Standard canthal anchoring techniques may result in upward clotheslining of lower lid and narrowing of orbital fissure (Fig. 38-8).
    ▶ Requires shifting point of fixation **inferiorly** and **internally** to accommodate

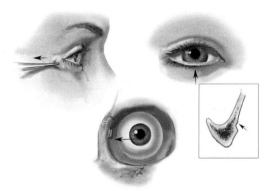

Fig. 38-8   Deep-set eye.

> **TIP:**   Deep-set or enophthalmic eyes present a unique challenge since the lateral commissure is usually at or near the orbital rim that requires supraplacement for any lower eyelid support that further narrows the vertical palpebral aperture, and the exaggerated (usually temporary) canthal tilt frequently lasts longer than one would expect.

- **Prominent eyes:** Standard canthal anchoring techniques may result in downward clotheslining of lower lid. This creates retraction of the lid, scleral show, and enlargement of the lateral **scleral** triangle (Fig. 38-9).

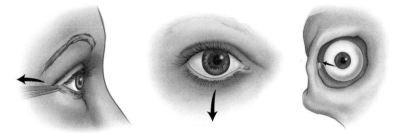

Fig. 38-9   Supraplaced canthoplasty.

> **TIP:**   Prominent eyes (i.e., high myopia, thyroid exophthalmos, large negative vectors) also present a challenge and more often require supraplacement (higher fixation at the lateral orbital tubercle). A more lateral placement of the suspension suture more often allows suspension without "clotheslining."

  ▶ Requires shifting point of fixation **superiorly** to accommodate

POSTOPERATIVE CARE

- Patients should be advised to expect a temporary change in the canthal positions, ecchymosis, chemosis swelling, and some difficulty on upward gaze.
- Patients should be counseled that they will look presentable 2-3 weeks after surgery.
- Lubricating drops should be used liberally.
- Ophthalmic antibiotic ointment should be used for routine incision care.

COMPLICATIONS

- **Lid malposition:** Most common
  - Scleral show
  - Ectropion
  - Lid retraction
- **Chemosis:** Also common and will usually resolve spontaneously
- See Chapter 35 for complete list of complications.

> **TOP TAKEAWAYS**
> ➤ Canthopexy or canthoplasty should be considered a routine component in aesthetic blepharoplasty procedures.
> ➤ Critical evaluation of each patient's periorbital morphology, lower lid laxity, and lower lid deformities is essential to determine the most effective lateral canthal anchoring procedure.

REFERENCES

1. Jelks GW, Jelks EB. Repair of lower lid deformities. Clin Plast Surg 20:417, 1993.
2. Fagien S. Algorithm for canthoplasty: the lateral retinacular suspension: a simplified suture canthopexy. Plast Reconstr Surg 103:2042, 1999.
3. Trussler AP, Rohrich RJ. MOC-PSSM CME article: Blepharoplasty. Plast Reconstr Surg 121(1 Suppl):S1, 2008.
4. Maffi TR, Chang S, Friedland JA. Traditional lower blepharoplasty: is additional support necessary? A 30-year review. Plast Reconstr Surg 128:265, 2011.
5. Flowers RS, Nassif JM, Rubin PA, et al. A key to canthopexy: the tarsal strap. A fresh cadaveric study. Plast Reconstr Surg 116:1752, 2005.
6. Tepper OM, Steinbrech D, Howell MH, et al. A retrospective review of patients undergoing lateral canthoplasty techniques to manage existing or potential lower eyelid malposition: identification of seven key preoperative findings. Plast Reconstr Surg 136:40, 2015.
7. Barton FE. Eyelids. In Barton FE, ed. Facial Rejuvenation. New York: Thieme Publishers, 2008.
8. Hamra ST. The role of septal reset in creating a youthful eyelid-cheek complex in facial rejuvenation. Plast Reconstr Surg 113:2124, 2004.
9. Hester TR Jr, Douglas T, Szczerba S. Decreasing complications in lower lid and midface rejuvenation: the importance of orbital morphology, horizontal lower lid laxity, history of previous surgery, and minimizing trauma to the orbital septum: a critical review of 269 consecutive cases. Plast Reconstr Surg 123:1037, 2009.
10. McCord CD, Boswell CB, Hester TR. Lateral canthal anchoring. Plast Reconstr Surg 112:222, 2003.

39. Blepharoptosis

Jason E. Leedy, Jordan P. Farkas

DEFINITION

Blepharoptosis is drooping of the upper lid margin to a position that is lower than normal. (Normal upper lid position is at the level of the upper limbus.)

ANATOMY[1] (Fig. 39-1)

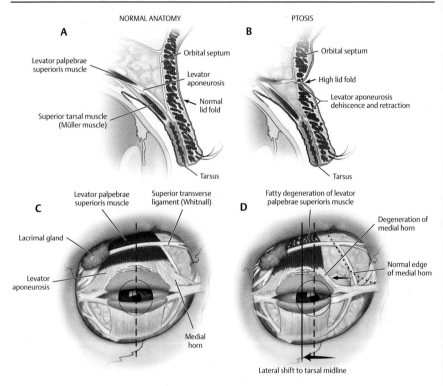

Fig. 39-1   Differences between normal and ptotic upper eyelid anatomy.

LEVATOR APONEUROSIS
- **Origin:** Lesser wing of the sphenoid
- **Insertion:** Orbicularis oculi, dermis, tarsus

- **Innervation:** Superior division of oculomotor nerve (CN III)
- **Action:** Provides 10-12 mm of eyelid elevation
- **Embryology:** Develops in the third gestational month from the superior rectus muscle
- Anterior lamella of the levator muscle forms aponeurosis
- Posterior lamella of the levator muscle forms Müller muscle
- Approximately 2-5 mm above the tarsus the anterior portion of the levator aponeurosis joins the orbital septum.

MÜLLER MUSCLE
- **Origin:** Posterior lamella of levator muscle
- **Insertion:** Superior border of tarsus
- **Innervation:** Sympathetics
- **Action:** Provides 2-3 mm of eyelid elevation

FRONTALIS MUSCLE
- **Origin:** Galeal aponeurosis
- **Insertion:** Suprabrow dermis
- **Innervation:** Frontal branch of facial nerve
- **Action:** Elevates brow and upper eyelid skin

ETIOLOGIC FACTORS/PATHOPHYSIOLOGY[2,3]

TRUE PTOSIS
- Intrinsic drooping of the affected eyelid

PSEUDOPTOSIS: CONDITIONS THAT MIMIC TRUE PTOSIS
- **Grave disease:** Retraction of contralateral lid can give appearance of ptosis on unaffected side
- **Hypotropia:** Downward rotation of the globe with accompanying lid movement
- **Duane syndrome:** Extraocular muscular fibrosis and globe retraction
- **Posttraumatic enophthalmos**
- **Contralateral exophthalmos:** Gives impression of ptosis on the unaffected side
- **Chronic squinting from irritation**

CONGENITAL PTOSIS[2,3]
- Developmental dysgenesis in the levator muscle
- Idiopathic persistent ptosis noticed shortly after birth
- Usually not progressive
- Signs confined to the affected eyelid(s)
- Decreased palpebral aperture with reduction of the pupil reflex to upper eyelid margin measurement (marginal reflex distance test [MRDI])
- Decreased levator excursion
  - Poor or absent levator function reflected in the absence of the supratarsal crease
- Ptotic eyelid generally higher than the normal eyelid during downgaze
- Inheritance pattern unclear
- Levator biopsies in congenital ptosis show absence of striated muscle fibers with fibrosis.

TIP: History alone usually can distinguish congenital from acquired ptosis, but if there is a question, lagophthalmos on downward gaze is characteristic of congenital ptosis, because levator fibrosis prevents downward lid migration.

- **Associated ocular abnormalities**
  - **Coexistent strabismus and amblyopia**
    - ▶ Caused by pupil occlusion
  - **Marcus Gunn jaw-winking syndrome**
    - ▶ Synkinesis of upper lid with chewing
    - ▶ Seen in 2%-6% of congenital ptosis
    - ▶ Caused by aberrant innervation from fifth cranial nerve
  - **Blepharophimosis syndrome**
    - ▶ Triad of **ptosis, telecanthus,** and **phimosis** of lid fissure
  - **Congenital anophthalmos or microphthalmos**
    - ▶ Hypoplasia of the lids, globe, and orbital bones
  - **Coexistent eyelid hamartoma**
    - ▶ Neurofibromas
    - ▶ Hemangiomas
    - ▶ Lymphangiomas

ACQUIRED PTOSIS[2,3]
- **Myogenic**
  - **Involutional myopathic (senile ptosis)**
    - ▶ *Most common type*
    - ▶ Stretching of the levator aponeurosis attachments to the anterior tarsus
    - ▶ Dermal attachments are maintained and therefore the supratarsal crease rises.
    - ▶ Levator function is usually good.
  - **Chronic progressive external ophthalmoplegia**
    - ▶ Progressive muscular dystrophy affects the extraocular muscles and levator.
    - ▶ 5% of cases involve the facial and oropharyngeal muscles.
- **Traumatic**
  - *Second most common type*
  - Allow recovery of myoneural dysfunction, resolution of edema, and softening of scar (approximately 6 months).
  - This can occur after cataract surgery from dehiscence of levator aponeurosis.
- **Neurogenic**
  - **Third nerve palsy:** Paralyzes levator muscle
  - **Horner syndrome:** Paralyzes Müller muscle
  - **Myasthenia gravis**
    - ▶ Primarily, young women and old men are affected.
    - ▶ Ptosis worsens with fatigue, at the end of the day.
    - ▶ Improvement with neostigmine or edrophonium is characteristic.
- **Mechanical**
  - Upper lid tumors
  - Severe dermatochalasis (excessive upper lid skin), brow ptosis

EVALUATION[2,3]

DETERMINATION OF CAUSE
- Congenital or acquired

> **TIP:** Evaluate for lagophthalmos during downward gaze. This indicates levator fibrosis, which is more commonly seen with congenital cases.

DEGREE OF PTOSIS (Table 39-1)
- Always compare with contralateral side.
- Measure amount of descent over upper limbus.
  - 1-2 mm: Mild
  - 3 mm: Moderate
  - 4 mm or more: Severe
- Record palpebral fissure height.

Table 39-1   *Degree of Ptosis*

Degree of Ptosis	Mild	Moderate	Severe
Lid descent over upper limbus	1-2 mm	3 mm	>4 mm

LEVATOR FUNCTION (Table 39-2)
- Measure from extreme downward gaze to extreme upward gaze while immobilizing the brow.
- >10 mm: Good
- 5-10 mm: Fair
- <5 mm: Poor

Table 39-2   *Levator Function*

Levator Function	Good	Fair	Poor
Levator excursion	>10 mm	5-10 mm	0-5 mm

PREOPERATIVE EVALUATION FOR DRY-EYE SYMPTOMS
- **Schirmer tests I and II** (see Chapter 34)
- **Bell phenomenon:** Upward rotation of globe when eyes forcibly opened, corneal protective mechanism during sleep
- **Tear film breakup and tear lysozyme electrophoresis:** Advanced ophthalmologic tests useful to further characterize causes of dry-eye symptoms

> **TIP:** General rule: If contact lenses can be worn, then tear production is adequate.

- **Assess lower lid position:** Scleral show or lower lid laxity—patient more prone to postoperative dry-eye symptoms and may benefit from lower lid procedure to improve position or tone in conjunction with ptosis correction

> **TIP:** All ptosis procedures cause lagophthalmos; therefore dry-eye symptoms must be evaluated preoperatively.

CONTRALATERAL EYE
- **Hering law[4]**
  - Levator muscles receive equal innervation bilaterally.
  - Severe ptosis on one side creates impulse for bilateral lid retraction. Therefore, if the severely affected side is corrected, innervation impulse for lid retraction diminishes, which may reveal ptosis of the contralateral side.
- **Hering test**
  - Attempt to reveal contralateral ptosis.
  - With brow immobilized in straightforward gaze, elevate affected lid with cotton-tipped applicator to alleviate ptosis; then examine for contralateral ptosis.

LID CONTOUR AND LID CREASE
- Evaluate contralateral lid contour and lid crease to determine proper postoperative lid crease on affected side.

OCULAR EXAMINATION
- Assess general ocular visual function and consider ophthalmologic consultation for formal examination.
- Consult with ophthalmologist preoperatively for baseline visual field testing.

COMPLICATING ISSUES[5,6]
- **Dry eyes**
  - Postoperative lagophthalmos with corneal exposure may threaten vision.
- **Hypoplastic tarsus**
  - This is seen in congenital cases. Ptosis repair can cause lid eversion.
- **Floppy upper lid**
  - Medial horn of levator aponeurosis is commonly dehisced and creates temporal shift of tarsus. Ptosis repair must recenter tarsus.
- **Asymmetrical ptosis**
  - Correction of ptosis in the severe eye can unmask ptosis in the contralateral eye.
- **Widened intercanthal distance**
  - Ptosis gives illusion of narrower intercanthal distance; if widened preoperatively, patient should be informed about possible appearance of telecanthus postoperatively.

ANESTHESIA FOR PTOSIS REPAIR
- IV sedation with local anesthetic
- Useful for mild to moderate degrees of ptosis correction in cooperative patients
- Most amenable to anterior-approach levator surgery
- Allows active patient participation with eye opening and closure so that precise correction can be achieved

TECHNIQUE

- Inject local anesthetic (use sparingly).
- Expose aponeurosis.
- Place key sutures.
- Have patient sit upright and focus on premarked spot on distant wall.
- Adjust key sutures until ptosis is corrected at appropriate level.

> **TIP:** Excess local anesthetic may impair levator function, which can markedly affect results.

CHOICE OF SURGICAL PROCEDURE[7] (Fig. 39-2)

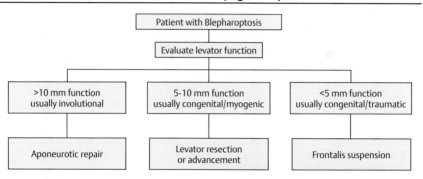

Fig. 39-2   Algorithm for ptosis repair.

- If **>10 mm** of levator excursion (excellent), then **aponeurotic surgery** or **müllerectomy**
- If **5-10 mm** of excursion (moderate), then **levator resection** or advancement
- If **0-5 mm** of excursion (poor), then **frontalis suspension** required

> **TIP:** In patients with mechanical ptosis, treat contributing factor(s) (e.g., brow ptosis, upper lid tumor).

- **The most important factor is the amount of levator excursion.**
  - Limit use of epinephrine in local anesthetic, because it stimulates Müller muscle, which gives 0.5-1 mm of temporary lid elevation. If using epinephrine with monitored anesthesia care, the operated side should be slightly overcorrected to compensate for postoperative relaxation of Müller muscle.

FASANELLA-SERVAT PROCEDURE[8] (Fig. 39-3)

- Conjunctival approach to excise tarsus, Müller muscle, and conjunctiva
- Should be considered only when levator function is excellent with minimal ptosis
- Avoids external incision—therefore cannot alter supratarsal crease
- Somewhat less predictable than external approaches
- Resection of tarsus can result in postoperative floppy lid with lid peaking and eversion.

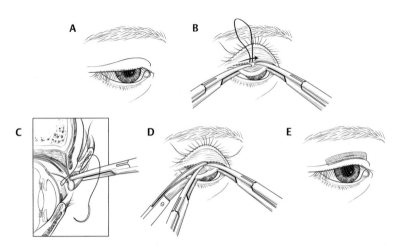

Fig. 39-3   The Fasanella-Servat (tarsal-conjunctival müllerectomy) procedure is indicated for patients with good levator excursion and mild ptosis.

MÜLLER MUSCLE–CONJUNCTIVAL RESECTION (PUTTERMAN PROCEDURE)[9,10]

- Appropriate candidates for surgery were tested with instillation of 2.5% phenylephrine hydrochloride drops into the conjunctival sac.
- Phenylephrine-stimulated contraction of the sympathetically innervated Müller muscle provided an excellent guide to the results of Müller muscle–conjunctival resection[10] (Table 39-3).
- 3.5-4.5 mm of folded Müller muscle conjunctiva complex is resected using a noncrushing vascular clamp. This corresponds to the 7-9 mm resection length determined by the phenylephrine evaluation.
- Double-armed catgut is placed in a running horizontal mattress fashion and then inserted from the conjunctiva through the external lid and tied loosely over the tarsal plate.

Table 39-3   *Phenylephrine Response Guideline*

Ptosis Response to Phenylephrine	Length of Müller Muscle–Conjunctiva to Resect (mm)
Excessive lid elevation	7-7.5
Perfect height	8
Inadequate lid elevation	9
No response	Müller muscle–conjunctival resection not indicated

LEVATOR APONEUROSIS ADVANCEMENT[11] (Fig. 39-4)

- Useful for mild to moderate ptosis
- Amenable to monitored anesthesia technique

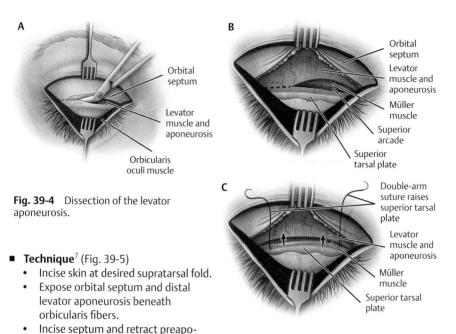

Fig. 39-4   Dissection of the levator aponeurosis.

- **Technique**[7] (Fig. 39-5)
  - Incise skin at desired supratarsal fold.
  - Expose orbital septum and distal levator aponeurosis beneath orbicularis fibers.
  - Incise septum and retract preaponeurotic fat to expose the aponeurosis, which can be identified by the vertically oriented vessels on its superior surface.
  - Incise distal aponeurosis at the superior tarsal border, and dissect it free from Müller muscle.
  - Place a central-lifting suture: Double-arm 6-0 suture passed into superior tarsus and levator aponeurosis. Tarsus will need to be recentered in cases of temporal displacement.

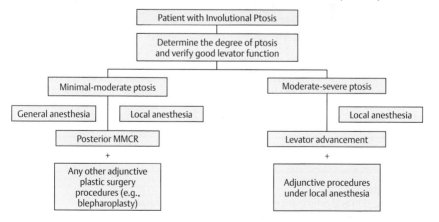

Fig. 39-5   Algorithm for treatment of involutional ptosis. (*MMCR*, Müller muscle–conjunctival resection.)

> **TIP:** In general, 4 mm of levator advancement is needed for every 1 mm of ptosis correction.

> **TIP:** If this patient is under general anesthesia, a gapping method can be applied, in which an advancement is performed until upper and lower eyelids are separated by an amount corresponding to preoperative levator excursion.

- • If levator excursion is 8-10 mm, upper lid should be slightly lower than the upper limbus after advancement; if it is 6-8 mm, it should be at the limbus; if it is 4-6 mm, it should be slightly higher than the limbus.
- • Additional medial and lateral sutures are placed.
- • Perform supratarsal crease fixation—"anchor blepharoplasty" or resection of orbicularis.
- ■ Alternatively, levator aponeurosis advancement can be performed by exposing levator muscle above Whitnall ligament and resecting muscle in ratio of 4:1 for desired correction.[11]
- ■ Levator plication has also been described using a 3:1 ratio without incision of aponeurosis, performed concurrently with aesthetic facial procedures under general anesthesia.[12]

EXTERNAL LEVATOR RESECTION[1,13] (Fig. 39-6)
- ■ Best used when levator function is fair
- ■ Sacrifices the viable levator muscle

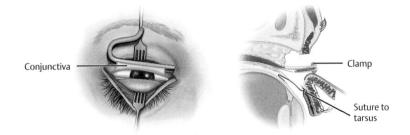

Conjunctiva   Clamp

Suture to tarsus

Fig. 39-6 Müller muscle–conjunctiva complex. The flap is everted exposing the conjunctiva. Conjunctiva is then dissected free from the overlying levator complex. It should be dissected in the fornix and reattached to the superior edge of the tarsus with absorbable sutures. This is then resected.

> **TIP:** Carraway and Vincent[11] espouse levator advancement over external levator resection because of improved results with less morbidity.

- ■ **Technique**
    1. Incise skin and orbicularis muscle at the desired supratarsal crease.
    2. Expose superior border of the tarsus.
    3. Incise full-thickness through superior tarsal attachments and place ptosis clamp.
    4. Dissect levator and Müller muscle complex from conjunctiva and orbital septum/ preaponeurotic fat; cut medial and lateral horns as necessary.

5. Remove full-thickness of levator aponeurosis/muscle and Müller muscle.
6. **Beard method:** If there are 1-2 mm of ptosis with 8-10 mm of levator function, resect 10-12 mm; if there are 2 mm of ptosis with 5-7 mm of levator function, resect 18 mm.
7. **Berke method:** Use the gapping method.

LEVATOR REINSERTION
- Only useful in true levator dehiscence, which is likely only after trauma
- Involves resuturing the dehisced end to the tarsus
- Uncommon procedure because of uncommon indication

FRONTALIS SUSPENSION[8] (Fig. 39-7)
- Required if levator function **poor** (<5 mm) (congenital cases, neurogenic cases)
- Can provide 1 cm of excursion; good result in straightforward gaze; may produce lagophthalmos while asleep, which requires ointment or nighttime patching
- Incorporates a sling (fascia lata, temporalis fascia, homograft fascia, silicone strips, Gore-Tex) from frontalis to lid
  - If eyes are dry preoperatively proceed with caution. Consider use of biologic or alloplastic material so level can be adjusted.
- For unilateral congenital cases, bilateral suspension performed to improve symmetry
- **Crawford technique**
  - Harvest 3 mm fascia lata strip.
  - Use three supralash incisions at medial, central, and lateral limbus and three brow incisions.
  - Thread fascia submuscularly from upper lid to brow.
- **Direct tarsal suturing with lid crease formation**
  - Creates supratarsal crease and fixation of sling material to tarsus to prevent late entropion seen with Crawford procedure

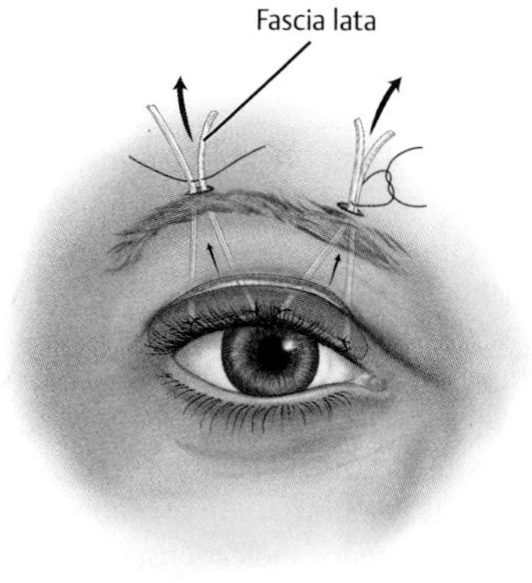

Fascia lata

Fig. 39-7 A frontalis sling tethers the upper eyelid to the frontalis muscle above by way of alloplastic or autologous material beneath the orbicularis oculi muscle.

COMPLICATIONS[12]
- Undercorrection
- Overcorrection
- Excessive lagophthalmos
- Corneal exposure or keratitis, dry-eye syndrome
- Eyelid contour abnormality, temporal overcorrection
- Eyelid crease asymmetry

- Eyelash ptosis or lash abnormalities
- Entropion or ectropion/eversion of the upper lid
- Extraocular muscle imbalance
- Conjunctival prolapse

TOP TAKEAWAYS
➤ Congenital ptosis usually requires frontalis suspension.
➤ Acquired ptosis is most often involutional.
➤ For correction of involutional ptosis, use levator advancement with monitored anesthesia and advance approximately 4 mm for every 1 mm of desired lid elevation.

REFERENCES

1. McCord CD Jr, Codner MA, eds. Eyelid & Periorbital Surgery. New York: Thieme Publishers, 2008.
2. McCord CD. The evaluation and management of the patient with ptosis. Clin Plast Surg 15:169, 1988.
3. McCord CD. Evaluation of the ptosis patient. In McCord CD Jr, Codner MA, Hester TR, eds. Eyelid Surgery: Principles and Techniques, ed 2. New York: Lippincott Williams & Wilkins, 2006.
4. Parsa FD, Wolff DR, Parsa MM, et al. Upper eyelid ptosis repair after cataract extraction and the importance of Hering's test. Plast Reconstr Surg 108:1527, 2001.
5. Carraway J. Correction of blepharoptosis. In Achauer BM, Eriksson E, Guyuron B, et al, eds. Plastic Surgery: Indications, Operations, and Outcomes, St Louis: Mosby–Year Book, 2000.
6. Carraway JH. Cosmetic and function considerations in ptosis surgery: the elusive "perfect" result. Clin Plast Surg 15:185, 1988.
7. Chang S, Lehrman C, Itani K, et al. A systematic review of comparison of upper eyelid involutional ptosis repair techniques: efficacy and complication rates. Plast Reconstr Surg 129:149, 2012.
8. Bentz ML, Bauer BS, Zuker RM, eds. Principles & Practice of Pediatric Plastic Surgery. New York: Thieme Publishers, 2008.
9. Guyuron B, Davies B. Experience with the modified Putterman procedure. Plast Reconstr Surg 82:775, 1988.
10. Liu MT, Totonchi A, Katira K, et al. Outcomes of mild to moderate upper eyelid ptosis correction using Müller's muscle-conjunctival resection. Plast Reconstr Surg 130:799e, 2012.
11. Carraway JH, Vincent MP. Levator advancement technique for eyelid ptosis. Plast Reconstr Surg 77:394, 1986.
12. de la Torre JI, Martin SA, De Cordier BC, et al. Aesthetic eyelid ptosis correction: a review of technique and cases. Plast Reconstr Surg 112:655, 2003.
13. McCord CD Jr. Complications of ptosis surgery and their management. In McCord CD Jr, Codner MA, Hester TR, eds. Eyelid Surgery: Principles and Techniques. New York: Lippincott-Raven, 1995.

40. Midface Rejuvenation

Sumeet Sorel Teotia, Sami U. Khan, Foad Nahai

The human "middle of the face," often called *midface,* is a loosely applied anatomic term that mainly focuses on the soft transition from the lower eyelid inferiorly toward the rounder, upper cheek as it transitions into the lateral face, upper lip, and soft tissue of the nasal sidewall. Thus a *midface* problem arises when any anatomic component within this region begins the aging process.

HISTORY

In the early twentieth century, surgical procedures to address facial aging consisted of skin and subcutaneous facelifts. These interventions had no effect on the midface.

RENAISSANCE ERA (1970s)[1]

- Early 1970s: Skoog[2] described subsuperficial musculoaponeurotic system (sub-SMAS) dissection.
- 1976: Mitz and Peyronie[3] defined SMAS.
- Late 1970s: Focus changed to dissecting, dividing, and repositioning the SMAS.
- These advances improved the appearance of the lower third of the face and neck, but not the midface.

DIFFERENT PLANES OF DISSECTION ERA (1980-1992)[1]

- Craniofacial surgeons, like Tessier,[4] introduced subperiosteal approaches to better reposition facial soft tissues.
  - "Mask lift": subperiosteal dissection of the malar region, zygomatic arches, and orbital region
  - Soft tissues dissected and redraped over the facial skeleton to rejuvenate the face
- 1984: Psillakis[5] attempted to reposition/elevate the soft tissues of the orbital and malar region by undermining the superficial temporofrontal fascia and fixing it to the aponeurosis of the temporalis.
- 1990: Hamra[6] introduced the deep plane rhytidectomy, combining a Skoog-type sub-SMAS dissection over the zygomaticus musculature and medially to fully release the nasolabial fold. This allowed total release of the all SMAS attachments. The flap was advanced laterally and fixed to the superficial temporal fascia.
- 1992: Hamra[7] refined his technique to improve midface rejuvenation with the "composite rhytidectomy." Through a transblepharoplasty incision, the orbicularis oculi was undermined, and this plane was connected to the facelift dissection plane. This created a composite flap of orbicularis muscle, cheek fat, and platysma, which, when repositioned, addressed the three major areas of soft tissue ptosis.

- 1992: Barton[8] provided a better understanding of the sub-SMAS plane and its relationship to the nasolabial fold. Anatomically, within the medial cheek the SMAS becomes the investing fascia of the zygomaticus major and minor.
  - Thus, simple SMAS manipulation does not significantly improve the appearance of the deepened nasolabial fold.
  - He recommended that, to address the fold, medial to the zygomaticus musculature the dissection must transition to skin–subcutaneous tissue plane to release the tethering effect of the SMAS.
- 1993: Owsley[9] defined the ***malar fat pad*** as a "discrete area of bulky subcutaneous fat, which overlies the maxillary zygomatic region." The fat pad is triangular in shape and has its base at the nasolabial fold. He advocated dissecting below the fat pad to completely mobilize it and then suspending it under tension to the subcutaneous fascia over the malar eminence with a vector perpendicular to the nasolabial crease (Fig. 40-1).

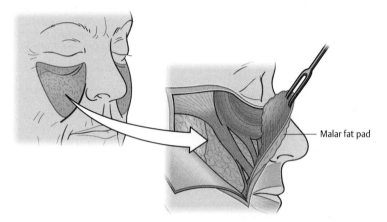

Fig. 40-1   Elevation and mobilization of the malar fat pad.

ADVANCED TECHNIQUES ERA (1992-1999)[2]
- 1992: Terino[10] described his concept of addressing the "fourth plane."
  - Advocated the use of alloplastic facial augmentation in conjunction with concepts of facial zonal anatomy to address volume loss in the midface
- 1993: Flowers[11] describes the ***tear trough deformity*** and used alloplastic implants for volumetric correction.
- 1994: Coleman[12] posed the question "Should we support and fill or should we excise and suspend?"
  - Popularized lipoinfiltration for soft tissue augmentation and lifting in the periorbital region through fat grafting
- 1994: Facial surgeons, including Fuente del Campo,[13] Isse,[14] and Ramirez,[15] started to incorporate the endoscope into facial rejuvenation.
  - 1995: Ramirez described six types of procedure combinations for rejuvenation of the upper and middle third of the face.
  - Types four through six addressed the midface and consisted of full open, full endoscopic, and biplanar combined procedures.

VECTORS AND VOLUME ERA (1999-PRESENT)[1]

- Concepts of volume management of the midface and correct vector of elevation/pull
- Little[15,16] described a volumetric approach to midface rejuvenation, both in the subcutaneous and subperiosteal plane.
- Significant anatomic studies refined the complex anatomy of the midface/periorbital region.
- Vectors of pull in rejuvenative surgery were reassessed, and a more **vertically oriented** direction of pull was advocated, especially for procedures addressing the midface.

PERTINENT ANATOMY

BASIC DEFINITION OF THE MIDFACE

- Portion of the cheek medial to a line extending from the frontal process of the zygoma to the oral commissure and from the lower lid above to the nasolabial fold below[17]
- Anatomically, the midface thus encompasses complex relationships of the lower lid, the nasolabial fold, the upper lip, and the malar eminence/cheek.

BASIC ANATOMY[18,19]

- **Skeleton**
  - Main determinant of contour of the midface, although the thickness of the soft tissue component is important, especially with changes in aging
  - Serves as platform for attachment of the overlying ligaments and muscles, which support the midface soft tissues
  - Upper/outer prezygomatic portion: Overlies the body of the zygoma
  - Lower/medial portion: Overlies the maxilla; covers the vestibule of the oral cavity
- **Soft tissue**
  - **Suborbicularis oculi fat (SOOF)**
    - ▶ Posterior to muscle
    - ▶ May require reduction, repositioning, or nothing
  - **Temporal fat pad**
    - ▶ Superior to zygoma between superficial and deep layers of temporal fascia
  - **Malar fat pad**
    - ▶ Main midface soft tissue structure
    - ▶ Triangular
    - ▶ Changes with age: Flattens, **loses projection, loses volume,** elongates, becomes narrower, and displaces inferiorly
  - **Buccal fat pad**
    - ▶ Superficial to the periosteum overlying the maxilla at the lateral buttress
    - ▶ Important support structure for the cheek mass
  - **SMAS**
    - ▶ Adipofascial layer superficial to the parotid fascia and mimetic muscles
    - ▶ Laterally anchored to the parotid fascia and at the osteocutaneous ligament of the zygoma and mandible
    - ▶ Midface elevation often achieved by elevating the SMAS in the midfacial region
    - ▶ Mainstay of SMAS facelift procedures for addressing facial aging in the midface region

- **Retaining ligaments**
  - Midface retaining ligaments[20] (Fig. 40-2)

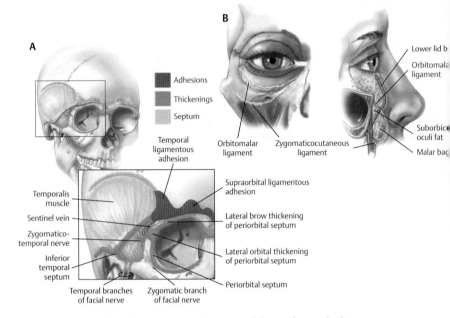

Fig. 40-2   Retaining ligaments of the midface and orbit.

- ◆ Orbicularis retaining ligament[21]
  - ◆ Zygomatic ligament
  - ◆ Upper masseteric ligament
- **Nasolabial fold** (see Chapter 43)
  - Confluence of SMAS, dermis, and muscle fascia overlying muscles of facial expression
  - Complex facial anatomic structure
  - Prominence adds to aged appearance
  - Contributes to midface aging
  - Surgical correction is complex and controversial as to the ideal procedure.
- **Tear trough** (see Chapter 37) (Fig. 40-3)
  - Also known as nasojugal groove
  - **Prominence increases with age**
  - Medial aspect of the lower eyelid
  - Becomes more prominent with loss of cheek volume and descent of midface structures; groove often accentuated by herniated orbital fat
    - ▶ Anatomic cause of groove is controversial.
      - ◆ Some surgeons think it is the prominence of the orbital rim after descent of the malar fat pad.

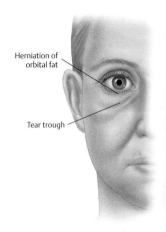

Fig. 40-3   Tear trough.

◆ Probably is **triangular confluence** of the inferomedial orbicularis oculi, levator alaeque nasi, and levator labii superioris, which is located inferior to the orbital rim and becomes apparent with volume loss in this area.

- **Muscles**
  - Orbicularis oculi
    - ▶ Most affected in midface lift procedures
    - ▶ Sphincteric muscle originating from the orbital bones and inserting into the soft tissues of the eyelids

TIP: Repositioning the lateral canthus and orbicularis oculi muscle, thus shortening the apparent length of the lower eyelid, is crucial to re-creating a youthful appearance of the periorbital region and midface.

- Zygomaticus major: Important for smiling
  - ▶ Major anatomic landmark in dissection of midface procedures
- Risorius: Important for smiling
- Levator labii superioris
- Orbicularis oris
- Masseter
- **Skin**
- **Blood supply**[18] (Fig. 40-4)

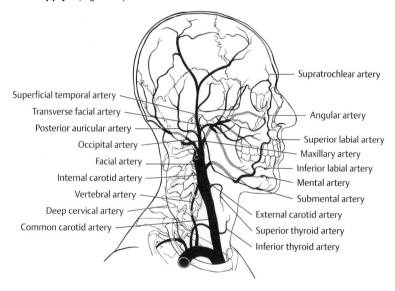

Fig. 40-4 Blood supply.

- Mainly from branches of the **external carotid artery**
- Significant anastomoses with the internal carotid artery system exist in the periorbital region
- Facial artery
- Internal maxillary artery

- Infraorbital artery
  - ▶ Supplies the lower eyelid and midcheek
  - ▶ May be injured during subperiosteal midface dissection as it exits its foramen
- Superficial temporal artery
  - ▶ Travels within the SMAS layer as it crosses the zygomatic arch
  - ▶ Protected in sub-SMAS dissection
- Transverse facial artery
  - ▶ Supplies lateral canthal region
- ▪ **Innervation**
  - Sensory: Branches of CN V_2 (trigeminal)
    - ▶ Infraorbital nerve
    - ▶ Zygomaticofacial nerve
    - ▶ Posterior maxillary nerve
  - Motor: Zygomatic and buccal branches of facial nerve (CN VII)
    - ▶ Orbicularis oculi is predominantly supplied by zygomatic branches that mainly enter near inferior lateral aspect entering on the posterior aspect of the muscle.
    - ▶ Lower lid receives additional innervation from a buccal branch from the midcheek, which passes deep to the zygomaticus major.
    - ▶ Additional buccal branches extend medially.
    - ▶ In general, in midface surgery, injury to a distal branch rarely results in a noticeable deficit.

APPLIED ANATOMY

- ▪ The midface is divided into an **anterior** and a **lateral** segment.
  - **Anterior** segment is called the ***midcheek***.[22]
  - Midcheek is the portion of the midface on the anterior aspect of the face, extending from the lower eyelid caudally to the nasolabial groove and upper lip[22] (Fig. 40-5, *A*).
  - The aesthetically pleasing fullness of the youthful cheek is produced by the midcheek.
- ▪ As a person ages, changes in the midcheek reveal that it comprises three distinct anatomic structures[22] (Fig. 40-5, *B*).
  1. Lid-cheek segment
  2. Malar segment
  3. Nasolabial segment

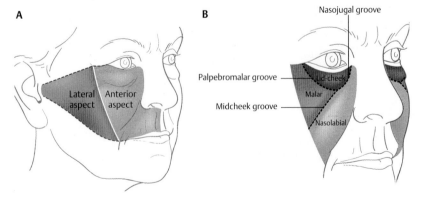

Fig. 40-5   Subcutaneous compartments of the midcheek.

- Understanding the influence of each of these structures and the changes affecting each during the aging process is important to adequately correct changes that occur over time.
  - As the aging process progresses and affects these three structures, the midcheek segments become separated by **three cutaneous grooves.**[22]
    1. **Palpebromalar groove:** superolaterally
    2. **Nasojugal groove:** Medially
    3. **Midcheek groove:** Inferolaterally
- These three grooves intersect to form an **obliquely oriented Y.**[22]
  - The *midcheek groove* runs essentially parallel to the nasolabial fold; cephalically, it extends into the *nasojugal groove.*
  - The *palpebromalar groove* extends laterally toward the lateral canthus at the cephalic limit of the midcheek.

Changes With Aging

- Loss of skin elasticity from decreased collagen
- Epidermal thinning and the development of rhytids
- Loss of fat volume
- Descent of soft tissues from attenuation of ligamentous structures, causing the development of prominent grooves and a gaunt look from volume loss
- Changes in the skeletal support structure of the midface
- Midface shape defined by specific shape and projection of the **orbital bones, zygoma, and maxilla**
  - May be the *most influential factor* creating individual variation of facial appearance
- Studies have shown the **changes in the bone structure** of the midface with age.
  - Pessa et al[23] suggested that age-related changes in bone structure led to posterior retrusion of the inferior orbital rim and the anterior maxilla.
  - Using facial CT scans to assess midface skeletal changes in male and female patients, Mendelson et al[24] found that the angle between the anterior maxilla and the orbital floor decreased in both sexes over time.
  - Yet, in contrast to previous reports, Mendelson found that the inferior orbital rim remained relatively fixed. Thus, the retrusion of the anterior maxillary wall in relation to the fixed inferior orbital rim leads to the **"negative vector"** appearance of the lid-cheek junction, as described by Jelks et al.[25]
  - Shaw and Kahn[26] also used CT evaluation to show significant decrease in the glabellar and maxillary angles with increasing age.
  - These studies all contrast the earlier notion that facial skeletal aging changes consisted of growth and expansion with advancing age.
  - Recent data intuitively make sense, because these skeletal structures serve as the foundation of the midface soft tissues and the site of attachment of the muscles of the lower lid and upper lip and the supporting/retaining ligaments of the midface.
  - Pessa et al[23] and Mendelson et al[24] showed greater changes in maxillary angles in males during aging. The posterior displacement of the anterior maxilla leads to loss of soft tissue support, which, in addition to soft tissue volume loss, accentuates the aging changes in the midface.
  - Skeletal support loss could explain the descent of the malar fat pad/soft tissues and their influence on deepening of the nasolabial fold, which is a fixed structure.

Midface Similarities With the Scalp
- The topographic anatomy of the scalp has been described in five layers:
  1. Skin
  2. Subcutaneous tissue
  3. Musculoaponeurotic layer
  4. Loose areolar tissue
  5. Fixed periosteum and deep fascia
- Anatomic structure of the midface can be equated with that of the scalp[22] (Fig. 40-6).

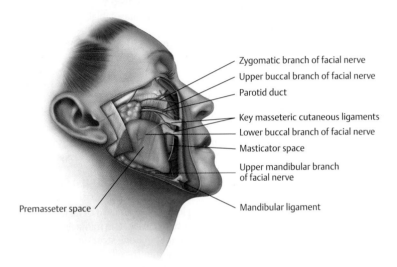

Zygomatic branch of facial nerve
Upper buccal branch of facial nerve
Parotid duct
Key masseteric cutaneous ligaments
Lower buccal branch of facial nerve
Masticator space
Upper mandibular branch of facial nerve
Mandibular ligament
Premasseter space

Fig. 40-6   Layers of the face.

- Retinacular cutis fibers traverse the subcutaneous tissue and attach the musculoaponeurotic layer to the skin.
  - ▶ Creates a mobile flap consisting of the first three layers (skin, subcutaneous tissue, and SMAS) that is freely mobile over the fifth layer (periosteum and deep fascia), which is fixed in place.
- **The fourth, loose areolar layer allows gliding movement of the upper three layers.**
- The scalp has no specific fixed points.
- In the midface and cheek, **layer three contains the mimetic muscles** within the SMAS layer. These muscles have more attachments to the overlying skin than to the underlying skeletal structures.

TIP: Intuitively, this makes sense, because the action of these muscles produces our facial expressions rather than movement of joints.

- *The key difference in anatomic arrangement of the scalp and midface lies in the fourth layer.* In the scalp this loose areolar layer acts as a simple glide plane. In the midface it retains this function but also contains the **facial retaining ligaments,** which serve as fixation points for the facial soft tissues (consisting of the top three layers).

- Midface retaining ligaments
  - Orbicularis retaining ligament
  - Zygomatic ligament
  - Upper masseteric ligament
- Within level four between the retaining ligaments are large areas **(spaces)** where there are no points of fixation, thus allowing movement of the soft tissues through the action of the mimetic muscles.[22]
  - The **roof** of these spaces is formed by the **underside of the SMAS.**
  - The **floor** is formed by the **deep fascia or periosteum.**
  - **Retaining ligaments** form the **walls.**
    - ▶ Within the walls pass the branches of the facial nerves and sensory nerves and the vascular structures.
- In the midface, the soft tissues overlie free space more than solid skeletal bone.
- **The four major midface spaces**[22] (Fig. 40-7):
  1. Preseptal
  2. Prezygomatic
  3. Masticator
  4. Oral cavity

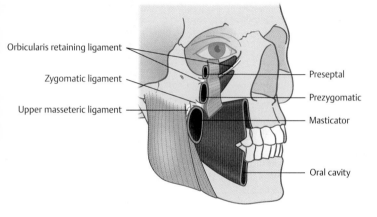

Fig. 40-7   Four major midface spaces.

- The ligaments fan out within the SMAS layer forming a perpendicular network of the retinacular cutis.
  - This network fixes the soft tissues to the dermis.
  - As the face ages, *facial bulges* arise as the fine ligaments within the SMAS layer lose their strength, allowing the soft tissues overlying the facial spaces to become distended. The strong ligamentous attachments to the dermis resist this distension and appear on the skin as *deep grooves.*[22]
  - These changes, coupled with the well-documented skin changes of aging, produce the characteristic aging of the midface.

ASSESSMENT OF THE MIDFACE

- Harmonious facial appearance defined as "balanced relationship among all tissues of the face"[27]
- Facial aging is the result of several factors, including:
  - Skin laxity
  - Ptosis of soft tissues
  - Volume loss within the soft tissues
  - Changes within the skeletal structure of the facial bones
- The process of facial aging progresses in a defined pattern.[28]
- Hester and Szczerba[19] defined the following **four most important changes** within the midface during the aging process:
  1. Gradual ptosis of the cheek skin below the inferior orbital rim with descent of the attenuated lower eyelid skin, creating a skeletonized appearance with infraorbital hollowness
  2. Descent of the malar fat pad, with loss of the malar prominence
  3. Deepening of the tear trough
  4. Exaggeration of the nasolabial fold
- Anatomic components of lower lid and midface aging include[19] (Fig. 40-8):

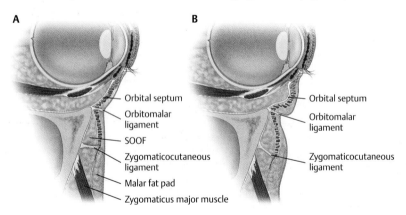

Fig. 40-8   Midsagittal anatomy of the midface. **A,** Youthful midface. **B,** Aged midface. (*SOOF,* Suborbicularis oculi fat.)

- Laxity and descent of the orbicularis oculi muscle
- Laxity of the orbital septum
- Descent of the lid-cheek junction
- Horizontal laxity of the tarsal plate component of the lower eyelid
- Descent of the cheek fat pad with laxity of the orbitomalar ligament
- Laxity of the zygomaticus muscles and other elevators of the upper lip
- Some degree of deepening of the nasolabial fold
- The cumulative effects of changes in all five anatomic soft tissue layers and skeletal structures of the midface, as described previously, lead to the observed midface changes of the aging process.

- Attenuation of the retaining ligaments at specific anatomic points causes a reduction in the fixation of the midcheek soft tissues.
- The classic loss of cheek volume is the result of three processes[18,29]
  1. Displacement (inferiorly) of soft tissue from ligamentous attenuation **(major)**
  2. Soft tissue and fat atrophy **(minor)**
  3. Skeletal changes and bone Loss **(minor)**

SURGICAL PRINCIPLES

- One of the greatest paradigm shifts in the approach to facial rejuvenation, in particular of the midface, occurred with the realization that simply undermining and redraping the facial skin flap under tension without addressing the deeper foundation structures of the face (i.e., soft tissue and facial skeletal support) did not adequately rejuvenate the midface.
- Recent advances, in particular the developments described by surgical anatomists, have led to a better understanding of midface rejuvenation, including:
  - Dissection planes
  - Volume augmentation
  - The concept of vectors and direction of lift[30]
- Mendelson[31] has advocated the following principles as paramount in achieving lasting results in addressing midface aging:
  - Adequate release of soft tissues
  - Appropriate vectors of elevation
  - Strength of fixation
- The concept of *fixation* in facial anatomy refers to the retaining ligaments of the face, which attach the dermis to the underlying facial skeleton, as previously described.
  - Functionally, these ligaments compartmentalize the face.[31]
  - As we age and the points of fixation become lax (allowing descent of soft tissues and the signs of facial aging), these changes occur within the confines of these compartments.
  - Surgical correction requires application of anatomically derived surgical principles of release of the fixation points **(ligamentous attachments),** which facilitates redraping and elevating of the soft tissues along appropriate vectors to achieve a more youthful position and appearance[31] (Fig. 40-9).

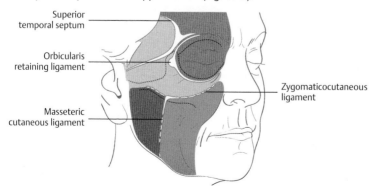

Fig. 40-9 Regions of the face.

- Full fixation release thus facilitates application of multiple vectors within a compartment, which allows complete repositioning of the soft tissues.
- Use of multiple sutures within a compartment decreases the load exerted on any one fixation point[31] (Fig. 40-10).

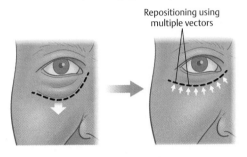

Repositioning using multiple vectors

Fig. 40-10   Principle of correction of laxity of the lower lid.

- This allows surgeons to reproduce the fixation points at the original ligamentous attachment to the facial skeleton and reduces tension on the SMAS flap and its potential distortion on the appearance of the face.

CHARACTERISTICS OF THE IDEAL MIDFACE LIFT

- Ramirez[32] described the following **concepts of the ideal midface rejuvenation** procedure:
  - Provides volumetric remodeling of the cheek
  - Allows management of the skeletal foundation by augmentation or reduction without additional incisions or alternative plane of dissection
  - Allows the injection of fat graft without the risk of migration or the need for fixation of alternative grafts
  - Corrects the fat pad herniation of the lower eyelid
  - Corrects the V deformity of the eyelid-cheek interface
  - Lifts the corner of the mouth
  - Potential for treating the skin layer in the same operative setting without the risk of skin necrosis or delay in healing
  - Minimizes facial edema
  - Minimizes facial numbness
  - Minimizes facial nerve injury

OPERATIVE TECHNIQUES

FAT GRAFTING[12,33] (see Chapter 23)

- Often used as an adjunct to a midface lift to address loss of volume
- Anatomic areas within the midface that often need soft tissue augmentation include:
  - Tear trough and infraorbital area
  - Malar eminence
  - Submalar region
  - Nasolabial crease
- The two most common areas that require volume augmentation are the **tear trough** (to re-create a youthful convex appearance) and the **nasolabial crease.**

- Neuber[34] first described use of fat to treat facial contour defects in 1893.
- Miller[35] described infiltration using a cannula in 1926, but the procedure did not gain widespread use.
- Coleman[12] popularized the use of **structural fat grafting.** He forwarded the notion of not only filling a defect, but of employing a three-dimensional approach to soft tissue augmentation and sculpting of the face using lipoinfiltration.
- Coleman's technique follows the sage advice of Miller, who stated that the end results in free fat transplantation depend, aside from various local and general factors, on the method and technique.
- Lipoinfiltration is performed in multiple planes, including, sub-SMAS, subperiosteal, and subcutaneous.

> **SENIOR AUTHOR TIP:**   Coleman cautioned against injection within muscles of the face (although previously advocated by other authors), because it can lead to edema, distortion, and undercorrection of the deficit, as well as muscle fibrosis and thickening, especially in the lip.

BARBED SUTURES[36-38]

- With the popularity of minimal (noninvasive) techniques for facial rejuvenation, barbed sutures were developed to allow suspension of facial soft tissues to create a more youthful appearance. Often, the results were disappointing or had only short-term results.
- The sutures can be placed at different levels or planes of the soft tissues of the face, including superficial, within the SMAS, and subperiosteal.
- Long-term results have shown that placement of barbed sutures within nondissected tissues produced dismal results.

ALLOPLASTIC IMPLANTS[39,40] (see Chapter 27)

- Terino[40] popularized the concept of alloplastic implants for facial augmentation, especially in the midface.
  - Developed the concept of **anatomic zones of the facial skeleton**
- The suborbital zygomatic region comprises two of the five distinct skeletal zones (Fig. 40-11).
  - **Zone 1: Major body of the malar bone**
    - ▶ Defined medially from the infraorbital nerve and extends laterally to the medial third of the zygomatic arch
  - **Zone III: Paranasal suborbital zone**
    - ▶ Extends from the lateral edge of the nasal bone to the infraorbital nerve. Within this zone lies the **"tear trough."**
- Traditional facial rejuvenation procedures focused on three different planes: skin, subcutaneous, and SMAS. These procedures produce two-dimensional changes. Alloplastic

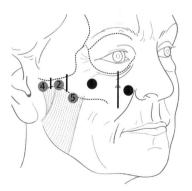

Fig. 40-11   Skeletal zones of the zygomatic region. *1,* Major body of the malar bone. *2,* Middle third of the zygomatic arch. *3,* Paranasal suborbital zone. *4,* Zone overlying the posterior third of the zygomatic arch. *5,* Submalar zonal triangle.

- implants focus on a fourth plane, the facial skeleton, thus producing three-dimensional changes through facial augmentation.
- Autologous techniques, like lipoinfiltration and dermal-fat or fascial grafts, also produce three-dimensional augmentation. Proponents of the alloplastic techniques cite the permanent effects created by these implants versus the potential for loss of volume over time with tissue augmentation techniques.
- Generally, alloplastic volume correction within the midface is combined with a subperiosteal midface lift. This facilitates suspension of the midface soft tissues and creation of subperiosteal pockets for anatomic fixation of the alloplastic implants, thus allowing volume correction of ptotic, atrophied midface soft tissues.[40]
- Surgical approaches for placement of alloplastic midface implants are through upper gingivobuccal sulcus, subciliary, or transconjunctival incisions, which can be used for a concomitant subperiosteal midface lift and/or lower blepharoplasty.

ENDOSCOPIC

- Hester and colleagues,[19,41,42] Byrd and Andochick,[43] Hunt and Byrd,[44] and Ramirez[15,32] popularized the endoscopic approach to midface rejuvenation. Each surgeon reviewed the specifics of his technique.
- Greatest advantage of the endoscopic approach is the **avoidance of traumatic dissection of the orbicularis oculi muscle,** thus preventing postoperative lower lid distortion.
- Because the pretarsal orbicularis oculi muscle is not dissected off the orbital septum, passive tightening of the orbicularis in a lateral direction passively tightens the orbital septum, thus reducing herniated orbital fat and eliminating the need for direct fat excision or repositioning.
- Ramirez outlined the **principles of endoscopic midface surgery:**
  - Wide subperiosteal and subfascial dissection
  - En bloc mobilization of midface structures
  - Periosteal release in the lower and medial boundaries of the cheek
  - Strong suspensory element to maintain the cheek in its elevated position
- Hester and colleagues used adjunctive procedures with endoscopic midface lift to address specific anatomic aging changes in some patients, including autologous fat grafting to address prominent nasojugal grooves and tear trough deformities and/or liposuction of the medial edge of a significantly prominent nasolabial fold.
- Byrd and Andochick and Hunt and Byrd emphasized the **deep temporal lift: a multiplanar, lateral brow, temporal, and upper facelift:**
  - Indicated for patients with aging of central and upper face and is ideal for patients with malar ptosis who simultaneously require periorbital rejuvenation
  - Exclusively useful for patients with the following features:
    - ▶ Young
    - ▶ Zygomatic hypoplasia
    - ▶ Lower lid bowing
    - ▶ Scleral show
    - ▶ Inferior displacement of lateral canthus
  - Zygomatic hypoplasia can be simultaneously addressed by hydroxyapatite augmentation.
  - Complex operation that emphasized sound knowledge of anatomy of the midface and upper lid

- Technique initially emphasized key dissection planes[43] (Fig. 40-12):
  - ► **Subgaleal** approach to forehead
  - ► **Subfascial** approach to temporal region
  - ► **Subperiosteal** approach to the zygomatic arch
  - ► **Suborbicularis** approach to the superior, lateral, and inferior orbital rim

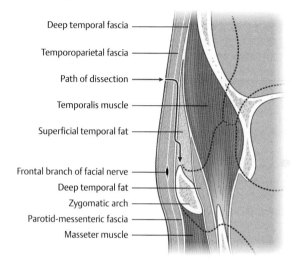

Deep temporal fascia
Temporoparietal fascia
Path of dissection
Temporalis muscle
Superficial temporal fat
Frontal branch of facial nerve
Deep temporal fat
Zygomatic arch
Parotid-messenteric fascia
Masseter muscle

Fig. 40-12   Dissection plane to the zygomatic arch.

- Byrd's technique evolved over a period of time to an endoscopic brow-midface lift from previously described deep temporal lift, although anatomic planes used were the same.[44]
- Dissection and suspension of the midface complex as a single unit in the **preperiosteal** planes allowed direct correction of the aging anatomy, with modification in brow fixation and zygomatic arch dissection.

TRANSPALPEBRAL MIDFACE LIFT
- Used by selective surgeons[41] and has high complication rates
- Midface and lower lid addressed simultaneously as a single unit using a lower blepharoplasty transcutaneous direct or endoscopic approach
- Generally reserved for the more aging midface with associated lower eyelid aging components

POSTOPERATIVE CARE
Generally directed toward prevention of complications and incorporates normal healing process
- Head elevation minimizes postoperative edema with limitation of fluid excess.
- Ice packs or cold compress can be applied to minimize edema.
- A temporary Frost suture can be used in immediate perioperative period to protect the lower eyelid from developing chemosis during early healing.

- Strict blood pressure control is important to prevent hematoma.
- Patient's general vision should be evaluated if surgical dissection involves the lower eyelid.
- Eye should remain lubricated with saline drops or lubricating ointment.
- Patients are instructed not to use contact lenses or cosmetic makeup on suture lines.
- Close follow-up postoperatively is necessary to reiterate patient instructions early in the healing phase.

SURGICAL COMPLICATIONS AND TREATMENT

- **Chemosis** is the most common **nonsurgical** complication from a **transpalpebral approach** to the midface.
  - Characterized by visible swelling of the conjunctiva
  - Symptoms include epiphora, irritation or foreign body sensation, and mild visual impairment.
  - It presents within 1 week of surgery and can last up to 4 weeks, even longer in rare circumstances
  - Prevention is the best treatment, starting with lubrication of the cornea in surgery, minimizing trauma and exposure.
  - **Temporary tarsorrhaphy** can reduce postoperative chemosis.
  - Treatment starts with eye lubrication with saline drops and ophthalmic lubricants.
  - Ophthalmic steroid drops (Tobradex) can be helpful.
  - Eye patches can be used if chemosis persists.
  - In severe cases or those lasting >2 weeks, conjunctivotomy at bedside with tarsorrhaphy should be considered.
- **Lower eyelid malposition**
  - Most common **surgical** complication from a **transpalpebral** approach
  - Causes include excessive skin or muscle removal, lower lid laxity, middle or posterior lamellar scarring, damage to pretarsal orbicularis oculi muscle, and even a small hematoma.
  - Characteristic features include lid retraction, scleral show, and ectropion.
  - Most common cause is vertical deficiency of anterior or posterior lamella in patients with laxity of the tarsus.
  - Patients who have **increased risks** are those with:
    - ► Lower lid laxity
    - ► Prominent eyes (as measured by Hertel exophthalmometer)
    - ► Negative vector
    - ► Negative canthal tilt
    - ► Preoperative scleral show
  - **Treatment of mild lower lid malposition**
    - ► Postoperative massage
    - ► External tape suspension laterally
    - ► Eye lubrication
  - **Failure of conservative treatment**
    - ► Surgical canthopexy or canthoplasty
    - ► Spacers may be included in surgery in rare instances.
    - ► Drill-hole canthal anchoring may be needed.

- **Severe lower lid malposition**
  - ▶ Immediate surgical correction may be necessary to prevent exposure keratopathy.
  - ▶ Drill-hole canthal anchoring is generally necessary.
- Epiphora is usually transient and resolves spontaneously.
- Infection is uncommon; however, it must be managed by antibiotics and vigilant follow-up to prevent facial or periorbital cellulitis.
- Hematoma needs to be addressed in accordance with its severity, and generally surgically.
- Corneal abrasions are uncommon but prevented by corneal lubrication.
- Minor visual changes such as diplopia are temporary and caused by edema.
- Nerve injuries are also generally temporary, resolving spontaneously in the perioperative period.
- Complications from using barbed sutures generally are attributed to asymmetry and suture migration or vector malposition, all of which usually require a surgical approach.
- Complications from alloplastic implants include malposition, rotation, asymmetry, bony resorption, local pain, and paresthesia; infection is rare. Treatment involves addressing the specific cause, possibly with surgical extraction.
- Fat grafting can overcorrect or undercorrect the deformity and may need to be repeated to achieve symmetry.

TOP TAKEAWAYS

- ➤ Detailed knowledge of the complex anatomy of the midface is crucial to successful midface rejuvenation.
- ➤ Accurate preoperative assessment of the contributing factors to facial aging is the foundation to build successful facial rejuvenation.
- ➤ Generalized facial aging is characterized by skin laxity, ptosis of soft tissue, volume loss within the soft tissues, and changes within the skeletal structure of the facial bones.
- ➤ The subunits of the face do not age independent of each other; rather, they each influence and complement each other in form and function. Therefore, to re-create a beautiful, harmonious face, correcting the changes that have occurred in each segment of the face is essential.
- ➤ The aging midface is characterized by soft tissue attenuation of retaining ligaments, leading to soft tissue ptosis. *Facial bulges* arise as the soft tissues overlying the facial spaces become distended. The strong ligamentous attachments to the dermis resist this distension and appear on the skin as *deep grooves.*
- ➤ Trauma to the lower eyelid is minimized by avoiding preseptal dissection.
- ➤ Midface vector pull is oriented vertically, not laterally.
- ➤ If present, correct horizontal lower lid laxity.
- ➤ Skeletal deficiencies should be addressed.
- ➤ Volume loss should be replaced, as needed.
- ➤ Successful surgical rejuvenation can be limited by inadequate or neglected skin rejuvenation.

REFERENCES

1. Paul MD, Calvert JW, Evans GR. The evolution of the midface lift in aesthetic plastic surgery. Plast Reconstr Surg 117:1809, 2006.
2. Skoog T. Plastic Surgery: New Methods and Refinements. New York: Thieme Publishers, 1974.
3. Mitz V, Peyronie M. The superficial musculo-aponeurotic system (SMAS) in the parotid and cheek area. Plast Reconstr Surg 58:80, 1976.
4. Tessier P. Facelifting and frontal rhytidectomy. In Transactions of Seventh International Conference on Plastic and Reconstructive Surgery, Rio de Janeiro, Brazil, Sept 1979.
5. Psillakis JM. Empleo de tecnicas de cirugia craniofacial en las ritidoplatias del tercio superior de la cara. Cirugia Plastica Ibero-Latino Americana 10:297, 1984.
6. Hamra ST. The deep-plane rhytidectomy. Plast Reconstr Surg 86:53, 1990.
7. Hamra ST. Composite rhytidectomy. Plast Reconstr Surg 90:1, 1992.
8. Barton FE Jr. The SMAS and the nasolabial fold. Plast Reconstr Surg 89:1054, 1992.
9. Owsley JQ. Lifting of the malar fat pad for correction of prominent nasolabial folds. Plast Reconstr Surg 91:462, 1993.
10. Terino EO. Alloplastic facial contouring: surgery of the fourth plane. Aesthetic Plast Surg 16:195, 1992.
11. Flowers RS. Tear trough implants for correction of tear trough deformity. Clin Plast Surg 20:403, 1993.
12. Coleman SR. The technique of periorbital lipoinfiltration. Oper Tech Plast Reconstr Surg 1:120, 1994.
13. Fuente del Campo A. Ritidectomia subperiostica endoscopia. Cirugia Plastica Ibero-Latino Americana 20:393, 1994.
14. Isse NG. Endoscopic facial rejuvenation. Clin Plast Surg 24:213, 1997.
15. Ramirez OM. Endoscopic facial rejuvenation. Perspect Plast Surg 9:22, 1995.
16. Little JW. Three-dimensional rejuvenation of the midface: volumetric resculpture by malar imbrication. Plast Reconstr Surg 105:267, 2000.
17. Mendelson BC, Muzaffar AR, Adams WP Jr. Surgical anatomy of the midcheek and malar mounds. Plast Reconstr Surg 110:885; discussion 897, 2002.
18. Harris PA, Mendelson B. Eyelid and midcheek anatomy. In Fagien S, ed. Putterman's Cosmetic Oculoplastic Surgery, ed 4. Philadelphia: Saunders Elsevier, 2008.
19. Hester TR, Szczerba S. Midface rejuvenation. In Nahai F, ed. The Art of Aesthetic Surgery: Principles and Techniques. New York: Thieme Publishers, 2005.
20. Owsley JQ, Roberts CL. Some anatomical observations on midface aging and long-term results of surgical treatment. Plast Reconstr Surg 121:258, 2008.
21. Muzaffar AR, Mendelson BC, Adams WP Jr. Surgical anatomy of the ligamentous attachments of the lower lid and lateral canthus. Plast Reconstr Surg 110:873; discussion 897, 2002.
22. Mendelson B, Jacobsen S. Surgical anatomy of the midcheek: facial layers, spaces, and the midcheek segments. Clin Plast Surg 35:395, 2008.
23. Pessa JE, Desvigne LD, Lambros VS, et al. Changes in globe-to-orbital rim position with age: implications for aesthetic blepharoplasty of the lower eyelids. Aesthetic Plast Surg 23:337, 1999.
24. Mendelson B, Hartley W, Scott M, et al. Age-related changes of the orbit and midcheek and the implications for facial rejuvenation. Aesthetic Plast Surg 31:419, 2007.
25. Jelks GW, Glat PM, Jelks EB, et al. the inferior retinacular lateral canthoplasty: a new technique. Plast Reconstr Surg 100:1262, 1997.

26. Shaw RB, Kahn DM. Aging of the midface bony elements: a three-dimensional computed tomographic study. Plast Reconstr Surg 119:675, 2007.
27. Psillakis JM, Rumley TO, Camargos A. Subperiosteal approach as an improved concept for correction of the aging face. Plast Reconstr Surg 82:383, 1988.
28. DeFatta RJ, Williams EF III. Evolution of midface rejuvenation. Arch Facial Plast Surg 11:6, 2009.
29. Moss CJ, Mendelson B, Taylor GI. Surgical anatomy of the ligamentous attachments in the temple and periorbital regions. Plast Reconstr Surg 105:1475, 2000.
30. Marten TJ. High SMAS facelift: combined single flap lifting of the jawline, cheek, and midface. Clin Plast Surg 35:569, 2008.
31. Mendelson B. Surgery of the superficial musculo-aponeurotic system: principles of release, vectors, and fixation. Plast Reconstr Surg 107:1545, 2001.
32. Ramirez OM. Three-dimensional endoscopic midface enhancement: a personal quest for the ideal cheek rejuvenation. Plast Reconstr Surg 109:329, 2002.
33. Coleman SR. Facial augmentation with structural fat grafting. Clin Plast Surg 33:567, 2006.
34. Neuber F. [Fat transplantation] Chir Kongr Verhandl Dsch Gesellch Chir 20:66, 1893.
35. Miller CG. Cannula Implants and Review of Implantation Techniques in Esthetic Surgery. Chicago: Oak Press, 1926.
36. Paul M. Barbed sutures for aesthetic facial plastic surgery: indications and techniques. Clin Plast Surg 35:451, 2008.
37. Lee S, Isse N. Barbed polypropylene sutures for midface elevation: early results. Arch Facial Plast Surg 7:55, 2005.
38. Sasaki GH. Personal approach to the aging lower lid and face. Clin Plast Surg 35:407, 2008.
39. Terino EO, Edward M. The magic of mid-face three-dimensional contour alterations combining alloplastic and soft tissue suspension technologies. Clin Plast Surg 35:419, 2008.
40. Terino EO. Alloplastic contouring for suborbital, maxillary, zygomatic deficiencies. In Fagien S, ed. Putterman's Cosmetic Oculoplastic Surgery, ed 4. Philadelphia: Saunders Elsevier, 2008.
41. Hester TR Jr, Codner MA, McCord CD, Nahai F, Giannopoulos A. Evolution of technique of the direct blepharoplasty approach for the correction of lower lid and midfacial aging: maximizing results and minimizing complications in a 5-year experience. Plast Reconstr Surg 105:393, 2000.
42. Hester TR Jr, Douglas T, Szczerba S. Decreasing complications in lower lid and midface rejuvenation: the importance of orbital morphology, horizontal lower lid laxity, history of previous surgery, and minimizing trauma to the orbital septum: a critical review of 269 consecutive cases. Plast Reconstr Surg 123:1037, 2009.
43. Byrd HS, Andochick SE. The deep temporal lift: a multiplanar, lateral brow, temporal, and upper face lift. Plast Reconstr Surg 97:928, 1996.
44. Hunt JA, Byrd HS. The deep temporal lift: a multiplanar lateral brow, temporal, and upper face lift. Plast Reconstr Surg 110:1793, 2002.

41. Perioral Rejuvenation

Alexey M. Markelov, Molly Burns Austin, Alton Jay Burns

INDICATIONS AND CONTRAINDICATIONS

INDICATIONS
- Congenital or acquired volume deficiency in the lips resulting from aging process
- Static and dynamic perioral skin lines
- Ptosis of the upper lip and deep nasolabial folds
- Patient's desire to improve aesthetic appearance of the lower face

CONTRAINDICATIONS
- Allergies to fillers or neuromodulators
- Congenital or medication-induced coagulopathy
- Body dysmorphic disorder
- Unrealistic expectations
- Active infection

PREOPERATIVE EVALUATION

ANATOMY (Fig. 41-1)
- The perioral region is bounded by:
  - Nasolabial creases
  - Labiomental crease
  - Nasal base

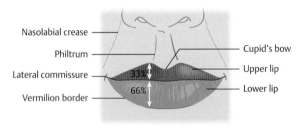

Fig. 41-1   The upper lip is smaller than the lower lip and is a third of the total lip volume.

Anatomic Landmarks of the Region
- Philtrum
- Philtral columns
- Philtral dimple
- Cupid's bow (a key anatomic feature of the upper lip)
- Nasolabial crease
- Labiomental crease

PATIENT EVALUATION

- The facial mimetics are studied in rest and in motion.
- With increasing age, facial asymmetries will become more prominent.
- The dental status is important.[1,2,3]

> **TIP:** Aesthetically, 2 to 3 mm of the upper incisors may show in repose, but the full length of the incisors should show while smiling.

- The findings and the treatment options should be discussed with patients.
- Treatment regimens should not be based on financial considerations alone, but surgeons should consider the most effective, economically feasible plan that will satisfy patients (Fig. 41-2).

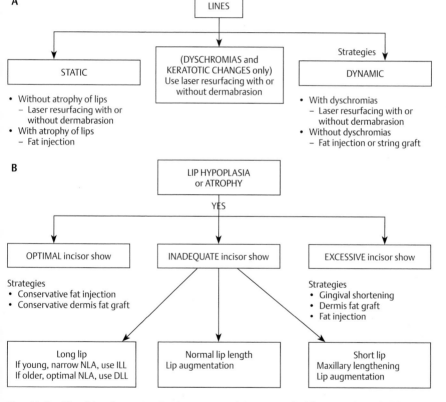

Fig. 41-2   Algorithm for perioral enhancement. (*DLL,* Direct liplift; *ILL,* indirect liplift; *NLA,* nasolabial angle.) © Oxford University Press.

> **TIP:** The mirror and camera are the most important tools to define, with the patient, what should be modified to obtain a better appearance.

TREATMENT OPTIONS
- Chemodenervation with neuromodulators
- Soft tissue fillers
- Fat grafting
- Laser resurfacing
- Chemical peels
- Surgical rejuvenation

INFORMED CONSENT
- Well-designed informed consent can help to improve communications when problems arise.
- Address preoperatively the possibility of **asymmetry** or **undercorrection.**
- Patients should be advised that filler longevity can vary based on their metabolism.
- Before performing ablative skin resurfacing, patients should be informed of the predicted immediate postoperative skin appearance, which can be temporarily disfiguring (see Chapter 17).

STRATEGIES AND TECHNIQUES

CHEMODENERVATION
- Best addresses perioral rhytids and depressed corners of the mouth
- Botulinum neurotoxin type A is the most widely used.

Technique (see Chapter 21)
- The **orbicularis oris** muscle and **depressor anguli oris** are targeted.
- 2-5 units are used on each side.
- The needle is inserted into peak of the Cupid's bow, 2 to 3 mm above the vermilion border.
- Injection of the depressor anguli oris muscle will cause elevation of the oral commissure.[4]
  - This muscle can be found by asking the patient to depress the lower lip or frown. The bulk of the muscle is palpable inferolateral to the oral commissure at the level of the mandible.

> **TIP:** Injecting 1 unit of botulinum toxin into the levator labii superioris muscle at its origin on the maxilla (superolateral to the ala) creates a weakness of the central aspect of the upper lip during smile, which eliminates gingival show.

SOFT TISSUE FILLERS (see Chapter 22)
- Hyaluronic acid–based filler (Restylane and Perlane, Galderma; Juvederm, Allergan)
- Poly-L-lactic acid (Sculptra, Galderma): Option for HIV patients with lipoatrophy
- Bovine collagen (Zyderm and Zyplast, Allergan): Concerns for hypersensitivity, requires skin test
- Human-based collagen (Cosmoderm and Cosmoplast, Allergan): Safer in terms of all allergic reactions, does not require skin testing

- Polymethylmethacrylate (Artecoll, Artefill): Permanent filler
- Calcium hydroxyapatite (Radiesse, Canderm Pharma): Long-lasting filler

Anesthesia
- For skin injections, topical anesthetic can be used.
- For lip injections, infraorbital and mental nerve blocks can be used, as well as fillers containing local anesthetic.
- Another option is to infiltrate local anesthetic in the upper or lower anterior vestibule from cuspid-to-cuspid region.

Application Techniques
- Linear threading
- Serial puncture (Fig. 41-3)

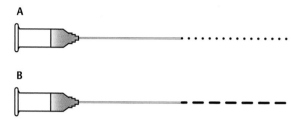

A

B

Fig. 41-3   A, Linear threading. **B,** Serial puncture.

Lips
- Cupid's bow or white roll can be augmented by filler injection to outline a "lazy M" configuration (Fig. 41-4).
- Cupid's bow becomes wider with age and should be made narrower.
- Approximately 10%-20% overcorrection is needed.
- The lip proper, from the wet-dry junction to the vermilion border, may be injected just deep to the mucosa within the orbicularis oris muscle.
- Placement posterior to the wet-dry junction along the wet mucosa may enhance the lip volume and projection.
- The depth of the mental fold increases with age and may require correction.
- Approximate volume for augmentation of the lips ranges from 0.5-1.0 ml per lip.

Fig. 41-4   Cupid's bow.

CAUTION: Radiesse and Sculptra should not be used for lip augmentation because of their high incidence of nodule formation.

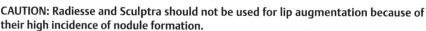

TIP: Use minimal volume in the upper lip above the vermilion border, because any added volume may cause lengthening of the upper lip.

Nasolabial Folds
- Filler is injected slightly medial to the actual fold (Fig. 41-5).
- The filler can then be massaged into the center of the fold.
- The filler can be placed at angles to the fold, and layering may be done to enhance longevity (cross-medial or cross-hatching technique).
- For very deep folds, more viscous products (Perlane, Cosmoplast, Zyplast) or permanent/semipermanent (Radiesse, Sculptra, Artefill) products may be placed deep under less viscous fillers such as Restylane, Juvéderm, and Cosmoderm.[5]
- Injection might require two or more syringes for each fold.[6]

SENIOR AUTHOR TIP: A reasonable goal is 50% correction of the depth of the nasolabial fold. Overfilling the fold will give patients an odd appearance when they animate or smile.

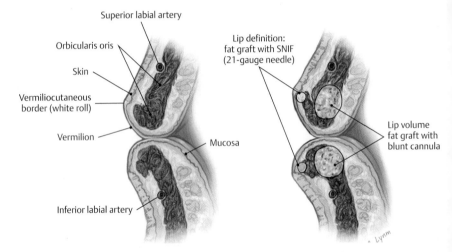

Fig. 41-5 Parasagittal section of the lips, before and after enhancement with microfat, illustrating the location of deep intramuscular lipofilling, in relation to labial arteries. (*SNIF,* Short needle intradermal fat.)

Marionette Lines
- The area to be filled is triangular, extending from the marionette line to the lower lateral lip vermilion to the superolateral aspect of the chin.
- More permanent viscous fillers are used for deeper correction.
- Less viscous, finer products such as Restylane should be used for more superficial correction.
- Radial fanning technique from two independent injection sites, superior and inferior, can lead to a smooth correction of the area.

■ Overcorrection should not be done, because it can lead to lumps that are visible or felt intraorally under the oral mucosa.[7]

Postprocedure Care
■ After filler or botulinum toxin injection, patients are able to resume their normal skin care and makeup routines almost immediately.
■ Exaggerated and repeated movements should be minimized during the first 3 days after a treatment to minimize product migration/displacement.
■ Swelling and bruising can be minimized by avoiding the use of anticoagulant medication and applying ice packs before and after a treatment, along with gentle pressure.

Complications
■ Acnelike skin eruptions
■ Overcorrection and undercorrection
■ Asymmetry, skin lumpiness, and visibility of filler material; migration of filler[8]
■ Skin necrosis
■ Infection (including viral)

TIP: As a general rule, nonpermanent, absorbable fillers can be injected more superficially, and more permanent fillers need to be injected more deeply.

TIP: Begin by injecting only temporary fillers.

FAT GRAFTING (see Chapter 23)
Besides increasing the volume, fat grafting immediately beneath the dermis can improve the quality of the skin, decreasing wrinkles, decreasing pore size, and even reducing scarring.

Anesthesia
■ Small areas of fat grafting can often be performed using local anesthesia.
■ Larger areas usually require sedation.

Technique
■ Fat is harvested using Coleman cannulas and 10 ml syringes.
■ The syringes are capped and centrifuged for about 3 minutes at 3000 rpm.
■ Serum and oil are drained.
■ Fat is transferred to 1 ml insulin syringes for further injection.
■ A 16-gauge needle is used to make incisions, with care not to push a core of skin into the subcutaneous plane.
■ Slightly curving the incisions makes them almost impossible to find once healed.
■ 17-gauge, blunt side-port Luer-Lok injection needles are used for fat grafting.
■ The fat is placed gently during the withdrawal of a blunt Coleman infiltration cannula, and it must be distributed in fine threads.

- At least 10 full-length needle passes per centimeter are made *("structural fat grafting" technique).*
- Approximately 1.2-1.5 ml should be injected into the upper lip and 1.5-2 ml into lower lip.
- Overcorrection is usually needed to account for partial absorption.

TIP: While injecting, fat must flow freely through the needle. Overcoming resistance by pushing harder will create a fat surge that will cause irregularity.

CHEMICAL PEELS (see Chapter 19)
- Most commonly used peels:
  - **20%-35% trichloroacetic acid (TCA)** (medium-level penetration, good safety profile)
  - **Jessner solution** (used mostly as a primer for TCA peel)
  - **88% phenol** (deepest penetration, but requires prolonged period of healing and has a potential for cardiotoxicity)

Anesthesia
- IV sedation is usually adequate.
- A cooling fan can be used to reduce the burning sensation.

Technique
- Facial subunits should be marked so that the peel can be applied evenly to each subunit.
- A cotton-tipped applicator should be used.
- The skin is disinfected and acetone is used to remove superficial skin scales.
- Peeling agent is applied homogenously over the entire surface with a consistent pressure.
- TCA application may be repeated several times, depending on the depth of the wrinkles, using light pressure.
- Each skin area is treated with the same intensity.
- The typical blanching, which is a sign that the treatment has started to take effect *(frost effect)*, begins before the treatment has been completed.
- Follow-up treatment with petrolatum will reduce the sensation of tautness.
- Herpes prophylaxis with acyclovir 400 mg three times daily is recommended for 3-5 days.

TIP: Pay special attention to the transition area between the facial skin and the lip, which is often inadequately peeled. Treatment of this area is facilitated by stretching and flattening the vermilion borders to provide even distribution over vertical rhytids along the lip.

DERMABRASION (see Chapter 20)

- Mechanically removes the epidermis and dermis, usually with a diamond-powered fraise
- Ideally performed in the operating room because of exposure

Anesthesia

- IV sedation
- Regional nerve block
- General anesthesia in some cases

Technique

- The operation site should be draped and disinfected carefully.
- A flat surface can be created by stretching the skin. This facilitates abrasion and allows the application of treatment at an exact depth.
- Skin tension must be maintained during the entire abrasion procedure.
- Abrasion should be moved over the surface of the skin against the rotation of the abrasion head at an angle of 90 degrees while applying light pressure.
- **Punctiform, superficial bleeding** is the most reliable indicator that the grinding procedure has reached the optimal depth.[9]
- Abrasion should not enter the subcutaneous plane.
- Dermabrasion is complete when an even wound surface with fine, punctiform/diffuse bleeding has been created.
- Gauze soaked with antibiotic ointment is placed over the wound.
- The dressing can be removed after 24 hours.
- The area should be treated with skin moisturizer for a further 8 days.
- The skin needs to be protected from the sun, or patients should avoid the sun, for 3 months (pigment abnormalities).

LASER ABLATIVE RESURFACING (see Chapter 17)
Carbon Dioxide Laser

- Protective eyewear and fire precautions must be strictly adhered to when using this modality.
- After disinfection of the operation site and anesthesia (e.g., blocking of the infraorbital nerve), the boundaries of the section to be treated by laser are defined.
- The laser is applied to the desired subunit, set at the recommended parameters for tissue ablation (10 J/cm^2).[10]
- The depth of ablation depends on the number of passes and the amount of cooling time allowed between passes.
- The clinical endpoint is a **pale yellow color** of the skin surface indicative that treatment has reached **mid-reticular dermis.**
- An occlusive dressing is applied after completion of the procedure (entire epidermis has been removed).

TIP: Insufficient cooling time can lead to thermal damage of the skin.

Erbium:YAG Laser
- Less thermal diffusion than CO_2 laser and usually shorter recovery time
- **Best for superficial and medium-depth wrinkles**
- The laser is guided evenly, section by section, over the area to be ablated.
- Slight overlapping will not be harmful.
- Wound discharge and crust formation are less pronounced after erbium:YAG laser treatment and do not persist for as long as with CO_2 laser treatment.[11]
- Less postoperative skin reddening occurs and reduces more quickly.
- **Complications**
  - Ablative resurfacing procedures can cause herpes simplex virus (HSV) activation, hyperpigmentation, and hypertrophic scarring.
  - Before the procedure, patients are placed on a prophylactic course of oral antiviral medications for 2 days.
  - Rarely, a patient will develop a herpetic outbreak; the antiviral medication is continued, at twice the prophylactic dose, for 1 week.

LIPLIFT (see Chapter 48)
Anesthesia
- Can be done using local anesthesia

Technique
- Patients are marked before injection and asked to review and approve the markings. (Even a 0.2 mm difference in vertical height can be noticed postoperatively.)
- The planned full-thickness skin resection is performed, starting from the vermilion border.
- To decrease the chances of hypertrophic scarring, the vermilion and skin directly within the philtral columns, corresponding to the prolabium, are not included in the resection.
- The wound is closed with interrupted fine monofilament sutures tied on the vermilion side of the wound.

SUBNASAL LIPLIFT
- Provides predictable increase in the vertical height of the red lip, without disruption of upper lid anatomy, and improves the red/white lip ratio.[12]

Anesthesia
Procedure can be performed using local anesthesia.

Technique (Fig. 41-6)
- The marked incision begins at the alar crease and traverses the vestibule of the nose within the nasal sill, following the subcolumellar–lip border bilaterally.
- Upper lip skin is excised in a bullhorn shape. No muscle is excised, and meticulous hemostasis is achieved.
- The wounds are closed with fine nonabsorbable monofilament sutures. One or two subcutaneous sutures might be necessary to reduce tension.

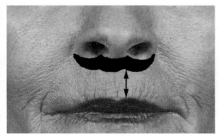

12 to 13 mm at phitral crest

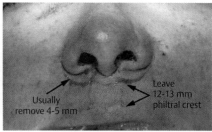

Usually remove 4 to 5 mm;
leave 12 to 13 mm philtral crest

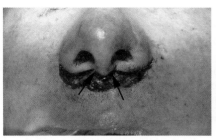

Crest points anchored to septal perichondrium;
do not take excision lateral to alar base

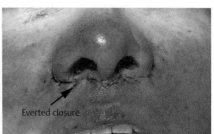

Everted closure

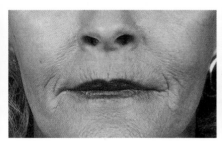

Preoperatively

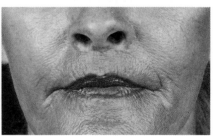

1 year postoperative

Fig. 41-6   Subnasal liplift surgical technique.

LIP IMPLANTS

■ Implants are mostly used for **vermilion augmentation**
■ **Implant materials**
   • Synthetic (Gore-Tex, PTFE, Tetrafluoroethylene tubes)
   • Biologic (AlloDerm, LifeCell; Surgisis, Cook Medical): AlloDerm is the most
     commonly used.[5]
   • Autologous (galeal fascia, palmaris longus)

Anesthesia
- Can be done with local anesthetic infiltration directly in the lip

Technique
- The implant is prepared according to manufacturer's specifications.
- Two small incisions are made in the corners of the mouth in the wet vermilion.
- A special passer is available for delivery of the graft, or a standard tendon passer can be used to bluntly tunnel from one incision to the other in the submucosal-subcutaneous plane.
- The implant sheet is grasped and carried through.
- Access incisions are closed with fine absorbable sutures.

> **TIP:** Massaging the graft smooths out the material and allows better placement.

COMPLICATIONS
- Hypertrophic scarring, asymmetry, numbness, and lumpiness
- Sensitivity to the implant material, extrusion, need for removal of the implant because of hardening, interference with lip function, and sensation changes

---

TOP TAKEAWAYS
- ➤ The mirror and camera are the most important tools to define, with the patient, what should be modified to obtain a better appearance.
- ➤ Well-designed informed consent can help to improve communications when problems arise.
- ➤ Radiesse and Sculptra should not be used for lip augmentation because of their high incidence of nodule formation.
- ➤ Fat grafting immediately beneath the dermis can improve the quality of the skin, decreasing wrinkles, decreasing pore size, and even reducing scarring.

REFERENCES
1. Agarwal A, Dejoseph L, Silver W, et al. Anatomy of the jawline, neck, and perioral area with clinical correlations. Facial Plast Surg 21:3, 2005.
2. Calhoun KH. Lip anatomy and function. In Calhoun KH, Stiernberg CM, eds. Surgery of the Lip. New York: Thieme Publishers, 1992.
3. Leveque JL, Goubanova E. Influence of age on the lips and perioral skin. Dermatology 208:307, 2004.
4. Loos BM, Maas CS. Relevant anatomy for botulinum toxin facial rejuvenation. Facial Plast Surg Clin North Am 11:439, 2003.
5. Monhian N, Ahn MS, Maas CS. Injectable and implantable materials for facial wrinkles. In Papel ID, ed. Facial Plastic and Reconstructive Surgery, ed 2. New York: Thieme Publishers, 2002.
6. Guyuron B. The armamentarium to battle the recalcitrant nasolabial crease. Clin Plast Surg 22:253, 1995.

7. Perkins SW, Sandel HD IV. Anatomic considerations, analysis, and the aging process of the perioral region. Facial Plast Surg Clin North Am 15:403, 2007.
8. Kanchwala SK, Holloway L, Bucky LP. Reliable soft tissue augmentation: a clinical comparison of injectable soft-tissue fillers for facial-volume augmentation. Ann Plast Surg 55:30, 2005.
9. Shpall R, Beddingfield FC III, Watson D, et al. Microdermabrasion: a review. Facial Plast Surg 20:47, 2004.
10. Schwartz RJ, Burns AJ, Rohrich RJ, et al. Long-term assessment of CO2 facial laser resurfacing: aesthetic results and complications. Plast Reconstr Surg 103:592, 1999.
11. Gregory R. Perioral laser rejuvenation. Semin Plast Surg 17:225, 2003.
12. Perkins NW, Smith SP Jr, Williams EF III. Perioral rejuvenation: complementary techniques and procedures. Facial Plast Surg Clin North Am 15:423, 2007.

42. Facelift

Adam H. Hamawy, Dino R. Elyassnia

PREOPERATIVE EVALUATION

- Consult with the patient to develop rapport while determining anatomic, psychological, and medical suitability.
- Establish baseline health and intercurrent illnesses, tobacco use, prior surgeries, and prior cosmetic treatments (i.e., botulinum toxin, lasers, and fillers). Carefully assess surgical risk based on medical history.
- Perform a systematic facial examination focusing on individual components and how they interact with the whole to give the appearance of facial aging.

ASSESSING THE AGING FACE[1]

- Facial aging is a function of soft tissue sagging, volume loss from atrophy, and skin surface changes.

SKIN QUALITY
- Skin thickness and elasticity are assessed.
- Dermal atrophy occurs with age and actinic damage.
- Thin, crêpey dermis is less elastic and less likely to maintain a smooth appearance after redundant skin has been removed.
- Trimming excess skin will address redundancy and reestablish some tone; however, the degree that can be maintained over time is **limited by the residual skin elasticity.**

SOFT TISSUE VOLUME
- Subcutaneous fat is distributed in discrete anatomic compartments.
- Facial fat compartments lose volume and deflate with time.[2]
- The superficial musculoaponeurotic system (SMAS) and platysmal laxity contribute to the downward migration of facial tissues that develops with aging.[3]
- Alteration in fat distribution and soft tissue laxity result in a morphologic change from a youthful "heart shape" to an aged, square appearance[4] (Fig. 42-1).

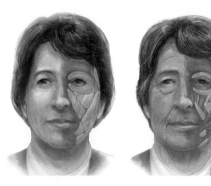

Fig. 42-1 The facial fat compartments and their aging changes. Aging leads to an inferior migration of the midfacial fat compartments and an inferior volume shift within the compartments. Deflation of the buccal extension of the buccal fat aggravates the inferior migration of the medial cheek fat, middle cheek fat, and suborbicularis oculi fat.

■ Restoring volume and proper redistribution of soft tissue can help to restore the appearance of youth.

SENIOR AUTHOR TIP: Patients with significant facial atrophy and age-related facial wasting will generally achieve suboptimal improvement from both surface treatments of facial skin and surgical lifts. Restoring lost facial volume using fat injections can produce a significant, sustained improvement in appearance that is unobtainable by other means. However, age-related facial atrophy rarely exists in isolation, and most patients troubled by it are not always appropriately treated by fat injections alone. Isolated fat injections are of questionable benefit to patients with significant facial sagging. Although aggressive filling of the sagging face can improve facial contour, it generally results in an unusually large, unnatural appearance. It is more logical to perform fat injections in conjunction with a facelift or after ptotic tissue has been treated.

SKELETAL SUPPORT
■ The facial skeleton loses volume and changes with age.[5]
■ Loss of skeletal support adds to the appearance of facial deflation and aging.
■ Skeletal augmentation can be an effective method to address changes of facial aging and establish support for overlying soft tissue (Fig. 42-2) (see Chapters 27 and 40).

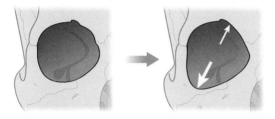

Fig. 42-2   The bony orbit of a young female subject on the left and an older female subject on the right. The aged orbit may be rejuvenated with volume augmentation.

FACIAL ANALYSIS
■ Assess and address the entire face as a whole to maintain facial harmony.
■ The key steps to consistent results are a thorough preoperative analysis and development of an operative plan to address individual aesthetic needs.

Forehead
■ Assess facial proportions. Forehead should represent the upper third of the face, measured from hairline to pupil.
■ Note the presence of active and passive wrinkles on the forehead from frontalis activation and on the glabella from contraction of the corrugators and procerus.
  • **Passive wrinkles (static rhytids) do not disappear with relaxation.** Passive wrinkles are best addressed by **skin resurfacing treatments** and will only be minimally improved by chemodenervation or surgical lifts.
  • **Active wrinkles (dynamic rhytids) occur with animation** and can be voluntary or involuntary. Active wrinkles can be improved with **chemodenervation** and possibly **browlifting.**

- Evaluate medial and lateral brow position in relation to orbital shape and upper lid.

> **NOTE:**   Lateral brow ptosis can give the appearance of excess upper lid skin and should be corrected with a browlift rather than a blepharoplasty.

Upper Eyelid
- Identify lid ptosis, characterized by **a low resting lid margin** and **high supratarsal crease.** Both brow and eyelid ptosis should be addressed in the surgical plan.
- Assess the amount of upper eyelid skin. Compensate for excess skin from lateral brow hooding by manual repositioning of the lateral brow.
- Assess periorbital fat, which will most often manifest as deflation and hollowing of the upper orbit.

Lower Eyelid
- Note the relationship of the orbital rim to the anterior surface of the globe (Fig. 42-3).
  - **Positive vector orbits** provide better support for lid suspension.
  - **Negative vector orbits** lack support and should be addressed by planning additional **lower lid support** or midface soft tissue augmentation.
- Globe prominence may indicate thyroid disease that should be treated appropriately.
- Assess lid tone and tarsal suspension using a lid snap-back test and lid distraction test.
- Determine skin laxity and quality. Trimming of excess lower eyelid skin must be very conservative to prevent complications.
- Assess for laxity of the orbicularis muscle, sometimes evident by the presence of festoons.
- Note bulging of fat, laxity of the orbital septum, and fat loss in the lower orbit.

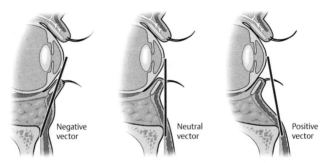

Fig. 42-3   Orbital vectors.

Cheek
- Examine skeletal proportions and the relationship of the bizygomatic diameter and maxillary height.
- Note the distribution of subcutaneous fat and tissue in relation to underlying bony structure.
- Assess depth and prominence of the nasolabial folds, which indicate volume loss and inferior migration of overlying tissue secondary to deflation of fat compartments.
- Jowls indicate shelving from ptotic cheek tissue or excess fat that may need to be addressed. Jowls can be accentuated by tethering at the mandibulocutaneous ligament that should be released or by volume loss along the jawline that should be replaced.

Perioral Area
- Note the presence of marionette lines from the oral commissures to the mandibular border.
- Assess for volume loss in the lips and lengthening of the upper lip. Note degree of upper incisor show at rest.
- The presence of a weak chin should be discussed with the patient and possibly addressed in the surgical plan.
- Deep perioral rhytids are important to note and will **not** improve with facelifting. Proper treatment will require skin resurfacing as an additional part of the surgical plan.

Neck
- Assess for presence of soft platysmal bands visible in repose, and hard bands visible with platysmal activation.
- Soft bands will respond to repositioning of lax platysma (i.e., platysmaplasty), whereas hard bands will require platysmal myotomy.
- Excess fat can be located superficial or deep to the platysma. Depending on the extent and location, this can be addressed by liposuction or direct excision.
- The amount of skin laxity is important to note; however, addressing the skin in isolation without considering the underlying structures will result in a modest improvement at best.

SENIOR AUTHOR TIP: For many patients, subplatysmal fat accumulation, submandibular salivary gland "ptosis," and digastric muscle hypertrophy will contribute significantly to their neck deformity. As patients age, fat stores generally shift from preplatysmal to subplatysmal, and the small amount of subcutaneous fat present in a typical patient presenting for a facelift is needed to preserve a soft, youthful neck. Excess subplatysmal fat is usually present in patients with firm, obtuse necks who have had lifelong cervicomental fullness. In these patients, partial subplatysmal lipectomy will be productive. Submandibular glands are usually palpable as firm, discrete masses in the lateral submental triangle, lateral to the anterior belly of the digastric muscle and medial to the mandibular border. Glands lying deep to the plane tangent to the inferior border of the mandible and ipsilateral anterior belly of the digastric muscle do not disrupt neck contour and will usually not require treatment. However, glands protruding inferior to this plane are likely to be problematic if excess cervical fat is removed and redundant skin excised. A small subgroup of patients will have digastric muscles with large, bulky anterior bellies that are evident as linear paramedian submental fullness. As in the case of large submandibular glands, large digastric muscles are frequently hidden by excess subplatysmal fat or lax platysma. In these patients, subtotal superficial digastric myectomy should be considered.

SURGICAL PLAN
- A surgical plan should include all the individual components of the face noted on facial analysis.
- Failure to address all the units comprehensively may lead to facial disharmony and less than optimal results.

- Although this chapter specifically focuses on facelift techniques, complete facial rejuvenation will often include surgery for the neck, brow, eyelids, and perioral region in addition to complimentary skin treatments.
- Preoperative photography is essential for planning and for documenting operative changes (see Chapter 3).

FACELIFT TECHNIQUES

There are as many facelift techniques as there are facelift surgeons. However, common themes allow generalization of certain methods and approaches. Rather than describing the technique attributed to each surgeon, the principles are listed below. Understanding the principles allows surgeons to compare methods and critically analyze "new" techniques as they are introduced.

TECHNIQUE PRINCIPLES
Skin Incisions
- **Preauricular (short-scar)** incision may extend onto the temporal hairline but does not extend posteriorly.
- **Postauricular extension** is needed to address skin redundancy in the neck.
- **Submental incision** may be required to directly address platysmal banding and deep-layer neck problems, i.e., subplatysmal fat, submandibular glands, and digastric muscles.
- **Temporal incisions** are used in a minimally invasive approach to the brow and midface.
- **Upper blepharoplasty incision** can be used to access the brow ligaments and corrugators, or for lower lid canthopexy.
- **Transconjunctival or subciliary blepharoplasty incisions** can be used as an alternative approach to lifting the midface.

SMAS Plication Versus Imbrication
- **Plication** involves placement of direct sutures to fold over and suspend the mobile SMAS to the immobile SMAS in a vector perpendicular to the line of suturing. No discrete flap is elevated. A common variation is excision of an intervening portion of SMAS (SMASectomy).[3]
- **Imbrication** involves elevating a discrete flap by making an incision, then elevating the SMAS to overlap and fixate or excise the redundant portion, and suturing end to end.

Vectors
- Ptotic facial soft tissue is ideally elevated by repositioning the SMAS in a vector perpendicular to the long axis of the zygomaticus major muscle.
- Redundant skin should only be trimmed in a slightly more horizontal vector.
- Excessive posterior traction can give an artificial "windswept" appearance postoperatively.

FACELIFT PLANES
Subcutaneous Facelifts
- A thick subcutaneous flap is raised and redraped while all redundant skin is excised.
- SMAS is addressed with a pure plication or with a partial SMAS resection and primary repair in the direction of the desired vector.
- A pure subcutaneous lift, without addressing the SMAS, is rarely performed today.

SENIOR AUTHOR TIP: Skin was meant to serve a covering function and not a structural or supporting one. Using skin as the vehicle to support sagging deep-layer tissue corrupts its function and results in abnormal tension and related secondary problems, including poor scars, tragal retraction, earlobe malposition, and a tight, unnatural appearance. Relying on the SMAS to lift sagging facial tissues circumvents this problem, because it is an inelastic structural layer capable of providing sustained support. Although skin is excised in SMAS procedures, only redundant tissue is sacrificed, and closure can be done under normal skin tension.

Sub-SMAS Facelifts
- A plane is developed deep to the SMAS to allow mobilization and imbrication in the desired vector.
- Degree of sub-SMAS plane development can vary; however, at a minimum, the fixed SMAS over the parotid and zygoma must be lifted to allow adequate mobilization.
- SMAS can be mobilized as an independent layer or with the overlying skin.
- Sub-SMAS dissection may result in more prolonged swelling and recovery from greater disruption of lymphatics.
- This technique is often referred to as a *deep plane lift,* although this term can be inaccurate, because deeper planes exist, which are described in the following text.

Supraperiosteal Facelift
- An avascular plane is developed between the periosteum and SMAS over the zygoma and periorbital rim.
- Approach is from a temporal incision to lift the upper face and midface as a single unit.
- Malar soft tissue is lifted and suspended independently from the temporal fascia.

Subperiosteal Facelift
- A subperiosteal plane is developed similarly to access dissection in craniofacial reconstruction.
- The skin, SMAS, and all overlying soft tissue are raised as a composite unit and fixed to achieve repositioning.
- Malar augmentation with soft tissue repositioning or by direct access and placement of implant is easily achieved.
- Neck and perioral region are not adequately addressed, and supplementation with another technique may be needed.

> **SENIOR AUTHOR'S PREFERRED TECHNIQUE:**   My preferred technique is a lamellar high-SMAS facelift. In a lamellar dissection, the skin and SMAS are elevated as separate layers and advanced bidirectionally along different vectors. This allows the skin and SMAS to be advanced by different amounts, along separate vectors, and suspended under differential tension. Each of these layers can be addressed individually, preventing skin tension, hairline displacement, and objectionable wrinkle shifts. Planning the upper border of the SMAS flap in a "high" position along the superior border of the zygomatic arch allows elevation of not only the lower cheek and jowl but also the midface and infraorbital regions.

ADJUNCTIVE PROCEDURES

To enhance the overall results, additional procedures can be performed in conjunction with a facelift. In addition to performing surgical lifts to address the forehead, eyelids, lips, and neck, the following adjunctive procedures are often required.

AUTOLOGOUS FAT GRAFTS
■ Volume is restored to deficient regions of the face through transferred autologous fat.
■ **Loss of 30%-50% of injected fat is expected.**
■ Results vary with surgeon and technique, and patients need to be informed that repeat injection may be necessary to achieve desired volume and contour.

SKELETAL AUGMENTATION
■ Bony prominences can be accentuated to achieve a youthful appearance by augmenting the skeleton.
■ Malar or mandibular augmentation can be achieved with silicone or porous polytheylene implants or subperiosteal placement of calcium hydroxyapatite.

SKIN RESURFACING
■ Improving the skin surface to address fine rhytids and dyschromia will enhance the structural changes achieved by the facelift.
■ Skin quality can be improved with controlled injury to the surface to promote new collagen deposition and reactive contraction.
■ Mechanism of injury is not as critical as depth to promote changes.
■ Laser, chemical peeling, and dermabrasion all work to achieve similar results.
■ **Dermabrasion** works by causing mechanical injury to ablate the surface layer (see Chapter 20).
    • Treatment of perioral rhytids is very effective.
    • Achieving uniform depth is technically difficult.
■ **Laser surgery** works by causing both ablation and heat injury (see Chapters 16 and 17).
    • Uniform treatment can be delivered with computer precision.
    • Treating different facial regions with variable depth is more difficult.
■ **Chemical peels** work by causing chemical injury (see Chapter 19).
    • Trichloroacetic acid (TCA) and phenol-croton oil are most commonly used.
    • Depth is determined by the concentration, time of application, and number of layers applied.

OPERATIVE AND FOLLOW-UP CARE

The care delivered in the operating room and during recovery is as essential to the final result as the specific techniques that are used. Attention to detail in every aspect of patient care will result in a smoother operative course, reduction in complications, and faster recovery.

ANESTHESIA
- If general anesthesia is used, endotracheal tube position should be adjustable during the procedure to allow access to all incision sites.
- The use of lidocaine with epinephrine injection during a facelift is nearly routine to provide pain control and hemostasis in a highly vascularized field.
- Tumescent fluid can allow facelift procedures to be performed with only oral or IV sedation, depending on the surgeon's and the patient's comfort level.

SENIOR AUTHOR TIP: I perform most facelifts with the patient under deep sedation given by an anesthesiologist using a laryngeal mask airway (LMA). This allows the patient to be heavily sedated without compromise of the airway. However, muscle relaxants are not given, and the patient can be allowed to breathe spontaneously. An LMA is less likely than an endotracheal tube to become dislodged during the procedure and to trigger coughing and bucking when the patient emerges from the anesthetic.

INTRAOPERATIVE MANAGEMENT
- A well-rehearsed plan of execution is necessary to maintain a steady surgical cadence to reduce operative time without compromising technical precision.
- Hair should be washed and can be prepped in the surgical field to give the surgeon an unobstructed view of the patient's entire face, neck, and scalp.
- Warming blankets should be used to maintain the patient's body temperature throughout the procedure.
- Injection of local anesthetic with epinephrine should be timed before making incisions or dissecting in a different facial region to ensure preemptive analgesia and maximum hemostatic effect.
- Tight blood pressure control can help to maintain a dry operative field and to reduce postoperative hematoma.
- Prevention of postoperative nausea is critical and treated with a multimodal approach of antiemetics given at the beginning of the procedure.
- A smooth extubation and emergence from anesthesia should be stressed.

POSTOPERATIVE CARE
- Head elevation can help prevent swelling but should not result in neck flexion.
- Cold compresses can be applied to the eyes 15-20 minutes each hour for the first 3 days.
- Postoperative hypertension can lead to a hematoma and should be prevented.
  - Clonidine patch (0.2 mg/day) placed preoperatively can offer sustained blood pressure control during and after surgery.
  - IV labetalol can be given in 5-10 mg boluses for breakthrough hypertension.
  - Chlorpromazine 25 mg every 4 hours is effective in controlling blood pressure and acts as a potent sedative antiemetic.

- Standing orders for antiemetic medications are given to control postoperative nausea and vomiting.
- Patients should ambulate the day of surgery if possible. The importance of staying mobile at home after discharge is emphasized.
- Salt and excessive intake of water, which can exacerbate swelling, are restricted.

SENIOR AUTHOR TIP: All patients are instructed to sleep flat on their back without a pillow. A small cylindrical neck roll is allowed if a patient requests it. This posture ensures an open cervicomental angle and averts dangerous folding of the neck skin flap and obstruction of regional lymphatics that inevitably occur if the patient is allowed to elevate the head on pillows. All patients are shown an elbow-on-knees position that ensures an open cervicomental angle while sitting. Patients should have a soft diet but avoid salty, sour, dry, and difficult to chew foods. They are instructed to abstain from alcohol for 2 weeks after surgery. Patients should begin showering and shampooing no later than 3 days after the procedure. The neck drain is left in place for 5 days, which reduces the likelihood that any small collections will form and speeds the overall resolution of edema and ecchymosis in the neck.

COMPLICATIONS

HEMATOMA
- More common in **males** than females
- Usually occurs within the **first 8 hours** postoperatively
- Large, expanding hematomas require **urgent evacuation** to prevent skin necrosis.
- **Risk factors**
  - Male sex
  - Preoperative hypertension
  - Postoperative rebound hypertension
  - Qualitative platelet disorders from medication or supplements
- Small (<5 ml) hematomas can be evacuated by needle aspiration.
- Hematomas >5 ml should be drained postoperatively to prevent secondary induration and prolonged distortion.

INFECTION
- Surgical site infections can occur in up to 2% of patients.
- The most common organisms are *Staphylococcus aureus* and *Pseudomonas aeruginosa*.
- Most appear at the **periauricular incision** about 5-7 days after surgery.
- They usually respond well to drainage and oral antibiotic therapy with minimal sequelae.

DELAYED WOUND HEALING
- Skin necrosis is more commonly seen with subcutaneous facelifts (4%) than with sub-SMAS dissections (1%).[3]
- Skin incisions should be designed to avoid long retroauricular flaps and undermining limited whenever possible.

- It is more likely to occur when **tension** is applied to skin closure.
- Risk is significantly increased in patients who **actively smoke** or **use nicotine products.**

NERVE INJURY

- The **great auricular nerve** is the most often recognized nerve injury after a facelift.
- Transient neurapraxia of the marginal mandibular or frontal branches of the facial nerve can occur.
- Most neurapraxias resolve within a few weeks, but can persist for several months.
- Injury to the buccal branch, although reportedly the "most common," can go unnoticed because of cross-covering branches.
- Permanent facial nerve injuries are rare and can be prevented by clearly understanding the anatomy and respecting the "danger zones" (Fig. 42-4).

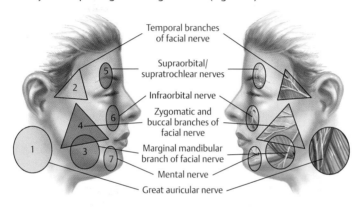

Temporal branches of facial nerve

Supraorbital/ supratrochlear nerves

Infraorbital nerve

Zygomatic and buccal branches of facial nerve

Marginal mandibular branch of facial nerve

Mental nerve

Great auricular nerve

Fig. 42-4   Facial danger zones: Motor and sensory nerves.

TOPICAL SKIN MAINTENANCE

- Topical skin care helps to maintain and preserve the longevity of facelift results and improves patient satisfaction.
- Counseling and recruiting patients to become active participants in their care is essential in implementing a successful regimen.
- Long-term benefits are seen with consistent, disciplined application.
- Successful skin care maintenance includes:
  - **Cleansing:** Nonsoap cleansers help to preserve natural lipid barriers between cells.
  - **Exfoliation:** Slow, gradual exfoliation can be achieved with alpha-hydroxy acids and retinols.
  - **Pigment control:** Melanin production and deposition can be inhibited using hydroquinone, kojic acid, or azelaic acid.
  - **Sun protection:** Use of a sunscreen and physical blockers with an SPF 30 or greater will absorb up to 97% of harmful radiation. Topical antioxidants such as vitamins C and E can also be applied to protect against photodamage.
  - **Cell stimulation:** Tretinoin is the only topical agent, other than chemical peels, that consistently results in clinically significant dermal stimulation.

TOP TAKEAWAYS
➤ Facial aging is a function of soft tissue sagging, volume loss from fat atrophy, and skin surface changes.
➤ Trimming excess skin will address redundancy and reestablish some tone; however, the degree that can be maintained over time is limited by the residual skin elasticity.
➤ Lateral brow ptosis can give the appearance of excess upper lid skin and should be corrected with a browlift rather than a blepharoplasty.
➤ For many patients, subplatysmal fat accumulation, submandibular salivary gland "ptosis," and digastric muscle hypertrophy will contribute significantly to their neck deformity.
➤ The care delivered in the operating room and during recovery is as essential to the final result as the specific techniques that are used.

REFERENCES

1. Gonyon DL, Barton FE. The aging face: rhytidectomy and adjunctive procedures. Sel Read Plast Surg 10:21, 2005.
2. Rohrich RJ, Pessa JE. The fat compartments of the face: anatomy and clinical implications for cosmetic surgery. Plast Reconstr Surg 119:2219, 2007.
3. Marten TJ. Lamellar high SMAS face and midface lift: a comprehensive technique for natural-appearing rejuvenation of the face. In Nahai F, ed. The Art of Aesthetic Surgery: Principles & Techniques, ed 2. New York: Thieme Publishers, 2010.
4. Gierloff M, Stohring C, Buder T, et al. Aging changes of the midfacial fat compartments: a computed tomographic study. Plast Reconstr Surg 129:263, 2012.
5. Shaw RB Jr, Katzel EB, Kolz PF, et al. Aging of the facial skeleton: aesthetic implications and rejuvenation strategies. Plast Reconstr Surg 127:374, 2011.

43. Nasolabial Fold

Sumeet Sorel Teotia, Maristella S. Evangelista

PERTINENT ANATOMY

The nasolabial fold is a combination of complex mechanisms consisting of skin, adjacent redundant cheek, the nasal ala, the lip, and dermal attachments of the various interacting and overlapping facial mimetic muscles with independent vectors of interaction, all affecting the modiolus, and thus the human smile.[1-8]

OBSERVATIONS ABOUT THE NASOLABIAL FOLD AFTER ANATOMIC DISSECTION

GROSS DISSECTION

- The fold is a **distinct fusion plane** that separates the fatty cheek from the dense upper lip.
- The nasolabial fold is a discrete unit with distinct anatomic boundaries.[9]
- Upper lip mimetic muscles insert into the orbicularis oris at the level of the fold.
- The *exact* arrangement of the muscular insertions into the dermis along the nasolabial fold is **unknown,** but perhaps this is what contributes to the uniqueness of every person's nasolabial fold.
- Little superficial fat covers the orbicularis oris, and in contrast, more fat is above the fold in the cheek region.
- The zygomaticus major and minor, levator labii superioris, and levator labii superioris alaeque nasi lie beneath the subcutaneous tissues.
- The levator anguli oris and buccinator muscles are deeper.
- The mimetic muscles abut the overlying dermis *only* when they reach the orbicularis oris border.
- Medial to the fold is a paucity of subcutaneous fat between the dermis and orbicularis oris, where skin is adherent to the sphincter directly.
- The upper lip levators are protected by a generous amount of subcutaneous fat from their origin on the zygoma and maxilla to their insertion into the orbicularis oris and modiolus.

- **The modiolus[6]:** Fibrovascular structure that forms a dense, compact, mobile mass.
  - Consists of interlacing arrays of terminal muscle fibers converging toward (labial tractors) or diverging away from (orbicularis oris) the center
  - Center is situated about 1.5 cm away from the labial commissure.
  - Texture, volume, and thickness (about 1 cm) can be palpated on bidigital examination.
  - Apex is covered by panniculus fibrosus.

TIP: The complex anatomy of nasolabial fold is well defined and must be understood in order to address clinical changes that occur and select appropriate and individualized treatment.

HISTOLOGIC OBSERVATIONS
- Responses to several publications[3,4,5-7,10] on microscopic anatomy around the nasolabial fold have overlapping, complementary elements:
  - The various mimetic muscles eventually insert into the entire perioral sphincter, composed of orbicularis muscle and modiolus.
  - The zygomaticus major and minor, modiolus, and levator labii superioris have cutaneous slips extending intermittently into the nasolabial fold dermis.
  - The nasolabial fold comprises (1) dense fibrous tissue, (2) muscle fibers branching from the levator muscles of the upper lip, and (3) striated muscle bundles originating in the fold fascia.
  - The lip elevator muscles and the "fold muscles" course down the lip to traverse the orbicularis oris and insert into the dermis of the (1) upper lip, (2) the cutaneous vermilion junction, and (3) the vermilion.
  - The muscle fibers of the levator superioris and zygomaticus major course down the cheek, with some muscle fibers separating from the main body to insert into the nasolabial fold fascia, traveling in many directions at the fold.

THE SMAS AND THE NASOLABIAL FOLD
Understanding the unique relationship between the nasolabial fold and the SMAS is critical to improving the aging face in this transitional zone of the central face. Histologic examinations elucidating the two have increased our understanding towards improving the nasolabial fold, whether surgically or nonsurgically.
- Complementary and supporting histologic evidence from various dissections gave rise to certain conclusions about the SMAS and the nasolabial fold.[3,11]
- The SMAS continues anteriorly up to the level of zygomaticus major muscle, at which point it seems indistinguishable from the investing fascia of the muscle.
- The attenuated SMAS also invests the undersurface of the zygomaticus muscle similar to its superficial coverage.
- A natural plane of dissection follows the deep surface of the SMAS behind the zygomaticus major muscle and into the buccal space.

- As it approaches the nasolabial fold, the SMAS anatomically divides into superficial and deep fascial leaves and envelops zygomaticus major and minor muscles.
- No separate subcutaneous extension of the SMAS appears to exist.

DYNAMICS OF THE NASOLABIAL FOLD

The movement of the nasolabial fold encompasses the complex anatomy and is a unique interaction between skin, the various facial mimetic muscles, adjacent fatty soft tissue (or the lack thereof), and the upper lip, all of which define the human smile and affect the expression of emotions. Following are some clinical observations[4,12]:

- Individual facial muscles retain their identity and can be stimulated to contract independently.
- Some muscles completely control a specific expression, whereas others incompletely control expressions, ranging from partial to full expression of the same emotion.
- Elevation of the upper lip (or smiling) deepens the nasolabial fold in all people.
- **Smirking** involves contracting single muscles and can produce discrete, unique dimples along the fold.
   • These discrete contour irregularities (dimpling) are the only sign of muscle action in a face that is in repose.
- Full smiling exaggerates dimpling.
- The dynamics of the fold move the upper lip to create different types of surface depressions.[4]
   • A comma-shaped crease lateral to commissure
   • A dimple above the modiolus
   • A narrow puckering along the fold in the upper lip (prominent at the beginning of the lip elevation but consumed by a full smile)
   • Shallow dimple next to the nasal ala in the upper fold
   • Some people have one dimple, and others none, but rarely are two dimples present in a person.

THE HUMAN SMILE (Fig. 43-1)

- Actions of the muscles surrounding the nasolabial fold and mouth give rise to the human smile, and one author noted the nasolabial fold as a keystone to the *smiling mechanism*.[10,13,14]
- The smile is formed in **stages.**
   • **First stage**
      ▶ The lip is raised to the fold by the levator muscles and the muscle bundles originating at the fold.
      ▶ The lip meets resistance at the fold because of the overlying fatty cheek mass.
   • **Second stage**
      ▶ Involves the levator muscles of the upper lip raising the lip and fold upward
- Paralysis of facial muscles effaces the nasolabial fold, confirming action of the mimetic muscles and their influence on deepening of the fold.
- In death, the nasolabial fold is retained.
- The fold is shallow in babies and deepest in elderly people.

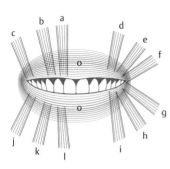

Elevators of upper lip (a-e):
a Caput annular of the levator labii superioris of the upper lip
b The rest of levator labii superioris
c Zygomaticus minor
d Zygomaticus major
e Upper part of the buccinator
f Caninus

Depressors of the angle of the mouth (g-i):
g The lower part of the buccinator
h Depressed angularis
i Risorius

Depressors of the lower lip (j-l):
j Platysma
k Depressor labii inferioris
l Mentalis

o Orbicularis oris circles the mouth

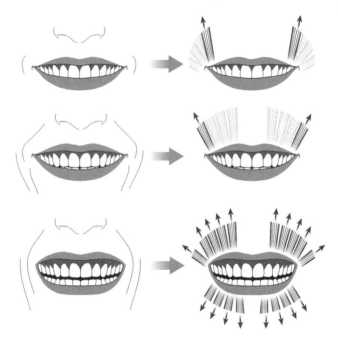

Fig. 43-1   Rubin's classic work on smiling.

WHAT DEEPENS THE NASOLABIAL FOLD?

■ Deep folds are a sign of aging, and the mechanism and dynamics of the fold contribute to the gradual deepening of the folds. The following factors contribute to the deepening of the folds[4]:
   • Redundant skin in the overlying cheek
   • Ptosis of the subcutaneous fat above the nasolabial fold

- Undercutting by the upper lip retractor muscles, particularly the levator labii superioris. Yousif et al[5] provided another perspective to the causes of the deepening nasolabial fold.
- The nasolabial fold is the point of juncture between two skin territories.
- Lateral to the fold, the territory contains no cutaneous muscle attachments, and thus is not supported by the muscles.
- Medial to the line of the nasolabial fold, the muscles insert on the skin and support this area against gravity and laxity of aging skin.
- During aging, the "unsupported" skin and cheek mass lateral to the fold descends at a much **greater rate** than the skin medial to the fold.

TIP: The discrepancy in the rate of descent of two adjacent skin territories creates and accentuates the nasolabial fold.

- Mendelson[15] compared cheek and lip contours separated by the nasolabial fold and noted the following effects of aging:
  - The contour of the youthful face becomes divided into a series of folds (convexities) and furrows (concavities).
  - In the midcheek, the round fullness of the youthful face is slowly lost, and hollowing appears as an obliquely oriented **midcheek furrow.**
  - The cheeks appear larger with aging, partly from the **nasolabial furrow** moving medially toward the lip.
  - Fullness and downward displacement of upper lip fold changes the commissure, which appears deeper and longer and droops to become the **marionette furrow.**
  - Lower lip loses its flatness to become more of a rounded fold that exaggerates depth of the marionette furrow.
  - Mental crease becomes deeper, longer, and downturned, as the **labiomental groove.**
- A **photogrammetric analysis** further defines the relationship with aging and deepening of the nasolabial fold.[16]
  - With aging, the cheek mass displaces **anteriorly, laterally,** and **inferiorly.**
    - ► This displacement deepens the nasolabial fold.
  - The relationship between the upper lip and fold remains constant.
  - The lateral commissure moves laterally, while the apparent angle of the nasolabial fold decreases.

TIP: Deepening of the nasolabial fold is caused by changes in the cheek mass and its support.

- In diseased states such as HIV lipodystrophy, overall facial fat atrophy deepens the nasolabial fold. **The following are observed in HIV patients:**
  - Atrophy of the fatty cheek above the fold
  - Ptosis of the "deflated" skin over the nasolabial fold
  - Continued action of upper lip retractor muscles to further the deepening by undercutting
  - Lack of significant atrophy of the upper lip, mainly from a paucity of subcutaneous fat
  - Massive-weight-loss patients have similar clinical findings.
  - These changes are additive with those of the aging process of the skin and subcutaneous tissue.

ASSESSING THE NASOLABIAL FOLD (Fig. 43-2)

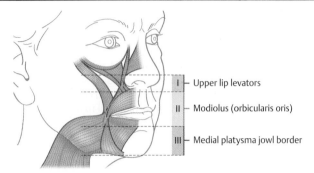

Fig. 43-2   Functional zones of the nasolabial fold according to Barton.

BARTON CLASSIFICATION
Barton[2] classified the nasolabial fold into **three functional zones,** as related to assessing rhytidectomy.
- **Zone I: Upper third of fold.** Influenced by contraction of levator muscles of the upper lip, particularly the levator labii superioris, levator anguli oris, zygomaticus minor, and to a lesser extent, zygomaticus major
- **Zone II: Area between oral commissure.** Affected by the skin attachment of modiolus and indirectly by muscles acting on it (zygomaticus major, orbicularis oris, and triangularis portion of depressor anguli oris)
- **Zone III: Between the commissure and mandibular angle.** Influenced by bony attachments of platysma to the mandible
- Each zone is an area of cutaneous wrinkling accentuated by actions of the underlying muscles.

ZUFFEREY CLASSIFICATION
Zufferey[6,17] noted three types of nasolabial folds and correlated them with the underlying anatomy, specifically the presence of superficial fibers from the zygomaticus major muscle.
- Three types of fold: **Convex, straight, and concave**
- The "fixed" fold is determined by the angle of articulation between the medial and lateral segments.
- This angle varies.

> **NOTE: Clinically, this classification is not helpful, but it reminds us that a guideline based on function and aging may be more appropriate.**

NAHAI CLASSIFICATION
Nahai[18] classified the nasolabial folds and marionette grooves based on the influence of aging. This classification is more clinically applicable (Fig. 43-3).

- **Grade I:** Visible folds on animation
- **Grade II:** Visible folds at rest
- **Grade III:** Visible folds at rest and deepening of folds on animation
- **Grade IV:** Deep folds at rest and deeper on animation
- **Grade V:** Overhanging folds

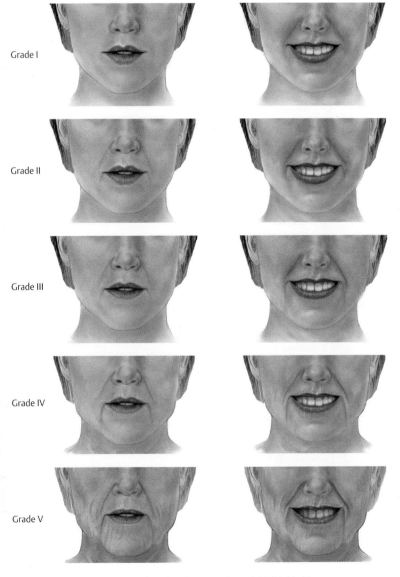

Fig. 43-3   Classification of nasolabial fold aging.

INFORMED CONSENT

- Before initiating treatment, goals should be discussed with the patient, including the inherent risks and benefits.
- Several treatment alternatives exist, from injection therapy to surgery, but not all modalities will be ideal for a particular patient or even for a group of patients.
- Intervention is chosen only after an honest conversation with the patient to define goals and expectations that can readily and safely be met.

MANAGEMENT OF THE NASOLABIAL FOLD (Fig. 43-4)

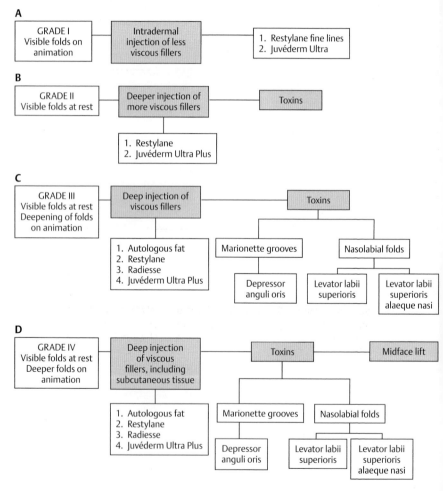

Fig. 43-4   Treatment options for nasolabial folds and marionette grooves. **A,** Grade I. **B,** Grade II. **C,** Grade III. **D,** Grade IV.

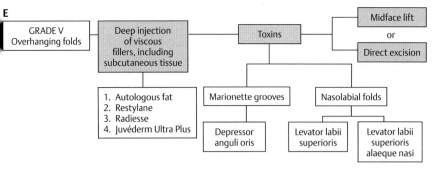

Fig. 43-4, cont'd   E, Grade V.

- Rejuvenation of the nasolabial fold begins with a careful assessment of the severity of the fold.
- Options range from "surface approaches" to "subsurface approaches"
  - Surface approaches: skin treatment and injections such as fillers and botulinum toxin
  - Subsurface approaches: lipectomy, excision, eversion, implantation, facelifts

INJECTIONS (see Chapter 21)

- Superficially placed materials (impermanent) can be injected in the dermis for effacement of the fold.
- This may be a first-line treatment for younger patients with minimal fold exaggeration.
- Various choices are available, and materials are constantly evolving.
- Examples include Restylane (Galderma), Juvéderm (Allergan), collagen, and fat injections and have variable longevity and success.
- Juvéderm Ultra Plus (Allergan) seems to correct nasolabial fold at least for 1 year.[19]
- **Nonhyaluronic acid fillers** are best avoided in the superficial plane; however, these fillers are longer-lasting than others if appropriately placed.[20]

CAUTION: Silicone injections are of historical interest and should never be placed anywhere in the human body.

- Carefully placed botulinum toxin is a useful adjunct to paralyze specific muscles (such as levator labii superioris or depressor anguli oris) and can serve to antagonize these muscles, which "undercut" and exaggerate the nasolabial fold. **Perioral neurotoxins should be injected with caution.**
- **Fat injections** have variable longevity, typically result in incomplete and short-lived correction, and may be best reserved for younger patients.
  - Rohrich[21] reported 81% improvement in the nasolabial fold using his lift-and-fill technique.
  - Marten[22] also reports excellent results with the combined technique; he describes a superficial subcutaneous injection to address nasolabial crease and a deep injection at the piriform to address maxillary recession in the upper nasolabial fold.

SENIOR AUTHOR TIP: When injecting hyaluronic acid fillers, inject gradually, usually in small amounts, one side at a time, and have patient assess improvement and symmetry as you go. This is a good gauge for postprocedure result and helps achieve patient buy-in.

DERMAL FAT GRAFTING (Fig. 43-5) (see Chapter 23)

- Adjunctive to a facelift and uses a dermal fat graft to smooth the nasolabial fold
- May be fashioned from a portion of redundant SMAS flap adequately freed
- Guyuron and Michelow[23] described their approach and note lasting results:
  1. Excess fat is debulked or repositioned in the nasolabial fold.
  2. Skin is undermined medial to the nasolabial crease to separate dermal attachments from underlying muscle and SMAS.
  3. A soft, supple graft is interpositioned at the site of the nasolabial crease to create a barrier to reattachment of muscle to dermis.
  4. Excess skin is eliminated, and skin and SMAS are redraped to reduce ptosis of subcutaneous structures.

> **NOTE: These grafts can be partially absorbed, leaving contour irregularities.**

- Dermal grafts should have symmetry and smoothness before insertion to prevent further palpable or visible irregularities.
- Grafts should be fixed by an absorbable suture (skin surface) to prevent migration or dislodgement.
- Graft should not be too bulky or scarring, and decreased absorption may contribute to palpable or visible irregularities.

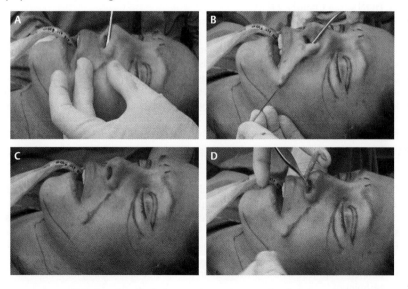

Fig. 43-5   A, A Tulip Biomed pickle fork is used to undermine the skin through a nasal vestibule incision. **B,** A Frasier suction cannula guides 4-0 plain suture percutaneously into the nose. **C,** The SMAS graft is attached to the suture. **D,** The graft is fed into its subdermal position by traction on the percutaneous suture.

NASOLABIAL LIPECTOMY

- Millard et al[24] presented their follow-up on nasolabial lipectomy through a facelift approach.
- The skin of the cheek is undermined in subcutaneous plane, with the scalpel turning deeper in the nasolabial region.
- Fat is pinched off the undersurface of the skin of the fold with scissors.
- The fold of the fat is further reduced with a right-angled scissors.

> **NOTE:** This approach is probably of historic interest; however, the results seem **long-lasting. It is another option in the surgical armamentarium.**

CAUTION: Inexperienced surgeons should avoid this approach unless comfortable with the surgical anatomy.

FACELIFT (see Chapter 42)

- The rationale for successful surgical effacement of the nasolabial fold from a facelift approach is anatomic and discussed previously. The procedure requires specific expertise and experience.
- Understanding the surgical anatomy is critical, because this approach is complex and carries the highest risk of complications if not used appropriately.
- The attachment of the SMAS to the zygomatic muscles should be severed[2,3] as one of the more effective surgical methods.
- The cheek flap medial to the zygomaticus major muscle must include only skin and subcutaneous tissue to free it from the underlying tether of the SMAS.[3]
- Thus, at the level of the **zygomaticus major** muscle, flap dissection should be carried *superficial* **to the SMAS**[3] **on the subcutaneous plane.**
- Releasing the SMAS flap from the muscle fascia allows the skin over the crease to move with the rest of the flap[3] (Fig. 43-6).

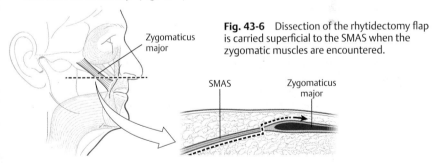

Fig. 43-6   Dissection of the rhytidectomy flap is carried superficial to the SMAS when the zygomatic muscles are encountered.

> **NOTE:**   When releasing the SMAS from the zygomaticus major muscle, transient orbicularis weakness should be expected, despite careful dissection, because of neurapraxia of the zygomatic branch of the facial nerve.

- An offshoot of the zygomatic branch of the facial nerve often crosses *over* the upper third of the belly of the zygomatic major muscle, then passes to the deep surface of the orbicularis oculi to provide innervations.[25] Thus **this branch is vulnerable to injury when the SMAS is separated from the zygomatic muscle.**

- SMAS, after release, can be manipulated and fixed in various combinations to provide an adequate vector and anchoring to efface the nasolabial fold.[2,15]
- The longevity of the improvement of the nasolabial fold using the surgical release method is clearly established.[2,15]

PRIMARY EXCISION (Fig. 43-7)

- This is the most direct method in eliminating the nasolabial fold and usually a **last resort.**
- In selected patients with overhanging nasolabial folds uncorrected or inappropriately corrected by procedures discussed previously, or combinations, can be managed by direct excision.
- The amount of redundancy should be substantial to justify the direct approach.
- Direct liposuction or excision of the deep fat through the facelift approach has failed and inadequately corrected persistent deformities.
- Methods of excision vary, but the scar must be placed for imperceptible healing.
- One approach is to reshape and reposition the ptotic cheek mass to smooth (not obliterate) the nasolabial fold during skin excision.[26]

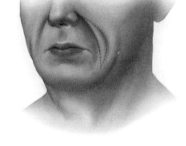

Fig. 43-7   If the nasolabial folds are very deep, particularly if there is an overlap of redundant skin, direct excision of the nasolabial folds should be considered.

- This approach is best performed in **men with sun-damaged skin**[27] and is highly effective, and in selected cases, it is better than any other method described.

ALTERNATIVE, NOVEL, AND OTHER APPROACHES

- Methods to correct the fold—at least noninvasive ones—will continue to evolve.
- Pessa[28] reported improvement of the medial nasolabial fold by selectively resecting the levator alae facial muscle, which was the first reported technique of modifying facial muscles to smooth the fold.
- Direct subcutaneous tissue that "forms the nasolabial fold" can be removed.[29]
- Noninvasive technologies, involving application of variable degrees of external thermal energy, exist and will continue to be explored and used as combination therapy with other types of treatments. Although these technologies may seem promising, most patient-reported and physician-reported improvement should be assessed appropriately.

POSTOPERATIVE CARE AND TREATMENT

- Injections with hyaluronic acids only need temporary topical treatment such as application of ice.
- Patients who tend to bruise could benefit from oral supplements of *Arnica,* although other major procedures may be more suitable.
- Local pain should be anticipated, and is generally treatable by NSAIDS or acetaminophen.
- Surgical procedures with incisions will require more postoperative vigilance than those using injectables.
- Patient follow-up is crucial to assess longevity of the result and appraise it honestly.

SURGICAL COMPLICATIONS AND TREATMENT

- Fillers causing visible and prominent asymmetry, when compared to the contralateral side, require early, in-office treatment with hyaluronidase injection, which is very effective and must be used very carefully. Zealous overinjection needs to be addressed with this treatment.
- Minor asymmetry is expected; therefore asymmetry noted preoperatively should be documented.
- Infections are unlikely but need to be addressed with antibiotic therapy urgently to prevent cellulitis.
- Venous drainage of the central nasofacial triangle is toward the cavernous sinus, and a very rare complication of **cavernous sinus thrombosis** can occur, which requires high vigilance of diagnosis and treatment.
- Minor asymmetry can be corrected within a week after primary injection of fillers.
- Scar improvement after direct excision can be enhanced by silicone tape; however, compliance is poor, and liquid silicone–based products containing an SPF will generally suffice.
- Dermal fat grafting can leave palpable and visible irregularities and firmness that could suggest necrosis, which is uncommon and needs to be addressed several months after the procedure. Aggressive massage and pressure therapy are important early postoperatively. Firmness should be expected early after the procedure.

TOP TAKEAWAYS

- ➤ Various anatomic and histologic studies confirm that the nasolabial fold is a distinct anatomic zone, and not simply a crease or a simple fold.
- ➤ The anatomy of the nasolabial fold continues to be refined.
- ➤ No one treatment, surgical or nonsurgical, completely corrects age-related deepening of the nasolabial fold.
- ➤ Whatever classification is used for managing the fold, one treatment may not be appropriate for all types of fold. A combination of treatments may be necessary and is usually more effective.
- ➤ Treatments may change during the course of a patient's life.
- ➤ When evaluating the various types of injectable materials to improve the nasolabial fold, surgeons should consider that they provide a temporary benefit to a long-term problem, while masking and perhaps distorting normal human anatomy.

REFERENCES

1. Mitz V, Peyronie M. The superficial musculo-aponeurotic system (SMAS) in the parotid and cheek area. Plast Reconstr Surg 58:80, 1976.
2. Barton FE Jr. Rhytidectomy and the nasolabial fold. Plast Reconstr Surg 90:601, 1992.
3. Barton FE Jr. The SMAS and the nasolabial fold. Plast Reconstr Surg 89:1054, 1992.
4. Barton FE Jr, Gyimesi IM. Anatomy of the nasolabial fold. Plast Reconstr Surg 100:1276, 1997.
5. Yousif NJ, Gosain A, Matloub HS, et al. The nasolabial fold: an anatomic and histologic reappraisal. Plast Reconstr Surg 93:60, 1994.
6. Zufferey J. Anatomic variations of the nasolabial fold. Plast Reconstr Surg 89:225; discussion 232, 1992.

7. Tonnard PL, Verpaele AM, Bensimon R. Centrofacial Rejuvenation. New York: Thieme Publishers, 2017.
8. Lightoller GH. Facial muscles: the modiolus and muscles surrounding the rima oris, with some remarks about the panniculus adiposus. J Anat 60:1, 1925.
9. Rohrich RJ, Pessa JE. The fat compartments of the face: anatomy and clinical implications for cosmetic surgery. Plast Reconstr Surg 119:2219, 2007.
10. Rubin LR, Mishriki Y, Lee G. Anatomy of the nasolabial fold: the keystone of the smiling mechanism. Plast Reconstr Surg 83:1, 1989.
11. Pensler JM, Ward JW, Parry SW. The superficial musculoaponeurotic system in the upper lip: an anatomic study in cadavers. Plast Reconstr Surg 75:488, 1985.
12. Pessa JE, Brown F. Independent effect of various facial mimetic muscles on the nasolabial fold. Aesthetic Plast Surg 16:167, 1992.
13. Jackson IT. Anatomy of the nasolabial fold: the keystone of the smiling mechanism [discussion]. Plast Reconstr Surg 83:9, 1989.
14. Rubin LR. The anatomy of the nasolabial fold: the keystone of the smiling mechanism. Plast Reconstr Surg 103:687; discussion 692, 1999.
15. Mendelson BC. Correction of the nasolabial fold: extended SMAS dissection with periosteal fixation. Plast Reconstr Surg 89:822, 1992.
16. Yousif NJ, Gosain A, Sanger JR, et al. The nasolabial fold: a photogrammetric analysis. Plast Reconstr Surg 93:70, 1994.
17. Zufferey JA. The nasolabial fold: an attempt at synthesis. Plast Reconstr Surg 104:2318, 1999.
18. Nahai F. Clinical decision-making for nonsurgical cosmetic treatments. In Nahai F, ed. The Art of Aesthetic Surgery: Principles & Techniques. New York: Thieme Publishers, 2005.
19. Lupo MP, Smith SR, Thomas JA, et al. Effectiveness of Juvéderm Ultra Plus dermal filler in the treatment of severe nasolabial folds. Plast Reconstr Surg 121:289, 2008.
20. Cohen SR, Berner CF, Busso M, et al. Five-year safety and efficacy of a novel polymethylmethacrylate aesthetic soft tissue filler for the correction of nasolabial folds. Dermatol Surg 33(Suppl 2):S222, 2007.
21. Rohrich RJ, Ghavami A, Constantine FC, et al. Lift-and-fill face lift: integrating the fat compartments. Plast Reconstr Surg 133:756e, 2014.
22. Marten TJ, Elyassnia D. Fat grafting in facial rejuvenation. Clin Plast Surg 42:219, 2015.
23. Guyuron B, Michelow B. The nasolabial fold: a challenge, a solution. Plast Reconstr Surg 93:522, 1994.
24. Millard DR, Mullin WR, Hunsaker RH. Evaluation of a technique designed to correct nasolabial folds. Plast Reconstr Surg 89:356, 1992.
25. Freilinger G, Gruber H, Happak W, et al. Surgical anatomy of the mimetic muscle system and the facial nerve: importance for reconstructive and aesthetic surgery. Plast Reconstr Surg 80:686, 1987.
26. Sen C, Cek DI, Reis M. Direct skin excision fat reshaping and repositioning for correction of prominent nasolabial fold. Aesthetic Plast Surg 28:307, 2004.
27. Rudkin G, Miller TA. Aging nasolabial fold and treatment by direct excision. Plast Reconstr Surg 104:1502, 1999.
28. Pessa JE. Improving the acute nasolabial angle and medial nasolabial fold by levator alae muscle resection. Ann Plast Surg 29:23, 1992.
29. Arrunategui C. Observations on a new concept for correction of the nasolabial fold in rhytidectomy. Aesthetic Plast Surg 24:97, 2000.

44. Necklift

Sumeet Sorel Teotia, Foad Nahai

VISUAL CRITERIA FOR A YOUTHFUL NECK[1] (Fig. 44-1)

- A distinct inferior mandibular border
- A visible subhyoid depression
- A visible thyroid cartilage bulge
- A visible anterior border of the sternocleidomastoid muscle
- A cervicomental angle of 105-120 degrees

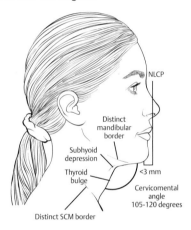

Fig. 44-1 Visual criteria for a youthful neck. (*NLCP*, Nose-lip-chin plane; *SCM*, sternocleidomastoid.)

> **SENIOR AUTHOR TIP:** Neck recontouring is an integral part of necklifting and often is all that is required.

- Thus, a corollary to a youthful neck comprises the visual criteria for an aging neck.

VISUAL CRITERIA FOR AN AGING NECK[2]

- An obtuse cervicomental angle, caused by:
  - Loose, excess skin
  - Excess subplatysmal fat
  - Excess preplatysmal fat
  - Low position of hyoid bone
- Cervical spinal compression changes related to age
- An aging chin
- An aging lower face
- Effacement of a sharp mandibular border

> **SENIOR AUTHOR TIP:**   In addition to thinking of the neck as youthful or aged, we must also consider its shape or contour. Some patients have a full neck with little contour despite normal skin elasticity with no excess skin. These are ideal candidates for recontouring only, with no skin alterations.

PREOPERATIVE EVALUATION[3]

Evaluating individual components of an aging neck guides toward an appropriate surgical algorithm.

SKIN

- **Skin quality,** with rhytids at rest and during animation, is evaluated in detail.

> **SENIOR AUTHOR TIP:**   I also look for the deep or etched transverse neck lines.

- **Apparent excess skin**
  - Redrapes after recontouring with no excision of skin usually necessary
  - Requires adequate elasticity to redrape
  - Local fat removal and platysmal plication often adequate
- **Real excess skin**
  - Extends below the thyroid cartilage
  - Extends posteriorly beyond sternocleidomastoid muscle
  - Excision of skin is necessary.
  - A retroauricular skin incision is necessary.
  - A submental skin incision is usually necessary.
- Evaluating skin excess helps to determine the final direction of skin flap redraping.
- Hairline distortions can be prevented by adequate skin evaluation.
- **Skin quality is inversely related to the length of the incision required.**

> **TIP:**   Adequate skin elasticity is essential for short-scar procedures. Skin damage and actinic changes require a full-length retroauricular incision because of the increased need to redrape.

FAT

- The difference between **subcutaneous (preplatysmal)** and **deep (subplatysmal)** fat is evaluated. (Fig. 44-2)
  - **Submental** fat can be pinched in the submental area at **rest.**
  - **Preplatysmal** and **subplatysmal** fat can be discerned by pinching the submental area during **contraction.**

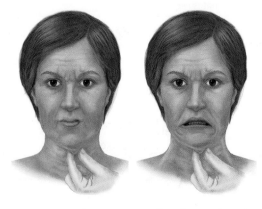

Fig. 44-2   Subcutaneous and deep fat is evaluated.

- If fat within the pinch diminishes on contraction of muscle, then significant fat lies deep to the muscle, and an **open approach** to the neck is needed.
- Fat removal has the most dramatic contouring effect.

PLATYSMA[4]

- **Static (passive)** or **dynamic (active)** platysmal banding is evaluated.

- Imperfections in the neck and jaw shadows are noted.
- Skin excess often accompanies platysmal banding.
- The neck and face interface is assessed, because platysma decussates above the youthful jawline.
- The location, direction, and distance between platsymal bands are noted.
- **Pathogenesis of platysmal banding** is controversial.[5-7]
  - A contracted platysma creates a hammock between the jawline and clavicle.
  - The contraction of muscle fibers creates a bow-string effect away from the tubular neck.
  - The bow-string effect is countered by superficial cervical fascia.
  - Age-related changes to the fascia allow contents of platysma (fat and other structures) to "bulge," creating bands (Fig. 44-3).

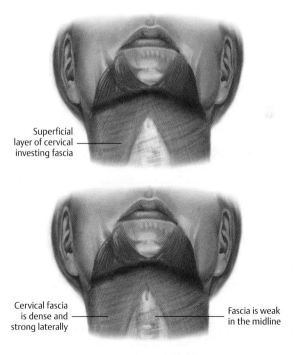

Superficial layer of cervical investing fascia

Cervical fascia is dense and strong laterally

Fascia is weak in the midline

Fig. 44-3   Platysmal banding.

Digastric Muscles[8]

- In a fatty neck, digastric muscles are not easily evaluated.
- In a thin neck, they can bulge below the inferior border of the mandible, creating a subtle but important irregular contour.
- A persistent bulge after submental fat excision can be caused by prominence of the digastric muscles.
- The status of digastric muscles is best evaluated intraoperatively, after removal of subcutaneous fat.

Submandibular Gland[9]

- Prominence of the gland below the mandibular rim within the submandibular triangle is evaluated.
- In a fatty neck, this is often not possible.
- Intraoperative evaluation is necessary in most cases.
- Flexing a patient's neck may help to accentuate a locally bulging deformity from the gland.

Mandibulocutaneous Ligament

- Jowls may result from tethering of the relaxing facial tissues at this ligament.
- The volume of jowling is evaluated with the patient in a supine position.
- Lower facial aging transmits its effects on the upper neck, and mandibular angle effacement is important to note posteriorly, along with inferior displacement of jowls.

Chin

- The chin should be evaluated in reference to facial proportions.
- Occlusion and the angle classification are noted.
- Demineralization of the lower jaw and teeth from age or pathological causes can influence the chin and overlying soft tissues, creating a shortened submental space and influencing anterior neck contour.
- Hypogenia or microgenia affects the ideal neck contour.
- An alloplastic chin implant or an osseous genioplasty may complement anterior neck contour.

SENIOR AUTHOR TIP: Look for the submental crease and assess chin ptosis (witch's chin).

INFORMED CONSENT

Before initiating treatment, the goals, inherent risks, and benefits of a particular treatment are discussed with the patient. An intervention is chosen only after an honest conversation with the patient to define goals and expectations that can readily and safely be met. A thorough knowledge of anatomy of the neck will help to prevent complications (see Chapter 30).

OPTIONS FOR NECK REJUVENATION

Developing an algorithm based on anatomy and clinical evaluation will help to improve neck contour. A logical, "layered" approach can help to plan steps in an operation and address each component of the neck.

- **Superficial tissues**
  - Skin
  - Subcutaneous fat
- **Intermediate tissues:** Platysmal muscle and banding
- **Deeper tissues**
  - Anterior belly of digastric muscles
  - Submandibular gland
  - Suprahyoid fascia
  - Subplatysmal fat pad

NONSURGICAL OPTIONS FOR NECK REJUVENATION

The role for injectable materials such as hyaluronic acid fillers and fat injections is not defined, particularly in primary neck rejuvenation. It may be reserved for secondary corrections.

> **SENIOR AUTHOR TIP:** Currently, injectables have a limited role as do nonsurgical skin-tightening technologies.

BOTULINUM TOXIN

- Use of **botulinum toxin** has been suggested.[10-12]
- May delay eventual surgical procedure
- May be useful supplement to surgery and for postsurgical defects of persistent banding
- Platysmal bands are injected with botulinum toxin.
- Technique involves grasping bands and distracting them away from the neck.
- Usual starting dose is 10-30 units in women, 10-40 units in men and women receive 2-12 injections per band and men receive 3-12 injections.
- A total of approximately 40-100 units is used (Botox).

> **SENIOR AUTHOR TIP:** The relatively large number of units required makes treatment with toxins very expensive, especially in the long term.

- **Best results in younger patients with active (rather than passive) bands**
- Not to be used where significant excess skin is present
- Not to be used in older patients with passive platysmal banding
- Requires firm, toned skin and youthful subcutaneous tissue
- Complications include dysphagia (rare).

ULTRASOUND SYSTEM

- A **microfocused ultrasound system** (Ulthera System, Merz) for improved skin laxity and tightening of the lower face has been reported[13]:
- Employs microfocused ultrasound to cause discrete focal heating of the dermis
- Stimulates neocollagenesis and elastin remodeling
- Largest clinical study to evaluate effectiveness of the technology
  - At day 90, improvements reported by two thirds of patients and nearly 60% of blinded reviews
  - Better outcomes in patients with BMI <30
  - Local anesthesia/sedation suggested, because patients report pain
- Technology requires judicial use in highly selected patients.

MEDICATION

In April 2015, the FDA approved an injectable drug (Kybella, Allergan) for treatment of submental fullness (also known as a *double chin*):

- **Deoxycholic acid,** given as an injection
- A naturally occurring molecule in the body that aids in breakdown and absorption of dietary fat
- Indicated for improving the appearance of moderate to severe convexity or fullness associated with submental fat in adults

CAUTION: Kybella should not be injected in patients with dysphagia; into or in close proximity to the marginal mandibular branch of the facial nerve; or close to the salivary glands, lymph nodes, or muscles.

- Causes injection site hematoma/bruising in most people (72% in clinical trials)
- The formulation is nonhuman and nonanimal.
- Causes destruction of fat cells when injected and cannot accumulate afterward
- Currently the first and only nonsurgical treatment approved by FDA for submental fullness
- Sold in Canada under the name Belkyra
- **Technique**
  - Injections are 2 mg/cm^2 per dose.
  - A single treatment consists of up to a maximum of 50 injections.
  - Each injection is 0.2 ml (up to a total of 10 ml), spaced 1 cm apart.
  - Up to six single treatments may be performed ≥1 month apart.
  - In clinical trials, 68% responded to improvement with Kybella compared with placebo, based on validated physician and patient measurements.

SURGICAL OPTIONS FOR NECK REJUVENATION

Several isolated and combination procedures are available, and each is best suited according to anatomy and clinical presentation.

LIPOSUCTION[14-20]

- **Indications**
  - Best for isolated, younger patients (generally 20-30 years of age)
  - Normal skin and subcutaneous quality with good tone
  - Localized excess submental subcutaneous fat
  - Not indicated for patients with subplastysmal fat (too deep for liposuction)
  - Skin and subcutaneous pinch test is best assessment for selecting candidates.
  - Should be no platysmal bands present at rest
  - Isolated method, and can improve a short, fatty neck
  - Can be combined with an open neck technique to ease subsequent surgical dissection
- **Technique**
  - General anesthesia is suggested, although local may be acceptable with caution.
  - Patient must be supine, with neck extended.
  - Incisions are in submental neck and/or (usually) behind earlobes.
  - Lidocaine with epinephrine should be added to the wetting solution.
  - A 2-3 mm single-hole cannula is adequate for suction-assisted liposuction (SAL).

- If ultrasonic suction (UAL) is used, a 2-3 mm solid probe set at 50% energy for no longer than 2-3 minutes is needed.
- UAL may be easier in thick, young, obtuse fatty neck.
- No drains are required if this is the only procedure.
- Jawline and lateral neck should be approached through earlobe incisions.

CAUTION: Stay above the platysma, or the marginal mandibular nerve may be injured by traction.

- **Preventing complications**[3]
  - Use short bursts of suction cannula strokes.
  - Fan out from submental incision (Fig. 44-4).
  - Avoid multiple passes in same direction.
  - Crisscross tunnels from earlobe incisions.
  - Preserving more fat is better than denuding fat.
  - **Do not skeletonize the subcutaneous tissue,** which can cause platysmal banding or visible underlying contour irregularities.
  - **Endpoint:** Use skin-pinch technique and observation of irregularities to ensure soft contour, leaving fat just under skin.
  - Oversuctioning may adhere the skin to underlying platysma, creating unnatural tethering and banding.

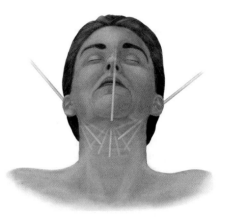

Fig. 44-4   Submental liposuction.

CAUTION: Do not carry the defatting over the mandibular border.

SUBMENTAL ANTERIOR NECKLIFT[17,21-24]

INDICATIONS
- Patients with anterior platysmal bands are good candidates.
- Undermining of the skin is necessary for neck contouring.
- It is performed as an isolated procedure (rare), or in combination with a facial procedure.
- Open neck approach is required in patients with platysmal banding or to access intermediate or deeper tissues.

GENERAL TECHNICAL POINTS
- Patient is placed in supine position, with the neck in extension.
- Local anesthetic infiltration assists in hemostatic dissection.
- Incision is made just **posterior** to the submental crease.

TIP: Avoid deepening the existing submental crease by making an incision on the crease.

- Crease is released anteriorly from underlying tissues.
- Dissection may be carried forward and laterally to release mandibular ligaments.
- Skin is undermined as much as needed to address the platysmal bands and the most inferior horizontal cervical crease.
- Dissection is carried laterally as needed to expose platysma.
- Fat is preserved in thin patients.
- Thick, fatty neck may benefit from cautious, direct defatting of the subcutaneous tissue under direct vision.
- Deeper structures can be addressed with this directed anterior approach.
- Platysmal procedures are performed using this approach.
- Platysmal muscle approximation is closed with nonabsorbable, permanent sutures (such as Mersilene or Prolene).

SPECIFIC TECHNICAL CONSIDERATIONS
- **Subplatysmal/interplatysmal fat excision**[25,26]
  - In an obtuse, fatty neck, some fat is always present beneath the platysma.
  - The fat lies in the midline and extends toward the submandibular gland.
  - The medial border of the platysma is elevated, and fat is excised between and deep to the platysma.
  - **Preserving an adequate subcutaneous layer of fat** is essential to prevent **submental depression.**
  - If a lymph node is present, it is included in the specimen.
  - The platysma is reapproximated at this level to prevent dehiscence from an insecured closure.
- **Digastric muscle excision**[8] (Fig. 44-5)
  - This should be considered a rare procedure.
  - After subplatysmal fat excision, the muscles are exposed through a submental incision.
  - The anterior belly of the digastric is tangentially excised, totally excised, or plicated in the midline.
  - A tangential excision is more common and starts anteriorly at the muscle origin.

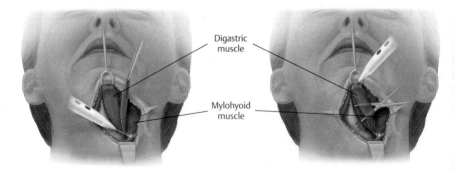

Fig. 44-5   Digastric muscle excision.

- **Submandibular gland**[9,27-28]
  - An enlarged submandibular gland is visualized after excision/retraction of the anterior digastrics.
  - The neck is flexed to assess the contour before the gland is removed.
  - Despite ptosis of the gland on preoperative assessment, addressing it surgically is uncommon.
  - Various methods have been described: Partial resection, suture suspension to mandibular border, and transcervical suspension.
  - Excision involves grasping with an Allis clamp and excising in piecemeal fashion with needletip cautery.
  - A drain should be placed if the gland is excised.
  - A rare **salivary gland fistula** may result, along with nerve injury.

ENDOSCOPIC NECKLIFT[29]

- This procedure is more of a historical interest, because visualization is improved using a lighted retractor, an appropriate retraction, and a small submental incision.
- Involves a 3-4 cm submental incision and 1 cm retroauricular incisions with the aid of fiberoptic visualization.
- No skin excision is performed with this technique.

SHORT-SCAR FACELIFT AND NECKLIFT[30] (Fig. 44-6)

- **Indications**
  - Ideally, patients with no excess neck skin
  - Presence of jowling
  - An aged neck-face interface
- **Technical points**
  - A vertical vector on the SMAS and slight diagonal vector on the skin will improve the jawline/upper neck.
  - The neck can be contoured using liposuction or through submental direct incision.
  - If the neck is opened, then the planes of face and neck dissection are connected in the subcutaneous plane.
  - Facial portion of the procedure is done through a prehairline incision below the sideburn and a preauricular retrotragal incision ending at the earlobe.
  - A skin flap is subcutaneously developed and extended to the posterior border of the sternocleidomastoid muscle.
  - A sub-SMAS dissection is performed at the junction of adherent and mobile SMAS to join a diagonal SMAS incision at the zygomatic prominence.
  - An SMAS-platysma flap is then dissected and pulled vertically in the face and posteriorly in the neck.
  - Alternative approaches, such as SMASectomy and SMAS plications, can be performed through this limited incision.
  - Permanent suture material (Mersilene) is used to plicate or fix the SMAS-platysmal flap.
  - Facial skin is directly pulled upward with a diagonal vector posteriorly.
  - Excess skin is trimmed, tailored, and inset.

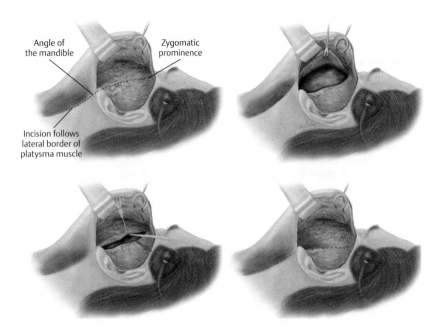

Fig. 44-6   Short-scar facelift and necklift.

FULL-SCAR FACELIFT AND NECKLIFT
- **Indications**
  - Aging changes of face and neck
  - Poorly defined neck-face interface
  - Inelastic and excess skin of face
  - Poor and excess skin of neck
  - Visible static platysmal bands down to inferior cervical neck crease below the thyroid
  - Visible submandibular gland
- **Technical points**
  - In unusually lax skin with significant excess in the lower neck, the **retroauricular incision** is continued **along the hairline** to prevent notching the occipital hairline and to remove more excess skin (Fig. 44-7).
  - Essentially, the concept of skin excess excision follows that of removal of a dog-ear along anatomic boundaries.
  - The key aspect is to **first align hairline,** then to remove skin.
  - The retroauricular sulcus is closed with a **three-point suture technique,** incorporating deep fascia to prevent scar migration.
  - The facelift approach is individualized and discussed in Chapter 40.
  - Platysma is treated according to anatomic findings.

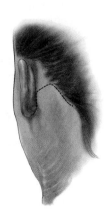

Fig. 44-7   Occipital hairline incision.

SKIN FLAP PROCEDURES[3]

- A **vertical vector** of pull is required for a youthful, harmonious necklift procedure.
- A **posterior and diagonal vector** is required when using the **retroauricular approach.**
- Managing the neck skin is different from managing the facial skin.

> **TIP:**   Avoid excising the skin before considering redraping and redistribution.

- If skin excision is necessary, then a retroauricular or hairline incision should be considered, according to amount requiring removal.
- **"Turkey-gobbler" neck deformity**[31]
  - In patients with severe and massive anterior neck redundancy, skin can be excised using a direct approach.
  - A **T-Z incision** can restore a youthful contour to the cervical angle.[32]
  - The initial procedure was done through a midcervical skin excision through which preplatysmal and subplatysmal fat was excised.[31]
  - Platysma is closed in the midline.
  - In men, persistent scarring in the neck is only occasionally acceptable in those who present with a very generous skin redundancy.[33]
  - This option is popular for patients who have had **massive weight loss.**
- Despite adequate analysis and treatment of excess skin, a **two-stage neck procedure** may rarely be necessary, and this should be discussed with patients.

PLATYSMAL PROCEDURES

The platysma can be **imbricated, plicated, incised, lengthened, or suspended.**[*] Once platysmal diastasis is addressed with any of the procedures discussed previously, either alone or in combination, the surrounding skin is recruited in the midline. This medial tightening leaves skin tethered laterally to the attachments of the lateral platysmal fascia, which is generally stronger. The skin is then allowed to contract or is excised laterally through a facelift approach. Specific methods for treating the platysma have been described.[21,35-39]

PLATYSMAL FLAP CERVICAL RHYTIDOPLASTY[7]

- Sectional myotomy of the medial edge of the platysma allows lateral rotation and advancement of the flap edges.
- Suturing the flaps to the mastoid fascia laterally prevents recurrence of the vertical banding.

> **TIP:**   When performing a myotomy, consider the ability of the thyroid cartilage to masculinize the neck. Some describe controlling the effect by performing the platysmal transection above or below the cartilage to camouflage or accentuate it.

---

*References 5, 6, 8, 20, 22, 34.

SUSPENSION SUTURES[40-42] (Fig. 44-8)

- Suspension sutures running along the inferior border of the mandible over the superficial fascia on the platysma can help to better define the jawline.
- Sutures are interlocked at the midline and tacked to the mastoid fascia.

PLATYSMAL MUSCLE SLING[8] (Fig. 44-9)

- A sling is made by dividing the platysma horizontally across the entire width.

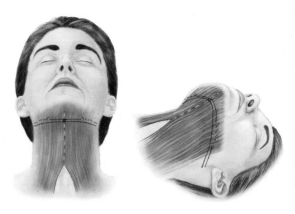

Fig. 44-8   Suspension sutures, interlocked at midline, run along the inferior mandibular border.

- A **potentially visible** wide gap is created, decreasing the popularity of the procedure.
- Muscle tissue bunches on the cephalad portion of the platysma, creating a phenomenon known as the **window-shading effect.**

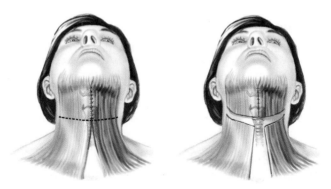

Fig. 44-9   Full transection of the platysma creates a wide gap and window-shading effect.

CORSET PLATYSMAPLASTY[38,39] (Fig. 44-10)

- An anterior open approach to the neck is required through a submental incision.
- The neck skin is elevated and medial edges of the platysma infolded using a permanent suture.
- The neck skin is shifted posteriorly, but the platysmal pull is forward and toward the midline anteriorly.
- The anterior pull of the platysma is a key element that is called **corset platysmaplasty.**
- No muscle is resected.
- The redundant neck skin can be allowed to contract, or it can be excised laterally.
- Occasionally, a very low 3-4 cm transection from the medial edge allows comfortable rotation of the muscle flaps to the midline for multilayered approximation.

- A multilayered seam approximates the full height of the midline platysma muscle edges, creating a "waistline" to the neck from an anterior plastysmal shift.
- Plication of the muscle medially continues to 3 fingerbreadths above the suprasternal notch.
- Crisscrossing and backtracking are advocated to maintain a straight seam.
- A nonabsorbable suture is used for plication (Mersiline or Prolene).
- This is a highly effective and popular technique for recontouring the submental area.
- If combined with lateral plication, midline plication of the platysma can define the jawline and neck-jaw transition beautifully. This is done with an occasional second row of running vertical oblique sutures.
- Additional submandibular suturing may be done to treat residual bulging in the area by creating a strong, flat pleat.

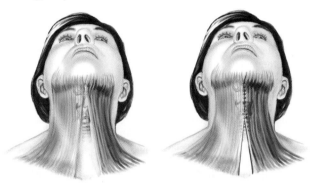

Fig. 44-10   Coaptation of decussated platysmal fibers in the midline creates a corset-type effect.

POSTOPERATIVE CARE[43]

- Analgesia control is routine, supplemented with sleeping pills, antiemetics, and instructions for their use.
- Patients are instructed not to use pillows that flex the neck to keep the cervicomental angle open (confirmed by an observer).
- The neck skin flaps should not be folded, which can contribute to edema by obstructing the neck lymphatics.
- Drains are used to eliminate serum and a small amount of blood, potentially reducing postoperative edema.
- Management of blood pressure is essential in preventing hematoma.
- Drains are removed as necessary on postoperative day 1 after the patient examination.
- Without applying pressure, cotton dressings or foam tape and an elastic garment are applied and left in place overnight to absorb oozing fluids.
- Operative dressings are removed on postoperative day 1 and replaced with a neck strap for ≤4 weeks.

NOTE: Some surgeons do not place dressings on the neck to prevent pressure necrosis.

- Patients are instructed to maintain an open neck angle, e.g., as when leaning forward while sitting, with the elbows on the knees, and looking straight ahead.
- Wounds are cleaned with half-strength hydrogen peroxide and coated with a topical antibiotic as needed.
- All nonabsorbable skin sutures are removed by day 7.
- Strenuous activity is restricted until week 6.
- Instructions for facelift recovery are similar to those for necklift recovery.

COMPLICATIONS AND SUBOPTIMAL RESULTS

- Postoperative problem areas result from **inappropriate patient evaluation** and **inappropriate choice of surgical procedure.**
- Any tissue level can result in an unpleasing appearance, including:
  - **Skin problems**
    - ▶ Contour irregularities and indentations related to overzealous treatment by suction or defatting subcutaneously, especially in the thin neck.
    - ▶ There is a tendency toward excessive removal of subcutaneous fat and deep subplatysmal fat.
    - ▶ Suboptimal contouring can result in suboptimal treatment of deeper structures such as subplatysmal fat, digastric muscle, and submandibular gland.
    - ▶ Most problems are caused by inadequate redraping of the skin because of insufficient undermining or poor skin quality.
    - ▶ Failure to correct jowls, the jawline, and the neck-face interface often is caused by undercorrection.
    - ▶ Revision with a facelift is often required.
    - ▶ Skin necrosis is more common if significant tension remains laterally at the retroauricular sulcus.
    - ▶ Skin slough is usually preceded by hematoma or infection, most commonly in the retroauricular area.
  - **Fat interface problems**
    - ▶ Usually from overexcision or underexcision
    - ▶ Overexcision is generally subcutaneous.
      - ◆ Can be prevented by using small cannulas, limiting passes of suction, and uniformly preserving 3-5 mm of subcutaneous fat
    - ▶ Underremoval of fat is often seen deep to the platysma and adjacent to submental incisions.
  - **Platysma**
    - ▶ Persistence of banding from failure of sutures or postoperative dehiscence is most common.
    - ▶ Absorbable sutures should generally **not** be used for plication.
    - ▶ Correction is often needed and requires opening the neck to replicate or resect as indicated.
    - ▶ Occasional use of botulinum toxin (discussed previously) should be specifically directed.
  - **Submandibular gland**
    - ▶ Postoperative bulging in the submental triangle is often from an enlarged gland.
    - ▶ This was usually present preoperatively and was not surgically addressed.
    - ▶ Correction entails opening the neck again and addressing the gland.

- **Digastric muscles**
  - ▶ The digastric muscle may be unmasked after removal of subcutaneous fat.
  - ▶ It is often seen as a persistent bulge along the submental area.
  - ▶ Correction is excision of the muscle belly through a repeat incision.
- **Inappropriate vectors**
  - ▶ Poor vector planning, especially in redundant skin with massive neck skin excess, can result in poor retroauricular or anterior tragal scars.
  - ▶ Excessive traction in any vector can lead to banding, bulging, or a hammock effect.
  - ▶ Correction requires reopening the neck with repositioning of the vectors.

TOP TAKEAWAYS
- ➤ The neck is a continuum of the face, adding a level of beauty while providing an important life function.
- ➤ Evaluating skin excess helps to determine the final direction of skin flap redraping.
- ➤ Adequate skin elasticity is essential for short-scar procedures.
- ➤ Kybella should not be injected in patients with dysphagia; into or in close proximity to the marginal mandibular branch of the facial nerve; or close to the salivary glands, lymph nodes, or muscles.
- ➤ **Stay above the platysma,** or the **marginal mandibular nerve** may be injured by traction.
- ➤ Postoperative problem areas result from **inappropriate patient evaluation** and **inappropriate choice of surgical procedure.**

REFERENCES
1. Ellenbogen R, Karlin JV. Visual criteria for success in restoring the youthful neck. Plast Reconstr Surg 66:826, 1980.
2. Vistnes AM, Souther SG. The anatomical basis for common cosmetic anterior neck deformities. Ann Plast Surg 2:381, 1979.
3. Nahai F, ed. The Art of Aesthetic Surgery: Principles & Techniques. New York: Thieme Publishers, 2010.
4. Cardoso de Castro C. The anatomy of the platysma. Plast Reconstr Surg 66:680, 1980.
5. Aston SJ. Platysma muscle in rhytidoplasty. Ann Plast Surg 3:532, 1979.
6. Guerrerosantos J. The role of platysma muscle in rhytidoplasty. Clin Plast Surg 5:29, 1979.
7. Guerrerosantos J. Neck lift. Simplified surgical techniques, refinements, and clinical classification. Clin Plast Surg 10:379, 1983.
8. Connell BF, Shamoun JM. The significance of digastric muscle contouring for rejuvenation of the submental area of the face. Plast Reconstr Surg 99:1586, 1997.
9. Singer DP, Sullivan PK. Submandibular gland I: an anatomic evaluation and surgical approach to submandibular gland resection for facial rejuvenation. Plast Reconstr Surg 112:1150; discussion 1155, 2003.
10. Brandt FS, Bellman B. Cosmetic use of botulinum A exotoxin for the aging neck. Dermatol Surg 24:1232, 1998.
11. Kane MA. Nonsurgical treatment of platysmal bands with injection of botulinum toxin A. Plast Reconstr Surg 103:656, 1999.
12. Matarasso A, Matarasso SL, Brandt FS. Botulinum A exotoxin for the management of platysmal bands. Plast Reconstr Surg 103:643, 1999.

13. Oni G, Hoxworth R, Teotia S, et al. Evaluation of a microfocused ultrasound system for improving skin laxity and tightening in the lower face. Aesthet Surg J 34:1099, 2014.

14. Jones BM, Grover R. Reducing complications in cervicofacial rhytidectomy by tumescent infiltration: a comparative trial evaluating 678 consecutive face lifts. Plast Reconstr Surg 113:398, 2004.

15. Courtiss EH. Suction lipectomy of the neck. Plast Reconstr Surg 76:882, 1985.

16. Tapia A, Ferreira B, Eng R. Liposuction in cervical rejuvenation. Aesthetic Plast Surg 11:95, 1987.

17. Zins JE, Fardo D. The "anterior only" approach to neck rejuvenation: an alternative to facelift surgery. Plast Reconstr Surg 1155:1761, 2005.

18. Gryskiewicz JM. Submental suction-assisted lipectomy without platysmaplasty: pushing the (skin) envelope to avoid a facelift for unsuitable patients. Plast Reconstr Surg 112:1393, 2003.

19. Mladick RA. Neck rejuvenation without facelift. Aesthet Surg J 25:285, 2005.

20. Knize DM. Limited incision submental lipectomy and platysmaplasty. Plast Reconstr Surg 101:473, 1998.

21. Connell BF. Cervical lifts: the value of platysmal muscle flaps. Ann Plast Surg 1:34, 1978.

22. Connell BF. Contouring the neck in rhytidectomy by lipectomy and a muscle sling. Plast Reconstr Surg 61:376, 1978.

23. Hamilton JM. Submental lipectomy with skin excision. Plast Reconstr Surg 92:443, 1993.

24. Gradinger GP. Anterior lipectomy with skin excision. Plast Reconstr Surg 106:1146, 2000.

25. Millard DR, Pigott RW, Hedo A. Submandibular lipectomy. Plast Reconstr Surg 41:513, 1968.

26. Robbins LB, Shaw KE. En bloc cervical lipectomy for treatment of the problem neck in facial rejuvenation. Plast Reconstr Surg 83:53, 1989.

27. Sullivan PK, Freeman MB, Schmidt S, et al. Contouring the aging neck with submandibular gland suspension. Aesthet Surg J 26:465, 2006.

28. Guyuron B, Jackowe D, Lamphongsai S. Basket submandibular gland suspension. Plast Reconstr Surg 122:938, 2008.

29. Eaves FE, Nahai F, Bostwick J. The endoscopic neck lift. Op Tech Plast Reconstr Surg 2:145, 1995.

30. Baker DC. Lateral SMASectomy. Plast Reconstr Surg 100:509, 1997.

31. Adamson JE, Horton CE, Crawford HH. The surgical correction of the "turkey gobbler" deformity. Plast Reconstr Surg 34:598, 1964.

32. Cronin TD, Biggs TM. The T-Z plasty for the male "turkey gobbler" neck. Plast Reconstr Surg 47:534, 1971.

33. Biggs TM, Koplin L. Direct alternatives for neck skin redundancy in males. Clin Plast Surg 10:428, 1983.

34. Fuente del Campo A. Midline platysma muscular overlap for neck restoration. Plast Reconstr Surg 102:1710; discussion 1715, 1998.

35. Labbe D, Franco RG, Nicolas J. Platysma suspension and platysmaplasty during neck lift: anatomic study and analysis of 20 cases. Plast Reconstr Surg 117:2001, 2006.

36. Fogli AL. Skin and platysma muscle anchoring. Aesthetic Plast Surg 32:531, 2008.

37. Guerrerosantos J. Managing platysmal bands in the aging neck. Aesthet Surg J 28:211, 2008.

38. Feldman JJ. Corset platysmaplasty. Plast Reconstr Surg 85:333,1990.

39. Feldman JJ. Neck Lift. New York: Thieme Publishers, 2006.

40. Giampapa VC, Bitzos I, Ramirez O, et al. Long-term results of suture suspension platysmaplasty for neck rejuvenation: a 13-year follow-up evaluation. Aesthetic Plast Surg 29:332, 2005.

41. Giampapa VC, Bitzos I, Ramirez O, et al. Suture suspension platysmaplasty for neck rejuvenation revisited: technical fine points for improving outcomes. Aesthetic Plast Surg 29:341, 2005.

42. Giampapa VC, Di Bernardo BE. Neck recontouring with suture suspension and liposuction: an alternative for the early rhytidectomy candidate. Aesthetic Plast Surg 19:214, 1995.

43. Meade RA. Neck lift. In Janis JE, ed. Essentials of Plastic Surgery. New York: Thieme Publishers, 2006.

45. Rhinoplasty

Ashkan Ghavami, Jeffrey E. Janis, Bahman Guyuron

FUNCTIONAL ROLE OF NOSE[1]

- Regulate airflow, humidification, olfaction, filtration
- Nasal airway: 50% of airway resistance
- Nasal cycle
  - Alternating constriction and dilation of nasal mucosa on each nasal side
  - Normal cycle is **4 hours.**
  - Abnormalities can be present from obstruction, allergies, or vasomotor irregularities (i.e., sensitivity to heat-cold changes).

RELEVANT ANATOMY

SKIN (Fig. 45-1)

- **Skin thickness** and **sebaceousness** are often underestimated components in predicting final nasal shape.[2]
- Skin is **thickest** in the **lower third** (tip, alae).
- Skin is **thinner** in the **upper and middle thirds,** with more gliding.
- Understanding the contractile properties of each patient's nasal skin is critical to the outcome.
  - Modifications of the underlying bony and cartilaginous frame (particularly at the paradomal and tip regions) may be obscured by thick, poorly contractile skin.
  - Debulking of skin and soft tissue can be an important maneuver.

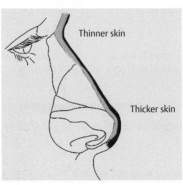

Fig. 45-1   Skin and soft tissue over the radix and tip region is typically thicker and less elastic than over the dorsum.

NASAL MUSCLES (Fig. 45-2)

- **Nasal superficial musculoaponeurotic system (SMAS)**
  - Includes **dilator nasi, transverse muscle fibers**
  - Flares nostrils
- **Levator labii superioris alaeque nasi**
  - Helps external valve to stay open
  - Elevates nostrils
- **Depressor septi nasi muscle**[3,4]
  - An important muscle in dynamic tip ptosis
  - Raises upper lip and pulls nasal tip down
  - Can be transpositioned or transected as part of rhinoplasty[5]
  - Can be chemodenervated for diagnostic or treatment purposes

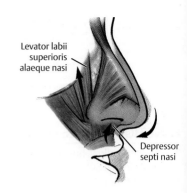

Levator labii superioris alaeque nasi

Depressor septi nasi

Fig. 45-2 The depressor septi nasi muscle and other musculature can affect nasal shape and the tip position.

BLOOD SUPPLY[5] (Fig. 45-3)

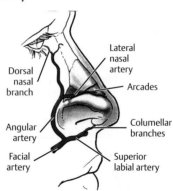

Dorsal nasal branch

Lateral nasal artery

Arcades

Angular artery

Columellar branches

Facial artery

Superior labial artery

Fig. 45-3 The lateral nasal artery is one of the most important vessels in nasal blood supply, and preserving it promotes healing and helps to prevent deleterious postoperative skin changes.

- Most blood supply is located within **subcutaneous plane.**

CAUTION: When debulking nasal soft tissue, do not violate the blood supply to the subdermal plexus.

- **Angular artery**
  - *Lateral nasal branch* arises from this artery 2-3 mm above alar groove.

NOTE: Stay below the alar groove during alar base resection to preserve this vessel.

▸ Supplies the subdermal plexus at nasal tip either unilaterally or bilaterally in 100% of cadaver specimens
• Excessive defatting of skin that violates subdermal plexus can compromise vascularity of tip/columellar skin.

> **TIP:** During secondary rhinoplasty, soft tissue debulking is more difficult because of scar tissue, and previously dissected nasal tip skin may be more prone to vascular compromise during dissection.

■ **Facial artery**
  • Branches: Superior labial artery and angular artery
    ▸ Supply nasal tip via columella
  • Dedicated columellar branch from superior labial artery
■ **Ophthalmic artery**
  • Gives off the following branches: Anterior ethmoidal, dorsal nasal, and external nasal arteries to sidewalls and upper third of nose

INTERNAL NASAL VALVE
■ Narrowest segment of nasal airway
■ Two thirds of airway resistance
■ Angle between caudal upper lateral cartilage (ULC) and septum should be **>10-15 degrees.**
■ Length, stability, and strength of ULC are important.

EXTERNAL NASAL VALVE
■ Dynamic structure: Mobile alar sidewalls and caudal septum
■ Alar arch, along with musculature, allows stenting effect with inspiration.
■ Internal nasal valve narrows while external valve opens during the negative pressure effect of inspiration.
■ Size, shape, strength, and orientation of lower lateral cartilage (LLC) help to determine external valve sufficiency.
■ **External nasal valve insufficiency**[1,6]
  • Flaccid or weak LLC
  • Slitlike nostril rims (vertical/narrow: iatrogenic or inherent)
  • Thin alar sidewalls
  • Malposition of LLC (cephalically oriented)
    ▸ Caudal edge of LLC is an excessive distance from nostril rim, so alar rim support is not provided during inspiration.

> **TIP:** External valve insufficiency is a significant contributor to postrhinoplasty airway complications. Diagnosis of potential external valve insufficiency is required, and preservation of at least a 6 mm rim strip of LLC, along with alar contour grafts and/or lateral crural strut grafts, may be necessary.

Nasal Vaults (Fig. 45-4)

- **Three nasal vaults:** Bony, upper cartilaginous, and lower cartilaginous

Bony Vault

- Paired nasal bones and ascending process of the maxilla
- Proximal third to half of nose
- Ethnic variations in length may exist.

Upper Cartilaginous Vault

- Known also as nasal midvault
- Paired ULCs
  - Underlap nasal bones 6-8 mm (keystone area)
    - ▶ Widest portion of nasal dorsum
  - *Scroll area:* Junction where ULCs underlap LLCs
  - *Internal nasal valve:* At junction of caudal ULC and septum
  - ULCs join the nasal septum at dorsum to form a T.
    - ▶ Affects dorsal aesthetic lines
    - ▶ Spreader grafts are placed at this junction.

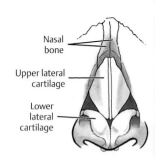

Fig. 45-4   The three nasal vaults are defined by the nasal bones (bony vault), upper lateral cartilage (midvault), and lower lateral cartilage (lower vault).

Labels on figure: Nasal bone; Upper lateral cartilage; Lower lateral cartilage

---

TIP: The "component dorsum reduction" technique helps to preserve the ULC-septal relationship through separation of the ULC from the adjacent mucoperichondrium and septum and incremental dorsal reduction.[7]

Lower Cartilaginous Vault

- Paired lower lateral, middle, and medial crura (cartilages)
- Responsible for nasal tip shape and external valve support

Nasal Tip

- Shape and position are critical in rhinoplasty.
- **Tripod concept:** LLC and medial crura act like legs of a tripod[8,9] (Fig. 45-5).
  - Variations in length and strength of each structure influence tip position and shape.
- Nasal tip supported by several **ligamentous attachments**[9-11] (Fig. 45-6):
  - Piriform ligament: LLC abutment with piriform aperture
  - Domal suspensory ligament

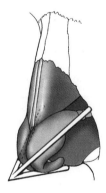

Fig. 45-5   The nasal tip "tripod concept" helps when trying to understand dynamic changes in nasal tip shape and position defined by the central medial crura and bilateral lower lateral cartilages.

- Fibrous attachments between ULC and LLC
- Medial crural ligaments
- Anterior septal angle

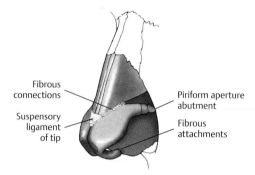

Fig. 45-6 The suspensory ligaments affect tip projection and are weakened in an "open" approach and with aging.

SEPTUM (Fig. 45-7)

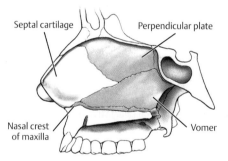

Fig. 45-7 All anatomic parts of the septum must be addressed in nasal airway obstruction, including the nasomaxillary and vomerine spicules that are often seen.

- Septal cartilage, perpendicular plate of ethmoid, and vomer
- Perpendicular plate of ethmoid is continuous with the cribriform plate.
  - Surgical or traumatic fractures of the perpendicular plate can result in **CSF rhinorrhea.**
  - Rhinoplasty fracture technique must be meticulous, gentle, and in a lateral direction to prevent cribriform injury.

INTERNAL NASAL VALVE (Fig. 45-8)

- Formed by junction of caudal ULC and nasal septum
- Normal valve angle is **10-15 degrees.**
- Angles <10 degrees can lead to nasal airway obstruction.
- Internal nasal valve provides **50%** of total airway resistance.
- True **spreader grafts** and **autospreader flaps** function through increasing the internal nasal valve angle.

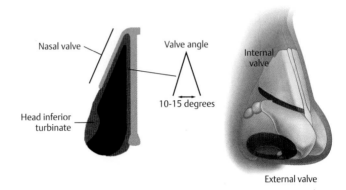

Fig. 45-8   The internal nasal valve is one of the most important aspects in septorhinoplasty and must be maintained open using spreader grafts and/or flaps.

EXTERNAL NASAL VALVE

- Formed by caudal edge of LLC, alar soft tissue, membranous septum, and nostril sill
- Dynamic structure
- Nasal muscles help to keep open during inspiration
- Alar contour grafts and lateral crural (alar) strut grafts can strengthen and reinforce external nasal valve.

TURBINATES

- Superior, middle, and inferior turbinates
- Extensions of lateral nasal cavity wall
- Anterior portion of middle and lateral turbinates project into airway and can affect airway resistance.
- **Inferior turbinate** is capable of up to **two thirds of airway resistance** at internal nasal valve region.

TIP: Often, a simple outfracture (micro or mini) of the inferior turbinate, with or without mucosal resection, is all that is needed to improve nasal airway obstruction caused by turbinate hypertrophy. A complete turbinectomy is rarely indicated and can result in an "open nose" deformity with imbalance in airway resistance.

NASAL OBSTRUCTION[1,6,12-14]

TYPES OF NASAL AIRWAY OBSTRUCTION
- **Allergic rhinitis:** Seasonal or obstruction related to dust, pollen, or other antigens
- **Bilateral obstruction:** Possible severe mucosal disease
- **Constant-fixed obstruction:** May be associated with a fixed abnormality such as septal deviation

NASAL OBSTRUCTION COMPLAINTS
- Nasal crusting
- Dry mouth (from mouth breathing, especially during sleep)
- Frequent sore throats
- Sinus problems

NASAL OBSTRUCTION HISTORY
- Time of onset
- Duration of obstruction
- Precipitating events
- Rhinorrhea (amount, duration)
- Epistaxis
- History of trauma or surgery
- Use of medications, nasal sprays
- Use of alcohol, tobacco, and drugs (especially cocaine)
- History of headaches, visual disturbances, and middle ear symptoms

> **TIP:** A deviated septum or other nasal obstruction can be a trigger for migraine headaches. Ask specifically about migraine headache history. Migraines that are triggered by this mechanism may be significantly improved with nasal obstruction correction.

PHYSICAL EXAMINATION
- Visual clues
  - Allergic shiners: Dark circles under eyes suggesting allergic rhinitis
  - Supraalar pinching or an excessively narrow midvault (inverted-V deformity) may have internal nasal valve insufficiency.
  - Watch midvault motion during nasal respiration.
    - ▶ If dynamic collapse occurs, midvault support will be needed.

> **SENIOR AUTHOR TIP:** Most patients who have breathing problems may not be aware of how else they can breathe, having been breathing through their mouth their entire life. Observation of lips being open and careful examination of the internal nose is crucial to prevent compounding the problems. Evaluation of the septum may reveal deviation, synechia, or perforation.

- **Cottle test**
  - Not specific because many will be positive, but is useful
  - Cottle maneuver: Hold unilateral cheek laterally to stabilize the nasal sidewall on one side while occluding the contralateral airway.
    - ▶ If significant improvement in the ipsilateral airway is noted on deep inhalation, then internal nasal valve narrowing may be present.
- **Alar rims**
  - Evaluate for notching or potential thereof, especially at soft triangle.
  - Dynamic notching may be a reflex of patient against external valve collapse.
  - Evaluate position of LLC ("parenthesis tip").
- **Intranasal examination**
  - Can use thumb to push up nostril rims to observe internal nasal valve angle without artificially stenting the valve open, which can occur with a nasal speculum
  - Use speculum and visualize septum, valve, turbinates with and without a vasoconstrictive agent.
  - Evaluate for polyps, crusting, mucosal color (excessive erythema suggests allergies).
  - In the septum look for spurs, deviation, perforations (postsurgical or from cocaine use).

MEDICAL THERAPIES

- Mucosal disease from common cold (viral rhinitis) most common cause
  - Bacterial rhinitis may complicate viral rhinitis.
  - Acute and chronic *bacterial* infection can be treated with a combination of:
    - ▶ Saline solution nasal irrigation
    - ▶ Short course of decongestant (spray and/or oral)
    - ▶ Nasal steroid spray
    - ▶ Mucolytic therapy
  - Check for concomitant sinus disease, because rhinosinusitis is common, with one aggravating the other.
- Allergic rhinitis
  - Allergen (environmental exposure) avoidance
  - Antihistamines
  - Intranasal steroid regimen
  - Allergy test
    - ▶ *Rhinitis medicamentosa:* Rebound vasodilation and nasal mucosa hypertrophy-hypersecretion
      - ◆ Caused by overuse of nasal decongestants (vasoconstrictive agents) like Neo-Synephrine and Afrin
      - ◆ True cause of nasal congestion must be treated to eliminate need for decongestants.
        - – Allergic rhinitis, nasal polyposis, septal deviation, turbinate hypertrophy
      - ◆ Treatment: Cessation of all decongestants, course of antihistamines, nasal steroids, and possibly an oral steroid taper
- Ozena: Primary atrophic rhinitis
  - Causes: Aggressive submucous septal resection, total turbinectomy
  - Squamous metaplasia of normal columnar mucosal cells
  - Treatment: Irrigation with saline solution, high-dose vitamin A, possible surgical closure of the nostrils

INDICATIONS AND CONTRAINDICATIONS

AESTHETIC

- Initiated by patient
- Proper patient selection is critical.
  - As with any aesthetic procedure, expectations must be realistic and achievable (see Chapter 1).
  - This becomes more of a challenge in secondary rhinoplasty patients (see Chapter 46).
  - **SIMON:** Acronym to describe male rhinoplasty patients
    - ▶ **S**ingle, **i**mmature, **m**ale, **o**bsessive, and **n**arcissistic
    - ▶ Used as a rough guide to remind surgeon of "problem rhinoplasty patients"
  - Good communication must assimilate surgeon's analysis and goals with those of patients.
    - ▶ If surgeon's and patient's goals are vastly different, proceeding with rhinoplasty may be imprudent.
    - ▶ Asking patients to list the top three things they want to have altered may be a good general idea (particularly for patients with nonspecific aesthetic goals and those unsure of their aesthetic goals).
  - Generally, rhinoplasty should address the imbalances between the nose and face.[12,15-17]
    - ▶ Specific desires and complaints should be addressed while pointing out other related deficiencies (when indicated), such as a deficient chin.
    - ▶ For example, a patient may have a wide nasal tip but only wants "the hump gone."
      - ◆ Dynamic relationships must be discussed with patients.
      - ◆ For example, significant hump reduction without elevation of a droopy tip will produce an imbalanced nose that appears flat and excessively droopy.

TIP: Much of the history of rhinoplasty is rooted in ethnic rhinoplasty. Ethnic patients may present a unique challenge. Clinically relevant variations in patient desires, nasofacial morphology, and anatomic nuances should be taken into account in preoperative evaluation and surgical planning.[2,12,15,18-20]

FUNCTIONAL

- This chapter does not focus on functional techniques; however, when performing a rhinoplasty, comprehensively addressing the nasal airway is critical.
- Patients without nasal airway obstruction before rhinoplasty may develop airway problems postoperatively unless preventative measures are taken.
  - For example:
    - ▶ Spreader grafts and flaps can help to reduce internal nasal valve narrowing when dorsal reduction and osteotomies are performed.[12,21]
    - ▶ *External valve dysfunction* can be prevented by placing lateral crural strut and/or alar contour grafts and recognizing alar malposition.

- Septoplasty[1,6,13,14,22]
  - Important to perform simultaneously
  - **Best source** of most grafts used in aesthetic rhinoplasty
  - **L-strut must be left intact with at least 1 cm (preferably up to 2 cm) dorsal and 1 cm caudal** (Fig. 45-9).
  - All bony protrusions and spicules should be excised to open airway effectively.
    - ▶ Most critical location is across from inferior turbinate.
    - ▶ A protuberant nasomaxillary crest is common and should be thoroughly addressed.

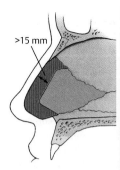

>15 mm

Fig. 45-9   L-strut.

TIP: A large elevator (Boies) or nasal speculum should freely pass, without resistance, into the bilateral nasal airway after septoplasty.

SENIOR AUTHOR TIP: Leaving a dorsal strut of <2 cm may result in sinking of the dorsum and development of a hump that was not present intraoperatively.

One of the most common reasons for unsuccessful straightening of a caudal nose deviation is failure to detect and reposition the dislodged caudal septum in the correct position on the nasal spine and maxillary crest. This requires removal of the redundant overlapping portion of the cartilage to facilitate repositioning the septum in the midline.

PREOPERATIVE EVALUATION[12,16,23,24]

TIP: The key component of a successful rhinoplasty is accurate, detailed, and thorough preoperative analysis. Rhinoplasty has evolved into a more predictable operation because of improvements in preoperative assessment of the nasal imbalances and aesthetic deformities. After proper preoperative analysis, a component-directed surgical plan can be developed to help guide the surgeon during rhinoplasty.

- Preoperative analysis requires an external examination of AP, lateral, and basilar views in addition to an internal airway examination.
- Ethnic variations should be taken into account, because anatomic variations in nasofacial morphology, as well as culture-specific goals, may not always be clear (see Chapter 47).
  - Racial incongruity should be prevented.
    - ▶ A nose that is off balance with the rest of the ethnic facial traits
    - ▶ Skin thickness and degree of sebaceousness are best seen in AP view.

TIP: Thick skin requires more aggressive cartilage frame modifications and conservative soft tissue debulking to reveal the true nasal shape.[2,18-20,23]

ANTEROPOSTERIOR VIEW
Symmetry and Nasal Deviation (Fig. 45-10)

- AP view of face can be divided into fifths to help evaluate proportion (Fig. 45-10, A).
  - Intercanthal width and alar base widths should coincide with measurements of fifths.
- A line can be drawn to bisect the nasal dorsum, upper lip, Cupid's bow, and central incisors to assess magnitude of nasal deviation (Fig. 45-10, B).
- Facial asymmetries are considered.
- Nasal deviation may be caudally located presenting a "twisted" appearance.
- Role of asymmetry in size and shape of nasal and malar bones is evaluated.

Aesthetic Lines and Measurements (Fig. 45-11)

- **Dorsal aesthetic lines** (Fig. 45-11, A)
  - Symmetry, deviation, width, and shape are important.
  - Should be gently diverging curvilinear lines extending from medial eyebrow (superciliary ridge) toward nasal tip–defining points
- **Width of bony base** (Fig. 45-11, B)
  - Should be **75%-80%** of alar base width
  - Asymmetries may exist from different angles of inclination of the nasal bones and ascending process of the maxilla.
  - Commonly, one side is wider (projecting more laterally) than the other.
- **Width of alar base** (Fig. 45-11, C)
  - Should coincide with **intercanthal width** (generally)
  - If wider than intercanthal width, then degree of alar flare will dictate operative plan

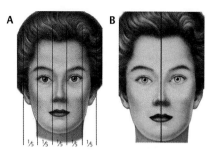

Fig. 45-10 A, Dividing the face into vertical fifths can help to guide overall nasal proportion in facial width. **B,** A vertical line drawn down the dorsum tip, Cupid's bow, and chin can help to determine nasal deviation, caudal deviation, and chin asymmetry.

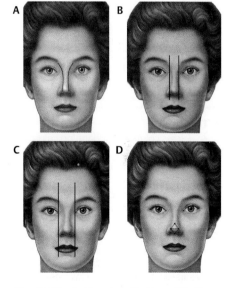

Fig. 45-11 A, Dorsal aesthetic contour lines are curvilinear in females and descend from the medial brow toward the tip-defining points. **B,** Nasal bones are generally narrower than the alar base width by about 20%-25%. **C,** Alar base width is generally equivalent to the medial canthi; however, many variations exist. **D,** Generally, aesthetically pleasing nasal tip highlights are diamond shaped.

- Evaluation:
  - ▶ Maximal alar flare width difference from width of alar base assessed
    - ◆ If >2 mm, then alar flaring is present.
    - ◆ If <2 mm, then the alar base itself is wide (excessive interalar distance).
- **Alar rims**[25-27]
  - Retraction or excess inherent "nostril show" is evaluated.
  - On lateral view, alar-columellar relationship should be balanced.
  - Should have a natural flare and inclination
  - Outline of infratip breakpoint should appear like a **"seagull in gentle flight."**
- **Nasal tip** (Fig. 45-11, *D*)
  - Four tip-defining points: One on each dome apex, a supratip break, and a columellar-lobule breakpoint
  - Lines can be drawn to assess asymmetry.
  - Domal angle and angle of domal divergence are assessed.
  - Imbalance in nasal tip aesthetic contour has various descriptions, such as bulbous, boxy, amorphous, and wide.

TIP: Evaluating tip aesthetics, as with other nasal proportions, requires careful attention to how the light reflects off the nose. External shadows and highlights on the nose provide important clues about the underlying framework. For example, asymmetry in the tip-defining point may reveal asymmetry in height, width, shape, and position of the lateral, middle, and medial crura.

SENIOR AUTHOR TIP: The intercanthal midline should be used as a reference (not the point bisecting the intereyebrow distance), because patients may pluck their eyebrows differently to reduce the impact of the nose deviation on the face.

- **Lobule**
  - Excess columella or hanging columella leads to excess infratip lobule.
  - Breakpoints should be in harmony making a diamond shape.
    - ▶ Caveat: Ethnic and gender variations should be considered.

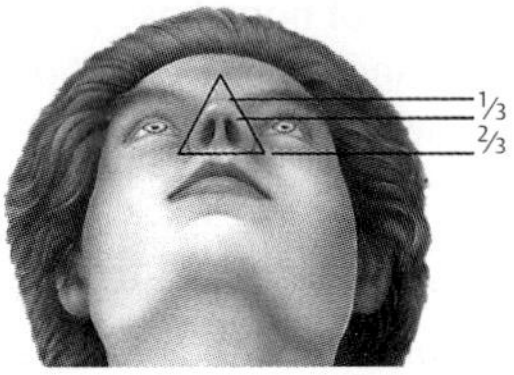

BASILAR VIEW[26,28,29] (Fig. 45-12)

- Alar rims should form an **equilateral triangle.**
- Nostril height (columellar length) to infratip lobule height ratio should be approximately **60:40,** respectively.
- Nostril inclination is approximately **60 degrees.**

Fig. 45-12   Nostril height is approximately 60%, whereas infratip height is 40%, of the basilar view height. Ethnic variations exist particularly relative to nostril length and shape.

NOTE: Ethnic features can vary significantly.

- Nostril has teardrop shape.
- Alar rims should not be excessively concave or convex, within the confines of an equilateral triangle.

LATERAL VIEW

- Multiple lengths and angles contribute to an aesthetically pleasing lateral view (Fig. 45-13).
- **Nasofrontal angle (NFA)**
  - Located at upper lash line and supratarsal crease (Fig. 45-14)
  - Formed by the intersection of the line between the glabella and the soft tissue nasion and the nasal dorsum tangent
  - NFA should be approximately **140 degrees.**
- **Dorsal curvature**
  - Determined by a line drawn from the radix at the NFA to the tip-defining point (Fig. 45-15)
  - Female dorsum should be **2 mm posterior** to this line.
  - Male dorsum should be **at or slightly anterior to this line**.
  - Angle of this line and where it begins can change the appearance of length.
    - ▶ Radix can be high or low.
    - ▶ Deep and inferiorly located radix has shortened nasal length (Fig. 45-16).

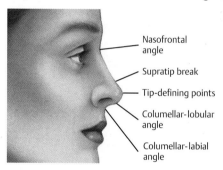

Fig. 45-13   Numerous breakpoints and angles help to define a pleasing lateral nasal view.

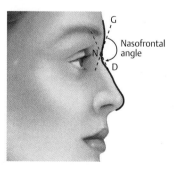

Fig. 45-14   The nasofrontal angle and position affect the appearance of the nasal length and femininity versus masculinity. (*D,* Dorsum; *G,* glabella; *N,* nasion.)

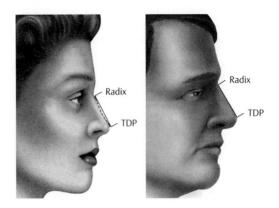

Fig. 45-15   The radix is often higher and the nasofrontal angle more obtuse in men versus women. (*TDP,* Tip-defining point.)

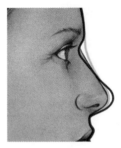

Fig. 45-16   Tip projection, dorsal curvature, and radix depth affect nasofacial balance, and variations are important to recognize in patient preference.

■ **Tip projection** (Fig. 45-17)[16]
  • Ideally tip projection should be **50%-60%** of the distance of a line drawn from the alar-cheek crease to the most anterior tip point (see Fig. 45-17, *A*).
  • Alternatively, tip projection is 0.67 × the nasal length.[5]
  • Can also be assessed on basilar view
  • Must be proportionate to chin and lip projection

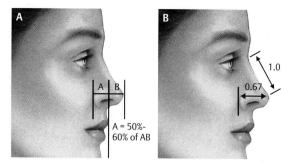

Fig. 45-17   Tip projection. **A,** The nasal tip is generally 50% of the total nasal projection from the alar-cheek junction. **B,** The nasal projection is approximately 67% of the nasal length (radix or nasal root to the most projected tip point). Morphological variations and preferences exist.

- **Tip rotation** (Fig. 45-18)
  - Draw line extending from anterior and posterior nostril rim.
  - Draw plumb line that is perpendicular to natural horizontal facial plane.
  - Angle between the nostril line and plumb line is the ***nasolabial angle*** **(NLA)** (see Fig. 45-18, *A*).
  - NLA is **95-110 degrees in females** and **90-95 degrees in males.**

> **NOTE:**   **Ethnic variations and racial congruity should be considered.**

- ***Columellar-labial angle:*** Junction of columella with upper lip; varies with degree of columellar fullness and "hang"
- ***Columellar-lobular angle:*** Junction of columella with the infratip lobule (30-45 degrees)

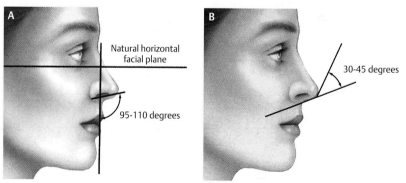

Fig. 45-18   Tip rotation. **A,** The angle between the nostril vertical line with the natural horizontal facial line is the nasolabial angle. **B,** The columellar-labial angle varies based on tip shape and breakpoints.

INFORMED CONSENT

Should include, but not be limited to, the following:

- **Swelling:** Varies depending on degree of undermining and soft tissue thickness. Patients with thick sebaceous skin may swell for a longer time, as do most secondary patients requiring multiple grafts. The nasal tip (shape and refinement) is the last location where edema subsides and the result is evident.
- **Ecchymosis:** Mostly limited to lower lid but can be completely periorbital
  - May not be seen if osteotomies are not performed
- Some darker-pigmented ethnic patients can show long-term "staining" of thin eyelid tissues.
- **Synechia, wound-healing delay, tissue loss, poor scarring**
  - Synechia in internal nasal valve region can be seen if component dorsal reduction with separation of ULC from septum is not performed before dorsal reduction.
  - Columellar incision almost always heals well but can be compromised in thin-skinned patients, smokers, and revision patients.
- **Infection:** Abscess is rare, usually a cellulitis that resolves with a short course of oral antibiotics
  - May be more common when multiple grafts used
  - Higher rate may be observed with nonautologous material.
- **Hematoma:** Septal hematoma or prolonged bleeding from mucosal surfaces is rare because of inherent drainage routes from surgery.
- **Poor cosmetic outcome, worsened or incomplete correction of asymmetries**
  - Recurrent deviations or new deviations created
  - Contour irregularities
  - Irregular or poor skin retraction
    - ▶ More common in patients with thick skin
- Worsening or new nasal airway obstruction
- Change in smell, taste, and cyclical rhinitis
  - Usually temporary
  - Nasal physiology may be changed forever, and nasal responses to inflammation, rhinitis, heat-cold alterations may be noticeably different.

EQUIPMENT

TIP: Scissors and osteotomes need to be sharp for accuracy.

KEY INSTRUMENTS
- **Scissors**
  - Converse angled
  - Long, Stevens-type scissors
  - Tissue scissors (small) for trimming mucosa, skin
  - Septal scissors

- **Elevators**
  - No. 9 oromaxillofacial elevator useful for dorsal subperiosteal dissection (is an ideal width)
  - Septal double-ended elevator (Cottle)
  - Freer
  - Boies ("butter knife")
- **Retractors**
  - Converse or other retractor for nasal skin retraction
  - Self-retaining retractors that have a chain or hanging weight are useful.
  - Ball-tip double-hook
  - Double- and single-hook
- **Forceps**
  - Adson-Brown
  - Small-tip Adson-type for skin closure
- **Osteotomes**
  - 2 mm
  - Curved 4 mm and 6 mm with guards
  - Straight 4 mm and 6 mm with lateral guards: For dorsal reduction
- **Special (other)**
  - Takahashi forceps
  - Glabellar and array of nasal dorsum rasps (Fomon downbiting)

SURGICAL TECHNIQUE: OPEN APPROACH

ADVANTAGES[11]
- Binocular vision
  - Can three-dimensionally assess incremental changes to nasal frame
- Evaluation of complete deformity and asymmetries without distortion
- Facilitates precise diagnosis and correction of deformities
- Use of both hands
- Increases options for original tissue and array of cartilage grafting techniques (with precise fixation)
- Direct control of bleeding with electrocautery

DISADVANTAGES
- External nasal incision (columella)
- Operative time prolonged
- Increased or prolonged tip edema
- Columellar incision problems (separation or delayed wound healing)
- Grafts need suture stabilization

GENERAL PRINCIPLES
- Bilateral infracartilaginous incisions made at caudalmost edge of LLCs
  - Incisions join bilaterally at internal edges of columella (along medial crura) where incision is continued to join transcolumellar incision.
- Transcolumellar incision can be stairstepped or made as an inverted-V.

> **TIP:** It may be safest and most predictable to work from lateral to medial in elevating the nasal skin. An assistant can use countertraction with a Brown forceps to help expose the caudal edge of the lower lateral crura. Inadvertent transection or laceration of cartilage is most likely to occur near the soft triangle at the middle crura (domal region).

- Cross-hatch incisions with the posterior edge of a No. 15 blade at various points to facilitate easy approximation at the end of the case.
- Elevate skin off the medial crura, and once elevation is off the domes, then apply countertraction with a double hook under each dome, pulling caudally.
  - "Hug" the perichondrium or go subperichondrially.
- Continue dissection to keystone using angled scissors, and perform subperiosteal elevation with a No. 9 elevator or Joseph elevator to radix.
- Dissect between medial crura to expose caudal septum and, if necessary, the anterior nasal spine.
  - This also allows efficient depressor septi nasi muscle transection or removal.

SURGICAL TECHNIQUE: CLOSED (ENDONASAL) APPROACH[12,15]

ADVANTAGES
- No external incision scar
- Dissection limited to areas of interest
- Precisely sized pockets can be created for graft placement, without fixation.
- Percutaneous fixation is possible with larger pockets.
- Postoperative edema lessened
- Operative time shorter
- Faster recovery
- Intact tip-graft pocket
- Allows composite grafting to the alar rim

DISADVANTAGES
- Need for experience and great reliance on preoperative diagnosis
- Does not allow simultaneous viewing by surgeon and student
- Does not allow direct visualization of nasal anatomy
- Difficult dissection of alar cartilages, especially if they are malpositioned

> **SENIOR AUTHOR TIP:** Although the endonasal approach has advantages, we think that in most cases, the ability to directly visualize the internal anatomy while dynamic and interrelated alterations are being made in the open technique outweighs the advantages of a closed approach. Throughout the years much of what we have learned in secondary rhinoplasty stems from the inadequacies of the closed approach. Precise surgical execution and experience are required for both approaches.

GENERAL PRINCIPLES
- Placement of incisions is related to type(s) of deformity.
- Preoperative diagnosis (as with open rhinoplasty) is essential.
- Translation of internal changes on the skin envelope must be assessed throughout the surgery.

Incision Types
- **Alar cartilage incisions** (Fig. 45-19)
  - **Intercartilaginous:** Between ULCs and LLCs
  - **Transcartilaginous:** Made within the LLCs (can be done in the region of the usual cephalic trim incision line)
    - ▶ Allows a cartilage-splitting approach
  - **Marginal:** Caudal to LLCs adjacent to alar rim
- **Cartilage delivery technique**
  - Intercartilaginous incision is made along with an infracartilaginous incision (or marginal incision), and the LLCs are "delivered" out of their anatomic pocket.
  - A retrograde or eversion approach can also be used.
  - Facilitates most tip-suturing techniques

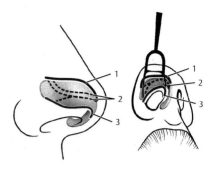

Fig. 45-19 Marginal incisions allow caudal access to the lower lateral crura and, when joined with a transcolumellar incision, provides the open approach to rhinoplasty. (*1,* Intercartilaginous; *2,* transcartilaginous; *3,* marginal.)

- **Septal incisions**
  - Transfixion incisions can be: Complete, partial (limited), hemitransfixion, or high septal
  - **Complete***:* A continuation of the intercartilaginous or transcartilaginous incision
    - ▶ Separates the caudal from the membranous septum and medial crura
    - ▶ Frees tip completely to expose nasal spine, depressor septi nasi muscle, and others
  - **Partial:** Attachments of medial crural footplates and caudal septum preserved
  - **Hemitransfixion**
    - ▶ Made unilaterally at junction of caudal septum and columella
    - ▶ Used to address deviation of caudal septum, and/or tip rotation or columellar treatment
  - **High septal:** Does not disrupt junction of caudal septum and medial crura or membranous septum

SURGICAL TECHNIQUES: NASAL DORSUM

> **NOTE:** Surgical techniques are described for the open rhinoplasty approach, but almost all are adaptable to the endonasal approach.

DORSAL HUMP REDUCTION
- First step in rhinoplasty, before tip work
- Dorsal osteocartilaginous frame exposed
- **Do *NOT* disrupt periosteum unnecessarily.**
- Using a **component dorsal reduction**[7,30]:
  - Separate the ULC from the septum during submucoperichondrial dissection.
  - Preserve the ULCs.
  - Trim dorsal septum with septal scissors and fine-tune with a No. 15 or No. 11 blade.
    - ▶ This is done incrementally.
    - ▶ Further trimming can be done after bony rasping and osteotomies.

- Use downbiting rasps to shave osseous hump. Use a double-guarded osteotome (4 or 6 mm) to reduce bony and septal humps as one unit (good for large humps)
- Perform three-finger palpation over redraped skin to check for irregularities.
- Fine-tune rasp any irregularities.

TIP: Do NOT think that the nose will look fine with time. It needs to look as good as possible before leaving the operating room. Correct all irregularities and contour problems in surgery. Evaluate the basilar view as well for any nostril discrepancies, which patients will notice and report. A ptotic tip that is corrected may reveal underlying nostril asymmetry that was not evident preoperatively.

- **ULC resection or autospreaders**[21]
  - ▶ Transverse portion of ULC resection can be *conservatively* performed.
  - ▶ Autospreader flaps of ULC can be turned in and can help to open the internal nasal valve while creating smooth dorsal aesthetic lines.
  - ▶ Autospreader flaps:
    - ◆ Require sufficient length (based on degree of dorsal septal reduction)
    - ◆ Can be turned in with or without scoring them
    - ◆ Not scoring them allows a more effective spring and functional flap.

SENIOR AUTHOR TIP: On deviated noses, the ULCs should not be trimmed or used as the spreader flaps until the osteotomy is completed and the nasal bones are repositioned because of the differential response by the ULCs to the osteotomy.

- **True spreader grafts**[12-14,31] (Fig. 45-20)
  - ▶ Typical dimensions (5-6 by 32 mm)
  - ▶ May be placed asymmetrically (in thickness and position) based on indications
  - ▶ Longer (extended spreader grafts) are used to lengthen a short nose.
  - ▶ Septal cartilage should be used to create spreader grafts between ULC and cartilaginous septum.
  - ▶ Role: Correct deviations (concave or collapsed midvault side can receive a convex, larger spreader graft than the contralateral side); straighten or buttress a deviated septum; maintain dorsal aesthetic lines

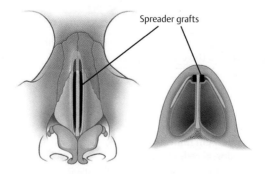

Spreader grafts

Fig. 45-20   Spreader grafts allow internal nasal valve patency.

OSTEOTOMIES[32,33] (Fig. 45-21)

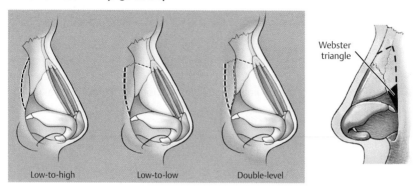

Fig. 45-21   Various starting points and endpoints of osteotomy patterns exist.

- Can be performed **before or after** tip work
  - Because it is related to dorsal aesthetics, osteotomies are performed along with all other dorsal work and before more delicate tip refinement.
- Average nasal bone length: **2.5 cm**
  - Asian and black patients may have very short nasal bones.
    - ▶ Osteotomies can be detrimental when bone is short and can collapse into bony vault if performed in these patients.
- **Indications**
  - To narrow wide nasal sidewalls
  - To close an open-roof deformity
  - To straighten a deviated nasal pyramid
- **Relative contraindications**
  - Ethnic patients with broad, short nasal bones
  - Elderly patients with thin bones
  - Heavy eyeglass wearers
  - Short nasal bones in general:
    - ▶ Caudal border is <1 cm below intercanthal line.
- Thicker nasal bone above medial canthus line at radix
- Thicker nasal bone region may be amenable to medial or "J-type" osteotomy configuration.
- Less force required at thinner caudal segments
- All bony "cuts" should be performed with a very sharp osteotome.
- **Types of lateral osteotomies**
  - **Low-high:** For minimally wide nasal base and/or small open roof; begins low (adjacent to piriform aperture, extending cephalad to intercanthal level, curving high on nasal sidewall)
  - **Low-low: Most common.** Good for excessive bony nasal width correction or large open roof; more bone recruited and medialized; allows more natural and smooth transition from native curve upward at ascending process of maxilla toward the nasal dorsum
  - Easily combined with a medial component or "J-type" extension at canthal level for a more controlled "transition" point

- **Double-level:** Good for asymmetry, especially with excessive convexity close to or at maxillary junction; lateral osteotomy near nasomaxillary suture is performed, followed by a low-to-low osteotomy; also useful for complex secondary nasal bone deformities
- **Internal versus percutaneous**[34,35]
  - **Internal:** May cause more disruption of internal mucosa and more edema/ecchymosis
  - **Percutaneous:** Uses a small imperceptible stab incision with a sharp 2 mm osteotome
    - ▶ Can be discontinuous or continuous
    - ▶ Well-controlled
    - ▶ Infiltrate area with lidocaine-epinephrine solution. (Inject before start of case and reinject during case, before osteotomy.)
    - ▶ Place 2 mm osteotome parallel to face of maxilla at midportion of nasal pyramid.
    - ▶ Exert gentle pressure on nasal bones to use bimanual palpation and spatial reference.
    - ▶ Sweep periosteum and angular vessel toward maxilla away from sidewall to limit bleeding.
    - ▶ Once subperiosteal, begin "tap-tap" osteotomy, starting from caudal to cephalad.
    - ▶ Keep the osteotome in contact with the nasal bones at all times.
    - ▶ Once cuts are all completed, use thumb and index finger to medialize bones.

TIP: The osteotomy path is marked on the skin preoperatively. Iced or a cold gauze is used as a compress, with the table in a reverse Trendelenburg position. The osteotome is angled so that one edge is in contact, increasing sharpness and control. One to two millimeters of bone can be left between each bony cut. Final fine rasping can be performed after the osteotomies, if the nasal bones remained stable, to smooth any raised bony edges from the repositioned nasal bones.

- **Medial osteotomies**
  - Helpful for reducing a narrow upper vault, thick or wide superior bony vault, high nasal deviations
  - Types: Medial oblique and paramedian
  - Must be performed caudal to intercanthal level
  - Bony cuts can be made from dorsal approach when osteocartilaginous exposure achieved
  - *Performing medial before lateral osteotomies facilitates a stable bony base.*

Dorsal Augmentation
- **Indications**
  - Low and/or wide dorsal height
  - Ethnic patients (Asian, black, Hispanic) with flattened dorsum
  - "Washed out," unrefined dorsal aesthetic lines requiring augmentation
  - Radix alone can be augmented when indicated.
    - ▶ In patients with a dorsal hump in whom dorsal height needs to be preserved or increased
- Can be combined with osteotomies to create narrowing appearance of dorsum
  - Requires appropriate nasal bone length

- **Augmentation sources**
  - Septal cartilage, conchal cartilage (suboptimal), autologous or irradiated rib cartilage, AlloDerm (LifeCell), Surgicel (Ethicon) or temporalis fascia–wrapped, diced cartilage (diced cartilage fascial graft), silicone
  - *Caveats:*
    - ▶ Irradiated rib grafts have a very high absorption rate.
    - ▶ Strongest source is autologous rib, but techniques to prevent warping are necessary.
      - ◆ Warping rates may be underreported, and when it occurs, reoperation is necessary.
    - ▶ Silicone must be fixed and placed under thick soft tissue because of possible future extrusion.
    - ▶ One of the most popular techniques currently is the use of diced cartilage fascia graft.
    - ▶ Human acellular dermal matrix can only be used for camouflaging (smoothing) effect or when minimal dorsal enhancement is required, but fascia-only techniques seem to be replacing this technique.
- **Septal cartilage**
  - Partial incisions (scores) made to allow bending into V-, U- (better for thin-skinned patients), and A-frame shapes (Fig. 45-22)
  - May be stacked and covered with temporal fascia or other fascia (mastoid, rectus)

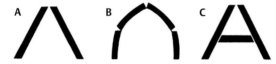

Fig. 45-22   Dorsal onlay grafts can be fashioned in different configurations but must be smooth in contour and without visible edges. **A,** V-frame. **B,** U-frame. **C,** A-frame.

- **Conchal cartilage**
  - Unpredictable and hard to keep a straight shape
  - Crushing and morselizing may help.
- **Costal (rib) cartilage**
  - Helpful when >3 mm augmentation required and in many secondary rhinoplasties in which dorsum has been overresected
  - Stabilization with sutures and threaded 0.028 K-wires recommended to prevent movement and warping
  - K-wire placed at dorsum and removed at 1 week
  - Threaded K-wire through the cartilage or perichondrial wrapping may reduce warping rates.
  - Secured to anterocaudal septum with sutures

SENIOR AUTHOR TIP: Place cartilage grafts in saline solution for 30 minutes to help predict warping characteristics. Use the Gibson principle of balanced cartilage carving.

- **Temporal fascia–wrapped dorsal graft**[36]
  - Developed after Surgicel-wrapped technique introduced[37]
  - Fascia-wrapped diced cartilage construct is becoming very widely used.

- Longevity data are promising.
- Short-term studies show excellent results.
- Malleable and aesthetically appealing
- Easy technique allowing the use of cartilage remnants
- Can be divided into its components
    ▶ Fascia-only onlay (camouflage)
    ▶ Varying size of diced grafts and how tightly the construct is wrapped can affect the aesthetic results.
    ▶ Advocates claim that worst case outcome is higher absorption than anticipated in long term, as opposed to worst case scenario for straight rib grafts which can require reoperation for warping.

SEPTOPLASTY
- See the section Surgical Techniques: Deviation and Nasal Airway Obstruction for details.
- Should be performed only after all dorsal work complete, including osteotomies
- Osteotomies affect dorsal aesthetic lines.
- Final dorsal resections may be necessary to smooth out dorsum after osteotomies.
- Dorsum needs to be finalized to determine how much septum can be removed to preserve a proper L-strut.
- Increasing septal and nasal length:
    - Various forms of septal extension grafts can be used to lengthen the central nose.[38]

SURGICAL TECHNIQUES: NASAL TIP[39-47]

TIP PROJECTION
- Support structures are important to tip shape, position, and projection.
    - Suspensory ligaments
    - Fibrous connections between the upper and lower lateral cartilage
    - Tip projection is decreased when the tip is dissected because of detachment of these support structures.

STRUCTURES INFLUENCING TIP PROJECTION
- Length and strength of the lower lateral crura and medial crura
    - Including the shape and position of the footplates
- Position of the entire tip complex can affect the degree of tip projection.
- Middle crura add minimally to overall tip projection but can be manipulated through tip-suturing techniques.
- Position of the anterior nasal spine

INCREASING TIP PROJECTION
- Graduated (incremental) approach (Fig. 45-23)
- Columellar strut aids in establishing and maintaining tip projection.
- Transdomal sutures can elevate and project tip minimally.
- Final placement of onlay grafts further shapes and increases projection.
    - Be aware of graft palpability and visibility in thin-skinned patients.

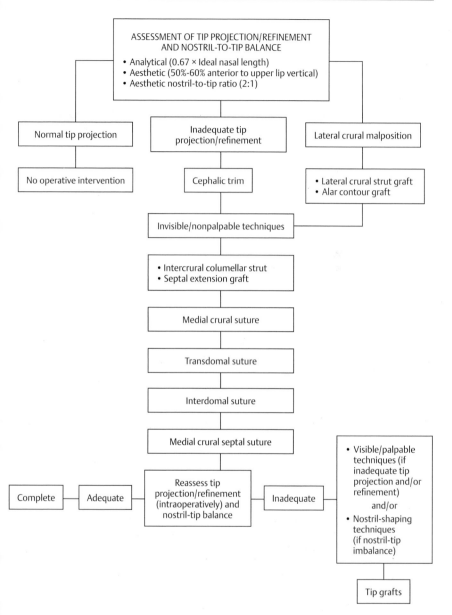

Fig. 45-23   Algorithm for sequencing tip shaping and position.

- **Columellar strut graft** (Fig. 45-24)
  - Placed between medial crura and sutured to medial crura
  - Maintains and/or increases tip projection
  - **Two types**
    - ▶ Type 1: Floating
      - ◆ Rests on soft tissue (2 mm) anterior to nasal spine region; mobile
      - ◆ Appropriate when only 1-2 mm increase in tip projection is required
    - ▶ Type 2: Fixed
      - ◆ Sutured or wired in place and relatively immobile
      - ◆ Indicated when >3 mm projection is necessary
      - ◆ Patient may feel the tip as being "too rigid."
      - ◆ Best reserved for complex revision cases

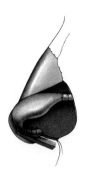

Fig. 45-24   A columellar strut graft reinforces proper tip projection and stability.

TIP-SUTURING TECHNIQUES[39-47] (Fig. 45-25)

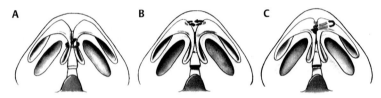

Fig. 45-25   Types of sutures. **A,** Medial crural sutures. **B,** Interdomal sutures. **C,** Transdomal sutures.

- Provide an additional 1-2 mm tip projection
- Projection can be increased by shaping the domes.

> **TIP:**   Nasal tip sutures are a critical tool in tip shaping. The degree by which they are tightened and the exact orientation, suture bite, distance, and suture material affect the cartilages in different ways. Finesse is required, and when a suture does not produce the desired effect, removal and replacement until the precise result is achieved is critical.

- **Medial crural sutures** (Fig. 45-26)
  - Placed to unify the medial crura
  - Often, at least two required
  - Columellar strut can be incorporated caudal or cephalad to this.
  - When medial crura are strong, strut may not be needed and suture unification alone provides the stable platform for tip position and projection.
- **Transdomal suture**
  - Horizontal mattress suture placed at lateral and medial genu of middle crura

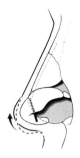

Fig. 45-26   Medial crural sutures can rotate the tip complex when placed high on the caudal septum or a columellar strut graft.

  - The more lateral this suture is placed on the LLC, the more lateral crura can be recruited into the tip complex, and more tip projection is provided.
  - Also helps to equalize domal and other tip asymmetries
  - The tighter the suture, the more sharp the dome shape and projection.

TIP: Tip projection and refinement are interlinked. Careful inspection of the shadows and highlights cast on the nasal skin preoperatively helps to detect tip asymmetries, details in tip shape, midvault bossing, and other irregularities. This allows more finesse in overall nasal shaping, along with improvement of asymmetries.

- **Interdomal suture**
  - Placed between the domes of each LLC
  - Depending on degree of tightness, the interdomal space is incrementally narrowed.
  - Assists in equalizing the domal positions based on differential suture placement to provide a "clocking" effect
- **Medial crural septal suture**
  - Attaches medial crura to septum
  - Assists in tip positioning, decreasing columellar show, and changing columellar and nasolabial angles
  - Very beneficial for droopy or aging nasal tips
  - Powerful suture in positioning nasal tip complex
  - Can increase tip rigidity

TIP GRAFTS (Fig. 45-27)

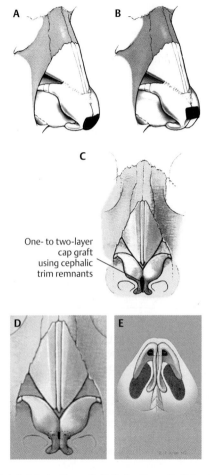

One- to two-layer
cap graft
using cephalic
trim remnants

Fig. 45-27 Tip grafts. **A,** Infralobular tip graft. **B,** Onlay tip graft. **C,** A soft cap graft can be placed on top of intercrural depressions or to soften tip-defining points and contour. **D** and **E,** A subdomal graft can reorient and stabilize the domes.

- **Infralobular graft** (see Fig. 45-27, *A*)
  - Improves infratip lobular shape and deficiencies in the middle crura
  - Provides appropriate infratip and supratip breakpoints when desired
  - These include variations on shield grafts.
  - A hexagonal or diamond shape is fashioned.
  - Scoring the diamond horizontally sharpens the breakpoint.

TIP: All grafts should be carefully constructed for their intended effect on nasal shape and projection. Edges should be beveled and softened. Grafts may be double layered, combined, or sutured together or to the native cartilage and soft tissues for added stability. Minimal crushing can minimize graft visibility and warping over time. Laying down skin after each graft is helpful to assess the resultant influence on tip contour.

■ **Onlay tip graft** (see Fig. 45-27, *B*)
  • Increases domal (tip) projection
  • Depending on shape, will influence tip shape
  • Width and length will alter tip contours.
  • Modification: Carve and remove a figure-of-eight shape and suture each oval to respective dome.
  • Double and triple layering may be indicated to further increase tip projection and angularity of the domal dimensions.
■ **Cap graft** (see Fig. 45-27, *C*)
  • Cephalic trim remnant
  • Thin, pliable, and not easily visible or palpable
  • Useful for camouflaging cartilage
■ **Subdomal graft**[48] (see Fig. 45-27, *D* and *E*)
  • Useful for correcting domal asymmetry and a pinched nasal tip
■ **Combined grafting**
  • Suturing multiple grafts together to improve nasal shape and control breakpoints
  • Useful in increasing tip projection and shaping in thicker-skinned patients with severely underprojected tips (e.g., black noses)

SENIOR AUTHOR TIP: A tip graft and a columellar strut cannot be used interchangeably. A strut is used when the columella is short. A tip graft is used when insufficient tip projection is the consequence of inadequate lobule volume.

DECREASING TIP PROJECTION
■ **Graduated technique**
  • Full transfixion incision
  • Release ligamentous attachments of lower lateral crura and medial crura.
  • This sets tip complex back in and on itself.
  • Transect lower lateral crus and suture it back to itself in a more posterior orientation.
  • Vestibular undermining is required.
  • Very effective
  • Can also correct convexities, which may be accentuated in overprojected noses
  • Transect medial crura if necessary (as described by Lipsett).[49]
  • Transect 2 mm posterior to junction of medial crura with middle crura ("medial genu").
■ **Closed approach**
  • Transfixion incision
  • Separate the lower lateral crura from the cartilaginous septum.
  • Undermine and transect lower lateral crura with overlapping of lateral segments.
  • Simultaneously corrects malposition
  • Transect medial crura and overlap

TIP: Consider the nasal tip as supported with a tripod, with the two lower lateral crura and medial crura representing the feet. The position and rotation of the tip can be adjusted by altering the length of the various crura incrementally and systematically.

BOXY NASAL TIP[44] (Fig. 45-28)

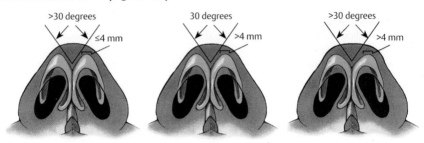

Fig. 45-28 Types I through III define degrees of the boxy tip based on angle of divergence between the domes and domal width within each dome.

■ Tip lacks definition and is broad and rectangular on basilar view. Three anatomic variations cause this morphology:
  • **Type I:** An increased angle of divergence (>30 degrees) between the domes. Interdomal sutures are required to close angle.
  • **Type II:** Wide domal arc but normal angle of divergence. Domal cephalic trim with transdomal sutures is needed.
  • **Type III:** Large angle of divergence and wide domal arc. Interdomal and transdomal sutures are required.
■ Caveat: Additional suturing and grafts may be required to enhance improvement, especially in thick-skinned patients.

SURGICAL TECHNIQUES: ALAR BASE AND NOSTRILS

CORRECTION OF WIDENED ALAR BASE (Fig. 45-29)

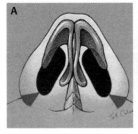 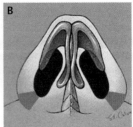

Fig. 45-29 **A,** Weir excisions correct flare. **B,** Extension into the sill will narrow the interalar distance and reduce the nostril aperture.

- Assess **alar flare**
  - Compare maximum alar width with width of ala at the base.
    - ▶ If difference is **>2 mm,** then the problem is **excessive flaring,** and a precisely measured **alar wedge** should be excised to **exclude** the vestibule (sill).
    - ▶ If the difference is **<2 mm,** then the problem is excessively **wide alar bases** (increased interalar distance).
      - ◆ Wedge excision, **including** vestibule-sill
  - **Technical steps**
    - ▶ Use No. 11 blade, 30-degree angle laterally, and preserve lip of tissue from lateral alar "flap" so that sill does not have tension.
    - ▶ Use "halving principle" to close without pleating.

ALAR RIM DEFORMITIES

- Commonly a result of overresection of the lower lateral crura or improper support during initial rhinoplasty
- Native, unfavorable morphology, such as alar-columellar discrepancies and lower lateral crural malposition can cause alar rim problem.
- **Alar contour graft**[25] (Fig. 45-30)
  - Indicated in secondary rhinoplasty with minimal vestibular lining loss and at least 3 mm of LLC remaining
    - ▶ Alar rim and soft triangle notching
    - ▶ As treatment or prevention
    - ▶ In addition to lateral crural strut graft in LLC malposition
- **Not** indicated when:
  - Excess lining loss
  - Severe alar scarring
  - Insufficient lower lateral crural remnant
- Technique: 6 by 2 mm (use wider grafts if indicated); septal cartilage preferred; subcutaneous and tight pocket in alar rim
  - Graft should not distort aesthetics of alar rim with nasal tip shape relation.

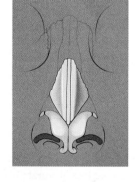

Fig. 45-30   Alar contour graft placed in a new "nonanatomic" subcutaneous position.

SENIOR AUTHOR TIP: When the alar retraction is significant, an internal V-Y advancement would provide a better means of correcting the deformity without having to harvest a composite graft. On patients with normal or thick skin, the use of a supratip suture, as described elsewhere, will eliminate the dead space and reduce the potential for a supratip deformity.

- **Lateral crural strut graft**[50] (Fig. 45-31)
  - Carved grafts from septum or conchal cartilage and sandwiched between vestibular skin and LLC remnant
  - Often extend to piriform area in a subcutaneous alar rim pocket
  - May be used with or without transecting/relocating the native lower lateral crura
  - **Indications**
    - ▶ Severe alar notching
    - ▶ Malpositioned and/or weak LLC
    - ▶ Alar retraction
    - ▶ Alar rim collapse
    - ▶ Concave LLC
  - **Technique**
    - ▶ After cephalic trim, vestibular skin is undermined.

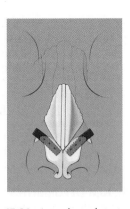

Fig. 45-31   Lateral crural strut grafts can be placed with or without transection and translocation of the lower lateral crura.

    - ▶ Strut (from septum or ear) is carved to be a straight 3-4 by 15-25 mm piece.
    - ▶ Placed and sutured to undersurface of LLC and extended to fit in a lateral subcutaneous pocket near piriform
    - ▶ Placed caudal to alar groove
    - ▶ Can be sutured laterally to LLC if transection of LLC required
    - ▶ Can be placed closer to tip-defining points to aid in projection
- **Lateral crural convexity control sutures**[51]
  - Horizontal mattress sutures placed 6 mm apart through lateral crura at most convex point
  - Can correct convexity of LLC by flattening the region where the sutures are placed
- **Lower lateral crural turnover flap**[52] (Fig. 45-32)
  - Location: Cephalic portion of lateral crura turned over onto the remaining caudolateral crura
  - Objective: Improve strength, position, and shape of lateral crura

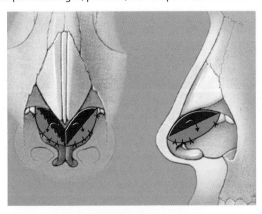

Fig. 45-32   Lower lateral crural turnover flap. Turning a cephalad flap over the lower lateral crura can correct convexity and concavities while creating a stronger bilaminate structure.

SURGICAL TECHNIQUES: DEVIATION AND NASAL AIRWAY OBSTRUCTION

NASAL DEVIATION[13,14,22]

- Causes: Deviated septum, ULC-deforming forces, asymmetrical nasal bones (including previous traumatic causes)

General Principles

- Wide exposure
- Release attachments to deviated segments.
- Separate deforming forces, such as LLC or ULC from septum (and scroll area).
- Septal deviation must be corrected, including straightening of concavities, tilts, and "off-center" connections to anterior nasal spine.
  - **Septal deviation**
    - ▶ L-strut creation with at least 10 mm caudally and dorsally preserved
    - ▶ Judicious use of spreader grafts (asymmetrical or bilateral) or autospreader flaps
      - ◆ May require extending grafts or fixation to a centralized, fixed columellar strut (more likely in secondary cases)
    - ▶ Reduction of caudal septum to anterior nasal spine with figure-of-eight suture to periosteum or using a drill hole
    - ▶ May need to create "swinging door" from caudal septum with vertical sectioning
      - ◆ If insufficient, excise small wedges from convex side with scoring on concave side.
    - ▶ If septal deviation is cephalad:
      - ◆ Shave convex side of deviation
      - ◆ Dorsal spreader graft to concave side
      - ◆ May need scoring techniques as well
    - ▶ If high dorsal deviation persists:
      - ◆ Full thickness, partial (<50%) cuts made to L-strut

CAUTION: Do not make cuts adjacent to the keystone, because the septum is vulnerable at its junction with the perpendicular ethmoid plate and may collapse.

      - ◆ Use spreader grafts
  - **Asymmetrical nasal bones**
    - ▶ Asymmetrical oblique rasping
    - ▶ Asymmetrical lateral and, if necessary, oblique (medial) osteotomies
    - ▶ Medial osteotomies required if nasal bones are asymmetrical
    - ▶ Consider double-level osteotomies in secondary and severe posttraumatic deformities.

SENIOR AUTHOR TIP: When the anterocaudal septum is deviated, a septal rotation suture, I have previously described, would move the septum to the midline.

NASAL AIRWAY OBSTRUCTION[1,6,13,14]

- Septal deviations must be corrected.
- Septoplasty is often required.
  - May unmask or worsen turbinate hypertrophy if turbinates not treated
- Wide medial crural footplates (Fig. 45-33)
  - Footplates resected or suture-cinched together (4-0 chromic), along with soft tissue excision between medial crura

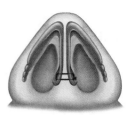

Fig. 45-33 Medial crural footplate sutures narrow the columellar base and can improve symmetry.

- Internal nasal valve collapse or narrowing
  - True spreader grafts or autospreader flaps
  - Alar batten grafts that support overresected or weakened area lateral to lateral crura
- External valve collapse
  - Lateral crural strut grafts and/or alar contour grafts
  - Lower lateral turnover flaps
  - LLC is repositioned, if severely malpositioned, and sutured to strut grafts laterally for lateral support and maintenance of position.
  - Lower lateral crura closest to the alar rim will provide improved external valve support.
    - ▶ Struts are indicated when the native crura are weak.
- Turbinate hypertrophy
  - In severe septal deviation, contralateral inferior turbinate undergoes hypertrophy to even out airway resistance *(compensated turbinate hypertrophy)*.
  - Correction of septal deviation may lead to worsened airway obstruction from turbinate on hypertrophied side.
  - Turbinate(s) may be outfractured laterally or reduced with submucosal cautery.[53-55]
    - ▶ May also make small incision and microfracture bony concha of turbinate with a 2 mm osteotome
  - Excessive turbinate resection should be avoided because can lead to *empty nose syndrome*
    - ▶ Exposed areas of the nasal mucosa not used to drying effects of airflow
    - ▶ Excess mucous evaporation (increased viscosity)
    - ▶ Increased bleeding and dysfunction of nasal cilia
    - ▶ Patients have open airways but feel as though they do not because of dysfunctions mentioned previously.
  - **Technique:** Submucous resection
    - ▶ Needletip cautery or coblation used to make small, 1.5 cm incision in anterior mucosa
    - ▶ Elevator lifts off anterior mucosa
    - ▶ Takahashi forceps used to resect exposed conchal bone (can also use 2 mm osteotome or a Cottle elevator to simply microfracture bony elements without removal)
    - ▶ Can outfracture with Boies elevator or long speculum to collapse and push turbinate elements laterally and out of the airway

TIP: Do NOT completely excise or perform complete inferior turbinectomy, because it can cause ozena, crusting, and atrophic rhinitis. Warn patients undergoing turbinate manipulation of possible prolonged malodor, nasal dripping, and more prolonged postseptorhinoplasty oozing.

POSTOPERATIVE CARE

Patients should be given instructions for postoperative care. Instructions should be fairly detailed, as shown below.

- Avoid smoking.
- For 2 weeks do not consume foods that require excess lip movement such as apples and corn on the cob. You will probably have bloody nasal discharge for 3-4 days and may change the drip pad under your nose as often as needed.
- Do not rub or blot your nose, as this will tend to irritate it.
- To prevent bleeding, do not sniff or blow your nose for the first 2 weeks after surgery.
- Try not to sneeze, but if you do, sneeze through your mouth.
- While the nasal splint is on, you may have your hair washed beauty-salon fashion.
- The nasal splint will be removed 6-7 days after surgery.
- After the splint is removed, do not wear glasses or allow anything else to rest on your nose for 4 weeks. Glasses should be taped to the forehead.
- Contacts can be worn as soon as the swelling has decreased enough for them to be inserted.
- Keep the inside edges of your nostrils and any stitches clean by using a cotton-tipped applicator saturated with half-strength hydrogen peroxide and then applying a thin coating of Polysporin or bacitracin ointment.
- You may advance the applicator into the nose as far as the cotton, but no farther.
- Protect your nose from excessive exposure to the sun for 6 months.
- Avoid strenuous activity (INCREASING YOUR HEART RATE ABOVE 100 BEATS PER MINUTE) for the first 3 weeks after surgery, such as aerobics, heavy lifting, and bending over.
- Avoid lifting anything heavier than 10 pounds for 3 weeks after surgery.
- After your sutures are removed and the internal/external splints are removed, we recommend using saline solution (salt water) (Ocean Spray or generic saline nasal spray) to gently remove crusty formation from inside your nose, especially if you had internal nasal surgery such as septal reconstruction or inferior turbinate resection.
- If you have increased nasal bleeding with bright red blood (with a need to change the nasal pad every 30-40 minutes) notify your doctor immediately. You should sit up and apply pressure to the end of your nose for 15 minutes, and you can use Afrin spray to stop the oozing in the interim. Bleeding usually stops with these maneuvers.
- It often takes approximately 1 year for the last 10% of the swelling to resolve. Your nose may feel stiff when you smile and not as flexible as before surgery. This is not noticeable to others, and things will gradually return to normal.

COMPLICATIONS

FUNCTIONAL-MEDICAL COMPLICATIONS

- These complications are generally less common than aesthetic or contour-related complications.

Bleeding

- Extreme epistaxis is rare and commonly stops in first 48 hours.
- Commonly from anterior septum (Kiesselbach triangle)
- More common with turbinate manipulation

- Various methods of tamponading, vasoconstriction, and blood pressure control are treatments.
- DDAVP injections have been reported to assist in both perioperative and postoperative recalcitrant epistaxis.[56]

Infection
- Rare
- Higher rates of methicillin-resistent *Staphylococcus aureus* (MRSA) in some regions in the United States may warrant prophylactic and postoperative use of mupirocin ointment on and inside the nares.
- More common with nonautologous implants
- Multiple grafts may lead to infection.
- Often, staphylococcal or other skin flora infection source
- Treated effectively with oral antibiotic therapy and/or mupirocin
- May require in-office irrigation multiple times using a catheter

Airway Obstruction
- Airway not addressed properly
- Deviations not corrected
- Internal nasal valve narrowing or synechia
- Excessive midvault narrowing or nasal bone collapse
- External nasal valve collapse or insufficiency
- Can often be assessed as early as 3 months when most edema has resolved

AESTHETIC COMPLICATIONS
- Most common complications are **aesthetic** and **contour related.**

Skin and Soft Tissue
- Poor contractile ability
  - More common in thick-skinned ethnic noses
- Excessive thinning from overzealous debulking and violation of subdermal plexus
  - Can create very difficult-to-treat superficial skin damage
  - May be corrected with soft tissue fillers
    - ▶ Supratip and infratip bulkiness from incorrect soft tissue filling with cartilage frame support
    - ▶ Unaesthetic shadowing or lines seen in paradomal and nasal sidewall region leading to an overoperated nasal appearance

Nasal Tip Contour Irregularities
- Excessive narrowing
  - Overzealous tip suturing (tightening, large bites) or excess/improper graft placement
- Asymmetrical domes, domal height, poor medial crural alignment
- Visible grafts and graft warping
- Overprojection or underprojection of nasal tip
- Unrefined nasal tip shape
  - Poor analysis and/or nasal tip–shaping techniques
  - Destructive maneuvers without support grafts and struts

Osteotomies

- Persistent deviations
- Asymmetries
- Visible osteotomy lines from too high a placement
- Excessive narrowing
- Collapse
- Inverted-V deformities

Improper Nasal Shape and Balance (Overoperated or Underoperated Appearance)

- Tip and dorsum disproportion
- Excess infratip lobule bulk
- Polly beak deformity
- Persistent droopy tip
  - Insufficient positioning of tip complex
  - Lack of columellar strut or nasal tip platform support maneuvers
  - Persistent depressor septi nasi muscle overactivity from lack of treatment
  - Insufficient caudal septal resection

TOP TAKEAWAYS

➤ During secondary rhinoplasty, soft tissue debulking is more difficult because of scar tissue, and previously dissected nasal tip skin may be more prone to vascular compromise during dissection.

➤ Often, a simple outfracture (micro or mini) of the inferior turbinate, with or without mucosal resection, is all that is needed to improve nasal airway obstruction caused by turbinate hypertrophy. Complete turbinectomy is rarely indicated and can result in an "empty nose" deformity with imbalance in airway resistance.

➤ Leaving a dorsal strut of <2 cm may result in sinking of the dorsum and development of a hump that was not present intraoperatively.

➤ On deviated noses, the ULCs should not be trimmed or used as the spreader flaps until the osteotomy is completed and the nasal bones are repositioned because of the differential response by the ULCs to the osteotomy.

➤ Higher rates of MRSA in some regions in the United States may warrant prophylactic and postoperative use of mupirocin ointment on and inside the nares.

REFERENCES

1. Beekhuis GJ. Nasal obstruction after rhinoplasty: etiology, and techniques for correction. Laryngoscope 86:540, 1976.
2. Ghavami A, Rohrich RJ. The ethnic rhinoplasty. In Aston SJ, Steinbrech DS, Walden JL, eds. Aesthetic Plastic Surgery. London: Saunders, 2009.
3. Rohrich RJ, Huynh B, Muzaffar AR, et al. Importance of the depressor septi nasi muscle in rhinoplasty: anatomic study and clinical application. Plast Reconstr Surg 105:376, 2000.
4. Ghavami A, Janis JE, Guyuron B. Regarding the treatment of dynamic tip ptosis using botulinum toxin A. Plast Reconstr Surg 118:263, 2006.

5. Rohrich RJ, Gunter JP, Friedman RM. Nasal tip blood supply: an anatomic study validating the safety of the transcolumellar incision in rhinoplasty. Plast Reconstr Surg 95:795, 1995.

6. Howard BK, Rohrich RJ. Understanding the nasal airway: principles and practice. Plast Reconstr Surg 109:1128, 2002.

7. Rohrich RJ, Muzaffar AR, Janis JE. Component dorsal hump reduction: the importance of maintaining dorsal aesthetic lines in rhinoplasty. Plast Reconstr Surg 114:1298, 2004.

8. Anderson JR. A reasoned approach to nasal base surgery. Arch Otolaryngol 110:349,1984.

9. Janeke JB, Wright WK. Studies on the support of the nasal tip. Arch Otolaryngol 93:458, 1971.

10. Adams WP Jr, Rohrich RJ, Hollier LH, et al. Anatomic basis and clinical implications for nasal tip support in open versus closed rhinoplasty. Plast Reconstr Surg 103:255, 1999.

11. Gunter JP. The merits of the open approach in rhinoplasty. Plast Reconstr Surg 99:863, 1997.

12. Sheen JH, Sheen A, eds. Aesthetic Rhinoplasty, ed 2. St Louis: CV Mosby, 1987.

13. Gunter JP, Rohrich RJ. Management of the deviated nose. The importance of septal reconstruction. Clin Plast Surg 15:43, 1988.

14. Rohrich RJ, Gunter JP, Deuber MA, et al. The deviated nose: optimizing results using a simplified classification and algorithmic approach. Plast Reconstr Surg 110:1509, 2002.

15. Joseph J, ed. Nasenplastick und Sonstige Gesichtsplastik Nebst Einen Anhang Ueber Mammaplastik. Leipzig: Curt Kabitzsch, 1931.

16. Byrd HS, Hobar PC. Rhinoplasty: a practical guide for surgical planning. Plast Reconstr Surg 91:642, 1993.

17. Toriumi DM. New concepts in nasal tip contouring. Arch Facial Plast Surg 8:156, 2006.

18. Rohrich RJ, Muzaffar AR. Rhinoplasty in the African-American patient. Plast Reconstr Surg 111:1322, 2003.

19. Daniel RK. Hispanic rhinoplasty in the United States with emphasis on the Mexican American nose. Plast Reconstr Surg 112:244, 2003.

20. Rohrich RJ, Ghavami A. Rhinoplasty for Middle Eastern noses. Plast Reconstr Surg 123:1343, 2009.

21. Byrd HS, Meade RA, Gonyon DL Jr. Use of the autospreader flap in primary rhinoplasty. Plast Reconstr Surg 119:1897, 2007.

22. Guyuron B, Behmand RA. Caudal nasal deviation. Plast Reconstr Surg 111:2449, 2003.

23. Guyuron B. Dynamics of rhinoplasty. Plast Reconstr Surg 88:970, 1991.

24. Janis JE, Ahmad J, Rohrich RJ. Clinical decision-making in rhinoplasty. Nahai F, ed. The Art of Aesthetic Surgery, ed 2. New York: Thieme Publishers, 2010.

25. Rohrich RJ, Raniere J J Jr, Ha RY. The alar contour graft: correction and prevention of alar rim deformities in rhinoplasty. Plast Reconstr Surg 109:2495, 2002.

26. Gunter JP, Rohrich RJ, Friedman RM. Classification and correction of alar-columellar discrepancies in rhinoplasty. Plast Reconstr Surg 97:643, 1996.

27. Guyuron B. Alar rim deformities. Plast Reconstr Surg 107:856, 2001.

28. Daniel RK. Rhinoplasty: large nostril/small tip disproportion. Plast Reconstr Surg 107:1874, 2001.

29. Guyuron B, Ghavami A, Wishnek SM. Components of the short nostril. Plast Reconstr Surg 116:1517, 2005.

30. Rohrich RJ, Muzaffar AR, Janis JE. Component dorsal hump reduction: the importance of maintaining dorsal aesthetic lines in rhinoplasty. Plast Reconstr Surg 114:1298; discussion 1309, 2004.

31. Sheen JH. Spreader graft: a method of reconstructing the roof of the middle nasal vault following rhinoplasty. Plast Reconstr Surg 73:230, 1984.

32. Guyuron B. Nasal osteotomy and airway changes. Plast Reconstr Surg 102:856, 1998.

33. Gruber R, Chang TN, Kahn D, et al. Broad nasal bone reduction: an algorithm for osteotomies. Plast Reconstr Surg 119:1044, 2007.
34. Rohrich RJ. Osteotomies in rhinoplasty: an updated technique. Aesthet Surg J 23:56, 2003.
35. Rohrich RJ, Janis JE, Adams WP, et al. An update on the lateral nasal osteotomy in rhinoplasty: an anatomic endoscopic comparison of the external versus the internal approach. Plast Reconstr Surg 111:2461; discussion 2463, 2003.
36. Daniel RK, Calvert JW. Diced cartilage grafts in rhinoplasty. Plast Reconstr Surg 113:2156, 2004.
37. Erol O. The Turkish delight: a pliable graft for rhinoplasty. Plast Reconstr Surg 105:2229, 2000.
38. Byrd S, Andochick S, Copit S, et al. Septal extension grafts: a method of controlling tip projection, rotation, and shape. Plast Reconstr Surg 100:999, 1997.
39. Gruber RP, Friedman GD. Suture algorithm for the broad or bulbous nasal tip. Plast Reconstr Surg 110:1752, 2002.
40. Ghavami A, Janis JE, Acikel C, et al. Tip shaping in primary rhinoplasty: an algorithmic approach. Plast Reconstr Surg 122:1229, 2008.
41. Behmand RA, Ghavami A, Guyuron B. Nasal tip sutures part I: the evolution. Plast Reconstr Surg 112:1125, 2003.
42. Guyuron B, Behmand RA. Nasal tip sutures part II: the interplays. Plast Reconstr Surg 112:1130, 2003.
43. Tebbetts JB. Shaping and positioning the nasal tip without structural disruption: a new systematic approach. Plast Reconstr Surg 94:61, 1994.
44. Rohrich RJ, Adams WP Jr. The boxy nasal tip: classification and management based on alar cartilage suturing techniques. Plast Reconstr Surg 107:1849; discussion 1864, 2001.
45. Tardy ME Jr, Cheng E. Transdomal suture refinement of the nasal tip. Facial Plast Surg 4:317, 1987.
46. Daniel RK. Rhinoplasty: creating an aesthetic tip. Plast Reconstr Surg 80:775, 1987.
47. Daniel RK. Rhinoplasty: a simplified, three-stitch, open tip suture technique. Part I: primary rhinoplasty. Plast Reconstr Surg 103:1491, 1999.
48. Guyuron B, Poggi JT, Michelow BJ. The subdomal graft. Plast Reconstr Surg 113:1037, 2004.
49. Lipsett E. A new approach to surgery of the lower cartilaginous vault. Arch Otolaryngol Head Neck Surg 70:52, 1959.
50. Gunter JP, Friedman RM. Lateral crural strut graft: technique and clinical applications in rhinoplasty. Plast Reconstr Surg 99:943, 1997.
51. Gruber RP, Nahai F, Bogdan MA, et al. Changing the convexity and concavity of nasal cartilages and cartilage grafts with horizontal mattress sutures: part II. Clinical results. Plast Reconstr Surg 115:595, 2005.
52. Janis J, Trussler A, Ghavami A. Lower lateral crural turnover flap in open rhinoplasty. Plast Reconstr Surg 123:1830, 2009.
53. Buyuklu F, Cakmak O, Hizal E, et al. Outfracture of the inferior turbinate: a computed tomography study. Plast Reconstr Surg 123:1704, 2009.
54. Lee DC, Jin SG, Kim BY, et al. Does the effect of inferior turbinate outfracture persist? Plast Reconstr Surg 139:386e, 2017.
55. Sinno S, Mehta K, Lee ZD, et al. Inferior turbinate hypertrophy in rhinoplasty: systematic review of surgical techniques. Plast Reconstr Surg 138:419e, 2016.
56. Faber C, Larson K, Amirlak B, Guyuron G. Use of desmopressin for unremitting epistaxis following septorhinoplasty and turbinectomy. Plast Reconstr Surg 128:728e, 2011.

46. Secondary Rhinoplasty

Richard Y. Ha, Lily Daniali, Cecilia Alejandra Garcia de Mitchell,
Bahman Guyuron

INDICATIONS
POSTOPERATIVE FUNCTIONAL OR AESTHETIC DEFORMITY
- Poor preoperative diagnosis
  - Failure to properly identify the structural problem resulting in functional compromise or aesthetic imbalance[1]
- Inappropriate surgical planning or inadequate technique resulting in distortion of supporting osteocartilaginous framework
- Problematic wound healing
  - Prolonged edema, ecchymosis, unfavorable scarring, obstructive or restrictive webbing, and occasionally hyperesthesia

PATIENT DISSATISFACTION
- Undesirable functional or aesthetic outcome
  - **Breathing difficulties** and **asymmetry** are most common complaints.[2]
- Inadequate preoperative counseling with regard to postoperative course, recovery time, desired and expected outcomes
- Unrealistic expectations
  - Even with appropriate preoperative counseling, some patients continue to have unrealistic expectations
  - If not identified, these patients will be dissatisfied with their results regardless of the outcome.[3,4]
- Postoperative deformity and patient dissatisfaction do not always correlate.

MOST COMMON DEFORMITIES OR PROBLEMS
- Displacement/deviation of anatomic structures
- Underresection by overly cautious surgeons
- Overresection by overly aggressive surgeons[5]
- Contour irregularities secondary to disruption of framework or unfavorable scarring
- Prosthetic complications including infection, extrusion, inflammation, palpability, or transillumination (e.g., in dorsal silicone implants)

SURGICAL OBSTACLES[6]

- Scarring of the subcutaneous tissues resulting in adherence to the underlying cartilaginous framework and destruction of tissue planes
- Osteocartilaginous distortion or damage requiring reconstruction for structural support
- Limited sources of cartilage grafts secondary to previous harvest of septal or conchal cartilage

CHANGES IN SKIN THICKNESS

- Thin skin in some patients, which is less forgiving of minor underlying deformities
  - Prone to graft extrusion
- Thick skin secondary to prolonged edema or scarring, which is less malleable and will not show desired framework changes as easily
- Compromised vascularity secondary to previous surgical incisions and scarring

SURGICAL APPROACHES

ENDONASAL/CLOSED APPROACH

- **Pros**
  - Decreased postoperative edema and scarring because limited dissection
- **Indications**
  - Isolated deformities that can be addressed independent of the overall framework
  - Severely scarred nose where vascularity is a significant concern

EXTERNAL/OPEN APPROACH

- *This is the preferred approach for secondary rhinoplasty.*[7]
- **Pros**
  - Provides maximal exposure for adequate visualization
  - Facilitates complete release of tissue attachments causing anatomic distortion
  - Facilitates precise diagnosis and correction of deformities under direct visualization
  - Allows direct hemostatic control
- **Cons**
  - Increased postoperative edema
- Placement of transcolumellar incision
  - If original scar is well hidden but at incorrect level of columella, ignore original scar and place second incision at appropriate location

PREOPERATIVE ASSESSMENT AND PLANNING

This is supplementary to the evaluation performed for a primary rhinoplasty, as presented in Chapter 45.

MEDICAL HISTORY

- All previous nasal surgeries
  - Obtain previous operative reports if possible to determine graft availability, presence of prosthetic material or hardware, and previous techniques or findings that may assist in evaluation and operative planning.

- History of trauma
- Allergies
- Cocaine/drug use
- Screen for **body dysmorphic disorder (BDD)** (see Chapter 1)
  - Mental disorder involving a distorted body image, defined as:
    - ▶ Preoccupation with an imagined physical deformity OR
    - ▶ Vastly exaggerated concern of a minimal physical deformity
  - **In 50% of patients with BDD, the nose is the primary complaint.**[8,9]
  - BDD occurs in secondary rhinoplasty consultations in about 12% of cases, and in 2%-7% of all primary cosmetic patient consultations.[8,9]
  - Plastic surgeons are often the first to encounter these patients; thus recognizing and addressing it are essential.
    - ▶ A **psychiatry consult** may be warranted.

CAUTION: Avoid reoperation in BDD patients.[10]

> **SENIOR AUTHOR TIP:** It is crucial to make sure that the secondary rhinoplasty patient's concerns are real and match what the surgeon sees in severity. Exaggerated concerns should be carefully assessed by asking the patient to rate the flaw on the scale of 1-10, 10 being the best. Disparity in rating beyond 3-4 points should be considered a red flag.

COMPREHENSIVE NASAL AND FACIAL ANALYSIS
- As described in the primary rhinoplasty chapter (Chapter 45), with special attention to common secondary deformities:
- **Bony pyramid**
  - Excessive narrowing or convexity
    - ▶ Secondary to inadequate alignment or splinting of bones after osteotomy
  - Irregularities/stairstep deformity
    - ▶ Because of unplanned fracture sites
  - Rocker deformity (Fig. 46-1)
    - ▶ Occurs from inadequate placement of medial osteotomy, resulting in a wide upper dorsum

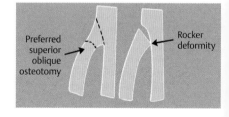

Fig. 46-1   Rocker deformity.

- **Midvault/upper lateral cartilages**
  - Asymmetry of dorsal aesthetic lines
  - Nasal deviation
  - Inverted-V deformity (Fig. 46-2)
    - ▶ Midvault collapse leading to visibility of the the caudal edge of the nasal bones
      - ◆ This edge or line forms an upside down or inverted V.
    - ▶ Results from overresection of the dorsal midvault and upper lateral cartilages or inadequate infracture of the nasal bones

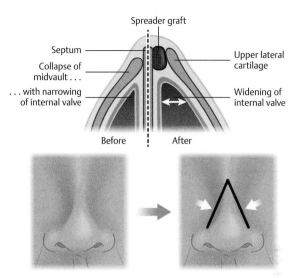

Fig. 46-2   Inverted-V deformity.

- Saddle nose deformity (Fig. 46-3)
  - ▶ Excessively depressed upper nasal and midvault regions secondary to overresection
- **Supratip area**
  - Polly beak deformity[11]
    - ▶ Convexity located just cephalad to the nasal tip
    - ▶ Secondary to overresection of the noncartilaginous caudal dorsum, underresection of the cartilaginous nasal dorsum and/or excessive scar formation in the dead space of the supratip area (Fig. 46-4)
- **Tip complex**[12,13]
  - Bulbous or boxy tip deformity
  - Pinched nasal tip deformity
    - ▶ Results from collapsed alar rims after disruption of lateral crural support

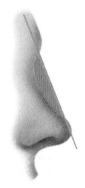

Fig. 46-3   Saddle nose deformity.

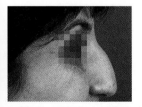

Fig. 46-4   Polly beak deformity. Postoperative profile view of a secondary rhinoplasty patient with a supratip deformity caused by both an underprojected tip and an underresected caudal dorsum.

- Loss of tip projection
  - ▶ From loss of tip support: Disruption of lower lateral cartilages (LLCs) and/or intercartilaginous attachments
- Overrotation
  - ▶ Obtuse nasolabial angle
- Asymmetry of tip-defining points
  - ▶ Secondary to inadequate placement of tip sutures or unrecognized damage to cartilage
- Infratip lobule
  - ▶ Excessive infratip lobule projection
    - ◆ From excessive length and buckling of middle crus or crura
  - ▶ Lack of definition
    - ◆ Middle crus too wide
  - ▶ Deformity may result from prominent caudal septum or obtuse septal angle.[14]

■ **Alae**
- Widened base
- Alar rim collapse resulting in impaired external valve competency (Fig. 46-5)
  - ▶ Loss of LLC integrity and failure to reconstruct framework at initial surgery
  - ▶ Clinically assessed by palpating preoperative resistance of alae to gentle compressive force
  - ▶ Weakness is useful for diagnosing either established or predisposition to alar collapse.
- Alar retraction
- Alar flaring
  - ▶ Widened base
- Notching
  - ▶ Secondary to inadequate placement or closure of previous incisions, scarring, and failure to place supporting grafts

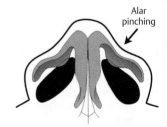

Alar pinching

Fig. 46-5   Alar rim collapse. Alar rim collapse caused by lack of lower lateral cartilage support.

■ **Columella**
- Retraction, deviation, and/or inferior bowing

■ **Intranasal**
- Airway occlusion most common underdiagnosed and untreated deformity in secondary rhinoplasty
  - ▶ Breathing difficulties most common complaint in patients presenting for revision[2]
- Septum
  - ▶ Deviation
  - ▶ Graft availability
- Turbinates
- Internal nasal valve competency
  - ▶ May have been medialized by osteotomy[15]

SENIOR AUTHOR TIP: History of septoplasty does not necessarily mean depletion of the cartilage in the septum. A thorough examination may result in discovery of sufficient cartilage in the septum.

FORMULATE TREATMENT PLAN

- Surgical approach
- Augmentation or resection
- Correction of distortion/displacement/irregularities
- Need for removal of prosthetic materials
- Source and quantity of structural graft materials
  - Rib cartilage
  - Ear cartilage
  - Septal cartilage
  - Iliac/calvarial bone
  - Alloplastic materials (controversial)
- Delay any secondary surgery for at least **12 months.**
  - Ensure maximal resolution of edema, scar maturation, and improved vascularity.
  - May consider early intervention within first **12 days** postoperatively only if gross abnormality present or significant technical error noted[16]
- Share preoperative analysis and treatment plan with patients.
  - Use visual imagery: Photos, computer imaging, or onlay tracing
  - Increases communication to establish realistic expectations and surgical goals

INFORMED CONSENT

NONSURGICAL TREATMENT

- Observation
- Injectable fillers for mild augmentation or contour irregularities

SURGICAL TREATMENT

- Open versus closed rhinoplasty

TECHNIQUE

- Reconstruction of the nasal osteocartilaginous framework is the foundation for successful secondary rhinoplasty.
- Keep in mind skin quality, graft availability, effects of scarring, and vascularity.

> **SENIOR AUTHOR TIP:** The most common reason for a residual caudal deviation after the primary and even secondary septorhinoplasty is failure to eliminate the redundant overlapping dislodged portion of the caudal anterior septum to allow repositioning the septum in the midline.

DISPLACED/DEVIATED ANATOMIC STRUCTURES

- **Nasal bones**
  - Secondary osteotomies to reposition
  - Occasional dorsal rasping to smooth contour
  - Postoperative external splint to maintain position

- **Midvault/septum**
  - Excise deviated bony or cartilaginous septum, maintaining L-strut for adequate support
  - Cartilage scoring to disrupt curving tendencies
  - Suture fixation to ensure placement
  - Spreader grafts: Unilateral or bilateral to maintain septal alignment, support upper lateral cartilages, and maintain integrity of internal nasal valve
  - Septoplasty
- **Tip**
  - Pinched tip
    - ► Alar spreader graft[17]
  - Bulbous or boxy tip
    - ► Refinement with interdomal and transdomal sutures
      - ◆ Keep in mind skin quality, because thick skin will require more dramatic framework changes to obtain the desired results.
    - ► Tip grafts
      - ◆ Can enhance definition and symmetry of tip-defining points when the lobule is small and suture refinement is insufficient
  - Deviated tip
    - ► Straighten caudal septum
      - ◆ Suture caudal septum to cartilage graft or nasal spine to maintain proper alignment.
      - ◆ Batten graft to provide necessary support and maintain position.
    - ► Columellar strut
      - ◆ Can be sutured to nasal spine or positioned with K-wire if greater strength needed
    - ► Infratip lobule
      - ◆ Excessive projection[14]: Medial crural sutures
      - ◆ Lack of definition: If broad middle crus with poor tip definition and asymmetry, consider partial resection of middle crus
      - ◆ May need to excise redundant caudal septum

UNDERRESECTION
- **Dorsal hump**
  - Component dorsal reduction (see Chapter 43)
- **Supratip**
  - Overfullness or polly beak deformity
  - A **differential height of 6-10 mm between tip and septum** must be present to have an appreciable supratip break for desirable results.[18]
  - Increase tip projection
    - ► Columellar strut
      - ◆ Septal cartilage graft if available
      - ◆ Rib cartilage if septum not available or if need more support

- ▶ Septal extension graft[18,19] (Fig. 46-6)
    - ◆ Spreader type
    - ◆ Batten type
    - ◆ Direct septal extension type

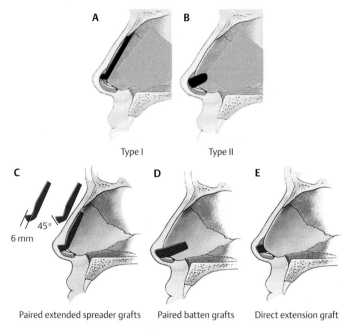

Fig. 46-6   Septal extension grafts. **A,** Septal extension graft type I. **B,** Septal extension graft type II. **C,** Spreader graft. **D,** Batten graft. **E,** Direct septal extension graft.

- ▶ Tip suturing
    - ◆ Transdomal
    - ◆ Interdomal
- ▶ Tip grafts if the lobule is small
    - ◆ Sheen shield graft[20]
    - ◆ Peck modified onlay graft[21,22]
- • Reduce dorsal septum further if the problem is an overprojected caudal dorsum.
- • Excessive scar tissue in the supratip area may be excised conservatively, keeping in mind potential vascular compromise.
- • If the skin in the supratip area is thick, a supratip suture from the subcutaneous tissue to the cartilage framework can be placed to increase definition in this area.[11]
- ■ **Tip**
    - • Persistent bulbous tip
    - • Cephalic trim
    - • Tip grafts
        - ▶ Sheen shield graft
        - ▶ Peck onlay tip graft

- Tip suturing
  - ► Transdomal
  - ► Interdomal
- **Alae**
  - Persistent hanging alae
  - Cephalic trim of the LLC
  - Marginal excision of soft tissue (controversial)
- **Soft tissue**
  - Excessive bulk
  - Debulking of tip, supratip, or alar soft tissues

SENIOR AUTHOR TIP: A columellar strut is used when the columella is short. A tip graft is used when the infratip volume is deficient. These should not be used interchangeably to restore tip projection.

CAUTION: This can be difficult and result in more scarring or prolonged edema with less predictable results. Be aware of further compromising vascularity.

OVERRESECTION
- **Dorsum**
  - Saddle nose or inverted-V deformity
  - Minor overresection requiring <3 mm augmentation for correction
    - ► Extended spreader grafts
  - Moderate to major overresection: Saddle nose or inverted-V deformity
  - Dorsal augmentation
    - ► Onlay rib graft
    - ► Septal cartilage grafts
      - ◆ A frame or V frame[7]
    - ► Cantilever bone grafts: Rib or split calvarial
    - ► Diced cartilage grafts wrapped in fascia
  - Revision nasal osteotomies
- **Midvault**
  - Internal nasal valve collapse and obstruction
    - ► Bilateral versus unilateral spreader grafts
      - ◆ Septal cartilage if available
- **Tip**
  - Short nose secondary to tip overrotation
    - ► Columellar strut graft
    - ► Extended spreader graft[18]
- **Alae**
  - Overzealous cephalic resection of the lateral crus or excessive tip suturing
  - Alar retraction
    - ► **Mild:** Minimal vestibular lining loss and at least 3 mm of residual LLC rim
      - ◆ This is an indication for an alar contour graft (ACG)[23] (Fig. 46-7)

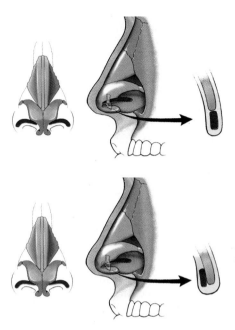

Fig. 46-7 Alar contour graft. A key element is proper placement and shape of the alar contour graft immediately above the alar rim and spanning the alar notched area.

- ▶ **Moderate:** Alar spreader graft or lateral crural strut graft[17]
- ▶ **Severe:** Significant skin or lining deficiency
  - ◆ Composite auricular cartilage graft is indicated for reconstruction of this multilayer defect.
  - ◆ May need intercartilaginous graft to span space between upper and LLCs and thus lengthen nasal sidewall as described by Gruber et al[24] (Fig. 46-8)
  - ◆ V-Y advancement described by Guyuron[15]
- • External nasal valve collapse: Secondary to weak or malpositioned LLC
  - ▶ Alar cartilage graft, alar spreader graft, or lateral crural strut graft
- • Notching
  - ▶ Alar cartilage graft: Can be used both to treat or prevent notching

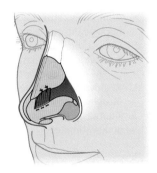

Fig. 46-8 Intercartilaginous graft. Insertion of a septal graft into the gap between the upper lateral cartilage and the lateral crus element. The cephalic end of it is sutured end-to-end to the upper lateral cartilage. The caudal end slips under (deep to) the edge of the lateral crus element.

> **SENIOR AUTHOR TIP:** It is crucial to eliminate the dead space after removal of any fibrofatty tissues from the supratip area using a supratip suture.

CONTOUR IRREGULARITIES

- Rasp mild bony deformities
- Secondary osteotomies for severe bony asymmetries
- Remove or replace displaced or partially resorbed tip or other visible grafts.
    - Onlay crushed cartilage for mild contour irregularities
- Mild irregularities can be corrected with injection of hyaluronic acid or calcium hydroxyapatite gel fillers.
    - Avoid particulate-based fillers, because the effects cannot be reversed with hyaluronidase if soft tissue ischemia occurs after injection.[25]
- Biologic skin substitutes (e.g., AlloDerm, LifeCell) can help to camouflage mild irregularities in patients with thin skin.[26]

PROSTHETIC COMPLICATIONS

- **Deviation**
    - *Most common alloplastic cause of revision rhinoplasty*[27]
        - ► From asymmetry or overdissection of the implant pocket
    - Correction: Removal of implant and surrounding capsule (as much as possible without damaging soft tissue envelope), correction of any untreated underlying nasal deviation, and use of autologous grafting techniques
- **Infection**
    - Antibiotic therapy for cellulitis and early removal of implant if infection persists
- **Extrusion, palpability, visibility**
    - Commonly caused by implant extension into tip with no intervening layer between implant and overlying soft tissue envelope
    - Correction: Removal of implant and augmentation of tip with autologous tissue only
        - ► Revision rhinoplasty to correct implant complications often requires removal of the prosthetic material.
    - Removal of the implant will uncover substantial underlying cartilage and bony atrophy.
- Amount of autologous graft material necessary for correction of deformity should not be underestimated.[27]

GRAFTS IN SECONDARY RHINOPLASTY

- **Autologous grafts** are preferred over alloplastic material because of the lower risk of infection or extrusion.
- To reconstruct the nasal osteocartilaginous framework, desirable grafts are those with **low resorption rates** and **adequate strength.**
- **Five potential donor sites** for autologous grafts in secondary rhinoplasty:
    - Iliac bone graft
        - ► Rarely used
        - ► Difficult to handle and unpredictable resorption

- Calvarial bone graft
  - ▶ Similar to iliac bone graft
- Auricular cartilage
  - ▶ Used occasionally as source of onlay grafting or reinforcement
  - ▶ Lacks sufficient rigidity for framework reconstruction[28]
- Septal cartilage
  - ▶ Preferred source because of location and strength. There is no significant donor site morbidity, and harvest does not require a separate incision site.
  - ▶ However, it is frequently inadequate because previously harvested or damaged
- Rib cartilage[29]
  - ▶ *Graft of choice in secondary rhinoplasty when septal cartilage unavailable*
  - ▶ Advantages: Abundance, versatility, adequate strength for necessary support
  - ▶ Harvest: Usually use **ninth** or **tenth** rib, because of ease of harvest and sufficient length and shape of cartilaginous portion
    - ◆ Use of fifth, sixth, or seventh rib for alternative approach[30]
    - ◆ Straight, long cartilaginous segment
    - ◆ Allows camouflage of incision several millimeters superior to the inframammary fold in female patients

DISADVANTAGES
- Additional donor site incision
  - In women the incision can be placed under the breast to be less conspicuous.
- Postoperative pain
  - Often relieved by injecting long-lasting local anesthetic into the donor site at the end of the operation
  - Some advocate using pain pumps.
- Risk of pneumothorax
  - Usually injury to parietal pleura only, not lung parenchyma
  - If detected, place red rubber catheter into cavity, close incision in layers, and remove catheter with suction while providing positive pressure ventilation.
    - ▶ Follow up with a postoperative upright radiograph.
- Potential to warp
  - K-wires may be placed through the graft to prevent distortion.
- Ossification in older patients
  - Some advocate a limited CT scan to evaluate cartilage availability in these patients.
  - Limited CT scan of ribs and sternum to evaluate cartilage availability
  - If extensive ossification renders autologous rib cartilage unusable, **irradiated donor cartilage** may be required.

POSTOPERATIVE CARE AND FOLLOW-UP
- Care is similar to that of primary rhinoplasty, with a few exceptions:
  - **Resolution of edema** may take much **longer.**
    - ▶ Patients should be counseled about this preoperatively and postoperatively.
    - ▶ Taping to address specific areas may be beneficial.
  - **Excessive scarring** may be treated with **steroid injections** in the subcutaneous tissues, avoiding the dermis.

SURGICAL COMPLICATIONS

MAJOR
- Devascularization of nasal tissue
- Infection
- Graft or implant resorption, loss, deviation, or extrusion
- Airway obstruction secondary to internal or external nasal valve collapse

MINOR
- Contour irregularity
- Soft tissue scarring

INCIDENCE
- Higher incidence of complications with increasing number of revision surgeries

COMMON TREATMENTS
- Implant removal if persistent infection
  - Autologous augmentation
- After soft tissue recovery from surgery (up to a year), consider revision surgery using previously described techniques.
  - Counsel patients to set appropriate expectations.
  - Use most supportive autologous cartilage available: rib cartilage.

TOP TAKEAWAYS
➤ The key requirements for successful secondary rhinoplasty are adequate preoperative evaluation and reconstruction of the nasal osseocartilaginous framework.
➤ Screen for BDD and avoid reoperating on these patients.
➤ Delay secondary surgery for at least 12 months from the last surgery.
➤ Five surgical obstacles in secondary rhinoplasty are scarring, framework disruption, limited graft donor sites, excessively thin or thick skin, and compromised vascularity.
➤ External or open rhinoplasty is the preferred approach to secondary rhinoplasty.
➤ Rib cartilage graft is the preferred donor material for secondary rhinoplasty.
➤ Postoperatively, resolution of edema may take much longer than after a primary rhinoplasty. Counsel patients accordingly.

REFERENCES
1. Constantian MB. Four common anatomic variants that predispose to unfavorable rhinoplasty results: a study based on 150 consecutive secondary rhinoplasties. Plast Reconstr Surg 105:316; discussion 332, 2005.
2. Lee M, Zwiebel S, Guyuron B. Frequency of the preoperative flaws and commonly required maneuvers to correct them: a guide to reducing the revision rhinoplasty rate. Plast Reconstr Surg 132:769, 2013.
3. Guyuron B, Bokhari F. Patient satisfaction following rhinoplasty. Aesthetic Plast Surg 20:153, 1996.

4. Gruber RP, Roberts C, Schooler W, et al. Preventing postsurgical dissatisfaction syndrome after rhinoplasty with propranolol: a pilot study. Plast Reconstr Surg 123:1072, 2009.
5. Gubisch W, Eichhorn-Sens J. Overresection of the lower lateral cartilages: a common conceptual mistake with functional and aesthetic consequences. Aesthetic Plast Surg 33:6, 2009.
6. Byrd HS, Constantian MB, Guyuron B, et al. Revision rhinoplasty. Aesthet Surg J 27:175, 2007.
7. Gunter JP, Rohrich RJ. External approach for secondary rhinoplasty. Plast Reconstr Surg 80:161, 1987.
8. Constantian MB. Identify BDD patients prior to rhinoplasty. Cosmetic Surgery Times, June 2001.
9. Constantian MB. Emotional matters. Presented at the Rhinoplasty Symposium at the Annual Meeting of the American Society for Aesthetic Plastic Surgery, New York, April 2007.
10. Sarwer DB, Wadden TA, Pertschuk MJ, et al. Body image dissatisfaction and body dysmorphic disorder in 100 cosmetic surgery patients. Plast Reconstr Surg 101:1644, 1998.
11. Guyuron B, DeLuca L, Lash R. Supratip deformity: a closer look. Plast Reconstr Surg 105:1140, 2000.
12. Constantian MB. The boxy nasal tip, the ball tip, and alar cartilage malposition: variations on a theme—a study in 200 consecutive primary and secondary rhinoplasty patients. Plast Reconstr Surg 116:268, 2005.
13. Constantian MB. The two essential elements for planning tip surgery in primary and secondary rhinoplasty: observations based on review of 100 consecutive patients. Plast Reconstr Surg 114:1571; discussion 1582, 2004.
14. Rohrich RJ, Liu JH. Defining the infratip lobule in rhinoplasty: anatomy, pathogenesis of abnormalities and correction using an algorithmic approach. Plast Reconstr Surg 130:1148, 2012.
15. Guyuron B. Nasal osteotomy and airway changes. Plast Reconstr Surg 102:856, 1998.
16. Gruber RP. Early surgical intervention after rhinoplasty. Aesthet Surg J 21:549, 2001.
17. Gunter JP, Rohrich RJ. Correction of the pinched nasal tip with alar spreader grafts. Plast Reconstr Surg 90:821, 1992.
18. Byrd HS, Andochick S, Copit S, et al. Septal extension grafts: a method of controlling tip projection shape. Plast Reconstr Surg 100:999, 1997.
19. Ha RY, Byrd HS. Septal extension grafts revisited: 6-year experience in controlling nasal tip projection and shape. Plast Reconstr Surg 112:1929, 2003.
20. Sheen JH. Tip graft: a 20-year retrospective. Plast Reconstr Surg 91:48, 1993.
21. Peck GC. The difficult nasal tip. Clin Plast Surg 1:478, 1975.
22. Peck GC. The onlay graft for nasal tip projection. Plast Reconstr Surg 71:27, 1983.
23. Rohrich RJ, Raniere J Jr, Ha RY. The alar contour graft: correction and prevention of alar rim deformities in rhinoplasty. Plast Reconstr Surg 109:2495; discussion 2506, 2002.
24. Gruber RP, Kryger G, Chang D. The intercartilaginous graft for actual and potential alar retraction. Plast Reconstr Surg 121:288e, 2008.
25. Kurkjian TJ, Ahmad J, Rohrich RJ. Soft-tissue fillers in rhinoplasty. Plast Reconstr Surg 133:121e, 2014.
26. Gryskiewicz JM, Rohrich RJ, Reagan BJ. The use of AlloDerm for the correction of nasal contour deformities. Plast Reconstr Surg 107:561; discussion 571, 2001.
27. Won TB, Jin H. Revision rhinoplasty in Asians. Ann Plast Surg 65:379, 2010.
28. Lee MR, Callahan S, Cochran S. Auricular cartilage: harvest and versatility in rhinoplasty. Am J Otolaryngol 32:547, 2011.
29. Marin VP, Landecker A, Gunter JP. Harvesting rib cartilage grafts for secondary rhinoplasty. Plast Reconstr Surg 121:1442, 2008.
30. Cochran CS, Gunter JP. Secondary rhinoplasty and the use of autogenous rib cartilage grafts. Clin Plast Surg 37:371, 2010.

47. Ethnic Rhinoplasty

Paul N. Afrooz, Dean M. Toriumi

- Rhinoplasty is becoming increasingly more common in nonwhite patients worldwide.
- Most patients desire an improvement in their appearance, with preservation of certain ethnic features.
  - This is accomplished through a highly individualized approach involving recognition of anatomic variations, familiarity with cultural aesthetics, an understanding of patients' preferences.
- **Surgical objectives include:**
  - Nasofacial harmony
  - Symmetry of the brow-tip aesthetic line
  - Appropriate dorsal line shape
  - Appropriate tip projection, rotation, and definition
  - Appropriate base width and alar flare
  - Functional breathing

PREOPERATIVE EVALUATION

- Patient consultation with discussion of aesthetic preferences and cultural concerns. Assess patient expectations and preferences, and determine whether the goal is for **Westernization of features** versus **maintenance of natural characteristics.**
- Complete problem specific and surgical history; history may greatly alter surgical plan
  - Trauma or prior nasal or sinus surgery
  - Previous alloplastic implant
  - Injectable fillers in the nose
  - Functional complaints
- Physical examination
  - Palpation of cartilaginous and bony structure, dynamic inspiration, endoscopy
- Standardized photography (frontal, lateral, three-quarter, basal views)[1] (see Chapter 3)
- Three-dimensional stereophotogrammetry facilitates objective comparison of preoperative and postoperative results.
- Digital image-morphing software[2,3] allows direct communication of proposed changes to all parameters (dorsal height, nasal length, tip rotation/projection, and base width). Patients may comment on desired modifications based on the morphed image.

> **TIP:**   The use of a computer-imaging program can demonstrate potential changes preoperatively and aid in communication between patients and surgeons regarding expectations and possible outcomes.[4]

- Facial analysis to assess for variation from the nonwhite aesthetic "norm." Similar differences exist among people of same ethnic group.
    - Recognition of each facial feature and how it relates to the nose is critical to achieve nasofacial harmony.
        - Forehead slope/glabellar prominence
        - Nasofrontal angle
        - Intercanthal distance
        - Upper lip length and contour
        - Premaxillary position
        - Dentition
        - Chin position

INFORMED CONSENT

- List exact procedure, including all planned types of grafts.
- Location and laterality of harvest site
- Possibility of banking unused cartilage behind the ear
- Alternatives to surgery
- Potential complications, including donor site morbidity and need for further surgery

PREPARATION

ANATOMIC VARIATIONS[5-9]

- Skin is usually **thicker,** more **sebaceous,** and relatively **inelastic** in ethnic patients.
- Fibrofatty layer is also thicker (2-4 mm) and more prominent over the lower lateral cartilages and between the medial crura. It plays a significant role in **lack of tip definition.** The soft tissue facet is often obtuse and filled with fat.

> **SENIOR AUTHOR TIP:**   Thick skin often requires making the nose larger (more projection) to stretch the envelope and allow underlying structure to provide definition.
>
> Thinning of the skin and soft tissue envelope is often necessary in ethnic patients. Fat is evenly removed from the undersurface while taking care to preserve the subdermal plexus.

- Alar base usually has an increased base width with insertion lateral to the medial canthal lines. There is excess flaring where the alae extend **more than 2 mm** lateral to the alar-facial groove.
- A wide spectrum of dorsal morphology exists (low height in black and Asian nose, hump in Middle Eastern nose). Nasal bone length can also vary widely (Table 47-1).

> **TIP:** Weak cartilaginous structure can lead to a more pronounced effect on tissue healing. This highlights the importance in creating strong support for long-term results.

Table 47-1   *Specific Ethnic Characteristics*

Ethnicity	Characteristics
Black nose	Short nasal bones Wide nose Low dorsum Wide bimalar distance Horizontally oriented nostrils, wide base Deficient premaxilla Limited septal cartilage
Asian nose	Thick sebaceous skin Low dorsum Weak lower lateral cartilage Less septal cartilage Deficient premaxilla Wide nasal base Retracted columella
Middle Eastern nose	Long nasal bones Low radix Large hump Hanging columella Septal deviation
Hispanic nose (types described by Daniel[10])	**Type I (Castilian):** Normal radix height, high bridge, normal tip projection **Type II (Mexican American)—most common:** Low radix height, near-normal bridge, dependent tip **Type III (Mestizo):** Broad base, thick skin, wide tip **Type IV (Creole)—predominantly black features:** Broad, flat lower third, short columella, transversely oriented nostrils, flaring alae

GRAFTING MATERIAL (see Chapter 27)

- Nasal septum, auricular cartilage
- Costal cartilage[11] is stronger; therefore it can be cut thinner with less bulk in the nose. It has a lower vascular demand making it less likely to resorb. Surgeons are able to harvest a larger volume of material. Pain at donor site is decreased (compared to the ear) because less cautery is used.

> **TIP:** Disadvantages to costal cartilage harvest (increased operative time, warping, and donor site morbidity) are minimized with experience.

- Bone grafts include iliac bone and split calvarial grafts.
- Irradiated rib may also be an option.

- Types of allografts include: Silicone, ePTFE, and porous polyethylene.
  - **Advantages:**
    - ▶ Ease of use
    - ▶ No additional surgical site
    - ▶ Minimal change in operative time
  - **Disadvantages:**
    - ▶ Increased lifetime risk of infection
    - ▶ Displacement/extrusion
    - ▶ Thinning of skin over implant site
    - ▶ Implant translucency and pain

TIP: Structural grafting can lead to nasal stiffness, which should be discussed with the patient during the initial consultation.

TECHNIQUE

PREOPERATIVE PLANNING

- General anesthesia with oral endotracheal intubation for airway protection from blood and secretions; also allows costal cartilage harvest if indicated
- Local anesthetic (1% lidocaine with 1:100,000 epinephrine) is injected before prepping and draping. This allows ample time for vasoconstriction. Injection also creates hydrostatic dissection for ease of elevation of mucoperichondrial flaps. Surgeons assess amount of available bony and septal cartilage by needle palpation at this time.
- Infection prophylaxis with first-generation cephalosporin and fluoroquinolone if costal or auricular cartilage to be harvested. The entire face and intranasal area are prepared with dilute povidone-iodine, and the patient is draped to maintain sterility throughout the procedure. If cartilage is to be harvested, surgeons must change gloves to prevent contamination.

OPENING THE NOSE

- Columellar (inverted-V, stairstep) incision made with a No. 11 blade. If deprojection is planned, incision is placed closer to tip lobule (below top of nostrils) (Fig. 47-1). For patients requiring increased projection, incision should be slightly below mid-columellar level and not close to the upper lip.

- Bilateral marginal incisions made with a No. 15 blade and connected to the extension of the columellar incision

- Tip exposure with sharp dissection (Converse scissors). *Avoid injury to soft tissue triangles, because they are difficult to repair.* Three-point retraction with sharp two-prong retractors is used to aid in dissection over the lower lateral cartilages.

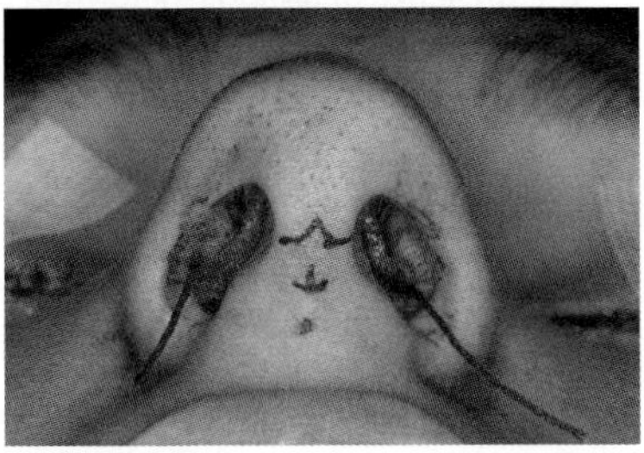

Fig. 47-1   Varying inverted-V columellar incision. Placed closer than normal to the tip lobule as the surgeon plans to deproject the nose.

- Dorsal exposure and elevation of periosteum over the nasal bones using a Joseph elevator. The extent depends on plan for augmentation/reduction/osteotomies.

- Septal exposure can be through a separate Killian incision or through lateral retraction and dissection between the medial crura. Raising bilateral mucoperichondrial flaps is important.
- Septal cartilage harvested after the upper third of the nose is addressed to prevent destabilization. A cartilaginous L-strut of **at least 10 mm** is preserved to ensure adequate support.

SENIOR AUTHOR TIP: Sharp dissection while opening the nose helps to preserve the subdermal plexus and prevent excessive swelling that occurs with tearing of the tissue during blunt dissection.

By limiting blunt dissection over the nasal dorsum, a tight subperiosteal pocket is preserved in anticipation of a secure dorsal augmentation graft.

Once the nose is open, the surgeon should evaluate the structural and contour deficiencies to plan for all subsequent grafts.

MANAGEMENT OF THE BONY VAULT

- Osteotomies are used to narrow the dorsum or to correct deviations or dorsal hump.[4] They are performed medial to lateral. Osteotomies should be avoided if major dorsal augmentation (large dorsal graft >3 mm in height) is planned to prevent tubular appearance and narrow-to-narrow look of the dorsum.

MANAGEMENT OF THE MIDDLE THIRD

- Spreader grafts increase the area of the internal nasal valve and provide foundation to prevent saddling and postoperative rotation/shortening. They also work to lengthen a short nose or retracted columella. Unilateral placement of a spreader graft is used to straighten the nose.
- Extended spreader grafts are typically 20-40 mm long, 4-6 mm wide, and 1-3 mm thick. If a strong L-strut exists, spreader grafts can be fashioned from curved cartilage. The presence of a saddle deformity or weak L-strut requires strong and straight grafts. They are placed between the divided upper lateral cartilages and the septum. They can also go in submucosal pockets in cases where the midvault is not opened. This helps to increase the internal nasal valve angle.
- To correct a concave midvault sidewall, surgeons may use multiple spreader grafts, batten grafts, or an onlay graft.

TIP: If curvature of the proposed spreader graft is a concern, place the concave sides toward the septum to prevent future asymmetry.

- Upper lateral cartilages must be secured to septum to prevent inverted-V deformity and pinching of the internal valve. Placement of a clocking suture can adjust for tilt in a crooked nose.

MANAGEMENT OF THE NASAL BASE

- Symmetry is evaluated from the head of the bed.
- The caudal septum is reset to midline with swinging-door maneuver or by shifting the nasal spine. This can be achieved with a 5 mm straight osteotome placed at a slight angle toward desired position. Once engaged, the osteotome acts as a lever to shift the spine. The septum or graft is secured to fibrous tissue lateral to the spine with a 4-0 PDS suture. Monitoring for change in dorsal line and projection after this maneuver is essential.
- The base is stabilized with a floating columellar strut, fixed/extended columellar strut, or a caudal septal extension graft (Fig. 47-2, A).
  - Caudal septal extension grafts increase tip projection to stretch amorphous skin and lengthen the short nose/retracted columella.
  - The grafts can be secured to septum end to end and flanked by[12,13] extended spreader grafts, slivers of cartilage, or 0.25 mm perforated PDS plates (Fig. 47-2, B and C).
  - Caudal septal replacement grafts also increase tip projection to stretch amorphous skin and often use less cartilage than when attempting to straighten a severely deviated L-strut[14] (Fig. 47-2, D).

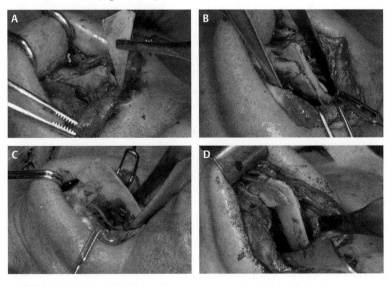

Fig. 47-2 **A,** Caudal septal extension graft. **B,** Graft secured with extended spreader grafts and slivers of cartilage. **C,** Graft secured with 0.25 mm perforated PDS plates. **D,** Caudal septal replacement graft.

TIP: Caudal septal extension/replacement grafts are the only cartilage grafts in structure rhinoplasty that must be straight. Septal cartilage may be preferred over costal cartilage in this case.

TIP: Caudal septal extension grafts or caudal septal replacement grafts are preferred, because they minimize postoperative loss of tip projection and help to control rotation and length.

DORSAL GRAFTING

- The **degree of augmentation** dictates grafting material used. Septal cartilage is used for small changes and costal cartilage for significant augmentation. Auricular cartilage is less favorable because of contour irregularities and potential to resorb.
- Serial carving with repeated soaking and drying will allow curvature to declare itself.

> **TIP:**   Apply cross-hatching and splinting techniques to modify identified tendencies of the cartilage to warp. Grafts should be placed concave side down (Fig. 47-3). Smoothing all edges of the graft and tapering cartilage for seamless transition at radix and supratip are essential. Perichondrium should be used to camouflage the transition of the graft.

- Three-point fixation of the graft is performed after the tip position has been set. A tight pocket at the cephalic edge of the dissection cavity (over nasal dorsum) is created. The cortical bone of the nasal dorsum is "roughened" while a segment of perichondrium is interposed between it and the cartilage graft to create an ossifying scar, accomplished through one of two methods:
  - To roughen the cortical bone and expose cancellous bone, 8-10 vertical perforations are made in the nasal bones using a 2 mm straight osteotome or the dorsum is rasped slightly.
- 5-0 PDS suture is placed bilaterally through the lower lateral aspect of the graft to the upper lateral cartilage as the second and third points of fixation.

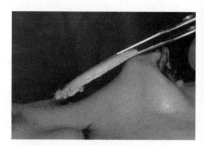

Fig. 47-3   Dorsal graft orientation. Placed with concave side down. If concave side is up, warping can occur resulting in fullness in the radix and supratip.

TIP CONTOURING[15]

- The medial crura are secured to the septal replacement or extension graft with a 4-0 plain gut suture on a straight (SC-1) needle. Several 5-0 PDS sutures are used to firmly attach the medial and intermediate crura to the septal extension graft. The medial crura are widely dissected to release and advance anteriorly on the caudal septal extension graft to create a more obtuse nasolabial angle and increase nasal tip projection.
- A shield graft is used to increase projection in thick-skinned patients for appropriate tip definition. The position of the graft augments the infratip and changes projection. Soft tissue can be placed over the shield graft to help camouflage the graft and prevent visibility (Fig. 47-4).

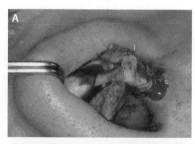

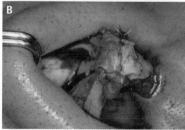

Fig. 47-4   A, Lateral crural grafts and tip shield graft, sutured in place. **B,** Perichondrium camouflages the graft edges.

- Tip onlay grafts are used when no change to the infratip is needed. Change in position and thickness alters projection, tip width, refinement, and supratip break. Soft material is preferred to prevent tip bossae.
- Lateral crural grafts (onlay) prevent alar collapse and control overrotation. They also prevent visibility of the shield graft. The surgeon bevels the cartilage at 45 degrees and attaches it to the posterior edge of the shield graft.
- Tip bulbosity can be corrected through alteration of the dome and the use of lateral crural strut grafts.
  - A dome suture is placed to flatten the domes, and interdomal sutures help with further narrowing.
  - Lateral crural strut grafts flatten convexity. The surgeon dissects the vestibular skin from the undersurface of lateral crura and creates a pocket extending toward the piriform aperture in same vector as the lateral crura. The medial edge of graft is beveled at 45 degrees and tucked into the dome apex. The graft is placed along cephalic edge of lower lateral cartilage. The concave side faces the airway to prevent nasal obstruction as a result of delayed warping. Graft dimensions are usually 25-30 mm by 4-5 mm by 1-2 mm.
- Malpositioned lateral crura and alar retraction are corrected through repositioning of asymmetrical or cephalically oriented lateral crura[16] (Fig. 47-5). Dissection of the lateral crura is the same as that mentioned previously, but the surgeon divides the lateral aspect of lower lateral cartilage at the areas of the sesamoid cartilage. Pockets are created in the most favorable vector for the patient.

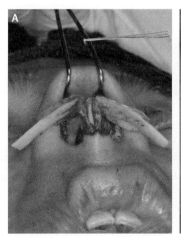 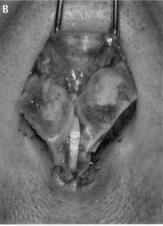

Fig. 47-5   A, Lateral crural strut grafts with repositioning. **B,** New, favorable orientation.

- The external valve is stabilized with alar batten grafts and alar rim grafts.
- Batten grafts strengthen the sidewall, especially if the lateral crura are repositioned. They also serve to improve asymmetries in the brow-tip aesthetic line.
- Alar rim grafts are used to smooth the transition between the tip lobule and alar lobule. They prevent valve collapse and pinching of the tip over time. They are placed by creating a small pocket immediately caudal to the marginal incision. The surgeon should taper the ends of the graft to prevent visibility (Fig. 47-6).

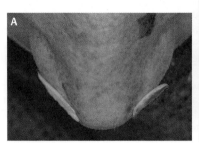
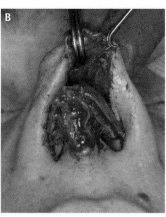

Fig. 47-6 A, Alar rim grafts before placement. **B,** Left alar rim graft placed in pocket caudal to the marginal incision.

> **TIP:** An individualized approach is crucial to tip management in ethnic patients. Repositioning of the lateral crus may be effective for flared nostrils caused by large convex lower lateral cartilages in Middle Eastern patients but may worsen the appearance in Asian patients with weak lower lateral cartilages and hanging alar lobules.

CLOSURE

- A single subcuticular 6-0 Monocryl suture in the midline of the collumelar incision is placed to relieve tension and align the skin/soft tissue envelope. This is followed by interrupted 7-0 nylon vertical mattress suture in at least seven places along the incision for slight eversion of the skin edges. The skin edge is further approximated with simple interrupted 6-0 fast-absorbing gut suture.

> **TIP:** In darker-skinned patients, the use of absorbable sutures will result in prolonged erythema and possible suture tracking.

- Marginal incisions are reapproximated with interrupted 5-0 chromic gut sutures. Ensuring the suture does not alter the alar margin is critical. If notching occurs, the surgeon may need a composite graft to address vestibular lining deficiency.
- Septal mucoperichondrial flaps are secured in place with 4-0 plain gut suture on a straight septal needle in running mattress fashion.
- Radiopaque 0.25 mm septal splints are placed if turbinate work is performed to prevent synechiae formation.
- Lateral wall splints[17] are placed if lateral crural strut grafts were used to ensure redraping of vestibular mucosa. They are fashioned from 0.25 mm bivalve splints.
- Tape is applied to the external nose before placement of a cast to protect skin.

> **SENIOR AUTHOR TIP:** I place a thermoplastic splint. This allows placement of adhesive remover through holes before removal.

BASE REDUCTIONS

- Performed after closure is complete. This provides the greatest potential to leave irreversible deformity if not done correctly.
- Types include internal alar base reduction used for treatment of the overlying large nostril and excessive nostril sill. External alar base reduction is needed in patients with excessive alar flare. Sliding alar flap involves the excision of both the nostril sill and alar lobule with medialization of the ala. This is employed for excess sill and flare. A cinching suture is placed as an adjunctive maneuver in patients with persistent alar base width.
- **Key steps to success**
  - Plan incision slightly adjacent to alar/facial or alar/vestibular junction.
  - Forego injecting local anesthetic, because it may deform anatomy.
  - Avoid all cautery.
  - Slightly bevel incisions to promote eversion of skin edges.
  - Close incisions meticulously.

> **TIP:** If performing a base reduction is questionable, the surgeon should defer this irreversible technique. The decision to forgo base reduction and possibly return at a later date should not be faulted.

POSTOPERATIVE CARE

- Oral second-generation cephalosporin is prescribed for 1 week and antibiotic soaks for 2 weeks postoperatively.
- Pain control is primarily with acetaminophen with narcotic prescription given for breakthrough pain. Patients are instructed to avoid aspirin- and ibuprofen-containing medications to decrease risk of epistaxis.
- Cast, splints, tape, and columellar sutures are removed about 1 week postoperatively. If base reduction is performed, sutures remain in place until postoperative day 10-14.
- Discharge instructions include: maintaining head elevation, consuming a low salt diet, using incentive spirometry if costal cartilage was harvested, and refraining from strenuous activity and heavy lifting for 1 month postoperatively.
- Lifelong follow-up and photodocumentation of results is critical to monitor for possible future change and to determine whether further intervention is indicated.

COMPLICATIONS

- Infection is managed aggressively to prevent graft resorption. These patients usually return to the operating room for washout and placement of drains. Broad-spectrum antibiotic coverage is crucial.
- Scarring is a potential complication. History of keloid formation should be determined. They are less likely to form on the face and are managed with massage and steroids.
- A widened scar is more probable if significant augmentation and stretch was required. This highlights the importance of the dermal suture at columellar incision.
- Visible grafts and warping should be managed during the initial procedure. Surgeons can determine the direction of warping with serial carving of the graft material and by allowing cartilage to soak and dry several times throughout the case for natural curvature to declare itself. Surgeons should be familiar with **cross-hatching** and **splinting** to minimize future warping.
- Asymmetry can occur after base reduction.

TOP TAKEAWAYS
➤ Knowledge of anatomic variations and differing aesthetic ideals is crucial to successful ethnic rhinoplasty.
➤ Patients' cosmetic concerns should be addressed while maintaining racial congruencies, if desired.
➤ Strong tip support mechanisms are established to increase projection while controlling rotation and length.
➤ Tip contouring techniques in ethnic patients vary from those used in whites.
➤ Costal cartilage harvest is often required for appropriate augmentation of the dorsum and tip.

REFERENCES

1. Afrooz PN, Amirlak B. Digital imaging and standardized photography. In Rohrich RJ, Adams WP Jr, Gunter JP, eds. Dallas Rhinoplasty: Nasal Surgery by the Masters, ed 3. New York: Thieme Publishers, 2014.
2. Dixon TK, Caughlin BP, Manaretto N, Toriumi DM. Three-dimensional evaluation of unilateral cleft rhinoplasty results. Facial Plast Surg 29:106, 2013.
3. Toriumi DM, Dixon TK. Assessment of rhinoplasty techniques by overlay of before-and-after 3D images. Facial Plast Surg Clin North Am 19:711, 2011.
4. Toriumi DM, Pero CD. Asian rhinoplasty. Clin Plast Surg 37:335, 2010.
5. Rohrich RJ, Muzaffar AR. Rhinoplasty in the African-American patient. Plast Reconstr Surg 111:1322; discussion 1340, 2013.
6. Kontis TC, Papel ID. Rhinoplasty on the African-American nose. Aesthetic Plast Surg 26(Suppl 1):S12, 2002.
7. Rohrich RJ, Ghavami A. Rhinoplasty for Middle Eastern noses. Plast Reconstr Surg 123:1343, 2009.
8. Bizrah MB. Rhinoplasty for Middle Eastern patients. Facial Plast Surg Clin North Am 10:381, 2002.
9. Beheri GE. Rhinoplasty in Egyptians. Aesthetic Plast Surg 8:145, 1984.
10. Daniel RK. Hispanic rhinoplasty in the United States, with emphasis on the Mexican American nose. Plast Reconstr Surg 112:244; discussion 257, 2003.
11. Toriumi DM, Asher SA. Primary rhinoplasty techniques: use of costal cartilage. In Cobo R, ed. Ethnic Considerations in Facial Plastic Surgery. New York: Thieme Publishers, 2015.
12. Park JH, Jin HR. Use of autologous costal cartilage in Asian rhinoplasty. Plast Reconstr Surg 130:1338, 2013.
13. Swanepoel PF, Fysh R. Laminated dorsal beam graft to eliminate postoperative twisting complications. Arch Facial Plast Surg 9:285, 2007.
14. Toriumi DM. Subtotal septal reconstruction: an update. Facial Plast Surg 29:492, 2013.
15. Toriumi DM. New concepts in nasal tip contouring. Arch Facial Plast Surg 8:42, 2006.
16. Gunter JP, Friedman RM. Lateral crural strut graft: technique and clinical applications in rhinoplasty. Plast Reconstr Surg 99:943; discussion 953, 1997.
17. Losquardro WD, Bared A, Toriumi DM. Correction of the retracted alar base. Facial Plast Surg 28:218, 2012.

48. Lip Augmentation

Michael Larsen, Robert K. Sigal

DEFINITION OF PROBLEM

THE AGING LIP
- Collagen framework loosens, dermis thins, orbicularis oris thins and loses curve, redistribution of volume, cumulative solar damage
- Contrary to previous teaching, there is **not** a loss of volume but **a redistribution from thickness to length.**[1,2]
- Resultant stigmata
  - Philtral flattening
  - Vermilion border flattening
  - Decreased pout
  - Cheiloptosis (elongated cutaneous upper lip)
  - Inverted vermilion (results in thin vermilion)
  - Minimal dental show
  - Attenuation and loss of Cupid's bow curvature
  - Downward tilt of oral commissures
  - Perioral wrinkle
- Congenital variations
  - Hypoplastic lip, long cutaneous upper lip, short cutaneous upper lip with excessive incisor or gum show, lack of ideal vermilion contours, asymmetries

GOALS OF TREATMENT

RESTORATION OR CREATION OF AESTHETIC LIP CHARACTERISTICS
- **Volume:** Projection of lips (upper lip in line with or in front of lower), central pout
- **Shape:** Defined philtral columns and Cupid's bow, projected "ski jump" transition at vermilion border[3]
- **Balance:** Upper cutaneous lip/upper vermilion ratio <3 (ideal 1.1-2.3), upper/lower vermilion ratio of 1:1.6 (see Fig. 48-1)

INDICATIONS AND CONTRAINDICATIONS TO TREATMENT

INDICATIONS
- Enhance lip volume, shape, balance
  - Improve self-image

CONTRAINDICATIONS
- Body dysmorphic disorder
- Emotional/psychological instability
- Unrealistic expectations
- Patient demands guarantees
- Pregnant or lactating

- Immunosuppression
- Bleeding disorders

PREOPERATIVE EVALUATION

PATIENT HISTORY
- Assess patient desires and expectations.
  - Ask patients to provide photos of their lips from when they were happy with them.
- Has the patient undergone prior lip augmentation?
  - Which fillers or methods were used?
  - Was the patient satisfied with those results?
- History of:
  - Bleeding disorders or immunosuppression
  - Allergies or history of anaphylaxis
    - ▶ Some products are impregnated with antibiotics.
  - Hypersensitivities or excessive scarring with previous allogeneics
  - Counsel patients to stop taking aspirin, NSAIDs, vitamin E, herbal supplements, and other anticoagulants or antiplatelets (if possible) at least 2 weeks before procedure to minimize bleeding and swelling.
  - Pregnancy or lactation
  - Smoking
    - ▶ Counsel the patient to stop a minimum of 2 weeks ahead of the procedure; permanent cessation is best.
  - Labial herpes
    - ▶ Counsel to take acyclovir or valcyclovir perioperatively (3 days before and 3 days after procedure)

PHYSICAL EXAMINATION
- Patient positioning: Upright and in repose
- Exclude a current perioral infection.
- Measure lip dimensions.

Ideal Lip Dimensions[4]
- Frontal view (Fig. 48-1)
  - The length of the lips should equal the distance from one medial corneal limbus to the other.
  - Ratio of upper/lower vermilion show should be 1:1.6 (golden ratio) (see Chapter 2).
  - Upper cutaneous lip/upper vermilion ratio <3 (ideal 1.1-2.3)
  - Interpupillary line and stomion (commissural line) should be parallel and horizontal.
- Aging leads to downward tilt of commissures (frown in repose).
  - Subnasale-stomion distance should be half of stomion-menton distance.

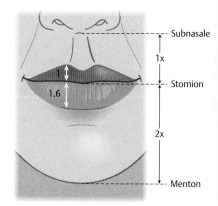

Fig. 48-1   Frontal lip view.

- Lips are sealed when in repose.
  - ▶ Incompetence can be caused by vertical maxillary excess, hypoplastic upper lip, open bite, or muscular dystrophy.
- With lips slightly parted, incisor show should be about 2 mm.
- When smiling, gum show should be minimal.
  - ▶ Excessive gum show can be caused by vertical maxillary excess, gum overgrowth (necessitating gingivectomy), hypoplastic upper lip, or overactive muscles.
- Cupid's bow forms a "gentle M" shape, the stomion forms a "lazy M," and the lower lip vermilion forms a "gentle W" with its peaks 2-3 mm lateral to the corresponding M peaks of the upper lip.
- Three thickenings of the upper lip: A central tubercle and lateral thickenings, which are separated from the central tubercle by arches
- Two paramedian thickenings of the lower lip, which correspond to and contour to the upper arches
- Profile view[5] (Fig. 48-2)
  - Nasolabial angle should be 85-105 degrees.
  - Slight eversion at the vermilion border with a projected "ski jump" transition[3]
  - Lips should project beyond line connecting subnasale and pogonion.
  - Upper lip either in vertical plane with lower lip, or slightly anterior (~2 mm)
  - Lower lip anterior to (~2 mm) soft tissue pogonion
  - Upper lip, lower lip, and chin should touch an imaginary line (Riedel line).
  - Chin should be within 1 mm of a vertical line drawn down from lower lip vermilion-cutaneous border (Frankfort plane).
  - Mid-nares to chin (Steiner line) should touch upper lip.
  - Labiomental groove ~4 mm deep

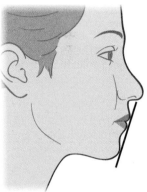

Fig. 48-2   Profile view of the lips. The red line depicts the Riedel line, connecting upper lip, lower lip, and chin.

- Note asymmetries and contour irregularities.
- Evaluate perioral region.
  - Assess vertical lip lines, nasolabial fold, labiomandibular fold (marionette lines), and prejowl sulcus.
  - Assess quality of rhytids (dynamic versus static).
  - Consider adjuvants for perioral rejuvenation (see Chapter 41) such as botulinum toxin, chemical or laser resurfacing, fillers, or implants.
- Assess structural/bony loss, dentition, and soft tissue volume loss.
- Take preprocedure photos with good lighting (frontal and profile views in repose, frontal and profile views with lips parted) to show the patient postoperative improvement (see Chapter 3).

Patient Counseling and Operative Planning[6]
- Outline aesthetic goals.
- Discuss various procedures and options (discussed later in the chapter).
  - There are many approaches to augmenting and enhancing the lips.
  - Whenever many techniques to solve a problem exist, a universally optimal solution is probably not available.

- Each option has advantages and disadvantages in various situations.
- Develop an individualized plan with the patient.
■ Manage expectations, emphasizing realistic aesthetic outcomes.
■ If a surgical intervention will be performed, inform patient of the risk of hypertrophic or depressed scarring.
■ Patients are often concerned about pain.
- Explain what they can expect during the procedure and the plan to minimize pain.
■ Explain the postoperative plan.

AUGMENTATION USING INJECTABLE FILLERS[7] (see Chapter 22)

ADVANTAGES
■ Minimally invasive
■ Reversible
■ Because fillers are temporary, they allow patients to "test-drive" lip augmentation before committing to an intermediate-duration or permanent treatment.

DISADVANTAGES
■ Good for **mild to moderate** volume needs, but not high-volume needs
■ Results are suboptimal in the aged, inelastic, ptotic lip.
■ Does not correct an elongated upper cutaneous lip.
- Can produce "duck bill" or "trout pout" lips in such patients
■ Should not be used in patients with a history of anaphylaxis, multiple severe allergies, or allergies to bacterial proteins

EXAMPLES
Collagen
■ **Bovine** (Zyderm and Zyplast, Allergan): 3%-5% have hypersensitivity reaction. **Must perform a skin test several weeks in advance**
■ **Human** (Cosmoderm and Cosmoplast, Allergan): **No** hypersensitivity reactions
■ **Porcine** (Evolence, Ortho-McNeil Pharmaceutical): Longer duration than other collagen (>6 months)
- **No** skin testing is required, but do not use it in patients with a history of anaphylactic or recurrent allergic reactions.
■ It has been reported to cause nodule formation.
■ Collagen injectables, in general, have a short duration (3-6 months).
■ Because of low viscosity, they are good for **superficial vertical lip lines** and the **vermilion border.**

Micronized Acellular Dermal Graft (Cymetra, LifeCell)
■ Short duration (3 months)
■ Rarely used

Hyaluronic Acid (HA) (Restylane, Galderma; Juvéderm, Allergan)
■ **Most commonly used** filler for lip augmentation
■ Natural constituent of extracellular matrix; hydrophilic nature draws in fluid volume.
■ Native human HA lasts only days, so synthesized products are **cross-linked** for increased stability and longevity.

- Rare complications
- Longer duration than collagen (6-12 months)
- Softer gels (Juvéderm) might be better for the lips, where the skin is thin.

Calcium Hydroxyapatite (Radiesse [formerly Radiance], Merz)

- High viscosity and elasticity
- Long duration (>12 months)
- Used for **deep creases** and **regional volume**
- Some experts use it along the vermilion border; however, many experts say to avoid its use in lips.
  - The lips are highly dynamic and can cause fillers to clump on animation.
  - This leads to lumps and nodules that are hard to treat when long-term or permanent fillers are used.

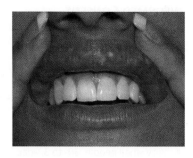

Fig. 48-3   Visible nodules after Radiesse injection into the lip vermilion.

> **SENIOR AUTHOR TIP:**   Do not inject Radiesse into the lip vermilion. Fig. 48-3 shows an example of the white clumps that often form after injection. These take a long time to disappear and need to be meticulously excised. Clear HA fillers, fat, and dermis are far better alternatives.

Poly-L-lactic Acid (PLLA) (Sculptra, Galderma)

- Injected into deep dermis and subcutaneous space
- **Mechanism of action:** Causes inflammatory reaction that leads to collagen deposition replacing filler
- Requires multiple treatments to achieve desired augmentation
- Long duration
- *Use in the lips is highly discouraged.*

Silicone (Silikon 1000, Alcon)

- Permanent
- Contraindicated in thin skin
- *Not intended for use in the lips*

Polymethylmethacrylate (PMMA) (Bellafill, Suneva Medical)

- PMMA microspheres suspended in 3.5% bovine collagen
  - Therefore skin testing for sensitivity is needed before use.
- Bovine collagen absorbed in 1-3 months, but the PMMA microspheres are surrounded by fibrous tissue and macrophages
- Permanent
- Can form nodules or granulomas
  - However, newer preparations have lower complication rates, ~0.01%.
- Successfully used in nasolabial fold, radial lip lines, and white roll
- Proper injection technique is vital.
  - Injected into deep dermis using linear tunneling method with constant pressure through a 26-gauge needle

- ▪ Not intended for use in the vermilion lip
  - • Many experts warn that it should not be used in this location because of a high risk of lump and nodule formation.

INFORMED CONSENT
- ▪ Needle marking, swelling, redness, ecchymosis, pain, itching
- ▪ Local reactions to filler or anesthetics
  - • These are usually self-limited.
- ▪ Asymmetries and contour irregularities
- ▪ Undercorrection or overcorrection
- ▪ Complications (as listed later in the chapter)

EQUIPMENT
- ▪ Good overhead lighting
- ▪ Very small needle, 30- to 32-gauge for low-viscosity products, or slightly larger (~27-gauge) for high-viscosity products
- ▪ Anesthetic
- ▪ Prepare filler.
  - • Powdered fillers should be reconstituted 2-4 hours before injection.

TECHNIQUE[8]
- ▪ The technique for HA or collagen injections is described here.
- ▪ Perform postprocedure massage (pinch and roll) if blending is needed.

Apply Anesthetic
- ▪ There are several viable approaches.
  - • **Cryoanalgesia:** Apply ice or a cold compress to the site before injection.
  - • **EMLA or other topicals:** Must apply 45-60 minutes before injection
  - • **Local anesthetic injections:** Avoid liberal infiltration, because it **distorts tissues.**
  - • Buffer the anesthetic with sodium bicarbonate because of the lips' great sensitivity.
  - • Inject along the vermilion border and areas to be augmented.
  - • Swelling should dissipate after 10 minutes.
  - • Some fillers come premixed with a local anesthetic.
    - ▶ For those that do not, a local anesthetic can be added.
- ▪ **Regional:** 0.5 ml of 1% lidocaine can be injected along the upper and 0.5 ml along the lower gingival sulci.
  - • Alternatively, topical benzocaine can be applied along the mucosal sulci using either a cotton-tipped applicator or a 2 × 2 gauze.
  - • Because of the rapid absorption through mucosal surfaces, the anesthetic only needs to be applied a few minutes before injecting filler.
- ▪ **Nerve blocks:** Inject ~0.25 ml at both the infraorbital and the mental foramina.
  - • This can prevent normal motion of the lips, compromising aesthetic outcome.
  - • Some think that this allows too-aggressive injections.

Sterile Technique
- ▪ Using sterile technique is imperative to prevent infections and biofilm: Remove makeup, prepare the injection site with antiseptic, and do not breach the mucosa.

Injection Technique

- **Injection techniques:** Anterograde linear threading, retrograde linear threading, radial fanning, serial puncture, and cross-hatching[9] (Fig. 48-4).

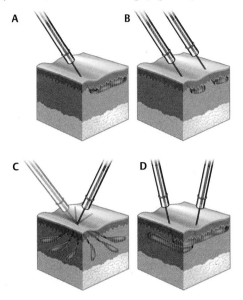

Fig. 48-4 Injection techniques. **A,** Linear threading. Filler is injected either as the needle is advanced (anterograde) or withdrawn (retrograde). **B,** Serial puncture. Filler is deposited in multiple, adjacent injections. **C,** Radial fanning. Filler is injected by linear threading but is redirected and advanced in a new radial direction before the needle is completely withdrawn. **D,** Cross-hatching. Filler is injected by linear threading along multiple parallel and perpendicular passes.

- Anterograde and retrograde linear threading and serial puncture are the techniques most used for lip augmentation.
- **Anterograde linear threading:** A thread of filler is pushed out ahead of the advancing needle.
  - ▶ Do not inject large boluses into one area.
- **Retrograde linear threading:** The needle is advanced to the desired location, then, as it is withdrawn, a thread of filler is injected.
- **Serial puncture:** The needle is inserted, and a small depot is deposited until resistance is met. The needle is withdrawn and then reinserted a short distance farther, and another small depot is deposited.
- Stretch or pinch the lip with nondominant hand to provide a firm, nonmobile surface.
- Position needle with bevel facing deep to prevent superficial deposition.
- **Aspirate before injecting to prevent intravascular deposition.**
- Inject vermilion lip, vermilion border, and philtral columns as needed for individualized enhancement, seeking to accentuate patient's anatomy.
  - A slow (<0.3 ml/minute) and gentle injection technique causes less pain. It also reduces the risk of vascular occlusion and other adverse effects.

- Pay careful attention to lip-defining structures.
  - Be conservative with the philtral columns. Minor alterations are visible.
  - Preserve the Cupid's bow. Small alterations are noticeable and can be distorting.
  - Avoid creating fullness above upper vermilion. This blunts the vermilion border and gives a flat "simian" look.
  - Accentuate the three upper lip and two lower lip thickenings.
- Overfilling effaces lip-defining structures, leading to "sausage" or "duck bill" lips.
- Taking a conservative approach, undercorrecting initially with gradual shaping over time, will lead to a more natural look.

Plane of Injection

- **Vermilion (mucosal):** Submucosal, just above orbicularis oris
- **Vermilion border:** Needle in potential space between red and white lip
  - ▶ Low resistance when in correct plane
  - ▶ This provides vermilion definition (ski jump transition).
- **Philtrum (cutaneous):** Mid-dermis[9] (Fig. 48-5)

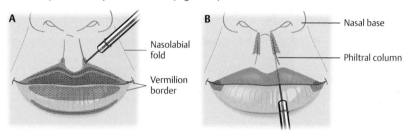

Fig. 48-5   Injection pattern. **A,** Young lips. **B,** Aging lips.

- **Young lips:** Inject caudal half of philtrum, central three fifths of upper and lower vermilion lips.
- **Senile lips:** Inject full philtrum and across entire vermilion lips.
- Some vermilion eversion and shortening of the cutaneous upper lip can be obtained by injecting submucosally in the wet vermilion.
- If using collagen, overcorrect by 10%-20%.
- Apply ice intermittently for swelling and cryoanalgesia.

Generic Augmentation Approaches

- Numerous generic augmentation approaches exist. Two are included here:
  - **Anterior flow or serial puncture technique**[3,10,11] (Fig. 48-6)
    - ▶ The patient is in an upright, sitting position.

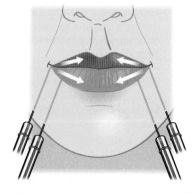

Fig. 48-6   Anterior flow or serial puncture technique. Inject vermilion from lateral to medial, inject corner of lips to create "supportive buttresses" from mandibular to lower lateral lip.

- ► Inject while standing at the patient's side. Intermittently reassess from frontal view.
- ► Inject from right to center and then from left to center.
- ► Stretch the lip to ensure the needle enters at the commissure (labiomandibular groove).
- ► Insert needle into potential vermilion space at 45-degree angle on mucosal side. Redirect it at 20-degree angle from lip.
- ► Inject filler, pushing ahead of the needle.
- ► When resistance is met and filler will not flow, injection is moved to next point.
- ► Finish half of lower lip. Then inject along the side of mouth, where lower and upper lip connect, thereby elevating the corner of lip and decreasing the labiomandibular groove.
- ► Inject upper lip.
- ► Inject from mandibular margin to lower lateral lip, creating "supportive buttresses" to reestablish vertical height (lost secondary to bone resorption).
- ► Repeat procedure on the other side.
- ► The total injected volume is ~1 cc into the upper lip and ~3 cc into the lower lip and buttresses.
- • **Six-step technique**[12] (Fig. 48-7)
  - ► 12 injections of ~0.1 cc each
  - ► Patient is in a supine position.
  - ► **Step 1: Define philtral columns.** Pinch philtral column with nondominant hand while injecting in retrograde threading fashion in dermis. Repeat procedure in other philtral column.

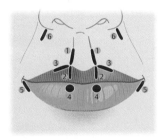

Fig. 48-7   Six-step technique. *1,* Define philtral columns. *2,* Cupid's bow. *3,* Define a portion of the vermilion-cutaneous junction. *4,* Lower lip paramedian tubercles. *5,* Support the oral commissures. *6,* Nasolabial fold.

  - ► **Step 2: Cupid's bow.** Insert needle at the base of the philtral columns and advance down to the wet-dry margin. Inject in a retrograde threading fashion, creating a strut for each Cupid's bow apex.
  - ► **Step 3: Define a portion of the vermilion-cutaneous junction.** Inject a thread along the vermilion-cutaneous junction from the apex of Cupid's bow laterally and halfway to the oral commissure. Repeat procedure on the other side.
- ► **Step 4: Lower lip paramedian tubercles.** With patient everting lower lip, insert needle into the wet-dry margin at about a third of the way from the midline to the commissure. Deposit 0.1 cc into the orbicularis oris muscle. Repeat procedure on the other side.
- ► **Step 5: Support the oral commissures.** Inject in the lateral lower cutaneous lip, just below the oral commissure. Repeat procedure on the other side.
- ► **Step 6: Nasolabial fold.** Inject superiorly in the nasolabial folds. This allegedly helps to evert the lip.

SENIOR AUTHOR TIP: When injecting lips with filler, microcannulas are a surgeon's best friend. Labial artery anatomy is notoriously variable.[13] The blunt tip of a 25-gauge microcannula introduced from each commissure and extending medially allows bruise-free volumization (Fig. 48-8, *A* and *B*). Philtral augmentation needs to be done sharply, however.

Numbing the sensitive vermilion is trivial and should be done with serial submucosal injections of lidocaine 1% with epinephrine at the sulcus. To make these relatively painless injections completely pain free, paint a topical anesthetic onto the mucosa 1-2 minutes before injections (Fig. 48-8, *C* and *D*). We use a combination of lidocaine 10%, prilocaine 10%, and tetracaine 4%. This technique prevents the problem of distorting the anatomy by direct injection of anesthetic into the lips.

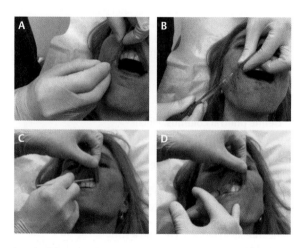

Fig. 48-8   A and **B,** The blunt tip of a 25-gauge microcannula introduced from each commissure and extending medially allows bruise-free volumization. **C** and **D,** Topical followed by local anesthetic for painless injections.

POSTPROCEDURE CARE
- Schedule next appointment (possibly for touch-ups in 2-4 weeks) to ensure patient retention.
- Little to no downtime
- Continue intermittent ice application for the next few hours.
- Avoid massaging perioral region, and minimize facial movements for the short-term.
- Sleep with head elevated for 1 night.
- Resume skin care and makeup application after 24 hours.
- Take postprocedure photos at follow-up visits.

COMPLICATIONS[14-17]
- Complications for HA and collagen injections are listed (Fig. 48-9).

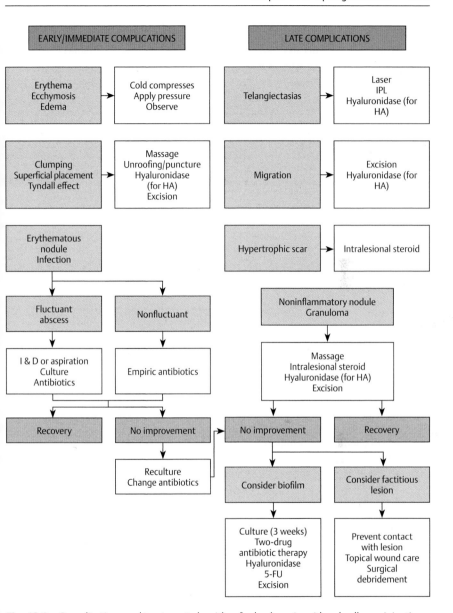

Fig. 48-9   Complications and treatment algorithm for hyaluronic acid and collagen injections. (*5-FU*, 5-fluorouracil; *HA*, hyaluronic acid; *I & D*, incision and drainage; *IPL*, intense pulsed light.) © Oxford University Press.

Minor

- Swelling (~73%-89% of cases), ecchymosis (~10%-61% of cases), erythema (~40%-93% of cases). These are self-limited, usually resolving within 7 days.
- Transient hyperpigmentation
- Infection (as high as 5%)
  - Treatment: Antibiotics
- Telangiectasias
  - Treatment: Pulsed dye laser
- Lumps or nodules (~11%)
  - These are caused by excessive or misplaced filler, migration with muscle movement.
  - **Treatment**
    - ▶ Massage the area and observe whether they resolve in a few days.
    - ▶ If it persists and is a solitary lesion, insert a 22- or 25-gauge needle and drain the fluid.
    - ▶ When multiple or deep lumps exist, or if a nodule persists, inject hyaluronidase (start with 150 IU and titrate up) and massage the area. This will dissolve the HA.
    - ▶ If lumps arise after patient leaves the office, abstain from manipulation for 12-24 hours, because these are often caused by swelling from needle entry.
- Delayed nodules
  - Biofilm purportedly plays a role.
  - Difficult to treat, because the bacteria's metabolism is slow and they secrete a protective matrix
  - **Treatment**
    - ▶ Hyaluronidase helps to break down protective matrix.
  - Consider antibiotics (fluoroquinolone AND third-generation macrolide), intralesional 5-FU, intralesional laser therapy.
- Bluish discoloration, or Tyndall effect, from injecting too superficially
  - **Treatment**
    - ▶ Hyaluronidase
    - ▶ Usually 15-50 IU is sufficient.
- Hypersensitivity reactions, local or systemic (angioedema, anaphylaxis)
  - Occurs in 3%-5% of cases with bovine collagen, and in <0.5% with HA
  - **Treatment**
    - ▶ 0.1% tacrolimus ointment
    - ▶ Local or systemic steroids plus antihistamines or cyclosporine
  - Granulomas
    - ▶ These are a type IV hypersensitivity reaction and appear weeks to months later.
    - ▶ Incidence is 0.01%-1.3% of cases.
    - ▶ **Treatment**
      - ◆ Intralesional steroids are effective.
      - ◆ Incision and drainage or excision

Severe

- Very rare, estimated to be <0.001% of cases
- Vascular occlusion
  - Caused by needle injury to vessels, intravascular embolism of filler, external vascular compression by filler

- Patients usually present with pain on injection, then develop blanching, duskiness, or ecchymosis.
- Delayed presentation can also occur, possibly from the volume of HA compressing vessels.
- Symptoms evolve over the next 1-2 days (erythema, edema, discoloration, constant pain)
- **Treatment**
  - ▶ Massage
  - ▶ Warm compress
  - ▶ Nitroglycerine paste
  - ▶ Hyaluronidase, regardless of filler type, because of its ability to reduce edema and associated pressure
  - ▶ Consider steroids to reduce inflammation and associated injury.

Tissue Necrosis
- A result of untreated vascular occlusion
- **Treatment**
  - Local wound therapy
  - Antibiotics
  - Debridement

AUGMENTATION WITH IMPLANTS (see Chapter 27)

ADVANTAGES
- Permanent
- Biocompatible: They have been used in medical devices for years.
- Reliable amount of bulk with little shrinkage
- Reversible

DISADVANTAGES
- Does not fully integrate: Possibility of migration or extrusion
- Does not treat a long cutaneous upper lip
- Carries the risk of inflammatory response and infection
- Although advertised as soft and pliable, many think that they have an unnatural feel.
  - This probably depends on which product is used.
- Some think they inhibit natural lip motion (in upper lip more than in lower).
- Expensive

SENIOR AUTHOR TIP: Implants to the lips are almost never a good idea. Objects placed into this highly mobile area, whether they integrate or not, are likely to distort the anatomy and become visible—most notably at extremes of expression. Because little or no shrinkage occurs over time, what might look proportional at 50 years of age will look overdone at 70 years of age. Finally, removing them is often not trivial. Integrating implants can be difficult to dissect free from investing tissue, and ones which do not integrate often leave capsules that are problematic in their own right.

EXAMPLES
Expanded Polytetrafluoroethylene (ePTFE)
- Earlier products (Gore-Tex, SoftForm, UltraSoft; Tissue Technologies) had low porosity, which did not allow adequate cellular ingrowth.
  - Surgeons and patients reported poor results, including hardening, palpability, and visibility of the implants.[18]
- Newer, dual-porosity products (Advanta, Atrium Medical) allow more cellular ingrowth and have a softer, more natural feel, and allow more natural lip movements.
  - These are reportedly three times softer than older constructs.
- Patient satisfaction with Advantra was 90% when implants were placed into nasolabial fold or lips.[19]
- Various shapes (round, oval) and diameters (1.8-5.0 mm); 15 cm length
- With or without preattached trocar

Saline (VeraFil, Evera Medical)
- The shell is composed of two membranes: An outer ePTFE shell and an inner silicone shell.
  - This supposedly allows some cellular ingrowth (to minimize migration) but is limited (to minimize hardening).
- Possibly softer than ePTFE
- Can rupture/deflate
- Lengths: 3, 4, 5 cm; diameters: 4.5, 5.5, 6.5 mm; 0.25-0.6 ml of saline fill

Silicone (Permalip, SurgiSil)
- No cellular ingrowth
- Possibly softer than ePTFE products
- Three diameters (3, 4, and 5 mm) and lengths (55, 60, and 65 mm)

INFORMED CONSENT
- Palpability, migration, and extrusion of implant
- Infection, with need for implant removal
- Contour irregularities, asymmetries
- Alterations in sensation, speech competence, oral competence; usually temporary
- Overcorrection or undercorrection: ~4% of patients require size adjustment.
- Swelling can take weeks to fully resolve.
- Expect ecchymosis, decreased motion of lips, and dysesthesia for weeks to months.
- Complications

EQUIPMENT
- Good overhead lighting
- 1% lidocaine with epinephrine
- Tenotomy scissors
- Bunnell tendon passer
- No. 11 or No. 15 blade
- Ruler
- Suture

TECHNIQUE[18]

- Measure the length of the lips while they are stretched or with the patient's mouth wide open.
- Choose appropriate implant size.
- Give anesthesia.
  - Usually a combination of blocks (infraorbital and mental), local anesthesia for vasoconstriction and hemostasis, and oral or IV sedation with agents (i.e., ketamine and valium) for patient comfort
- Preoperative and postoperative antibiotics
  - Some surgeons soak the implant in antibiotic solution before implantation.
- Make 3-5 mm stab incisions bilaterally a few millimeters medial to the oral commissures on the upper lip.

NOTE: The incision must be lateral enough so that the implant is not placed directly under the incision.

- Using tenotomy scissors or a Bunnell tendon passer, create a submucosal or intramuscular tunnel across the vermilion.
  - Some perform this along the course of the wet and dry lip margin, whereas others place the tunnel at the vermilion border.
  - If an implant is placed too high, it can cause a ridge or blunt the vermilion-cutaneous junction, whereas if placed too low, it can cause a retracted appearance.
- Different practitioners advocate differing levels of tunneling: submucosal, intramuscular, or submuscular.
  - If placed too superficially, the implant will be palpable and may extrude.
  - Some think that when placed intramuscularly, the implants tend to migrate.
- Ensure uniform depth of the tunnel across the lip.
- Insert the implant using a tendon passer.
- Touch-free technique: Avoid touching the implant or allowing it to touch mucosa (oral flora) or skin.
- If one implant is used to span the entire upper lip, bow-stringing or abnormal motion on animation can result.
  - Using two implants in series (one for each hemilip) can lead to more natural lip motion.
  - The lower lip can be spanned with one implant.
- Repeat procedure for the lower lip.
- Multiple implants can be added for more volume.
- Some implants (Advanta) are preloaded with a trocar and placed percutaneously.
- Some implants come tapered; others should be cut so that the ends taper.
- Bimanual palpation is done to confirm proper placement.
- Suture the stab wounds.

POSTPROCEDURE CARE

- Antibiotics for 5-7 days
- Cold compress for first 48 hours
- Limit talking/chewing (soft diet) for a couple days and facial animation (smiling, laughing, puckering) for 1-2 weeks.

- Sleep with head elevated for several days.
- Avoid strenuous activity for 1-2 weeks.
- Good oral hygiene
- Vaseline or lip moisturizer

COMPLICATIONS[18-22]
- Bleeding, hematoma
- Infection (0.2%-4.2%)
  - Treatment: Antibiotics
  - Removal of implant
- Shrinkage (0.2%-3% of cases with newer products, ~16% for older products)
- Migration, capsular contracture, palpability, stiffness, asymmetry
  - 1.5%-10% revision rate, except VeraFil revision rates have been reported as high as 25%
  - 0.8%-7.5% of patients request removal of an implant. Rates of removal of older products (Gore-Tex, SoftForm, UltraSoft) are much higher, with some reports as high as 100%.
- Numbness
  - Usually self-limited
- Allergic reaction (very rare)
- Granuloma: Rare
- Ulcers
- Extrusion (~1%)

AUGMENTATION WITH GRAFTS

ADVANTAGES
- Biocompatibility
- Full integration
- Quite natural feel
- If complicated by an infection, the graft does not usually need to be removed.

DISADVANTAGES
- Variable rates of resorption, results not completely predictable
- A graft does not fix a long cutaneous upper lip.

EXAMPLES
Allograft[23]
- Human dermal matrix (Alloderm, LifeCell), human tensor fascia lata (Fascian, Fascia Biosystems), human collagen matrix (Dermalogen, Collagenesis), porcine collagen matrix (Surgisis)
- Acceptable longevity 1-3 years: ~80% survival at 1 year
- No need for donor site
- Must document allergies preoperatively, because many of these products are antibiotic impregnated

- Very expensive
- ~4% complication rate

Autologous Grafts

- Inexpensive if harvested during a concurrent procedure (e.g., blepharoplasty, facelift, liposuction); otherwise, expensive in OR costs and materials, and leaves an additional scar

SENIOR AUTHOR TIP: Fat grafting can be done using a local anesthetic in the office.

- Varying resorption rates
- Various autografts can be used:
  - **Muscle, fascia:** Orbicularis oculi, superficial musculoaponeurotic system (SMAS), temporalis fascia, postauricular fascia, galea, palmaris longus, sternocleidomastoid
    - ▶ Muscle will atrophy.
    - ▶ Fascia shrinks 20% over 4-6 weeks through a process of compaction, not resorption.
- **Fat:** Fat injections and core fat grafts
  - Natural feel
  - The lips are the *worst recipient site* compared with other facial subunits. Nondynamic recipient areas are better.[24]
    - ▶ Varying levels of longevity have been reported
    - ▶ Eremia et al[25] showed total resorption at 8-9 months regardless of multiple treatments.
    - ▶ Churukian[26] found that long-term results were possible with >5 treatments.
    - ▶ Colic[27] reported <20% resorption when injected intramuscularly into orbicularis oris.
      - ♦ Resorption was also correlated to age, with more resorption in older patients.
  - Dermal-fat graft
    - ▶ Less resorption than fat alone
    - ▶ Harvested during other procedures, from existing scars or from discrete areas (e.g., lower abdomen; subiliac crest; or suprapubic, gluteal, or inframammary folds)

SENIOR AUTHOR TIP: Dermal-fat grafts are a wonderful way to restore volume to lips that need more than just fat grafting. When harvesting a strip of dermis, make sure to deepithelialize first. (This will not be possible after skin is harvested!) Take almost twice the amount needed if harvesting from the abdomen, and if working near the pubis, be careful of engrafting hair follicles.

Remove as much fat as possible from the underside of the dermis before threading between the commissural incisions. (I like to weight each end of the dermis with a small clamp and drape it over my nondominant hand/finger to expose the fat.) Once the dermis is passed through the lip, center it and then pull the lip away from the face to maximize its length. This maneuver will pull as much dermis as possible into the lip. Trim the excess, but leave 2 mm to insert into the incision at closure. I use 5-0 chromic gut, making sure to capture the dermal edge into the commissural closure to anchor the dermis in place.

INFORMED CONSENT
- Undercorrection or overcorrection
- Lips will appear overcorrected for a short period because of the expected resorption.
- Contour irregularities, asymmetries
- Need for multiple treatments to approach permanency
- Secondary procedures to correct imperfections or increase volume
- Expect ecchymosis, decreased motion of lips, and dysesthesia for weeks to months.
- Complications

EQUIPMENT
- Same as equipment used for implant augmentation (see previous description)
- Fine-tipped coagulator/cautery

TECHNIQUE
- Measure length of lips while they are stretched.
- **Apply anesthesia**
  ► Similar to that used for implant augmentation

Allograft, Muscle, Fascia, or Dermal-Fat Grafting Technique
- Harvest graft from donor site. Ensure hemostasis.
  - If using a dermal-fat graft, deepithelialize the graft.
- If using human acellular dermal matrix, a 3.5 by 7 cm graft usually suffices for both lips.[28]
  - Rehydrate product as per instructions, if necessary.
- Trim the graft to the desired size and shape.
  - Usual dimensions range is 3-5 by 5-10 by >10 cm.
  - Some experts simply make strips rather than contouring the graft, because they think such contouring leads to asymmetries and surface irregularities.
- Allograft can be inserted either as a rolled construct or as flat, multiple, thin (2-5 mm) strips.
- Some advocate two grafts for the upper lip (one for each hemilip) with ~3 mm of overlap, thereby enhancing or creating the natural central tubercle.
- Insert graft into a submucosal or intramuscular tunnel with a tendon passer in a similar manner as for implants.

Percutaneous Graft Insertion
- A 14- or 16-gauge angiocatheter is inserted into the vermilion border just medial to the oral commissure, tunneled submucosally, and brought out at the midline.
- A stylet from a 5 Fr suction device is passed through the catheter, hooked to the graft, and withdrawn back through the tunnel to properly seat the graft.
- This is repeated on the other side.
- The lower lip can be augmented with one pass extending from one side to the other.

Fat Grafting Technique
■ See Chapter 23 for greater detail.
■ **Fat injections**[29]
  • Fat is harvested using dry or tumescent technique.
  • Possible donor sites include periumbilical region, inferior buttock, trochanter, flank, or thigh.
  • Atraumatic harvesting technique is employed.
    ▶ Large cannula (17-gauge), low negative pressure, and gentle passes of the cannula.
  • The aspirate can be processed with centrifugation or gravity separation.
    ▶ The middle fat layer is used.
  • Using an injecting cannula, fat is injected into the lips, either intramuscularly or into the submucosal tissue.
  • To decrease the risk of complications (e.g., vascular occlusion, fat emboli, hematoma), epinephrine, deposition of small aliquots, and large blunt cannulas are employed.
  • Small aliquots (0.1-0.2 ml) of fat are injected as the cannula is withdrawn to decrease the force needed for deposition and thereby minimize adipocyte trauma.
  • Multiple passes, making new tracts each time, are performed.
  • Typical injection volumes: 1-2 ml into the upper lip and 1.5-3 ml into the lower lip
  • Significant overcorrection (~30%) is needed because of resorption.
■ **Core fat grafts**[30]
  • The donor region (usually inferior buttock or periumbilical region) is infiltrated with 0.5% lidocaine hydrochloride with epinephrine 1:100,000.
  • The tip of a 1 ml syringe is cut off at an oblique angle.
  • A 5 mm incision is made at the donor site.
  • The oblique end of the syringe is inserted into the subcutaneous fat using a boring motion (rotation and advancement), while simultaneously gently pulling back on the syringe piston to make room in syringe for the fat core.
    ▶ Suction should not be created.
  • The syringe is inserted into a deep mucosal lip tunnel, and while the syringe is withdrawn, the piston is gently pushed to insert the fat core into the tunnel.
  • The lips should be overcorrected by ~10%-15%.

POSTPROCEDURE CARE
■ Similar to augmentation with implant
■ Antibiotics are not needed.
  • Antimicrobial ointment can be applied over the incisions.

COMPLICATIONS
■ Hematoma
■ Infection
  • Treatment: Antibiotics
  • Usually do not need to remove graft

- Graft fibrosis, hardening, and stiffening
- Graft exposure
- Fat necrosis (fat grafting or dermal-fat graft)
- Epidermal cysts (dermal-fat graft)
- Oil cysts, fibrosis (fat grafting)
    - Animal studies have shown less inflammatory reaction and fewer oil cysts when platelet-rich plasma (PRP) is added to the fat graft.
- Arterial occlusion (fat injection)
    - Treatment: Can try approach similar to that used with injectable fillers
    - Fat embolization with resultant stroke or blindness (two known case reports from fat injections into lower third of face)

AUGMENTATION WITH V-Y ADVANCEMENT

ADVANTAGES
- Augmentation with one's own tissue (no concern for hypersensitivity reactions)
- Permanent
- Nonvisible scars

DISADVANTAGES
- Can have unwanted philtral protrusion
- Does not change cutaneous upper lip length
- Advancements can lead to poor lip motion postoperatively.
- Can have poor results with thin, aged lips
    - Results are better in people <40 years of age with good elastic tissues.
- Steep learning curve for mastery

INFORMED CONSENT
- Expect lip dryness
- Asymmetry
- Paresthesia
- Philtral protrusion
- Prolonged severe edema leading to difficulty eating, articulating, or pursing lips
- Complications

EQUIPMENT
- Good overhead lighting
- 1% lidocaine with epinephrine
- No. 15 blade
- Tenotomy scissors
- Ruler
- Suture

TECHNIQUE
- Apply anesthesia.
- One of the many V-Y advancement patterns is chosen (Fig. 48-10).
    - **Vertical V-Y:** A wide V pattern is incised with the base of the V facing the labial sulcus and the tips pointing toward the wet-dry margin.
        - This flap is advanced and closed in a Y pattern.
        - This creates more vermilion show by advancing mucosa forward.

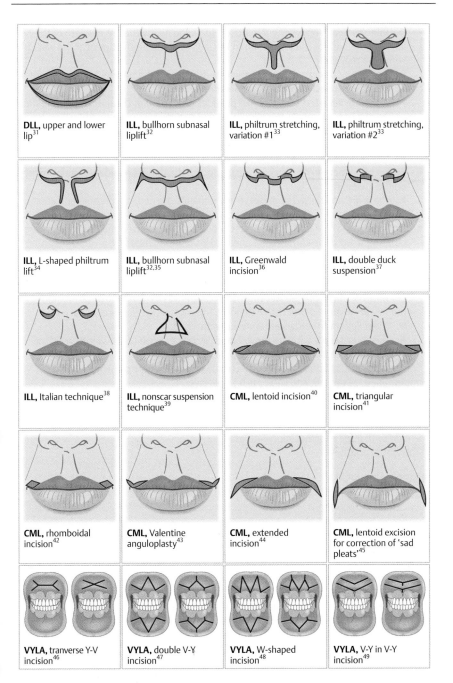

Fig. 48-10 V-Y advancement patterns. The areas shaded *red* indicate incisions or areas to be resected. (*CML,* Corner of the mouthlift; *DLL,* direct liplift; *ILL,* indirect liplift; *VYLA,* V-Y lip augmentation.)

- **Double-vertical V-Y:** A large V is incised spanning nearly the entire width of the lip, with the base of the V pointing to the labial sulcus and the tips near the wet-dry vermilion margin.
  - ▶ A smaller V is incised closer to the wet-dry margin and parallel to the previous V, but its width just covers the middle third of the lip.
  - ▶ When advanced, the large V flap provides protrusion of the entire lip, while the small V flap augments the middle third of the lip.
- **W-plasty:** One or two W patterns are incised in the wet mucosa with bases pointing toward labial sulcus and tips toward wet-dry margin.
  - ▶ This plasty does not preserve the natural contour of lips.
- **Series of vertical V-Ys:** Three Vs are incised on the upper lip and two can be incised on the lower lip.
  - ▶ These are positioned to preserve and enhance the natural contours and areas of fullness; namely, the central tubercle and the lateral thickenings.
- **Horizontal V-Y[50]:** A horizontal V is incised laterally in the wet mucosa with its base pointing toward the commissure and the tips pointing medially.
  - ▶ When the flap is advanced to the Y, lateral tissue is moved to create medial fullness.
  - ▶ This shortens the transverse length of the lip.
- **Double Y-V plasty:** In the wet mucosa, a central 12-15 mm horizontal incision is made with V-shaped branches extending toward the commissures at each end.
  - ▶ The resultant four flaps are widely undermined.
  - ▶ The two lateral V flaps are moved medially toward each other, slightly overlapping.
  - ▶ This shortens the transverse length of the lip.
- The mucosa and submucosa are incised to the level of the muscle. The flaps are undermined, advanced, and closed in a single layer.
- The orbicularis oris can be plicated for added thickness.

POSTOPERATIVE CARE
- Similar to that for augmentation with grafts
- Antiseptic mouthwash

COMPLICATIONS[51]
- Debilitating edema >3 weeks (9.4%)
- Asymmetry (2.8%-25%)
- Undercorrection (4%-21%)
- Overcorrection (3%)
- Paresthesia (12%)
- Infection
- Dehiscence (6%)

SENIOR AUTHOR TIP: The learning curve for V-Y mucosal advancements is steep, and there is very little call for them in senile (thin, long) lips. We rarely do them in our practice, their place taken by combinations of volumization and direct skin excisions.

ADJUVANT SURGERIES

- Augmentation with fillers can remedy lip volume and shape.
  - However, one aspect of senescent lips remains—the elongated cutaneous upper lip.
  - Imaging studies have given evidence that the senescent lip is not actually volume depleted, but that the *volume is redistributed over now-elongated tissue.*
- Lip augmentation alone can lead to an unnatural "duck bill" or "trout pout" look.
- Liplifts are the only intervention that shortens an elongated cutaneous upper lip.[52]
- Liplifts fell out of favor because of noticeable scars.
  - However, with modifications that seek to minimize scar visibility, they seem to be making a comeback.

INDIRECT LIPLIFT (ILL), SUBNASAL LIFT, "BULLHORN LIPLIFT"

ADVANTAGES
- Decrease the length of the cutaneous upper lip by resecting a portion of the upper lip just below the nose.
- Accentuate pout.
- The scar can be well hidden and is least noticeable in patients with a wide nostril base, flat philtrum, and obvious nostril sill.

DISADVANTAGES
- Shorten the upper lip mainly centrally.
  - Can be combined with a corner mouthlift to balance the lip
- Overcorrection results in excessive upper incisor show.

INFORMED CONSENT
- Risk of noticeable scar
- Expect ecchymosis and dysesthesia for weeks to months.
- Overcorrection or undercorrection
- Complications

EQUIPMENT
- Same as that used for V-Y advancement

TECHNIQUE
- Give anesthesia.
  - Often done under a regional (infraorbital nerve) block with local anesthetic for vasoconstriction
  - Sedation can be added, based on patient comfort.
- Using a fine-tipped pen, a curvilinear (bullhorn-shaped) marking is made along the nasal crease below the nostril sill (see Fig. 48-10 for variations).
  - The incision can be extended inferolaterally along the nasolabial fold to reduce droopy nasolabial fold.
  - The skin below the columella can be spared.
    - ▶ The incision starts at the nasal ala, curves into the nostril, and continues up toward the footplate of the medial crus as a transfixion incision.
    - ▶ The columella is dissected off of the nasal septum.

▶ This technique can be combined with a lip suspension.
▶ This variation makes the scar less conspicuous.

SENIOR AUTHOR TIP: It is extremely difficult to make this liplift variant look natural, and it is best left to only the most experienced surgeons.

NOTE: Any incision crossing the philtral columns increases scar noticeability.

- The medial aspect of the incision can be extended inferiorly along philtral columns to accentuate or create the Cupid's bow.
- A midline triangular or a wide vertical excision can be added to either narrow a wide philtrum or treat an absent Cupid's bow.
- The incision can be made to stairstep up into the nasal sill.
■ The height of the skin to be excised should be ~3-5 mm.
  - Ensure that the height from nasal base to Cupid's bow is at least 12 mm, regardless of incisor show, or else the lip will look too short.
■ The skin and subcutaneous tissue down to the orbicularis oris fascia are excised.
■ Either no undermining, or wide undermining of the upper cutaneous lip almost down to vermilion border can be performed.
  - Not undermining will shorten the upper lip more.
  - Wide undermining will decrease cutaneous lip/vermilion ratio more (increases vermilion height).
■ Meticulous two-layer closure with 6-0 suture

SENIOR AUTHOR TIP: Patient selection is critical for any direct excision around the mouth, but particularly for liplifts. Particular attention should be paid to the acuity of the labiocolumellar angle (the sharper the better), the ratio of the width of the nose to the width of the mouth (the larger the better), and to the individual anatomy at the nostril sill. Some sills lend themselves to bullhorn excisions (e.g., the lip skin seems to move into the nostril), and others are more linear with an abrupt change from nostril to labial skin at the sill.

Vertical components added to the liplift are powerful ways to narrow a wide, simian senile upper lip. The vertical component can be taken down all the way to the vermilion, if necessary, where the dog-ear can help to re-create the pout at the center of Cupid's bow.

Be very cautious in undermining the upper lip skin. Any postoperative bleeding (in this vascular area) not evacuated from beneath the skin flap will at best become lumpy and at worst turn the lip to "concrete" for an extended period.

POSTOPERATIVE CARE
■ Same as that for augmentation with grafts
■ Early removal of sutures 5-7 days postoperatively

COMPLICATIONS[51,53,54]
■ Prolonged edema >1 month 10%, and >3 months 8.3%
■ Undercorrection (2.4%)

- Infection (1.6%-2.1%)
- Hypertrophic scarring (5.3%), or scar needing correction with dermabrasion (20%)

LIP SUSPENSION[39]

ADVANTAGES
- No visible scar
- Increases nasal tip projection
- Minimal operative time
- Easily reversed by removing the suspension suture

DISADVANTAGES
- Possibly unwanted changes to nasal tip

INFORMED CONSENT
- Can have ecchymosis, decreased motion of lips, and dysesthesia for a period of time
- Complications

EQUIPMENT
- No. 15 blade
- Tenotomy scissors
- Fine-tipped cautery
- 3-0 monofilament, nonabsorbable, suspension suture

TECHNIQUE
- An incision is made starting at the nasal floor, continuing up the septum (transfixion incision separating lower lateral cartilages from nasal septum), and then finishing as an intercartilaginous incision (separating lower lateral from upper lateral cartilages).
  - This is done bilaterally.
- Using tenotomy scissors, the subcutaneous tissues are dissected off of the orbicularis oris.
  - This extends horizontally the width of the base of the nose, and inferiorly halfway to the vermilion-cutaneous border.
- Through the intercartilaginous aspect of the incision, the nasal tip and dorsum are undermined so that the columella and lower lateral cartilages move freely as a subunit.
  - If the medial footplates flare causing external valve obstruction, they should be resected.
- A 3-0 suspension suture is passed through the inferior portion of the incision and down halfway to the vermilion-cutaneous border.
  - The suture is passed through orbicularis oris muscle and fascia and brought back up and secured to the anterior nasal spine.
- The upper lip skin is pulled up as the suture is tightened, redistributing the skin into the nasal vestibule (where excess tissue can be excised), as well as up through the columella and nasal tip, which rotates and projects the tip.
- A tip rhinoplasty can be done for patients with excessive nasal tip projection.
  - Likewise, a resection of caudal septum can be done for patients with a hanging columella.
- The columella is sutured to the septum, and the incision is closed.

> **SENIOR AUTHOR TIP:**   We have no experience with this technique and would urge caution when depending on long, permanent sutures—especially mobile ones—to indefinitely modify soft tissues.

POSTOPERATIVE CARE
- Same as that for augmentation with grafts
- Early removal of sutures 5-7 days postoperatively

COMPLICATIONS
- Synechia
- Nasal stenosis
- Loosening of suspension suture (1%)
- Suture abscess (2%)
- Paresthesias
- Undercorrection
  - Only 85% of patients had shortened total lip height.
  - 79% had increased sagittal projection pout.
  - 74% had increased incisor show, and 25% had increased vermilion show.

DIRECT LIPLIFT, GULL-WING LIPLIFT, VERMILION LIPLIFT

ADVANTAGES
- Allow optimal control of the desired vermilion placement by incising along the vermilion and directly advancing it
- Shortens the cutaneous upper lip and increases vermilion height

DISADVANTAGES
- Risk of losing the white roll
- The scar usually fades to become less noticeable, but this can take years.
- Usually reserved for patients >50 years of age, because scarring is more noticeable in young skin.

INFORMED CONSENT
- Scar will likely be quite noticeable for months.
- Risk of effacement of the vermilion border
- Expect ecchymosis, dry lips, decreased motion of lips, and dysesthesia for weeks to months.
- Complications

EQUIPMENT
- Same as that used for V-Y advancement

TECHNIQUE
- Using a very-fine-tipped pen, mark the midline and Cupid's bow peaks with a vertical line.
- Trace vermilion border (or ~0.25 mm above white roll).

- Mark the new Cupid's bow peaks (usually 3-5 mm higher than the original) and the new central portion (usually 2-3 mm higher than the original).
  - Preserve and exaggerate the Cupid's bow.
- The tissue medial to the Cupid's bow can be spared to make the scarring less noticeable.
  - This is essentially a corner mouthlift.
- Continue the marking from the peaks laterally and parallel to the vermilion, tapering down toward the lateral vermilion near the commissure.
- Overcorrect the upper lip by 1 mm, because tissues will settle and descend ~1 mm by 6 months postoperatively.
- Extension to or beyond the commissures can lead to lateral scars that are noticeable.
- Infiltrate the upper lip with lidocaine with epinephrine 1:100,000.
- Excise the marked skin.
  - Some surgeons excise down to muscle.
  - Others advocate simply excising immediately subdermally, keeping as much subcutaneous tissue as possible to preserve or create a natural ridge at the vermilion border.
- Some surgeons undermine 1-2 mm, whereas others do not.
- Meticulous closure with 6-0 suture is crucial.
  - Closing Cupid's bow peak and trough points with vertical mattress sutures promotes an everted edge.
  - For the rest of the incision, a subcuticular suture can be run, and if further eversion is desired, a simple running suture can be implemented.
- Dermabrasion or laser resurfacing along incision decreases scar noticeability.

> **SENIOR AUTHOR TIP:** Whereas lower lip advancement (i.e., excision of the lip skin at the vermilion border all the way across the lip) is a tried and true technique in our hands, we long ago abandoned the technique for the upper lip. The problem was stricture that was unfixable in 4 of the first 14 patients.
>
> It is far safer to extend the corner mouthlift only to the peaks of Cupid's bow and leave the central lip skin intact. The central part of the lip can then be shortened by a liplift.

POSTOPERATIVE CARE
- Same as that for augmentation with grafts
- Early removal of sutures 5-7 days postoperatively
- Some surgeons think that Micropore paper tape on the incision for >6 weeks can decrease scarring.
- Use lipstick or cosmetic tattooing to cover scar.

COMPLICATIONS[51,55,56]
- Asymmetry, contour irregularities, obliteration of ski jump transition
- Overcorrection
- Undercorrection (6.25%-26%)
- Hematoma
- Asymmetry (5%-13%)
  - Revisions done in ~10% of patients
- Hypertrophic scarring (3%-27%)
- Infection (~5%)

CORNER MOUTHLIFT, ANGULOPLASTY
- Similar to the direct liplift, but the excision stays lateral to the Cupid's bow apices

ADVANTAGES
- It can be used for downturned corners or combined with an indirect liplift (which lifts centrally) to balance the mouth.

DISADVANTAGES
- Similar to direct liplift
- Can lead to permanent smirk if overcorrected

INFORMED CONSENT
- Scar can be noticeable
- Risk of effacement of the lateral vermilion border
- Complications

EQUIPMENT
- Same as that used for V-Y advancement

TECHNIQUE
- Infiltrate lip using lidocaine with epinephrine.
- Many marking patterns (see Fig. 48-10)
  - The original technique involved marking a lentoid shape at the lateral lip, but resulted in a scar that extended laterally past the commissure.
  - A triangle pattern at the lateral lip is useful when the commissures are to be lifted (eliminate frown).
    - ▶ This can lead to excess skin wrapped around into lower lip margin.
  - Spearhead and rhomboidal shapes similarly can tilt the commissures upward.
  - A lentiform pattern can be used that extends laterally then inferiorly to incorporate the marionette folds.
  - A simple ellipse along the lateral lip is the most used pattern.
    - ▶ This is essentially a direct liplift that is kept lateral to the Cupid's bow peaks.
  - Excise skin.
  - Meticulous closure with 6-0 suture

POSTOPERATIVE CARE
  - Similar to that for direct liplift

COMPLICATIONS [39,51]
- Scar hypertrophy and erythema occurred early postoperatively (18.8%), and all resolved with time.
- Misplaced scar above vermilion
  - Treatment: Surgical revision with repositioning of scar along the vermilion border
- Infection (~3.7%)
- Undercorrection (4%)

- Hypertrophic visible scar (15%)
  - Six months postoperatively, 22.3% of patients were satisfied with scars while not wearing makeup, and 84% were satisfied when makeup was applied.
  - After 1 year, 87.5% were satisfied without makeup, and 89.5% were satisfied when makeup was applied.
- Depressed scar (7%)

SENIOR AUTHOR TIP: Corner mouthlifts are extremely useful techniques when sculpting senile vermilion. They have gone through three iterations in our practice:

The first involved an excision of the lateral lip skin past the commissure, which left the scar mentioned above. It remains the most powerful lift of the three variants we use frequently, but has the downside of a "whisker-like" scar that is present 20% of the time. It is reserved for only the most downturned corners.

A wraparound corner mouthlift extends the incision around the commissure onto the vermilion border of the lower lip for a distance long enough to eliminate the dog-ear. It has medium power to lift, but can blunt the commissure.

A simple skin excision that stops at the commissure and tapers medially is our most common corner mouthlift. Its downside is that it does not lift the commissure, but the scar should be minimal >95% of the time.

TOP TAKEAWAYS

➤ Although perioral rejuvenation is scary in that many of the techniques involve direct excisions that are "right out front," it is crucial in achieving a harmonious facial rejuvenation. Indirect approaches to the mouth (facelifts, midface lifts) have no effect inside the nasolabial folds. Mastery of at least some of the techniques described in this chapter is crucial.

➤ The good news is that all of these techniques, although best done at the time of a broader facial rejuvenation, can be done using local anesthesia in the office. Thus, if patients happy with their facelift return concerned about their long upper lip or downturned corners, surgeons can offer these procedures at minimal cost. This is a great advantage, because surgeons have already developed a trusting rapport with their patients.

REFERENCES

1. Iblher N, Kloepper J, Penna V, et al. Changes in the aging upper lip—a photomorphometric and MRI-based study (on a quest to find the right rejuvenation approach). Plast Reconstr Surg 61:1170, 2008.
2. Iblher N, Stark GB, Penna V. The aging perioral region—do we really know what is happening? J Nutr Health Aging 16:581, 2012.
3. Klein AW. In search of the perfect lip: 2005. Dermatol Surg 31:1599, 2005.
4. Raphael P, Harris R, Harris SW. Analysis and classification of the upper lip aesthetic unit. Plast Reconstr Surg 132:543, 2013.

5. Guyuron B, Eriksson E, Persing J, eds. Plastic Surgery: Indications and Practice. Philadelphia: Elsevier, 2009.
6. Ali MJ, Ende K, Maas CS. Perioral rejuvenation and lip augmentation. Facial Plast Surg Clin North Am 15:491, 2007.
7. Sarnoff DS, Saini R, Gotkin RH. Comparison of filling agents for lip augmentation. Aesthet Surg J 28:556, 2008.
8. Barton FE Jr, Carruthers J, Coleman S, et al. The role of toxins and fillers in perioral rejuvenation. Aesthet Surg J 27:632, 2007.
9. Hilinski JM, Cohen SR, eds. Techniques in Aesthetic Plastic Surgery Series: Facial Rejuvenation with Filler. Philadelphia: Elsevier, 2009.
10. Carruthers J, Klein AW, Carruthers A, et al. Safety and efficacy of nonanimal stabilized hyaluronic acid for improvement of mouth corners. Dermatol Surg 31:276, 2005.
11. Aston SJ, Steinbrech DS, Walden JL, eds. Aesthetic Plastic Surgery. Philadelphia: Elsevier, 2009.
12. Sarnoff DS, Gotkin RH. Six steps to the "perfect" lip. J Drugs Dermatol 11:1081, 2012.
13. Edizer M, Magden O, Tayfur V, et al. Arterial anatomy of the lower lip: a cadaveric study. Plast Reconstr Surg 111:2176, 2003.
14. de Vries CG, Geertsma RE. Clinical data on injectable tissue fillers: a review. Expert Rev Med Devices 10:835, 2013.
15. DeLorenzi C. Complications of Injectable Fillers, part I. Aesthet Surg J 33:561, 2013.
16. Glogau R, Bank D, Brandt F, et al. A randomized, evaluator-blinded, controlled study of the effectiveness and safety of a small gel particle hyaluronic acid for lip augmentation. Dermatol Surg 38:1180, 2012.
17. Ozturk CN, Li Y, Tung R, et al. Complications following injection of soft-tissue fillers. Aesthet Surg J 33:862, 2013.
18. Clymer MA. Evolution in techniques: lip augmentation. Facial Plast Surg 23:21, 2007.
19. Truswell WH. Using permanent implant materials for cosmetic enhancement of the perioral region. Facial Plast Surg 15:433, 2007.
20. Maloney BP, Truswell W, Waldman SR. Lip augmentation: discussion and debate. Facial Plast Surg 20:327, 2012.
21. Narsete T, Ersek R, Narsete MP. Further experience with permafacial implants for lip augmentation: a review of 100 implants. Aesthet Surg J 31:488, 2011.
22. Niamtu J. Advanta ePTFE facial implants in cosmetic facial surgery. J Oral Maxillofac Surg 64:543, 2006.
23. Brown C, Watson D. Lip augmentation utilizing allogenic acellular dermal graft. Facial Plast Surg 27:550, 2011.
24. Mojallal A, Shipkov C, Braye F, et al. Influence of the recipient site on the outcomes of fat grafting in facial reconstructive surgery. Plast Reconstr Surg 124:471, 2009.
25. Eremia S, Newman N. Long-term follow-up after autologous fat grafting: Analysis of results from 116 patients followed at least 12 months after receiving the last of a minimum of two treatments. Dermatol Surg 26:1150, 2000.
26. Churukian M. Red lip augmentation using fat injections. Clin Facial Plast Surg 5:61, 1997.
27. Colic MM. Lip and perioral enhancement by direct intramuscular fat autografting. Aesthetic Plastic Surgery 23:36, 1999.
28. Rohrich RJ, Reagan BJ, Adams WP Jr, et al. Early results of vermilion lip augmentation using acellular allogeneic dermis: an adjunct in facial rejuvenation. Plast Reconstr Surg 105:409; discussion 417, 2000.
29. Metzinger S, Parrish J, Guerra A, et al. Autologous fat grafting to the lower one-third of the face. Facial Plast Surg 28:21, 2012.

30. Guyuron B, Majzoub RK. Facial augmentation with core fat graft: a preliminary report. Plast Reconstr Surg 120:295, 2007.
31. Meyer R, Kesserling UK. Aesthetic surgery in the perioral region. Aesthet Plast Surg 1:61, 1976.
32. Cardoso AD, Sperli AE. Rhytidoplasty of the upper lip. In Hueston JT, ed. Transactions of the fifth international congress of plastic and reconstructive surgery, 1971 Feb 22–26. Melbourne, Australia, Butterworhts, Sydney, Australia (1971).
33. Austin HW. The lip lift. Plast Reconstr Surg 77:990, 1986.
34. González-Ulloa M. The aging upper lip. D. Marchac, J.T. Hueston (Eds.), Transactions of the sixth meeting of the international confederation for plastic and reconstructive surgery and the international society of aesthetic plastic surgery, Masson, Paris (1975), pp. 443-446.
35. Marques A, Brenda E. Lifting of the upper lip using a single extensive incision. Br J Plast Surg 47:50, 1994.
36. Greenwald A. The lip lift. Plast Reconstr Surg 79:147, 1987.
37. Cardim VLM, Dos Santos A, Lucas R, et al. Double duck nasolabial lifting. Rev Bras Cir Plast 26:466, 2011.
38. Santachè P, Bonarrigo C. Lifting of the upper lip: personal technique. Plast Reconstr Surg 113:1828, 2004.
39. Echo A, Momoh AO, Yuksel E. The no-scar lip-lift: upper lip suspension technique. Aesthet Plast Surg 35:617, 2011.
40. Greenwald A. The lip lift: cheiloplexy for cheiloptosis. Am J Cos Surg 2:16, 1985.
41. Austin HW. Rejuvenating the aging mouth Semin Plast Surg 8:27, 1994.
42. Perkins SW. The corner of the mouth lift and management of the oral commissure grooves. Facial Plast Surg Clin N Am 15:471, 2007.
43. Ching S, Flowers RS. Perioral rejuvenation using the valentine anguloplasty. Paper presented in American society for aesthetic plastic surgery annual meeting. 2005 Apr 28–May 3 (2005).
44. Parsa FD, Parsa NN, Murariu D. Surgical correction of the frowning mouth. Plast Reconstr Surg 125:667, 2010.
45. Borges AF. Sad pleats. Ann Plast Surg 22:74, 1989.
46. Delerm A, Elbaz JS. Cheiloplastie des lèvres minces. Proposition d'une technique. Am Chir Plast 20:243, 1975.
47. Aiache AE. Augmentation cheiloplasty. Plast Reconstr Surg 88:222, 1991.
48. Ho LCY. Augmentation cheiloplasty. Br J Plast Surg 47:257, 1994.
49. Mutaf M. V-Y in V-Y procedure: new technique for augmentation and protrusion of the upper lip. Ann Plast Surg 56:605, 2006.
50. Lassus C. Surgical vermilion augmentation—different possibilities. Aesth Plast Surg 16:123, 1992.
51. Moragas JSM, Vercruysse HJ, Mommaerts MY. "Non-filling" procedures for lip augmentation: a systematic review of contemporary techniques and their outcomes. J Craniomaxillofac Surg 42:943, 2014.
52. Ponsky D, Guyuron B. Comprehensive Surgical Aesthetic Enhancement and Rejuvenation of the Perioral Region. Aesthet Surg J 31:382, 2011.
53. Holden PK, Sufyan AS, Perkins SW. Long-term analysis of surgical correction of the senile upper lip. Arch Facial Plast Surg 13:332, 2011.
54. Knize DM. Lifting of the upper lip: Personal technique [discussion]. Plast Reconstr Surg 113:1836, 2004.
55. Yoskovitch A, Fanous N. Correction of thin lips: a 17-year follow-up of the original technique. Plast Reconstr Surg 112:670, 2003.
56. Weston GW, Poindexter BD, Sigal RK, et al. Lifting lips: 28 years of experience using the direct excision approach to rejuvenating the aging mouth. Aesthet Surg J 29:83, 2009.

49. Genioplasty

Ashkan Ghavami, Bahman Guyuron

RELEVANT ANATOMY

MUSCLES (Fig. 49-1)
- Mentalis
  - Conelike, vertical fibers from incisive fossa to overlying skin
  - Can cause wrinkling, and if hyperdynamic, may be visible under lower lip
  - Midline void between fibers seen when chin dimple present
- Orbicularis oris (lower fibers)
- Depressor anguli oris
- Quadratus (depressor) labii inferioris
- Geniohyoid, genioglossus, mylohyoid, and anterior belly of digastric
  - Attach to lingual (posterior) aspect of chin

BONY LANDMARKS
- Mental foramen
- Digastric fossa
- Mental protuberance
- Mental spines
- Submandibular fossa

NERVE SUPPLY
- **Inferior alveolar nerve** and **mental nerve** (terminating branch exiting mental foramen)
  - **Mental nerve:** Located at base of first or second bicuspid
  - **Inferior alveolar nerve**
    - Risk of injury during genioplasty procedures
    - Osteotomies should be **5-6 mm** below mental foramen to prevent injury to nerve branches or tooth apices.

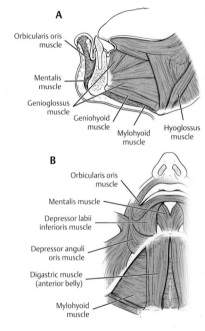

A
- Orbicularis oris muscle
- Mentalis muscle
- Genioglossus muscle
- Geniohyoid muscle
- Mylohyoid muscle
- Hyoglossus muscle

B
- Orbicularis oris muscle
- Mentalis muscle
- Depressor labii inferioris muscle
- Depressor anguli oris muscle
- Digastric muscle (anterior belly)
- Mylohyoid muscle

Fig. 49-1 Relevant muscular anatomy for genioplasty.

NOTE: The inferior alveolar nerve can be absent or distorted in patients with hemifacial microsomia or other facial deformities.

BLOOD SUPPLY

- **Labial branch** (dominant supply) of facial artery
- Inferior alveolar artery

SIGNIFICANT CEPHALOMETRIC POINTS (Fig. 49-2)

- **Pogonion (Pog):** Most projecting portion of mandible. Denotes chin excess or deficiency in relation to other structures (i.e., nasion and lip position)
- **Menton (Me):** Lowest (most caudal) portion of chin
- **Subspinale (A):** Columellar-labial junction
- **Supramentale (B):** Deepest point between pogonion and incisor
- **Nasion (N):** Nasofrontal junction

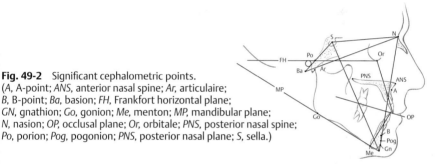

Fig. 49-2   Significant cephalometric points. (*A*, A-point; *ANS*, anterior nasal spine; *Ar*, articulaire; *B*, B-point; *Ba*, basion; *FH*, Frankfort horizontal plane; *GN*, gnathion; *Go*, gonion; *Me*, menton; *MP*, mandibular plane; *N*, nasion; *OP*, occlusal plane; *Or*, orbitale; *PNS*, posterior nasal spine; *Po*, porion; *Pog*, pogonion; *PNS*, posterior nasal plane; *S*, sella.)

INDICATIONS AND CONTRAINDICATIONS

OSSEOUS GENIOPLASTY

- **Indications**
  - Horizontal asymmetries of any magnitude
  - Excess deficiency or excess in both vertical and sagittal planes
    - ▶ Moderate to severe microgenia
  - Secondary cases after osseous or alloplastic genioplasty
  - Adjunct to formal orthognathic surgery
    - ▶ Alloplastic genioplasty is rarely, if ever, combined with formal orthognathic lower or upper jaw surgery.
- **Contraindications**
  - Inadequate bone stock (i.e., elderly patients, bone pathology)
  - Abnormal dentition or significant dental pathology
  - Patient preference to not have osteotomy
- Contrary to common belief, can be a relatively simple and efficient procedure
- More versatile procedure versus alloplastic augmentation
  - Allows **multidimensional chin correction,** including reduction

ALLOPLASTIC AUGMENTATION
■ **Indications**
  • Mild isolated sagittal deficiencies
  • Need to increase only the labiomental fold depth
  • Relative: Concomitant necklift/facelift
    ▶ Easily facilitates alloplastic augmentation as a concomitant procedure
■ **Contraindication**
  • Excess horizontal deficiency
  • Any vertical deficiency
  • Mandibular asymmetry
  • Secondary cases with bony erosion
  • Malocclusion: Orthognathic surgery required

TIP: Generally, alloplastic augmentation should be used only in patients with mild to moderate chin deficiency in the sagittal plane and a shallow labiomental fold.[1-4]

■ **Caveat:** Aesthetic surgery patients seem to prefer alloplastic augmentation, and tend to shy away from osteotomies.
  • Facelift/necklift procedures often include a submental incision that can easily be used for placing a chin implant.
  • Popular media has shown a bias toward alloplastic augmentation and present any "cuts in the bone" as very "invasive."
■ Malocclusion requires consideration of orthognathic surgery and a more extensive workup (cephalometric analysis, occlusion models) and possible collaboration with an oromaxillofacial surgeon.
■ Significant microgenia usually requires an osseous genioplasty, because a very large implant can appear awkward.

PREOPERATIVE EVALUATION
■ **Medical comorbidities**
  • Diabetic and immunosuppressed patients: Not good candidates for alloplastic chin implantation
    ▶ Osteotomy site(s) may heal poorly.
  • Age: Higher-age patients may have osteopenic bone—not good candidates for osseous genioplasty
■ **Occlusion type** (Fig. 49-3)
  • **Normal occlusion (Angle class I)**
    ▶ Mesiobuccal cusp of maxillary first molar occludes into the buccal groove of the mandibular first molar (Fig. 49-3, A).
  • **Angle class II malocclusion**
    ▶ Mesiobuccal cusp of maxillary first molar occludes medial to the buccal groove (Fig. 49-3, B).

- ▶ *Most common malocclusion in North American whites.*
- ▶ Class II is often an indication for further evaluation and possibly orthognathic surgery with maxillary and mandibular osteotomies.
- **Angle class III malocclusion**
  - ▶ Mesiobuccal cusp of the maxillary first molar occludes distal to the buccal groove of the mandibular first molar (Fig. 49-3, *C*).

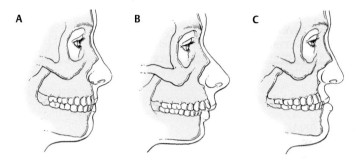

Fig. 49-3 Occlusion types. **A,** Angle class I. **B,** Angle class II. **C,** Angle class III.

TIP: Obtaining previous orthodontic history is important; because occlusion may have been corrected without addressing maxillary and mandibular disharmonies (deformity becomes masked).

- ■ **Dentition**
  - • Before 15 years of age, permanent dentition may not be fully erupted.
    - ▶ Greater risk of injury during osteotomies
  - • Elderly patients may have retruded alveolar ridge (if edentulous), which contributes to chin pad ptosis.
    - ▶ Presence of little bone stock
    - ▶ May be better candidates for alloplastic augmentation
  - • Patients with **poor dentition** or **infected dentition** are **very poor candidates** for any form of genioplasty until fully treated.

LIFE-SIZE PHOTOGRAPHS[2]
- ■ Bilateral sagittal view, frontal views, and bilateral oblique (three-quarter) views

MIDFACE HEIGHT
- ■ **Vertical maxillary excess:** Especially important when accompanied by a deep labiomental fold
  - • Patient better served by formal orthognathic correction, with or without a genioplasty

NOSE-CHIN-LIP EVALUATION (Fig. 49-4)

- Nasofacial harmony is linked with chin dimensions and vice versa.
- Chin projection should be 3 mm posterior to nose-lip-chin plane (NLCP).[5]
- Nasal length: Two thirds of midfacial height and exactly equal to chin vertical length[5]

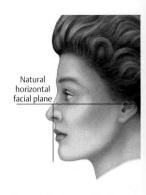

Symmetry of Lower Third of Face

- Right-to-left asymmetries of the mandible and chin may require multiple osteotomy configurations to centralize chin or canting of the osteotomy line and differential plate bending.
- Difficult to correct with alloplastic augmentation alone

Fig. 49-4   Nose-chin-lip evaluation.

SOFT TISSUE ANALYSIS

- **Soft tissue pad:** Normally **9-11 mm** thick
  - Palpated at pogonion and off midline with patient in repose and then when smiling
  - Soft tissue contribution can predict effects of augmentation.
- **Stomion:** Junction between upper and lower lip in repose
- **Upper/lower lips:** Lower lip eversion from deep bite, excess lip bulk, or excess overjet may deepen labiomental fold.[4]
- **Labiomental fold**
  - Indentation or crease between lower lip and lowest point of mandible (menton) best seen on **sagittal view**
  - Fold aesthetics dependent on vertical proportion of mandible and facial length[3]
    - ▶ Example: Deep fold may look good on longer faces.[3]
  - Evaluate for height (when stomion-to-menton is divided into thirds, fold often falls at junction of upper and middle third).
    - ▶ If fold is too low, augmentation may only address chin pad.[4]
  - Depth
    - ▶ Fold depth approximately **6 mm** in **men** and **4 mm** in **women**[6]
    - ▶ If deep, horizontal vector, chin augmentation may result in an awkward exaggerated deep fold and an overprojected chin
    - ▶ If shallow, may be further effaced by vertical augmentation
- **Riedel line:** A line drawn vertically down facial plane on sagittal view, tangential to anterior upper and lower lip (Fig. 49-5)
  - Lower lip should be 2-3 mm posterior to upper lip projection.
  - Pogonion should never project beyond this line and should be slightly posterior to it (or just touching it).

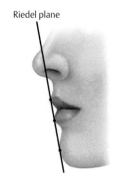

Fig. 49-5   Riedel plane is a simple line that connects the most prominent portion of the upper and lower lip, which on a balanced face should touch the pogonion.

SENIOR AUTHOR TIP: The simplest and most useful means for assessing the chin projection disharmony is Riedel line, which connects the upper to the lowermost projected points and should touch the pogonion.

DYNAMIC AND STATIC CHIN PAD ANALYSIS[4]

- A **thin chin pad** on smiling: Potential for increased pad effacement with increased bony prominence (i.e., native or from augmentation)
  - Burr reduction or osteotomy setback may be required.
- A **thick pad** may increase submental soft tissue fullness and worsen the cervicomental angle if bony setback performed

WITCH'S-CHIN DEFORMITY

- **Definition:** Ptosis of soft tissue caudal to menton and an exaggerated submental crease
- Correction requires soft tissue/muscle resection and/or repositioning.
- Augmentation can exaggerate deformity.

TIP: Mentalis muscle fixation superiorly is critical to preventing any soft tissue descent. Secondary cases may require soft tissue fixation with a Mitek device (DePuy Synthes) to prevent ptosis recurrence.[7]

CERVICOMENTAL ANGLE

- Angle between chin and neck on sagittal view should not be very obtuse or acute **(105-120 degrees).**
- Adjunct neck soft tissue contouring techniques: Submental lipectomy, platysmaplasty, anterior digastric resection, and/or submandibular gland resection or suspension can further enhance chin aesthetics.

IMAGING

- Cephalograms and/or Panorex
  - Always indicated for secondary cases
  - Required: If maxillary/mandibular imbalance or malocclusion suspected
  - Obtain Panorex if any concern for nerve malposition or uncertain apical teeth location and/or dental pathology

SOFT TISSUE RESPONSE/OSSEOUS MOVEMENT RATIO

- **Osteotomy and alloplastic augmentation: Approximately** 0.8-0.9:1.0
- **Ostectomy: Approximately** 0.25-0.50:1.0

CLASSIFICATION OF CHIN DEFORMITY (Fig. 49-6)

- **Microgenia:** Small chin
- **Macrogenia:** Large chin

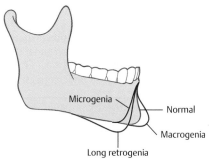

Fig. 49-6 Chin deformity.

- **Combined deformities:** Short or long macrogenia/microgenia
  - Horizontal (off-center) asymmetries can also exist.
- Classification system proposed by Guyuron et al[8] can serve as a guide for operative planning (Table 49-1).

Table 49-1 *Classification System for Chin Deformity and Correction*

Type	Deformity	Vector and Surgical Treatment
Class I	Macrogenia	Horizontal: Osteotomy with setback or osteotomy Vertical: Osteotomy and resection Both horizontal and vertical: Osteotomy, resection, and setback
Class II	Microgenia	Horizontal: Osteotomy with advancement, autogenous or alloplastic augmentation Vertical: Osteotomy and lengthening, with or without graft Both horizontal and vertical: Osteotomy, lengthening, and advancement, with or without graft
Class III	Combined	Horizontal macrogenia with vertical microgenia: Osteotomy with lengthening and setback Horizontal microgenia with vertical macrogenia: Osteotomy with resection of horizontal segment and advancement
Class IV	Aysmmetrical	Short anterior lower face: Addition of wedge of bone to short side Normal lower facial height: Removal of wedge of bone from long side; add to short side Long anterior facial height: Removal of wedge of bone based on long side
Class V	Witch's-chin	Soft tissue correction
Class VI	Pseudomacrogenia	Soft tissue adjustment (not predictable)
Class VII	Pseudomicrogenia	Maxillary osteotomy

INFORMED CONSENT

Should include, but not be limited to, the following:
- Possible injury to nerves in the area with subsequent temporary versus permanent changes in sensation
  - Neurosensory changes in chin and lips
- Asymmetry and palpable bony step-offs
- Malunion, nonunion, plate/hardware extrusion and need for later removal (for osseous genioplasty)
- Implant malposition, extrusion (exposure), palpability, need for later removal, and the possibility of bone resorption under the implant should be described (for alloplastic augmentation genioplasty)
- Overcorrection versus undercorrection

> **TIP:** Preoperative asymmetries should be pointed out to patients, but guarantees of their corrections should not be made.

EQUIPMENT AND IMPLANT MATERIAL

ALLOPLASTIC CHIN AUGMENTATION: GENERAL EQUIPMENT

- For alloplastic augmentation, fixating the implant with either bone anchor suture or clear nylon suture (3-0 to 4-0 caliber) that is passed through the implant is recommended.
  - Many implants have preplaced holes; silicone implants allow suture to easily pass through the implant.
  - Ideal fixation should be performed **centrally** and **one fixation point laterally** to either bone or periosteum.
  - Craniofacial screws (and therefore drills and appropriate screw applicators) can be used to directly screw in the implant and is best indicated for polyethylene implants, which are firmer.
- Colorado needletip cautery and 9 mm periosteal elevator for pocket dissection (alloplastic and osseous techniques)

ALLOPLASTIC IMPLANT TYPES[9]

- **Synthetic**
  - **Silicone (polysiloxane):** Available in smooth or textured
    - ▶ Vulcanized form of polysiloxane
    - ▶ Extended anatomic implants developed by Terino[10,11]
      - ◆ **Terino**[10,11]**:** Developed system based on zonal anatomy with chin implants that have lateral tapered edges, which can also augment the mandibular body (midlateral-ML) to widen the anterior jawline (Fig. 49-7)
    - ▶ **Advantages:** Easy to sterilize by steam or irradiation, easy to carve, can be stabilized with screw or sutures (Mitek Bone Anchor System), allergic reaction extremely rare, no ingrowth, which allows easy removal
    - ▶ **Disadvantages:** Causes resorption in underlying bone (increased with malposition), potential for migration, visibility if thin skin
  - **Porous polyethylene (Porex, Porex Corporation or Medpor, Stryker):** Contains 125-250 µm diameter pores that cause tissue ingrowth, and incorporation of implant versus encapsulation (as with silicone and nonporous implants)
    - ▶ **Advantages:** Firm consistency but malleable and carvable, infection rate may be lower than silicone-based implants (perhaps because of vascular ingrowth),

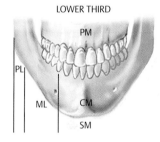
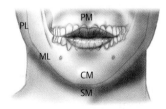

Fig. 49-7 Zonal anatomy of the premandibular jawline aesthetic facial segment. (*CM*, Central mentum; *ML*, midlateral; *PL*, posterolateral; *PM*, premaxilla; *SM*, submandibular.)

less tendency to migrate and erode underlying bone, easily fixed with screws or sutures

    ▶ **Disadvantages:** Requires larger soft tissue pocket, placement more difficult than for smoother implants, implant removal is more difficult than for smooth silicone prosthesis, usually has large dimensions and requires trimming/customizing intraoperatively

• Custom-made (silicone- or polyethylene-based) implants based on three-dimensional modeling (perhaps, more useful if multiple facial implants required) are available.

BIOLOGIC CHIN AUGMENTATION
■ Autologous cranial bone
■ Rib or conchal cartilage grafts
■ Irradiated cartilage sources

OSSEOUS GENIOPLASTY: SPECIAL EQUIPMENT
■ A limited orthognathic or genioplasty tray with reciprocating sagittal saw (side-cutting) is preferred.
■ A four-hole low-profile step plate (2.0 mm plate and screw system)
■ Two plates sometimes needed if correcting horizontal asymmetry or performing a jumping genioplasty

SURGICAL TECHNIQUES: OSSEOUS GENIOPLASTY (Fig. 49-8)

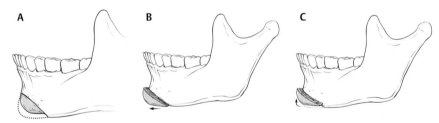

Fig. 49-8   Common types of osseous genioplasty. **A,** Reduction genioplasty. **B,** Sliding genioplasty. **C,** Jumping genioplasty.

> **TIP:**   Excess inferior/posterior stripping may devascularize the lower bone segment after an osteotomy is performed. Only lateral exposure is required to visualize mental nerves.

> **SENIOR AUTHOR TIP:**   Regarding patients with long face deformity and horizontal microgenia, it is crucial to realize that should the patient not undergo a maxillary vertical reduction advancement of the chin to an optimal position, this may result in a longer appearing face and in major potential patient dissatisfaction. Under this condition, the chin advancement should be conservative.

REDUCTION GENIOPLASTY

- **Indication:** To correct increased vertical height or sagittal excess
- Zide et al[11] have developed an evaluation system that does not require cephalometrics.
  - Highlights of the preoperative evaluation and technique include:
    - ▶ Evaluating the **thickness of the chin pad** with patient smiling. Thinner-padded patients may reveal exaggerated chin prominence when smiling. This requires a more aggressive reduction.
    - ▶ **Chin pad percentage:** A higher chin pad percentage means greater chin size appearance and a greater reduction is needed.
    - ▶ **Lower lip white roll-to-labiomental fold inclination:** Chins with similar bony projection but different lip-to-fold inclination require different amounts of chin reduction.
      - ◆ As the inclination becomes more oblique, greater reduction is warranted.
- Angling osteotomy inferiorly will produce a vertical reduction.

NOTE: Excess vertical height of mandible requires formal orthognathic procedures, commonly with a simultaneous genioplasty.

- Ostectomy
  - Indication: Significant height reduction

TIP: Genioplasty results can be enhanced with submental soft tissue procedures: liposuction, lipectomy, and/or platysmaplasty.

SLIDING GENIOPLASTY

- **Indication:** Standard operation for **horizontal (sagittal) deficiency**
- **Two-tier genioplasty:** Two segments advanced anteriorly
  - Rarely necessary, used for extreme sagittal and/or vertical deficiency

TIP: Dissection that is carried obliquely and anteriorly or at a right angle to bone will provide a small cuff of intact mentalis muscle to facilitate soft tissue approximation when closing.

JUMPING GENIOPLASTY

- **Indication:** Very minor chin height excess
- Inferior fragment "jumped" over superior segment as an onlay

INTERPOSITIONAL BONE GRAFTS (OR HYDROXYAPATITE)

- **Indication:** To add more vertical length
- Added to osteotomy segment that has been angled superiorly

CENTRALIZING GENIOPLASTY
- **Indication:** To correct asymmetries
- Wedges of autologous bone graft or hydroxyapatite often needed

CORRECTION OF LONG, NONPROJECTING CHIN[12]
- Presents a unique challenge and can be successfully treated with both a one-cut in situ contoured jumping genioplasty and extraoral vertical reduction/sagittal augmentation genioplasty, which:
  - Reduce excess chin height, control sagittal advancement, provide pogonion projection, and prevent the risks of a standard wedge ostectomy.

> **SENIOR AUTHOR TIP:**   Leaving minimum 10 mm mucosa and muscle attached to the cephalic portion of the lip incision facilitates reattachment of the soft tissues and reduces the potential for the lip ptosis.

SURGICAL TECHNIQUE: GENIOPLASTY
- 3-4 cm transverse incision (needletip electrocautery) in anterior gingivobuccal sulcus (>1 cm anterior), **leaving adequate gingival cuff for closure**
- Mucosa incised and dissection carried oblique anterior or at right angle to bone, **leaving small cuff of mentalis muscle**
- Subperiosteal dissection of symphysis, only inferior enough to do osteotomy (excess inferior/posterior stripping may devascularize lower bone segment after osteotomy performed); exposure continued laterally to *mental nerves;* posterior dissection inferior to molar roots
- Burr or saw is used to make midline vertical hash mark as a reference
- Reciprocating osteotomy saw used to make horizontal osteotomy, at least 5-6 mm inferior to mental foramen, cut posteriorly
  - Orientation/angle of cut (oblique) guides direction of mobility and degree of correction (see previous TIP)
- Mobilization of segment (digastric muscle disinsertion may be needed) assessed intraoperatively with measurements obtained previously for amount of advancement, side-to-side repositioning or reduction needed
- **Bone grafting** if required
- **Fixation:** Single plate in midline. Asymmetry correction, multisegments, or jumping genioplasty requires two plates. (Some surgeons prefer biodegradable screw/plate systems.)
- Irrigation, muscle repair *(mentalis fixation is critical to preventing soft tissue ptosis),* and appropriate, high fixation; secondary cases may require Mitek soft tissue fixation to prevent soft tissue ptosis recurrence.[7]
- Mucosal closure (with 4-0 chromic gut) with incorporation of muscle layer or, preferably, closure of muscle layer with 4-0 Vicryl or 4-0 clear nylon suture and 1-inch Microfoam tape compression dressing and/or a chin strap garment

> **SENIOR AUTHOR TIP:**   The osteotomy plane should be 5 mm below the mental foramen to reduce the potential injury to the nerve.

SURGICAL TECHNIQUE: IMPLANT GENIOPLASTY

APPROACH: ADVANTAGES AND DISADVANTAGES
- **Extraoral**
  - Submental exposure allows more precise placement.
  - Possibly fewer cases of malposition and mental nerve injury
  - Soft tissue/muscle closure should be strong to prevent soft tissue ptosis.
  - Relatively indicated with concomitant facelift and/or necklift
- **Intraoral**
  - No visible scars
  - Similar infection rate
  - Improper implant position (often too superior)—no direct visualization of pocket
  - May have higher chance of plate/screw extrusion

FIXATION
- **Methods**
  - Screws[13]
  - Sutures,[4,7,14] Mitek
- If no fixation, **precise pocket dissection** and soft tissue approximation becomes even more important

> **TIP:** Securing the implant is well worth the time. Bone holes are not needed. By preserving strategically located cuffs of soft tissue and periosteum, suture fixation with 3-0/4-0 clear nylon or 3-0/4-0 PDS is adequate.

IMPLANT POSITION
- **Proper position:** Directly over **pogonion** is **critical**
- Superior positioning
  - Can increase bone and/or tooth root resorption/erosion, movement, and asymmetries
    - This may be more likely with the intraoral approach.
- Superficial placement
  - Implant may be visible, palpable, and show irregularities.
  - Place subperiosteally
  - Polyethylene (Porex) may be more likely to show.

> **TIP:** Creating too large a pocket can increase malposition rates. A larger pocket is required in polyethylene implants, which should be directly fixated.

> **SENIOR AUTHOR TIP:** On edentulous patients the mental nerve is often significantly malpositioned and it is closer to the alveolar ridge.

IMPLANT REMOVAL/SECONDARY CASES
- Will often require:
  - Replacement with a smaller implant with fixation or an osseous genioplasty
  - Osseous genioplasty will effectively fill soft tissue void.

- Soft tissue/muscle manipulations (resection, repositioning) to prevent:
  - ► Soft tissue pad "balling"
  - ► Chin pad ptosis
  - ► Fasciculations or menton dimpling—not preventable but can be treated with botulinum toxin A injections[7]
- A recent study has demonstrated the efficacy of a *textured fixed implant* in both primary and secondary cases.[15]
  - ► **Primary indications:** Tension chin and wide interlabial gap (>3 mm), concern about implant movement/malposition, patients do not want silicone prosthesis
  - ► **Secondary indications:** Replacement after malposition and/or bony erosion, patients do not want osteotomy
  - ► **Technical caveats:** Conscious sedation with field block used; drill holes necessary, pogonial and implant midline scored, implant custom carved to fit in precise pocket

POSTOPERATIVE CARE

DRESSING
- Microfoam tape (if used) removed in 3-4 days, along with the chin strap, to examine contour and incision
- Patients instructed to wear elastic chin support garment for 24 hours a day for the first 5-7 days and then at night for the next 1-2 weeks

POSITION AND ACTIVITY
- Patients instructed to limit activity that increases heart rate for 5-7 days
- Head of bed up (45 degrees) for 3-5 days
- Sleep supine as much as possible for the next 1-2 weeks.

DIET
- Can resume previous diet as tolerated
  - Some patients may benefit from protein shake supplements if reluctant to mobilize early
- After osseous genioplasty, avoid hard foods such as apples for the first 3 days.
- Rinse mouth after each meal with water and/or Peridex.
- Limit salt intake.

PROPHYLACTIC ANTIBIOTICS
- One dose of first-generation cephalosporin is given before incision; thereafter oral dose continuation for 3-5 days every 8 hours is all that is needed.
- If intraoral approach used, a 3-day regimen of Peridex oral rinse solution is helpful, scheduled every 8 hours and as a rinse after each meal

STEROIDS
- Recommended to decrease edema
- IV dose should be given perioperatively.
- A steroid taper regimen is recommended postoperatively (i.e., Solu-Medrol 5-day taper)

HERBS, OTHER POSTOPERATIVE MEDICATION
- *Arnica montana* orally for 3-5 days postoperatively may be beneficial, along with *Bromelain* (high-dose pineapple extract).

COMPLICATIONS

AESTHETIC RESULTS
- **Poor aesthetic result:** Likely most common "complication"
  - However, dissatisfaction rate is very low.
  - **Satisfaction rates[16]:**
    - ▶ **Osseous genioplasty:** 90%-95%
    - ▶ **Alloplastic augmentation:** 85%-90%
- *Overcorrection:* More common in women; may result in overprojection and masculinization
- *Implant versus osseous genioplasty:* Very controversial with limited reports
  - One study showed slightly higher satisfaction and self-esteem improvement rates with osseous genioplasty.[16]
- *Asymmetries:* Related to technique of improper soft tissue/muscle (mentalis) dissection and fixation/reapproximation
  - Bony asymmetries with osseous genioplasty: Increase chance if osteotomy not posterior enough

HEMATOMA
- Rare; commonly at lateral osteotomy site
- Responds to simple aspiration and antibiotics; cover for oral flora

INFECTION
- Uncommon (<5% for implants (Proplast, Vitek), approximately 3% for osseous)[1,16]
- More likely with hematomas in osseous techniques
- Overall may be more common in alloplastic implantation (may require implant removal)
- Some surgeons report no infections.[13]
- Implant extrusion: Very rare, related to infection and high placement

MALPOSITION
- More common with intraoral implant placement
- Leads to increased *bone resorption* rates
- May be best treated with a textured secured implant or osseous technique

BONE RESORPTION
- Seen most often with malposition and a nonsecured smooth silicone implant
- Treat with textured secured implant
- Osseous procedures usually not adequate because of inadequate bone stock

NERVE INJURY
- **Neurapraxia:** Often a retraction injury and resolves in 2-6 weeks
  - Permanent: Extremely rare and probably results from direct transection or avulsion during dissection or unrecognized implant pressure directly on the mental nerve
  - If significant paresthesia occurs and implant suspected to be compressing nerve, then must **reoperate ASAP**

> **TIP:** Limit retraction and manipulation of mental nerves as much as possible.

■ **Lower lip paresthesias:** 5%-6% rate
  • Temporary drooling may be present. If >6 weeks, consider removal, trimming of implant.
  • Permanent deficits extremely rare; often related to improper osteotomy technique and damage of inferior alveolar nerve as it courses caudally

---

TOP TAKEAWAYS
➤ The inferior alveolar nerve can be absent or distorted in patients with hemifacial macrosomia or other facial deformities.
➤ Some patients have an imbalance in chin projection, height, and/or asymmetry relative to other facial features.
➤ Generally, alloplastic augmentation should be used only in patients with mild to moderate chin deficiency in the sagittal plane and a shallow labiomental fold.[1-4]
➤ Preoperative asymmetries should be pointed out to patients, but guarantees of their corrections should not be made.

REFERENCES
1. Cohen SR. Genioplasty. In Achauer BM, Eriksson E, Guyuron B, et al, eds. Plastic Surgery: Indications, Operations, and Outcomes, vol 5. St Louis, Mosby–Year Book, 2000.
2. Guyuron B, ed. Genioplasty. Boston: Little Brown, 1993.
3. Rosen HM. Osseous genioplasty. In Aston SJ, Beasley RW, Thorne CN, eds. Grabb and Smith's Plastic Surgery, ed 5. Philadelphia: Lippincott-Raven, 1997.
4. Zide BM, Pfeifer TM, Longaker MT. Chin surgery: I. Augmentation—the allures and the alerts. Plast Reconstr Surg 104:1843, 1999.
5. Byrd HS, Hobar PC. Rhinoplasty: a practical guide for surgical planning. Plast Reconstr Surg 91:642, 1993.
6. Michelow BJ, Guyuron B. The chin: skeletal and soft tissue components. Plast Reconstr Surg 95:473, 1995.
7. Zide BM, Boutros S. Chin surgery III: revelations. Plast Reconstr Surg 111:1542; discussion 1551, 2003.
8. Guyuron B, Michelow BJ, Willis L. Practical classification of chin deformities. Aesthetic Plast Surg 19:257, 1995.
9. Yaremchuk MJ. Facial skeletal augmentation. In Mathes SJ, Hentz VR, eds. Plastic Surgery: The Head and Neck, ed 2. Philadelphia: Saunders Elsevier, 2006.
10. Terino EO. Alloplastic facial contouring by zonal principles of skeletal anatomy. Clin Plast Surg 19:487, 1992.
11. Zide BM, Warren SM, Spector JA. Chin surgery IV: the large chin—key parameters for successful chin reduction. Plast Reconstr Surg 120:530, 2007.
12. Warren SM, Spector JA, Zide BM. Chin surgery V: treatment of the long, nonprojecting chin. Plast Reconstr Surg 120:760, 2007.
13. Yaremchuk MJ. Improving aesthetic outcomes after alloplastic chin augmentation. Plast Reconstr Surg 112:1422, 2003.
14. Zide BM, Longaker MT. Chin surgery: II. Submental ostectomy and soft-tissue excision. Plast Reconstr Surg 104:1854, 1999.
15. Warren SM, Spector JA, Zide BM. Chin surgery VII: the textured secure implant—a recipe for success. Plast Reconstr Surg 120:1378, 2007.
16. Guyuron B, Raszewski RL. A critical comparison of osteoplastic and alloplastic augmentation genioplasty. Aesthetic Plast Surg 14:199, 1990.

50. Otoplasty

Joseph M. Brown, Jeffrey E. Janis, Charles H. Thorne

NORMAL EAR ANATOMY AND DEVELOPMENT[1-5] (Fig. 50-1)

- Lateral skin (scapha) is adherent and thin with little subcutaneous tissue.
- Medial skin is loose, fibrofatty, and thick.
- The ear is **85%** of its adult size by the **sixth** year of life.
- Average length of 10-year-old male ear is 60 mm.
- Ear cartilage becomes stiffer and more brittle with age.
- Neonatal cartilage is malleable and softer.

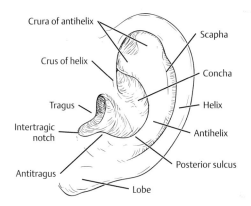

Fig. 50-1 Anatomy of the external ear.

TIP: Good outcomes have been achieved by molding techniques if implemented within the first few weeks of life while circulating maternal hormones remain elevated.

EMBRYOLOGY

Ear begins to protrude approximately 3-4 months of gestation.

VASCULARITY (Fig. 50-2)

- **External carotid** gives off two terminal branches to the ear:
  - Posterior auricular artery
  - Superficial temporal artery

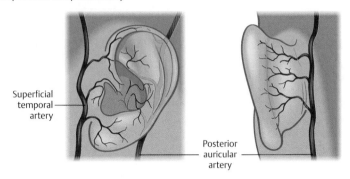

Fig. 50-2   Vascularity of the external ear.

INNERVATION

- **Auriculotemporal nerve (CN V)**
  - Innervates tragus and crus helicis
- **Great auricular nerve (C2-3)**
  - Divides into anterior and posterior branches
  - Innervates remaining scapha and lobule
- **Arnold nerve (CN X)**
  - External acoustic meatus and medial conchal bowl
- **Lesser occipital nerve (C2-3)**

CARTILAGINOUS ANATOMY (Fig. 50-3)

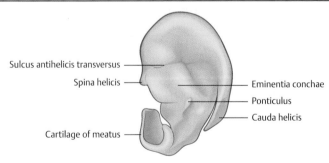

Fig. 50-3   Cartilaginous anatomy (posterior view).

■ Posterior surface has two important landmarks:
  • **Ponticulus** is the site of attachment to the auricularis posterior muscle.
  • Must be dissected and removed before conchamastoid sutures (Furnas technique)
  • **Cauda helicis** serves as possible transition point from posterior dissection to an anterior dissection in the subperichondral plane without violating the lateral skin envelope.

NORMAL PROPORTIONS OF THE AESTHETIC EAR[4,6] (Fig. 50-4)

■ The long axis of the ear inclines posteriorly approximately 20 degrees from vertical.
■ The ear axis does not normally parallel the bridge of the nose.
  • Usually a 150 degrees differential
■ The ear is positioned approximately one ear length (5.5-7 cm) posterior to the lateral orbital rim between horizontal planes that intersect the eyebrow and columella.
■ The width is approximately 50%-60% of the length.
  • Width 3-4.5 cm
  • Length 5.5-7 cm
■ The anterolateral aspect of the helix protrudes at a 21-30 degree angle from the scalp.
■ The anterolateral aspect of the helix is approximately 1.5-2 cm from the scalp.
  • There is a large amount of racial and gender variation.
■ The lobule and antihelical fold lie in a parallel plane at an acute angle to the mastoid process.
■ The helix should project 2-5 mm more laterally than the antihelix in frontal view.

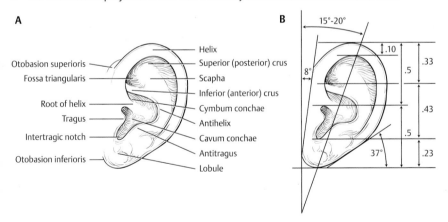

Fig. 50-4   Proportions of the ear. **A,** The normal ear and its parts. **B,** The ear's critical proportions.

EPIDEMIOLOGY/PATHOLOGY[6-9]

- Autosomal dominant trait
- Incidence in whites is about 5%.
- **Three major contributing factors to the abnormal morphology:**
  1. **Underdeveloped antihelical fold**
     - ► Obtuse conchoscaphal angle (>90 degrees)
     - ► Scapha and helical rim protrude causing prominent upper and middle third of ear.
  2. **Prominent concha**
     - ► Either excessively deep conchal wall (>1.5 cm)[10] or obtuse conchamastoid angle
     - ► Causes prominent middle third of ear
  3. **Protruding earlobe**
     - ► Causes prominent lower third of the ear
- Multiple studies[5,6,11,12] indicate protruding ears may lead to teasing and bullying that can result in emotional and behavioral problems in the long term.
- Recent literature emphasize that, performed in the correct patients, otoplasty can positively affect patients' self-esteem, psychological well-being, and quality of life.

GOALS OF SURGICAL TREATMENT[9]

- All upper-third ear protrusion must be corrected.
- The helix of both ears should be visible beyond (lateral to) the antihelix from an anterior view.
- The helix should have a smooth and regular contour along its course.
- When viewed from behind, the contour of the helical rim should be a straight line.
- The postauricular sulcus should not be markedly decreased or distorted.
- The helix-to-mastoid distance should be in the normal range of **10-12 mm** in the upper third, **16-18 mm** in the middle third, and **20-22 mm** in the lower third.
- The position of the lateral ear border to the head should match within **3 mm** at any point between the two ears.

PREOPERATIVE EVALUATION[13]

- A thorough history should be obtained.
  - • The history should include the motivations and desires of the patient, as well as any indication of psychological stress.
- Examination should focus on the following:
  - • Degree of antihelical folding
  - • Depth of the conchal bowl
  - • Plane of the lobule and deformity, if present
  - • Angle between the helical rim and the mastoid plane
  - • Quality and spring of the auricular cartilage
    - ► To assess likelihood of necessity of cartilage scoring

> **SENIOR AUTHOR TIP:**   First question: Are the protruding ears of normal shape or are they protruding AND of abnormal shape (e.g., constricted ear, Stahl ear).

- Preoperative photographs should be obtained. Spira[14] recommended taking two frontals, right and left lateral views, and a modified worm's-eye view.
  - Two frontal views help to accommodate the patient's blink reflex.
  - Worm's-eye view helps to determine the degree of the deformity that may otherwise be masked by lighting/shadows.

> **SENIOR AUTHOR TIP:**   I think the posterior view is critical and perhaps more important than some of the views mentioned previously.

INDICATIONS/CONTRAINDICATIONS

- **Contraindications**
  - **Surgical intervention should not be performed before patients are 4 years of age.** In the neonatal period, nonoperative management can be very effective, as elevated circulating estrogen levels keep auricular cartilage malleable and responsive to molding casts.
- The ear is nearly fully developed by **6-7 years of age,** at which time surgery should be considered in appropriate candidates.

> **NOTE:**   However, it is important to address timing of surgery on a patient-to-patient basis, because some patients may experience significant bullying at an even younger age, and earlier intervention may be necessary.

  - Balogh and Millesi[15] have shown that auricular growth was not halted after a 7-year mean follow-up in 76 patients who underwent cartilage excision otoplasty for prominent ears.
  - Patients with prominent ears generally do not care if a little growth inhibition results from the surgery.

INFORMED CONSENT

- Addressing specific concerns for each patient and setting appropriate expectations are essential.
- Although the goal of this surgery is to improve self-image through correction of the deformity, it does not guarantee a "better life."
- Risks include undercorrection, overcorrection, unnatural or sharp contours, hematoma, infection, chondritis, recurrent deformity (early and/or late), persistent asymmetry with the contralateral ear, and protrusion of permanent sutures through the medial skin.

EQUIPMENT

- A Dingman otoabrader or half of an Adson-Brown Tissue forceps may be used for cartilage scoring.
- Aside from this, no special equipment is required for this surgery.
- Methylene blue is a useful tool for transposing landmarks on the anterolateral surface of the ear to the cranial surface through the use with a 25-gauge needle.

SURGICAL TECHNIQUES

- **Most common**
  - **Mustardé**[16]: Cartilage shaping
  - **Furnas**[17]: Cartilage shaping
  - **Converse–Wood-Smith**[18]: Cartilage breaking
- **Others**
  - **Stenstroem**[19]: Cartilage scoring
  - **Chongchet**[20]: Cartilage scoring

NOTE: Cartilage-scoring techniques are based on the observation that cartilage curls away from a cut surface because of release of "interlocked stresses" when the perichondrium and outermost layer of chondrocytes are incised.[21,22]

TIP: Even when performing a unilateral otoplasty, draping both ears into the field for intraoperative assessment for symmetry is encouraged. To prevent asymmetry after the procedure, performing an otoplasty on both ears should be considered, even if only one appears particularly prominent.

- Younger patients should undergo general anesthesia in an appropriate facility.
- Older patients may tolerate corrective surgery under local anesthesia in an office setting. Adults can almost always undergo the procedure under local anesthesia.

MUSTARDÉ TECHNIQUE (Fig. 50-5)

- Used to correct a poorly defined antihelical fold
- Used to correct upper-third deformities
- **Almost never performed in isolation;** almost always performed in combination with other maneuvers

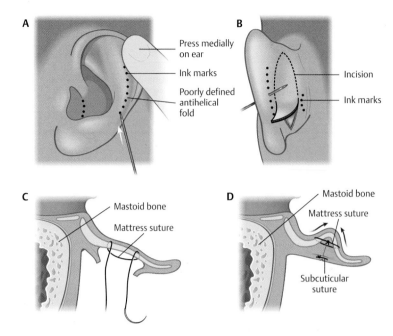

Fig. 50-5   The Mustardé technique. **A,** Several pairs of ink marks are made on the concha and outer aspect of the antihelix. **B,** Several 25-gauge needles dipped in ink are used to transfer the ink marks to the postauricular skin. **C,** The skin excision is carried down to cartilage. After hemostasis is obtained, several sutures are placed through the full thickness of cartilage. Usually only two or three well-placed sutures are required. **D,** The sutures are tied simultaneously. A subcuticular 4-0 nylon suture is used for closure.

■ **Procedure**

• Press medially on the scapha to create the proposed antihelical fold and superior crus.

▶ Mark the outer boundaries of these structures.

▶ Use a 25-gauge needle to transpose the lateral markings to the cranial surface of the ear.

▶ Bathe the needle with a methylene blue–soaked cotton-tipped applicator.

▶ Remove the needle to tattoo the skin and cartilage.

TIP: Scratching the needle with a Bovie pad may help to remove the outer silicone layer of the needle and allow a better hold of the methylene blue and leave more pronounced markings.

- On the cranial surface of the ear, mark the postauricular skin excision as an ellipse between the tattooed markings.

SENIOR AUTHOR TIP: Excising skin may not be needed in some cases.

- 1% lidocaine with epinephrine 1:100,000 is infiltrated with a 30-gauge needle, using hydrodissection in the subperichondrial plane.
  - ▶ The cranial surface, lateral surface of the concha, and scapha should be infiltrated, as well as the conchal bowl.
- Undermine in a subperichondrial plane using sharp dissection.
  - ▶ Extend along the cranial surface almost to the helical rim from the cauda helicis (see Fig. 50-3) to the cephalicmost portion of the scapha.
  - ▶ If cartilage is to be scored, access to the anterior surface of the scapha may be obtained by dissecting a window between the cauda helicis and the conchal cartilage. This is done with sharp dissecting scissors.
  - ▶ Subperichondrial dissection on the anterior surface is performed with a Joseph elevator.

TIP: Undermine only the area intended for cartilage scoring, because this will minimize the dead space on the anterior surface of the auricle.

- Place permanent mattress sutures (4-0 clear nylon or 4-0 Mersilene) full thickness through the cartilage along the tattooed marks, making sure to capture the anterior perchondrium without piercing anterior skin. When each half of the Mustardé mattress suture is placed, the lateral skin should be examined to rule out a full-thickness bite, *before the needle is removed* for the next bite.

NOTE: Be diligent to ensure the anterior skin has not been penetrated.

TIP: The placement of the mattress sutures in the scapha should be wider than the placement in the concha. These should span like spokes on a wheel, unlike parallel mattress sutures (see Fig. 50-5). This will create a more curvilinear, natural-appearing antihelix.[23]

- Place all mattress sutures before tying (four to six mattress sutures are usually required).
  - ▶ Once placed, tie sutures down to effect.
  - ▶ This may require "floating" sutures or purposeful "air knots."
- The skin is then approximated with interrupted 5-0 plain gut.

FURNAS TECHNIQUE (Fig. 50-6)
- Used to correct deformities of the middle third by addressing conchal excess
- **Almost never performed in isolation;** almost always performed in combination with other maneuvers such as Mustardé sutures and correction of lobular prominence; may be combined with other techniques (e.g., Mustardé technique for correcting an absent antihelical fold)

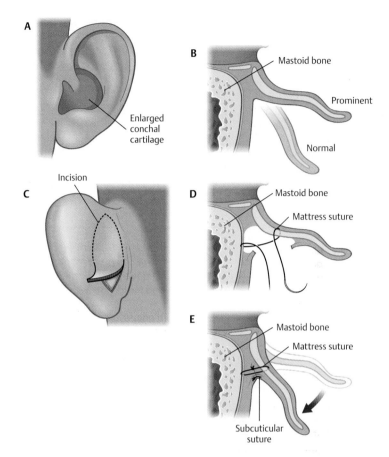

Fig. 50-6   The Furnas technique. **A,** The Furnas technique is best used for patients with prominence of the superior two thirds of the ear. **B,** The deeply cupped and enlarged conchal cartilage of the prominent ear is contrasted with normal conchal cartilage in cross section. **C,** An ellipse of skin is excised in the postauricular sulcus, exposing the posterior auricular muscles and ligaments. These are divided and resected. **D** and **E,** Several mattress sutures are used to attach conchal cartilage to the mastoid fascia. The mattress sutures should be placed through the full thickness of the conchal cartilage. The sutures are tied simultaneously.

■ **Procedure**
   • Take care to extend the dissection medially across the auriculocephalic angle onto the mastoid fascia.
   • Dissection should extend medially along the conchal cartilage until the ponticulus is identified, which is the insertion of the auricularis posterior.
      ▶ This muscle should be identified and resected to allow placement of conchamastoid sutures.
      ▶ Resection of this muscle, as well as fibrofatty tissue, over the mastoid fascia allows accentuation of the setback.[24]

CAUTION: Some terminal branches of the great auricular nerve will be inevitably divided.

- Dissection should also extend to ~2 cm over the mastoid region.
- A segment of mastoid fascia is resected to expose the underlying perichondrium. *Mastoid fascia is preserved intact so that sutures can be placed into it.*
- The ear is then depressed medially until a desirable effect is obtained.
- One or two permanent mattress sutures (4-0 clear nylon or 4-0 Mersilene) are then placed.
  - ▶ Full-thickness cartilaginous bites of the concha are taken, incorporating both the posterior cartilaginous surface and the anterior perichondrium, while sparing the anterior skin.
  - ▶ The sutures should incorporate strong bites of the mastoid fascia to prevent pull-through.
- Sutures are tied down to desired effect. This may require "floating" sutures.

TIP: In cases of excessively large conchae, anterior displacement of the medial aspect of the concha may narrow the external auditory canal (Fig. 50-7). In this situation, a laterally based 1 cm wide flap of perichondrium and underlying cartilage may be elevated and sutured to the mastoid region to obtain similar results (Fig. 50-8).[14]

- The skin may be approximated with a running 5-0 chromic gut suture.

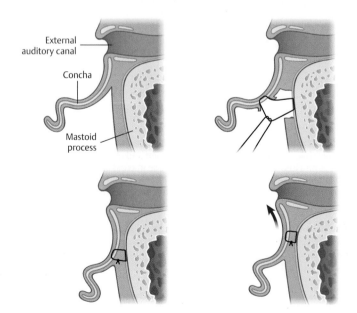

Fig. 50-7   Narrowing of the external auditory canal from anterior displacement of the medial aspect of the concha.

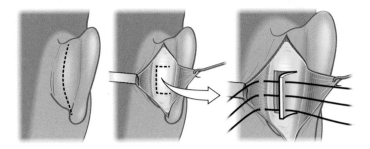

Fig. 50-8   Perichondrium and underlying cartilage elevated and sutured to the mastoid region.

CONVERSE–WOOD-SMITH TECHNIQUE (Fig. 50-9)

- A **cartilage-breaking technique,** rather than cartilage-molding technique, as in the previously discussed examples
- Useful for correcting very severe prominent ear deformities (when the entire ear is involved)
- **Drawback:** May cause cartilaginous ridging, sharp edges, or overdefinition of the antihelix and superior crus that may leave a "postoperative" appearance
- **Procedure**[18]
  - Press medially on the auricle to create an antihelical fold in the desired location, in a fashion similar to that described for the Mustardé technique.
  - Mark the superior rim of the triangular fossa, the upper border of the superior crus, and the junction of the helix and scapha.
  - Mark the full length of the conchal rim.
  - Transpose these markings with a 25-gauge needle, mark an ellipse of skin to be excised, infiltrate with local anesthesia, and dissect down to raw cartilage, similar to the fashion described for the Mustardé technique.
  - Incise cartilage full thickness with a scalpel, sparing the lateral skin.
  - Create the antihelix by placing full-thickness mattress sutures with permanent suture (4-0 clear nylon or 4-0 Mersilene) and tie them down to effect.
  - Estimate the amount of conchal excess by pressing inward on the newly created antihelix, and excise the appropriate amount.
  - Approximate the newly cut edges of the concha and antihelix with permanent suture.

TIP: Avoid everting the edges, because doing so will cause permanent ridging.

  - The skin may be approximated with a running 5-0 chromic gut suture.

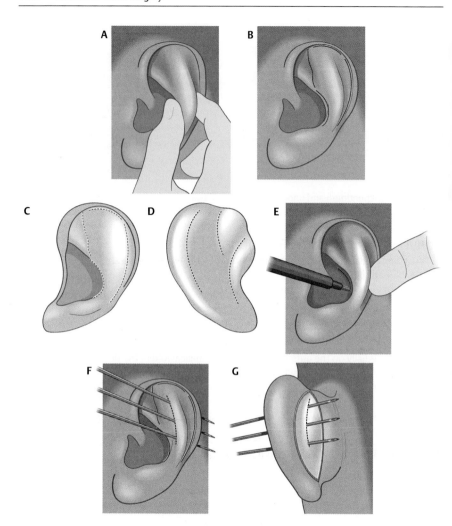

Fig. 50-9   The Converse–Wood-Smith technique. **A,** The pinna is folded back to define the superior crus of the antihelix, as well as the crural junction. **B,** The anterior and posterior borders of the antihelix, the superior border of the superior crus, and the conchal rim are outlined with ink. **C** and **D,** The planned cartilaginous incisions. **E,** Conchal rim definition may be facilitated with pressure applied to the scapha. **F** and **G,** The center line of the superior crus and antihelix is marked by 25-gauge needles. An ellipse of skin is fashioned to incorporate these and excised.

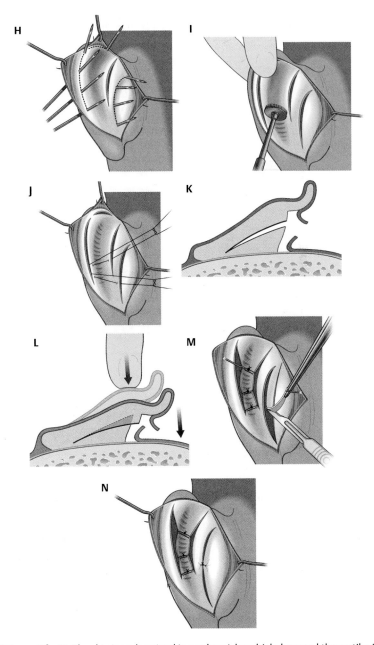

Fig. 50-9, cont'd   H, The skin is undermined in a subperichondrial plane and the cartilaginous segments marked with needles. The cartilage is incised full thickness, without merging the incisions. **I,** If necessary, a wire brush may be used to thin thick and rigid cartilage. **J,** Mattress sutures are placed to form the superior crus and body of the antihelix. **K,** The conchal rim is incised. **L,** Digital pressure is used to assess the amount of conchal excess. **M** and **N,** The appropriate amount of conchal cartilage is excised, and the antihelix and conchal rim are approximated with a single suture.

CORRECTION OF LOBULE PROMINENCE (LOWER THIRD) (Fig. 50-10)
■ Corrected using the **modified fishtail excision** (Wood-Smith)[25]

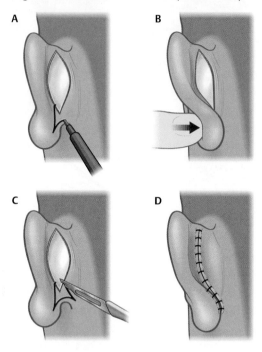

Fig. 50-10 Correction of a prominent lobule using a modified fishtail excision. **A,** A V extension of the posterior auricular incision is drawn on the posterior surface of the lobule. **B,** While the ink is still wet, the lobule is pressed against the mastoid skin. **C,** The mirror impression of the V is transposed to the mastoid skin. All skin within the borders of the modified fishtail design is excised. **D,** Closure is performed with a running 4-0 nylon suture.

■ **Procedure**
  • Mark a "V extension" from the inferior aspect of the postauricular incision used for correction of prominent ear deformity (e.g., Furnas or Mustardé).
  • Transpose the marking to the mastoid skin while the ink is still fresh, forming a mirror image pattern in the shape of a fishtail.
  • Excise skin and excess fibrofatty tissue along the demarcated lines.
  • Approximate skin.

CORRECTION OF A PROMINENT HELICAL ROOT[10]

- A prominent helical root that overprojects laterally may be addressed with a **Hatch suture** (Fig. 50-11).
- **Procedure**
  - An incision is made in the sulcus where the root of the helix abuts the scalp with a No. 15 blade scalpel.
  - The skin is undermined medially to the deep temporal fascia and laterally to the cartilage of the root of the helix.
  - A permanent (4-0 clear nylon or 4-0 Mersilene) mattress suture is placed between the deep temporal fascia and the cartilage, which is tied down to effect.

Temporalis fascia

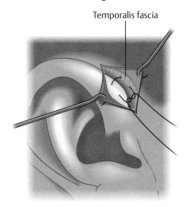

Fig. 50-11   The Hatch suture. An incision is made down to cartilage and deep temporal fascia. These two structures are then approximated with a single mattress suture and tied down to effect.

ADJUNCTIVE TECHNIQUES FOR SPECIFIC FINDINGS

- **Darwin tubercle:** A pointed thickening at the junction of the upper and middle third of the helix in approximately 10% of all patients. Full-thickness excision of the excess skin and cartilage can be performed so that scar is inconspicuous at the transition from lateroanterior to medioposterior. Helical contour is improved, and apparent prominence is further reduced (Fig. 50-12).
- **Stahl ear:** The presence of the third and/or horizontal superior crus with a pointed upper helix. Results in upper- and middle-third prominence. A variety of techniques exist, including combination approaches.[26] Because of high relapse rate, the upper pole prominence at a minimum should be addressed.
- **Mastoid prominence:** Soft tissue between the concha and mastoid can be resected to prevent the effect of a prominent mastoid on the projection of the concha. Alternatively, a burr can be used to carefully remove mastoid cortical bone.

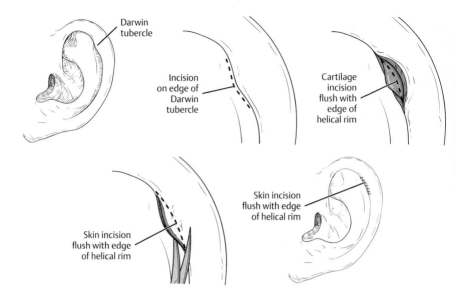

Fig. 50-12   Darwin tubercle.

POSTOPERATIVE CARE

- Postoperative care usually involves a bulky, protective dressing.
- Spira[14] sees his patients for their first postoperative visit within 48 hours to assess for hematoma, extreme pain, and general well-being.
  - The dressings are removed at 7-10 days and the incisions cleaned with dilute peroxide.
  - Spira has patients take a 5-day regimen of oral antibiotic (usually cephalexin).
  - The external sutures dissolve spontaneously.

COMPLICATIONS

HEMATOMA

- **The most immediate and pressing postoperative complication**
- Sudden onset of persistent, unilateral pain should alert surgeons of a possible hematoma.
- Management
  - Dressing removal
  - Suture removal
  - Evacuation of clot
  - Reapplication of dressings with mild compression
- Should be done in operating room for reexploration and hemostasis if active bleeding encountered

INFECTION
- Uncommon
  - Suspect if sudden increased unilateral pain on postoperative day 3 or 4
- Usually from *Staphylococcus* or *Streptococcus,* occasionally *Pseudomonas*
- **Sulfamylon** useful in preventing spread of infection and chondritis
- Some advocate liberal use of hospital admission and IV antibiotics after culture and sensitivity for purulent infection to prevent progression to chondritis.[14]

CHONDRITIS
- Surgical infection that requires prompt identification and debridement of necrotic cartilage

LATE DEFORMITY
- Usually manifests within 6 months of surgery
  - Recurrence after 1 year is rare.
- More often operator dependent than technique dependent
- Tan[27] found:
  - 24% of patients undergoing the Mustardé technique require "reoperation."
  - 10% of patients undergoing the Stenstroem technique required "reoperation."
    - Reason: Presence of sutures resulted in sinuses and wound infection in 15% of cases.
  - Cartilage-breaking techniques (e.g., Luckett, Converse, and Wood-Smith) leave more "sharp edges" and "contour irregularities" than do noncartilage-breaking techniques (e.g., Mustardé and Stenstroem).

TIP: Surgeons need to "break the ring of cartilage" to prevent telephone ear deformity.

TOP TAKEAWAYS
- ➤ The endpoint of a procedure is a straight helical contour when the ear is viewed from behind. A straight contour ensures harmonious setback of the upper, middle, and lower thirds of the ear.
- ➤ Do not excise skin, except for the triangle behind the lobule, for lobule repositioning.
- ➤ Make absolutely sure that no sutures have penetrated the lateral skin. They will inevitably cause a granuloma or inflammation requiring removal.

REFERENCES
1. Allison GR. Anatomy of the external ear. Clin Plast Surg 5:419, 1978.
2. Tan ST, Abramson DL, MacDonald DM, et al. Molding therapy for infants with deformational auricular anomalies. Ann Plast Surg 38:263, 1997.
3. Tan ST, Shibu M, Gault DT. A splint for correction of congenital ear deformities. Br J Plast Surg 47:575, 1994.

4. Farkas LG, Posnick JC, Hreczko TM. Anthropometric growth study of the ear. Cleft Palate Craniofac J 29:324, 1992.

5. Adamson JE, Horton CE, Crawford HH. The growth pattern of the external ear. Plast Reconstr Surg 36:466, 1965.

6. Macgregor FC. Ear deformities: social and psychological implications. Clin Plast Surg 5:347, 1978.

7. Hao W, Chorney JM, Bezuhly M, et al. Analysis of health-related quality-of-life outcomes and their predictive factors in pediatric patients who undergo otoplasty. Plast Reconstr Surg 132:811e, 2013.

8. Braun T, Hainzinger T, Stelter K, et al. Health-related quality of life, patient benefit, and clinical outcome after otoplasty using suture techniques in 62 children and adults. Plast Reconstr Surg 126:2115, 2010.

9. McDowell AJ. Goals in otoplasty for protruding ears. Plast Reconstr Surg 41:17, 1968.

10. Campobasso P, Belloli G. [Protruding ears: the indications for surgical treatment] Pediatr Med Chir 15:151, 1993.

11. Bradbury ET, Hewison J, Timmons MJ. Psychological and social outcome of prominent ear correction in children. Br J Plast Surg 45:97, 1992.

12. Janz BA, Cole P, Hollier LH Jr, et al. Treatment of prominent and constricted ear anomalies. Plast Reconstr Surg 124(1 Suppl):27e, 2009.

13. Ellis DA, Keohane JD. A simplified approach to otoplasty. J Otolaryngol 21:66, 1992.

14. Spira M. Otoplasty: what I do now—a 30-year perspective. Plast Reconstr Surg 104:834, 1999.

15. Balogh B, Millesi H. Are growth alterations a consequence of surgery for prominent ears? Plast Reconstr Surg 89:623, 1992.

16. Mustardé JC. The correction of prominent ears using mattress sutures. Br J Plast Surg 16:170, 1963.

17. Furnas DW. Correction of prominent ears by conchamastoid sutures. Plast Reconstr Surg 42:189, 1968.

18. Converse JM, Wood-Smith D. Technical details in the surgical correction of the lop ear deformity. Plast Reconstr Surg 31:118, 1963.

19. Stenstroem SJ. A "natural" technique for correction of congenitally prominent ears. Plast Reconstr Surg 32:509, 1963.

20. Chongchet V. A method of antihelix reconstruction. Br J Plast Surg 19:276, 1966.

21. Gibson T, Davis W. The distortion of autogenous cartilage grafts: its cause and prevention. Br J Plast Surg 10:257, 1958.

22. Fry HJ. Interlocked stresses in human nasal septal cartilage. Br J Plast Surg 19:276, 1966.

23. Thorne C, Wilkes G. Ear deformities, otoplasty, and ear reconstruction. Plast Reconstr Surg 129:701e, 2012.

24. Elliott RA. Complications in the treatment of prominent ears. Clin Plast Surg 5:479, 1978.

25. Wood-Smith D. Otoplasty. In Rees T, ed. Aesthetic Plastic Surgery. Philadelphia: Saunders, 1980.

26. Weinfeld AB. Stahl's ear correction: synergistic use of cartilage abrading, strategic Mustarde suture placement, and anterior anticonvexity suture. J Craniofac Surg 23:901, 2012.

27. Tan KH. Long-term survey of prominent ear surgery: a comparison of two methods. Br J Plast Surg 39:270, 1986.

PART VIII

Breast Surgery

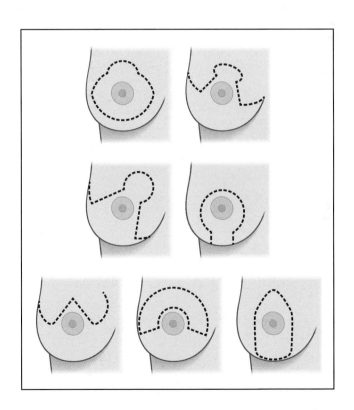

Breast Surgery

51. Breast Anatomy

Melissa A. Crosby, Glyn Jones

EMBRYOLOGY, DEVELOPMENT, AND PHYSIOLOGY

EMBRYOLOGY
- The breast is **ectodermally derived.**
- From week 8-10 of embryologic development, breast growth begins with differentiation of cutaneous epithelium of pectoral region.
- In week 6, milk ridge develops extending from axilla to groin.
- From week 7 of gestation to birth, mammary anlage on chest wall develops into an epithelial bud with 15-20 ducts, and nipple develops into circular smooth muscle fibers.
- First 7 weeks after birth, clear fluid similar to colostrum ("witch's milk") containing water, fat, and cellular debris may be secreted from the neonatal breast, stimulated by maternal hormones.
- Normal breast development in anterolateral pectoral region at level of fourth intercostal space
- Supernumerary breasts *(polymastia)* and nipples *(polythelia)* can occur along milk ridge.
  - Most common location for polymastia is **lower left chest** wall below the inframammary crease.
  - **Polythelia** is the **most common congenital breast anomaly,** occurring in **2%** of the population.
- Abnormal regression of milk line can lead to underdevelopment of breasts (hypoplasia).
- Complete absence of breast (amastia) usually associated with hypoplasia of ipsilateral pectoralis musculature and chest wall (Poland syndrome).

DEVELOPMENT
- Puberty begins at 10-12 years of age as a result of hypothalamic gonadotropin-releasing hormones secreted into the hypothalamic-pituitary portal venous system.
- Anterior pituitary secretes follicle stimulating hormone (FSH) and luteinizing hormone (LH).
- FSH causes ovarian follicles to mature and secrete estrogens.
- Estrogens stimulate longitudinal growth of breast ductal epithelium.
- As ovarian follicles become mature and ovulatory, the corpus luteum releases progesterone, which, in conjunction with estrogen, leads to complete mammary development.
- **Stages of breast development described by Tanner[1]:**
  - *Stage 1:* Preadolescent elevation of nipple only; no palpable glandular tissue or areolar pigmentation
  - *Stage 2:* Presence of glandular tissue in the subareolar region; nipple and breast project as single mound
  - *Stage 3:* Further increase in glandular tissue with enlargement of breast and nipple but continued contour of nipple and breast in single plane

- *Stage 4:* Enlargement of areola and increased areolar pigmentation with secondary mound formed by nipple and areola above level of breast
- *Stage 5:* Final adolescent development of a smooth contour with no projection of the areola and nipple
- **Normal variants in breast development**
  - **Infantile hyperplasia of breast**
    - ▶ Result of transplacental estrogen from maternal-placental unit
    - ▶ Occurs in both sexes and may be associated with secretion of colostrum
    - ▶ Found in more than half of newborns
  - **Pubertal gynecomastia**
    - ▶ Occurs in 70% of boys
    - ▶ May be unilateral or bilateral
    - ▶ Tender
    - ▶ Can persist for up to 2 years
  - **Premature thelarche**
    - ▶ Breast development beginning before 8 years of age in girls without other signs of puberty or skeletal maturation
    - ▶ Most often bilateral but can be unilateral
    - ▶ Usually noted with first 2 years of life and ends after 3-5 years
  - **Delayed maturation**
    - ▶ Absence of breast development by 14 years of age in absence of chronic illness or endocrine abnormality
    - ▶ Family history of delayed maturation typical
    - ▶ Because relatively uncommon, need to rule out primary ovarian failure by testing for abnormal gonadotropin levels

MENSTRUAL CYCLE
- *Premenstrual:* Estrogen peak, breast engorgement, breast sensitivity
- *Follicular phase* (days 4-14): Mitosis and proliferation of breast epithelial cells
- *Luteal phase* (days 5-28): Progesterone levels rise, mammary ducts dilate, and alveolar epithelial cells differentiate into secretory cells; estrogens increase blood flow to breast
- *Menstruation:* Breast involution and decrease in circulating hormones
- *Breast engorgement and tenderness* (at a minimum 5-7 days after menstruation): Palpation is most sensitive for detecting masses and most comfortable for patient at this time.

PREGNANCY AND LACTATION
- Marked ductal, lobular, and alveolar growth occurs under influence of estrogen, progesterone, placental lactogen, prolactin, and chorionic gonadotropin.
- *First trimester:* Estrogen influences ductal sprouting and lobular formation, early to late breast enlargement ensues, superficial veins dilate, and pigmentation of nipple-areola complex (NAC) increases.
- *Second trimester:* Lobular events predominate under influence of progestins, and colostrum collects within the lobular alveoli.
- *Third trimester:* By parturition, breast size triples from vascular engorgement, epithelial proliferation, and colostrum accumulation.
- Withdrawal of placental lactogen and sex hormones with delivery results in breast being **predominantly influenced by prolactin.**

- **Anterior** pituitary secretion of **prolactin** influences milk production and secretion.
- **Posterior** pituitary secretion of **oxytocin** leads to breast myoepithelial contraction and milk ejection.
- Prolactin and oxytocin secretion is stimulated by nursing infant's tactile stimulation of nipple.
- Postlactational involution occurs during the 3 months after cessation of nursing; regression of extralobular stroma is a primary feature.

Menopause
- Involves loss of glandular tissue and **replacement with fat**
- Some lobules remain, but postmenopausal breast consists mainly of fat, connective tissue, and mammary ducts.

VASCULAR SUPPLY[2] (Fig. 51-1)

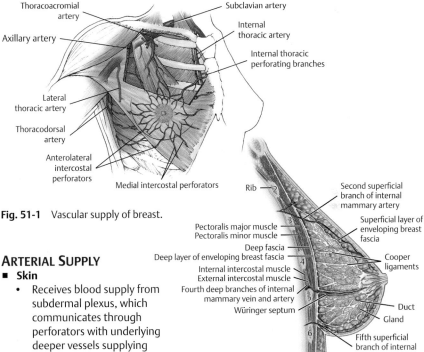

Fig. 51-1   Vascular supply of breast.

Arterial Supply
- **Skin**
  - Receives blood supply from subdermal plexus, which communicates through perforators with underlying deeper vessels supplying the breast parenchyma.
- **Parenchyma**
  - Supplied by:
    - ▶ Perforating branches of internal mammary artery
    - ▶ Lateral thoracic artery
    - ▶ Thoracodorsal artery
    - ▶ Intercostal perforators
    - ▶ Thoracoacromial artery

- **Nipple-areola complex**
  - Receives both parenchymal and subdermal blood supply

VENOUS DRAINAGE
- Follows the arterial supply

INNERVATION[2] (Fig. 51-2)

- Dermatomal in nature
- Derived from the anterolateral and anteromedial branches of the thoracic intercostal nerves T3-5
- Supraclavicular nerves from lower fibers of cervical plexus also provide innervation to the upper and lateral portions of the breast.
- Nipple-areolar sensation is derived from the anteromedial and anterolateral **T4** intercostal nerve.
- Intercostal brachial nerve courses across axilla to supply upper medial arm and is often injured during axillary dissection, resulting in anesthesia and paresthesia.

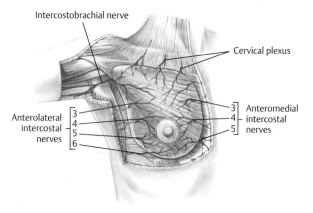

Fig. 51-2   Innervation to breast.

ANATOMIC STUDIES
- **Schlenz et al[3]**
  - 28 unilateral breast dissections in female cadavers
  - **Found consistent innervation of the NAC by the anterior and lateral cutaneous branches of the third through fifth intercostal nerves**
  - Lateral cutaneous branch (LCB) supplied innervations through posterior innervations of the nipple in 93%.
    - Fourth LCB provided posterior innervations in 93% of cases and was the only source 79% of the time.

- Anterior cutaneous branch (ACB) had superficial course to supply medial aspect of NAC.
  - ▶ Third and fourth ACB combined to provide innervations in 57% of cases.
- **Würinger et al**[4,5]
  - 28 anatomic dissections and 14 arterial injection studies of female cadavers
  - Defined a "brassierelike" connective tissue suspensory system
  - **Found neurovascular supply to the nipple runs along this well-defined suspensory apparatus**
    - ▶ Vertical ligaments originated from the pectoralis minor (laterally) and sternum (medially)
  - Defined parenchymal borders and carried corresponding neurovascular structures
  - Horizontal septum originated from the pectoral fascia along the fifth rib: **Würinger septum** (Fig. 51-3).
    - ▶ It merged with the lateral and medial vertical ligaments.
    - ▶ Breast parenchyma was bipartitioned as the septum ran anteriorly to the NAC.
    - ▶ Cranial aspect carried thoracoacromial and lateral thoracic arterial branches.
    - ▶ Caudal aspect carried branches of the fourth through sixth intercostal arteries.
    - ▶ *Main contributory nerve to the nipple (LCB of fourth intercostal) was always found within septum.*

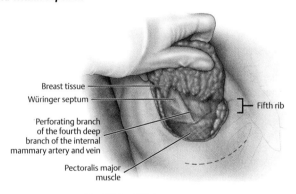

Breast tissue
Würinger septum
Perforating branch of the fourth deep branch of the internal mammary artery and vein
Pectoralis major muscle
Fifth rib

Fig. 51-3   Würinger septum.

- **O'Dey et al**[6]
  - Injection study of seven female cadavers with arterial distribution patterns mapped for 14 breasts
  - **Outlined four distinct arterial zones**
  - Largest territory supplied by branches of the internal mammary (zone 1) and lateral thoracic (zone 2)
  - Evaluated safety of eight different pedicles based on vascular reliability and regularity to the NAC
  - Concluded that pedicles with a **lateral** or **medially based** component may be **safer** strictly based on regularity of arterial anatomy
  - Study did not account for added safety with greater breast width.

SKIN AND PARENCHYMA[2] (Fig. 51-4)

- Adult breast extends from the second to the seventh rib in the midclavicular line and from the sternocostal junction medially to the midaxillary line laterally.
  - Also extends into the axilla, providing breast teardrop shape (axillary tail of Spence)

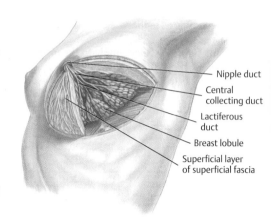

Nipple duct
Central collecting duct
Lactiferous duct
Breast lobule
Superficial layer of superficial fascia

- Adult mammary gland comprises multiple lobules connected and drained by 16-24 main lactiferous ducts.
- **Lobule** is the functional unit of breast.
  - Each lobule is composed of hundreds of **acini.**
    - ► Each acinus has secretory potential and is connected to the lactiferous ducts by its own interlobular ducts.
  - Lobules are situated in radial distribution.

Fig. 51-4   Lobules are situated in a radial distribution.

- Each main lactiferous duct dilates as it approaches the nipple, forming a sinus **(lactiferous sinus or central collecting duct),** which functions as reservoir for milk storage.
- Nipple contains orifices to drain each lactiferous duct; these may act as conduits for bacteria.
- **Morgagni tubercles** are elevations formed by openings of ducts of **Montgomery glands** and are located near periphery of areola.
- *Montgomery glands* are large sebaceous glands capable of secreting milk; they represent an intermediate stage between sweat and mammary glands.
  - Montgomery glands also act to lubricate the areola during lactation.
- Fat content varies but is responsible for most of bulk, contour, softness, consistency, and shape of breast.
  - Fat content increases as glandular component subsides, i.e., after lactation or during menopause.
- Breast is supported by layers of **superficial fascia.**
  - **Superficial layer of superficial fascia** is located near dermis and is difficult to distinguish unless patient is thin.
  - **Deep layer of superficial fascia**—on deep surface of breast: A loose areolar plane exists between this layer and deep fascial layer that overlies underlying musculature.
- *Cooper ligaments* penetrate deep layer of superficial fascia into parenchyma breast to dermis; ptosis results from attenuation of these attachments.
- The inframammary fold (IMF) is the lower border of the breast and is a distinct anatomic structure that should be preserved whenever possible. **It represents fusion of the deep and superficial fascia with the dermis.** Distinct fibers crisscross, holding the skin in place (similar to the gluteal fold).[7]

UNDERLYING MUSCULATURE (Fig. 51-5)

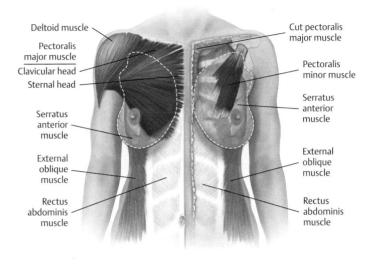

Fig. 51-5   Underlying musculature.

PECTORALIS MAJOR
- **Origin:** The medial clavicle, sternum, anterior ribs (second through sixth), external oblique, and rectus abdominis fascia
- **Insertion:** Upper humerus 10 cm from humeral head on lateral side of intertubercular sulcus
- **Function:** Adduction and medial rotation of arm
- **Blood supply:** Internal mammary perforators, thoracoacromial, intercostal perforators, lateral thoracic artery
- **Innervation:** Medial (sternal portion) and lateral (clavicular portion) pectoral nerves *(named for brachial plexus cord from which it originates)*
- Upper medial portion of breast located over pectoralis major
- Absence of sternal head of pectoralis major seen in Poland syndrome

PECTORALIS MINOR
- **Origin:** Enterolateral surface of third through sixth ribs
- **Insertion:** Coracoid process of scapula
- **Function:** Draws scapula down and forward
- **Blood supply:** Pectoral branch of thoracoacromial, lateral thoracic artery, direct branch of axillary artery
- **Innervation:** Medial pectoral nerve

TIP: The pectoralis minor serves as a landmark during axillary dissection, because the lateral margin divides the superficial from the deep axillary nodes.

SERRATUS ANTERIOR
- **Origin:** Anterolateral aspects of upper eight ribs
- **Insertion:** Anterior surface of medial aspect of scapula
- **Function:** Stabilizes scapula against chest wall during abduction and elevation of arm in horizontal direction; pulls scapula forward and laterally
- **Blood supply:** Lateral thoracic artery, branches of thoracodorsal artery
- **Innervation:** Long thoracic nerve

RECTUS ABDOMINIS MUSCLE
- **Origin:** Pubic base
- **Insertion:** Third through seventh costal cartilages
- **Function:** Flexes the vertebral column and tenses the abdominal wall
- **Blood supply:** Superior and inferior epigastric artery and vein, subcostal and intercostal perforators
- **Innervation:** Segmental motor nerves from seventh through twelfth intercostal nerves

EXTERNAL OBLIQUE
- **Origin:** External surface of lower anterior and lateral ribs
- **Insertion:** Iliac crest and medial abdominal fascial aponeurosis
- **Function:** Compression of abdominal contents
- **Blood supply:** Inferior eight intercostal arteries
- **Innervation:** Seventh through twelfth intercostal nerves

LYMPHATIC DRAINAGE[2] (Fig. 51-6)

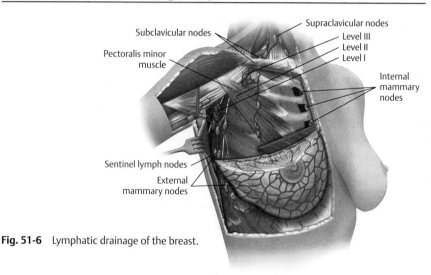

Fig. 51-6   Lymphatic drainage of the breast.

- Extensive lymphatic network of both **superficial** and **deep** lymphatic drainage
- **Superficial lymphatic drainage** originates from periareolar lymphatic plexus that accompanies venous drainage.

- **Deep lymphatic drainage** begins as individual lymphatics that drain each lactiferous duct and lobule and then penetrate through the deep fascia of the underlying musculature.
- Lymphatic drainage from the upper outer quadrant passes around pectoralis major to deep pectoral nodes or directly to subscapular nodes.
- Lymphatic efferent vessels of breast travel to central axillary nodes to apical axillary nodes to supraclavicular nodes.
- Medial lymphatic channels run with internal mammary perforating vessels and drain to parasternal nodes.
- **Most of the lymph from the breasts drains into axillary nodes. Three levels identified:**
  - *Level I:* Lateral to lateral border of pectoralis minor
  - *Level II:* Behind pectoralis minor and below axillary vein
  - *Level III:* Medial to medial border of pectoralis minor
- *Rotter nodes:* Between pectoralis major and minor

BREAST SHAPE AND AESTHETICS[8] (Fig. 51-7)

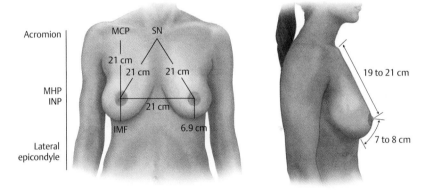

Fig. 51-7 Ideal breast measurements. (*IMF*, Inframammary fold; *INP*, ideal nipple plane; *MCP*, midclavicular point; *MHP*, midhumeral plane; *SN*, sternal notch.)

- Less full above areola (upper pole) and fuller below (lower pole)
- Ideally in harmony with proportions of the chest, torso, and buttocks
- NAC: 19-21 cm from the sternal notch, 9-11 cm from midline, and 7-8 cm from IMF
- Medial cleavage: Function of medial origin of the pectoralis major and the medialmost extent of the breast parenchyma
- Ideally symmetrical in size, shape, volume, and ptosis
- Ptosis: Nipple position relative to IMF and breast parenchyma (see Chapter 53)

> **TIP:** Perfect symmetry is rare and should be noted and documented preoperatively. Women desiring full medial cleavage without bra support are often disappointed with aesthetic and reconstructive efforts. Preoperative counseling is helpful.

BREAST FOOTPRINT[9] (Fig. 51-8)

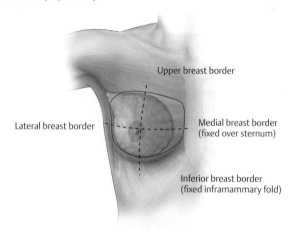

Fig. 51-8   Breast footprint.

- The breast footprint on the chest wall consists of four landmarks:
  1. Upper breast border
  2. Inframammary fold
  3. Medial breast border
  4. Lateral breast border

BREAST EXAMINATION[2,10]

- Patient medical history, including prior breast problems, surgery, routine screening, family history, menstrual history, and reproductive history important
- Examination is easiest to perform **during week after menses,** when tenderness and engorgement are minimal.
- Begin with palpation of supraclavicular and anterior and posterior cervical lymph node chains.
- Next, inspect and compare breasts.
  - Minor size differences (up to 10%) are normal.
  - Observe for skin changes, dimpling, or nipple abnormalities.
  - Abnormalities in lower quadrants may be accentuated by patient raising arms or contracting pectoralis muscle.
  - Location of breasts/nipple and breast width compared to chest wall width is important.
- Location of inframammary crease and axillary fold fullness should be assessed.
- Breasts should be palpated while patient is in **upright** and **supine** positions, including palpation of **axilla** and **lymph nodes.**

TIP: Placement of patient's ipsilateral hand behind head while supine allows pull of the lateral quadrants and tail of the breast into the chest wall for easier and more complete examination.

- Assess for scoliosis or asymmetrical chest wall.
- Confirm patient performs monthly breast self-examination and receives routine mammograms.
- Perform appropriate measurements and photographs (Fig. 51-9), depending on plastic surgery procedure to be performed (see Chapter 3).

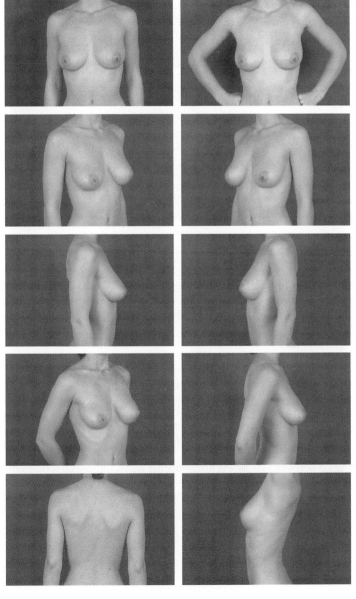

Fig. 51-9   Standard photographic views of the breast.

TOP TAKEAWAYS

➤ Although breast parenchyma generally gives way to a fibrofatty breast with menopause and age, some women retain their baseline dense glandular breast, which can make rotation of breast pedicles during reductions more difficult.

➤ The fourth intercostal nerve appears to be the primary supply for nipple sensation; however, every attempt should be made to protect all lateral intercostal nerves during augmentation mammaplasty to minimize sensory loss.

➤ During a mastectomy, the second and third internal mammary perforators should be preserved, because they are the most significant vessels for medial breast perfusion.

➤ The nipple areolar complex is innervated by the anterolateral branch of the fourth intercostal nerve.

➤ Supernumerary nipples and breasts can occur along the milk line from the axilla to the groin.

➤ Attenuation of Cooper ligaments leads to ptosis and increased breast mobility.

➤ Injury to the intercostal brachial nerve results in paresthesia/anesthesia of the upper medial arm.

➤ Three levels of axillary lymph nodes exist.

➤ Poland syndrome results in absence of the sternal head of the pectoralis major.

REFERENCES

1. Tanner JM, ed. Growth at Adolescence, ed 2. Oxford: Blackwell Scientific, 1978.
2. Bostwick J III. Anatomy and physiology. In Bostwick J III, ed. Plastic and Reconstructive Breast Surgery, ed 2. New York: Thieme Publishers, 2000.
3. Schlenz I, Kuzbari R, Gruber H, et al. The sensitivity of the nipple-areola complex: an anatomic study. Plast Reconstr Surg 105:905, 2000.
4. Würinger E, Mader N, Posch E, et al. Nerve and vessel supplying ligamentous suspension of the mammary gland. Plast Reconstr Surg 101:1486, 1998.
5. Würinger E, Tschabitscher M. New aspects of the topographical anatomy of the mammary gland regarding its neurovascular supply along a regular ligamentous suspension. Eur J Morphol 40:181, 2002.
6. O'Dey DM, Prescher A, Pallua N. Vascular reliability of nipple-areola complex-bearing pedicles: an anatomical microdissection study. Plast Reconstr Surg 119:1167, 2007.
7. Muntan CD, Sundine MJ, Rink RD, et al. Inframammary fold: a histologic reappraisal. Plast Reconstr Surg 105:549, 2000.
8. Jones G, ed. Bostwick's Plastic and Reconstructive Breast Surgery, ed 3. New York: Thieme Publishers, 2010.
9. Hall-Findlay EJ, ed. Aesthetic Breast Surgery: Concepts & Techniques. New York: Thieme Publishers, 2011.
10. August DA, Sondak VK. Breast. In Greenfield LJ, Mulholland M, Oldham KT, et al, eds. Surgery: Scientific Principles and Practice, ed 2. Philadelphia: Lippincott-Raven, 1997.

52. Breast Augmentation

Evan B. Katzel, Thornwell H. Parker III, Jeffrey E. Janis, Dennis C. Hammond

BACKGROUND

- Breast augmentation is the **second most common** cosmetic surgery (after liposuction).[1]
- Silicone implants were introduced in 1964.
- Saline implants were introduced in 1970s as an alternative to silicone.
- The U.S. FDA placed a moratorium on silicone implants in 1992 for primary augmentation because of concerns about autoimmune and connective tissue disease.
  - In 1999 the NIH Institute of Medicine and the National Academy of Sciences reviewed 17 epidemiologic studies and were **unable to detect any link between silicone and systemic, autoimmune, or prenatal disease.**
  - Studies found silicone in local macrophages, lymph nodes, and breast tissue.
  - Studies did not demonstrate elevated systemic levels (normal liver, lung, and spleen).[2]
- Saline implants increased in popularity during the 1990s because of silicone scare.
- Silicone implants have evolved through different generations (Table 52-1).

Table 52-1   *Generations of Silicone Gel–Filled Breast Implants*

Implant Generation	Production Period	Characteristics
First	1960s	Thick shell (0.25 mm average) Thick viscous gel Dacron patch
Second	1970s	Thin shell (0.13 mm average) Less viscous gel No patch
Third	1980s	Thick, silica-reinforced barrier coated shells
Fourth	1992-present	Stricter manufacturing standards Refined third-generation devices
Fifth	1993-present	Cohesive silicone gel–filled devices Inner laminar layer to prevent gel bleed Form-stable devices

NOTE: Some consider the introduction of textured surfaces and anatomic shapes to represent fourth or fifth generations.

- Restriction on use of silicone gel implants for primary breast augmentation was lifted in November 2006.
  - Before this change, silicone implants were approved only for breast reconstruction, silicone implant exchange, and replacement of saline implants with complications.[3,4]

- **Cohesive gel implants** are considered to offer significant advantages.
  - In Europe since 1995
  - In Canada since 2000
  - **Advantages:** More natural shape, less rippling, limited gel migration in event of rupture
  - **Disadvantages:** Larger incision, more expensive, stiffer

INDICATIONS AND CONTRAINDICATIONS

INDICATIONS
- Increase breast size
- Restore prelactation breast appearance
- Correct breast asymmetry
- Enhance breast shape and volume
- Improve body image, symmetry, and balance
- Improves fit of clothing
- Provide the appearance of a breast lift and increased cleavage
- Rejuvenation after postpartum deflation

CONTRAINDICATIONS[5]
- Significant breast disease (e.g., severe fibrocystic disease, ductal hyperplasia, breast cancer)
- Collagen vascular disease
- Body dysmorphic disorder
- Psychological instability
- Social instability (e.g., divorce or separation, searching for a relationship)
- Patient responding to pressure from friends, family, or partner
- Patient <18 years of age
- **Silicone implants are not FDA approved for women <22 years of age** (see Chapter 1).
- The following situations require mindfulness[6]:
  - After obtaining the history, the surgeon does not like the patient.
  - Patient desires an outcome the surgeon cannot deliver.
  - Patient desires an outcome outside the surgeon's aesthetic sense of normal.
  - Patient is critical of previous surgeons or praises the current surgeon excessively.
  - Patient lies, provides a false history or information.
  - Patient refuses to be examined or photographed.
  - Patient is a perfectionist and wants a guarantee of results.
  - Patient is paranoid, delusional, or depressed.
  - Patient fails to communicate or is unable to understand what informed consent entails.

PREOPERATIVE EVALUATION

HISTORY/INTERVIEW
- Begins with open-ended questions
- The patient talks and the surgeon listens.
- Assessment:
  - Motivation for surgery
  - Psychological state of mind and stability
  - Level of understanding

- Expectations
- Self-esteem

MEDICAL HISTORY

- Full medical history
  - Personal or family history of breast disease or cancer
  - Pregnancy history and plans for future pregnancies
  - Breast size before, during, and after pregnancy
  - Mammography history (recommended for patients >35 years of age and those with significant breast cancer risk)
  - Patients without significant history should have a mammogram every 2 years starting at 40 years of age, and every year beginning at 50 years of age.[7]
  - Previous surgeries or procedures on breasts
  - Previous cosmetic procedures
  - Tobacco or nicotine replacement use, drug use
  - Anticoagulation use
  - Current breast size
  - Desired breast size (many patients will bring pictures to clinic)

PHYSICAL EXAMINATION

- **Breast examination**
  - Masses, dimpling, discharge, lymph nodes
  - Cancer screening
- **Skin quality**
  - Stretch marks, tone, elasticity
- **Asymmetries:** Chest wall, scoliosis, breast
  - Difference in breast volume
  - Difference in inframammary fold (IMF) height
  - Difference in nipple-areolar complex (NAC) height
- **Soft tissue pinch test**
  - <2 cm, may obtain a better result with a submuscular implant placement
  - Ptosis (see Chapter 53)
  - Mild ptosis is improved by augmentation.
  - Moderate to severe ptosis may require mastopexy.
- **Measurements** (patient sitting up straight)
  - Breast width at its widest point
  - Breast height
  - Intermammary distance
  - Mark true midline of the chest
  - Mark IMF
  - Height, weight, body frame (small to large)
  - Sternal notch to nipple (SN-N)
  - Nipple to inframammary fold (N-IMF) during stretch
  - Base width (width of breast base)
  - Parenchymal coverage (pinch test)
  - Superior pole
  - Lower pole
  - Anterior-pull skin stretch (centimeters of anterior stretch with pull at edge of areola)
  - Parenchymal fill (percentage of skin envelope filled by parenchyma)

- **Photographs** (all jewelry and identifying markers removed) (see Chapter 3)
  - Chin to below navel
  - Front, lateral, oblique, with arms at rest and elevated
- **Point out and document**
  - Chest wall deformities
  - Spinal curvature
  - Asymmetries (nipple shape and size, nipple position, IMF position, breast size, breast ptosis)

INFORMED CONSENT

- ***Not just signing a paper***
- **Photographic review**
  - Note asymmetries, ptosis, cleavage.
  - Note that asymmetries, ptosis, and cleavage are often unchanged or even accentuated by breast augmentation alone.
- **Implant selection**
  - Review and discuss risks and benefits of implant type, texture, volume, positioning, and access incisions.
  - Review and discuss previous restrictions on silicone implants.
- **The patient must be thoroughly informed about:**
  - Risks and complications
  - Bleeding
  - Infection
  - Capsular contracture
  - Change in nipple and skin sensation
  - Scarring
  - Breast calcifications
  - Breast implant-associated anaplastic large cell lymphoma (BIA-ALCL)
  - Seroma
  - Hematoma
  - Breast venous thrombosis
  - Implant failure
  - Implant extrusion
  - Changes in mammography detection
  - Implant visibility and palpability
  - Implant wrinkling or rippling
  - Implant malposition or displacement
  - Leakage of filling substance
  - Rare difficulties with breast-feeding
  - Chest wall deformation
  - Animation deformities (if submuscular)
  - Limitations of high-impact activity
  - Unsatisfactory result
  - The need for additional surgeries
    - ▶ Many insurance carriers do not cover cosmetic operations, correction of complications that may arise from surgery, and changes that necessitate revision surgery.

- Implant weight, aging, weight loss or gain, and pregnancy will result in expected changes in breast appearance.
- Benefits
  - ▶ Enhances natural body contour
  - ▶ Corrects loss of volume after pregnancy and lactation
  - ▶ Balances asymmetries
  - ▶ Replaces ruptured or displaced implants
- Alternatives
  - ▶ Silicone versus saline
  - ▶ Fat grafting
  - ▶ Autologous tissue transfer
  - ▶ No surgery
- ■ Can use official ASPS informed consents
- ■ Document desired implant type, size, and shape discussed with patient.

EQUIPMENT

INSTRUMENTATION
- ■ Double hooks
- ■ Lighted breast retractor versus headlight
- ■ Army-Navy retractors
- ■ Extended Bovie tip
- ■ Endoscopic retractor (transaxillary approach, transumbilical augmentation)
- ■ Closed-loop saline-filled setup (saline-filled implants)
- ■ Implant sizers (if applicable)
- ■ Triple antibiotic solution
  - 50,000 units bacitracin, 1 g cefazolin, 80 mg gentamicin per 500 ml saline solution (may reduce infection rate and capsular contracture)[8]
- ■ Keller funnel (Allergan)
  - Allows no-touch insertion of silicone implant through minimal-sized incision
- ■ Implants

FILLER MATERIAL
Saline
- ■ **Advantages**
  - Historically lower contracture rates
  - Adjusts quickly to body core temperature
  - Leaks easily detected and safely absorbed by body
  - Size more customizable—easier to adjust for size and correct breast asymmetry
- ■ **Disadvantages**
  - Wrinkling
  - Less natural look and feel
  - Complete deflation with leak
- ■ **Construction**
  - Silicone shell filled with physiologic saline solution

Silicone
- ■ **Advantages**
  - More natural feel and appearance than saline implants

- **Disadvantages**
  - Historically higher contracture rate
  - Must be ≥22 years of age to receive silicone implant per FDA
  - Adjusts slowly to temperature change (e.g., implants remain cold after swimming)
  - Ruptures more difficult to detect and can cause local inflammation and granulomas
  - MRI recommended 3 years after surgery, then every 2 years to monitor for rupture, as per FDA
  - More expensive
- **Construction**
  - Silicone shell with silicone filler
  - Silicone: Polymer of dimethylsiloxane. Longer chains with greater interchain cross-linking lead to increased viscosity.

Double-Lumen (Becker Implant, Mentor)
- **Advantages**
  - Natural feel of silicone
  - Allows postoperative adjustments to inner-lumen saline volume
  - Useful for asymmetry and for patients uncertain of desired size
- **Disadvantages**
  - Fill port temporarily implanted, requiring second procedure to remove
  - Possible fill valve failure
- **Construction**
  - Outer and inner silicone shell: Outer lumen filled with silicone, and adjustable inner lumen filled with saline

VOLUME
- **Patient preference**
  - Sizers put in bra to establish desired volume (not recommended)
  - Photos of other women
  - Digital imaging
- **Surgeon's experience**
  - 125-150 cc to increase by one cup size
  - Larger body frames require larger implant volumes to increase cup size
- **Breast analysis**
  - **High Five system**[9]
  - Objective measures to determine optimal implant and volume
  - Volume based on breast base width
  - Add or subtract volume based on skin stretch, breast envelope fill, and N-IMF
- **Intraoperative breast sizers**
- **Pitfalls of large implant volume**
  - Stretching and stressing of tissues
  - Atrophy and thinning of parenchyma and skin
  - Increased palpability
  - Traction rippling

CAUTION: Large implant can have detrimental effects on overlying soft tissues.

TEXTURE

SMOOTH
- **Advantages**
  - Thinner capsule formed
  - Less palpable: Preferable for patients with thin coverage
- **Disadvantages**
  - Higher contracture rates
  - Requires larger pocket dissection
  - Requires displacement exercises to prevent contracture

TEXTURED
- **All shaped implants are textured to prevent malposition.**
- **Advantages**
  - Lower contracture rate (surface disorients collagen deposition)
  - Less migration and implant rotation
- **Disadvantages**
  - Require precise pocket dissection
  - More palpable
  - Traction rippling more common
  - Greater association with BIA-ALCL based on current data
- **Technique**
  - Intraoperative positioning of implant is critical, because textured surface resists migration or movement in pocket.
  - Base must be properly oriented along IMF.

POLYURETHANE-COVERED
- **Advantage**
  - Dramatically low contracture rates (<1% over 10 years)
- **Disadvantage**
  - Pulled from U.S. market, because polyurethane breaks down as a carcinogenic compound, although levels likely insignificant
- **Construction**
  - Polyurethane coating separates over weeks to months and becomes incorporated into the capsule, helping to disperse contractile forces.
  - Textured implants were developed to mimic the effect of polyurethane on the capsule.

SHAPE/DIMENSION

ROUND (CIRCULAR IMPLANT)
- **Advantages**
  - Offered in many different projections and sizes
- **Disadvantages**
  - Less natural appearance
- Low-profile
- Moderate-profile
- Moderate-plus-profile

- High-profile
  - Increased projection for given base width
  - Increased projection with less volume
  - Advantage with a constricted lower pole or a narrow breast base width

SHAPED/ANATOMIC
- Implant height different than width
- Increased implant height and projection for a given base width
- Upper pole tapered; fuller lower pole, reducing upper pole collapse and filling out lower pole of breast
- Most textured to maintain position
- **Advantages**
  - Designed to give more natural appearance
  - Less upper pole fullness
  - More natural upper pole contour
- **Disadvantage**
  - Must be oriented properly and symmetrically
  - More prone to malposition
  - Fewer available implant sizes in the United States

SIZE
- **Based on:**
  - Patient's desired size and projection
  - Breast base width
  - Implant should be slightly narrower than the patient's breast width
  - Dimensions and compliance of the patient's breast
- **High-volume implants (>400 cc) are more prone to complications.**
  - Many surgeons have special consent forms for such implants.
  - Rule of thumb: 125-150 cc per cup size increase

> **SENIOR AUTHOR TIP:**   While the anatomically shaped implants may help with the creation of natural breast contours, the real advantage of these devices is that they are wrinkle resistant. As a result of the anatomic shape of the shell combined with the more cohesive gel, these devices resist collapse and wrinkle formation which greatly reduces stress on the shell resulting from fold flaw failure. As a result, the rupture rates at 10 years for these devices are impressively low which can make these implants an attractive option for patients and surgeons alike.

TECHNIQUE

MARKINGS
- IMF
- True midline
- Incisions

POCKET POSITION
- **Pocket dissection is based on type of implant** (Fig. 52-1).
  - Smooth gel implants can use larger pockets and displacement exercises to prevent capsular contracture formation.
  - Textured implants are placed in and are only slightly larger than the footprint of the implant to minimize malposition.

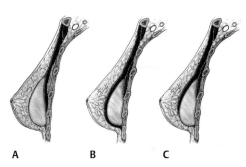

Fig. 52-1   Pocket plane and dissection.
A, Subglandular augmentation.
B, Submuscular augmentation.
C, Biplanar augmentation.

A   B   C

Subglandular/Subfascial
- **Subglandular:** The implant rests under the breast gland.
- **Subfascial:** The implant is placed under the anterior pectoralis major fascia and the pectoralis major muscle.
- **Advantages**
  - Avoids implant distortion with pectoralis activity and in muscular patients
  - More anatomic
  - Better implant projection
- **Disadvantages**
  - Higher capsular contracture rate
  - Visible implant wrinkling or rippling, especially if paucity of native breast tissue
  - Implant edges may be palpable
  - Interference with mammography
- **Technique**
  - Dissection on top of pectoralis major, below gland
  - **If pinch test is greater than 2 cm,** the implant can safely be placed in the subglandular/subfascial plane.
    - ▶ Thin parenchymal coverage if upper pole pinch test is <2 cm

Total Subpectoral
- Rarely performed in cosmetic surgery
- **Advantages**
  - Lowest capsular contracture rates (<10%)
  - Thick soft tissue coverage
  - Good preservation of nipple sensation

- **Disadvantages**
  - Implant shifts with pectoralis activity
  - "Dancing breasts" during pectoralis contraction
  - Implant malposition over time (superiorly and laterally)
  - Difficult to control upper pole fill
- **Relative contraindication**
  - Muscular or active patient
- **Technique**
  - Dissection below pectoralis major but above pectoralis minor
  - The implant is placed completely under the pectoralis major muscle
  - *Does not disrupt inferior attachments of pectoralis if "total subpectoral"*

Dual Plane[10]

- The origin of the pectoralis major is completely divided from its origin at the level of the IMF, stopping at the medial aspect of the IMF.
- The **upper pole** of the implant is placed **under the pectoralis,** and the **lower pole** is placed **subglandularly.**
- The attachments of the pectoralis to the breast parenchyma are selectively divided. (The amount of dissection differentiates dual plane type I, II, and III.)
- **Advantages**
  - Decreases implant displacement caused by pectoralis contraction
  - Provides thick upper pole soft tissue coverage with subpectoral placement
  - Lower capsular contracture rates than with subglandular placement
  - Increased control of IMF position compared to submuscular
  - The breast parenchyma and the pectoralis can be dissected apart to adjust for differing types of breasts.
  - Low contracture rate
  - Increases implant-parenchymal interface, which expands lower pole and prevents double-bubble deformity
- **Disadvantage**
  - Usually restricted to IMF incision when performing dual plane II and III
- **Contraindication**
  - IMF pinch test <0.4 cm
- **Rationale**
  - Complete muscle coverage restricts expansion of inferior pole, forcing implant superiorly and laterally.
  - Especially with ptotic and loose breast parenchyma, breast tissue may slide inferior to the axis of the implant while implant remains fixed higher on the chest wall, causing a type A double-bubble deformity.
  - Dual plane techniques release inferior pectoralis attachments, allowing some pectoralis retraction superiorly.
  - This maximizes implant contact with lower pole breast parenchyma, with the advantage of upper pole coverage by the pectoralis.
- **Dual plane type I**[10] (Fig. 52-2)

PARENCHYMA-MUSCLE INTERFACE
SEPARATION

PECTORALIS MUSCLE
DIVISION

PECTORALIS MUSCLE POSITION
RELATED TO IMPLANT

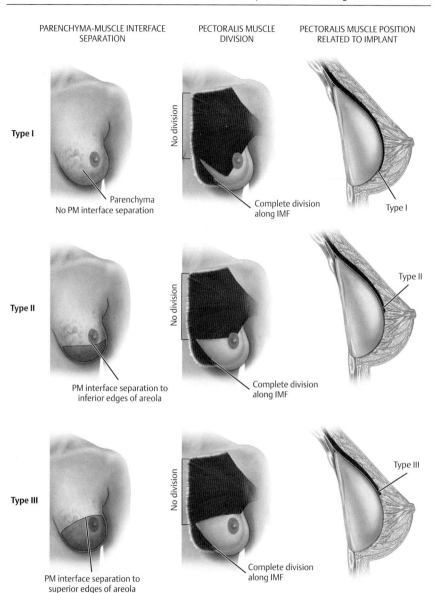

Type I

Parenchyma
No PM interface separation

No division

Complete division
along IMF

Type I

Type II

No division

PM interface separation to
inferior edges of areola

Complete division
along IMF

Type II

Type III

No division

PM interface separation to
superior edges of areola

Complete division
along IMF

Type III

Fig. 52-2   Dual plane augmentation techniques. The extent of dissection at the parenchyma-muscle (PM) (*top*). The position of the inferior edge of the divided pectoralis origins (*center*). The pectoralis position relative to the implant (*bottom*). (*IMF*, Inframammary fold.)

- Complete division of the pectoralis from its origin at level of IMF, stopping at the medial aspect of the IMF, in addition to subpectoral dissection
- **No dissection in the retromammary plane to free the breast parenchyma-muscle interface**
- Indications: Most "routine breasts"
- All breast parenchyma located above the IMF
- Tight attachments at the parenchyma-pectoralis interface
- Minimally stretched lower pole (NAC-IMF distance 4-6 cm)

■ **Dual plane type II**
- Complete division of the pectoralis from its origin at level of IMF, stopping at the medial aspect of the IMF
- Pectoralis separated from breast parenchyma in the retromammary plane **to level of inferior NAC**
- Indications: "Highly mobile parenchyma"
- Most of the parenchyma located above IMF
- Looser parenchyma-pectoral attachments (breast tissue much more mobile relative to pectoralis major)
- Moderate lower pole stretch (NAC-IMF distance 5.5-6.5 cm)

■ **Dual plane type III**
- Complete division of the pectoralis from its origin at level of IMF, stopping at the medial aspect of the IMF
- Separation of pectoralis from parenchyma in the retromammary plane is continued **to level of superior NAC.**
- Indications: "Glandular ptotic" and "constricted lower pole breasts," including tuberous breasts
  ▶ Breasts with glandular ptosis or true ptosis when a third or more of parenchyma is below the projected IMF
  ▶ Very loose parenchyma-pectoral attachments (parenchyma readily slides off pectoralis surface)
  ▶ Markedly stretched lower pole (NAC-IMF distance 7-8 cm)
  ▶ Tight, constricted lower breast with short, tight IMF
  ▶ Parenchymal maldistribution, tightly concentrated centrally leading to narrow base width
- Short NAC-IMF distance (tuberous breasts) (2-5 cm)
- Use radial and concentric scoring through breast parenchyma

SENIOR AUTHOR TIP: It is possible to consider an even more aggressive release of the muscle, essentially separating the breast from the muscle along its leading edge all the way up into the axilla. This allows the muscle to further "window shade" to a location above the NAC. This could be thought of as a dual plane type IV, or as the senior author calls it, a "combination pocket" and results in a great reduction in postoperative breast animation and yet still provides contour softening in the upper inner quadrant of the breast.

INCISION CHOICE (Table 52-2)

Table 52-2 *Incision Options for Breast Augmentation*

Factor	Axillary	Periareolar	Inframammary	Transumbilical*
Implant Plane				
Submuscular	+	+	+	–
Subglandular	–	+	+	+
Implant Type				
Saline, round	+	+	+	+
Saline, shaped	–	+	+	–
Silicone, round or shaped	–	+	+	–
Preoperative Breast Volume				
High (>200 g)	+	+	+	+
Low (<200 g)	+	+	–	+
Preoperative Breast Base Position				
High	+	+	+	+
Low	–	+	+	+
Breast Shape				
Tubular	–	+	–	–
Glandular ptosis	+	+	+	+
Ptosis (grades I and II)	–	+	–	–
Areolar Characteristics				
Small diameter	+	–	+	+
Light or indistinct	+	–	+	+
Inframammary Fold				
None	+	+	–	+
High	+	+	–	+
Low	+	+	+	+
Secondary Procedure	–	+	+	–

*Included for completeness, but generally not recommended.
+, Applicable; –, not generally recommended.

Inframammary Incision
- **Advantages**
  - Well hidden with mild ptosis or well-defined IMF
  - Best control
  - Complete visualization of subglandular or submuscular pocket
- **Disadvantages**
  - Leaves visible incision scar on breast
- **Technique**
  - Incision is placed **in projected IMF** rather than in existing one.
  - Incision is made along IMF lateral to nipple.
  - Most (two thirds) of incision is **lateral to nipple,** because it is more visible when placed medially.
  - **Saline** implants can be placed through incisions **<3 cm.**
  - **Silicone** implants may require incisions **up to 5 cm** based on implant size.
  - Dissection proceeds through Scarpa fascia.
  - Pectoralis fascia is identified.
  - Dissection continues either subglandularly, or the origin of the pectoralis major is completely divided from its origin at the level of the IMF, stopping at the medial aspect of the IMF for dual plane technique.
  - For subpectoral placement, initial dissection is carried out laterally to identify the lateral border of the pectoralis major.
  - Be mindful of medial intercostal perforators, which should be prospectively coagulated using insulated forceps.
  - Lateral intercostal cutaneous nerves are preserved to maintain NAC sensation.
  - Loose areolar connective tissue under the pectoralis major is divided, *avoiding lifting of the pectoralis minor.*
  - Once the pocket is dissected, sizers can be used (if surgeon preference)
  - Patient is placed in sitting position to 90 degrees to evaluate symmetry and implant position.
  - Corrections are made and hemostasis obtained.
  - Pocket is thoroughly irrigated with triple antibiotic solution.
  - Gloves are changed.
  - Skin reprepared with Betadine.
  - Implant is inserted using "no-touch" technique or the Keller funnel.
  - Closure is completed in multiple layers.

Periareolar Incision
- Placed in the **areolar-cutaneous junction**
- Subglandular or submuscular plane
- **Advantages**
  - Well hidden at interface of NAC and skin
  - Allows adjustment of IMF
  - Good access if areolar diameter **>3.5 cm**
- **Disadvantages**
  - Limited exposure
  - Transection of parenchymal ducts, leading to possible *Staphylococcus epidermidis* colonization
  - Possible nipple sensitivity changes

- Visible scar: White or hypopigmented scar when placed within areola
- Potential for visible hypertrophic scarring
- May traverse and scar a cancer-prone organ
- Should not be used if areolar diameter **<3.5 cm**

■ **Technique**
- Incision is placed around the lower half of the areola precisely at the junction of areola and breast skin.
- Incision is limited to a **maximum of 3 o'clock to 9 o'clock position on the areola.**
- Dissection proceeds through breast parenchyma to the pectoralis fascia.
- Dissection of a subglandular, dual plane or submuscular pocket is then the same as for an IMF incision, and the implant is placed in the standard fashion.
- For inferior pole constricted breasts, **radial scoring** of the parenchyma is used to redrape the soft tissues over the implant.

■ **Dissection options:**
- **Direct dissection**
  - ► Through breast parenchyma
  - ► Discouraged because of possible bacterial contamination from ducts and may scar breast parenchyma
- **Stairstep dissection**
  - ► After cutting through the skin, dissection continues inferiorly following the subcutaneous plane to the inferior edge of the breast mound, and a pocket is created.
  - ► This technique is preferred, because less parenchyma is disrupted.

Transaxillary Incision
■ **Advantages**
- Can perform bluntly or with endoscope
- Endoscope allows precise dissection and release of pectoralis major inferior attachment for dual plane technique and precise hemostasis.
- Avoids breast scars
- Saline or silicone implant in submuscular, subglandular plane or dual plane

■ **Disadvantages**
- Need for second incision for any revision surgery
- Precise implant placement can be difficult
- Without endoscope, difficult to fully visualize pocket
- Potential scar visibility when sleeveless and raising arms
- Silicone implants are sometimes difficult to insert.

■ **Technique**
- Patients arm fully adducted, and anteriormost point of the axilla marked (limit of the incision)
- Arm abducted to 90 degrees
- Incision made and dissection carried out to the lateral border of the pectoralis major to prevent injury to the intercostal nerve
- Subglandular, dual plane, or submuscular pocket dissected either bluntly with a Montgomery dissector or using an endoscope for visualization and standard electrocautery dissection
- Implant placed in the standard fashion
- Incisions closed in layers

Transumbilical Incision
- **Advantages**
  - Single, hidden incision
  - Scar hidden and distant from breast
- **Disadvantages**
  - Difficult, blind dissection
  - Difficult to make adjustments or corrections
  - Can only use saline implant
  - Hemostasis and implant positioning very difficult
  - High or asymmetrical placement
  - Revision surgery requires second incision
  - Additional specialized equipment required
- **Technique**
  - Additional preoperative mark from umbilicus to the medial border of the NAC while patient supine
  - 2-3 cm horizontal incision at highest point of axilla, 1 cm behind border of pectoralis
  - Dissection medially in superficial subcutaneous plane, and continuing to posterolateral border of pectoralis, incising vertically to enter subpectoral or subglandular plane
  - Incision in the umbilicus large enough to fit the operator's index finger
  - Endotube with blunt obturator passed above rectus fascia
  - Pocket dissected bluntly
  - For subglandular implants, force directly upward at IMF level
  - Tunnel stops just cephalad to the NAC
  - Obturator removed and endoscope used to evaluate pocket and hemostasis
  - Endoscope and endotube removed and rolled expander is moved up the tunnel
  - Expander filled to 150% of the final implant volume
  - Expander removed using traction on fill tube
  - Permanent saline implant inserted in similar fashion
  - Incision closed in layers
- Blind procedure in the early 70s, now significantly advanced by endoscopic technique[11]

TECHNICAL POINTS[12]
- **Perioperative antibiotics**
  - First-generation cephalosporin 30-59 minutes before incision
- Pocket irrigated with **triple antibiotic solution (TAB)**[8]
  - 1 g cefazolin, 80 mg gentamicin, 50,000 units bacitracin per 500 ml saline
  - Pocket soaked for 5 minutes
  - In 2000 FDA banned povidone iodine (Betadine) contact with implants because of complications when used intraluminally (implant delamination and leakage), but there is no scientific evidence that extraluminal contact is harmful.[13]
- Precise dissection
- Meticulous hemostasis
- Hand-switched monopolar cautery
- Deep closing sutures placed before implant inserted, with knots away from implant
- Skin wiped with antibiotic solution
- Only talc-free gloves used
- Change gloves before the implant is handled or placed.

- **"No-touch technique"** always used
  - Prevents implant contamination from skin[14]
- Only sterile saline through a closed system used to fill saline implants (if applicable)

> **TIP:** Avoid deep dissection in axilla; intercostobrachial and median brachial cutaneous nerves are vulnerable.

TREATMENT OF INFRAMAMMARY FOLD

- Appropriate IMF height centers the axis of the implant behind or just below the NAC.
- N-IMF length should correspond to implant volume (Table 52-3).
  - Approximately 7 cm at 250 cc, 8 cm at 300 cc, 8.5 cm at 350 cc, 9 cm at 375 cc, and 9.5 cm at 400 cc
  - Areola-IMF distance: Should approximate radius of implant and half of breast base width

Table 52-3 *Relationship of Implant Volume and Nipple–Inframammary Fold Length*

Implant Volume	250 cc	300 cc	350 cc	375 cc	400 cc
N-IMF length (cm)	7	8	8.5	9	9.5

> **TIP:** The IMF can be carefully lowered when a significant discrepancy exists between implant size and N-IMF distance, or when asymmetry exists.

POSTOPERATIVE CARE

- Outpatient procedure

MEDICATIONS

- Acetaminophen or NSAIDS preferred for routine pain control
  - Narcotics only as needed for severe pain
- Carisoprodol (Soma, Vanadom): Helps pectoralis relax
- No data to support routine antibiotic use, but many surgeons provide 3 days of oral antibiotics

BRASSIERE AND DRESSING

- Steri-Strips for 6 weeks
- Brassiere optional
  - No underwire or push-up bras for 6 weeks

ACTIVITY

- Patients may shower 24 hours postoperatively.
- For smooth implants, displacement exercises are initiated between postoperative day 1 and day 3 or when they do not cause pain.
  - Push implant medially and superiorly
  - Ten pushes three times a day for 1 month, then once daily
- Aerobic activity is restricted for 2-3 weeks.

- Heavy lifting is restricted for 6 weeks.
- Postoperative visits are scheduled for 1-3 days, 2 weeks, 4-6 weeks, 3 months, and 1 year.
- Photos should be taken at each postoperative visit.

COMPLICATIONS

PERIOPERATIVE
Altered Nipple Sensation[15,16]
- **15%** have permanent sensory changes.
- Hyperesthesia/anesthesia
- Secondary to traction or transection of lateral intercostal cutaneous nerve
- Incidence and severity are the same with all techniques.

Seroma
- Most surgeons do not use drains for cosmetic breast implant cases.
- Most seromas resorb within the first week, if present.
- Persistent seromas should be drained under ultrasound visualization.

Hematoma
- Rare: 0.5% of patients
- Can lead to pain, asymmetry, and capsular contracture

Infection
- <1% of patients
- Most often cultured organism *S. epidermidis*
- Implant generally removed

Galactorrhea[17]
- Rare
- Thought to be secondary to transection of the thoracic nerves
- Treated with bromocriptine

Asymmetry

DELAYED COMPLICATIONS
Synmastia[18]
- Secondary to **migration** of one or both implants across midline
- **Result of:**
  - Overdissection of the medial pocket
  - Excessively large implants
  - Disproportionately wide implants compared to chest wall

Chest Wall Deformities
- Thoracic hypoplasia, pectus excavatum
- Simultaneous augmentation and mastopexy
- Very difficult to correct

Rippling
- **Secondary to underfilling or traction**
- Seen in upper pole of underfilled implants
- Prevented by filling saline implants to recommended fill or overfill
- Traction rippling seen in textured implants
  - Prevented by ensuring adequate soft tissue over implant and matching pocket size with implant

Leak or Rupture
- **Saline**
  - 2%-5% rate at 5 years, 5%-10% rate at 10 years, or 1% per year[19]
  - **Risk factors**
    - ▶ Underfilling >25 cc
    - ▶ Intraluminal antibiotics or steroids
  - Requires implant exchange
- **Silicone[20]**
  - True incidence difficult to assess
    - ▶ 30% at 5 years
    - ▶ 50% at 10 years
    - ▶ 70% at 17 years
  - **Intracapsular rupture:** When silicone rupture is contained within the implant capsule
  - **Extracapsular rupture:** When silicone leaks outside of the capsule (also called *extrusion*)
  - Often leads to granuloma formation
  - FDA recommends MRI 3 years after surgery and then every 2 years to monitor for rupture ("linguine sign").
- **Etiologic factors**
  - Fold flaw
  - Underfilling
  - Manufacturing flaws
  - Technical errors
  - Higher problem rates with thin-shell implants (second generation)
- **Diagnosis**
  - **Physical examination**
    - ▶ Asymmetry
    - ▶ Obvious deflation (less obvious with silicone)
  - **Radiographs/mammogram**
    - ▶ Low sensitivity
    - ▶ Moderate specificity
    - ▶ Expense low
  - **Ultrasound**
    - ▶ Findings: Snowstorm, stepladder appearance
    - ▶ Moderate sensitivity
    - ▶ Moderate specificity
    - ▶ Expense moderate

- **MRI**
  - ► Findings: *Linguine sign,* silicone extrusion
  - ► High sensitivity
  - ► High specificity
  - ► High expense
- **Treatment**
  - Treatment as soon as possible to prevent further distortion of the deflated breast, contraction of the capsules, and local inflammation and granulomas with silicone leak
  - Removal of implant and residual implant material
  - Capsulotomy (or capsulectomy) as needed
  - Possible replacement of implants

Capsular Calcification[21]
- Related to implant age
- 0% occurrence for implants <10 years old
- 100% occurrence for implants >23 years old
- Remove by capsulectomy

Migration and Tissue Changes
- **Bottoming out**
  - Increased N-IMF distance, less than half of base width
  - Related to poor tissue characteristics, large implant size, and overdissection of IMF

> **SENIOR AUTHOR TIP:** Bottoming out of the breast implant can be prevented by suturing Scarpa fascia down to the chest wall with 3-0 Prolene sutures after the implant has been placed. This maneuver must be done with patient at least 60 degrees in the upright position to prevent inadvertent overelevation of the fold. By closing off the very loose deep subscarpal space, proper support of the fold is provided, thus ensuring a stable implant position.

- **Double-bubble deformity type A ("waterfall deformity")** (Fig. 52-3)
  - Implant is **above** breast mound.
  - Implant is held high on chest wall by total pectoral coverage or contracture, and loose parenchyma slides off pectoral muscles inferior to axis of the implant.
- **Double-bubble deformity type B**
  - Implant is **below** breast mound.
  - With significant overdissection of IMF, implant can slide caudal to the breast mound and create a second IMF below the native IMF and breast mound.

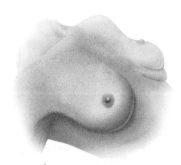

Fig. 52-3   Double-bubble deformity appearance.

Capsular Contracture
- The body naturally forms capsules around all implants.

- *Capsular contracture* is tightening of the capsule, with compression and distortion of the implant.
  - Can lead to asymmetry, pain, and implant rupture
- **Baker classification**[22]
  - **Grade I:** No palpable capsule. The augmented breast feels as soft as an unoperated breast.
  - **Grade II:** Minimal firmness. The breast is less soft, and the implant can be palpated but is not visible.
  - **Grade III:** Moderate firmness. The breast is harder, the implant can be palpated easily, and it (or distortion from it) can be seen.
  - **Grade IV:** Severe contracture. The breast is hard, tender, and cold. Associated with **pain.**
    - ▶ Distortion is often marked.
- **Treatment**
  - **Capsulectomy**
    - ▶ Indications[23]
      - ◆ For Baker grade III and IV
      - ◆ Calcified or thick capsule
      - ◆ Ruptured silicone implant
      - ◆ Silicone granulomas
      - ◆ Infection around implant
      - ◆ Polyurethane implant
      - ◆ Need to replace previous implant with larger-volume implant
      - ◆ New plane needed (e.g., subglandular changes to subpectoral)
    - ▶ Advantages
      - ◆ Low contracture recurrence
      - ◆ Removal of potential contaminants
    - ▶ Disadvantages
      - ◆ Hemostasis more difficult
      - ◆ Anteriorly: Thins soft tissue coverage
      - ◆ Posteriorly: Risk of pneumothorax (if previous subpectoral implant)
    - ▶ Technique
      - ◆ Complete capsulectomy preferred in the subglandular plane, but caution is needed anteriorly with thin soft tissue coverage
      - ◆ Anterior capsulectomy alone, if in the subpectoral plane and posterior capsule is densely adherent to chest wall, to avoid entering chest cavity
      - ◆ Implant plane changed (subglandular to submuscular)
  - **Open capsulotomy**
    - ▶ Controlled scoring of the existing capsule
    - ▶ Concentric and radial
    - ▶ High recurrence rates (37%-89%)
  - **Closed capsulotomy**
    - ▶ Manual external compression (squeezing and compressing) to disrupt the capsule
    - ▶ No longer widely used because of risk of implant rupture and extremely high recurrence rates (31%-80%)
  - **Breast massage and displacement exercises**
    - ▶ Early: <2 weeks postoperatively
  - **Pharmacotherapy**
    - ▶ Leukotriene inhibitors (e.g., zafirlukast [Accolate]): Potential for rare liver toxicity
    - ▶ Papaverine hydrochloride (Pavabid)

- ▶ Oral vitamin E
- ▶ Intraluminal steroids: Reduces contracture, but higher rate of implant rupture, skin erosion, atrophy, and ptosis
- ▶ Cyclosporine (Neoral, Sandimmune), mitomycin C (Mutamycin)

- ■ **Etiologic factors**
  - Subclinical infection[24-27]
  - Correlation well established, but causal relationship uncertain
  - *S. epidermidis* most common, but many other types of bacteria implicated
  - Hypertrophic scar hypothesis
- ■ **Time course**
  - Most contractures occur **within 1 year.**
  - Late occurrence may be secondary to systemic bacterial seeding or capsular maturation.
- ■ **Historical rates and risk factors**
  - **Pocket location**[20]
    - ▶ Subglandular: 32% contracture rate
    - ▶ Subpectoral: 12% contracture rate
  - **Filler**[28]
    - ▶ Silicone: 50% contracture rate
    - ▶ Saline: 16% contracture rate
  - **Implant surface**[29,30] (Fig. 52-4)
    - ▶ Smooth: 58% contracture rate at 10 years
    - ▶ Textured: 11% contracture rate at 10 year

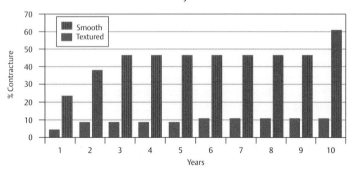

Fig. 52-4   Ten-year development of subglandular capsular contracture in smooth versus textured implants.

- ■ **Current data AFTER FDA reinstatement 2006** (Boxes 52-1 and 52-2)[31-37]
  - With significantly lower contracture rates, data have shown less correlation between implant texture, filler, or pocket choice.
  - Saline trial: 2001, Mentor Corporation (Santa Barbara, CA)[32]
    - ▶ 9% contracture rate with primary augmentation
    - ▶ 30% contracture rate with reconstruction
  - Saline trial: 2001, Inamed (Allergan) Corporation (Irvine, CA)[33]
    - ▶ 9% contracture rate with primary augmentation
    - ▶ 25% contracture rate with reconstruction
  - Silicone gel premarket approval trial: Mentor 2006, Allergan (previously Inamed) 2006, Sientra (Santa Barbara, CA) 2012[34]

Box 52-1   *2006 DATA BY MANUFACTURER*

Mentor (3-year data)

- Primary augmentation (551 patients)
  - Overall complication rate 36.6%
  - Overall reoperation rate 15.4%
  - Capsular contracture III/IV 8.1%
  - MRI cohort rupture 0.5% (0% in non-MRI cohort)
- Revision augmentation (146 patients)
  - Overall complication rate 50%
  - Overall reoperation rate 28%
  - Capsular contracture III/IV 18.9%
  - MRI cohort rupture 7.7% (0% in non-MRI cohort)

Allergan (4-year data)

- Primary augmentation (455 patients)
  - Overall complication rate 41.3%
  - Overall reoperation rate 23.5%
  - Capsular contracture III/IV 13.2%
  - MRI cohort rupture 2.7% (0.4% in non-MRI cohort)

- Revision augmentation (147 patients)
  - Overall complication rate 56.9%
  - Overall reoperation rate 35.3%
  - Capsular contracture III/IV 17.0%
  - MRI cohort rupture 7.7% (0% in non-MRI cohort)

Sientra (3-year data)

- Primary augmentation (1115 patients)
  - Overall complication rate 20.2%
  - Overall reoperation rate 12.6%
  - Capsular contracture III/IV 6.0%
  - MRI cohort rupture 2.5% (0% in non-MRI cohort)
- Revision augmentation (362 patients)
  - Overall complication rate 26.3%
  - Overall reoperation rate 20.3%
  - Capsular contracture III/IV 5.2%
  - MRI cohort rupture 0% (0.4% in non-MRI cohort)

Box 52-2   *FDA UPDATE 2011 DATA*

Mentor Core Study (8-year data)

- Large study (2007-2009) data (3-year follow-up)
- 41,900 patients silicone, 1030 saline
- Primary augmentation rupture rate 10.1%
- Revision augmentation rupture rate 6.3%
- Reoperation rate primary augmentation 10.8%
- Reoperation rate revision augmentation 14.6%
- Rupture rate primary augmentation 0.2%
- Rupture rate revision augmentation 1.0%
- Capsular contracture III/IV primary augmentation 5.3%
- Capsular contracture III/IV revision augmentation 11.8%

Allergan Core Study (10-year data)

- Large study (2007-2010) data (2-year follow-up)
- 41,342 patients silicone, 15,646 saline
- Primary augmentation rupture rate 13.6%
- Revision augmentation rupture rate 15.5%
- Reoperation: 6.5% silicone augmentation; 4.5% saline augmentation
- Rupture silicone 0.5%
- Saline deflation 2.5%
- Capsular contracture III/IV: 5.0% silicone; 2.8% saline

BREAST IMPLANT-ASSOCIATED ANAPLASTIC LARGE CELL LYMPHOMA (BIA-ALCL)[38,39]

- BIA-ALCL is a rare and treatable type of T-cell lymphoma that can develop around breast implants. *BIA-ALCL is not a cancer of the breast tissue itself.*
- The current lifetime risk of BIA-ALCL in the United States is estimated to be 1:30,000 women with textured implants based upon current confirmed cases and textured implant sales data over the past two decades.
- It is important to differentiate BIA-ALCL from primary lymphoma of the breast which is predominantly a B-cell lymphoma with an incidence of approximately 1:4 million.
- BIA-ALCL should continue to be discussed with any patient considering breast implants as part of the informed-consent process.[38]
- The lag time between implant insertion to diagnosis of BIA-ALCL has been from 2 to 28 years, with a median of 8 years.
- *No cases of BIA-ALCL have been definitively associated with patients who have only had smooth implants.* However, it is not possible to exclude the appearance of BIA-ALCL in association with smooth implants at this time.
- The association of BIA-ALCL textured implants may be related to the increased surface area of the texturing; however, this has not yet been definitively proven. The variation in surface texturing among manufacturers may mean there are variable risks for the development of BIA-ALCL, although the number of cases to date remain too low to make any significant distinctions between the various forms of texturing.
- The disease has been associated with both silicone and saline implants in aesthetic as well as reconstructive patients.
- The majority of patients present as a delayed seroma. Diagnosis is based on ultrasound-guided fine needle aspiration of the periimplant fluid, which is assessed with immunohistochemistry for CD30-positive and ALK-negative T-cell lymphocytes.
- PET-CT and MRI scans are investigations performed following a positive diagnosis. Mammograms are not helpful.
- Consideration should be given to a multidisciplinary approach including, when required, an oncological breast surgeon and an oncologist specializing in lymphoma.
- Incomplete capsular resection has been associated with both recurrence and significantly lower survival.
- The majority of patients can be cured of their disease by bilateral total capsulectomy and implant removal. Rare patients will present with a mass and have an increased risk of requiring radiotherapy and chemotherapy. Treatment approach should follow international guidelines established by the National Comprehensive Cancer Network (NCCN) for BIA-ALCL, available at *www.nccn.org.*
  - 93 percent of patients are disease-free at 3-year follow-up, which is an excellent prognosis when treated appropriately.
- Current treatment recommendation is for bilateral complete capsulectomy and implant removal, as a small number of women have had contralateral disease found incidentally.[39]

- The FDA recommends that any suspected or confirmed cases of BIA-ALCL be reported to the PROFILE registry, the MAUDE database, and the device manufacturer. To submit a case to PROFILE, go to *ThePSF.org/PROFILE*. To submit a case to the FDA's Manufacturer and User Facility Device Experience (MAUDE) database, which collects medical device reports (MDRs) of suspected device-associated deaths, serious injuries and malfunctions, visit *www.accessdata.fda.gov*.

REOPERATION
- Large-scale prospective studies (2004 FDA hearings about Inamed Corporation data)[28-30]
- Current 3-year reoperation rate: 13% for saline and 21% for silicone

CANCER SURVEILLANCE
- Implants cause interference with normal mammogram imaging.
- **Eklund mammogram views** displace breast and implant to increase parenchymal imaging after breast augmentation.
- With appropriate imaging, no increased risk for cancer is found; diagnosis not later; no difference in survival or recurrence.[40,41]

> **SENIOR AUTHOR TIP:** The preoperative consult must determine the precise goals of the patient.
>
> Three variables must be measured during the preoperative evaluation, including implant base diameter, volume, and projection.
>
> Visualization tools such as external bra sizers, computer-generated images, and virtual reality technology can help to ensure physicians understand fully the goals of their patients.
>
> The IMF should be lowered only in selected circumstances, because lowering of the fold can lead to distortion.
>
> In lieu of lowering the fold, the use of a smaller implant can help to reduce the risk of fold distortion.
>
> Aggressive dual or combination plane dissection can help to reduce distortion along the fold.
>
> Implants that resist wrinkling, such as anatomically shaped cohesive gel devices, lead to longer-term performance with reduced 10-year rupture rates.
>
> Anatomic implants can help to prevent the need for a mastopexy in selected patients.

Top Takeaways

➤ Early mammograms are recommended for patients undergoing breast surgery (by age 30-35 years).

➤ Eklund mammographic views improve radiographic imaging of breast tissue after augmentation.

➤ During preoperative evaluations, asymmetries should be noted and discussed with the patient. If asymmetries are present before surgery, asymmetries will be present afterward.

➤ Mild ptosis is improved with augmentation. However, patients whose N-IMF distance is >9.5 cm should undergo mastopexy.

➤ Subglandular augmentation is not recommended with thin upper pole coverage (superior pole pinch test is <2 cm).

➤ Larger implants increase long-term detrimental effects on the breast.

➤ Historically, higher contracture rates occur with smooth implants, silicone implants, and subglandular placement.

➤ Textured implant surfaces disorient collagen deposition, thereby reducing contracture.

➤ Subglandular placement potentially increases risk of implant contamination, subclinical infection, and subsequent contracture.

➤ The use of antibiotic irrigation, and other techniques, dramatically reduces contracture rates.

➤ The dual plane (biplanar) technique takes advantage of extra upper pole pectoralis coverage while maximizing the implant-parenchymal interface in the lower pole.

➤ MRI is the most sensitive and specific test for implant rupture or leakage.

➤ BIA-ALCL should be suspected in late developing seromas, especially if history of textured implant.

References

1. American Society of Plastic Surgeons. Procedural statistics trends 1992-2004. Available at *www.plasticsurgery.org/public_education/Statistical-Trends.cfm.*

2. Barnard JJ, Todd EL, Wilson WG, et al. Distribution of organosilicon polymers in augmentation mammaplasties at autopsy. Plast Reconstr Surg 100:197, 1997.

3. Silicone gel-filled breast implants approved. FDA Consum 41:8, 2007.

4. Tillman DB. Department of Health and Human Services, Food and Drug Administration. Letter to Mentor Corporation, Department of Clinical and Regulatory Affairs re: Silicone Gel-Filled Breast Implants, November 17, 2006.

5. Rohrich R. Streamlining cosmetic surgery patient selection—just say No! Plast Reconstr Surg:104:220, 1999.

6. Gorney M. Patient selection criteria. Medico-legal issues in plastic surgery. Clin Plast Surg 26:37, 1999.

7. National Breast Cancer Foundation. Early detection. Available at *http://www.nationalbreastcancer.org/early-detection-of-breast-cancer.*

8. Adams WP, Rios JI, Smith SJ. Enhancing patient outcomes in aesthetic and reconstructive breast surgery using triple antibiotic breast irrigation: six-year prospective clinical study. Plast Reconstr Surg 117:30, 2006.

9. Tebbetts JB, Adams WP. Five critical decisions in breast augmentation using five measurements in 5 minutes. The high five decision support process. Plast Reconstr Surg 116:2005, 2005.

10. Tebbetts JB. Dual plane breast augmentation: optimizing implant-soft-tissue relationships in a wide range of breast types. Plast Reconstr Surg 107:1255, 2001.

11. Price CI, Eaves FF III, Nahai F, et al. Endoscopic transaxillary subpectoral breast augmentation. Plast Reconstr Surg 94:612, 1994.

12. Rohrich RJ, Kenkel JM, Adams WP. Preventing capsular contracture in breast augmentation: in search of the Holy Grail. Plast Reconstr Surg 103:1759, 1999.

13. Wiener TC. Betadine and breast implants: an update. Aesthet Surg J 33:615, 2013.

14. Mladick RA. "No-touch" submuscular saline breast augmentation technique. Aesthetic Plast Surg 17:183, 1993.

15. Courtiss EH, Goldwyn RM. Breast sensation before and after plastic surgery. Plast Reconstr Surg 58:1, 1976.

16. Mofid MM, Klatsky SA, Singh NK, et al. Nipple-areola complex sensitivity after primary breast augmentation: a comparison of periareolar and inframammary incision approaches. Plast Reconstr Surg 117:1694, 2006.

17. Rothkopf DM, Rosen HM. Lactation as a complication of aesthetic breast surgery successfully treated with bromocriptine. Br J Plast Surg 43:373, 1990.

18. Spear SL, Bogue DP, Thomassen JM. Synmastia after breast augmentation. Plast Reconstr Surg 118(7 Suppl):S168, 2006.

19. Gutowski KA, Mesna GT, Cunningham BL. Saline-filled breast implants: a Plastic Surgery Educational Foundation multicenter outcomes study. Plast Reconstr Surg 100:1019, 1997.

20. Biggs TM, Yarish RS. Augmentation mammoplasty: a comparative analysis. Plast Reconstr Surg 85:368, 1990.

21. Peters W, Smith D. Calcification of breast implant capsules: incidence, diagnosis, and contributing factors. Ann Plast Surg 34:8, 1995.

22. Baker JL Jr. Augmentation mammaplasty. In Owsley JQ Jr, Peterson RA, eds. Symposium on Aesthetic Surgery of the Breast, vol 18. St Louis: CV Mosby, 1979.

23. Young VL. Guidelines and indications for breast implant capsulectomy. Plast Reconstr Surg 102:884, 1998.

24. Virden CP, Dobke MK, Stein P, et al. Subclinical infection of the silicone breast implant surface as a possible cause of capsular contracture. Aesthetic Plast Surg 16:173, 1992.

25. Dobke MK, Svahn JK, Vastine VL, et al. Characterization of microbial presence at the surface of silicone mammary implants. Ann Plast Surg 34:563, 1995.

26. Burkhardt BR, Dempsey PD, Schnur MD, et al. Capsular contracture: a prospective study of the effect of local antibacterial agents. Plast Reconstr Surg 77:919, 1986.

27. Burkhardt BR. Effects of povidone iodine on silicone gel implants in vitro: implications for clinical practice. Plast Reconstr Surg 114:711, 2004.

28. Gylbert L, Asplund O, Jurell G. Capsular contracture after breast reconstruction with silicone gel and saline-filled implants: a 6-year follow-up. Plast Reconstr Surg 85:373, 1990.

29. Collis N, Coleman D, Foo IT, et al. Ten-year review of a prospective randomized controlled trial of textured versus smooth subglandular silicone gel breast implants. Plast Reconstr Surg 106:786, 2000.

30. Marotta JS, Widenhouse CW, Habal MB, et al. Silicone gel breast implant failure and frequency of additional surgeries: analysis of 35 studies reporting examination of more than 8000 explants. J Biomed Mater Res 48:354, 1999.

31. U.S. Food and Drug Administration. Center for Devices and Radiological Health. FDA update on the safety of silicone gel-filled breast implants, June 2011. Available at *www.fda.gov/downloads/medicaldevices/productsandmedicalprocedures/implantsandprosthetics/breastimplants/ucm260090.*

32. Mentor Corporation. Saline implant premarket approval information, 2001. Available at *http://www.fda/gov/downloads/medicaldevices/productsandmedicalprocedures/implantsandprosthetics/breastimplants/ucm232436.pdf.*

33. Allergan Corporation. Saline implant premarket approval information, 2001. Available at *www.fda.gov//downloads/medicaldevices/productsandmedicalprocedures/implantsandprosthetics/breast-implants/ucm064457.pdf.*

34. Mentor, Allergan, and Sientra Corporations. Silicone breast implant premarket approval information, 2003, 2005, 2012. Available at *www.fda.gov/medicaldevices/productsandmedicalprocedures/implantsandprosthetics/breastimplants/ucm063871.htm.*

35. Mentor Corporation. Saline implant premarket approval information, 2001. Available at *http://www.accessdata.fda.gov/scripts/cdrh/cfdocs/cfpma/pma.cfm?start_search=1&sortcolumn=do_desc&PAGENUM=500&pmanumber=P990075.*

36. Inamed Corporation. Saline implant premarket approval information, 2001. Available at *http://www.accessdata.fda.gov/scripts/cdrh/cfdocs/cfpma/pma.cfm?start_search=1&sortcolumn=do_desc&PAGENUM=500&pmanumber=P990075.*

37. Inamed Corporation. Silicone breast implant premarket approval information, 2003 and 2005. Available at *http://www.accessdata.fda.gov/scripts/cdrh/cfdocs/cfpma/pma.cfm?start_search=1&sortcolumn=do_desc&PAGENUM=500&pmanumber=P990075.*

38. Clemens MW, Miranda FN, Butler CE. Breast implant informed consent should include the risk of anaplastic large cell lymphoma. Plast Reconstr Surg 137:1117, 2016.

39. Clemens MW, Medeiros LJ, Butler CE, et al. Complete surgical excision is essential for the management of patients with breast implant-associated anaplastic large-cell lymphoma. J Clin Oncol 34:160, 2016.

40. Hoshaw SJ, Klein PJ, Clark BD, et al. Breast implants and cancer: causation, delayed detection, and survival. Plast Reconstr Surg 107:1393, 2001.

41. Jakubietz M, Janis JE, Jakubietz R, et al. Breast augmentation: cancer concerns and mammography: a review of the literature. Plast Reconstr Surg 113:117e, 2004.

53. Mastopexy

Joshua Lemmon, Smita R. Ramanadham, James Christian Grotting

NATURAL HISTORY AND CLASSIFICATION[1,2]

BREAST CHANGES: MULTIFACTORIAL
- The amount of breast parenchyma changes with **age, body weight, pregnancy,** and **hormonal changes.**
  - The skin envelope is stretched when the parenchyma enlarges.
  - Supporting ligaments and ductal structures are also stretched.
  - **Ptosis** results when the parenchymal volume decreases, and the skin envelope and supporting structures do not retract.
    - ▶ As a consequence, the breast assumes a lower position on the chest wall, and the youthful breast contour is lost.

REGNAULT CLASSIFICATION[1] (Fig. 53-1)
- *Describes ptosis by the relative position of the nipple-areola complex (NAC) and the inframammary fold*
  - **Grade I ptosis (mild ptosis)**
    - ▶ NAC is **at** the level of the inframammary fold.
  - **Grade II ptosis (moderate ptosis)**
    - ▶ NAC lies **below** the level of the inframammary fold, but remains above the most dependent part of the breast parenchyma.
  - **Grade III ptosis (severe ptosis)**
    - ▶ NAC lies **well below** the inframammary fold and at the most dependent part of the breast parenchyma along the inferior contour of the breast.
  - **Pseudoptosis or glandular ptosis**
    - ▶ NAC is **above or at** the level of the inframammary fold, but most of the breast parenchyma has descended **below** the level of the fold.
    - ▶ Nipple-to-inframammary fold distance has increased.

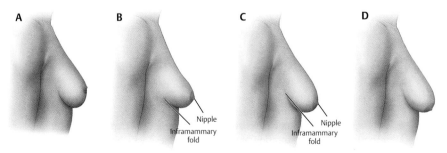

Fig. 53-1   Regnault classification of breast ptosis. **A,** Pseudoptosis. **B,** Grade I ptosis. **C,** Grade II ptosis. **D,** Grade III ptosis.

INDICATIONS AND CONTRAINDICATIONS[3-5]

INDICATIONS
- Women who desire an improvement in breast contour without a change in volume
- Women who seek a more lifted, "perky," youthful breast appearance and aim to correct upper pole deflation, ptosis of the areolar complex and breast tissue, and laxity of skin envelope

CONTRAINDICATIONS
- Active smoking
- Women who desire volume change

PREOPERATIVE EVALUATION[2, 6]

HISTORY
- **Age:** Involution of breast after menopause
- **Breast history:** Lactation, pregnancy changes, size changes with weight loss/gain, tumors, previous procedures, family history of breast cancer, recent mammogram
- **Patient goals**
- **Medications,** including psychotropic, oral contraceptive, and hormone replacement[6]

MEASUREMENTS
- **Sternal notch-to-nipple distance:** Allows detection of asymmetry in nipple position
- **Nipple-to-inframammary fold distance:** A measurement of the redundancy of the lower pole skin envelope
- **Classification of ptosis severity** (see Fig. 53-1)

OTHER CONSIDERATIONS
- **Breast position on chest wall:** Patients with low breast position without significant ptosis will not benefit from mastopexy.[7]
- **Skin quality and amount:** Presence of striae reflects the inelastic quality of affected skin; degree of skin laxity
- **Parenchymal quality:** Fatty, fibrous, or glandular parenchyma and overall volume
- **Areolar shape and size:** Areola are often stretched and large with asymmetries.

PHOTOGRAPHS
- **AP, lateral,** and **oblique** photographs should be obtained (see Chapter 3).

PATIENT EXPECTATIONS
- **Breast size**
  - Mastopexy techniques combine small amounts of parenchymal resection (<300 g traditionally in literature[3]) and redistribution with reduction of the skin envelope—this can result in a reduction in breast size.
    - ▶ **Average decrease of one cup size postoperatively:** *Important in patient counseling.*[3]
  - Many patients desire restoration of upper pole fullness, which may necessitate the placement of an implant simultaneously.
    - ▶ Mastopexy, augmentation-mastopexy, and reduction all increased breast and upper pole projection with significantly greater boost when implants were combined with mastopexy.[8]

- Volume-deficient patients may often require augmentation-mastopexy as well[7] (see Chapter 54).
- **Scar position**
  - Mastopexy procedures trade scars for improved contour.
  - Patients should be informed in detail preoperatively about scar placement and scar quality.
- **Other considerations**
  - Thorough patient education regarding procedural complications, use of drains, and recurrence of ptosis are essential components of preoperative preparation.

INFORMED CONSENT

Recommend items to be included in the informed consent:
- A general description of the procedure and location of incisions and the potential need for placement of drains
- A sufficient description of potential risks
  - Bleeding and hematoma
  - Infection
  - Delayed healing and wound separation
  - Change in nipple and skin sensation
  - Potential changes in breast-feeding
  - Asymmetry and poor cosmetic result
  - **Poor scar quality**

> **TIP:** Postoperative scars are a frequent source of litigation; therefore they are an essential component of the informed consent process. However, breast shape should not be compromised to reduce the scar burden.

MASTOPEXY TECHNIQUES

- Historically, mastopexy was based on primary skin excision; however, since the mid-1990s, internal shaping of tissue using various supportive materials or parenchymal pillars has also been emphasized.[4]
- Technique depends on degree of ptosis.

PERIAREOLAR TECHNIQUES

GENERAL
- Incisions are made and closed around the areola.
- Scars are therefore camouflaged at the areolar-skin junction.

PATIENT SELECTION
- Useful with **mild** and moderate ptosis
- Skin quality should be reasonable without striae, and parenchyma should be fibrous or glandular.

TECHNIQUES
- **Simple periareolar deepithelialization and closure**
  - Breast parenchyma is **not** repositioned; therefore only useful with mild ptosis
  - Permits **nipple repositioning**
  - Limited ellipitical techniques can elevate the NAC approximately **1-2 cm.**[2]
- **Benelli technique**[9] (Fig. 53-2)
  - A periareolar technique that can be applied to patients with larger degrees of breast ptosis
  - Allows parenchymal repositioning
  - Areolar sizers are used to mark the new areolar diameter, and a wider ellipse is marked to reposition the NAC and resect redundant skin envelope.
  - Undermining separates the breast gland from the overlying skin.
  - The breast parenchyma is then incised leaving the NAC on a superior pedicle.
  - Medial and lateral parenchymal flaps are mobilized and crossed or invaginated in the midline, narrowing the breast width and coning the breast shape.
  - The periareolar incision is closed in a purse-string fashion with permanent suture.

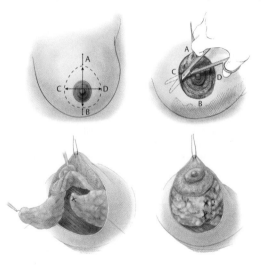

Fig. 53-2   Benelli periareolar mastopexy. Markings, undermining, and parenchymal coning.

- **Other periareolar techniques**
  - Variations on the technique discussed above include use of mesh to support the parenchyma[10] or routine use of breast implants to reduce the amount of skin resection required.[11,12]

ADVANTAGES
- Short scar
- Scar position camouflaged at border of pigmented areola and nonpigmented skin

DISADVANTAGES
- Scar and areolar widening occur frequently.
- Breast projection can be flattened.
- Purse-string closure results in skin pleating that takes several months to resolve.

> **SENIOR AUTHOR TIP:**   If periareolar purse-string suture remains palpable, it can be removed in a simple office-based procedure after 6 weeks.

VERTICAL SCAR TECHNIQUES

GENERAL
- Vertical mastopexy techniques are variations of vertical reduction mammaplasty techniques.
- Incisions are closed around the areola and inferiorly toward the inframammary fold.
- Techniques rely on parenchymal support inferiorly to narrow and cone the breast.

PATIENT SELECTION
- Techniques can be applied to patients with all degrees of ptosis.

TECHNIQUES
- **Vertical mastopexy without undermining (Lassus)**[13] (Fig. 53-3)
  - Skin incised (see Fig. 53-4, *A*)
  - The inferior, ptotic skin; fat; and gland are resected en bloc, and the nipple is transposed superiorly without undermining.
  - Medial and lateral breast pillars are closed.

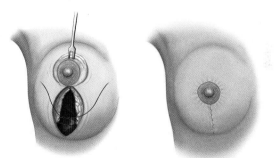

Fig. 53-3   Vertical mastopexy without undermining. Inferior skin, fat, and gland are resected en bloc. The nipple is transposed to the desired position. The medial and lateral breast pillars are closed vertically.

- **Vertical mastopexy with undermining and liposuction (Lejour)**[14]
  - Skin incision (see Fig. 53-4, *B*)
  - Liposuction is performed in larger breasts to reduce parenchymal volume and facilitate mobilization of the superior dermal-parenchymal pedicle.

▶ Inferior skin, fat, and gland are resected.
▶ Wide undermining is performed, and medial and lateral breast pillars are closed inferiorly.
▶ Skin is closed in a single vertical line with redundant skin left as fine wrinkles between the inferior sutures.
- **Short-scar periareolar inferior pedicle reduction mammaplasty (Hammond)**[15]
  ▶ Skin incision (see Fig. 53-4, C)
  ▶ NAC is transposed to desired location based on an inferior pedicle.
  ▶ Nipple is transposed and supported with parenchymal suspension sutures.
  ▶ Inferior skin is tailor-tacked to create the desired contour and closed in a vertical pattern.

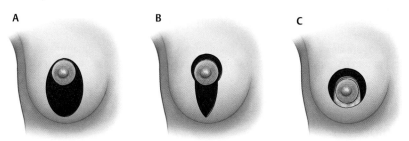

Fig. 53-4   Vertical scar mastopexy techniques. **A,** Lassus. **B,** Lejour. **C,** Hammond.

- **Medial pedicle vertical mammplasty (Hall-Findlay)**[16]
  ▶ Medial pedicle is designed, carrying the NAC.
  ▶ Lateral and inferior tissue is removed or repositioned superiorly.
  ▶ Nipple is transposed to desired position.
  ▶ Breast pillars are closed inferiorly to provide parenchymal support.
  ▶ Skin is closed in vertical fashion.
  ▶ Redundant skin is gathered along vertical closure.

MODIFICATIONS
■ **Inferior chest wall–based flap**[17]
  - Vertical mastopexy technique is performed, but inferior dermoglandular flap is tunneled superiorly **under a sling of pectoralis major muscle** to secure it in place.
  - Designed to restore upper pole fullness and increase breast projection

ADVANTAGES
■ Limited vertical scar without horizontal inframammary fold incision
■ Parenchymal closure inferiorly provides additional support to limit recurrent ptosis.

DISADVANTAGES
■ Immediate postoperative result frequently displays pronounced upper pole fullness that settles over time.
■ Skin redundancy inferiorly will occasionally not retract, requiring horizontal excision at a later date.

> **TIP:** In an attempt to limit the redundancy in the inferior pole skin, the vertical closure can be brought obliquely laterally (creating an L-shape). This eliminates excessive inferior skin redundancy and still prevents a medial horizontal scar.

VERTICAL AND HORIZONTAL SCAR TECHNIQUES (INVERTED-T)

GENERAL
- Incisions are closed around the areola, vertically to the inframammary fold, and horizontally within the fold itself.

PATIENT SELECTION
- Employed for **severe ptosis**
- Should also be considered for mastopexy in patients with both **very poor skin quality** and **fatty parenchyma**

TECHNIQUES
- Most frequently a Wise-pattern skin incision technique is used because of the popularity of the Wise-pattern breast reduction technique.
- Other skin excision patterns exist (Fig. 53-5), which attempt to reduce the length of the horizontal scar.

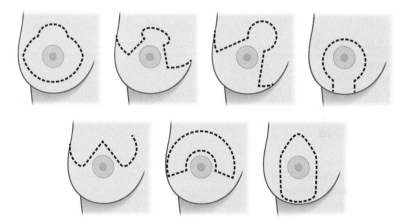

Fig. 53-5   Several skin incision patterns for inverted-T mastopexy techniques.

- Parenchymal resection is indicated in hypertrophic breasts.
- In most mastopexy patients, parenchymal support can be obtained with **inferior closure of medial and lateral breast pillars.**
- Inferior parenchyma can be repositioned superiorly to restore superior pole fullness or used to support the inferior pole of the breast.
  - Tunneled under a pectoralis sling[17]
  - Folded under a superior pedicle and secured to the pectoralis fascia[18]
  - Folded over to create a supportive sling for the lower pole[19]

> **TIP:** In traditional inverted-T mastopexy techniques, breast shape is maintained only by the skin envelope. Modern variations rely heavily on parenchymal support to lend longevity to the result.

ADVANTAGES
- Surgeon familiarity with technique because of widespread use in reduction techniques[20]
- Predictable results

DISADVANTAGES
- Scar burden
- Recurrent ptosis occurs frequently if parenchymal support not used

POSTOPERATIVE CARE
- If drains are placed, they are removed within the first 1-3 postoperative days.
- Postoperative pain is treated with oral analgesics.
- A supportive bra is required for 6 weeks postoperatively for full support during the healing process.
- Scar treatment begins 3 weeks postoperatively with the surgeon's preferred technique.
- If scar revisions are necessary, they are performed after 1 year.

COMPLICATIONS[2,6]
- **Hematoma**
  - Relatively infrequent
  - Patients should not take aspirin and antiplatelet medications for 10 days preoperatively.
  - Tight hematomas require urgent reoperation for evacuation, hemostasis, and closure.
- **Infection**
  - Also uncommon
  - Limited perioperative antibiotics are used routinely to reduce the risk of infection.[21]
- **Wound-healing problems**
  - Mostly present in inferior-T–designed procedures
  - More common among smokers. Mastopexy should not be performed on active smokers for this reason.
- **Nipple and breast asymmetry**
  - Patients should be counseled preoperatively that absolute breast symmetry will never be achieved.
  - Vast asymmetries in nipple position, areolar size, and breast shape require revision surgery.
- **Scar deformities**
  - Periareolar scar widening and medial horizontal inframammary fold scars are a source of frequent patient dissatisfaction.
  - Scar revisions can be performed 1 year after the initial surgery.
- **Recurrent ptosis**
  - Gravity and aging continue to affect the breast after mastopexy.

- Inferior parenchymal (not dermal) support is thought to decrease the likelihood of recurrent ptosis.
- Mastopexy is a temporary procedure, and long-term results usually reveal some recurrence of the deformity.[2]

SPECIAL CONSIDERATIONS

AUGMENTATION-MASTOPEXY (see Chapter 54)
- The loss of upper pole fullness with breast ptosis has led many surgeons to advocate placement of subglandular or subpectoral breast implants during mastopexy procedure.[2,6,12]
- Augmentation and mastopexy techniques work against each other.[22]
  - Mastopexy is designed to reposition the nipple, reshape the breast without tension to limit scarring, and reduce the size of the redundant skin envelope.
  - Augmentation increases the size of the skin evelope, increases the mass of the breast subjecting it to a greater force of gravity, and increases the tension of wound closure.
- Surgeons should consider **staging** augmentation and mastopexy in patients with moderate or severe ptosis.

MASTOPEXY AFTER EXPLANTATION
- Many patients with previously placed silicone gel implants now present for explantation for various reasons, including rupture, fear of rupture, and capsular contracture.
- Often these patients benefit from simultaneous breast contouring procedures during the capsulectomy and implant exchange.[23,24]
  - Preexplantation ptosis is rarely corrected without formal mastopexy.
  - Good candidates are nonsmokers, with mild to moderate ptosis, and adequate (>4 cm) soft tissue coverage over the implant.
  - In patients with sparse soft tissue coverage or severe ptosis, mastopexy should be staged 3 months following explantation.

TIP: Avoid mastopexy in all smokers.

- Choice of mastopexy technique depends on preoperative classification of ptosis (Table 53-1).

Table 53-1 *Breast Contouring Techniques by Ptosis Classification*

Ptosis Type	Characteristics	Technique
Pseudoptosis	Adequate volume Good nipple position Nipple-to-inframammary fold: 6 cm	Inframammary fold wedge excision
Grade I	Nipple repositioned <2 cm Areola: <50 mm diameter	Periareolar mastopexy Vertical mastopexy
Grade II	Nipple repositioned 2-4 cm	Wise-pattern mastopexy
Grade III	Nipple repositioned >4 cm <4 cm breast thickness	Delayed mastopexy (3 months, smoker)

TUBEROUS BREAST DEFORMITY[25]
- **Definition**
  - A spectrum of deformity with variable severity[26]
  - Deficient breast development in vertical and horizontal dimensions
    - ▶ Constricted (narrowed) breast base
    - ▶ High inframammary fold
    - ▶ Breast parenchyma herniation into the areola resulting in disproportionately large areola
- These patients often present in consultation desiring mastopexy or augmentation.

> **SENIOR AUTHOR TIP:** Distinguishing these patients is essential. They are often unaware of their anatomic abnormalities, and typical mastopexy techniques are not adequate.

- **Treatment goals**[27]
  - Expand breast circumference.
  - Expand skin envelope in the lower pole.
  - Release constriction at the breast-areolar junction.
  - Lower the inframammary fold.
  - Increase breast volume (when appropriate).
  - Reduce areolar size and correct herniation.
  - Correct nipple location and breast ptosis.
- **Treatment options**[26]
  - **Periareolar mastopexy** techniques can be used to reduce the areolar size and reposition the NAC on the breast mound.
  - The breast parenchyma usually requires modification with **inferior pole radial scoring,** mobilization, or division.
  - Augmentation with permanent implants or expandable permanent implants is usually required to restore parenchymal volume.

OUTCOMES[28]

- **Long-term nipple position**
  - Ahmad and Lista[29] reviewed 1700 vertical scar procedures and evaluated measurements over time to determine position of the NAC.
    - ▶ Compared with preoperative markings, the NAC was 1.3 cm higher on postoperative day 5 and 1 cm higher at 4 years.
    - ▶ Distance from the IMF to the inferior border of the NAC did not lengthen over time, and pseudoptosis did not occur.
  - Swanson[28] reviewed 82 publications on mastopexy and reduction and various assessments on measurements such as breast projection, upper pole projection, nipple level, and breast convexity.
    - ▶ Techniques reviewed included inverted-T (with superior/medial, central, and inferior pedicles), vertical, periareolar, inframammary, and lateral.
    - ▶ Breast projection and upper pole projection were not increased significantly by any of the mastopexy or reduction procedures.

► Nipple overelevation was common (41.9%), and teardrop areola deformity (53.8%) was significantly higher in patients with open nipple placement techniques.

► Methods to increase upper pole fullness or projection, such as fascial sutures and autoaugmentation, generally did not maintain shape in the long term.[30]

SURVEY COMPARISON OF VARIOUS TECHNIQUES

■ Based on a survey of board-certified plastic surgeons, **periareolar techniques** had the **highest rate of surgeon dissatisfaction**[31] and the **highest rate of revision.**

■ Although most popular, **the inverted-T group** reported a significantly greater frequency of bottoming out ($p = 0.043$) and **excess scarring along the inframammary fold** ($p = 0.001$), compared with the short-scar and periaroeolar groups.

> **SENIOR AUTHOR TIP:** Tissue expansion is necessary in patients with severe inferior pole skin deficiency with staged placement of a permanent breast prosthesis.

TOP TAKEAWAYS

➤ Classification of breast ptosis is determined by the nipple-areolar position relative to the inframammary fold.

➤ Modern mastopexy techniques rely on inferior parenchymal support to elevate the gland on the chest wall and limit recurrent ptosis.

➤ Mild ptosis can be corrected with periareolar techniques alone.

➤ Moderate and severe ptosis require vertical or vertical/horizontal skin excision.

➤ Mastopexy and augmentation procedures have contradicting properties and should be combined with caution.

➤ Identifying patients with tuberous breast deformities is essential, because specific techniques must be employed in treatment.

REFERENCES

1. Regnault P. Breast ptosis. Definition and treatment. Clin Plast Surg 3:193, 1976.
2. Bostwick J III. Mastopexy. In Bostwick J III, ed. Plastic and Reconstructive Breast Surgery, ed 2. New York: Thieme Publishers, 1999.
3. Weichman K, Doft M, Matarasso A. The impact of mastopexy on brassiere cup size. Plast Reconstr Surg 134:34e, 2014.
4. Nahabedian MY. Breast deformities and mastopexy. Plast Reconstr Surg 127:91e, 2011.
5. Ibrahim AM, Sinno HH, Izadpanah A, et al. Mastopexy for breast ptosis: utility outcomes of population preferences. Plast Surg (Oakv) 23:103, 2015.
6. Grotting JC, Chen SM. Control and precision in mastopexy. In Nahai F, ed. The Art of Aesthetic Surgery: Principles and Techniques. New York: Thieme Publishers, 2005.
7. Hidalgo DA, Spector JA. Mastopexy. Plast Reconstr Surg 132:642e, 2013.
8. Swanson E. Prospective photographic measurement study of 196 cases of breast augmentation, mastopexy, augmentation/mastopexy, and breast reduction. Plast Reconstr Surg 131:802e, 2013.

9. Benelli L. A new periareolar mammaplasty: the "round block" technique. Aesthetic Plast Surg 14:99, 1990.
10. Goes JC. Periareolar mammaplasty: double skin technique with application of polyglactin or mixed mesh. Plast Reconstr Surg 97:959, 1996.
11. Spear SL, Giese SY, Ducic I. Concentric mastopexy revisited. Plast Reconstr Surg 107:1294, 2001.
12. Kirwan L. Augmentation of the ptotic breast: simultaneous periareolar mastopexy/breast augmentation. Aesthet Surg J 19:34, 1999.
13. Lassus C. A 30-year experience with vertical mammaplasty. Plast Reconstr Surg 97:373, 1996.
14. Lejour M. Vertical mammaplasty and liposuction of the breast. Plast Reconstr Surg 94:100, 1994.
15. Hammond DC. Short scar periareolar inferior pedicle reduction (SPAIR) mammaplasty. Plast Reconstr Surg 103:890, 1999.
16. Hall-Findlay EJ. A simplified vertical reduction mammaplasty: shortening the learning curve. Plast Reconstr Surg 104:748, 1999.
17. Graf R, Biggs TM, Steely RL. Breast shape: a technique for better upper pole fullness. Aesthetic Plast Surg 24:348, 2000.
18. Flowers RS, Smith EM Jr. "Flip-flap" mastopexy. Aesthetic Plast Surg 22:425, 1998.
19. Svedman P. Correction of breast ptosis utilizing a "fold over" de-epithelialized lower thoracic fasciocutaneous flap. Aesthetic Plast Surg 15:43, 1991.
20. Rohrich RJ, Gosman AA, Brown SA, et al. Current preferences for breast reduction techniques: a survey of board-certified plastic surgeons in 2002. Plast Reconstr Surg 114:1724, 2004.
21. Platt R, Zucker JR, Zaleznik DF, et al. Perioperative antibiotic prophylaxis and wound infection following breast surgery. J Antimicrob Chemother 31(Suppl B):43, 1993.
22. Spear S. Augmentation/mastopexy: "Surgeon, beware." Plast Reconstr Surg 112:905, 2003.
23. Rohrich RJ, Beran SJ, Restifo RJ, et al. Aesthetic management of the breast following explantation: evaluation and mastopexy options. Plast Reconstr Surg 101:827, 1998.
24. Rubin JP, Toy J. Mastopexy and breast reduction in massive-weight-loss patients. In Nahai F, ed. The Art of Aesthetic Surgery: Principles and Techniques, ed 2. New York: Thieme Publishers, 2011.
25. Rees TD, Aston SJ. The tuberous breast. Clin Plast Surg 3:339, 1976.
26. von Heimburg HD, Exner K, Kruft S, et al. The tuberous breast deformity: classification and treatment. Br J Plast Surg 49:339, 1996.
27. Versaci AD, Rozzelle AA. Treatment of tuberous breasts utilizing tissue expansion. Aesthetic Plast Surg 15:307, 1991.
28. Swanson E. A retrospective photometric study of 82 published reports of mastopexy and breast reduction. Plast Reconstr Surg 128:1282, 2011.
29. Ahmad J, Lista F. Vertical scar reduction mammaplasty: the fate of nipple-areola complex position and inferior pole length. Plast Reconstr Surg 121:1084, 2008.
30. Jones GE. Mastopexy. In Jones GE, ed. Bostwick's Plastic & Reconstructive Breast Surgery, ed 3. New York: Thieme Publishers, 2010.
31. Rohrich RJ, Gosman AA, Brown SA, et al. Mastopexy preferences: a survey of board-certified plastic surgeons. Plast Reconstr Surg 118:1631, 2006.

54. Augmentation-Mastopexy

Purushottam A. Nagarkar

GENERAL PRINCIPLES

- Augmentation-mastopexy is a technique used to simultaneously correct low volume and skin excess.
- **Augmentation** alone corrects relative **deficiency of volume.**
- **Mastopexy** alone corrects relative **excess of skin.**
- If volume deficiency and skin excess are significant enough that either procedure alone will result in a persistent relative mismatch, combined procedure is needed.
- **The revision rate is high (8%-20%).**[1-3]
- Gonzales-Ulloa[4] described the technique in 1960, followed by Regnault[5] in 1966.
- Surgical planning depends on relative locations of nipple and inframammary fold (IMF) (i.e., ptosis). Regnault described three categories[6,7] (Fig. 54-1):

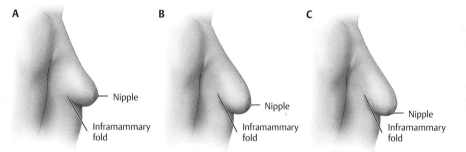

Fig. 54-1   Regnault classification of breast ptosis. **A,** Grade I. **B,** Grade II. **C,** Grade III.

- **Grade I:** Nipple at IMF
- **Grade II:** Nipple below IMF
- **Grade III:** Nipple at the lowest point on breast
- **Pseudoptosis:** Nipple at or above IMF but breast parenchyma below IMF[8] (Fig. 54-2, A)
- **Glandular ptosis:** Excess gland in the lower pole of the breast[8] (Fig. 54-2, B)

A
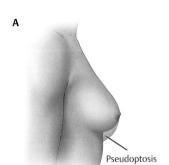

B
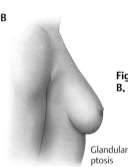

Fig. 54-2 A, Pseudoptosis. **B,** Glandular ptosis.

Pseudoptosis

Glandular ptosis

ALTERNATIVES

AUGMENTATION ALONE
- Use if skin excess is minimal: i.e., minimal gland below IMF, minimal ptosis, AND
- Augmentation alone can provide appropriate projection and adequately correct ptosis by decreasing *relative* skin excess.

MASTOPEXY ALONE
- Use if volume deficiency is minimal, AND
- Skin resection alone will appropriately raise the nipple position and adequately correct projection by decreasing *relative* volume deficiency.

INDICATIONS
- Ptosis (skin excess) combined with significant volume deficiency
- Periareolar mastopexy with augmentation requires[9]:
  - Nipple no more than 2 cm below the fold
  - Nipple-areola complex (NAC) at or above breast border, not pointing inferiorly
  - No more than 3-4 cm of associated breast ptosis
- More significant ptosis will require a vertical or Wise-pattern mastopexy.

SINGLE-STAGE VERSUS TWO-STAGE PROCEDURE[10]

SINGLE-STAGE PROCEDURE
- Thought to be unpredictable, with higher revision rate than that of both procedures combined[11]
- **One of the most common causes for malpractice claims**[12]
- **Contraindications**[13,14]**:**
  - Constricted breast or skin deficiency
  - Unclear whether both procedures will be necessary
    - For example, no mastopexy required if patient has[13]:
      - No ptosis and no pseudoptosis (<2 cm of breast parenchyma below the IMF)
      - Alternatively, per Lee, Unger, and Adams,[15] skin stretch <4 cm and nipple-to-IMF (N-IMF) distance <10 cm

- Significant asymmetry that is going to require an asymmetrical mastopexy for correction
- Significant vertical skin excess that will require a large skin resection

TWO-STAGE PROCEDURE

- Per Lee, Unger, and Adams,[15] **vertical excess >6 cm** is indication for staging procedure.
  - If primary goal is ptosis correction, perform mastopexy first, and stage augmentation.
  - If primary goal is improved projection or upper pole fullness, place implant first, and stage the mastopexy.

OUTCOMES (see Tables 54-1 and 54-2)

- Multiple large series have shown ~8%-20% reoperation rate for one-stage procedures.[1-3]
- Using his algorithm to select patients for two-stage procedures, Adams achieved:
  - ▶ 6.5% reoperation rate for one-stage procedures
  - ▶ 7% reoperation rate for two-stage procedures

PREOPERATIVE EVALUATION

- Mammogram within the last year for selected patients: AMA and ACOG[16] guidelines
  - Age over 40 years, or
  - Age over 35 years with high risk for breast cancer, or
  - Personal history of breast cancer
- Detailed breast history, including previous breast surgery
- Understand goals. Does the patient want
  - Greater volume?
  - Greater projection?
  - A "lift" (i.e., nipple and glandular elevation)?
- **Set expectation that asymmetry is common at baseline;** therefore it is common at endpoint as well.
- Set expectation of reoperation rate of up to 20%.

SURGICAL PLANNING AND TREATMENT

- Measurements (tissue-based planning)[15,17]
  - Pinch thickness in the superior pole of the breast: Results useful for choosing implant.
  - Skin stretch (SS): Nipple excursion on light traction; provides information on laxity in the anteroposterior dimension[15] (Fig. 54-3, A and B)
  - Nipple-to-IMF (N-IMF) distance on maximal stretch: Laxity in vertical dimension[15] (Fig. 54-3, C).
  - Vertical excess (VE): Anticipated excess skin/parenchyma to be resected
  - Base diameter (BD): Used to choose implant and define ideal N-IMF
- **Determine whether procedure needs to be staged**[15] (Fig. 54-4).
- **Choose appropriate implant material, shape, volume, location, approach.**
  - Material: Silicone versus saline; usually based on preference of patient and surgeon
  - Tissue-based planning to guide choice of implant volume and tissue plane
    - ▶ Higher risk of complications with subglandular implants in general
    - ▶ Risk increased when combined with mastopexy because of increased dissection, soft tissue disruption

- Incision: Depends on choice of mastopexy incision
  - ▶ Inferior periareolar incision
  - ▶ IMF incision for vertical or Wise-pattern mastopexy

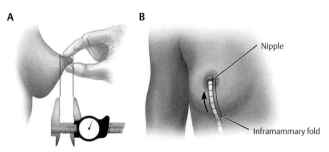

Fig. 54-3   A, Skin stretch. **B,** Nipple-to-IMF stretch.

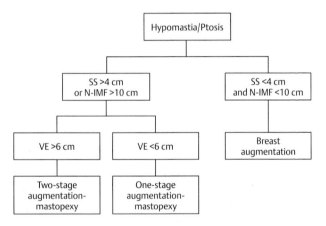

Fig. 54-4   Algorithm for selecting mastopexy, one-stage augmentation-mastopexy, or two-stage mastopexy. (*N-IMF,* Nipple-to-IMF distance; *SS,* skin stretch; *VE,* vertical excess.)

- ▪ **Choose mastopexy incision**[9,18]
  - Periareolar for patients with:
    - ▶ Minimal ptosis: Nipple <2 cm below IMF, AND
    - ▶ NAC at or above breast border, not pointing inferiorly, AND
    - ▶ No more than 3-4 cm of associated breast ptosis
  - Vertical for patients with:
    - ▶ Nipple >2 cm below IMF, AND
    - ▶ Horizontal skin excess
    - ▶ Minimal vertical skin excess
  - Wise pattern for patients with:
    - ▶ Nipple >2 cm below IMF
    - ▶ Both vertical and horizontal skin excess

- **Intraoperative details**
  - Markings
    - ▶ Details vary based on choice of mastopexy incision (see Chapter 53)
    - ▶ Midline, IMF, breast meridian
  - Place implant first, then perform mastopexy.
    - ▶ Determine whether augmentation provides adequate ptosis correction.
    - ▶ Tailor-tacking helps to determine final skin excision and prevents skin from being short.[19]

POSTOPERATIVE CARE

- Consider covering incisions with semipermeable dressing (e.g., Tegaderm) or skin adhesive (e.g., Dermabond).
- Surgical brassiere is worn while upright to provide support and off-load incisions.
- No stress should be placed on internal and external incisions for 6 weeks to allow healing.

OUTCOMES AND COMPLICATIONS[1,3,15] (Tables 54-1 and 54-2)

Table 54-1 *Complication Rates for One-Stage Augmentation-Mastopexy*

Complication	Rate for Stevens et al[1] (321 patients) (%)	Rate for Calobrace et al[3] (235 primary augmentation-mastopexy patients) (%)
Reoperation	14.6	20
Tissue related	3.7	11.5
Implant related	10.9	8.5
Implant rupture	3.7	0.4
Unattractive scarring	2.5	2.1
Recurrent ptosis or bottoming out	2.2	3.0
Nipple malposition or asymmetry	2.2	3.0
Capsular contracture	1.9	3.8
Breast asymmetry	1.6	2.1
Infection	1.3	0.4
Loss of nipple sensation	1.2	NA
Nipple loss or depigmentation	0.6	2.6
Implant malposition	0.3	0.4
Hematoma	0.6	1.3
Seroma	NA	0.4

Table 54-2 *Comparison of Complication Rates*

Procedure	Number	Complication Rate (%)	Reoperation Rate (%)
One-stage augmentation-mastopexy	91	10	6.5
Two-stage augmentation-mastopexy	14	7	7
Mastopexy alone	71	14	1.4

TOP TAKEAWAYS
➤ The goal of augmentation-mastopexy is to correct ptosis while increasing volume.
➤ This can be a difficult and unpredictable technique, because two opposing breast characteristics and forces are treated simultaneously.
➤ Augmentation-mastopexy requires excellent patient selection and meticulous technique.
➤ Generally, if performing a single-stage procedure, place the implant first and then reassess to prevent being skin-short.

REFERENCES

1. Stevens WG, Freeman ME, Stoker DA, et al. One-stage mastopexy with breast augmentation: a review of 321 patients. Plast Reconstr Surg 120:1674, 2007.
2. Spear SL, Boehmler JH IV, Clemens MW. Augmentation/mastopexy: a 3-year review of a single surgeon's practice. Plast Reconstr Surg 118(7 Suppl):S136, 2006.
3. Calobrace MB, Herdt DR, Cothron KJ. Simultaneous augmentation/mastopexy: a retrospective 5-year review of 332 consecutive cases. Plast Reconstr Surg 131:145, 2013.
4. Gonzales-Ulloa M. Correction of hypotrophy of the breast by exogenous material. Plast Reconstr Surg Transplant Bull 25:15, 1960.
5. Regnault P. The hypoplastic and ptotic breast: a combined operation with prosthetic augmentation. Plast Reconstr Surg 37:31, 1966.
6. Regnault P. Breast ptosis: definition and treatment. Clin Plast Surg 3:193, 1976.
7. Kirwan L. Augmentation of the ptotic breast: simultaneous periareolar mastopexy/breast augmentation. Aesthet Surg J 19:34, 1999.
8. Hall-Findlay EJ, ed. Aesthetic Breast Surgery: Concepts & Techniques. New York: Thieme Publishers, 2011.
9. Davison SP, Spear SL. Simultaneous breast augmentation with periareolar mastopexy. Semin Plast Surg 18:189, 2004.
10. Nahai F, ed. The Art of Aesthetic Surgery: Principles & Techniques, ed 2. New York: Thieme Publishers, 2011.
11. Spear SL. Augmentation/mastopexy: "surgeon, beware." Plast Reconstr Surg 118(7 Suppl):S133, 2006.
12. Gorney M. Ten years' experience in aesthetic surgery malpractice claims. Aesthet Surg J 21:569, 2001.
13. Spear SL, Giese SY. Simultaneous breast augmentation and mastopexy. Aesthet Surg J 20:155, 2000.
14. Spear SL, Dayan JH, Clemens MW. Augmentation mastopexy. Clin Plast Surg 36:105, 2009.
15. Lee MR, Unger JG, Adams WP Jr. The tissue-based triad: a process approach to augmentation mastopexy. Plast Reconstr Surg 245:215, 2014.
16. American College of Obstetricians-Gynecologists. Practice bulletin no. 122: breast cancer screening. Obstet Gynecol 118(2 Pt 1):372, 2011.
17. Tebbetts JB, Adams WP. Five critical decisions in breast augmentation using five measurements in 5 minutes: the high five decision support process. Plast Reconstr Surg 116:2005, 2005.
18. Kirwan L. A classification and algorithm for treatment of breast ptosis. Aesthet Surg J 22:355, 2002.
19. Jones GE, ed. Bostwick's Plastic and Reconstructive Breast Surgery, ed 3. New York: Thieme Publishers, 2010.

55. Breast Reduction

Joshua Lemmon, Michael R. Lee, Daniel O. Beck, Elizabeth Hall-Findlay

PATHOPHYSIOLOGY

- Breast hypertrophy is thought to be an abnormal end-organ response to circulating estrogens.[1,2]
- Normal number of estrogen receptors and normal levels of circulating estrogens have been found in women with hypermastia; thus an increased *sensitivity* to the hormone is suspected.[3]
- Hypermastia typically begins within the hormonal milieu of puberty or pregnancy.
- With the increasing obesity epidemic, breast hypertrophy is often from **excess adipose tissue** rather than glandular hyperplasia.
- Studies suggest that fat accounts for **46%-61%** of modern breast reduction specimens.[4,5]

INDICATIONS FOR SURGERY

Breast reduction has an **extremely high patient satisfaction rate** and has been shown to **improve self-image.**[6,7]

MEDICAL INDICATIONS

- Neck pain
- Back pain
- Shoulder pain
- Bra strap grooving
- Persistent or recurrent intertriginous infections, rashes, maceration, and irritation
- Chronic headaches
- In extreme cases, degenerative arthritis of the cervical and thoracic spine

EVIDENCE

- **Netscher et al**[8]
  - Symptomatic hypermastia is better defined by symptom complex than by volume of tissue removed.
- **Kerrigan et al**[9,10]
  - Symptomatic hypermastia affects quality of life on par with other significant chronic medical conditions (e.g., kidney transplant, living with moderate angina pectoris).
  - Symptoms are more important than volume in determining health burden and surgical benefit.
  - Weight loss, special bras, and medical treatments are not successful.

AESTHETIC INDICATIONS
- Women with hypermastia frequently report aesthetic dissatisfaction with breast size and shape.
- Complaints include pendulous appearance and wide nipple-areola complex.
- Excessive size may limit clothing selection and athletic participation.

> **TIP:** Determining the aesthetic or medical necessity of reduction mammaplasty is ambiguous and nonstandardized by health insurance carriers in the United States.

PREOPERATIVE EVALUATION
PATIENT HISTORY
- Age (>50 years of age with higher complication rate, according to Shermak et al[11])
- Medical history of comorbid disease(s), clotting disorders
- Surgical history pertaining to breast
- Social history of smoking or nicotine use
- Familial history of breast disease, anesthesia problems, deep vein thrombosis (DVT)
- Breast history of lactation, changes with pregnancy and weight fluctuations, tumors
- Previous medical or therapeutic treatment for hypermastia

PHYSICAL EXAMINATION
- **Sternal notch-to-nipple distance:** Allows detection of asymmetry in nipple position
- **Nipple-to-inframammary fold distance:** Serves as a measurement of the redundancy of the lower pole skin envelope
- **Base width:** Allows detection of asymmetrical breast footprint
- **Areolar diameter:** Widening of the areola is very common in patients with hypermastia (normal areolar diameter is 38-45 mm).
- Classification of **ptosis** severity (see Chapter 52)
- Breast examination for **mass** or **lymphadenopathy**

ADDITIONAL CONSIDERATIONS
- **Skin quality:** Presence of striae indicates the inelastic quality of affected skin.
- **Parenchymal quality:** Fatty, fibrous, or glandular parenchyma

MAMMOGRAM
- When indicated

PHOTOGRAPHY (see Chapter 3)
- Anteroposterior (AP), lateral, and oblique photographs should be obtained.
- Photographs of shoulder grooving and rashes, when present.

PATIENT EXPECTATIONS
- **Breast shape**
  - Reduction mammaplasty will not result in a virginal breast.
  - Most techniques will naturally result in a pendulous, mature-looking breast, but with a size more proportionate to the body habitus of the patient.
- **Breast size**
  - The desired postoperative breast size can vary widely between patients and should be dicussed at length at the initial consultation.

- Inform patients that complications with breast reduction are more common in larger reductions (>700 g) and in patients with a higher BMI.[12]

TIP: Although surgeons and patients frequently discuss bra-cup size, surgeons can better determine patients' wishes by asking them to find representative photographs of the desired postoperative size in magazines or professional portfolios.

INFORMED CONSENT

Recommend items to be included in the informed consent:
- A general description of the procedure and location of incisions
- A sufficient description of potential risks
  - Bleeding and hematoma
  - Infection
  - Delayed healing and wound separation
  - Nipple necrosis, complete or partial
  - Change in nipple and skin sensation
  - Potential changes in breast-feeding
  - DVT and pulmonary embolism (significant risk with BMI >30[13])
  - Asymmetry and poor cosmetic result
  - Poor lactation (70% of patients can lactate after surgery, but many require supplementary feeding.)[14,15,16]
  - Poor scar quality

SURGICAL OPTIONS

- Most techniques described in Chapter 53 were initially developed for breast reduction. Most patients with hypermastia also have breast ptosis. For detailed information on short-scar techniques, please see Chapter 53.
- Liposuction has been described as an additional or sole treatment for reduction mammaplasty.
- Reduction mammaplasty by excision can be thought to include the following four elements:
  1. Selecting a pedicle to provide vascularity and innervation to the nipple-areola complex (NAC)
  2. Determining the quadrants of the breast from which to resect tissue
  3. Excising excess skin after removal of breast parenchyma
  4. Creating an overall aesthetic breast shape.[17]

SUCTION LIPECTOMY

- Liposuction is often used in combination with excisional techniques to limit scar burden but can be used alone to reduce breast size.[18]

PATIENT SELECTION/INDICATIONS
- Ideal candidates:
  - Have a normally positioned NAC
  - Good skin quality
  - Predominantly fatty breasts.

■ A useful technique in **elderly patients** with significant symptoms of hypermastia and insignificant cosmetic concerns[19]

ADVANTAGES
■ Smaller scars
■ Preserves lactation and vascular supply to the NAC
■ Preserves existing sensation
■ Can be easily performed with local and intravenous sedation

DISADVANTAGES
■ Most surgeons agree that **breast ptosis cannot be adequately treated** with suction lipectomy alone and may be worsened in patients with poor skin quality.
■ Postoperative edema and induration often take months to resolve.
■ The evacuated breast tissue **cannot effectively be sent for pathological evaluation.**
   • Unexpected breast malignancy may go undetected.[20,21]
   • The absence of adequate pathological evaluation has brought controversy.[15,22-24]

TECHNIQUE
■ Lateral and medial inframammary fold (IMF) stab incisions are used.
■ Wetting solution is infiltrated.
■ 3-5 mm cannulas are used to treat both superficially and deep.
■ Postoperative compressive bras are worn for 6 weeks.

> **NOTE:**   Ultrasound-assisted liposuction has been used in the breast, but surgeons are advised to obtain exhaustive informed consents from their patients, discussing the unknown effects of ultrasonic energy on breast tissue.

EXCISIONAL TECHNIQUES

PEDICLE SELECTION
■ Options include inferior pedicle, superior/superomedial pedicle, and central mound technique.

Inferior Pedicle (Fig. 55-1)
■ Has been the preferred method (in the United States) and is easily teachable[25]
■ NAC maintained on an inferior dermal-parenchymal pedicle
■ Lateral, medial, and superior breast tissue can be removed.
■ Usually paired with an inverted-T skin excision
■ May use short-scar periareolar inferior pedicle (SPAIR) introduced by Hammond[26]
■ **Advantages**
   • Large parenchymal resections can be done safely.
   • Reliable neurovascular supply
   • Lactation preserved in most patients[14,15]
   • Low complication profile (11.4%)[27]

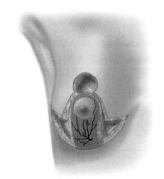

Fig. 55-1   Inferior pedicle technique.

- **Disadvantages**
  - When nipple to fold is >18 cm, the pedicle becomes bulky, limiting extent of reduction.
  - Passive creation of breast shape from tailoring skin around parenchyma
  - Often creates a boxy breast
  - High rate of bottoming out

Superior/Superomedial Pedicle (Fig. 55-2)

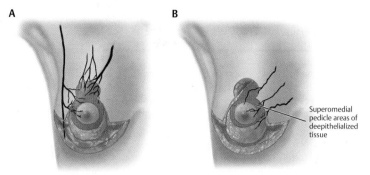

A   **B**

Superomedial pedicle areas of deepithelialized tissue

Fig. 55-2   **A,** Superior pedicle. **B,** Superomedial pedicle.

- Lassus[28,29] is credited with introduction of the superior pedicle technique.
- Lejour[22,30] is credited with refinements and popularization of the technique.
- Hall-Findlay[31] popularized the superomedial pedicle.
- Nahabedian and Mofid[32] and Lista and Ahmad[33] made contributions.
- Modifications include Strombeck horizontal bipedicle technique.[34]
- NAC is maintained on a superior or superomedial dermal-parenchymal pedicle.
- Lateral, medial, and inferior breast tissue can be removed.
- **Advantages**
  - Large parenchymal resections can be done safely, and involve resection of the ptotic tissue.
  - Pedicle is created from main blood supply of NAC.[35]
  - Pedicle is superior, where fullness is commonly desired.
  - Allows creation of inferior pillar support to limit bottoming out
  - Ease of use with short-scar techniques
  - Nipple-areolar sensation reliably maintained
- **Disadvantages**
  - Learning curve for technique
  - Creates dead space at dependent part of breast, where fluid may accumulate

Central Mound Technique (Fig. 55-3)

- NAC is maintained on a central parenchymal pedicle (without dermis).

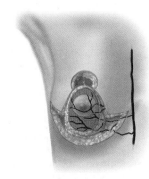

Fig. 55-3   Central pedicle/mound.

- Breast tissue can be excised laterally, medially, superiorly, and inferiorly, leaving a central glandular component.
- **Advantages**
  - Less reliable nipple-areolar neurovascular supply
  - Ideal to preserve lactation
  - Allows variable resection of parenchyma in multiple quadrants
- **Disadvantages**
  - Underresection is common.
  - Safety issues with undermining pedicle as blood supply comes from chest wall.
  - Breast shape/support largely dependent on dermal support
  - Possible bottoming out.

> **TIP:**   With all pedicle patterns, nipple viability should be checked before thinning the breast flaps. If the NAC is ischemic, the operation can be converted to a free nipple graft and the pedicle debrided to the appropriate level without compromising breast volume.

SKIN RESECTION PATTERNS
- Mastopexy procedures (or very small reductions) allow periareolar incisions and skin resection alone, but this is inappropriate for use in patients with true hypermastia.

Vertical Pattern (Fig. 55-4)

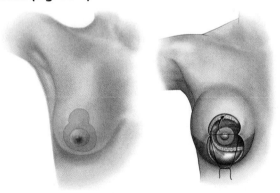

Fig. 55-4   Vertical pattern.

- Allows excision of lax skin in horizontal dimension
- With lateral (lazy-J) extension lax skin in the vertical dimension[36,37]
- Some authors advocate tailor-tacking to facilitate incision placement.
- Once desired shape and skin contour are obtained, the "tailored" resection pattern is marked and excised.
- Other techniques avoid a transverse scar by gathering the skin in the vertical closure, leaving a dog-ear in the inframammary fold (IMF).[31] This skin redundancy requires delayed excision in approximately **5%** of patients.
  - More recent evidence, however, cautions against the use of gathering sutures[38]
    - ▶ Significantly reduce the incision length in the operating room but do **not** change the areola-to-IMF distance or pucker revision rate.
    - ▶ Gathering negatively influences skin vascularity and wound healing.

SENIOR AUTHOR TIP: If the remaining dog-ear appears exceptionally large in the IMF, do not hesitate to excise it with a small horizontal excision. A small horizontal incisional scar is usually preferable to a revision procedure, even if done in the office.

Inverted-T (Wise) Pattern (Fig. 55-5)

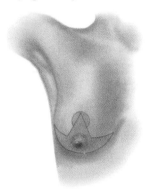

Fig. 55-5   Inverted-T pattern.

- Skin excision includes both a vertical and horizontal excision.
- **Horizontal excess** is removed through the **vertical incision.**
- **Vertical excess** is removed with the **horizontal excision** placed in the inframammary fold.
- Especially useful in large reductions with excessive amounts of skin redundancy
- Wound separation is fairly common at the intersection point in the IMF.

SURGICAL TECHNIQUES

INFERIOR PEDICLE WITH INVERTED-T SKIN RESECTION[39] (Fig. 55-6)

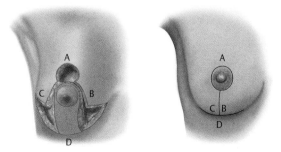

Fig. 55-6   Inferior pedicle with inverted-T skin resection.

Markings
- **Step 1:** Place patient in an upright position.
- **Step 2:** Mark the midline.
- **Step 3:** Mark the breast meridian to determine a new horizontal nipple position.
- **Step 4:** Mark the vertical nipple location (Pitanguy point) by transposition of IMF to front of breast.
- **Step 5:** Mark the IMF position, elevating mark a few millimeters onto the breast. This keeps the IMF scar on the breast and not on the chest, because the base of the breast is narrowed during reduction.
- **Step 6:** Measure bilaterally from notch to nipple and from midline to ensure symmetry.
- **Step 7:** Mark the vertical limbs, which should measure approximately 7-8 cm under tension.
  - Long limbs can always be shortened on the operating table; short limbs may result in closure under tension, which may compromise shape and skin viability.
  - The angle of divergence determines amount of skin resection.
- **Step 8:** Connect vertical limbs to the medial and lateral aspects of the IMF marking, following a lazy-S pattern.
- **Step 9:** Mark the pedicle approximately 10-12 cm from the midline.
- **Step 10:** Mark the areola at 42 mm; replace at 38 mm to minimize traction and distortion on the areola.
- **Step 11:** Mark all areas to be liposuctioned.

Technical Tips
- Develop the pedicle before raising skin flaps. To prevent undercutting, bevel away from pedicle.
- Place the patient in a sitting position and tailor-tack, as needed, to achieve desired shape.
- Hidalgo[40] reviewed the inverted-T pattern markings, along with modifications to improve aesthetic outcome.

SUPEROMEDIAL PEDICLE WITH INVERTED-T SKIN RESECTION[39] (Fig. 55-7)

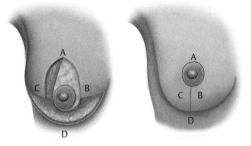

Fig. 55-7 Superomedial pedicle with inverted-T skin resection.

Markings

- **Step 1:** Place patient in an upright position.
- **Step 2:** Mark the midline.
- **Step 3:** Mark the upper breast border.
- **Step 4:** Mark the position of the IMF.
- **Step 5:** Confirm that the new nipple position is 8-10 cm below the upper breast border at the intersection of the breast meridian.
- **Step 6:** Mark the top of the areolar opening 2 cm above the new nipple position.
- **Step 7:** Extend areolar markings to create 4 cm diameter opening on closure.
- **Step 8:** Mark the vertical limbs by rotating the breast medially and laterally.
- **Step 9:** Join the vertical limbs at the meridian 2-4 cm above the IMF.
- **Step 10:** Design the pedicle with a 6-10 cm base; carry base slightly lateral to the meridian if a superomedial pedicle is desired.
- **Step 11:** Mark areas to be liposuctioned.

Technical Tips

- Creating a V pattern rather than a U when joining the vertical limbs above the IMF will prevent skin pucker on closure.
- After parenchyma is excised, approximate breast pillars, inset the NAC, and close the vertical incision in a gathering fashion, as needed.
- **Refer to Hall-Findlay[31,41] for an excellent review of this technique.**

> **TIP:** Symmetry in final breast shape and size is determined by what is left behind, not by what is removed.

BREAST REDUCTION IN ADOLESCENTS

Patients should generally have stable breast size for 12-24 months. Surgery is performed earlier only if patients have severe physical or psychological symptoms.

- **McMahan et al[42]**
  - Study included 48 women whose average age was 17.8 years at reduction.
  - 94% reported satisfaction (i.e., would recommend the surgery to a friend).
  - 60% complained of a prominent scar.
  - 35% reported changes in nipple sensation.
  - About 80% had relief of pain.
  - 72% had some regrowth of tissue; only one had reoperation for hypermastia.

SECONDARY BREAST REDUCTION

- Causes include recurrence and inadequate primary reduction.
- Revision must be tailored to the presenting deformity, cause of deformity, previous surgical technique, and patient expectations.
- Published evidence is controversial on using same pedicle.[43]

- Algorithm for the workup and treatment of recurrent mammary hypermastia[44] (Fig. 55-8)
    - Rule out malignancy as a possible cause.
    - With inadequate primary excision, surgical approach is dictated by the amount of tissue to be resected and knowledge of primary pedicle.

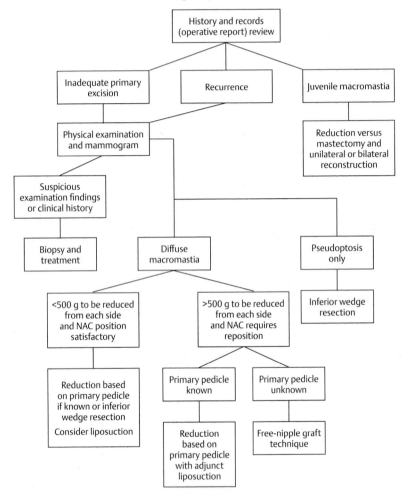

Fig. 55-8   Algorithm for workup and treatment of recurrent mammary hypermastia.

DATA DEMONSTRATED MIXED OUTCOMES FROM USE OF TRANSECTED PEDICLES

- **Hudson and Skoll**[45]
  - 2 patients had previous pedicle transected; both developed NAC compromise.
  - 1 of 5 developed healing complications when pedicle was not transected.
  - Authors recommended free-nipple graft if primary pedicle is unknown.
- **Losee et al**[46]
  - Two thirds of patients with transected pedicles had a complication that healed conservatively.
  - Authors concluded that it was safe to change pedicles.
- **Mistry et al**[43]
  - Breast re-reduction can be performed safely and predictably, even when the previous technique is not known.
  - Four key principles were developed:
    - ▶ (1) Nipple-areola complex can be elevated by deepithelialization rather than re-creating or developing a new pedicle.
    - ▶ (2) Breast tissue is removed where it is in excess, usually inferiorly and laterally.
    - ▶ (3) Resection complemented with liposuction to elevate the bottomed-out inframammary fold.
    - ▶ (4) Skin should not be excised horizontally below the inframammary fold.

REDUCTION OF IRRADIATED BREASTS

- **Spear et al**[47]
  - No complications in three cases
  - Waited 6 months between cessation of radiation and surgery
  - Minimized pedicle length and flap undermining
- **Parrett et al**[48]
  - 12 patients had bilateral reduction; mean 86 months after lumpectomy and radiation.
  - 42% complication rate in irradiated breasts
    - ▶ Seroma, fat necrosis, wound dehiscence, and cellulitis
  - 25% postoperative asymmetry
  - Four of 12 had secondary surgery: two for complications and two for asymmetry.

BREAST INFILTRATION

Infiltration with dilute epinephrine-containing solutions (e.g., liposuction wetting solution) reduces operative blood loss.

- **Wilmink et al**[49]
  - 41 reductions performed after injecting infiltration solution versus 29 performed without
  - Infiltration solution: 0.25% prilocaine + 1:800,000 epinephrine
  - 40 ml to each breast: 20 ml injected to retroglandular space + 20 ml injected along incision markings
  - Reduction patterns: Superomedial pedicle, inferior pedicle, or McKissock (bipedicle)
  - Average resection in each group approximately 1000 g

- Blood loss significantly reduced in epinephrine-treated group as measured by:
  - ► Total blood loss (ml)
  - ► Ratio of blood loss to tissue excised (g)
  - ► Postoperative drop in hematocrit/hemoglobin
  - ► Trend toward shorter hospital stay in treated group
  - ► No significance between groups in skin flap viability, postoperative drainage, or operation time
- **Samdal et al**[50]
  - 12 bilateral reductions performed with infiltration solution in one breast
  - No infiltration of contralateral breast
  - Infiltration solution: 1:1,000,000 epinephrine
  - 200 ml injected to retroglandular space + 40 ml injected along incision markings
  - Reduction patterns: Superomedial pedicle or inferior pedicle
  - Mean resection: 685 g (infiltrated breast) and 669 g (noninfiltrated breast)
  - Epinephrine use significantly reduced mean intraoperative blood loss to <50% of the untreated contralateral control.
  - Epinephrine use significantly reduced operative time.
  - There was no significant difference in skin flap viability or postoperative drainage.

TECHNICAL REFINEMENTS

The following are suggestions for improving postoperative breast shape and ultimate aesthetic result.

NIPPLE POSITION

- Appropriate postoperative nipple position is critical to the final result.
  - The nipple should be slightly lower in mature, fatty breasts.
  - The nipple should be slightly higher in young patients with firm, glandular breasts.

> **SENIOR AUTHOR TIP:** In superior pedicle vertical reductions, the nipple will move higher in the larger breast on closure of the pillars, *so mark the location slightly lower than on the larger side.*

- *The nipple should not be placed too high; this is a difficult problem to correct.*

INVERTED-T SKIN EXCISION

- As the superior keyhole angle widens, the skin margins at the inferior aspect of the T become increasing difficult to approximate.
  - This is especially true in patients with firm, glandular breasts, leading to wound-healing problems and scar widening.
    - ► Wide angles (>60 degrees) should therefore be avoided in these patients.
  - An excessively wide angle can also lead to postoperative flattening of the lower pole.[51]
- Short vertical limbs were encouraged in the past as a method to minimize inferior parenchymal descent, but relying on dermal support for long-term shape is now outdated.
  - Short limbs increase tension in the T region.
  - Vertical limbs should be kept **at least 7 cm** in length, and limbs of 8-10 cm may be necessary for safe closure in patients with firm, fibrous breast tissue.

> **TIP:** Some suggest leaving a small wedge of skin at a three-cornered closure of the inverted-T to reduce the final tension of closure (Fig. 55-9).

VERTICAL SKIN EXCISION

- A more difficult operation than the inverted-T because of the required tailoring
- Tension should be on **parenchymal pillars** and not on skin.
- Avoid horizontal bunching, because this can cause train-track scars.
- **Boxing sutures** can be useful to shorten the nipple-to-fold distance.
- If lazy-J extension is needed, make sure it curves up with the new breast fold.

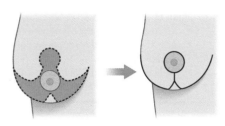

Fig. 55-9   A small wedge of skin at the site of closure limits tension at the final closure.

AXILLARY FULLNESS

- Hypertrophic breasts are typically wider than normal.
- Also exhibit a poorly defined lateral mammary fold
- The breast appears to extend upward and laterally into the axilla and the midaxillary line.
- Subcutaneous fat can be directly excised in this region and the overlying skin sutured.
- Liposuction can be used, but poor skin elasticity in this location limits its usefulness.

POSTOPERATIVE DRAINS

- Studies do **not** demonstrate lower complication or hematoma rates attributable to drain use.
  - **Wrye et al**[52]
    - ▶ 49 consecutive patients with inferior pedicle reductions
    - ▶ One drained and undrained breast, per patient, chosen by randomization
    - ▶ *No difference in complications or hematomas*
  - **Corion et al**[53]
    - ▶ 107 patients with superomedial pedicle reductions
    - ▶ Prospective randomization to receive drains or not after bilateral reduction
    - ▶ No statistical difference in hematoma rate complications
    - ▶ *Overall complication rate higher in patients with drains (40% versus 23%)*
  - **Matarasso et al**[54]
    - ▶ Purpose: To determine rate of complications in reduction mammaplasty performed without drains
    - ▶ 50 patients: 84% superomedial pedicle, 14% inferior pedicle, 2% amputation-style reduction
      - ◆ Average total resection 953 g
    - ▶ Six total complications in 3 of 50 patients
      - ◆ Fat necrosis (4%), wound disruption (4%), hematoma (2%), partial nipple loss (2%)
    - ▶ No cases of infection or total nipple loss

- ▶ No statistical difference in complication rate versus previously reported studies in patients with drains
- ▶ *Concluded that routine use of closed suction drainage after reduction mammaplasty is unnecessary*
- **Ngan et al**[55]
  - ▶ Retrospective review of reduction mammaplasty in 182 patients (333 breasts)
  - ▶ Age >50 years and resection weight >500 g associated with increased total drain output
  - ▶ Pedicle choice and BMI had no influence on drain output.
  - ▶ *Concluded that patients <50 years of age with reductions <500 g may not need postoperative drains*

OUTCOME STUDIES

- **Miller et al**[56]
  - 93% of patients reported decrease in symptoms.
  - 62% of patients reported increase in activity.
- **Dabbah et al**[57]
  - 97% of patients reported symptom improvement (59% had complete elimination of symptoms).
- **Davis et al**[6]
  - Patients reported 87% overall satisfaction rate.
  - Main sources of dissatisfaction were breast size, shape, and scars.

CANCER DETECTION

- Recommendations for preoperative mammography vary widely.
  - At a minimum, follow American Cancer Society guidelines.
  - Many surgeons recommend mammography for reduction patients >25 years of age.[58]
  - Send all specimens to a pathologist.
  - Incidence of cancer in reductions is reported at 0.06%-1.8%.
  - Obtain new baseline mammograms 1 year postoperatively.
  - Fat necrosis may trigger necrotic changes that are difficult to differentiate from breast carcinoma.
  - CT or MRI can be used when routine screening is unclear.

SPECIAL CONSIDERATIONS

FREE-NIPPLE GRAFTING

- **Relative indications**
  - Patients with severe hypermastia in which traditional pedicles will too greatly limit the ability of the surgeon to reduce the breast to the desired size
  - Patients with systemic illnesses that may impair vascular supply to the NAC (e.g., diabetes mellitus)
  - Patients requiring short anesthesia times

- **Procedure**
  - NAC is removed at the beginning of the procedure.
  - NAC is defatted like a skin graft.
  - The redundant skin and breast tissue is then excised and shaped into a new breast mound. (Inverted-T pattern skin resection is used almost exclusively.)
  - Often, autoaugmentation (i.e., inferior flap)[59] can be performed to improve volume or projection, because many of these patients have a flat upper pole.
  - NAC is grafted at the desired nipple position.
  - Bolster is placed over graft.
- **Disadvantages**
  - Complete loss of lactation potential can occur.
  - Sensory recovery is poor.
  - Patchy hypopigmentation occurs routinely.
  - Breast shape is rarely ideal.

> **NOTE:** This technique is included for completeness. It is not recommended for aesthetic surgery patients.

POSTOPERATIVE CARE

- Drains, when used, are usually removed within the first 1-3 postoperative days.
- Drains are not required for all breast reductions.
- Postoperative pain is treated with oral analgesics.
- Scar treatment begins 3 weeks postoperatively with the surgeon's preferred technique.
- Scar revisions, when necessary, are performed after 1 year.

COMPLICATIONS

VASCULAR COMPROMISE OF THE NIPPLE-AREOLA COMPLEX
- A devastating complication of breast reduction is loss of the NAC.
- Nipple-areolar compromise: Less than 1% of patients
- More common in patients with systemic illness, tobacco use, very large breasts, and patterns closed under excessive tension
- Although noninvasive monitoring options are available (laser Doppler flowmeter), clinical examination is the most commonly used method to assess intraoperative viability.

What to Do if the Nipple Turns Blue or Dies[60]
- During flap elevation or pedicle formation:
  1. Stop dissection.
  2. Ensure patient has adequate blood pressure (BP), urinary output, and temperature.
  3. Observe for 10-15 minutes for red bleeding from areola or pedicle borders.
  4. Consider conversion to free-nipple graft if clear venous congestion without resolution and fear of complete nipple compromise; be sure nonviable parenchyma underlying nipple is also resected.

- During closure:
    1. Open flaps and inspect.
    2. Evacuate hematoma if present.
    3. Check pedicle for kinking.
    4. Ensure patient has adequate BP, urinary output, and temperature.
    5. Resect more tissue to decrease pressure on pedicle with flap closure if needed.
    6. If nipple returns to normal color, close.
    7. Options are available if nipple is compromised with reclosure.
- Convert to free-nipple graft.
- Loosely approximate, allow 2-3 days for edema resolution, then attempt closure.
- Postoperatively:
    - If hematoma is obvious, release periareolar suture and return to operating room.
    - If no hematoma is obvious, release periareolar suture(s).
        - If nipple returns to pink, leave wound open and close when edema resolves.
        - If nipple remains blue, return to operating room and use previous algorithms.

CHANGES IN NIPPLE SENSIBILITY
- After reduction mammaplasty, the nipple-areolar sensibility may be lost, decreased, and even become more sensitive[51] (thought to be from relief of chronic neural traction).
- Altered nipple sensation: 9%-25% of patients
- Increased rates with increased amounts of resection
- Improved sensation in patients with gigantomastia; probably from reduced traction on nerves to NAC
- Larger resections are associated with greater loss of sensation[61-63] (up to 52% in very large reductions).
- Some studies indicate that areolar sensibility is better maintained with an inferior pedicle design, compared with medial[32] or superior[64] pedicles.

NOTE: Although studies are designed with highly sensitive measures of nipple sensation, patients often do not complain of decreased sensibility even when objective measurements show a decline in sensation. Clinically significant changes are probably less common than studies indicate.

OTHER COMPLICATIONS
- **Unsatisfactory scarring:** 4% of patients
- **Wound-healing complications:** Up to 19% of patients; more prevalent in larger reductions, especially if closed with excessive tension

BREAST-FEEDING
- **Aboudib et al**[65]
    - 91% of patients reported normal lactation postoperatively.
- **Sandsmark et al**[66]
    - 65% of patients could breast-feed.
    - Supplemental feeding was needed in all cases.

- **Brzozowski et al**[15]
  - 69% of patients could breast-feed.
  - 18% needed supplemental feeding.
- **Other complications**
  - Fat necrosis, hypertrophic scarring and scar widening, asymmetry, underresection or overresection, persistent pain, infection, change in breast shape over time, hematoma (incidence is not decreased with placement of drains; more common in patients with hypertension)

TOP TAKEAWAYS

➤ Excessive breast size in proportion to body habitus may result in unsatisfactory breast aesthetics and the medical and physical complications of hypermastia.

➤ Breast reduction has an **extremely high patient satisfaction rate** and has been shown to **improve self-image.**

➤ Determining the aesthetic or medical necessity of reduction mammaplasty is ambiguous and nonstandardized by health insurance carriers in the United States.

➤ Although noninvasive monitoring options are available (laser Doppler flowmeter), clinical examination is the most commonly used method to assess intraoperative viability.

REFERENCES

1. Pang S. Premature thelarche and premature adrenarche. Pediatr Ann 10:29, 1981.
2. Root AW, Shulman DI. Isosexual precocity: current concepts and recent advances. Fertil Steril 45:749, 1986.
3. Jabs AD, Frantz AG, Smith-Vaniz A, et al. Mammary hypertrophy is not associated with increased estrogen receptors. Plast Reconstr Surg 86:64, 1990.
4. Lejour M. Evaluation of fat in breast tissue removed by vertical mammaplasty. Plast Reconstr Surg 99:386, 1997.
5. Cruz-Korchin N, Korchin L, González-Keelan C, et al. Macromastia: how much of it is fat? Plast Reconstr Surg 109:64, 2002.
6. Davis GM, Ringler SL, Short K, et al. Reduction mammaplasty: long-term efficacy, morbidity, and patient satisfaction. Plast Reconstr Surg 96:1106, 1995.
7. Glatt BS, Sarwer DB, O'Hara DE, et al. A retrospective study of changes in physical symptoms and body image after reduction mammaplasty. Plast Reconstr Surg 103:76, 1999.
8. Netscher DT, Meade RA, Goodman CM, et al. Physical and psychosocial symptoms among 88 volunteer subjects compared with patients seeking plastic surgery procedures to the breast. Plast Reconstr Surg 105:2366, 2000.
9. Kerrigan CL, Collins ED, Striplin D, et al. The health burden of breast hypertrophy. Plast Reconstr Surg 108:1591, 2001.
10. Kerrigan CL, Collins ED, Kneeland TS, et al. Measuring health state preferences in women with breast hypertrophy. Plast Reconstr Surg 106:280, 2000.
11. Shermak MA, Chang D, Buretta K, et al. Increasing age impairs outcomes in breast reduction surgery. Plast Reconstr Surg 128:1182, 2011.

12. Nahai FR, Nahai F. MOC-PSSM CME article: breast reduction. Plast Reconstr Surg 121(1 Suppl):1, 2008.
13. Young VL, Watson ME. Patient safety: the need for venous thromboembolism (VTE) prophylaxis in plastic surgery. Aesthet Surg J 26:157, 2006.
14. Harris L, Morris SF, Freiberg A. Is breast feeding possible after reduction mammaplasty? Plast Reconstr Surg 89:836, 1992.
15. Brzozowski D, Niessen M, Evan HB, et al. Breast-feeding after inferior pedicle reduction mammaplasty. Plast Reconstr Surg 105:530, 2000.
16. Cruz-Korchin N, Korchin L. Breast-feeding after vertical mammaplasty with medial pedicle. Plast Reconstr Surg 114:890, 2004.
17. Hammond DC, Loffredo M. Breast reduction. Plast Reconstr Surg 129:829e, 2012.
18. Matarasso A. Suction mammaplasty: the use of suction lipectomy alone to reduce large breasts. Clin Plast Surg 29:433, 2002.
19. Lejour M. Reduction mammaplasty by suction alone [discussion]. Plast Reconstr Surg 92:1285, 1993.
20. Brown MH, Weinberg M, Chong N, et al. A cohort study of breast cancer risk in breast reduction patients. Plast Reconstr Surg 103:1674, 1999.
21. Colwell AS, Kukreja J, Breuing KH. Occult breast carcinoma in reduction mammaplasty specimens: 14-year experience. Plast Reconstr Surg 113:1984, 2004.
22. Lejour M. Vertical mammaplasty and liposuction of the breast. Plast Reconstr Surg 94:100,1994.
23. Goldwyn RM. Outcome study in liposuction breast reduction [discussion]. Plast Reconstr Surg 114:61, 2004.
24. Brauman D. Reduction mammaplasty by suction alone. Plast Reconstr Surg 94:1095, 1994.
25. Courtiss EH, Goldwyn RM. Reduction mammaplasty by the inferior pedicle technique: an alternative to free nipple and areolar grafting for severe macromastia or extreme ptosis. Plast Reconstr Surg 59:500,1977.
26. Hammond DC. Short scar periareolar inferior pedicle reduction (SPAIR) mammaplasty. Plast Reconstr Surg 103:890, 1999.
27. Mandrekas AD, Zambacos GJ, Anastasopoulos A, et al. Reduction mammaplasty with the inferior pedicle technique: early and late complications in 371 patients. Br J Plast Surg 49:442, 1996.
28. Lassus C. A technique for breast reduction. Int Surg 53:69, 1970.
29. Lassus C. Breast reduction: evolution of a technique—a single vertical scar. Aesthetic Plast Surg 11:107, 1987.
30. Lejour M. Vertical mammaplasty: early complications after 250 personal consecutive cases. Plast Reconstr Surg 104:764, 1999.
31. Hall-Findlay EJ. A simplified vertical reduction mammaplasty: shortening the learning curve. Plast Reconstr Surg 104:748, 1999.
32. Nahabedian MY, Mofid MM. Viability and sensation of the nipple-areolar complex after reduction mammaplasty. Ann Plast Surg 49:24, 2002.
33. Lista F, Ahmad J. Vertical scar reduction mammaplasty: a 15-year experience including review of 250 consecutive cases. Plast Reconstr Surg 117:2152, 2006.
34. Strombeck JO. Mammaplasty: report of a new technique based on the two pedicle procedure. Br J Plast Surg 13:79, 1960.
35. Michelle le Roux C, Kiil BJ, Pan WR, et al. Preserving the neurovascular supply in the Hall-Findlay superomedial pedicle breast reduction: an anatomical study. J Plast Reconstr Aesthet Surg 63:655, 2010.

36. Bozola AR. Breast reduction with short L scar. Plast Reconstr Surg 85:728, 1990.
37. Chiari Júnior A. The L short-scar mammaplasty: a new approach. Plast Reconstr Surg 90:233, 1992.
38. Matthews JLK, Oddone-Paolucci E, Lawson DM, Hall-Findlay EJ. Vertical scar breast reduction: does gathering the incision matter? Ann Plast Surg 77:25, 2016.
39. Jones G, ed. Bostwick's Plastic and Reconstructive Breast Surgery, ed 3. New York: Thieme Publishers, 2010.
40. Hidalgo DA. Improving safety and aesthetic results in inverted T scar breast reduction. Plast Reconstr Surg 103:874; discussion 887, 1999.
41. Hall-Findlay EJ, Shestak KC. Breast reduction. Plast Recontr Surg 136:531e, 2015.
42. McMahan JD, Wolfe JA, Cromer BA, et al. Lasting success in teenage reduction mammaplasty. Ann Plast Surg 35:227, 1995.
43. Mistry RM, MacLennan SE, Hall-Findlay EJ. Principles of breast re-reduction: a reappraisal. Plast Reconst Surg 139:1313, 2017.
44. Rohrich RJ, Thornton JF, Sorokin ES. Recurrent mammary hyperplasia: current concepts. Plast Reconstr Surg 111:387,2003.
45. Hudson DA, Skoll PJ. Repeat reduction mammaplasty. Plast Reconstr Surg 104:401, 1991.
46. Losee JE, Cladwell EH, Serletti JM. Secondary reduction mammaplasty: is using a different pedicle safe? Plast Reconstr Surg 106:1004, 2000.
47. Spear SL, Burke JB, Forman D, et al. Experience with reduction mammaplasty following breast conservation surgery and radiation therapy. Plast Reconstr Surg 102:1913, 1998.
48. Parrett BM, Schook C, Morris D. Breast reduction in the irradiated breast: evidence for the role of breast reduction at the time of lumpectomy. Breast J 16:498, 2010.
49. Wilmink H, Spauwen PH, Hartman EH, et al. Preoperative injection using a diluted anesthetic/adrenaline solution significantly reduces blood loss in reduction mammaplasty. Plast Reconstr Surg 102:1913, 1998.
50. Samdal F, Serra M, Skolleborg KC. The effects of infiltration with adrenaline on blood loss during reduction mammaplasty: an early survey. Scand J Plast Reconstr Hand Surg 26:211, 1992.
51. McKissock PK. Reduction mammaplasty with a vertical dermal flap. Plast Reconstr Surg 49:245, 1972.
52. Wrye SW, Banducci DR, Mackay D, et al. Routine drainage is not required in reduction mammaplasty. Plast Reconstr Surg 111:113, 2003.
53. Corion LU, Smeulders MJ, van Zuijlen PP, et al. Draining after breast reduction: a randomized controlled inter-patient study. J Plast Reconstr Aesthet Surg 62:865, 2009.
54. Matarasso A, Wallach SG, Rankin M. Reevaluating the need for routine drainage in reduction mammaplasty. Plast Reconstr Surg 102:1917, 1998.
55. Ngan PG, Iqbal HJ, Jayagopal S, et al. When to use drains in breast reduction surgery? Ann Plast Surg 63:135, 2009.
56. Miller AP, Zacher JB, Berggren RB, et al. Breast reduction for symptomatic macromastia: can objective predictors for operative success be identified? Plast Reconstr Surg 95:77, 1995.
57. Dabbah A, Lehman JA Jr, Parker MG, et al. Reduction mammaplasty: an outcome analysis. Ann Plast Surg 35:337, 1995.
58. Lemmon JA. Reduction mammaplasty and mastopexy. Sel Read Plast Surg 10(19), 2007.
59. Ribeiro L, Accorsi A, Buss A, et al. Creation and evolution of 30 years of the inferior pedicle in reduction mammaplasties. Plast Reconstr Surg 110:960, 2002.
60. Hall-Findlay EJ, ed. Aesthetic Breast Surgery: Concepts & Techniques. New York: Thieme Publishers, 2011.
61. Gonzalez F, Brown FE, Gold ME, et al. Preoperative and postoperative nipple-areola sensibility in patients undergoing reduction mammaplasty. Plast Reconstr Surg 92:809, 1993.

62. Makki AS, Ghanem AA. Long-term results and patient satisfaction with reduction mammaplasty. Ann Plast Surg 41:370, 1998.
63. Greuse M, Hamdi M, DeMey A. Breast sensitivity after vertical mammaplasty. Plast Reconstr Surg 107:970, 2001.
64. Hamdi M, Greuse M, DeMey A, et al. A prospective quantitative comparison of breast sensation after superior and inferior pedicle mammaplasty. Br J Plast Surg 54:39, 2001.
65. Aboudib JH Jr, de Castro CC, Coelho RS, et al. Analysis of late results in postpregnancy mammoplasty. Ann Plast Surg 26:111, 1991.
66. Sandsmark M, Amland PF, Abyholm F, et al. Reduction mammaplasty: a comparative study of the Orlando and Robbins methods in 292 patients. Scand J Plast Reconstr Hand Surg 26:203, 1992.

56. Gynecomastia

Ronald E. Hoxworth, Kuylhee Kim, Dennis C. Hammond

INDICATIONS AND CONTRAINDICATIONS

- Typically, **neonatal** and **pubertal cases** resolve with expectant management.[1]
  - Neonatal cases: Resolved within several weeks
  - Pubertal cases: 75% of cases resolved within 2 years without treatment[2]
- Drug-related cases can resolve with removal of the offending agent before the development of breast tissue fibrosis.
- Pathological causes necessitate formal medical evaluation with special attention to the associated comorbidities.
  - Patients with Klinefelter syndrome (karyotype 47, XXY) have a 50× higher incidence of male breast cancer. (The prevalence of Klinefelter syndrome in males with breast cancer is 7.5%.)[3,4]
- The presence of hypertrophic breast tissue for >12 months typically warrants surgical treatment because of fibrotic transformation.[5,6]

DEMOGRAPHICS

- Reported incidence: Up to 36% in general population[7]
- 65% of pubertal boys affected (up to 75% bilateral)[8]

ETIOLOGIC FACTORS

- Often **multifactorial,** involving *excess estrogens, decreased androgens,* and/or *androgen receptor defects.*

CLINICAL CLASSES
- **Idiopathic: Most common (25%)**
- **Physiologic**
  - Neonatal: Influence of maternal estrogens
  - Pubertal: Elevated estradiol/estrogen ratio
  - Senile: Peripheral conversion of testosterone to estrogen by aromatase
- **Pathological:** Cirrhosis, kidney failure, testicular/adrenocortical/pituitary tumors, hypogonadism, hyperthyroid, adrenal hyperplasia, and bronchogenic carcinoma
- **Pharmacologic:** Estrogens, gonadotropins, androgens, antiandrogens, chemotherapy agents, calcium channel blockers, ACE inhibitors, digitalis, CNS agents, antituberculosis medications, and drugs of abuse

HISTOLOGY[5]
- Represents the cellular changes seen with prolonged gynecomastia
- **Florid:** Symptoms <4 months; cellular stroma and ducts increased
- **Intermediate:** Symptoms present 4-12 months; mix of florid and fibrous patterns
- **Fibrous:** Gynecomastia present >1 year; minimal ducts but extensive stromal fibrosis

PREOPERATIVE EVALUATION

HISTORY
- Age of onset
- Duration
- Additional symptoms
- Current/recent medications
- Illicit drug use
- Past medical history
- Family history (breast cancer)

> **SENIOR AUTHOR TIP:**   Be certain to note whether or not the presence of the excess breast tissue causes pain. This can be an important symptom that may determine whether or not insurance coverage will be extended for treatment.

PHYSICAL EXAMINATION
- Breast: Fatty versus fibrosis, ptosis grade, masses, skin excess, unilateral versus bilateral, milky discharge (prolactin-secreting tumor)
- Testicular examination: Size, masses, firmness
  - Ultrasound examination for abnormal findings (i.e., masses)
- Organomegaly: Liver, thyroid, abdominal viscera
- Feminine features
- Absence of masculine attributes (i.e., hair pattern)

LABORATORY TESTS
- Beta-human TSH/free thyroxine, chorionic gonadotropin, follicle-stimulating hormone, luteinizing hormone, serum testosterone, and estradiol levels to correlate abnormal physical findings
- Consider liver function tests for hepatomegaly.
  - Endocrine consult and chromosomal analysis when indicated

IMAGING
- Breast imaging through mammography or ultrasonography: May be controversial, because gynecomastia is much more common than male breast cancer
- Mammography: When breast cancer is suspected.[9] Helpful for assessing the quality of breast tissue (fatty versus fibrous)

> **TIP:**   Completion of a testicular exam needs to be documented in the medical record. If there is any concern for potential scrotal mass or inconsistency in testicular exam, ultrasound imaging of the scrotum/testicles is indicated.

STAGING[10]
- **Grade I:** Minimal hypertrophy (<250 g) and no ptosis
- **Grade II:** Moderate hypertrophy (250-500 g) and no ptosis
- **Grade III:** Severe hypertrophy (>500 g) and grade I ptosis
- **Grade IV:** Severe hypertrophy (>500 g) and grade II or III ptosis

INFORMED CONSENT

- If surgery is indicated, the planned incisions and appearance are discussed.
  - Pictures/diagrams are used to reinforce the discussion.
- Both the general and the most relevant potential complications (see preceding section) are included.
- Asymmetry, contour irregularities, and the need for further procedures are discussed, especially when liposuction is used alone or staged excision is planned.

TECHNIQUE

NONOPERATIVE

- **Expectant management** is recommended for neonatal (weeks to months), pubertal (up to 2 years), and idiopathic cases.
- Offending agents (medications, drugs) are removed or changed if pharmacologic source suspected.
- Hormonal therapy is considered where appropriate.
  - Testosterone, antiestrogens (tamoxifen), and danazol show limited efficacy.
- For pathological causes, the underlying disease or source (i.e., testicular tumor; liver, pituitary, or thyroid disease) is treated.
- Gynecomastia present for >12 months typically will not spontaneously regress because of **dense fibrosis** and **hyalinization.**

OPERATIVE

> **SENIOR AUTHOR TIP:**   If at any time the condition begins to adversely affect the normal social development of the patient resulting in social withdrawal, avoidance of normal sports activities, or embarrassment in situations where the chest is exposed as in swimming, a low threshold for operative treatment should be instituted.

- Markings are made while patients are standing.
  - Boundaries for treatment are outlined.
  - A topographic technique is employed involving concentric circles extending outward from areola.
- The breast is palpated to identify parenchyma (fibrous) versus fat deposits.
- The IMF is identified and may need to be undermined and redraped after liposuction.
  - Zones of adherence along the periphery are noted and undermined and released as needed.
- The procedure is performed with the patient under general anesthesia or local anesthesia with IV sedation in the operating room or a licensed surgery center.
- A standard instrument tray is used for surgical excision and includes lighted breast retractors or a headlight.

> **TIP:**   Disruption of the IMF is a key technical consideration in redraping of the soft tissue for cosmesis. This is a distinguishing feature between female breast surgery where obliteration of the IMF would be considered technically improper.

SURGICAL EXCISION

- Still referred to as the mainstay of treatment for excessive and refractory cases (grades III and IV), although many think surgery has become less indicated
- **Skin-sparing:** Excess glandular tissue without skin excess
  - **Incisions:** Inferior areolar semicircle (preferred), transverse transareolar, radial/hemitransverse areolar (last resort)
  - Dense subareolar glandular tissue resected with any adipose tissue
  - Creation of "saucer deformity" with overresection prevented by **leaving small cuff of gland under areola**
- **Skin resection:** Skin and glandular removal both required
  - Reduction-pattern mammaplasty with dermal pedicle or mastectomy with free nipple grafts
  - Extensive resections may necessitate drainage.

> **TIP:**   While creation of a "saucer deformity" is considered technically incorrect, some overresection of the subareolar tissue is often performed in order to meet patient expectations for removal of "all" the symptomatic tissue.

> **SENIOR AUTHOR TIP:**   In cases of severe skin excess, a horizontal ellipse is the best pattern to use to resect the redundant skin. This avoids the vertical scar and places the surgical scar in the inframammary fold. The blood supply to the NAC is preserved via an inferior pedicle.

ULTRASOUND-ASSISTED LIPOSUCTION (UAL)

- The point is marked as described previously.
- General anesthesia or local with IV sedation is used.
- The patient is placed in a supine position with arms abducted.
- 3 to 4 mm stab incisions are made with a No. 11 blade scalpel along the lateral IMF for optimal access to all treatment areas. (Some authors advocate similar exposure through superior axillary and periareolar incisions.)
- An ultrasound generator (Mentor or Lysonix), a 5 mm blunt-tip titanium cannula or a 4 mm golf tee cannula, and a surgical aspirator are needed.
- Uniform, subcutaneous infiltration of wetting solution is performed using a 3.0 mm cannula and infiltration pump.
  - A "superwet" technique is used.
  - All injected volumes are recorded for comparison between sites.
- Ultrasound emulsification is performed with the generator at appropriate settings, and the cannula is used to create deliberate uniform strokes in a radial pattern, concentrating on the areas of interest based on the preoperative markings.
  - A Mentor generator is set at an energy level between 70% and 90%. 90% is most effective for dense fibrous tissue (subareolar).
  - A Lysonix generator is set at energy level between 5 and 7, and intensity is adjusted to tissue density and treatment response.
  - A bimanual technique is recommended to guide the cannula and to assess depth of treatment.
- The subareolar region requires more treatment because of the concentration of fibrous tissue.
- The IMF should be thoroughly obliterated to allow redraping of the overlying skin.

- The time for each treatment area is recorded.
  - Endpoints for treatment are **time** and **loss** of resistance.
- The emulsified fat is evacuated with a suction cannula.
  - Volumes from distinct areas are recorded for comparison between sides.
- Final contouring and feathering should be performed with a 3.7 mm cannula (or smaller based on surgeon preference).
  - Irregularities are smoothed, disrupting the IMF and avoiding adherence zones except for final contour issues.
  - Bimanual palpation can aid in this final step.
- Incisions are closed with fast-absorbable sutures.
- Dressings are applied.

SUCTION-ASSISTED LIPOSUCTION (SAL)
- SAL employs the same preparation and approach as outlined previously.
- After infiltration with "superwet" or "tumescent" technique, standard suction lipectomy is undertaken with a 2.7 to 5.2 mm cannula.
  - Treatment is initiated with small cannula to feather and break up fibrous tissue.
  - Larger cannulas are used for more dense and resistant tissue.
- A bimanual technique is necessary for SAL, because the nondominant hand is used to grasp and elevate the breast tissue being treated.
  - Endpoints are determined by **pinch test** and **contour assessment.**
  - A greater degree of resistance is noted with the treatment of the dense subareolar area.
- Radial patterns are again employed.
- Incisions are closed and dressed as with UAL.

COMBINED/STAGED APPROACH
- Some authors advocate a combination of both liposuction and excision based on the degree of fibrosis and clinical stage.[11,12]
- **Usually, the dense subareolar tissue is refractory to UAL or SAL,** and the remaining bud needs direct excision.
  - This is usually best seen after the liposuction portion.
  - It can be performed using a limited-incision "pull-through approach."[11]
- Some authors advocate delayed excision until final skin contraction after liposuction.
  - The delay may preclude the need for surgery or lessen the extent of resection if contraction is significant.

POSTOPERATIVE CARE
- If drains are placed after excision technique, the patient should be counseled regarding drain care and output recording.
  - Removed when output <25 cc/24 hours
- Dressings: External support with compression vest or tight "T-shirt" is needed at all times for first 4 weeks, then at night for next 2 weeks.
- Perioperative prophylactic antibiotics are given.
- Histopathologic evaluation: According to a literature review, the possibility of accrual breast cancer in adolescents with gynecomastia is 1% (maximum).[13] Some authors argue that routine histopathologic examination incurs negative productivity costs.[14] However, the prevalence of malignancies in gynecomastia specimens increases with

patient age.[15] Histologic evaluation is recommended for all patients with pathologic gynecomastia.

> **SENIOR AUTHOR TIP:**   Standard post-operative vests are often ill-fitting and uncomfortable. It is instead recommended that the patient purchase a snug-fitting athletic compression shirt before surgery and bring this garment with him to surgery. In this fashion, a properly fitted compression garment can be applied after surgery that the patient can wear comfortably, thus enhancing compliance.

COMPLICATIONS
- Complication and revision rates vary widely, depending on the techniques and author.
- Complications typically range from 10% to 25%[16,17] and include hematoma, seroma, underresection/overresection, scarring (hypertrophic scar, nipple retraction), areolar hypopigmentation, and cicatricial alopecia of chest hair.
- Revision rates vary from 0% to 42%, depending on the source and technique.
- The presence of skin excision, whether at the initial procedure or delayed, is associated with increased complication rates, from 14% to 40% in some studies.

OUTCOMES
- **Liposuction and excision**[18]
  - Comparison of liposuction only (16 patients) versus combination (liposuction and excision) therapy (48 patients)
  - Retrospective comparison of 64 patients
  - Improved outcomes and patient satisfaction for combined treatment group
  - *Recommended combination approach as the "standard of care"*
- **Excision**[19]
  - Management based on different body types
  - Patient expectations predicated on body types
  - All underwent subcutaneous mastectomy
  - *Increased patient satisfaction when body type/expectations addressed*
  - Complications: 312 cases; 6 seromas (2%), 3 hematomas (1%)
- **Excision**[6]
  - Overresection in 18.7% of cases
  - Poor scarring in 18.7% of cases
  - Hematomas in 16% of cases
  - Seromas in 9% of cases
  - Underresection in 22% of cases
- **UAL (Gingrass and Shermak)**[20]
  - No hematomas, skin necrosis, or other complications
  - Results uniformly good to excellent at 4-year follow-up
- **UAL**[10]
  - 61 patients
  - *Ultrasound-assisted liposuction (UAL) was more effective than suction-assisted liposuction (SAL) at treating the dense, fibrous tissue common in persistent (12 months) gynecomastia.*

- Overall, 87% of patients required only UAL.
- Staged skin excision was required by 33% of stage III and 57% of stage IV patients.
- Staged skin excision was performed 6-9 months after UAL to allow maximal skin retraction.
- **UAL with excision**[11]
  - No nipple-areola complex (NAC) necrosis, hematoma, or infection
  - One patient each with scar retraction, seroma, access port skin burn, epidermolysis, or decreased NAC sensation
  - All patients pleased with results
- **SAL with excision**[12]
  - Treated 20 patients who used anabolic steroids
  - Resulted in two hematomas, two seromas, three recurrences
- **Liposuction with tissue shaver**[21]
  - 76 patients of 226 treated with combination liposuction and tissue shaver for gynecomastia
  - Resulted in two seromas, one hematoma, one ultrasound burn, one skin buttonhole, four operations for recurrence
  - No significant difference in complication rate compared with patients undergoing single therapy (excision or liposuction)
  - *Objective conclusion of better patient satisfaction with liposuction plus shaver*

TOP TAKEAWAYS

➤ Approximately 75% of pubertal gynecomastia cases resolve without treatment. The presence of hypertrophic breast tissue for >12 months typically warrants surgical treatment because of fibrotic transformation.

➤ The cause of gynecomastia is unknown in around 25% of cases.

➤ Gynecomastia can be caused by medication and pathological conditions such as tumor and chronic disease. A thorough medical history should be obtained and an extensive physical examination performed.

➤ Various techniques such as direct excision, conventional liposuction, UAL, SAL, and a combination of excision and liposuction can be used for treatment of gynecomastia.

➤ Delayed skin excision after liposuction leaves a minimal scar and can preclude the need for extensive excision.

REFERENCES

1. Wise GJ, Roorda AK, Kalter R. Male breast disease. J Am Coll Surg 200:255, 2005.
2. Shulman DI, Francis GL, Palmert MR, et al; Lawson Wilkins Pediatric Endocrine Society Drug and Therapeutics Committee. Use of aromatase inhibitors in children and adolescents with disorders of growth and adolescent development. Pediatrics 121:e975, 2008.
3. Hultborn R, Hanson C, Köpf I, et al. Prevalence of Klinefelter's syndrome in male breast cancer patients. Anticancer Res 17:4293, 1997.
4. Brinton LA. Breast cancer risk among patients with Klinefelter syndrome. Acta Paediatr 100:814, 2011.
5. Banyan GA, Hajdu SI. Gynecomastia: clinicopathologic study of 351 cases. Am J Clin Pathol 57:431, 1972.

6. Courtiss EH. Gynecomastia: analysis of 159 patients and current recommendations for treatment. Plast Reconstr Surg 79:740, 1987.
7. Nuttall FQ. Gynecomastia as a physical finding in normal men. J Clin Endocrinol Metab 48:338, 1979.
8. Niewoehner CB, Nuttal FQ. Gynecomastia in a hospitalized male population. Am J Med 77:633,1984.
9. Mathew J, Perkins GH, Stephens T, et al. Primary breast cancer in men: clinical, imaging, and pathologic findings in 57 patients. AJR Am J Roentgenol 191:1631, 2008.
10. Rohrich RJ, Ha RY, Kenkel JM, et al. Classification and management of gynecomastia: defining the role of ultrasound-assisted liposuction. Plast Reconstr Surg 111:909, 2003.
11. Hammond DC, Arnold JF, Simon AM, et al. Combined use of ultrasonic liposuction with the pull-through technique for the treatment of gynecomastia. Plast Reconstr Surg 112:891, 2003.
12. Babigian A, Silverman RT. Management of gynecomastia due to anabolic steroids in bodybuilders. Plast Reconstr Surg 107:240, 2001.
13. Kwan D, Song DH. Discussion. Breast cancer incidence in adolescent males undergoing subcutaneous mastectomy for gynecomastia: is pathologic examination justified? A retrospective and literature review. Plast Reconstr Surg 127:8, 2011.
14. Senger JL, Chandran G, Kanthan R. Is routine pathological evaluation of tissue from gynecomastia necessary? A 15-year retrospective pathological and literature review. Can J Plast Surg 22:112, 2014.
15. Lapid O, Jolink F, Meijer SL. Pathological findings in gynecomastia: analysis of 5113 breasts. Ann Plast Surg 74:163, 2015.
16. Weisman IM, Lehman A Jr, Parker MG, et al. Gynecomastia: an outcome analysis. Ann Plast Surg 53:97, 2004.
17. Li CC, Fu JP, Chang SC, et al. Surgical treatment of gynecomastia: complications and outcomes. Ann Plast Surg 69:510, 2012.
18. Kim DH, Byun IH, Lee WJ, et al. Surgical management of gynecomastia: subcutaneous mastectomy and liposuction. Aesthetic Plast Surg 40:877, 2016.
19. Innocenti A, Melita D, Mori F, et al. Management of gynecomastia in patients with different body types: considerations on 312 consecutive treated cases. Ann Plast Surg 78:492, 2017.
20. Gingrass MK, Shermak MA. The treatment of gynecomastia with ultrasound-assisted lipoplasty. Semin Plast Surg 12:101, 1999.
21. Petty PM, Solomon M, Buchel EW, et al. Gynecomastia: evolving paradigm of management and comparison of techniques. Plast Reconstr Surg 125:1301, 2010.

PART IX

Body Contouring

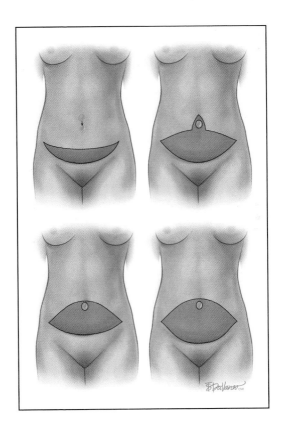

Part IX

Body Contouring

57. Liposuction

Cedric L. Hunter, Rohit K. Khosla, Jeffrey R. Claiborne, Simeon H. Wall, Jr.

- First recorded attempt at lipectomy is attributed to the French surgeon **Dujarier,** who, in the 1920s, attempted to remove fat from a dancer's calves using a uterine curette.[1]
  - Vascular damage resulted in amputation of the leg.
- In the mid-1970s **Giorgio Fischer** and his father, **Arpad Fischer,** developed the "cellusuctiotome," an instrument made of a hollow curette and blade attached to a suction pump. This method had a high rate of bleeding complications.
- **Yves-Gerard Illouz** and **Pierre Fournier** improved on the prior techniques by replacing the sharp curettes of the 1970s with a cannula and suction system, the introduction of a "wetting solution" containing saline solution and hyaluronidase, and the use of a "crisscross" technique.
  - These methods decreased bleeding and contour-associated complications.
- In the 1980s a dermatologist, **Jeffrey Klein,** introduced the tumescent technique.
  - *Tumescent technique*: Subcutaneous infiltration of a large volume of diluted lidocaine and epinephrine that expands the fat compartment causing it to become swollen and firm, or tumescent
  - Provides local anesthesia and reduces blood loss

ANATOMY

SUBCUTANEOUS LAYERS (Fig. 57-1)

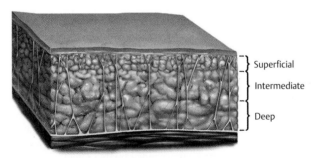

Superficial

Intermediate

Deep

Fig. 57-1 Differences in subcutaneous tissues in various areas of the body.

- Subcutaneous adipose tissue is divided into **superficial** and **deep** layers throughout the body by Scarpa fascia or the superficial fascial equivalent.[2]

- For purposes of body contouring, the subcutaneous fat is arbitrarily divided into **three layers.**[3]
  - **Superficial**
    - ▶ Dense fat, adherent to overlying skin
    - ▶ *Aggressive, avulsive, or thermal liposuction methods should be used with great caution in this layer to prevent contour irregularities and skin damage.*
  - **Intermediate**
    - ▶ **Safest** layer
    - ▶ Most commonly suctioned layer
  - **Deep**
    - ▶ Loose and less compact layer
    - ▶ Can be removed safely in most areas

ZONES OF ADHERENCE (Fig. 57-2)

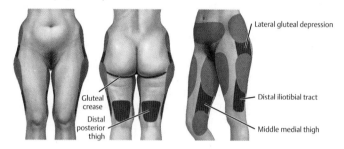

Fig. 57-2   Zones of adherence.

- Distal iliotibial tract
- Gluteal crease
- Lateral gluteal depression
- Middle medial thigh
- Distal posterior thigh

CAUTION: Be very cautious removing fat from zones of adherence. The stiff fibrous network predisposes these areas to postoperative contour deformities.

> **SENIOR AUTHOR TIP:**   The rigid fibrous connections at zones of adherence can be relaxed using an exploded tip cannula without suction (i.e., separation and equalization). The tissue will become more pliable to allow smooth transitions into surrounding areas and enable these zones to be traversed or treated safely.

CELLULITE (GYNOID LIPODYSTROPHY)

- *Peau d'orange* and mattresslike deformity seen primarily in women and obese patients
- **Two types**[4]
  - **Primary or cellulite of adiposity:** Results from *hypertrophic fat cells* in the superficial fat between the septa of the superficial fascial system

- ▶ Typically present when supine and erect, seen in younger women
- ▶ Generally not improved with skin-tightening procedures
- **Secondary or cellulite of laxity:** Results from *increased skin and superficial fascial system laxity*
  - ▶ Present when erect but not supine, usually >35 years of age
  - ▶ Treated with skin- and superficial fascial system–tightening procedures

PREOPERATIVE EVALUATION

PHYSICAL EXAMINATION
- ■ Check for deviation from ideal contour (Fig. 57-3).

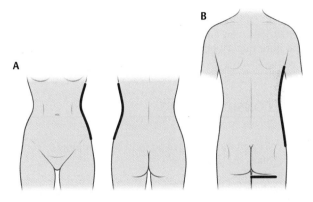

Fig. 57-3 Ideal contour. **A,** Female. **B,** Male.

- **Female ideal contour**
  - ▶ Concavity below the rib cage that changes to a convexity over the hips and thighs
  - ▶ Medial and lateral thighs have mild convexities.
  - ▶ The buttock crease blends laterally with thigh.
- **Male ideal contour**
  - ▶ More linear silhouette, less concavity and convexity below rib cage and over thighs
  - ▶ The buttock crease is squared and linear.
  - ▶ Flat anterior infraumbilical region
- Note any of the following:
  - ▶ Asymmetries
  - ▶ Dimpling/cellulite
  - ▶ Location of fat deposits
  - ▶ Areas of adherence
  - ▶ Hernias and myofascial diastasis
- Check skin **laxity.**
- Examine spine for **scoliosis.**
  - ▶ May cause **asymmetry**
- Assess for **hernias/diastasis.**

MEDICAL HISTORY

- Agents that interfere with coagulation should be avoided.
  - Aspirin
  - NSAIDs
  - St. John's wort
  - Vitamin E
  - Herbal supplements
  - Other anticoagulants
- Note personal and family history of deep venous thrombosis or clotting disorders.
- Photographs
  - Standard photographs of areas to be treated should be obtained.
  - See Chapter 3 for further details on photography.

> **SENIOR AUTHOR TIP:** Patient selection is critical. Common pitfalls include: redundant and poor quality skin, obesity with excess intraabdominal fat and unreasonable expectations.

PERIOPERATIVE CONSIDERATIONS

PREOPERATIVE

- Complete blood cell count if expecting to perform **large-volume** (>5 L total lipoaspirate) procedure
- Perioperative IV antibiotics
- Deep venous thrombosis prophylaxis
  - Intermittent pneumatic compression devices should be used intraoperatively.
  - Chemoprophylaxis may be given to those at higher risk (see Chapter 11).

HYPOTHERMIA

- Forced-air warming blankets
- Consider circulating warm water mattresses
- Cover exposed body areas.
- Warm intravenous fluids.
- Warm operating room.
- Warm wetting solutions.

POSITIONING

- Pad all pressure points.
- Prone position
  - Protect face, breasts, and genitals.
  - Soft hip roll beneath iliac crest
- Supine position
  - Arm abduction <90 degrees to prevent brachial plexus injury
  - Hips and knees flexed at 30 degrees with a pillow

SENIOR AUTHOR TIP: Using multiple patient positions allows for target areas to be treated thoroughly, without the distortion and compression from the operating table seen when using a single supine position, or even in supine/prone positioning. Three positions: Supine, lateral decubitus, and the opposite lateral decubitus allow for complete exposure of the body circumferentially while avoiding the more onerous and time-consuming prone position. As a caveat, if the operating surgeon is strongly one-handed, adding the prone position to the standard three position routine can help intraoperative assessment and prevent asymmetries. Additionally, multiple patient positions allow cross-hatching and help ensure complete treatment. It also reduces the risk of creating iatrogenic contour deformities.

MARKINGS (Fig. 57-4)
- Patients should be marked when they are in an upright position or standing.
- Use marker to outline areas to be treated.
- Mark zones of adherence and other areas to be avoided with parallel lines or cross-hatch marks.

INCISIONS
- Longer for ultrasound-assisted liposuction (UAL) compared with suction-assisted liposuction (SAL) (6-8 mm versus 2-3 mm, respectively).
- Incisions can be placed anywhere adjacent to areas being treated.
- Multiple incisions are used for access to target areas, and ideally they are strategically located to allow **crisscross suctioning.**
  - Liposuction from a single access incision may lead to contour deformity.
- **Locations** (Fig. 57-5; Box 57-1)

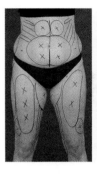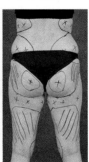

Fig. 57-4 Markings. Circled *Xs* are over zones of prominence, and lines are over zones of adherence.

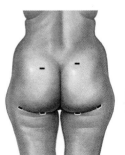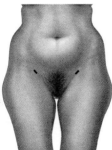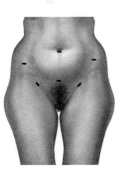

Fig. 57-5 Incisions for buttocks, medial thighs, and abdomen.

Box 57-1 *INCISION LOCATIONS FOR LIPOSUCTION*

- Breast (male): Anterior axillary fold and/or periareolar
- Lateral back: Lateral bra line
- Vertical back: Midline
- Flank/hip: Sacral, groin crease, midaxillary line in panty line
- Abdomen: Lateral lower abdomen/suprapubic/umbilical
- Buttock: Sacral, midaxillary line in panty line
- Lateral thigh: Midaxillary line in panty line
- Posterior thigh: Midaxillary line in panty line
- Medial thigh: Medial groin crease and inguinal crease
- Anterior thigh: Inguinal crease
- Upper arm: Anterior and posterior axillary folds, olecranon radial elbow crease

LIPOSUCTION CANNULAS[5]
- Most tips are **blunt** with multiple openings set back from the end to allow suctioning of fat with passage of the cannula.
  - Blunt tips limit risks of penetration of unwanted structures such as fascia, peritoneum, vessels, and nerves.
- Suction cannulas range from 1.8 mm up to 1 cm in diameter (typical use for liposuction is 2.5-5.0 mm) with varying cannula lengths.
  - **Larger** suction cannulas are typically used for **deeper** tissue.
  - As suction cannula size increases, the rate of fat removal with each pass increases, as does the risk of contour irregularities.

PHYSICS AND THEORY OF LIPOSUCTION[6]
- SAL removes fragmented fat through a cannula and tubing into a receptacle.
- **Fragmentation of fat**
  - "Jackhammer effect": The cannula striking fatty tissue
  - The avulsion of fat into the islets of the cannula as the cannula moves in and out
- **Rate of fat aspiration**
  - Directly proportional to the diameter of the cannula and suction tubing
  - Directly proportional to vacuum pressure
  - Inversely proportional to the length of the cannula
  - Poiseuille law concepts
    - $R = (L/r^4) \times K$, where R is the resistance, r is the radius of the tube, L is the length of the tube, and K is a constant factor

WETTING SOLUTIONS

PURPOSES
- Volume replacement
- Hemostasis
- Analgesia

- Enhance cavitation (UAL)
- Dissipate heat
- **Constituents vary, examples:**
  - 1000 ml of lactated Ringer solution at 21°C
  - 30 ml of 1% lidocaine plain (15 ml if large volume)
  - 1 ml of 1:1000 epinephrine
- **Klein recipe**[7]
  - 1000 ml normal saline solution
  - 50 ml 1% lidocaine plain
  - 1 ml 1:1000 epinephrine
  - 12.5 ml of 8.4% sodium bicarbonate
    - ▶ Alkalization may decrease pain with infiltration, but is not needed with general anesthesia.

WETTING SOLUTION TECHNIQUE[8] (Table 57-1)

Table 57-1 *Wetting Solution Infiltrate and Estimated Blood Loss by Technique*

Technique	Infiltrate	Estimated Blood Loss (as % volume)
Dry	None	20-45
Wet	200-300 ml/area	4-30
Superwet	1 ml infiltrate:1 ml aspirate	<1
Tumescent	3-4 ml infiltrate:1 ml aspirate	<1

Infiltrate may contain lidocaine, epinephrine, and/or sodium bicarbonate, depending on surgeon's preference.

LIDOCAINE IN WETTING SOLUTION[7,9-11]

- Analgesia is provided for up to **18 hours** postoperatively.
- Recommended maximum is **7 mg/kg** in the presence of epinephrine (**4 mg/kg** in the absence of epinephrine).
- The estimated maximum safe lidocaine dosage using the **tumescent technique** is **35 mg/kg.**
  - Peak plasma concentration is 10-14 hours after infiltration.
  - Klein's original study noted doses up to 52 mg/kg with no adverse effect; this has been confirmed in other studies.
  - Objective signs of lidocaine toxicity at plasma concentration >5 μg/ml
- **Use of high quantities of lidocaine made possible because of:**
  - Diluted solution
  - Slow infiltration
  - Vasoconstriction of epinephrine
  - Relative avascularity of fatty layer
  - High lipid solubility of lidocaine
  - Compression of vessels by infiltrate

NOTE: **The wet environment may be lost after 20-30 minutes.**

LIDOCAINE TOXICITY[12] (Table 57-2)

Table 57-2 *Plasma Lidocaine Levels and Symptoms of Toxicity*

Plasma Level (µg/ml)	Symptoms
3-6	Subjective (circumoral numbness, tinnitus, drowsiness, lightheadedness, difficulty focusing
5-9	Objective (tremors, twitching, shivering)
8-12	Seizures, cardiac depression
12-14	Unconsciousness, coma
15-20	Respiratory arrest
>20	Cardiac arrest

LIPOSUCTION TECHNIQUES

SUCTION-ASSISTED LIPOSUCTION (SAL)[8,13]
- Surgeon's arm provides energy.
- Movement of cannula results in mechanical disruption and avulsion to allow fat cell aspiration.
- External source of suction to facilitate fatty tissue removal (usually 300-600 mm Hg)

ULTRASOUND-ASSISTED LIPOSUCTION (UAL)[13-16]
- First described by Zocchi[15] in 1992
- Piezoelectric crystals in the probes convert electric energy into high-frequency sound waves that interact with tissue to create interstitial cavities and cellular fragmentation—a process termed, *"cavitation."*
  - Adipose is more susceptible than muscle, fascia, or neural tissue.
  - The emulsified fat is then removed through the cannula.
  - Heat is generated as a byproduct.
- Use a hollow cannula or a solid probe.
- UAL with improved contouring over SAL for **fibrous areas** such as:
  - Upper abdomen
  - Back
  - Flanks
  - Gynecomastia
- **Three-stage technique**
  - *Stage I*: Subcutaneous infiltration with wetting solution
  - *Stage II*: Ultrasound treatment to emulsify fat
  - *Stage III*: Evacuation of emulsified fat and final contouring with SAL
- **Key factors to UAL**
  - The **stroke rate is slower** than with traditional SAL to allow time for cavitation.
  - The dry technique should **never** be used with UAL (minimum superwet environment).
  - The cannula/probe must be **moving at all times** to limit thermal injury.
  - The endpoint is a **loss of resistance** to probe advancement (Table 57-3).

Table 57-3   *Surgical Endpoints for UAL and SAL/PAL*

Endpoint	UAL	SAL/PAL
Primary	Loss of tissue resistance Blood aspirate	Final contour Symmetrical pinch test
Secondary	Treatment time Treatment volume	Treatment time Treatment volume

PAL, Power-assisted liposuction; *SAL,* suction-assisted liposuction; *UAL,* ultrasound-assisted liposuction.

- **Complications of UAL**
  - Thermal injury (burn or blisters of skin)
  - Seroma
  - Hyperpigmentation
- **Superficial UAL**
  - Can result in increased skin retraction but at the risk of increased contour deformities
  - Power settings and suction should be decreased compared to those used in deeper planes.
  - *Be careful to prevent thermal skin injury.*
- **UAL advantages**
  - Decreased surgeon fatigue in more fibrous tissues
  - May improve skin tightening
- **UAL disadvantages**
  - Equipment cost
  - Slightly larger incisions
  - Longer operative times
  - Increased risk of thermal injury to skin
  - Increased scarring in adipose tissue bed
  - Cannula misguidance due to diminished cannula resistance

POWER-ASSISTED LIPOSUCTION (PAL)[5,13,17,18]

- Augmented SAL with externally powered reciprocating cannula replicating the to-and-fro motion of the operator's arm[19]
- Approximately 2 mm motion at rates of up to 4000-6000 cycles/minute
  - Electric energy source or medical grade compressed air
  - **Less wetting solution** is required compared to UAL.
- **PAL advantages**
  - Decreased surgeon fatigue
  - Large volumes
  - Revision liposuction
  - Shortened procedure times
- **PAL disadvantages**
  - Operator discomfort induced by vibrating handpiece
  - Noise generation
  - Equipment cost

LASER-ASSISTED LIPOSUCTION (LAL)[5,17,20]

- Technique involves subcutaneous insertion of a laser fiber via a small skin incision.
  - Fiber is either housed with a cannula or as a single fiber.
- Most commonly used wavelengths in the United States
  - 924/975 nm, 1064 nm, 1319/1320 nm, and 1450 nm
- Laser acts to disrupt cell membranes and emulsify fat by photothermolysis.
  - Different wavelengths vary in their effectiveness to preferentially target adipose cells and photocoagulation of small vessels while excluding surrounding structures.
- Previously marketed for skin-tightening effect (mostly anecdotal)
  - Theory: Heating of the subdermal tissue contributes to possible skin-tightening effect.
  - Studies have shown **no difference** between LAL and conventional techniques.
- **Four-stage technique**
  - *Stage I*: Subcutaneous infiltration with wetting solution
  - *Stage II*: Application of energy to the subcutaneous tissues with laser probe
  - *Stage III*: Evacuation of emulsified fat with SAL
    - ► Some advocate skipping this stage in smaller regions (neck) and allowing the body to absorb the liquefied contents.
  - *Stage IV:* Subdermal skin stimulation
- **LAL advantages**
  - Decreased intraoperative blood loss
  - Decreased postoperative ecchymosis
  - Possible skin tightening (not confirmed)
- **LAL disadvantages**
  - Potential thermal injury to skin
  - Equipment cost
  - Prolonged procedure time
  - Increased scarring in adipose tissue bed
  - Cannula misguidance due to diminished resistance

WATER-ASSISTED LIPOSUCTION (WAL)[21,22]

- Technique uses a **dual-purpose cannula** to emit pulsating, pressurized, fan-shaped jets of wetting solution with simultaneous suctioning of the fatty tissue and instilled fluid.
  - Injected fluid loosens fat cells while minimizing surrounding soft tissue damage.
- Can be done in office setting under local anesthetic
- **Two-stage technique**
  - *Stage I*: Subcutaneous preinfiltration with wetting solution
    - ► A standard wetting solution for local anesthesia and vasoconstriction
  - *Stage II*: Simultaneous infiltration of "rinsing solution" and aspiration
    - ► Lower infiltration setting and lower lidocaine concentration
  - *Endpoint*: Final contour and pinch test
- **WAL advantages**
  - Reduced pain for patient
  - Decreased need for general anesthesia
  - Patient awake and able to change positions
- **WAL disadvantages**
  - Equipment cost
  - Prolonged procedure time

RADIOFREQUENCY-ASSISTED LIPOSUCTION (RFAL)[23,24]

- Technique uses **bipolar radiofrequency energy** to disrupt the adipose cell membrane and facilitate lipolysis.
  - A hollow cannula allows simultaneous aspiration of liquefied fat.
- Allows a constant treatment depth
- Controlled thermal injury at subdermal surface may lead to skin-tightening effect.
- The external electrode has a thermal sensor that measures skin temperature to prevent thermal injury.
  - Once the skin reaches 38°-42° C, thermal heating is complete and completion SAL or PAL contouring is then performed.
  - Approximately 30% of aspiration occurs during RFAL.[17]
- **Three-stage technique**
  - *Stage I*: Subcutaneous infiltration with wetting solution
  - *Stage II*: Radiofrequency energy treatment to emulsify fat
  - *Stage III*: Evacuation of emulsified fat and final contouring with SAL or PAL
  - *Endpoint*: Loss of resistance to forward motion rather than pinch or palpation
- **RFAL advantages**
  - Decreased surgeon fatigue, especially in fibrous areas
  - Decreased ecchymosis
  - Possible skin-tightening effect
- **RFAL disadvantages**
  - Potential thermal injury
  - Equipment cost
  - Prolonged procedure time

> **TIP:** Thermal methods of liposuction (laser, ultrasonic, radiofrequency, and others) dramatically reduce cannula resistance within the tissues indiscriminately, narrowing the resistance differential between targeted and unwanted tissues. Thereby, surgeon precision is compromised as the tactile feedback is blunted. Additionally, these devices create a significant scar burden, and as the skin redrapes postoperatively, the fibrosis generated predisposes the patient to dermal adherence to underlying tissues, which can result in contour deformities and unnatural contours.

SEPARATION, ASPIRATION, AND FAT EQUALIZATION LIPOSUCTION (SAFELIPO®)[25,26]

- First described by Wall in 2004, published in 2010
- A nonthermal, multistep process approach for comprehensive fat management that includes reduction (SAFELipo), equalization, and augmentation (expansion vibration lipofilling)
- Developed in response to the unique challenges presented by revision liposuction cases and correcting contour deformities
- Allows more aggressive or complete treatment with a lower contour deformity risk profile
- **3-step process**: Separation, aspiration and fat equalization
  - **Step 1: Separation**—expanded tip, multiwinged cannula without suction
    - ▶ Emulsifies and liquefies the targeted adipose tissue preferentially prior to suction
    - ▶ Exploits the resistance differential between the targeted tissue and critical structures to allow greater control, precision, and safety
    - ▶ 40% of treatment time

SENIOR AUTHOR TIP: Simultaneous separation and tumescence (SST) with a PAL device is utilized in order to provide immediate vasoconstriction and separation of targeted fat, dramatically reducing operative time.

- **Step 2: Aspiration**—multiport, non-expanded, blunt cannula with suction
  - ▸ The low resistance, separated (liquefied) fat is preferentially aspirated without causing avulsion injury to blood vessels and stromal network
  - ▸ 40% of treatment time
- **Step 3: Fat equalization**—expanded tip, multiwinged cannula without suction (Fig. 57-6)
  - ▸ After all separated fat has been aspirated, residual areas of uneven fat removal are equalized, with treatment undertaken in a significantly wider area than the original area of excess, in order to maximize skin retraction.
  - ▸ Equalizing effectively separates more fat, all of which will remain and serve as local fat grafts to fill in any imperfections and prevent adhesions.
  - ▸ Corrects any tissue thickness irregularities
  - ▸ *This phase is more critical in thinner patients when small discrepancies in tissue thickness become more readily visible externally*
  - ▸ 20% of treatment time

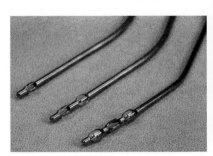

Fig. 57-6 Examples of angled, multi-winged wall cage cannulas used for fat separation, fat equalization, and expansion vibration lipofilling. The expanded "wings" of the cannula, in combination with rapid movement (vibration) create high and low pressure zones in the subcutaneous fat, causing the relatively low-resistance solid fat to liquefy, while allowing the relatively higher resistance unintended structures (blood vessels, stromal support structures) to remain intact and undamaged.

- ▪ Separation and equalization soften the deep septal stromal network that runs throughout the subcutaneous layer and loosen fascial adherences.
- ▪ Rigid subcutaneous adherences tether the skin and are one etiology of contour irregularities.
- ▪ Angled cannulas are used exclusively in SAFELipo processes in order to gain a wider field of coverage and provide enhanced control.
- ▪ **Expansion vibration lipofilling (EVL)** allows for simultaneous equalization and fat grafting, utilizing the same principles as the reductive phase of SAFELipo.
- ▪ **SAFELipo advantages**
  - • Reduced incidence of contour deformities
  - • Enhanced skin-tightening effect
  - • Ability to treat areas completely, widely or circumferentially, beyond areas of excess, or through zones of adherence without fear of creating a contour deformity
  - • Decreased ecchymosis
  - • Enhanced precision, with ability to combine with fat shifting and expansion vibration lipofilling to treat areas comprehensively
- ▪ **SAFELipo disadvantages**
  - • Increased operative time to properly execute the technique

> **TIP:** by relaxing the attachments of the skin to underlying structures, the skin can be predictably manipulated and redistributed as needed from areas of excess into areas of deficiency.

FLUID RESUSCITATION DURING LIPOSUCTION[27,28]

- 1 L of isotonic fluid is absorbed from the interstitium in **167 minutes.**
- Any infiltrate not removed through aspiration is slowly reabsorbed and mobilized by normal homeostatic mechanisms.

CAUTION: As volume of aspiration increases, so does the potential for extreme fluid shifts that could result in volume overload.

- **Superwet infiltration technique**[29] is preferred over tumescent technique with equivalent blood loss and decreased potential of volume overload and congestive heart failure.
- **IV (using superwet infiltration)**
  - Crystalloid IV at maintenance rate (adjust to urine output and vital signs)
    - ▶ Foley catheter should be placed for patients undergoing large-volume liposuction (>5 L total aspirate)
  - Replacement IV of 0.25 ml/kg of aspirate over 5 L
  - Intraoperative fluid ratio goals

  Ratio = (Vol. of intraop fluid + Vol. of lipoaspirate + Vol. of superwet solution) / Aspiration vol.

  - **Small-volume liposuction: 1.8**
  - **Large-volume liposuction: 1.2**
    - ▶ Continue maintenance IV postoperatively until oral intake is adequate.

GENERAL DETAILS OF TRADITIONAL LIPOSUCTION STAGES[30]

STAGE I: INFILTRATION
- Subcutaneous infiltration with wetting solution
- Record delivered amount to each area.
- Endpoint is uniform blanching and skin turgor.
- Allow at least 7-10 minutes for maximal vasoconstriction from epinephrine.

> **SENIOR AUTHOR TIP:** Simultaneous separation and tumescence (SST) allows a more efficient distribution of infiltrate, and the time needed for maximum vasoconstriction to take effect is drastically reduced.[31]

STAGE II: UAL TREATMENT (OMIT IF PERFORMING SAL/PAL ONLY)
- Place access incisions asymmetrically.
- Use port protector and wet towels to protect skin.
- Treat posterior areas first (can treat **70%-80%** of the circumference from this position).
- Withdraw to within 3 cm of incisions to redirect and minimize torque.
- Move from superficial to deep (in contrast to SAL, which goes from deep to superficial).

STAGE III: EVACUATION AND FINAL CONTOURING[32]
- Set aspirator to 60%-70% of usual suction.
- Begin with deep layer and move superficially.

> **SENIOR AUTHOR TIP:**   The use of angled cannulas can reduce skin abrasions, improve manipulation and "driveability" of cannulas, allow for more thorough coverage of an area, and decrease operator fatigue. A rolling pinch test can check for tissue thickness discrepencies at treatment completion.

LIPOSUCTION BY AREA[33,34]

HIPS AND FLANKS
- **Flank (males)**
  - Begins in paraspinous area
  - Widest just above iliac crest
  - Anteriorly blends with lower abdominal adiposity of lateral rectus sheath
  - Begins at convexity below flare of rib cage: becomes convex and full over the iliac crests
  - Inferiorly defined by zone of adherence lying along the iliac crest
- **Hips (females)**
  - Similar areas as the flank, only more inferior so that its bulk is centered over the iliac crests
  - Ends lower than the flank
- **Gluteal depression**
  - Convexity between the hips and above the lateral thigh below
  - Also known as the *"saddlebag"* area
- **Technical details**
  - Jackknife when prone
  - Average infiltration volumes: 500-800 ml in the hip
  - Avoid violation of the lateral gluteal depression.

THIGHS
- Thigh should be a shallow convex arc on both anterior and posterior surfaces.
- Lateral thigh extends from the gluteal depression to the knee.
- Buttock extends from the sacrum to the inferior gluteal fold.
- *"Banana roll"* is the fullness from inferior gluteal fold to the posterior upper thigh zone of adherence.
- There should be an unbroken curve from the iliac crest to the distal thigh.
- Medially there should be a slight convexity of the upper third of the medial thigh; middle to distal third is flat or slightly concave.
- **Technical details**
  - Prone position allows operator to work on both sides and assess symmetry of lateral and posterior thighs.
  - *"Frog leg"* position is used to treat the medial thigh area.
  - Suction both deep and intermediate planes.
  - Suctioning in superficial plane can worsen preexisting contour irregularities.

BUTTOCKS
- **Ideal buttock**
  - Slightly convex
  - Nonptotic
  - Firm with a slight lateral gluteal depression

- In **women** the buttocks are **rounded** and flow into lateral thigh.
- **Male** buttocks are more angular and almost **squared laterally** (more muscle, less fat, more firm).
- **Technical details**
  - Area should be approached with caution, because an aesthetically pleasing buttock varies across age groups, geography, and ethnicity.
  - *Avoid deep aggressive suctioning* to preserve the integrity of the inferior gluteal crease.
  - Overtreatment of the deep or superficial plane may result in buttock ptosis.
  - Excessive suctioning of the lateral proximal posterior thigh may result in extension of gluteal fold in female patients and masculinization of the gluteal area.

ABDOMEN
- **Borders**
  - Xiphoid superiorly
  - Pubic ramus inferiorly
  - Laterally extends to the anterior iliac crest along the inguinal ligament
- Clearly delineated linea alba depression from top to bottom
- Requires careful evaluation of the hips/flanks for circumferential improvement.
- **Anteriorly**
  - Slight supraumbilical concavity
  - Infraumbilical convexity
- **Women**
  - Highlighted by bilateral concavities (hourglass shape), as defined by the flank from rib to the iliac crest
- **Men**
  - Do **not** have bilateral concavity
  - **No flare** at the iliac crest
  - Infraumbilical region should be **flat**
- **Technical details**
  - Short, controlled strokes should be used to prevent inadvertent fascial perforation.
  - Suctioning of the deep two thirds of the fat is safe and effective.

ARMS
- Ideal arm is lean and has an anterior convexity of the deltoid merging with a convexity of the biceps.
- Posterior surface of the arm should be slightly convex from axilla to elbow.
- Patients with at least 1.5 cm of fat by the pinch test are good candidates.
- **Technical details**
  - When patient is prone: Incision placed in posterior axillary fold, and SAL incision at radial elbow
  - Along the distal third of arm and elbow region, the **basilic vein** and **medial antebrachial cutaneous nerve** are superficial to the deep fascia and vulnerable to injury.
  - Long radial strokes to prevent waviness/contour deformity

CAUTION: Perform UAL from radial incision only to prevent ulnar nerve injury.

BACK
- Prone jackknife positioning is preferred.
- Very dense and fibrous fat

- Lipodystrophy along bra line responds well to UAL, allowing the fold to be broken up and excess fat removed.
- Technical details
  - Place incisions in bra/bathing suit line.
  - Avoid forceful excursion to prevent unsafe cannula redirection by dense tissue.

NECK
- Patient is positioned with the neck hyperextended on a shoulder roll.
- Overzealous suctioning can lead to hollowing and skeletonizing of the neck or potential neuropraxia of the marginal mandibular nerve.

> **SENIOR AUTHOR TIP:** The senior author prefers a full-body prep and three positions for most body cases—supine and both lateral decubitus positions. Prone positioning is usually unnecessary. Minimizing incisions and keeping all incisions in hidden areas has been made possible by the use of long, angled cannulas in association with the SAFELipo process approach. All access incisions are left open to drain, minimizing chance of seroma. Careful analysis and planning is required in order to avoid feminization of the male silhouette. Concurrent expansion vibration lipofilling in association with most liposuction procedures has shown improved results, and can be easily incorporated into SAFELipo procedures. Avoiding gluteal crease incisions in liposuction of the lateral thighs can prevent buttock collapse and other severe contour deformities of the thighs and buttocks. Most "banana rolls" are actually bulging posterior pillars of support of the buttock, and are not improved with liposuction. Instead, they can be treated with EVL of the buttocks and posterior thigh in order to enhance thigh and buttock support, minimizing the bulging and improving the "banana roll."

DRAINS
- Not routinely used, except in large-volume liposuction of the circumferential trunk
- Consider for liposuction procedures combined with resection

ACCESS SITE MANAGEMENT
- Massage out excess fluid.
- May close or leave open to drain.
- Cover with antibiotic ointment, gauze, and paper tape or adhesive dressing.
- Place compression garment that is customized based on surgeon's preference and procedure performed.
  - Compression foam may be used under the garment for the first week to assist with contouring.

POSTOPERATIVE CARE
- Begin ambulating the day of surgery.
- May shower 1-2 days postoperatively

- Postoperative compression garment
  - Based on surgeon's preference, no consensus on regimen
  - Example: Patient should wear compression garment at all times for 2 weeks then at night for 2 additional weeks.
- Patients return to work 3-5 days after small-volume procedures.
- After a large-volume procedure, patients may require 7-10 days before returning to work.
- Full activities are resumed in 3-4 weeks as tolerated.
- Patients should expect some weight gain postoperatively from fluid shifts; this resolves over time.

> **SENIOR AUTHOR TIP:** The senior author prefers that all liposuction access sites are treated with fat equalization to minimize any contour depression, and all are left open to drain. Half-inch or one-inch foam is utilized postoperatively for several weeks, with a minimally compressive compression garment only serving to hold the foam in place.

> **NOTE:** There are no data to support a maximum volume of safe liposuction. Pay attention to state regulations, where applicable.

- Regardless of the anesthetic route, **large-volume liposuction** (>5 L total aspirate) should be performed in an acute-care hospital or in a facility that is either accredited or licensed.
- Vital signs and urinary output should be monitored postoperatively, and patients should be monitored overnight in an appropriate facility by qualified staff familiar with the perioperative care of liposuction patients.[35]

HEALING COURSE

- **Days 1-3:** Access incisions drain until healed.
- **Days 3-5:** Edema peaks and drainage slows.
- **Days 7-10:** Ecchymosis resolves.
- **Weeks 4-6:** Edema resolves.
- **Weeks 8-10:** Induration in large-volume areas
- **Months 3-6:** Final aesthetic result (revision liposuction cases will take a year to equilibrate.)

COMPLICATION PREVENTION AND INTERVENTION

SAFETY GUIDELINES IN LIPOSUCTION

- Appropriate patient selection (ASA class I, within 30% of ideal body weight)
- Use of superwet infiltration technique
- Meticulous monitoring of volume status (urinary catheter, noninvasive hemodynamic monitoring, communication with anesthesiologist)
- Judicious fluid resuscitation per protocol
- Overnight monitoring of large-volume (>5 L of total aspirate) liposuction patients in an appropriate health care facility
- Use of pneumatic compression devices in patients under general anesthesia or if case lasts >1 hour
- Maintenance of total lidocaine doses <35 mg/kg (wetting solution)

LOCAL ANESTHETIC SYSTEM TOXICITY TREATMENT (LAST)[36]

■ Infuse **20% lipid emulsion.**
- Bolus 1.5 ml/g (lean body mass) intravenously over 1 minute.
- Provide continuous infusion at 0.25 ml/kg/minute.
- Repeat bolus once or twice for persistent cardiovascular collapse.
- Double the infusion rate to 0.5 ml/kg/minute if blood pressure remains low.
- Continue infusion for at least 10 minutes after circulatory stability is achieved.

■ Recommended upper limit is approximately 10-12 ml/kg lipid emulsion over the first 30 minutes.

TOP TAKEAWAYS

➤ Consider whether the correct procedure has been chosen: liposuction versus skin resection.

➤ Mark patients while they are awake and standing; allow them to provide guidance in choosing the areas to be treated.

➤ Thermal methods of liposuction diminish cannula resistance and reduce surgeon fatigue, but can burn the patient, resulting in uncorrectable contour deformities.

➤ Perform repeated assessments of progress to prevent contour deformities.

➤ Underresection is preferable to an overtreatment leading to contour deformities that are difficult to correct.

➤ Superficial plane liposuction requires careful attention to prevent contour deformities.

➤ Use of compression garment in the postoperative setting is essential to prevent contour deformities and chronic seroma formation and provides patient comfort in the acute healing period.

REFERENCES

1. Grazer FM. Suction-assisted lipectomy, suction lipectomy, lipolysis, and lipexeresis. Plast Reconstr Surg 72:620, 1983.
2. Lockwood TE. Superficial fascial system (SFS) of the trunk and extremities: a new concept. Plast Reconstr Surg 87:1009, 1991.
3. Rohrich RJ, Smith PD, Marcantonio DR, et al. The zones of adherence: role in minimizing and preventing contour deformities in liposuction. Plast Reconstr Surg 107:1562, 2001.
4. Lockwood TE. Superficial fascial system (SFS) of the trunk and extremities: a new concept. Plast Reconstr Surg 87:1009, 1991.
5. Neligan P, Warren RJ, eds. Plastic Surgery, vol 2, ed 3. Philadelphia: Saunders Elsevier, 2013.
6. Young VL, Brandon HJ. The physics of suction-assisted lipoplasty. Aesthet Surg J 24:206, 2004.
7. Klein JA. Tumescent technique for local anesthesia improves safety in large-volume liposuction. Plast Reconstr Surg 92:1085; discussion 1099, 1993.
8. Iverson RE, Pao VS. MOC-PS(SM) CME article: liposuction. Plast Reconstr Surg 121(4 Suppl):S1, 2008.
9. Achar S, Kundu S. Principles of office anesthesia: part I. Infiltrative anesthesia. Am Fam Physician 66:91, 2002.
10. Ostad A, Kageyama N, Moy RL. Tumescent anesthesia with a lidocaine dose of 55 mg/kg is safe for liposuction. Dermatol Surg 22:921, 1996.

11. Lozinski A, Huq NS. Tumescent liposuction. Clin Plast Surg 40:593, 2013.
12. Matarasso A. Lidocaine in ultrasound-assisted lipoplasty. Clin Plast Surg 26:431, 1999.
13. Berry MG, Davies D. Liposuction: a review of principles and techniques. J Plast Reconstr Aesthet Surg 64:985, 2011.
14. Rohrich RJ, Beran SJ, Kenkel JM, et al. Extending the role of liposuction in body contouring with ultrasound-assisted liposuction. Plast Reconstr Surg 101:1090; discussion 1117, 1998.
15. Zocchi M. Ultrasonic liposculpturing. Aesthetic Plast Surg 16:287, 1992.
16. Kenkel JM, Janis JE, Rohrich RJ, et al. Aesthetic body contouring: ultrasound-assisted liposuction. Oper Tech Plast Reconstr Surg 8:180, 2002.
17. Shridharani SM, Broyles JM, Matarasso A. Liposuction devices: technology update. Med Devices (Auckl) 7:241, 2014.
18. Rebelo A. Power-assisted liposuction. Clin Plast Surg 33:91, 2006.
19. Fodor PB. Power-assisted lipoplasty versus traditional suction-assisted lipoplasty: comparative evaluation and analysis of output. Aesthetic Plast Surg 29:127, 2005.
20. Badin AZ, Gondek LB, Garcia MJ, et al. Analysis of laser lipolysis effects on human tissue samples obtained from liposuction. Aesthetic Plast Surg 29:281, 2005.
21. Sasaki GH. Water-assisted liposuction for body contouring and lipoharvesting: safety and efficacy in 41 consecutive patients. Aesthet Surg J 31:76, 2011.
22. Man D, Meyer H. Water jet-assisted lipoplasty. Aesthet Surg J 27:342, 2007.
23. Paul M, Mulholland RS. A new approach for adipose tissue treatment and body contouring using radiofrequency-assisted liposuction. Aesthetic Plast Surg 33:687, 2009.
24. Theodorou SJ, Paresi RJ, Chia CT. Radiofrequency-assisted liposuction device for body contouring: 97 patients under local anesthesia. Aesthetic Plast Surg 36:767, 2012.
25. Wall SH Jr. SAFE circumferential liposuction with abdominoplasty. Clin Plast Surg 37:485, 2010.
26. Wall SH Jr, Lee MR. Separation, aspiration, and fat equalization: SAFE liposuction concepts for comprehensive body contouring. Plast Reconstr Surg 138:1192, 2016.
27. Rohrich RJ, Leedy JE, Swamy R, et al. Fluid resuscitation in liposuction: a retrospective review of 89 consecutive patients. Plast Reconstr Surg 117:431, 2006.
28. Commons GW, Halperin B, Chang CC. Large-volume liposuction: a review of 631 consecutive cases over 12 years. Plast Reconstr Surg 108:1753; discussion 1764, 2001.
29. Rohrich RJ, Janis JE. Discussion of article by Cardenas-Camarena: lipoaspiration and its complications: a safe operation. Plast Reconstr Surg 112:1442, 2003.
30. Kenkel JM, Gingrass MK, Rohrich RJ. Ultrasound-assisted lipoplasty. Basic science and clinical research. Clin Plast Surg 26:221, 1999.
31. Wall SH Jr, Del Vecchio D. Expansion vibration lipofilling (EVL)—concepts and applications of a new paradigm in large volume fat transplantation. Seventeenth Annual Dallas Cosmetic Surgery Symposium, Dallas, TX, Mar 2014.
32. Zocchi ML. Ultrasonic assisted lipoplasty. Technical refinements and clinical evaluations. Clin Plast Surg 23:575, 1996.
33. Stephan PJ, Kenkel JM. Updates and advances in liposuction. Aesthet Surg J 30:83, 2010.
34. Koehler J. Complications of neck liposuction and submentoplasty. Oral Maxillofac Surg Clin North Am 21:43, 2009.
35. Iverson RE, Lynch DJ; American Society of Plastic Surgeons Committee on Patient Safety. Practice advisory on liposuction. Plast Reconstr Surg 113:1478; discussion 1491, 2004.
36. Weinberg GL. Lipid emulsion infusion: resuscitation for local anesthetic and other drug overdose. Anesthesiology 117:180, 2012.

58. Brachioplasty

Tyler M. Angelos, Jeffrey E. Janis, Constantino G. Mendieta

INDICATIONS

- Excess skin and/or subcutaneous tissue of the arm refractory to conservative treatment such as diet and exercise

CONTRAINDICATIONS

ABSOLUTE

- Neurological or vascular disorders of the upper extremity
- Collagen-vascular disorders (Ehlers-Danlos syndrome, progeria, elastoderma)
- Lymphedema of the arms
- Unrealistic patient expectations

RELATIVE

- Severe comorbid conditions (including heart disease, thromboembolic disease, diabetes)
- Unstable weight gain or loss
- Expecting future pregnancy
- Active smoker
- Patients with a history of keloids or hypertrophic scars

ANATOMY (Fig. 58-1)

- **Skin:** The skin covering the shoulder and arm is smooth and very mobile over the underlying structures.
  - It is thin on medial aspect and progressively thicker laterally.
- **Subcutaneous tissue:** Fat accumulates on the inferoposterior aspect of the arm, with a minimal amount medially.
- **Superficial fascia:** The superficial fascia both circumferentially and longitudinally encases the fat of the arm from the axilla to the elbow.
  - This fascia weakens with age and weight gain, causing ptosis of the posteromedial arm.
- **Deep fascia:** The deep fascia invests all muscles and important neurovascular structures.
  - This layer should **never be violated** during brachioplasty or suction-assisted lipectomy.

> **TIP:** Along the distal third of the arm and in the region of the medial elbow, the basilic vein and medial antebrachial cutaneous nerve run together and are superficial to the deep fascia and vulnerable to injury, especially where they pierce the deep fascia an average of 14 cm proximal to the medial epicondyle.[1]

TIP: The only nerves found superficial to the deep investing fascia are branches of the **medial brachial cutaneous nerve** and the **intercostobrachial nerve.** All other important neurovascular structures are deep to the investing fascia.

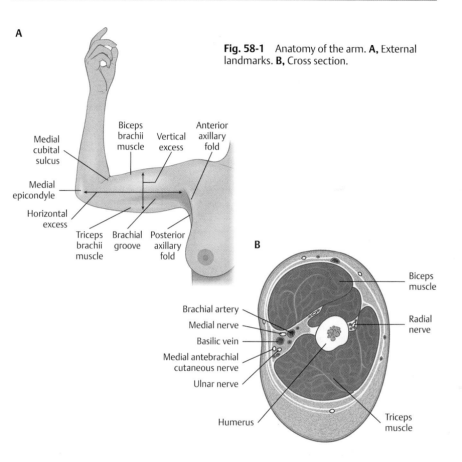

Fig. 58-1 Anatomy of the arm. **A,** External landmarks. **B,** Cross section.

PREOPERATIVE EVALUATION

■ Obtain a complete medical history, paying specific attention to weight gain/loss, weight stability, tobacco use, and scarring.

TIP: Weight should be stable for 6-12 months before performing any body contouring procedure on a massive-weight-loss patient.

■ Physical examination should focus on **the amount of excess skin, excess subcutaneous tissue,** and degree of ptosis present in the arm.
■ Patients can then be stratified into one of three groups (Table 58-1).
■ An algorithm (Fig. 58-2) can then be used to help guide surgeons to the procedure that is best suited to achieve optimal results.[2]

Table 58-1   *Classification of Upper Arm Contouring*

Type	Skin Excess	Fat Excess	Location of Skin Excess
I	Minimal	Moderate	n/a
IIA	Moderate	Minimal	Proximal
IIB	Moderate	Minimal	Entire arm
IIC	Moderate	Minimal	Arm and chest
IIIA	Moderate	Moderate	Proximal
IIIB	Moderate	Moderate	Entire arm
IIIC	Moderate	Moderate	Arm and chest

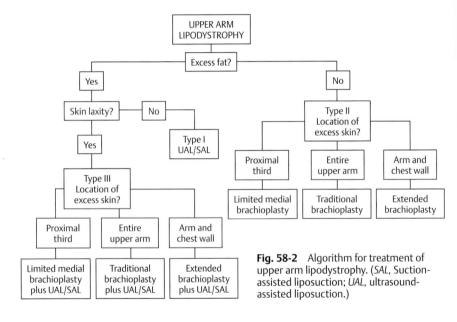

Fig. 58-2   Algorithm for treatment of upper arm lipodystrophy. (*SAL,* Suction-assisted liposuction; *UAL,* ultrasound-assisted liposuction.)

INFORMED CONSENT

- Patients need to be informed that, with a brachioplasty, they are trading a more pleasing shape and contour of the arm for a scar.
- The **scar is not inconsequential** and will be visible depending on the type of clothing worn.
- Scars may stay thick and heavy for a prolonged period of time.
- *The brachioplasty scar is likely the most noticeable scar in all of aesthetic surgery.*

SENIOR AUTHOR TIP: In the preoperative consult, use a skin marker to draw the potential scar on the patient's arms to help them understand the procedure and to align their expectations with reality. Document this in their medical record.

TIP: Photographs are imperative when discussing brachioplasty outcomes.

- Common brachioplasty complications include widened hypertrophic scar, wound dehiscence, seroma, infection, paresthesias/numbness, scar tethering across the axilla, and recurrent skin laxity.

EQUIPMENT
- No special equipment is needed to perform a brachioplasty unless concomitant liposuction is performed.
  - In this case, wetting solution and liposuction equipment are required.

TECHNIQUE

MARKINGS
- An area of debate for surgeons performing brachioplasty is where to place the arm scar.
- Many place the scar within the **brachial groove, whereas** others prefer a **posteriorly positioned scar.**
- A survey of plastic surgeons and the general public showed that a **medial,** straight brachioplasty scar is more acceptable than a **posterior** straight scar.[3]
- Brachioplasty markings depend on the type of brachioplasty performed.
- The type of brachioplasty performed depends on the location of the excess skin (see Table 58-1).
  - **Type I:** Minimal skin excess, moderate fat excess
    - ▶ If skin tone is good, this is best treated with suction-assisted lipectomy alone.
  - **Type IIA:** Moderate proximal skin excess, minimal fat excess
    - ▶ A minibrachioplasty[4] is used, which is isolated to the axillary fold.
    - ▶ If the skin excess is purely horizontal, then a vertically oriented wedge or ellipse is placed in the axillary fold (Fig. 58-3, *A*).
    - ▶ If skin excess is horizontal and vertical, a T-shaped excision is used (Fig. 58-3, *B*).

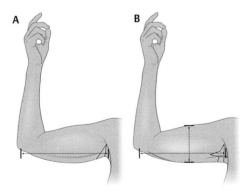

Fig. 58-3   Type IIA markings. **A,** Markings for proximal horizontal excess only. **B,** T-shaped resection markings for proximal vertical and horizontal excess.

- **Type IIB:** Moderate skin excess of the entire arm (axilla to elbow), minimal fat excess
  - ▶ A traditional brachioplasty is used placing the scar in the brachial groove.
  - ▶ If there is vertical skin excess only, then use a linear horizontal incision (Fig. 58-4, A).
  - ▶ If there is vertical and horizontal skin excess, add an L-shaped extension to the linear horizontal incision in the axilla (Fig. 58-4, B).

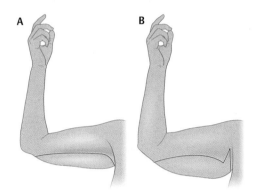

Fig. 58-4   Type IIB markings. **A,** Markings for vertical excess only. **B,** L-shaped excision markings for horizontal and vertical excess.

- **Type IIC:** Moderate skin excess of the arm and chest, minimal fat excess
  - ▶ An extended brachioplasty is needed, which extends the excision onto the chest wall.
  - ▶ These are typically **massive-weight-loss patients.**
  - ▶ A horizontal incision is made in the brachial groove and carried through the axilla down onto the chest wall.
  - ▶ This excision often passes distal to the elbow (Fig. 58-5).
- **Type IIIA:** Moderate proximal skin excess, moderate fat excess
- **Type IIIB:** Moderate skin excess of the entire arm, moderate fat excess
- **Type IIIC:** Moderate skin excess of the arm and chest, moderate fat excess
  - ▶ In these cases (type III), fat excess is moderate and skin excess is moderate.
  - ▶ Options for treatment include further weight loss before surgery, staged liposuction followed by skin resection, or concomitant liposuction and brachioplasty.
  - ▶ Skin-resection brachioplasty patterns are the same as for type II subtypes.

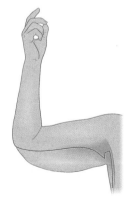

Fig. 58-5   Type IIC markings for excess along the upper arm and chest wall. A Z is made in the axilla to prevent scar contracture.

TWO-ELLIPSE TECHNIQUE[5] (Fig. 58-6)

- Outer ellipse based on tissue redundancy
- Inner ellipse adjusted to allow for closure
  - Avoids potential issues with overaggressive resection, vascular compromise
- Steps
  - Patient is marked seated with arm abducted and elbow at 90 degrees.
  - Amount of redundancy marked using pinch test on medial and lateral arm from the axillary crease to the elbow (Fig. 58-7, A).
  - Inner ellipse is designed by cheating in one-half X, where X is pinch thickness (Fig. 58-7, B).
  - Orientation marks made for guidance of closure techniques (Fig. 58-7, C)

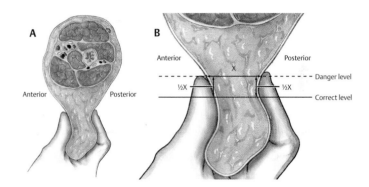

Fig. 58-6   A, Amount of tissue resection based on pinch thickness does not take into account the distance between the surgeon's fingers. **B,** To account for this discrepancy, the amount of resection is reduced by one-half X on each side.

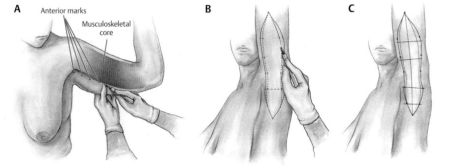

Fig. 58-7   A, Tissue is pinched below the underlying muscle mass, and anterior and posterior marks are made. Marks can continue to the distal end of the upper arm to eliminate excess tissue. **B,** Marks continue around the upper arm to the axillary crease. These marks are used to create the inner ellipse but serve as the actual resection line. **C,** A line through the midline is marked to orient the resection and allow placement of retraction clamps. Cross-hatched marks guide alignment at closure.

NOTE: There is a commonly debated concept regarding scar placement posteriorly versus medially. A medial scar lies in a less visible area (only seen when the arm is externally rotated and abducted); however, the poor dermal quality of the skin here creates an often wider scar. A posteriorly placed scar can be a fine-line scar because of better dermal quality, but this will be visible from behind when the patient wears sleeveless clothing.

NOTE: In a newer concept, the scar is placed at a happy medium between the true posterior and true medial (bicipital groove) area at the posteromedial aspect of the arm. This allows better dermal alignment without the high visibility of a posterior scar. It requires slight variation in determining possible resection. Conservative resection is advised when learning this technique to prevent overly tight closures (Kenkel, JM, personal communication, 2012).

OPERATIVE PROCEDURE

- Intravenous catheters and blood pressure cuffs should be placed **distal to the elbows** or on the **lower extremities.**
- The arm is circumferentially prepped extending onto the chest wall.
- The hand and distal forearm are wrapped in a sterile towel to allow full mobility of the arm.
- If concomitant liposuction is desired, it is then performed.
- The previously marked skin excision pattern is again marked.
  - Three to five vertical cross-hatches are evenly placed to ensure proper alignment after resection (Fig. 58-8).
  - The inferior line of the incision is estimated by a simple pinch test and marked.
- The brachial groove is marked, followed by the superior anchor line of the incision.
  - This is drawn with downward tension placed on the skin to simulate skin excursion.
  - The superior anchor line is typically 1-2 cm superior to the brachial groove.
- The superior anchor line is incised sharply along with the anterior aspect of the chest wall extension (if needed) and a skin/subcutaneous flap is elevated in an inferior direction, taking care not to violate the deep investing fascia.
- If the dissection is carried within 5 cm of the medial epicondyle, care is taken to identify and preserve the **medial antebrachial cutaneous nerve** often running with the basilic vein.
- The skin flap should be raised inferior to the proposed inferior line of the resection, as determined preoperatively by the pinch test.
  - This will allow greater skin mobility for final closure.

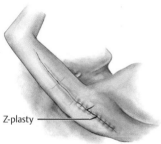

Z-plasty

Fig. 58-8   Brachioplasty marked with vertical cross-hatches. Note the Z-plasty used to prevent contracture across the axilla.

- The tissues of the upper arm are redraped to ensure they are not tethered before the margins of resection are estimated.
- A penetrating towel clamp or heavy forceps is then used to pull the skin flap in a superior direction to estimate how much tissue can be safely removed.
- The flap is divided sharply down the most medial cross-hatched line until the maximum amount of tolerated tension is reached.
  - This point is then secured to the superior incision line with suture or a towel clamp.
  - This is repeated, moving laterally along the remaining three to four cross-hatched lines, removing the tissue in a segmental manner.

TIP: Sequential resection/closure allows safe closure of the wound and prevents overresection in light of the expected edema. The edema can be severe, and wound closure likely will not be possible if performed after dissection of the entire wound.

- The superficial fascia of the medial aspect of the inferior skin flap is anchored to the clavipectoral fascia with a 0 braided nylon suture to keep the tissue suspended in the axilla.[6]
- The dermis is then closed in layers over a closed-suction drain. Aligning the skin edges as soon as possible is essential so the edema does not prevent wound closure.
- After wound closure, a gentle compressive wrap is placed on the arm.
- The most catastrophic complication directly related to brachioplasty is **overresection and inability to close the wound.**
  - If this happens one could attempt liposuction to debulk the remaining arm; however, split-thickness skin grafting using the resected tissue as the donor site may be necessary.

CAUTION: Use caution with barbed sutures during a brachioplasty, because the dermis of the medial arm is very thin and barbed sutures can present problems with wound healing.[7]

TIP: If the incision crosses the axilla, a Z-plasty should be added to the skin excision to prevent contracture across the axilla (see Fig. 58-8).

LIPOSUCTION

- In **type I** arms (minimal skin excess, moderate fat excess), **liposuction alone** is the treatment of choice.
- In **type III** arms (moderate skin excess, moderate fat excess), one option is to perform **liposuction concurrently with brachioplasty.**
- Opinions differ on whether liposuction should be performed concurrently with brachioplasty or at an earlier stage.
- All agree that edema in the arms can be very problematic for skin closure.
- Liposuction of the arm can be performed safely and effectively outside the region of excision during the brachioplasty.[8,9]
- A thicker arm—specifically, along the posterior aspect—typically requires liposuction to assist with general debulking and smooth contouring into the region in which excision is performed.

- Those who perform liposuction at the same time as the brachioplasty suggest operating on each arm separately in this order:
  - Infiltrate wetting solution (1:1 ratio of fluid infiltrated to the volume of aspirate removed).
  - Wait 5 minutes.
  - Perform suction-assisted lipectomy.
  - Resect tissue immediately.
  - Close the wound.
- Liposuction cannula is typically placed over the olecranon process and/or in the axilla in the medial aspect of the purposed incision.

TIP: Avoid placing the liposuction incisions at the medial epicondyle to prevent ulnar nerve injury.

SENIOR AUTHOR TIP: Patients who present with excessive skin and a rather "deflated" arm will not benefit from the addition of liposuction.

POSTOPERATIVE CARE

- After wound closure over a closed-suction drain, a compressive wrap is placed around the entire arm to decrease swelling.
  - Make sure this wrap starts distally at the hand and extends up to the shoulder.
- The wrap is typically removed after 48 hours, and the wounds are checked.
- Patients are then allowed to shower; however, they are encouraged to keep the arms wrapped (or in surgical sleeves) as much as possible for the first 2 weeks.
- Patients should be instructed not to raise their arms or abduct their shoulders for 2 weeks.
  - After 2 weeks, gentle range of motion exercises begin.
- The drains are typically removed within the first week.

COMPLICATIONS

- By far the most common complaint after brachioplasty is **widened, unsightly scars.**
- Counseling patients preoperatively that the scar will not reach maturity until 12 months postoperative is critical.
- Common brachioplasty complications include widened hypertrophic scar, wound dehiscence, seroma, infection, paresthesias/numbness, scar tethering across the axilla, residual standing cone of tissue deformities, and recurrent skin laxity.
- Complication rates after brachioplasty range from 25%-40% and revision rates range from 3%-25%.[10-12]
- Zomerlei et al[13] showed that 8.3% of the brachioplasty patients needed a revision because of scarring.
- The most common complication not related to the scar is **seroma formation** (6%-70%).[10,13]
  - These are typically aspirated in the office.

Top Takeaways

➤ The most common postsurgical complaint is the scar; therefore, remember to mark patients using a red marker during consultation to show them where the scar will be. Have them leave the consultation with the markings to see if they can get used to it.

➤ Identify your preferred scar placement, and use anatomic landmarks for its placement.

➤ Combining liposuction with brachioplasty will enhance the overall result.

➤ Use towel clamps to reconfirm skin resection before making an incision.

➤ Consider intraoperative drain placement.

References

1. Knoetgen J, Moran S. Long-term outcomes and complications associated with brachioplasty: a retrospective review and cadaveric study. Plast Reconstr Surg 117:2219, 2006.

2. Appelt EA, Janis JE, Rohrich RJ. An algorithmic approach to upper arm contouring. Plast Reconstr Surg 118:237, 2006.

3. Samra S, Sawh-Martinez R, Liu YJ, et al. Optimal placement of brachioplasty scar: a survey evaluation. Plast Reconstr Surg 126:77, 2010.

4. Abramson DL. Minibrachioplasty: minimizing scars while maximizing results. Plast Reconstr Surg 114:1631, 2004.

5. Aly AS, ed. Body Contouring After Massive Weight Loss. New York: Thieme Publishers, 2006.

6. Lockwood T. Brachioplasty with superficial fascial system suspension. Plast Reconstr Surg 96:912, 1995.

7. Shermak MA, Mallalieu J, Chang D. Barbed suture impact on wound closure in body contouring. Plast Reconstr Surg 126:1735, 2010.

8. Bossert RP, Dreifuss S, Coon D, et al. Liposuction of the arm concurrent with brachioplasty in the massive weight loss patient: is it safe? Plast Reconstr Surg 131:357, 2013.

9. Baroudi R. Body sculpturing. Clin Plast Surg 11:419, 1984.

10. Gusenoff JA, Coon D, Rubin JP. Brachioplasty and concomitant procedures after massive weight loss: a statistical analysis from a prospective registry. Plast Reconstr Surg 122:595, 2008.

11. Cannistra C, Valero R, Benelli C, et al. Brachioplasty after massive weight loss: a simple algorithm for surgical plane. Aesthetic Plast Surg 31:6, 2007.

12. Knoetgen J III, Morgan SL. Long-term outcomes and complications associated with brachioplasty: as retrospective review and cadaveric study. Plast Reconstr Surg 117:2219, 2006.

13. Zomerlei TA, Neman KC, Armstrong SD, et al. Brachioplasty outcomes: a review of a multipractice cohort. Plast Reconstr Surg 131:883, 2013.

59. Buttock Augmentation

Sammy Sinno, Constantino G. Mendieta

BACKGROUND[1]

- Buttock augmentation rapidly increasing in popularity
  - 58% increase in 2014 in the United States according to the American Society for Aesthetic Plastic Surgery
  - Over 35,000 patients have had gluteal implants placed in the United States and Brazil.
  - Approximately 10,000 patients per year undergo buttock augmentation with fat grafting in the U.S.
  - Celebrity and social media attention to gluteal augmentation has attracted even more interest in the general population.
- **Three major methods of augmentation**
  - Autologous fat grafting
  - Silicone implants
  - Autologous flap augmentation (in massive-weight-loss patients)

INDICATIONS[2-4]

- Ideal for patients in good health who desire improved gluteal shape and contour
- Thin patients typically have very dramatic results.
- Overweight patients require additional liposuction to improve contour.
- Slightly overweight patients are excellent candidates for autologous fat grafting.
  - Excellent results seen for patients with excess sacral, lower back, and posterior triangle fat

> **SENIOR AUTHOR TIP:** The choice of operation, autologous fat grafting versus silicone implants for gluteal augmentation is typically based on amount of fat available. If the patient has enough fat, a fat grafting is performed. If not, a gluteal implant is performed. To date, no systematic reviews exist that compare overall safety and efficacy of these two strategies (particularly for implants).

CONTRAINDICATIONS

- Pregnancy
- Neoplasm
- Severe comorbid conditions

PREOPERATIVE EVALUATION

- Understand the anatomy of the gluteus maximus muscle (Fig. 59-1).
  - Origin along lateral sacrum and continues upward to posterior iliac spine
  - Attaches to superior iliac crest
  - Inserts into iliotibial tract and greater trochanter

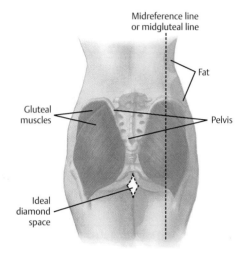

Fig. 59-1 Gluteus maximus muscle anatomy.

- Divide each buttock into four quadrants.

TIP: Ideally, each quadrant should have equal volume.

- Understand key anatomic landmarks (discussed below).

TIP: The lower inner gluteal fold ideally is diamond shaped.

- Evaluate the buttock laterally.
  - Presacral area should have a lazy-S shape.
- Preoperative pinch test to evaluate donor fat areas

SENIOR AUTHOR TIP: For autologous fat grafting, ensure patients have enough donor fat, because the amount of fat needed can range from 450-1800 cc or greater per side.

INFORMED CONSENT

- Fat grafting patients should be informed that lipoharvest, not liposuction, for removal is goal.
- Silicone implant patients should be informed of risk of wound dehiscence, implant exposure, capsular contracture, infection, seroma, extrusion, and displacement.
- Patients should be encouraged to avoid any medications that may promote bleeding before surgery.
- Enema is given day before surgery.
- Preoperative antibiotics are commonly given.

> **SENIOR AUTHOR TIP:** Keep in mind that aesthetic ideals for gluteal augmentation may vary between ethnic groups.

EQUIPMENT

AUTOLOGOUS FAT GRAFTING[2,5]

- Large-bore cannula (4 mm and 5 mm)
- Several techniques for processing, including centrifugation, can be used but are time consuming.

> **TIP:** A metal strainer can be used to irrigate and purify autologous fat.

- Large-volume syringes (60 cc), Autoinfusion systems do not exist.

SILICONE IMPLANTS

- Lighted retractors
- Long instruments
- Implant selection (silicone)
  - High cohesive gel–filled texturized
  - High cohesive gel–filled polyurethane surface cover
  - Elastomer solid implant
  - Can be anatomic, oval, or round shaped

TECHNIQUE

AUTOLOGOUS FAT GRAFTING (MENDIETA)[6-10]

- Conceptualizing the 10 aesthetic units of the posterior region is essential.
- Respecting these aesthetic units is crucial to obtain a smooth contour (Fig. 59-2).

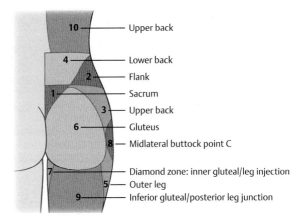

Fig. 59-2   Mendieta's 10 aesthetic units or zones. (*1*, Sacrum; *2*, flank; *3*, upper back; *4*, lower back; *5*, outer leg; *6*, gluteus; *7*, diamond zone: inner gluteal/leg injection; *8*, midlateral buttock point C; *9*, inferior gluteal/posterior leg junction; *10*, upper back.)

- General or IV sedation
- Patient marked standing; all zones
- Landmark areas identified
  - Posterior superior iliac spine (marks gluteal muscle height)
  - Presacral "V" (superior point of intergluteal fold and posterior iliac dimples)
    - ▶ Zone 1
    - ▶ When liposuctioned creates desirable contour
  - Midlateral buttock contour
    - ▶ Ideally has no depression
- Can give preoperative steroids for swelling, antibiotics, antireflux medications (patient will be in prone position)
- Wetting solution injected
- Supine position
- Fat harvest through 5 mm cannula in deep layers and 4 mm cannula in superficial layers
  - Most fat in buttock removed from zones 1, 2, 3, and 4

TIP: Typically, liposculpt zones 1 through 4, carefully liposuction in zone 5, and remember that fat transfer is difficult in zone 8 because of the paucity of muscle.

- Suctioning can be performed with patients in either lateral decubitus or prone positioning, depending on zones targeted.

TIP: It is helpful to have sterile straps to move patients frequently on the operating table.

- Fat is strained in metal strainer.
- Fat is loaded into larger syringes and injected.
  - Goal is to add volume and improve contour.

- Fat injections should be performed with patients in supine, lateral decubitus, and prone positions.
- Penrose drains can be placed to reduce occurrence of seromas but are not necessary.

SILICONE IMPLANTS[11,12]
- **Four possible planes (Fig. 59-3): Subcutaneous** (rarely used), **submuscular, intramuscular, subfascial**
  - Submuscular approach has potential for sciatic nerve injury
  - Intramuscular approach has disadvantages of difficult dissection and seroma incidence, although it is more commonly used in the United States.
- de la Peña described anatomic basis of subfascial technique, capable of securing implant with little associated morbidity.[13]
  - Requires textured gel implants

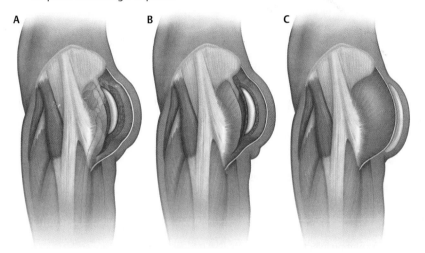

Fig. 59-3   Common locations for silicone implant placement for gluteal augmentation: **A,** submuscular, **B,** intramuscular, and **C,** subfascial.

- General or epidural anesthesia
  - Paramedial incisions are marked 1 cm lateral to midline.
  - Markings must respect gluteal shape (Fig. 59-4).

TIP: Preserve the sacral triangle and infragluteal fold.

  - Incision begins 4 cm above the anus and extends superiorly for 6-7 cm.
  - Dissection is above presacral fascia, then proceeds laterally to sacral bone.
  - 8-10 cm incision is made parallel to lateral sacrum in gluteal aponeurosis, to the subfascial space.

TIP: Hydrodissection under the gluteal aponeurosis can help to identify the avascular plane.

- Sharp dissection is performed between aponeurotic expansions.
- Superior and inferior gluteal artery perforators are ligated, if encountered.
- Sterile sizer is used before selecting final implant.
- Meticulous hemostasis is achieved and drain placed.
- Definitive implant is inserted using no-touch technique.
- Closure with aponeurosis reinsertion is performed using 2-0 Monocryl.
- Superficial and deep subcutaneous fascia are closed with 4-0 Monocryl.
- Skin is closed distinctly and skin glue applied.
- Long-acting local anesthetic is injected for pain.

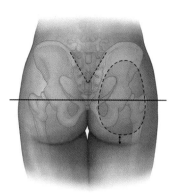

Fig. 59-4   Skin markings.

Intramuscular Placement (Vergara and colleagues)[14,15]
- One incision is made in gluteal cleft or two incisions separated within the cleft.
- Fascia is opened along muscle fibers for 5 cm.
- Muscle is entered with tonsil.
- Using alternate spreading achieves muscle depth of 2.5-3 cm.
- Muscle is opened along entire length of fascial incision.
- Deaver retractors are used to create a pocket intramuscularly.
  - No defined pocket exists, but keep 3 cm thickness.
- Curve deeper as dissection proceeds laterally.

TIP: A special muscle dissector can be used to help define the pocket.

- Wound is packed with lap pads for hemostasis.

Autologous Fat Augmentation ("Autoaugmentation") (Colwell and Borud)[16]
- Massive-weight-loss patients have excess skin and fat between the iliac crest and superior gluteal margin.
  - Also have dropping of central crease and inferior gluteal crease
- Patient is in standing position while marked.
- Anatomic zones are marked as detailed previously.
- L5 dimple is noted, and low point of V is marked 5 cm below.
- Upper incision is made just above posterior superior iliac spine and continued laterally just above the gluteus medius muscle.
- Upper flap is immobile.

TIP: Design the incision to have a final scar in the boundary between the gluteal region and the back.

- Lower incision is within the upper margin of the central crease.

- Doppler probe is used for identification of perforators.
- Flap is designed around two perforators 6-9 cm from midline on each side (Fig. 59-5).

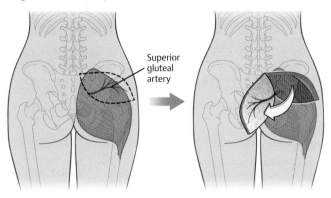

Superior gluteal artery

Fig. 59-5   Flap design with inferomedial rotation.

- Midline tissue that does not contain perforators is excised to reduce fullness.
- Flaps are deepithelialized.
- Gluteal pocket is created above gluteus muscle, allowing inferomedial rotation of flap, which is tacked to fascia with 0 PDS suture.
- Inferior gluteal skin is advanced superiorly.
- Incisions are closed in layers.
- Two drains are placed.

POSTOPERATIVE CARE

- Similar for all techniques of gluteal augmentation
  - Precise details vary from surgeon to surgeon.
- Compressive garments worn for 1 month
- Sitting restricted to bathroom only for 2 weeks
- Otherwise, pressure on buttocks avoided for 6 weeks
- Normal activity resumed at 2 weeks
- Refrain from exercise for 3 months, refrain from bicycle or horseback riding for 3-6 months (risk of wound dehiscence).

COMPLICATIONS[17,18]

- **Autologous fat:** Less common
  - Skin irregularities
- Infection: 2%
  - Pain or sciatica: 2%
  - Seroma: 3%
  - Fat resorption
  - Oil cysts
  - Wound-healing problems

- Fat embolus syndrome and macroscopic fat embolism
  - Complications that occur when fat enters bloodstream
  - Fat can be introduced into the **inferior gluteal vein,** which drains into the iliac veins then into the inferior vena cava.
  - More likely to occur with increased volumes, intramuscular placement, and injection near the piriformis muscle (location of gluteal vessels)
  - Maintain high index of suspicion if patients show signs of **confusion, petechiae, fever, or respiratory distress** postoperatively.
  - Can result in major complications including **death**
  - Can be avoided by keeping injection cannula parallel (not perpendicular) to patient and injections subcutaneous, avoiding excess volumes of injection, and maintain hydration

TIP: A review of the literature showed an approximately 8% complication rate with autologous fat injection.

- **Silicone implants**: More common[19]
  - Implants have been shown to cause muscle atrophy in CT and three-dimensional volume studies.
  - Wound dehiscence: 10%
  - Seroma: 5%
  - Infection: 2%
  - Paresthesia: 1%
  - Implant exposure
  - Capsular contracture
  - Chronic pain

TIP: A review of the literature showed an approximately 20%-40% complication rate with silicone implants.

Top Takeaways
- Buttock augmentation is rapidly increasing in popularity.
- Three major methods of augmentation are autologous fat grafting, silicone implants, and autologous flap augmentation.
- The choice of operation for gluteal augmentation—autologous fat grafting versus silicone implants—is typically based on available fat.
- Know and understand Mendieta's 10 gluteal region zones; zones 1-4 are typically liposculpted.
- Hydrodissection under the gluteal aponeurosis can help to identify the avascular plane.
- Autoaugmentation can be used for gluteal contouring in massive-weight-loss patients.
- In the available literature, gluteal augmentation with implants appears to be associated with a higher overall complication rate compared with augmentation using autologous fat. Fat is the preferred reshaping and augmentation method.
- Implant augmentation is reserved for patients who do not have enough fat available for transfer.

REFERENCES

1. American Society for Aesthetic Plastic Surgery. Statistics, surveys, and trends. Available at *http://www.surgery.org/media/news-releases/statistics-surveys-and-trends.*
2. Tardif M, de la Peña JA. Gluteal augmentation. In Aston SJ, Steinbrech DS, Walden JL, eds. Aesthetic Plastic Surgery. Philadelphia: Saunders Elsevier, 2009.
3. Cádenas-Camarena L, Arenas-Quintana R, Robles-Cervantes JA. Buttocks fat grafting: 14 years of evolution and experience. Plast Reconstr Surg 128:545, 2011.
4. Centeno RF, Young VL. Clinical anatomy in aesthetic gluteal body contouring surgery. Clin Plast Surg 33:347, 2006.
5. Guerrerosantos J. Autologous fat grafting for body contouring. Clin Plast Surg 23:619, 1996.
6. Mendieta CG. Classification system for gluteal evaluation. Clin Plast Surg 33:333, 2006.
7. Mendieta CG. Gluteal reshaping. Aesthet Surg J 27:641, 2007.
8. Mendieta CG. Gluteoplasty. Aesthet Surg J 23:441, 2003.
9. Nahai F. The Art of Aesthetic Surgery: Principles & Techniques. New York: Thieme Publishers, 2005.
10. Peren PA, Gomez JB, Guerrerosantos J, et al. Gluteus augmentation with fat grafting. Aesthetic Plast Surg 24:412, 2000.
11. Robles JM, Tagliapietra JC, Grandi MA. Gluteoplastia de augmento: implante submuscular. Cirplast Ibero Latinoam 10:365, 1984.
12. Serra F, Aboudib JH, Marques RG. Intramuscular technique for gluteal augmentation: determination and quantification of muscle atrophy and implant position by computed tomographic scan. Plast Reconstr Surg 131:253e, 2013.
13. de la Peña JA. Subfascial technique for gluteal augmentation. Aesthet Surg J 24:265, 2004.
14. Vergara R, Amezcua H. Intramuscular gluteal implants: 15 years' experience. Aesthet Surg J 23:86, 2003.
15. Vergara R, Marcos M. Intramuscular gluteal implants. Aesthet Plast Surg 20:259, 1996.
16. Colwell AS, Borud LJ. Autologous gluteal augmentation after massive weight loss: aesthetic analysis and role of the superior gluteal artery perforator flap. Plast Reconstr Surg 119:345, 2007.
17. Bruner TW, Roberts TL, Nguyen K. Complications of buttocks augmentation: diagnosis, management, and prevention. Clin Plast Surg 33:449, 2006.
18. Sinno S, Chang JB, Brownstone ND, et al. Determining the safety and efficacy of gluteal augmentation: a systematic review of outcomes and complications. Plast Reconstr Surg 137:1151, 2016.
19. Mofid MM, Gonzalez R, de la Peña JA, Mendieta CG, et al. Buttock augmentation with silicone implants: a multicenter survey review of 2226 patients. Plast Reconstr Surg 131:897, 2013.

60. Abdominoplasty

Wesley N. Sivak, Luis M. Rios, Jr., James Christian Grotting

ANATOMY

- **The abdominal wall is composed of seven layers.**
  1. Skin
  2. Subcutaneous fat
  3. Scarpa fascia (the superficial fascial system of the abdomen)
  4. Subscarpal fat
  5. Anterior rectus sheath
  6. Muscle
  7. Posterior rectus sheath

SKIN

- The skin of the abdominal wall receives a rich vascular supply from multiple muscle and fascial perforating vessels.
- The skin of the abdominal wall can vary in quality depending on a person's genetics, age, previous pregnancies, and history of weight gain and loss.
- The skin of the abdominal wall may feature multiple **striae,** which are evidence of **attenuated or absent dermis.**

FAT

- The abdominal wall has **two** layers of fat, **superficial and deep,** separated by Scarpa fascia (Fig. 60-1).

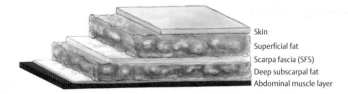

Skin
Superficial fat
Scarpa fascia (SFS)
Deep subscarpal fat
Abdominal muscle layer

Fig. 60-1   Layers of fat. (*SFS,* Superficial fascial system.)

- The **superficial layer** of fat is thicker, more dense, more durable, and has a heartier blood supply.
- The **deeper layer** of fat is less dense and receives most of its blood from the subdermal plexus and underlying myocutaneous perforators.

SENIOR AUTHOR TIP: Because the blood supply to the deeper fat is distinct from the blood supply to the skin, it can be more easily excised when thinning the abdominal wall flap in an abdominoplasty. By contrast, thinning the superficial layer of fat may lead to vascular compromise of the overlying skin.

- There are **four paired muscle groups** of the abdominal wall.
  1. Rectus abdominis
  2. External oblique
  3. Internal oblique
  4. Transversus abdominis
- The aponeurotic portions of the transversus muscle and the two oblique muscles envelop the rectus abdominis muscles, forming the anterior and posterior rectus sheaths and meeting in the midline to form the linea alba.
- The **arcuate line** represents a transition point.
  - **Above the arcuate line,** there are distinct anterior and posterior rectus sheaths.
  - **Below the arcuate line,** contributions from the internal oblique and transversus abdominus join contributions from the external and internal obliques to form a single anterior rectus sheath with no posterior rectus sheath.
  - The arcuate line is roughly halfway between the umbilicus and symphysis pubis.

VASCULARITY OF THE ABDOMINAL WALL

- Huger[1] divided the vascular supply to the abdominal wall into **three zones** (Fig. 60-2).

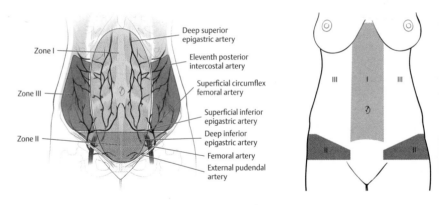

Fig. 60-2   Huger vascular zones.

- **Zone I**
  - Between the lateral borders of the rectus sheath from the costal margin to a horizontal line drawn between the two anterior superior iliac spines (ASIS)
  - Supplied primarily by superficial branches of the **superior and inferior epigastric systems**
- **Zone II**
  - Below the horizontal line between the two ASISs to the pubic and inguinal creases
  - Supplied by the superficial branches of the **circumflex iliac** and **external pudendal vessels**
- **Zone III**
  - Superior to zone II and lateral to zone I
  - Supplied by **intercostals, subcostals,** and **lumbar** vessels
- Sensation to the abdomen is from **intercostal nerves T7-12.**

NERVES AND THE ABDOMINAL WALL

LATERAL CUTANEOUS BRANCHES
- Perforate the intercostal muscles at the midaxillary line
- Travel within the subcutaneous plane

ANTERIOR CUTANEOUS BRANCHES
- Travel between the transversus abdominus and internal oblique muscles to penetrate the posterior rectus sheath just lateral to the rectus
- Eventually enter the rectus muscles and then pass to the overlying fascia and skin

LATERAL FEMORAL CUTANEOUS NERVE (Fig. 60-3)
- Innervates the skin in the lateral aspect of the thigh
- Emerges close to the ASIS

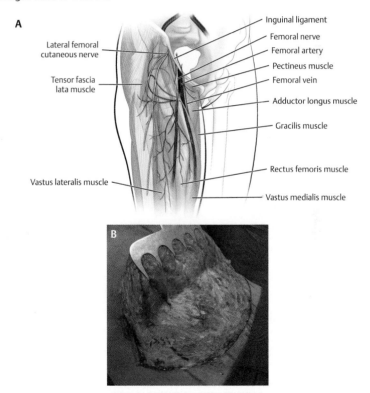

Fig. 60-3 Lateral femoral cutaneous nerve. **A,** Diagram of the nerve anatomy. **B,** Location of the ASIS in relation to the umbilicus.

TIP: To prevent injury, a layer of fat should be left over the ASIS.

- The umbilicus is located **on or near the midline at the level of the iliac crest.**
    - The umbilicus is located exactly in the midline of the body in only 1.7% of patients.[2]
    - An **aesthetically pleasing umbilicus** has the following characteristics[3]:
        ▶ Superior hooding
        ▶ Inferior retraction
        ▶ Round or ellipsoid shape
        ▶ Shallow
    - **Blood supply to the umbilicus** (Fig. 60-4) **is from:**
        ▶ Subdermal plexus
        ▶ Right and left deep inferior epigastric artery (DIEA)
        ▶ Ligamentum teres
        ▶ Median umbilical ligament

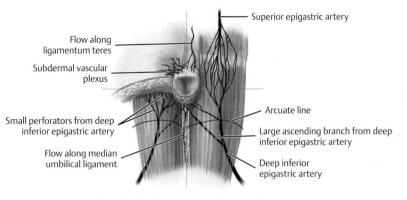

Fig. 60-4   Blood supply to the umbilicus.

AESTHETIC ASPECTS OF ABDOMINOPLASTY[4]

- Incision should be low and symmetrical
- Umbilicus
    - Inverted scar
    - Superior hooding
    - Circular or ellipsoid
- Scaphoid abdominal wall
- Smooth transition at the incision
- Aesthetic appearance of mons pubis

INDICATIONS AND CONTRAINDICATIONS

- Due to the number of variations of the abdominoplasty procedure, it is key to select the appropriate technique for each patient to minimize morbidity and deliver the intended result (Table 60-1).[5] Selection of appropriate technique is based on the patient's expectations and physical examination.

Table 60-1   *Indications*

Procedure	Excess Fat	Excess Skin	Skin Tone	Diastasis
Liposuction[6]	Mild	None	Good	None
Liposuction and endoscopic repair	Mild	None	Good	Present
Miniabdominoplasty	Infraumbilical	Infraumbilical	Good	Present
Traditional or lipoabdominoplasty	Significant and not confined to infraumbilical region	Significant and not confined to infraumbilical region	Fair to poor	Present
Circumferential	Mild to moderate	Extends to back	Fair to poor	Present
High-lateral-tension	Mild to moderate	Lateral abdominal area and thigh	Poor	Present
Fleur-de-lis	Mild to moderate	Vertical and horizontal	Fair to poor	Present
Reverse abdominoplasty	Mild to moderate	Upper abdomen	Fair to poor	Present

CONTRAINDICATIONS
- **Absolute**
  - Significant health risks, unrealistic surgical goals, and body dysmorphic disorder are **primary** contraindications for an abdominoplasty.
- **Relative**
  - Right, left, or bilateral upper abdominal scars
  - Severe comorbid conditions (e.g., heart disease, diabetes, morbid obesity [BMI >40], cigarette smoking)
  - Plans for future pregnancy
  - A history of thromboembolic disease
  - **Subcostal scars** are particularly concerning, and many of these patients are not optimal candidates for a traditional abdominoplasty.
    - ▶ These scars represent an interruption in the blood supply upon which the abdominoplasty flap will rely postoperatively.
- Patients with a disposition to **keloid** formation or **hypertrophic scars** have to be accepting of the poor scarring associated with these conditions.
- **Gross deformity in adjoining areas** may lead to disfiguring results and poor patient satisfaction.
  - Most massive-weight-loss patients are not candidates for abdominoplasty alone and will require circumferential procedures.
- **Increased intraabdominal pressures** can lead to serious problems postoperatively, possibly resulting in abdominal compartment syndrome.
  - In cases of elevated intraabdominal pressure, the abdominal wall elevates above a line between the costal margin and iliac crest in the supine position.
  - Abdominoplasty procedures with or without rectus plication have to be performed cautiously in the nonscaphoid abdomen.

PREOPERATIVE EVALUATION

- Assessment must include a detailed medical history with specific focus on:
  - Prior cesarean section or other abdominal surgeries
  - Pregnancy history
  - Weight fluctuations and stability
  - Prior liposuction in the abdominal area
  - Thromboembolic risk
  - Smoking status
  - Hormone use
  - History of postoperative nausea and vomiting (PONV)

> **TIP:** Abdominoplasty is an enormous stressor in terms of blood supply to the abdominal wall. To minimize complications, avoid operating on active smokers. If a patient has a history of smoking, insist that the patient quit smoking prior to the procedure. A thorough discussion of the increased risk of complications associated with smoking must occur. In certain cases, a urine nicotine test may be warranted preoperatively and postoperatively should complications occur.

- Other patient factors to consider include:
  - Weight fluctuations and constancy
  - Exercise routine
  - Gastrointestinal history including irritable bowel syndrome or constipation
  - Cardiac and pulmonary history (including obstructive sleep apnea)
  - Desire for future pregnancy (patients should be encouraged to wait)
- Physical examination must explore the existence and localization of vertical and horizontal abdominal tissue excess and its relation to the underlying abdominal wall; deformity present in adjoining areas must be noted as they affect the final result.

> **TIP:**   If the patient is examined only in the standing or supine positions, one may be fooled into thinking there is little to no excess skin. The patient must be examined while standing, sitting, and supine.

- Musculofascial laxity must be thoroughly assessed (Fig. 60-5).
  - A **diver's test** can be performed with the patient first standing and flexing at the waist; worsening of lower abdominal fullness indicates significant laxity (see Fig. 60-5).
  - The **pinch test** can also be performed. If tensing the abdominal wall significantly decreases the amount of fullness, significant laxity is present.
  - Midline **rectus diastasis** must be assessed by palpation of a tensed abdominal wall in the supine position.

> **TIP:**   Nearly all patients who have been pregnant have some degree of musculofascial laxity of the abdominal wall in addition to excess skin.

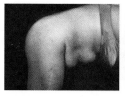 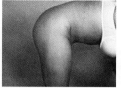 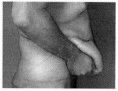

Fig. 60-5   The classic "diver's test" demonstrating the extent of abdominal wall laxity.

- Preoperative identification of any existing **ventral** or **umbilical hernia** is imperative. Examination should include evaluation for incisional, epigastric, periumbilical, and inguinal hernias—especially in patients with prior abdominal surgeries and massive weight loss.

TIP: The importance of a thorough hernia examination cannot be overstated. Preoperative knowledge of hernias can help the surgeon avoid bowel injury during dissection. Depending on the site of the hernia and the comfort level of the plastic surgeon, preoperative knowledge of a hernia may allow repair to be coordinated with a general surgeon. In cases of uncertainty, a computed tomography (CT) scan is indicated.

- The presence of **scars** represents alterations to the blood supply of the abdominal wall and must be thoroughly assessed.
  - ▸ **Upper midline scars** may limit the inferior movement of the abdominal skin flap; they may require release at the time of abdominoplasty.
  - ▸ **Subcostal scars** represent an interruption of the superolateral blood supply that the abdominoplasty flap relies upon postoperatively (these patient are at highest risk of complications).

CAUTION: To prevent wound-healing complications, the abdominal wall skin flap must not be undermined beneath a subcostal incision. The limitations of undermining, limited results, and high risk of complications must be discussed with these patients. Many are not candidates for abdominoplasty.

- Examine for **rashes** or **excoriations** on the abdominal wall, especially under the pannus in obese and massive-weight-loss patients.
- Photographic documentation consisting of eight views should be obtained preoperatively and postoperatively: anterior, oblique anterior, side, oblique posterior, posterior, anterior sitting position, bending position (both front and side views) (see Chapter 3).
  - ▸ Views with the patient's abdominal wall contracted and relaxed may also prove beneficial in surgical planning.
  - ▸ Views with the patient grasping and holding up excess abdominal tissue in the central and waist areas may also prove useful.

INFORMED CONSENT

- In addition to the standard risks of surgery, the surgeon must discuss the location and length of **scars** with the patient. Considerations include:
  - Standard lower abdominal transverse scar
  - Standard circumumbilical scar
  - Potential need for a midline vertical scar
  - Potential for cutaneous deformities or "dog-ears" at the lateral ends of the abdominoplasty incision
- Abdominal **striae** located inferior to the umbilicus may be removed as part of the abdominoplasty. Above the umbilicus, striae will not be removed and *may become more prominent* as a result of abdominoplasty.
- Wound-healing complications must be discussed as both the transverse incision at the waist and the umbilicus are at risk due to the blood supply to these regions following the abdominoplasty procedure.
- **Loss or malposition of the umbilicus** must be discussed; patient should be reminded that the structure is truly midline in only **1.7%** of patients.[2,7]
- Risk of postoperative **seroma** formation should be discussed; the need and purpose for postoperative drains should be thoroughly explained (if used).
- Comprehensive postoperative care instructions should be fully discussed. The use of any additional recommended materials such as compression garments or specialized dressings and the associated costs should be fully disclosed.
- Potential need for secondary revision surgeries or additional procedures must be discussed.

> **TIP:** Most patients requesting abdominoplasty have at least some degree of fat excess in the hips, flanks, or thighs. These areas will become more noticeable postoperatively. The patient should be made aware of this and should be encouraged to consider concomitant or staged liposuction procedures. Failure to disclose this preoperatively will result in an unhappy patient with a less than optimal result.

- Financial arrangements and the patient's responsibilities for procedures should be explained and agreed upon preoperatively. The discussion should include fee structures for secondary procedures.
- Patients must understand that they may not be able to walk fully erect for several days following the procedure. They must be agreeable to 2 weeks off from work and a minimum of 6 weeks without strenuous exercise or lifting.
- The patient must be warned of the risk and life-threatening nature of venous thromboembolism. Fully detail strategies utilized to minimize this risk (e.g., early ambulation, pneumatic compression devices, chemoprophylaxis)[8] (see Chapter 11).

> **TIP:** SCD must be applied and started prior to induction of anesthesia.

■ **Infection:** Risk in the literature is 0% to 0.8%. The Surgical Care Improvement Project (SCIP) identifies areas to reduce the risk of infection (Box 60-1).

Box 60-1   *SCIP PROTOCOL*

Shaving is not required. Do not use razors.
IV antibiotics given 30-59 minutes before the incision
24 hours of postoperative antibiotics
Elective surgery with Hgb A1C <7
Avoid intraoperative hypothermia
Foley catheter out within 24 hours

TECHNIQUE

TRADITIONAL ABDOMINOPLASTY
Preoperative Markings

TIP: Patients should be encouraged to wear their undergarments of choice the day of surgery to aid in planning of the incisions and scar placement.

■ Preoperative markings begin with identification of the pubic bone and the anterior superior iliac crest.
■ The planned incision should be marked transversely at the level of the pubic bone.
   • At least **5 cm** must be left between this incision and the top of the vulval commissure to prevent postoperative deformity.
■ The planned incision should extend laterally below the anterior superior iliac spine (ASIS).
■ If possible, keep the incisions low in order to prevent visibility of the scar.
■ With the patient standing, the lateral aspects of the abdominal folds are marked. This is a guide to the lateral extension of the incision.
■ A pinch test should be performed to determine how much skin could be comfortably resected and a proposed upper incision is marked.
■ Areas for concomitant liposuction should be marked at this time.

Surgical Technique
■ Orientation of the umbilicus can be done with placement of two traction sutures 180 degrees apart.
■ The umbilicus is incised circularly, and dissecting scissors are used to separate the umbilicus from the subcutaneous fat all the way down to the rectus sheath.

TIP: Leave a small cuff of fat around the umbilical stalk, as skeletonizing the umbilical stalk can lead to compromised vascularity of the umbilicus and postoperative necrosis.

■ The inferior incision is carried out bilaterally and dissection is taken through Scarpa fascia.

> **TIP:** Leave a small amount of fat on the musculofascia in the region of the ASIS to prevent injury to the lateral femoral cutaneous nerve. Injury to this nerve can cause significant pain, numbness and dysesthesia in the hip and medial thigh (a condition known as *meralgia paraesthetica*). van Uchelen et al found a 10% incidence of injury in their review of abdominoplasty procedures[9] (see Fig. 60-3, *B*).

■ The skin and fat of the abdominal wall is elevated from the underlying fascia in a loose areolar plane up to the costal margins and the xiphoid process.
■ Limited undermining is done from the umbilicus to the xiphoid.

> **TIP:** As dissection proceeds along the musculofascia centrally, be careful not to transect the umbilical stalk. A number of periumbilical perforators present serve as warning to the surgeon to slow dissection and preserve the umbilical stalk.

■ Once the abdominal flap is elevated, any rectus diastasis or hernia repair is performed (Fig. 60-6). Rectus plication should be performed with **permanent or long-acting resorbable sutures**[10]
  • A cotton-tipped applicator is used to apply methylene blue to the rectus sheath in an elliptical area to be imbricated.
  • The rectus sheath is imbricated by placing interrupted sutures along the borders of the elliptical area.
  • Reinforcing sutures should be run from the xiphoid process to the umbilicus and from the umbilicus to the pubis.
  • Horizontal plication sutures are used if necessary.

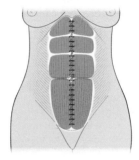

Fig. 60-6 Plication sutures of abdomen, including horizontal sutures.

> **TIP:** It is vital to begin rectus plication at the level of the xiphoid process. Failure to do so can result in a postoperative bulge in the epigastric area.

■ Surgical drains, if used, should be brought out through the lateral incision, thus avoiding unsightly scars in the mons pubis. Drains should be affixed at the exit site with permanent suture.
■ The bed is then flexed to a beach chair position with the hips flexed approximately 30 degrees. The amount of skin and fat that can safely be removed and allow for a tension-free closure is marked.
■ Excess skin and subcutaneous fat are resected.
■ Copiously irrigate the wound and temporarily tack the skin closed.

SENIOR AUTHOR TIP: In order to avoid "dog-ears," advance the flaps medially. If necessary, do not hesitate to extend the scar laterally

- Interrupted 2-0 Vicryl progressive tension sutures can be placed to secure the flap to the abdominal wall (which may obviate drain placement).
- The level of the umbilicus is transposed with a marking pen to the overlying skin of the abdominal wall; the umbilicus is inset.
- The superficial fascial system (i.e., Scarpa fascia) is closed with interrupted sutures, followed by closure of the deep dermal and subcuticular layers. Surgical cyanoacrylate glue may also be applied.

TIP: If surgical cyanoacrylate glues are used, be sure to allow adequate drying time prior to applying a gauze dressing.

- A gauze dressing is placed and held in place with an abdominal binder. The patient is transferred to a hospital bed in the flexed position.

PROGRESSIVE TENSION SUTURES[11-13] (Fig. 60-7) (see Chapter 28)

- The abdominal flap is sutured and advanced onto the musculofascia using interrupted 2-0 Vicryl or running continuous barbed suture.
- As the flap is advanced, progressive tension is exerted on each suture and away from the incision.
- Decreased tension on the incision prevents necrosis and hypertrophic scars.
- The dead space is closed, preventing hematoma and seroma formation.
- Sutures can be used in lipoabdominoplasty, other forms of abdominoplasty, and body contour surgery.
- Running barbed sutures have also been effectively used as PTS sutures.[13]

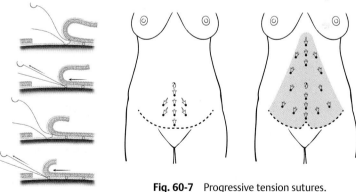

Fig. 60-7   Progressive tension sutures.

LIPOABDOMINOPLASTY[14]

- The areas for liposuction are marked, usually avoiding liposuction of the upper midline.
- Superwet technique is used.
- Ultrasonic or traditional suction-assisted liposuction (SAL) is safe.
- A thin layer of fat is left on the abdominal wall to preserve lymphatic supply. At least 17% of lymphatics are preserved below Scarpa fascia.[15]
- Selective undermining of the flap is limited to the central area that will require plication, most commonly to the lateral border of the rectus[3,16] (Fig. 60-8).

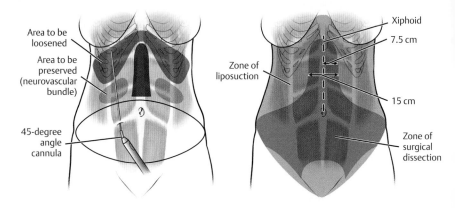

Fig. 60-8   Central (selective undermining) of abdominoplasty flap.

- The abdominal perforators at the lateral aspect of the rectus muscle are preserved.[8]
- Progressive tension sutures (PTS) and/or drains can be used.
- Saldanha et al[14] theorized that 80% of blood supply, nerves, and lymphatics are preserved with this technique, thus contributing to their low rate of seroma (0.4%), dehiscence, necrosis, and hematoma. The incidence of DVT and PE remain the same.
- Roostaeian et al[17] showed, via laser fluorescence imaging, that lipoabdominoplasty maintained flap perfusion as well as wide undermining. The authors concluded lipoabdominoplasty was as safe as traditional abdominoplasty.

> **SENIOR AUTHOR TIP:**   Lipoabdominoplasty is safe if selective undermining principles are followed. Flap perfusion is equivalent in traditional lipoabdominoplasty compared to traditional abdominoplasty.

MINIABDOMINOPLASTY

- The miniabdominoplasty is indicated in patients with primarily an excess of *isolated infraumbilical skin and fat*.[3,16] This is not a very common procedure.
- A **shorter scar** is planned than for traditional abdominoplasty; the scar should be **12-16 cm** in length.

- The umbilicus remains attached to the abdominal flap. If necessary, the umbilical stalk is transected at the level of the anterior rectus sheath.
    - The fascial defect created by umbilical transection **must** be repaired.
- Rectus diastasis, if present, is repaired using **permanent** or **long-acting resorbable sutures.**
- Excess skin and fat is resected; this is a much more conservative resection than performed for traditional abdominoplasty (Fig. 60-9).
    - The umbilicus will generally move **2 cm inferiorly** using this technique.
- Liposuction is frequently added to the miniabdominoplasty to improve overall abdominal contour, especially in the supraumbilical region.

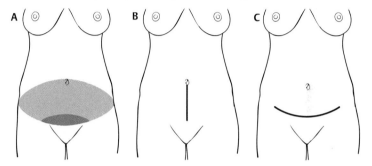

Fig. 60-9   Miniabdominoplasty. **A,** Skin elevated and skin cut out. **B,** Musculofascial repair. **C,** Scar.

HIGH-LATERAL-TENSION ABDOMINOPLASTY

- Lockwood high-lateral-tension abdominoplasty is indicated in patients with excess skin infraumbilically that is primarily **vertical** in nature and excess skin in the epigastric region that is primarily **horizontal** in nature.[18]
    - Lockwood believed that the skin of the epigastrium develops horizontal laxity due to strong superficial fascial attachments to the linea alba, limiting vertical descent of the skin.
    - During the procedure, less skin is taken centrally and more is resected laterally, resulting in an **oblique vector** of pull.
    - Undermining is only performed centrally in an area that allows for rectus plication.
- The procedure also has the advantage of performing a lift of the anterior and lateral thighs; it also allows for liposculpture of the abdominal wall.
- Patients must be aware the scars are typically longer and higher in this procedure.
- **Preoperative markings**
    - Marking begins with a suprapubic mark 7.0 cm superior to the vulvar commissure or base of the penis.
    - The ASIS is marked bilaterally and connected to the suprapubic mark.
    - The vertical excess of infraumbilical skin is then pulled taut and the edge of the skin meeting the inferior incision line is marked.
    - Excess skin laterally is tested using a pinch test and marked; this is then connected to the inferior edge of the vertical excess.

- The proposed incision should lie below the level of the umbilicus centrally and above the level of the umbilicus laterally.
- Proposed areas of liposuction are then marked both centrally and laterally.
■ **Surgical technique**
  - The lower incision is opened and the skin and fat are elevated off the rectus fascia centrally just enough to allow for rectus plication; rectus plication is performed.
  - Laterally the abdominal skin flap remains connected to the underlying rectus fascia but is loosened by discontinuous undermining using vertical spreading with Mayo scissors, the surgeon's finger, an oversized suction cannula, or a Lockwood Underminer.
  - The amount of skin and fat that can be resected centrally and laterally is confirmed using a pinch test.

TIP: Remember, the more skin and fat should be resected laterally than centrally when utilizing this technique.

- The umbilical stalk can be left in place or transected and left to float in place. Alternatively, it can also be excised and translocated as in a traditional abdominoplasty procedure.
- The wound is temporarily tacked closed and then liposuction is performed.
- Drains are placed and secured.
- The superficial fascial system (i.e., Scarpa fascia) is repaired with intermittent sutures, followed by closure of the deep dermis and the skin.

FLEUR-DE-LIS ABDOMINOPLASTY (Fig. 60-10)

■ The *fleur-de-lis* technique allows for excision of both lower abdominal skin and fat and supraumbilical horizontal excess skin through a transverse incision.[19]
■ The vertical midline incision can be taken as high as the xiphoid process and as low as the mons pubis, depending upon the areas of skin laxity.

TIP: It is paramount to leave the skin flaps attached to the underlying fascia, except in areas contained within the fleur-de-lis excision, to maximize vascularity.[3]

■ This procedure can cause powerful changes to the abdominal contour not available with other techniques. The resulting scars must be discussed with the patient because they can be rather significant.

Fig. 60-10   Fleur-de-lis abdominoplasty.

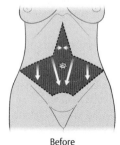 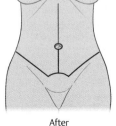

Before   After

REVERSE ABDOMINOPLASTY (Fig. 60-11)

- A transverse upper abdominal incision is made roughly at the level of the inframammary fold, and redundant superior abdominal tissue is pulled up to meet this incision and excised.[20]
- The principal indication for this procedure is the correction of redundant tissue left superiorly after lower abdominoplasty; rarely a patient will present with isolated excess skin and abdominal protuberance in the epigastric region of the abdomen.
- The reverse abdominoplasty can be combined with breast procedures (e.g., a Wise-pattern reduction of mastopexy) as the inframammary fold incision can be used for both procedures.

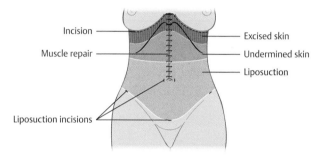

Incision

Muscle repair

Excised skin

Undermined skin

Liposuction

Liposuction incisions

Fig. 60-11   Reverse abdominoplasty.

POSTOPERATIVE CARE

- Operations can be performed in either outpatient or inpatient setting.
  - Miniabdominoplasty can easily be performed on an outpatient basis.
  - Traditional abdominoplasty can be safely performed as an outpatient procedure in healthy patients.[21]
  - Patients with preexisting scars should be observed for possible disturbances of blood supply.
- **Early ambulation is mandatory;** frequent breathing exercises and use of incentive spirometer should be encouraged to prevent postoperative atelectasis.
- Drains, if used, are left in place until discharge is <30 ml in two-consecutive 24-hour periods; showering is permitted following drain removal.
- The patient should rest in a flexed position (approximately 30 degrees of flexion at the hip joint) for 2-3 weeks postoperatively to ensure tension-free healing.
- Postoperative follow-up examinations should evaluate for seroma formation.
- Patients should be asked about bowel function; stool softeners should be provided to avoid constipation and straining with defecation (especially when plication or hernia repair has been performed).
- Silicone sheeting or steroid impregnated tape may be applied to the incisions once healed for a period of 3 months, which may improve the appearance of the scars.

■ Strenuous activities should be avoided for a minimum of 6 weeks postoperatively (8 weeks in the case of hernia repair or plication).
■ An abdominal binder is worn until the drains are removed. At this time the patient is switched to compression garments. Often times, patients enjoy the compression and security of the garments and elect to wear them a few months after surgery.
■ Patients should be advised to avoid sunbathing or tanning beds for 1 year postoperatively to avoid pigment changes in the remodeling scar. Sunblock should be liberally applied when sun avoidance is not possible.
■ Any complaint of shortness of breath should be taken seriously and venous duplex ultrasound should be considered on stable patients.

COMPLICATIONS

■ Patients can routinely expect postoperative pain and soreness, numbness of the abdominoplasty flap, bruising, fatigue, and discomfort due to increased abdominal tension for weeks following the procedure.
■ **Local (minor) complications include**[22-25]:
  • Hematoma (0.6%-1.3%)
  • Seroma (5.0%-15.4%)
  • Wound infection (0.3%-3.5%)
  • Fat necrosis (2.0%)
  • Wound dehiscence (2%)
    ▶ Minor wound dehiscence is common and normally self-limiting
    ▶ Major wound dehiscence may be due to excess tension or marginal wound necrosis
  • Paresthesias and persistent numbness
■ **Systemic (major) complications include**[22-25]:
  • **Deep vein thrombosis/pulmonary embolism** (0.3%-0.8%) (see Chapter 11)
  • The Caprini risk assessment model is a helpful tool to determine a patient's risk for deep vein thrombosis (Fig. 60-12).
  • Respiratory compromise and abdominal compartment syndrome
  • Systemic infections
■ Surgeons should be aware that abdominoplasty, especially when combined with other procedures such as liposuction, has a higher systemic complication rate than any other type of routine aesthetic surgical procedure.
■ If chemoprophylaxis used, administer for 7 days postoperative.
■ Any patient with complaints of postoperative shortness of breath should have a venous ultrasound.
■ PE is evaluated with CT scan.
■ Future studies still needed to determine indications, dosage, timing and length of prophylaxis

Choose All That Apply

Each Risk Factor Represents 1 Point
☐ Age 41-60 years
☐ Minor surgery planned
☐ History of prior major surgery (<1 month)
☐ Varicose veins
☐ History of inflammatory bowel disease
☐ Swollen legs (current)
☐ Obesity (BMI >25)
☐ Acute myocardial infarction
☐ Congestive heart failure (<1 month)
☐ Sepsis (<1 month)
☐ Serious lung disease incl. pneumonia (<1 month)
☐ Abnormal pulmonary function (COPD)
☐ Medical patient currently at bed rest
☐ Other risk factors _____

Each Risk Factor Represents 3 Points
☐ Age over 75 years
☐ History of DVT/PE
☐ **Family history of thrombosis***
☐ Positive factor V Leiden
☐ Positive prothrombin 20210A
☐ Elevated serum homocysteine
☐ Positive lupus anticoagulent
☐ Elevated anticardiolipin antibodies
☐ Heparin-induced thrombocytopenia (HIT)
☐ Other congenital or acquired thrombophilia
If yes:
Type _____
*most frequently missed risk factor

Each Risk Factor Represents 2 Points
☐ Age 60-74 years
☐ Arthroscopic surgery
☐ Malignancy (present or previous)
☐ Major surgery (>45 minutes)
☐ Laparoscopic surgery (>45 minutes)
☐ Patient confined to bed (>72 hours)
☐ Immobilizing plaster cast (<1 month)
☐ Central venous access

Each Risk Factor Represents 5 Points
☐ Elective major lower extremity arthroplasty
☐ Hip, pelvis, or leg fracture (<1 month)
☐ Stroke (<1 month)
☐ Multiple trauma (<1 month)
☐ Acute spinal cord injury (paralysis) (<1 month)

For Women Only (Each Represents 1 Point)
☐ Oral contraceptives or hormone replacement therapy
☐ Pregnancy or postpartum (<1 month)
☐ History of unexplained stillborn infant, recurrent spontaneous abortion (≥3), premature birth with toxemia or growth-restricted infant

Total Risk Factor Score ☐

Fig. 60-12   Caprini risk assessment model.

Top Takeaways

➤ An abdominoplasty is considered a major surgical procedure and must be approached systematically to avoid complications.

➤ It is mandatory to analyze any suspected skin tumor in the area of excised tissues.

➤ Be precise in determining the best procedure for the patient based on preoperative expectations and physical examination.

➤ Avoid operating on BMI >40 and try to operate on candidates with BMI <30 if possible.

➤ Examine abdominal wall for scars, rashes, and hernias.

Continued

> ➤ Consider CT scan of abdominal wall if ventral hernias are suspected.
> ➤ Examine abdominal wall in a supine position to measure if it is scaphoid and amenable to plication.
> ➤ To get best results, encourage liposuction of lower back and mons pubis if needed.
> ➤ Preoperative medical evaluation is imperative before operating.
> ➤ Have policies for operating on smokers and diabetics.
> ➤ Address constipation and consider a laxative, such as polyethylene glycol 3350, preoperatively and postoperatively.
> ➤ Have patients clean umbilicus daily starting the week before surgery.
> ➤ Determine history of postoperative nausea and vomiting and be proactive to prevent this complication.
> ➤ DVT risk assessment for all patients and strategy for high-risk patients
> ➤ Consider using the SCIP protocol to decrease surgical site infections (SSIs).
> ➤ Try to keep incisions low.
> ➤ Intraoperative photos to document results and tissue resected
> ➤ Extend the incision to get rid of "dog-ears."
> ➤ Try to achieve an aesthetic umbilicus and mons pubis.
> ➤ Do not overuse antibiotics. Get cultures of wounds to guide treatment.
> ➤ Any postoperative patient with shortness of breath gets evaluated for venous thromboembolism.

REFERENCES

1. Huger WE Jr. The anatomic rationale for abdominal lipectomy. Am Surg 45:612, 1979.
2. Rohrich RJ, Sorokin ES, Brown SA, et al. Is the umbilicus truly midline? Clinical and medicolegal implications. Plast Reconstr Surg 112:259, 2003.
3. Nahai F. The Art of Aesthetic Surgery: Principles & Techniques. New York: Thieme Publishers, 2005.
4. Patronella C. Redefining abdominal anatomy: 10 key elements for restoring form in abdominoplasty. Aesthet Surg J 35:972, 2015
5. Hunstad JP, Repta R. Atlas of Abdominoplasty. Philadelphia: Elsevier Health Sciences, 2008.
6. Rohrich RJ, Beran SJ, Kenkel JM, et al. Extending the role of liposuction in body contouring with ultrasound-assisted liposuction. Plast Reconstr Surg 101:1090, 1998.
7. Florman LD. Is the umbilicus truly midline? [Correspondence and Brief Communications] Plast Reconstr Surg 113:1089, 2004.
8. Friedland JA, Maffi TR. MOC-PS(SM) CME article: abdominoplasty. Plast Reconstr Surg 121:1, 2008.
9. van Uchelen JH, Kon M, Werker PM. The long-term durability of plication of the anterior rectus sheath assessed by ultrasonography. Plast Reconstr Surg 107:1578, 2001.
10. Nahas FX, Ferreira LM, Augusto SM, et al. Long-term follow-up of correction of rectus diastasis. Plast Reconstr Surg 115:1736, 2005.
11. Pollock H, Pollock T. Progressive tension sutures: a technique to reduce local complications in abdominoplasty. Plast Reconstr Surg 105:2583, 2000.
12. Pollock T, Pollock H. Progressive tension sutures in abdominoplasty: a review of 597 consecutive cases. Aesthet Surg J 32:729, 2012.

13. Rosen A. Use of absorbable barbed suture and progressive tension technique in abdominoplasty: a novel approach. Plast Reconstr Surg 125:1024, 2010.
14. Saldanha OR, Federico R, Daher PF, et al. Lipoabdominoplasty. Plast Reconstr Surg 124:934, 2009.
15. Friedman T, Coon D, Kanbour-Shakir A, et al. Defining the lymphatic system of the anterior abdominal wall: an anatomical study. Plast Reconstr Surg 135:1027, 2015.
16. Landfair AS, Rubin JP. Applied anatomy in body contouring. In Nahai F, ed. The Art of Aesthetic Surgery: Principles & Techniques. New York: Thieme Publishers, 2005.
17. Roostaeian J, Harris R, Farkas JP, et al. Comparison of limited-undermining lipoabdominoplasty and traditional abdominoplasty using laser fluorescence. Aesth Surg Journal 34:741, 2014.
18. Lockwood T. High-lateral-tension abdominoplasty with superficial fascial system suspension. Plast Reconstr Surg 96:603, 1995.
19. Dellon AL. Fleur-de-lis abdominoplasty. Aesthetic Plast Surg 9:27, 1985.
20. Baroudi R, Keppke EM, Carvalho CG. Mammary reduction combined with reverse abdominoplasty. Ann Plast Surg 2:368, 1979.
21. Spieglman J, Levine RH. abdominoplasty: a comparison of outpatient and inpatient procedures shows that it is a safe and effective procedure for outpatients in an office-based surgery clinic. Plast Reconstr Surgery 118:517, 2006.
22. Stewart KJ, Stewart DA, Coghlan B, et al. Complications of 278 consecutive abdominoplasties. J Plast Reconstr Aesthet Surg 59:1152, 2006.
23. Alderman AK, Collins ED, Steu R, et al. Benchmarking outcomes in plastic surgery: national complication rates for abdominoplasty and breast augmentation. Plast Reconstr Surg 124:2127, 2009.
24. Winocour J, Gupta V, Ramirez JR, et al. Abdominoplasty: risk factors, complication rates, and safety of combined procedures. Plast Reconstr Surg 136:597e, 2015.
25. Neaman KC, Armstrong SH, Baca ME, et al. Outcomes of traditional cosmetic abdominoplasty in a community setting: a retrospective analysis of 1008 patients. Plast Reconstr Surg 131:403e, 2013.

61. Medial Thigh Lift

Wendy Chen, Jeffrey A. Gusenoff

ANATOMY

- The medial thigh has a relatively thin outer layer of epidermis and dermis.
- Beneath the dermis are two layers of fat separated by a relatively weak superficial fascial system.
- Deep to the subcutaneous fat lies the strong, thick **Colles fascia**.[1-4]
  - Attaches to the ischiopubic rami of the bony pelvis, to Scarpa fascia of the abdominal wall, and to the posterior border of the urogenital diaphragm
  - Has an especially strong area at the junction of the perineum and the medial thigh
  - Provides the anatomic shelf that defines the perineal thigh crease
  - Best found intraoperatively by dissecting at the origin of the adductor muscles on the ischiopubic ramus and retracting the skin and superficial fat of the vulva medially
  - Lies just at the deepest and most lateral aspect of the vulvar soft tissue[5]
- The **femoral triangle** lies lateral to the Colle fascia dissection (Fig. 61-1).
  - Midinguinal point between the pubic symphysis and anterior superior iliac spine
  - Borders
    - ▶ Superior: Inguinal ligament
    - ▶ Medial: Adductor longus
    - ▶ Lateral: Sartorius

NOTE: Surgeons must be aware of the femoral triangle and avoid entering it to prevent major vascular or nerve injury and disruption of the lymphatic channels.

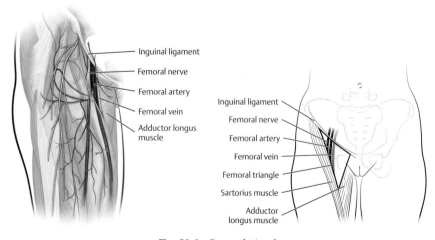

Inguinal ligament
Femoral nerve
Femoral artery
Femoral vein
Adductor longus muscle

Inguinal ligament
Femoral nerve
Femoral artery
Femoral vein
Femoral triangle
Sartorius muscle
Adductor longus muscle

Fig. 61-1 Femoral triangle.

INDICATIONS AND CONTRAINDICATIONS

INDICATIONS

- The indication for a medial thigh lift is the presence of **skin laxity.** Without skin laxity, thigh contouring may be achieved with liposuction alone.
- Accurately classifying the deformity is critical for guiding treatment (see Tables 61-1 through 61-3).

CONTRAINDICATIONS

- Contraindications for performing a medial thigh lift are similar to those for any elective or aesthetic procedure and include the following:
  - The presence of modifiable risk factors, including residual obesity
  - Unresolved depression
  - Unrealistic expectations
  - Unwillingness to accept a lengthy scar or likelihood of common complications
  - Massive-weight-loss (MWL) patients with unstable chronic illnesses, cardiovascular disease, postphlebitic syndrome, or lymphedema

PREOPERATIVE EVALUATION: HISTORY AND PHYSICAL EXAMINATION

- A complete history is obtained, with special attention to the following:
  - Smoking status
  - Nutrition status, with adequate protein and vitamin supplementation in bariatric patients
  - Weight history, especially weight stability
  - Surgical history, i.e., previous body contouring procedures
  - Psychiatric evaluation
  - Plans for other body contouring procedures and priority problem areas for the patient
- A complete physical examination is performed, with special attention to the following:
  - Presence, location, and degree of skin ptosis—drape, bulges, tension, the pattern of sagging (i.e., proximal versus distal)
  - Skin tone and the relationship of skin to the underlying adipose
  - Context of the remaining thigh and lower body deformity
    - ▶ Presence or absence of extra subcutaneous fat in the medial and lateral thighs, lower body, which may be addressed with liposuction during surgery
- Standardized photographs should be taken (see Chapter 3).

CLASSIFICATION SYSTEMS
Non-Massive-Weight-Loss Patients (Table 61-1)

Table 61-1 *Classification and Surgical Recommendations for Non-Massive-Weight-Loss Patients*

Classification	Description	Treatment
Type I	Lipodystrophy with no sign of skin laxity	Liposuction alone
Type II	Lipodystrophy and skin laxity confined to the upper third of the thigh	Liposuction and a horizontal skin incision in the medial thigh
Type III	Lipodystrophy and moderate skin laxity that extends beyond the upper third of the thigh	Both liposuction and horizontal and vertical skin excision in the medial thigh
Type IV	Moderate skin laxity that extends the length of the thigh	Longer vertical resection than type III
Type V	Severe medial thigh skin laxity with lipodystrophy	Staged procedure: First stage: Aggressive liposuction Second stage: Excisional medial thigh lift

Massive-Weight-Loss Patients (Table 61-2)

Table 61-2 *Classification and Surgical Recommendations for Massive-Weight-Loss Patients*

Classification	Description	Treatment
Type I	Deflated: Skin laxity over the entire thigh without significant residual lipodystrophy	Horizontal vector thigh lift
Type II	Nondeflated: Skin laxity and significant lipodystrophy	Staged suction lipectomy and horizontally based medial thigh lift

Pittsburgh Rating Scale[6] (Table 61-3)

Table 61-3 *Pittsburgh Rating Scale*

Classification	Description	Treatment
0	Normal	None
1	Excessive adiposity	UAL and/or SAL ± excisional lifting procedure
2	Severe adiposity and/or severe cellulite	UAL and/or SAL ± excisional lifting procedure
3	Skin folds	Excisional lifting procedure

SAL, Suction-assisted liposuction; *UAL,* ultrasound-assisted liposuction.

> **TIP:**   Careful evaluation of each patient's deformity is needed to determine the best treatment.

> **SENIOR AUTHOR TIP:**   Careful evaluation of the lower leg preoperatively is essential. Many patients after weight loss will present with **lipedema,** which should be differentiated from preexisting lymphedema. The feet and ankles should be photographed preoperatively so that patient concerns of postoperative swelling can be assessed in comparison with the baseline examination.

> The thigh can be addressed in thirds, regardless of whether patients have had massive weight loss. Skin laxity in the upper third can be treated by a medial thighplasty (crescent thighplasty) with the scar completely hidden in the groin crease. Laxity to the middle third can be treated with a short-scar vertical thighplasty. Laxity down to the knee and encompassing the entire thigh can be treated with a full-length vertical thighplasty. Global thigh adiposity is best treated with staged procedures: debulking liposuction first, followed by an excisional procedure. Patients with outer thigh skin laxity may be best treated with a circumferential lower body lift or Lockwood type 1 body lift first, which will allow some skin relaxation to occur postoperatively. Tissues will relax in a medioinferior direction; thus a staged medial thigh lift can help to correct any of the residual laxity after the initial body lift. If a patient had a prior abdominoplasty or panniculectomy, medial thighplasty can be combined with a lower body lift in a Lockwood type 2 procedure.

INFORMED CONSENT

- The informed consent should include the likely possibility of wound complications and the possibility for extension of the incision/scar.

> **SENIOR AUTHOR TIP:**   Thighplasty can have most of the complications seen in body contouring. Because the rate of minor wound-healing complications is very high with this procedure, they should be discussed in detail with patients before surgery to prevent postoperative dissatisfaction. Complications include seroma, hematoma, delayed wound healing, scar migration, prolonged pain, swelling or change in the shape of the genital region, tissue relaxation, leg swelling (which may be permanent and require chronic care [lymphedema]), unsatisfactory thigh contour and shape, incomplete correction of loose skin at the knee, and risk of deep vein thrombosis (DVT) or pulmonary embolism.

EQUIPMENT

- The medial thigh lift is a procedure with various methods of patient positioning and can be combined with other body contouring procedures, requiring lengthy operating times.

■ In addition to liposuction equipment, sequential compression devices for venous thromboembolism (VTE) prophylaxis, drains, warming blankets, and compression garments, surgeons also require equipment for appropriate patient positioning and padding.

TECHNIQUES

■ The preoperative marking process helps to reinforce and inform patients regarding scar length and expectations. Markings may be made on the same day or the night before surgery.
■ Given the biomechanics of skin excess, this procedure may also be combined with lower body lift and abdominoplasty.

CLASSIC MEDIAL THIGH LIFT WITH TRANSVERSE SKIN EXCISION/UPPER THIGH CRESCENT EXCISION

■ **Preoperative markings**
  • The patient is in a standing position with knees apart.
  • Skin is retracted medially and posteriorly and marked for excision.
  • Areas of excess fat are marked for liposuction.
  • The femoral triangle is marked to prevent damage to neurovascular and lymphatic structures.
  • The incision is marked from the level of the ischium along the inner surface of the buttock's fold medially and inferiorly to the labia majora (female).
  • Skin laxity beyond the upper third of the thigh is examined (pinch test) for the need to add a vertical component to the incision (Fig. 61-2).
  • Patients may also be in a recumbent position for marking (Fig. 61-3).

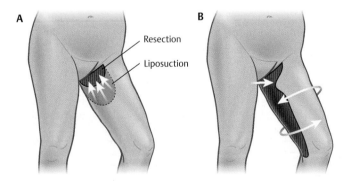

Fig. 61-2   A, Classic Lockwood medial thighplasty. **B,** Vertical incision thighplasty. (*Dark gray shading* indicates liposuction; *red shading* indicates resection; *arrows* indicate vectors of pull.)

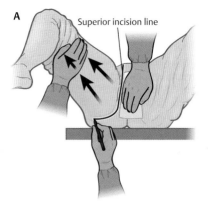

Fig. 61-3 Upper medial thighplasty. **A,** The patient flexes the hip and abducts the thigh. As an assistant pushes the loose thigh skin toward the knee, the superior incision is drawn between the labia majora and thigh. **B,** The point of maximal resection along the mid-medial thigh is determined with the thigh flexed and adducted. **C,** As the thigh is again abducted, the crescent-shaped inferior incision line is extended from this inferior resection mark anterior to the outer mons pubis line and posterior to the buttock-thigh junction line.

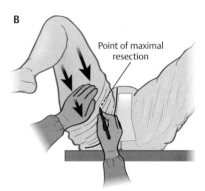

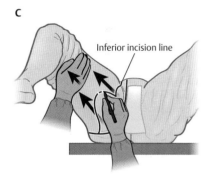

SENIOR AUTHOR TIP: Patients should be marked while they are in a frog-leg position. This will allow surgeons to determine a safe amount of tissue to resect to prevent labial distortion postoperatively when the patients spread their legs. Overestimating a resection when patients are standing can lead to overresection and labial distortion when the legs are spread.

All medial thighplasty scars are placed close in the pubic region to frame it and to prevent visible scars on the thighs, which can migrate inferiorly over time. I typically mark patients 4 cm lateral to the vulval commissure to keep the scar in close.

■ **Technique**
  • The surgery begins with the patient in the prone position; liposuction of the hip and thighs is performed, followed by excision of the posterior portion of skin and fat. This wound is closed in layers.
  • The patient is then placed in a supine position; further liposuction is performed.
  • The legs are placed in a frog-leg position. The proximal incision is made, with care to not violate the femoral triangle, followed by undermining down to the caudal incision.

- Colles fascia is identified near the origin of the adductor muscles on the ischiopubic ramus.
  - ▶ Lateral traction aids in identification of the fascia.
  - ▶ During dissection, the fascia and the soft tissue bundle between the mons pubis and femoral triangle are preserved, to prevent lymphatic complications.
  - ▶ Anchoring sutures are placed to incorporate Colles fascia with the superficial fascial system of the medial thigh skin.
- Drains are placed, and the skin is closed with deep dermal and subcuticular layers. Skin glue and Steri-Strips may also be used.

> **SENIOR AUTHOR TIP:**   Liposuction is completely optional in thighplasty procedures. Some evidence shows that liposuction outside the zone of resection can lead to an increase in infection postoperatively. Care should be taken to avoid liposuction in the banana roll of the buttocks to prevent contour deformity.
>
> Dissection is superficial in the femoral region to the adductor longus tendon. All anchoring sutures are placed distal to the adductor longus to prevent injury to lymphatics and other structures in the femoral region. Three 2-0 absorbable braided sutures are placed from the superficial fascial system of the thigh to Colles fascia in the groin to prevent labial distortion. These sutures are placed when the patient is in a frog-legged position and tied when the leg is adducted into a supine position. Care should be taken to not grab any of the thigh muscle or muscle fascia when placing these sutures, because movement after surgery can cause them to tear and lead to bleeding.

MEDIAL THIGH LIFT FOR MASSIVE-WEIGHT-LOSS PATIENTS

- ▪ Medial thigh lift in MWL patients must address the unique **horizontal laxity** and increased risk for recurrent ptosis seen in these patients.
  - Compared to the classic method, this is achieved by a **longitudinal medial thigh incision** that accomplishes the thigh lift through a horizontal vector.
    - ▶ The horizontal incision is limited to excision of cutaneous deformities (dog-ears).

> **SENIOR AUTHOR TIP:**   All thighplasty procedures have Colles fascia sutures placed to prevent scar migration and labial distortion.
>
> The transverse excision in the groin crease is usually not very robust and acts to remove the dog-ears at the end of the large, full-length vertical thighplasty excision.

- ▪ **Preoperative markings**
  - The patient is standing with knees apart.
  - Areas of excess fat in the distal third of the thigh are marked for liposuction.
  - The desired placement of the vertical incision is marked at the medial thigh.
  - Skin and tissue are gathered to meet this incision line, first posteriorly then anteriorly, to determine the amount of skin to be resected. This wedge is marked for resection (Fig. 61-4, *B*).
  - Patient may also be marked while they are in a recumbent position (Fig. 61-4).

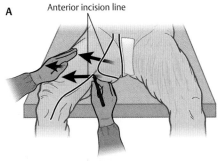

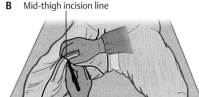

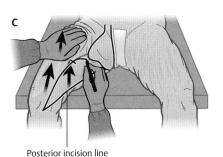

Fig. 61-4   Vertical band excision.
A, With the leg on the bed, and superior and medial drag on the anterior thigh skin, the anterior excision line is drawn. **B,** The width of maximal resection at the mid-thigh is gathered and marked. **C,** From this mid-thigh mark, a widening posterior incision line is drawn from below knee to the ischial tuberosity. The angle between this vertical limb and the upper crescent excision is widened by edging the superior portion of the anterior line posteriorly. After marking, the patient stands. Adjustments are made as needed.

■ **Technique**
- Type II MWL patients (nondeflated) require a staged procedure, with the first stage being aggressive liposuction. Resection is performed 3-6 months later.
- The patient is positioned supine, with legs in a frog-leg position.
- Liposuction is performed as needed.
- The anterior incision is made to the level of the deep fascia.
  ▶ Lymphatic structures and the great saphenous vein are preserved.
- The dissection is carried posteriorly to meet the posterior markings. The posterior incision is then made.
- Skin is excised from distal to proximal, with segmental closure with staples to minimize tension and edema and to optimize wound closure.
- Drains are placed. The wound is closed in layers (superficial fascial system, deep dermal, subcuticular). Cyanoacrylate skin glue and Steri-Strips may also be used.

SENIOR AUTHOR TIP: The dissection plane should be deep to the superficial fascial system, thereby avoiding even seeing the great saphenous vein if possible.

Dissection near the knee should be more superficial.

Care should be taken to prevent injury to the saphenous vein, which is associated with increased risk of lymphedema.

FASCIOFASCIAL SUSPENSION TECHNIQUE IN MEDIAL THIGH LIFTS (Fig. 61-5)

- Given the complications associated with medial thigh lifts, the goals of this technique are to minimize subcutaneous undermining and maximize fascial suspension.
    - These are achieved by placing the tension of the thigh lift on **the overlap of gracilis and adductor longus fascia** rather than on the Colles fascia or the skin flap.

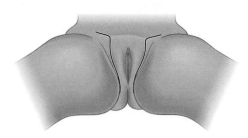

- **Preoperative markings**
    - The patient is in a standing position when marked.
    - The transverse incision is medial to the groin crease. Superiorly it extends bilaterally on the pubis and ends with a Burow triangle. Inferiorly, the incision runs

Fig. 61-5 Fasciofascial suspension technique. Preoperative marking of skin incisions. A Burow triangle is drawn to allow outward rotation of the thigh flap.

along the perineal-thigh crease, extending posteriorly into the medial gluteal fold.
- **Technique**
    - Skin and fat are undermined to the fascia of the gracilis and adductor longus muscles.
    - The fasciae are horizontally incised and dissected from the underlying muscle.
    - The fasciae are advanced with the skin and fat resection and secured cranially. As a result, the inferior fasciocutaneous thigh flap is advanced maximally with minimal tension on the skin closure.

SPIRAL LIFT: MEDIAL AND LATERAL THIGH LIFT WITH BUTTOCK LIFT (SOZER ET AL[7]) (Fig. 61-6)

- Patients with a pear-shaped body contour deformity often have buttock ptosis and posterior thigh laxity, which present a surgical challenge that cannot be corrected with liposuction alone.
- **Preoperative markings**
    - With the patient in a prone position, legs are abducted to assess lateral resection.
    - Symmetry is evaluated while the patient is standing.
    - A line is drawn from the inferior gluteal fold medially toward the upper inner thigh, to the pudendal region, along the inguinal line, through the anterior iliac spine to the posterior iliac crest, above the buttocks, ending in a V at the sacrum to adjoin with the marking from the contralateral side.
    - Pinch test is used to assess the amount of skin resection.
- **Technique**
    - With the patient in a prone position with legs abducted, liposuction of the thighs and flanks is performed.
    - The marked wedges are resected down to fascia and the gluteal flap deepithelialized.
    - By undermining, a pocket is created for the flap.
    - Liposuction is performed with the patient in a supine position with legs abducted.

- A crescent of tissue joining the previous excision sites is resected at the superior medial thigh.
- The inferior skin flap is suspended from the superficial fascial system to Colles fascia of the perineum medially, to the inguinal ligament anteriorly, and the periosteum of the anterior superior iliac spine laterally.
- The wound is closed in layers.

> **TIP:**   To prevent recurrence of thigh ptosis, anchor the closure to Colles fascia or use fasciofascial suspension of the adductor and gracilis muscles.

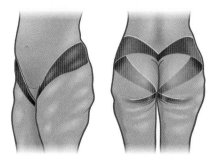

Fig. 61-6   Spiral lift. Excised tissue extends from the inner inside crease of the buttocks along the inguinal crease and anterior iliac spine, spiraling above the buttocks and meeting the contralateral incision at the sacrum.

> **SENIOR AUTHOR TIP:**   To help prevent delayed wound healing in the groin near the T-point closure, permanent sutures are used from the T point distally. This aids in preventing problems postoperatively when patients are in a sitting position either on a chair or the toilet, which can place significant pressure on the suture line.

POSTOPERATIVE CARE

- Pain control with a multimodal analgesia
- Early ambulation (POD 0)
- Given the long duration of body contouring cases and fluid administration during such cases, attention to postsurgical total body fluid retention is critical. If natural diuresis has not occurred within 3 days, then oral diuretics should be prescribed.
- Drains may be removed when daily output is sufficiently low (i.e., 30-50 ml, usually POD 10).
- Compression garments may be started immediately postoperatively or after 2 weeks, according to surgeon's preference regarding the effect of compression garments on incision line healing and hygiene.
- Given the location of the wound and likelihood for wound complications, meticulous hygiene and care of the suture line are important.
- Patients are usually discharged from the hospital POD 1-4.

- Sequential compression devices, such as Lympha Press (Lympha Press USA), are used for a month to minimize swelling.
- Noninvasive mechanical body contouring, such as Endermologie (LPG Systems), are used within 2 weeks to minimize edema and improve skin quality.

> **SENIOR AUTHOR TIP:**   Patients are placed in ACE wraps postoperatively until the drains are removed (POD 7-14). Patients are then encouraged to wear a compression garment that extends down to the ankles. They are instructed to elevate their legs for the first week after surgery when not ambulating. Swelling tends to increase 2-3 weeks after surgery as patients become more active. If swelling in the feet is noted, wrapping should start immediately. If edema persists, early referral to a physical therapist who specializes in lymphedema management is encouraged. Patients are reassured that edema usually is limited and resolves over time.

COMPLICATIONS

- The original technique described by Lewis[8] did not gain widespread acceptance because of problems of inferior wound migration, widening of scars, lateral traction deformity of vulva, early recurrence of ptosis.
- In current practice, complication rates vary with technique, ranging from **43% to 67%.**[9,10] Complications include the following:
  - Seroma
    - ▶ Tense or ballotable asymmetrical swellings
    - ▶ May form after premature removal of drains
    - ▶ An incidence of 9.4% has been cited.[9]
    - ▶ Treated with large-bore needle aspiration and compression garments; in recurrent cases, reinserting a drain may be necessary. If a scarred cavity has formed, treatment may require sclerosing agents or surgical excision with quilting.
  - Lymphatic complications
    - ▶ Lymphedema or lymphoceles
    - ▶ Lymphoceles are firm, deep, slightly tender masses containing straw-colored, watery fluid that can quickly reaccumulate after aspiration.
    - ▶ Lymphoceles may form because of iatrogenic disruption of lymphatic channels during dissection of the femoral triangle.
    - ▶ Moreno et al[11] have reported an incidence of 30.8% of abnormal lymphoscintigraphy after medial thigh lift.
    - ▶ Lymphoceles are treated with prolonged closed suction drainage. Small residual masses may be observed, because they usually proceed to fibrosis.
  - Incision line wound complications, such as skin necrosis, suture line dehiscence
    - ▶ An incidence of 20.8% has been cited for dehiscence, 5.7% for infection, 1.9% for partial skin necrosis.[9]
    - ▶ Wound complications may be prevented by meticulous wound care and hygiene.
    - ▶ Wound complications may be treated with local wound care.

- Cutaneous deformities (dog-ears), skin irregularities, and depressions
- Hypertrophic scars, scar migration (17% incidence[9])
- Flattening of the buttocks from tension of wound closure
- Recurrence of thigh ptosis
- Prolonged nonlymphatic edema
- Contour deformity of the mons pubis; descent of labial thigh scars and distortion of labii
  - ▶ Unless a result of overresection of medial thigh skin, this can be prevented by placement of a Colles fascia stitch.
  - ▶ If severe, this complication may require split-thickness skin grafting or tissue expansion.

TIP: Surgeons should carefully dissect and identify the femoral triangle to prevent lymphedema.

TOP TAKEAWAYS

➤ When I mark patients, they are placed in the frog-leg position. I estimate the transverse excision component by pushing up on the thigh tissues to reach the groin crease. A line is drawn from the palpated adductor longus tendon down to the knee. Holding the marking pen on this line, the tissues are repeatedly mobilized medially and laterally to mark the planned estimated area of resection. I do this multiple times to verify the resection. Hash mark lines are used as reference points to align the medial and lateral incisions. Symmetry is checked between the thighs to make sure the estimates are appropriate.

➤ A dilute epinephrine solution of 1:100,000 is injected. Excision is performed by making the anterior and groin crease incisions first and elevating to the estimated line of resection. No undermining is performed beyond this. A rat-tooth pickup and pen are used to verify the estimated resections along the hash marks. The tissues are serially resected to prevent overresection. The T point is verified multiple times to prevent overresection.

➤ Closed suction drains are brought out in the pubic region to prevent additional scars near the knee and for ease of maintenance.

➤ Because of the discomfort and difficulty ambulating after surgery, patients are typically instructed to stay 2 nights in the hospital and are given a patient-controlled analgesia (PCA) for the first 24 hours after surgery.

➤ Lymphoceles that are resistant to serial drainage or even to resection can be treated with marsupialization or negative-pressure wound therapy.

➤ Medial thighplasty involves an extensive recovery, and appropriate postoperative care at home is required for a successful outcome. Patients should arrange to have assistance at home for at least the first week after surgery.

Continued

➤ Some surgeons advocate for excision site lipectomy, in which the area of resection is defatted with liposuction before excision. This will decrease the injury to lymphatics and prevent long-term complications. No prospective randomized controlled trials have been conducted to prove this technique is effective. If this modality is used, surgeons should stay at least 1-2 cm inside the zone of resection to prevent damage to the skin edges, which can lead to wound-healing problems.

➤ Judicious liposuction near the knees during thighplasty can aid in contouring these difficult areas.

➤ For patients with laxity of the skin in the lower leg, the medial thighplasty incision can be carried further onto the leg; however, the scar appearance may be suboptimal.

➤ Large-volume liposuction of the thighs for debulking can require significant compression afterward to reduce edema. Standard ACE wraps may be inadequate for compression, and referral to physical therapy for stiffer compression wraps may be required.

REFERENCES

1. Lockwood TE. Fascial anchoring technique in medial thigh lifts. Plast Reconstr Surg 82:299, 1988.
2. Lockwood TE. Transverse flank-thigh-buttock lift with superficial fascial suspension. Plast Reconstr Surg 87:1019, 1991.
3. Lockwood T. Lower body lift with superficial fascial system suspension. Plast Reconstr Surg 92:1112; discussion 1123, 1993.
4. Lockwood TE. Maximizing aesthetics in lateral-tension abdominoplasty and body lifts. Clin Plast Surg 31:523, 2004.
5. Mathes DW, Kenkel JM. Current concepts in medial thighplasty. Clin Plast Surg 35:151, 2008.
6. Candiani P, Campiglio GL, Signorini M. Fascio-fascial suspension technique in medial thigh lifts. Aesthetic Plast Surg 19:137, 1995.
7. Sozer SO, Agullo FJ, Palladino H. Spiral lift: medial and lateral thigh lift with buttock lift and augmentation. Aesthetic Plast Surg 32:120, 2008.
8. Lewis JR. Correction of ptosis of the thighs: the thigh lift. Plast Reconstr Surg 37:494, 1966.
9. Bertheuil N, Thienot S, Huguier V, et al. Medial thighplasty after massive weight loss: are there any risk factors for postoperative complications? Aesthetic Plast Surg 38:63, 2013.
10. Gusenoff JA, Coon D, Nayar H, et al. Medial thigh lift in the massive weight loss population: outcomes and complications. Plast Reconstr Surg 135:98, 2015.
11. Moreno CH, Neto HJ, Junior AH, et al. Thighplasty after bariatric surgery: evaluation of lymphatic drainage in lower extremities. Obes Surg 18:1160, 2008.

62. Body Contouring in Massive-Weight-Loss Patients

Jeff Chang, Rohit K. Khosla, Joseph Hunstad

CLASSIFICATION OF MORBID OBESITY[1,2] (Table 62-1)

- **Obesity:** Body mass index (BMI) >30 kg/m^2
- **Severe obesity:** BMI >35 kg/m^2
- **Morbid obesity:** BMI >40 kg/m^2. Morbidly obese patients exceed their ideal body weight (IBW) by >100 pounds or are >100% their IBW.
- **Super obesity:** BMI >50 kg/m^2. These patients exceed their IBW by >225%.

Table 62-1 *National Institutes of Health Classification of Overweight and Obesity*

	BMI (kg/m^2)	Obesity Class
Underweight	<18.5	
Normal	18.6-24.9	
Overweight	25.0-29.9	
Obese	30.1-34.9	I
Severely obese	35.0-39-9	II
Extremely obese	40.0+	III

COMORBIDITIES OF MORBID OBESITY[1,2]

- Osteoarthritis
- Obstructive sleep apnea
- Gastroesophageal reflux
- Lipid abnormalities
- Hypertension
- Diabetes mellitus
- Congestive heart failure
- Asthma

SENIOR AUTHOR TIP: Following massive weight loss (MWL), 70% of patients experience a significant reduction in self-image due to the deflated nature of their tissues.

COMPLICATIONS OF SKIN REDUNDANCY

- Intertriginous infections/rashes
- Musculoskeletal pain
- Functional impairment, especially with ambulation, urination, and sexual activity
- Psychological issues such as depression and low self-esteem

BARIATRIC SURGERY TECHNIQUES[2]
- Performed through traditional open techniques or laparoscopic techniques. **Laparoscopic techniques** substantially reduce the morbidity from postoperative wound infections, dehiscence, and incisional hernias.

RESTRICTIVE PROCEDURES
- Manipulate the **stomach only**
- Reduce caloric intake by decreasing the quantity of food consumed at a single meal
  - **Vertical banded gastroplasty (VBG):** Not very effective, because >50% of patients unable to maintain weight loss
  - **Laparoscopic adjustable gastric band (lap band):** Achieves approximately 50% reduction of excess weight
  - **Gastric sleeve**
    - ▶ Gastric tube created by resecting greater curvature of stomach
    - ▶ 70% remission of type 2 diabetes, which is less than with gastric bypass[3]
    - ▶ Mean excess weight loss 50% at 6 years[3]
  - **Orbera weight loss balloon** (Apollo Endosurgery)
    - ▶ Fluid-filled intragastric balloon to decrease gastric capacity

COMBINATION RESTRICTIVE AND MALABSORPTIVE PROCEDURES[2,3,4]
- *Superior for weight reduction and decreases in comorbidities* (Fig. 62-1)

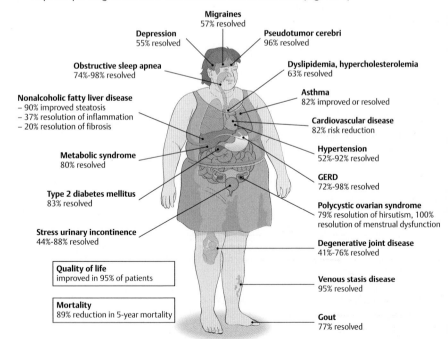

Migraines
57% resolved

Depression
55% resolved

Pseudotumor cerebri
96% resolved

Obstructive sleep apnea
74%-98% resolved

Dyslipidemia, hypercholesterolemia
63% resolved

Nonalcoholic fatty liver disease
– 90% improved steatosis
– 37% resolution of inflammation
– 20% resolution of fibrosis

Asthma
82% improved or resolved

Cardiovascular disease
82% risk reduction

Metabolic syndrome
80% resolved

Hypertension
52%-92% resolved

GERD
72%-98% resolved

Type 2 diabetes mellitus
83% resolved

Polycystic ovarian syndrome
79% resolution of hirsutism, 100% resolution of menstrual dysfunction

Stress urinary incontinence
44%-88% resolved

Degenerative joint disease
41%-76% resolved

Quality of life
improved in 95% of patients

Venous stasis disease
95% resolved

Mortality
89% reduction in 5-year mortality

Gout
77% resolved

Fig. 62-1   Comorbidity reduction after bariatric surgery.

- The malabsorptive component limits the absorption of nutrients and calories from ingested foods by bypassing the duodenum and other specific lengths of the small intestine.
  - **Biliopancreatic diversion (BPD):** Achieves nearly **75%-80%** reduction of excess weight, produces significant nutritional deficiencies
  - **BPD with duodenal switch:** Approximately **73%** of excess weight loss
  - **Roux-en-Y gastric bypass (RYGB):** This is the most common bariatric procedure performed and is considered the benchmark. It achieves excess weight loss **>50%.** Vitamin and mineral deficiencies present in 30%-40% of patients.

> **SENIOR AUTHOR TIP:**   Space-occupying balloons are becoming more popular in the United States and worldwide. They have been shown to be effective for achieving weight loss, particularly for the low and moderate BMI patients. Laparoscopic adjustable bands are losing popularity because of subsequent weight gain that is frequently seen.

FUNDAMENTALS OF BODY CONTOURING AFTER MASSIVE WEIGHT LOSS[1,4,5]

LIPOSUCTION
- **Not effective as a sole modality** in massive-weight-loss patients
- Can be used in areas of mild contour irregularities as an **adjunct** to excision procedures
- Can be performed after recovery from major excisional procedures for refinement of contour
- Can be performed at the excision or as a staged surgery. Table 62-2 presents the pros and cons of liposuction in massive-weight-loss patients.[6]

Table 62-2   *Pros and Cons of Single or Multiple Procedures*

	Pros	Cons
Single procedure	Elimination of additional surgery Areas are treated one at a time, which allows the area to be rejuvenated in one sitting	Significant edema may compromise the results/scarring Potential to compromise vascularity of the flaps
Separate procedures	Requires additional surgical stage Debulking is completed prior to excision Avoids edema associated with liposuction	Additional surgical stage is necessary Cost of additional surgery Additional recovery time Tissues may stiffen and make later advancement more difficult

TIMING OF BODY CONTOURING AFTER BARIATRIC SURGERY[1,4,5,7]
- Delay surgery until the patient's weight has **stabilized for at least 6 months.** This corresponds to **~12-18 months after gastric bypass.**
- Reasons to delay surgery until stable weight achieved:
  - Patients have time to achieve metabolic and nutritional homeostasis.
  - The period of rapid weight loss is detrimental to wound healing.

- The risk of surgical complications decreases significantly from around **80% to 33%** when patients approach their IBW.
- Aesthetic outcomes are better for patients near their IBW.
- Most patients will settle at a **BMI of 30-35 kg/m²** after bariatric surgery.
  - Consider motivated patients in this category for an initial panniculectomy or breast reduction to improve comfort during exercise.
  - This may facilitate lifestyle changes that will result in further weight loss and provide better aesthetic outcomes with subsequent surgery.
- **The best candidates for extensive body contouring after massive weight loss will have a BMI of 25-30 kg/m².**

> **SENIOR AUTHOR TIP:** Massive-weight-loss patients can be considered either "complete" or "incomplete," based on residual subcutaneous fat. Most massive-weight-loss patients fall in the "incomplete" category, requiring reduction of subcutaneous tissue in addition to skin resection.

PREOPERATIVE EVALUATION[1,4,8]

- Record greatest and presenting BMI.
- Assess stability of medical comorbidities and psychiatric problems.
  - **40%** of bariatric patients are treated for psychiatric diagnoses.
- Determine smoking history.
- Common nutritional deficiencies
  - Iron deficiency anemia
  - Vitamin B_{12}
  - Calcium
  - Potassium
  - Zinc
  - Fat-soluble vitamins (A, D, E, K)
  - Protein deficiencies
- Preoperative laboratory tests should include complete blood cell count (CBC), electrolytes, blood urea nitrogen (BUN), creatinine, uric acid, liver function tests, glucose, calcium, ferritin, total protein, albumin/prealbumin, B_{12}/folate, prothrombin/partial thromboplastin time (PT/PTT), fat-soluble vitamins.

> **SENIOR AUTHOR TIP:** "Complete" weight-loss patients are more likely to have had a significant bypass procedure resulting in anemia, protein, and other deficiencies. Preoperative evaluation and treatment is imperative for proper wound healing.

SURGICAL STRATEGY

- The goals of surgery are to alleviate the functional, aesthetic, and psychological impairments from skin redundancy.
- Determine the priorities of the patient. However, general sequence should be:
  1. Trunk, abdomen, buttocks, lower thighs
  2. Upper thorax/breasts, arms
  3. Medial thighs
  4. Facial rejuvenation

STAGING CONSIDERATIONS[9]

- Body contouring surgery in patients requiring several areas of correction is **multistaged** to best minimize complications, pain, and need for blood transfusions.
- Solo surgeon versus team approach
  - The team approach can accomplish more in one stage.
  - **Patient safety is paramount.**
  - Longer operative times will increase likelihood of morbidities (e.g., hypothermia, anemia, thromboembolism, and wound complications).
  - Design operating times that are patient-, surgeon-, and practice-specific.
- The greater the drop in BMI, usually the greater the deflation.
- Generally, more resection can be accomplished at one time with greater deflation or lower BMI.
- Determine patient's ability to tolerate long procedures.
- Evaluate patient's assistance at home for recovery process.
- Patients should be back to their preoperative health status before returning to the operating room. Recovery of at least **3 months** is usually required before performing additional stages.

> **SENIOR AUTHOR TIP:**   A sequence of three procedures is usually required to complete body contouring following massive weight loss. This can often require 1 year or more.

PHYSICAL EXAMINATION

- Assess body habitus of patient.
- Evaluate regional fat deposition.
- Evaluate laxity of the skin envelope.
- Evaluate quality of skin-fat envelope, which depends on degree of deflation.
- Estimate extent of tissue resection using a pinch test.
- Assess "translation of pull," which is the extent that distant tissue is affected with region of resection.
- Evaluate for old scars.
- Anticipate location of scars and expect scar migration.

TISSUE CHARACTERISTICS AND SURGICAL TECHNIQUES

TRUNK/ABDOMEN[1,6,7,10]

- The abdomen usually has the greatest deformity in massive-weight-loss patients.
- Most tissue descent is seen along the lateral axillary lines.
- The truncal tissues take on an appearance of an inverted cone (Fig. 62-2).
- The mons pubis will have varying degree of ptosis.
- **Surgical goals**
  - Flatten contour.
  - Tighten abdominal wall with fascial plication.
  - Repair ventral hernia, if present.
  - Elevate the mons pubis.

Preoperative Evaluation of the Trunk/Abdomen

- Identify locations of old scars on the abdomen.
- Determine the extent of the panniculus and descent of abdomen onto lateral thighs.
- Identify any presence of hernias.
- Assess extent of mons ptosis.
- Assess for presence/extent of midback or lower back rolls.
- Assess for buttock ptosis and contour. Determine if patient may benefit from buttock autoaugmentation.

Surgical Approach to the Trunk/Abdomen[1,6,7,10]

- *Traditional abdominoplasty* techniques fail to maximally improve body contour in this patient population, because they do not address the lateral tissue laxity.
- Fleur-de-lis abdominoplasty (Fig. 62-3) can be performed for patients without back and lateral thigh ptosis.
- *Circumferential belt lipectomy/lower body lift* (Fig. 62-4) addresses the circumferential nature of the tissue ptosis seen in the trunk.[7]
  - Allows resection of the entire lower section of the inverted-cone deformity
  - Allows elevation of the buttocks and lateral thighs to produce a comprehensive additional lower body lift

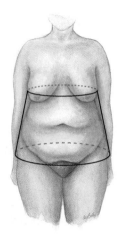

Fig. 62-2 Truncal body contour after massive weight loss. The trunk takes on the form of an inverted cone. The soft tissue is narrow at the rib cage and wider at the pelvic rim. A belt lipectomy eliminates the inferior aspect of the cone.

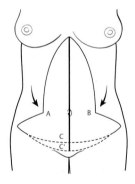

Fig. 62-3 Markings for a fleur-de-lis abdominoplasty. Redundant vertical tissue above the umbilicus is removed as a triangle connected to the redundant skin in the lower abdomen, which is marked as a standard abdominoplasty. Points *A* and *B* will join as an inverted-T closure in the midline at the pubic symphysis (point *C*). In patients with significant mons ptosis, point *C′* is marked 4-6 cm below to resect additional inferior redundancy and to elevate the mons.

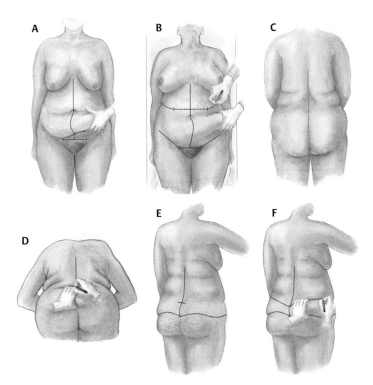

Fig. 62-4 Markings for a belt lipectomy. **A,** The midline is marked initially. The horizontal pubic incision is marked below the natural hairline to allow elevation of the mons. The inferior midline of the closure should be level with the pubic symphysis. The pannus is elevated superiorly and medially in the direction of the arrows to allow marking of the lateral extension of the inferior incision to just below the anterior superior iliac spine (ASIS). **B,** The superior markings are made anteriorly using a pinch technique to determine the extent of resection. **C,** The midline of the back is marked with the inferior point at the coccyx. **D,** The patient is slightly bent at the waist, and the pinch test is used to estimate the superior extent of resection. **E** and **F,** The superior and inferior back marks are made to meet the abdominal marks laterally.

- Patients with **BMI >35** have higher risks for complications after belt lipectomy/lower body lift.[1]
- **Key components of surgical technique**
  - Mark patient as shown (see Fig. 62-4).
  - Start with the patient prone. Make superior incision first on back and dissect inferiorly.
  - The posterior resection should be taken down deep to the superficial fascia to maintain a layer of fat on the deep fascia. This will minimize seroma formation.
  - Perform liposuction on lateral thighs to release zones of adherence, which allows lateral thigh elevation.
  - Align final scars below pelvic rim (horizontal level across the superior aspect of iliac crests). This will keep scars hidden under most undergarments and bikinis.
  - Make inferior incision on the abdomen, similar to traditional abdominoplasty technique.

- Perform an umbilicoplasty to shorten the umbilical stalk flush with the newly contoured abdominal skin, regardless of the contouring technique used.
- Prevent excess tension on the mons, which can elevate the clitoris and urethral meatus.
- Widely drain anteriorly and posteriorly to prevent seroma formation.

TIP: Perform markings in the office on the day before surgery for patient comfort and to prevent time delays on day of surgery.

Mark the anterior/inferior incision at the level of the pubic bone, generally 4-7 cm above the introitus or base of the penis.

Minimize posterior skin resection to prevent competing anterior and posterior tension forces.

Be more aggressive with lateral and anterior resections, because these are most visible areas to the patient.

Contour the mons in two stages to prevent distortion of the clitoris and urethral meatus.

SENIOR AUTHOR TIP: The addition of a vertical resection (fleur-de-lis procedure) can be combined with an abdominoplasty or a body lift. Vertical resection is important when significant transverse or horizontal laxity is present. Many patients have a pre-existing vertical scar which facilitates this. Mons hypertrophy and ptosis is often very significant and a significant upper portion resection is necessary to achieve normal hygiene and appearance.

WAIST AND LATERAL THIGHS[1,7]
- Massive weight loss creates a contour that lacks waist and hip definition.
- Lack of definition is caused by ptosis of the abdomen, lateral thighs, and buttocks.
- Maximum vertical relaxation occurs along lateral body contours. Tissue excess descends in an anteroposterior direction and spirals down the thigh.
- **Surgical goals**
  - Narrow waist as much as possible, especially in women.
  - Create a smooth, natural curve from rib cage through waist and down onto hips.

Surgical Approach to the Waist and Lateral Thighs[1,7]
- The lateral thigh is structurally dependent on truncal tissues. Effective elevation of the thighs is not possible if the trunk remains lax.
- Circumferential belt lipectomy/lower body lift is an effective modality to define the waist and lateral hips in a single-stage procedure.

TIP: Use independent leg extensions on the OR table that will allow hip abduction while patients are prone and supine. This eliminates tension on the lateral thigh advancement.

Suture the superficial fascial system (SFS) on both skin flaps in a three-point configuration to the deep fascia with permanent suture to maintain elevation of the lateral thigh, effectively establishing a new zone of adherence at the level of the final scar.

Buttocks[1,5,7]

- Lack definition as the back and buttocks tend to blend together. This gives the appearance of a long vertical buttock height.
- The central buttock crease descends, leaving minimal soft tissue coverage over the coccyx.
- The lateral inferior buttock creases lie in a more horizontal direction without a shapely curve.
- **Surgical goals**
  - Define the buttocks by creating a line of demarcation from the back to the buttocks. Align the final scar following the superior gluteal curve in a central gull-wing pattern.
  - Elevate the buttocks, including the central crease.
  - Cover coccyx with additional soft tissue if a deficiency is present.
  - Develop an upward curve of the inferior buttock crease.

Surgical Approach to Buttocks[1,5,7,11,12]

- The goals of buttock definition are effectively achieved with the circumferential belt lipectomy/lower body lift.
- However, consider autologous gluteal augmentation to enhance buttock contour, especially with central buttock projection.
- Autologous gluteal augmentation can be performed with fat grafting, dermal/fat flaps, split myocutaneous flaps or perforator flaps.
  - Design the dermal/fat flap based on which area of the buttock needs further augmentation. The flap can be superior, medial, central or inferiorly based (Fig. 62-5).

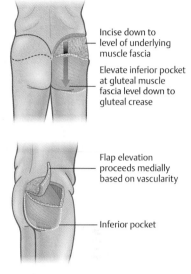

Incise down to level of underlying muscle fascia

Elevate inferior pocket at gluteal muscle fascia level down to gluteal crease

Flap elevation proceeds medially based on vascularity

Inferior pocket

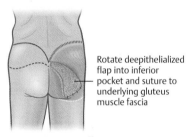

Rotate deepithelialized flap into inferior pocket and suture to underlying gluteus muscle fascia

Fig. 62-5   The design and inset of a medially based gluteal flap.

Back[1,5,7]

- Massive weight loss can lead to upper and lower back rolls.
- Upper back rolls are typically singular and may be an extension of the lateral breast.
- Lower back rolls may be multiple and can be oriented in a horizontal or upward-sweeping direction.
- **Surgical goals**
  - Resect as many rolls as possible.
  - Create a flat contour to the back.

Surgical Approach to the Back[1,5,7]

- Circumferential belt lipectomy/lower body lift is effective for the resection of lower back rolls.
- The upper back roll requires liposuction and/or direct excision in a separate staged procedure from the belt lipectomy (Fig. 62-6).

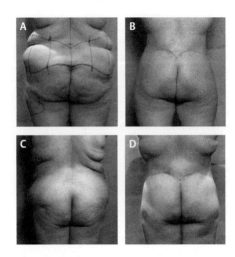

Fig. 62-6   **A** and **B,** Lower back folds corrected after lipectomy. **C** and **D,** Upper back folds may require direct excision.

TIP: Align transverse and posterior scars along the bra line in women.

MEDIAL THIGHS[1,6]

■ Most massive- weight-loss patients have more **horizontal** skin excess of thighs relative to vertical excess of thighs.

■ Vertical medial thigh lift is more effective than horizontal medial thigh lift in these patients (Fig. 62-7).

■ Most patients will require vertical excision with some horizontal component.

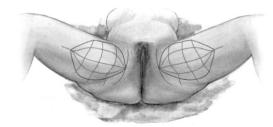

Fig. 62-7   Medial thigh markings.

■ **To reduce potential for labial spreading, do not place tension on the horizontal scar.**

■ Medial thigh lift should be performed in a separate staged procedure after addressing the lateral thighs.

■ This can be combined with liposuction of the medial, anterior, and posterior thigh as an adjunct for mild contour irregularities.

■ **Contraindications to medial thigh lift**
  • Preexisting lymphedema
  • History of lower extremity deep vein thrombosis (DVT)
  • Presence of varicose veins. Obliterate varicosities prior to medial thigh lipectomy.

■ **Surgical goals**
  • Create a flat contour to the medial thigh.
  • Minimize labial spreading.

Surgical Approach to the Medial Thigh[1,6]

- Mark the perineal crease on the inner thigh as the superior extent of the vertical ellipse.
- Perform a pinch test in a superior-to-inferior direction to estimate the extent of resection.
- **Preserve the superficial saphenous vein** during resection.
- To reduce potential for labial spreading, **do not place tension on the horizontal scar.**
- Superior dog-ear can be worked out along the posterior inferior buttock crease or anterior inguinal crease as a horizontal component.
- Carry excisions below the knee if skin redundancy extends inferior to the knee.

> **TIP:** Wait 6-12 months after lower body lift to minimize tension on the medial thigh procedure.
>
> To preserve inguinal lymphatics, resect only skin if the incision is taken anteriorly.
>
> Suture the SFS of the thigh to the Colles fascia with nonabsorbable sutures if a horizontal medial thigh lift performed.
>
> A sequential resection and closure technique prevents overresection and excess tension on the skin closure.

> **SENIOR AUTHOR TIP:** Inner or medial thigh lift is usually an inadequate procedure for the massive-weight-loss patient. Vertical thigh lift is almost always necessary to correct the significant transverse laxity of the thigh. The extent of the vertical thigh lift is based on the deformity and patient desires. The vertical excision can extend down to the calf if indicated. Following bimanual palpation, aggressive, thorough, complete liposuction of the intervening area will eliminate all residual subcutaneous tissue volume and allow for an incision and avulsion method of the skin, which completely preserves and protects all neurovascular and lymphatic structures. This has reduced the complication of lymphocele commonly seen in the knee region following traditional methods of vertical thigh lift.

BREASTS[1,5,6]

- The volume and characteristics of breast tissue will be highly variable after massive weight loss.
- Critically evaluate amount of breast parenchyma, and location of the inframammary fold.
- The lateral inframammary fold is often poorly defined and displaced inferiorly.

Surgical Approach to the Breast[1,5]

- Reduction mammaplasty is indicated for patients with persistent macromastia.
- No single reduction technique is superior in this patient population.
- Mastopexy or augmentation is indicated for patients with grade I/II ptosis.
- Mastopexy with or without augmentation is indicated for patients with grade III ptosis.
- Consider local dermal/fat flaps for breast autoaugmentation as an alternative to breast implants for volume restoration.
- Revisions are usually required to optimize results.

SENIOR AUTHOR TIP: The deflated breast following massive weight loss usually has a very medialized nipple which should not be used to identify the breast meridian. The breast meridian should be based on the center of the breast extending superiorly to a point somewhere between 6 cm and the midline of the clavicle.

Massive-Weight-Loss Mastopexy[13]

- Significant deflation with skin excess after MWL resulting in ptosis with loss of upper pole fullness
- Patients may require an **implant** to restore upper pole fullness.
- Scars are often long.
- **Breast characteristics** (Fig. 62-8)
  - Poor shape, projection, and skin elasticity
  - Severe ptosis and volume loss
  - Flattening of breast
  - Distorted, ptotic nipples, often inferomedially translocated

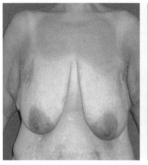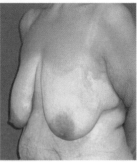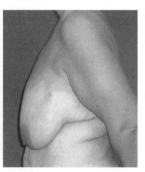

Fig. 62-8   Breast appearance after massive weight loss.

- **Goals**
  - Correct nipple position.
  - Reshape skin envelope.
  - Eliminate lateral fat roll, creating a defined lateral breast curvature.
- **Treatment principles**
  - Tailored based on breast shape, volume loss, and degree of ptosis
- **Grading**
  - **Severity grade 1** (ptosis grade I or II or macromastia)
    - ▶ Traditional mastopexy (vertical technique preferred)
    - ▶ Standard breast reduction techniques
    - ▶ Augmentation-mastopexy
  - **Severity grade 2** (ptosis grade III, moderate volume loss or constricted breast)
    - ▶ Traditional mastopexy (often Wise pattern)
    - ▶ Augmentation-mastopexy
  - **Severity grade 3** (severe lateral roll and/or severe volume loss with excess skin)
    - ▶ Parenchymal reshaping with dermal suspension
    - ▶ Autoaugmentation
    - ▶ Avoid implant if existing volume is sufficient.

Dermal Suspension Autoaugmentation-Mastopexy (Fig. 62-9)

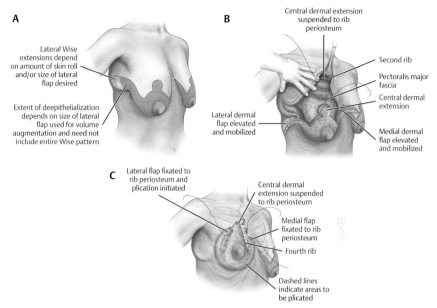

Fig. 62-9   **A,** Wise-pattern markings. *Shading* indicates areas to be deepithelialized. **B,** Medial and lateral areas of breast are rotated to create the appropriate shape. **C,** The breast is anchored to rib periosteum, and gland is reshaped.

- **Technique**
  - For patients with sufficient parenchyma
    1. Mark a Wise pattern, including the lateral roll of tissue.
    2. Deepithelialize the Wise pattern.
    3. Deglove the parenchyma.
    4. Elevate medial and lateral parenchymal flaps.
    5. Suspend flaps to rib periosteum.
    6. Plicate dermis to shape the breast.
    7. Place sutures to define the lateral edge of the breast curvature.
    8. Redrape the skin.
    9. Release any skin tethering.
    10. Close the skin.

Male Breast[6,9]

- Difficult to treat because of varying ptosis, nipple malposition, excessive parenchyma-fat relationship, loss of definition and shape.
- Lower body procedures may tighten the chest sufficiently to preclude additional breast surgery.
- Most men with greater weight loss will require excisional techniques.
- Scars are extensive and visible.
- An inverted-T mastopexy is effective for skin redundancy only.
- Consider free-nipple grafting in cases with severe nipple malposition or nipple ptosis.

UPPER ARMS[1,6]

- Severely ptotic skin of the upper arm develops that extends from the olecranon across the axilla onto the chest wall.
- The excess arm skin is contiguous with the posterior axillary fold on the lateral chest.
- Ideal candidates for brachioplasty have deflated upper arms with a small amount of residual fat.
- **Surgical goals**
  - Eliminate horizontal upper arm excess.
  - Eliminate lateral thoracic skin excess.
  - Create a smooth transition from the lateral chest onto the upper arm.
  - Minimize scar visibility and contracture.

Surgical Approach to the Upper Arm[1,6]

- Brachioplasty techniques that place the incisions **posterior to the bicipital groove** are less noticeable to patients and less visible to others when viewed from the front. However, there is varied opinion and literature on this.
- Scars placed along the bicipital groove tend to widen and take longer to mature.
- Resect the entire subcutaneous tissue down to the muscular aponeurosis.
- Identify and prevent injury to the ulnar nerve during resection.
- The incision should be carried onto the axilla with a Z-plasty to reduce axillary ptosis and to restore a more natural dome shape to the axilla.

> **TIP:** Patients with significant remaining upper arm fat will benefit from liposuction as a staged procedure before excisional lipectomy.
>
> A sequential resection and closure technique prevents overresection and excess tension on the skin closure.

> **SENIOR AUTHOR TIP:** Following bimanual palpation, the intervening area of tissue of the arm can be infiltrated and very thoroughly liposuctioned to eliminate all subcutaneous fat. The skin pattern can be rechecked, incised, and avulsed immediately at the subdermal level. This protects all important neurovascular and lymphatic structures, in particular the medial antibrachial cutaneous sensory nerve that resides in the bicipital groove.

FACE AND NECK[6,14]

- Skin redundancy exceeds that of the superficial musculoaponeurotic system (SMAS) laxity after massive weight loss.
- An appearance of **premature aging** develops.
- More volume loss occurs in the midface relative to nonmassive-weight-loss patients.
- An "aged" facial appearance may be more displeasing to a young patient than redundant skin elsewhere. Patients are able to camouflage skin redundancy elsewhere with clothing.
- **Surgical goals**
  - Redrape the skin over the face and neck to restore a normal-appearing jaw and neckline.
  - Harmonize facial appearance with the contouring of the rest of the body.

Surgical Approach to the Face and Neck[6,14]

- Correction of facial skin redundancy requires more skin undermining to produce a smooth contour relative to a typical rhytidectomy.
- More aggressive skin resection is required.
- Fig. 62-10 demonstrates vectors for facial rejuvenation for varying portions of the face.
- Consider midline skin excision of neck if redundancy is too severe for lateral pull.
- Less elevation of SMAS is required, because laxity at this tissue level is not the structural problem. Normal SMAS plication is performed.
- Perform platysmaplasty if platysmal banding is present.
- Perform suction-assisted or direct lipectomy of remaining fat deposits of jowls and submental triangle.
- The skin incision can enter the temporal hairline above the helical root if the planned vector of facial elevation is posterior and superior.
- Carry the incision around the earlobe and onto the conchal bowl posteriorly.
  - The vector of elevation on the neck can be mostly superior, which prevents an incision across the occipital hairline.
  - Use a traditional postauricular incision with occipital hairline extension if skin laxity of the neck is severe.
- Consider volume replacement to the midface with fat grafting or long-acting fillers.

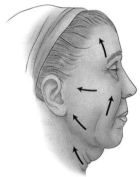

Fig. 62-10   Vectors of facial rejuvenation.

SAFETY CONCERNS IN BODY CONTOURING SURGERY[9]

ANESTHESIA ISSUES (see Chapter 7)
- **Intubation**
  - Anatomic variability. Fiberoptic intubation may be helpful.
  - Many patients have **obstructive sleep apnea.**
  - Patients who have had manipulation of the gastroesophageal junction may be at increased risk for **reflux** and aspiration.
- **Hypothermia**
  - Body temperatures can fall rapidly because of large, exposed areas during surgery and long operative times.
  - Body temperature should be maintained **>35° C.**
- **Maneuvers to prevent hypothermia**
  - Warming blankets
  - Warmed infiltration fluid and intravenous fluid
  - Warming preparatory solutions
  - Covering patients during position changes
  - Keeping room temperatures elevated
- **Fluid management:** Attention to IVF fluid resuscitation during the perioperative period is essential in large-volume excisional surgeries (e.g., belt lipectomy).
  - Intraoperative fluid management should consist of maintenance fluid + 10 ml/kg/hr.
  - Closely monitor urine output during the first 24-48 hours postoperatively with continued IVF resuscitation as needed.

ANEMIA
- **50%** of massive-weight-loss patients are anemic.[8]
- Recognize and treat anemia preoperatively.
- Transfuse intraoperatively and postoperatively as necessary.

THROMBOEMBOLISM (see Chapter 11)
- Obesity is a risk factor for DVT/PE and pulmonary embolism (PE).
- Risk of DVT/PE is <0.1%.
- Higher risk during truncal lipectomies. Increased intraabdominal pressure leads to decreased venous return from lower extremities.
- **Prophylaxis**
  - Heparin or low-molecular-weight heparin before surgery and during hospitalization may reduce risk.
  - Epidural analgesia decreases incidence of DVT/PE, according to orthopedic literature.[15] Benefits unknown in body contouring.
  - Sequential compression devices are placed before induction of general anesthesia and maintained postoperatively.
  - Patients should start ambulating with assistance starting the day of surgery.
  - Incentive spirometry

COMPLICATIONS OF BODY CONTOURING SURGERY[1,4,5,9]

HEMATOMA (1%-5%)
- Typically occurs in the immediate postoperative period
- Requires operative evacuation and exploration

SEROMA (13%-37%)
- Higher incidence in patients with BMI >35, primarily in lower back after belt lipectomy/lower body lift
- Maintain drains until output <30 ml over 24 hours.
- Drain seromas early before capsule formation.
- Aspiration can be performed in the office. Serial aspiration may be needed.
- Large seromas can be drained by percutaneously placed closed suction drains.
- Inject cavity with doxycycline to sclerose walls. Wait at least 4-7 days after surgery to minimize pain associated with earlier infusion.

> **TIP:** Obliterate dead space with progressive tension sutures and three-point sutures at the level of the skin closure.
>
> The preservation of a thin layer of fat on the deep fascia may diminish the risk of seroma by maintaining some lymphatic drainage.
>
> Fibrin sealants may help to reduce the incidence of seromas.

LYMPHOCELE
- Prevent occurrence by tying off both channels to a lymph node when they are encountered.
- Seen primarily in the inguinal region from aggressive resection into femoral triangle
- Perform serial aspiration.
- Percutaneous drainage with placement of closed suction drain

- Doxycycline injection
- Requires operative exploration and ligation of leaking lymphatic channels if nonoperative management fails

> **SENIOR AUTHOR TIP:**   Direct resection of the tissues of the medial thigh in a vertical thigh lift is commonly associated with a lymphocele formation in the area of the knee. Thoroughly liposuctioning the areas of tissue excess identified with bimanual palpation and then removing the skin using an avulsion technique will protect all neurovascular and lymphatic structures, dramatically reducing the incidence of lymphocele. Eliminating a lymphocele commonly requires excision and space-obliterating sutures.

WOUND COMPLICATIONS
- **Dehiscence** (22%-30%)
  - Most often occur within first few days of surgery
  - Early dehiscence from excess tension or movement, often seen in the posterior closure of the body lift
  - Late dehiscence often results from underlying seroma.
- **Skin necrosis** (6%-10%)
- **Wound infection/cellulitis** (1%-7%)
- **Suture extrusion**
- **Factors that increase incidence of wound complications:**
  - Tobacco use. Wait at least 1 month after cessation of smoking to perform surgery.
  - Diabetes
  - Active systemic steroid use
  - BMI >40 kg/m^2

> **TIP:**   Mark body lift patients when they are in a sitting or slightly flexed position.
>
> Avoid permanent or long-lasting absorbable sutures superficial to the SFS.
>
> Ensure that patients are awake and alert before postoperative movement. Cooperative patients can determine which movements place excess tension on their incisions.
>
> Have caregivers assist with postoperative activities, such as showering and removal of compression garments, that can cause orthostasis and fainting, resulting in falls.

TOP TAKEAWAYS
- RYGB is the most common, reproducible, and effective bariatric operation performed today.
- Start body contouring surgery when patients have stabilized their weight for at least 6 months.
- The best aesthetic outcomes with the least perioperative risks will occur with patients near their IBW or with a BMI of 25-30 kg/m^2 after bariatric surgery.
- The abdomen demonstrates the greatest deformity, and most tissue ptosis is appreciated along the lateral axillary lines.
- Assess for nutritional deficiencies before initiation of body contouring surgery.
- Treat the trunk, lateral thigh, and buttocks as a single aesthetic unit.

Continued

- ➤ Circumferential belt lipectomy/lower body lift provides resection of excess truncal tissue and elevates the buttocks and lateral thighs.
- ➤ Perform liposuction on the lateral thighs during a belt lipectomy to release the zones of adherence, which allows more effective elevation of the lateral thigh.
- ➤ Massive-weight-loss patients may require breast reduction or mastopexy, depending on the amount of breast volume loss.
- ➤ Patients develop premature facial aging because of skin redundancy rather than SMAS laxity.
- ➤ Liposuction techniques can be used as an adjunct during or after excisional operations for additional refinement of contour.
- ➤ Complication rates increase with higher BMI.

REFERENCES

1. Aly AS. Body Contouring After Massive Weight Loss. New York: Thieme Publishers, 2006.
2. Rubin JP, Nguyen V, Schwentker A. Perioperative management of the post-gastric-bypass patient presenting for body contouring surgery. Clin Plast Surg 31:601, 2004.
3. Taylor J, Shermak M. Body contouring following massive weight loss. Obes Surg 14:1080, 2004.
4. Hamad GG. The state of the art in bariatric surgery for weight loss in the morbidly obese patient. Clin Plast Surg 31:591, 2004.
5. Gilbert EW, Wolfe BM. Bariatric surgery for the management of obesity: state of the field. Plast Reconstr Surg 130:948, 2012.
6. Kenkel J. Marking and operative techniques. Plast Reconstr Surg 117(1 Suppl):45S; discussion 82S, 2006.
7. Aly AS, Cram AE, Heddens C. Truncal body contouring surgery in the massive weight loss patient. Clin Plast Surg 31:611, 2004.
8. Kenkel J. The physiological impact of bariatric surgery on the massive weight loss patient. Plast Reconstr Surg 117(1 Suppl):14S; discussion 82S, 2006.
9. Kenkel J. Safety considerations and avoiding complications in the massive weight loss patient. Plast Reconstr Surg 117(1 Suppl):7S; discussion 82S, 2006.
10. Fernando da Costa L, Landecker A, Manta A. Optimizing body contour in massive weight loss patients: the modified vertical abdominoplasty. Plast Reconstr Surg 114:1917; discussion 1924, 2004.
11. Colwell A, Borud L. Autologous gluteal augmentation after massive weight loss: aesthetic analysis and role of the superior gluteal artery perforator flap. Plast Reconstr Surg 119:345, 2007.
12. Sozer SO, Agullo FJ, Palladino H. Split gluteal muscle flap for autoprosthesis buttock augmentation. Plast Reconstr Surg 129:766, 2012.
13. Rubin JP, Toy J. Mastopexy and breast reduction in massive-weight-loss patients. In Nahai F, ed. The Art of Aesthetic Surgery: Principles and Techniques, ed 2. New York: Thieme Publishers, 2011.
14. Sclafani AP. Restoration of the jawline and the neck after bariatric surgery. Facial Plast Surg 21:28, 2005.
15. Moran MC. Benefits of epidural anesthesia over general anesthesia in the prevention of deep vein thrombosis following total hip arthroplasty. J Arthroplasty 10:405, 1995.

63. Female Genital Aesthetic Surgery

Phillip D. Khan, Christine Hamori

- Incidence of female genital aesthetic surgery has increased as the quest for the aesthetic "ideal" becomes more popular.
  - Fivefold increase in the number of patients seeking cosmetic surgery of the vaginal region.[1]
- Often, the balance of aesthetic beauty and functional optimization, particularly in terms of sexual intercourse, has played hand in hand.
- Genital beauty is **culturally defined and dependent.**[2] (Table 63-1)
  - In Japan, the "winged butterfly" appearance of the small labia is popular.
  - In Western society, protruding inner labia are considered less desirable.
  - In part of Africa, in a ritual known as Kudenga, the inner labia are stretched from a young age in the belief it optimizes sexual intercourse.

Table 63-1 *Female Genital Aesthetic Surgery Terms and Definitions*

Term	Synonyms/Definition
Vulvovaginal plastic surgery	Umbrella term encompassing all procedures defined below
Vaginal rejuvenation	Not recommended for use as a proprietary term for medical terminology
Labiaplasty/nymphoplasty	Reduction of the labia minora
Clitoral hood reduction	Reduction of the clitoral hood
Labia majora reduction	Reduction of the labia majora
Vaginoplasty	Repair of the vagina to correct vaginal relaxation
Perineoplasty	Excision of excess introital and perineal tissue and repair of the perineal musculature
Vaginal tightening (colpoperineoplasty)	Both perineoplasty and some degree of posterior vaginal repair for vaginal restoration
Hymenoplasty	Repair/reconstruction of the hymen so as to mimic the virginal state

- Labiaplasty has become the cornerstone of this multiarea concern
  - Aesthetic and functional concerns drive this trend.
  - Reasons in Westernized women[3]:
    - ▶ Media
    - ▶ Internet
    - ▶ Brazilian waxing
    - ▶ Functional issues like rubbing and hygiene

- Media influence may increase pressure for women to improve their appearance.[4]
  - Small, hardly visible, symmetrical labia minora have become the norm, with commercial images being altered to reduce the size.[4,5]
  - Growing habit of shaving the genital area, and even the availability of pornography, may influence this ideal image.[4]
- A series from Alter[6] revealed the following reasons for surgery:
  - 85.5% aesthetic reasons, with some discomfort with clothing, exercise, or sexual intercourse
  - 13.3% aesthetic reasons alone
  - 1.2% medical reasons
- **Ideal aesthetic traits for each segment**[2,7]:
  - Labia minora that is symmetrical and does not protrude past the labia majora on standing
  - Full labia majora that conceals the labia minora completely with minimal bulkiness in tight clothing
  - Inconspicuous clitoral hood
  - Mons fat pad that does not protrude in clothing

LABIA MINORA ENLARGEMENT

- Labia enlargement is classified by measurement (Table 63-2).[8]

Table 63-2   *Felicio Classification of Labia Minora Enlargement*

Type	Measurement (cm)
I	<2
II	2-4
III	4-6
IV	>6

CONDITIONS AND CAUSES

- Enlargement or hypertrophy in both length and width[9-16] (Box 63-1)
  - Most feel that 5 cm in length, measured from the base of the minora to the labial edge, is the upper limit of normal.[4]
  - Some have suggested that those seeking reduction have a mean labial width of 3.52 ± 0.71 cm[8,9]
  - Felicio classification[8] (see Table 63-2)

Box 63-1   *CAUSES OF LABIA MINORA ENLARGEMENT*

Congenital

Most common

Acquired

Pregnancy, birth control pills, aging, exogenous hormones[7,11]
Topical estrogen[12]
Stretching or weight attachment of the labia[13]
Dermatitis secondary to urinary incontinence[14]
Vulvar lymphedema from infections with filarial sanguinous[14]
Myelodysplastic disease[15]
Repetitive stretching from pregnancy, sexual intercourse, chronic masturbation[16]

- Atrophy or hypoplasia
- **Issues driving correction**
  - **Aesthetic**
    - ▶ Loss of self-esteem/social embarrassment
- **Functional**
  - Interference with intercourse
  - Chronic local irritation
  - Hygiene problems
    - ▶ Almost 50% of patients seeking correction report difficulty performing adequate local hygiene[10]
  - Discomfort during walking, cycling, sitting, wearing more formfitting pants

CLITORIS AND CLITORAL HOOD[1,17]

NOTE: Clitoral hood conditions may develop either separately or along with labia minora hypertrophy.

- Excessive, unattractive skin from preputial fold hypertrophy
  - Can occur in the horizontal and vertical dimension
  - Parallel folds lateral to the clitoral hood
  - Drape-like folds that separate the anterior vulvar commissure on standing[1]
  - May protrude to give the appearance of a small penis
  - Apparent hypertrophy of hood after aggressive edge trim labiaplasty[17]
  - "Buries" the clitoris

NOTE: This quite often becomes noticeable after a labiaplasty that does not address the clitoral hood concomitantly or after aggressive trimming of the labia minora. *Hood redundancy is the most common reason patients seek revision surgery.*[18]

- Phimotic clitoral hood over the clitoris
- Clitoral glans hypertrophy
  - ► Elongation or general size
  - ► Primary or secondary from hormonal changes
  - ► Genetic abnormalities such as disorders of sexual development
  - ► Clitoral hood **varies greatly** and is **commonly asymmetrical.**[19]
    - ◆ Length of 2-6 cm measured from the midline of the anterior labial commissure to the distal clitoral prepuce
    - ◆ Smooth or with multiple folds
    - ◆ May have a parallel fold lateral to the main clitoral hood
    - ◆ Variable thickness depending on the amount of subcutaneous tissue (dartos fascia)
    - ◆ May protrude, if enlarged, to give the appearance of a small penis

LABIA MAJORA
- Primary hypertrophy[2]
  - Volume excess
  - Fatty infiltration of the labia majora and ptosis of the anterior labial commissure[20]
- Secondary hypertrophy
  - Volume loss, creating excess skin
- Fat and skin excess
  - Creates overhang and droop, often with a central crease from the introitus
  - Protuberance
    - ► Creates two concerns:
      - ◆ Overly fatty, full labia majora
      - ◆ Fat deficient, stretched labia majora with skin excess
- **Issues driving correction**
  - Same as those for labia minora reduction
  - Aesthetic concern
  - Functional concern
    - ► Discomfort, fitting of clothes, hygiene, secondary sexual dysfunction, chronic irritation
  - Weight-related issues are key concerns.
    - ► Weight gain and obesity with resultant fat and skin enlargement
    - ► Secondary to weight loss or time after pregnancy
    - ► Ptosis of mons from massive weight loss, creating majora laxity and skin excess

MONS PUBIS
- Lipodystrophy
- Descent of tissue
  - Massive weight loss
- Excess skin
  - Massive weight loss

NOTE: Mons hypertrophy or redundancy is seen in both the transverse and vertical dimension.[21]

KEY POINT: Enlarged mons fat is usually associated with large, protuberant labia majora as a result of fat excess and stretched skin and is rarely eliminated by weight loss.[7,20,22]

GOALS OF TREATMENT

- Varies across cultures, particularly in relation to the labia minora
- Aesthetically desirable result, addressing any functional issues
- Preserving sensory innervation and physiology is critical.

LABIA MINORA

- Create an aesthetically pleasing labia minora while addressing functional concerns[4,6]
- Reduction of the hypertrophic labia minora
  - Thin and straight labia
  - Light colored, with optimal color and texture match of the labial edges
  - Nonredundant edges
  - Symmetry

> **NOTE:** This has been a topic of debate with some feeling that the minora are not perfectly symmetrical, citing a functional advantage of one labia being larger than the other as a sealing mechanism for protection against vaginitis (see below).[8]

  - Preservation of the introitus
  - Maintenance of neurovascular supply
  - Preservation of sensitivity to the labium and labial edge
    - ▶ Malinovsky et al[23] reported several different groups of nerve endings involved in sexual sensitivity with labial hypertrophy
- Improve volume of the atrophic or hypoplastic labia minora[8]
  - Aesthetic
  - Some point out a functional aspect
    - ▶ May provide greater comfort for some with sexual intercourse
    - ▶ May provide more shock absorption as well as aid in tightening of the vaginal space

CLITORIS AND CLITORAL HOOD

- Reduce excess skin
- Release entrapment
- Resuspend to the pubic symphysis

LABIA MAJORA

- Reduce excess skin redundancy and tissue descent
- Reduce fat volume
- Enhance contour
- Augment atrophy

MONS PUBIS

- Lift and tighten
  - Decrease protuberance of excess fat
  - Lift descent
  - Contour excess or ptotic skin
  - Smooth transition from the lower abdomen to pubic area

- Correct ptosis of the anterior labial commissure
- Increase visibility of the genitalia
- Decrease pressure on urinary bladder and sense of urinary urgency

PERTINENT ANATOMY[3,7,24,25] (Fig. 63-1)

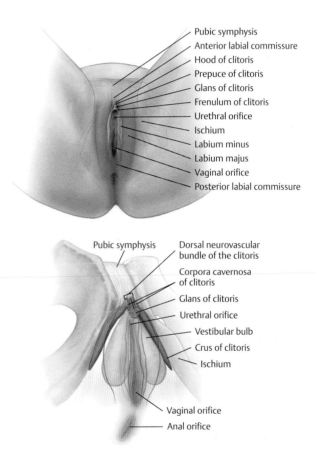

Pubic symphysis
Anterior labial commissure
Hood of clitoris
Prepuce of clitoris
Glans of clitoris
Frenulum of clitoris
Urethral orifice
Ischium
Labium minus
Labium majus
Vaginal orifice
Posterior labial commissure

Pubic symphysis

Dorsal neurovascular bundle of the clitoris

Corpora cavernosa of clitoris

Glans of clitoris
Urethral orifice
Vestibular bulb
Crus of clitoris
Ischium

Vaginal orifice
Anal orifice

Fig. 63-1   Pertinent anatomy.

CLITORAL REGION
- Clitoris, prepuce, frenulum, clitoral hood

Clitoris
- Erectile organ typically 2 cm in length and <1 cm in diameter
- Attached to the pubic symphysis by the suspensory ligament of the clitoris
- Consists of a **root, body,** and **glans**

- Body
  - ▶ Composed of two corpora cavernosa and two crura which diverge inferiorly and laterally to attach bilaterally to the ischium
  - ▶ Corpora cavernosa enclosed within the fibroelastic tunica albuginea
- Glans
  - ▶ **Most highly innervated organ of the area**
- Covered by thinly cornified stratified squamous epithelium devoid of sebaceous, apocrine, or sweat glands
- The subcutaneous tissue (dartos fascia) of the hood is superficial to the deeper Buck fascia.
- Dorsal neurovascular bundle travels at the 11 o'clock and 1 o'clock positions at the junction of the glans and body.
  - Travels within the deep Buck fascia directly on the tunica albuginea

Prepuce
- Covers the glans
- Formed from folds of the labia minora that pass dorsal (anterior) to the glans

Frenulum
- Extends from ventral (posterior or deeper) glans bilaterally
- Meets with an extension of the hood to form the labia minora

Clitoral Hood
- Appearance varies and is frequently **asymmetrical**[19]
  - Length 2-6 cm
  - Smooth or corrugated
  - Parallel folds
  - Variable thickness
  - Protrusive if hood is thickened or clitoris enlarged

LABIA MINORA[3]
- Other names include *nymphae* or *labium minus* pudenda.
- Two longitudinal, hairless cutaneous folds
  - Varying in size and devoid of fat
  - Internally situated between the labia majora
  - Paired folds surrounding the vestibule of the vagina
- Skin is smooth, pigmented, and mildly rugose at the edges.
  - The dermis has a comparatively thick connective tissue component.
    - ▶ Composed mainly of elastic fibers and small blood vessels, making up erectile tissue
  - The dermis is similar in thickness to eyelid dermis. This varies patient to patient. Some patients have very thick dermis of the labia minora.[16]
- Core of spongy connective tissue
  - Contain erectile tissue and many small blood vessels and sensory nerve endings
  - Contribute significantly to engorgement and thickening during sexual stimulation
- Inner surfaces of each labium have numerous sebaceous and eccrine glands, along with sensory nerve endings.
  - Pink color of mucus membranes

- The posterior ends may be joined across the midline by a fold of skin (frenulum labiorum pudendi, fourchette, or posterior commissure of the labia minora).
- Anteriorly
  - Each labium divides into upper (anterior or dorsal) and lower (posterior or ventral) parts
    - ▶ Upper part passes above the clitoris to meet the contralateral side.
      - ◆ Creates an overhang known as the *preputium clitoridis* (prepuce)
      - ◆ Often asymmetrical
    - ▶ Lower part passes below the clitoris to meet the contralateral side, forming the frenulum of the clitoris.
- Notable sensibility
  - Highly innervated for the entire edge, which is notable for sexual response[10,26-30]
  - Genital corpuscles for erogenous sensibility, as well as Pacinian and Meissner corpuscles[26,31]

Labia Majora[25]
- Prominent folds of skin surrounding the pudendal cleft
- Each contains:
  - Loose subcutaneous tissue with smooth muscle
  - The termination of the round ligament of the uterus
  - Membranous fat, which is continuous with the superficial perineal fascia
- Externally, covered with pigmented skin (variable), sebaceous glands, crisp pubic hair
- Internally, pink and hairless

Mons Pubis
- Rounded, fatty prominence anterior to the pubic symphysis, pubic tubercle, and superior pubic rami
- Mass of fatty subcutaneous tissue
  - Typically increases at puberty, decreases at menopause
- Surface continuous with the anterior abdominal wall

Vestibule
- Space between the labia minora containing openings of the urethra, vagina, and ducts of the greater and lesser vestibular glands
- Urethral orifice is located 2-3 cm posterior to the glans of the clitoris.
- **Bulbs of the vestibule**
  - Paired masses of elongated erectile tissue (~3 cm in length) along the sides of the vaginal orifice
  - Covered by the bulbospongiosus muscles
  - Homologous to the bulb of the penis and corpus spongiosum
- **Vestibular glands**
  - **Greater vestibular glands** are partially overlapped posteriorly by the vestibular bulbs.
    - ▶ Open in the vestibule on either side of the vaginal orifice
    - ▶ Secrete mucus during sexual intercourse

- **Lesser vestibular glands**
  - ▶ Open into the spaces between the urethra and vaginal orifice
  - ▶ Secrete mucus into the vestibule to moisten the labia
- **Superficial perineal muscles**
  - Superficial transverse perineal
  - Ischiocavernosus
    - ▶ Attaches to the ischial ramus and partly surrounds the crus of the clitoris
    - ▶ Contraction during arousal creates blood flow to the corpora cavernosa and compression of deep dorsal veins, contributing to clitoral engorgement (erection).[26]
  - Bulbospongiosus
    - ▶ Arises from perineal body to pass around the vagina
    - ▶ Inserts into the clitoris
    - ▶ Covers the bulb of the vestibule and the greater vestibular glands
    - ▶ Weak constrictor of the vagina when acting together

SENSORY INNERVATION
- **Anterior labial nerves**
  - Ilioinguinal nerve
  - Genital branch of the genitofemoral nerve
  - Perineal branch of the posterior cutaneous nerve of the thigh
- **Posterior labial nerves**
  - Run posterior to anterior toward the mons
  - Pudendal nerve
    - ▶ Perineal branches
    - ▶ Posterior labial branches
  - Terminal branches of the posterior cutaneous nerve of the thigh
- **Autonomic innervation from the pelvic and hypogastric plexus**
  - Increases vaginal secretion
  - Erection of the clitoris
  - Engorgement of erectile tissue in the bulbs of the vestibule
- Malinovsky et al[23] demonstrated multiple different groups of sensory nerve endings in hypertrophy of the labia minora involved in sexual sensitivity.

VASCULAR SUPPLY[19,32]
- Extensive collaterals
  - External superficial pudendal artery branches
    - ▶ External superficial pudendal artery anastomosis with the posterior labial artery (branch of the internal pudendal artery)
      - ◆ Supplies much of the labia majora
      - ◆ This arch gives rise to multiple arches supplying labia minora
  - Internal pudendal artery branches
    - ▶ Perineal, posterior labial, dorsal clitoral arteries
  - Internal circumflex artery

PREOPERATIVE EVALUATION

■ A thorough discussion regarding patient's aesthetic and functional goals is essential.
■ Examine in both **standing** and **lithotomy** positions.
■ Evaluate area as a unit comprising the mons, pubic area, labia minora and majora, clitoral hood and clitoris, introitus.

NOTE: Patients should use a mirror while pointing out areas of concern in each position. Surgeons can identify areas of resection or proposed lift.

LABIA MINORA[6,7]
■ Protrusion
    • Length (base to most projecting point)
    • Length in anteroposterior direction
■ Thickness
■ Symmetry
■ Skin quality
■ Skin color
■ Relationship of the introitus
    ▶ High posterior lip
    ▶ Opened introitus from previous episiotomy

LABIA MAJORA
■ Excess of loose skin
■ Excess or lack of fat
■ Projection in the anteroposterior direction
■ Anterior labial commissure in relation to the pubic symphysis
    • *This is a guide point, particularly in procedures with a planned pubic lift*
■ Must evaluate alongside mons pubis descent and pubic lipodystrophy

NOTE: Evaluating the labia majora with the legs abducted and adducted is critical. The relationship to the inner thighs is noted here. This helps to prevent possible overresection of the labia majora and secondary tethering of skin, a complication that can lead to vaginal splaying.

CLITORIS AND CLITORAL HOOD
    • Evaluate patients while they are in standing and lithotomy position.
    • Note protrusion, symmetry, hyperkeratotic or darkened skin, extra folds (horizontal and vertical), clitoral gland size, and degree of clitoral exposure.
    • Hood deformities are best noted with patient standing.

NOTE: Alteration of the minora may affect the appearance of the clitoral hood.

Mons Pubis

- Mons descent
- Observe the related enlargement, descent, or protrusion of the labia majora.
  - Assess the labia majora with simulated elevation of the pubic fat pad, noting the amount of inferior labial protrusion.
  - Examine the majora with the mons lifted.
- Panniculus
  - Determine the amount of pubic skin above the hairline that will need to be excised transversely.
  - Simulating a possible lift, note the position of the anterior labial commissure.
    - ► Should be at the pubic symphysis
    - ► Reference point for magnitude of lift and subsequent amount of skin to be excised

NOTE: **The skin excision extent may vary with fat removal.**

INFORMED CONSENT

- Postoperative course and complications
- Labial swelling
  - Labia minora and clitoral hood edema
- Change in position of the anterior labial commissure
- Inadequate reduction
- Pain
- Color change
  - Suture line may create a contrast between lighter and darker tissue or between coarse and finer hair.
  - Seen in all forms of labia minora and labia majora reduction
- Reduction of one area of the total complex may result in prominence of other areas.
  - Reduction of the labia majora alone may result in more prominence of the labia minora or clitoral hood.
- Sexual dysfunction
- Change in position, sensation, or even tethering of the vaginal introitus
- Exposure of the clitoral glans
- Vaginal dryness
- Changes in sexual sensation
- Scarring—widened, hypertrophic, painful
- Hematoma
- Infection
- Transient dyspareunia
- Fistula or major wound dehiscence

TECHNIQUES

All techniques are performed with patients in the lithotomy position. Markings are made, and local anesthesia is injected.

LABIA MINORA
Volume Reduction (Fig. 63-2)

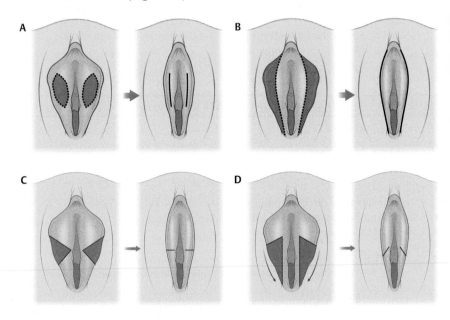

Fig. 63-2   Labiaplasty. **A,** Deepithelialization; central portion of labial mucosa deepithelialized and reapproximated. **B,** Direct excision; full-thickness excision using contoured excision parallel to each labia minora, sparing the fourchette. **C,** Central wedge resection; central wedge of excess tissue excised and labium reapproximated. **D,** Inferior wedge resection with superior flap; inferior wedge of tissue is resected and labium reapproximated.

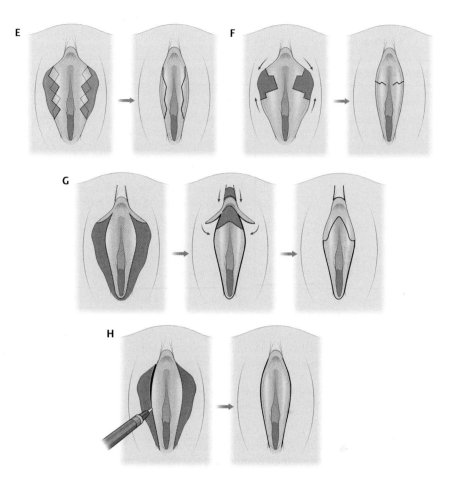

Fig. 63-2, cont'd   **E,** W-plasty excision (zigzag technique); complementary, running, W-shaped resections along medial and lateral aspects of each labium minus, sparing clitoris and fourchette. Interdigitating reapproximation of tissue. **F,** Z-shaped wedge resection; Z-shaped incisions to excise central wedge of tissue with approximation of each labium minus. **G,** Composite reduction; curved excision with narrow, superiorly based pedicled flaps and frenulum clitoris preserved. Crescent of tissue below clitoris removed to an extent to which the clitoris will move caudally. Central, rectangular skin segment cranial to the clitoris excised and reapproximated. **H,** Laser excision; laser used to excise tissue similar to direct excision and wedge resection.

■ **Labiaplasty (labia minora reduction)**
  • Edge trim (most common) [3]
  • Wedge resection patterns, as originally described by Alter[6,18-20] or a variant of such techniques
  • Bilateral deepithelialization technique
  • Composite reduction[33]
  • Laser excision technique[9,34]

■ **Edge resection**
  • **Elliptical incisions**[12,13,17,35,36] (Box 63-2)

Box 63-2   *LABIA MINORA REDUCTION TECHNIQUES–ELLIPTICAL EXCISION: PROS AND CONS*

Pros	Cons
Edge irregularities are reduced. Techniques are powerful for those with extreme hypertrophy.[35] Removal of pigmented edge. Debulks thick leading edge of labia minora.	A scarred, stiff suture line subject to tenderness and scar retraction remains. Potential for excess tissue resection, especially if minora retracted laterally during marking and subsequent excision. Some pigmentation may remain depending upon location and amount of labial hypertrophy. The transition zone between the labium, frenulum, and clitoral hood may become distorted, resulting in an abrupt-ending clitoral frenulum and large, noticeable, overhanging clitoral hood.

► **Markings**
  ◆ Traction is placed over the most prominent portion of the labia.
  ◆ The most anterior portion of the resection is kept to within 1 cm of the clitoral hood and does not include the frenulum.
  ◆ Posteriorly, the markings are stopped **before they cross the midline** of the posterior fourchette.
  ◆ Anteriorly, markings are stopped within 1 cm of the urethral opening to avoid distortion.
► **Technique**
  ◆ Full-thickness edge resection of minora
  ◆ Closure with interrupted or running absorbable suture. Avoid excess tension on suture line to avoid suture track scarring.
  • **Zigzag technique** (Maas and Hage[37]) (Box 63-3)

Box 63-3   *ZIGZAG TECHNIQUE: PROS AND CONS*

Pros	Cons
Preservation of natural border Elimination of the labia minora edge scar, thus creating a more rounded lateral edge.	Color mismatch or asymmetry. Pigmentation is lost along the labial edge.[3] Excess bulk from Z-plasty[35]

► **Markings** (Fig. 63-3)
  ◆ Similar to basic elliptical markings in terms of area resected and guidelines
  ◆ Medial aspect of the resection is marked in a running W-shaped resection pattern.
  ◆ Corresponding lateral markings are made.
► **Technique**
  ◆ Skin incision is made on the medial border, then on the corresponding lateral border. Medial and lateral flaps are created in the process.
  ◆ The lateral cutaneous and medial mucosal edges are approximated in interdigitating fashion with interrupted 6-0 absorbable suture.

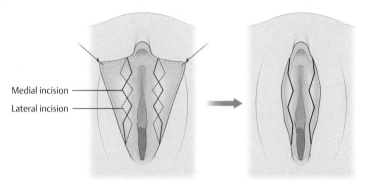

Medial incision
Lateral incision

Fig. 63-3 Zigzag technique. The uninterrupted line indicates the marking of the running W-shaped incision on the medial aspect, and the interrupted line indicates the complementary marking on the lateral aspect of each labium minus.

• Felicio[8] described free edge amputation technique with the use of an S-type incision to decrease the chance of scar contracture.
■ **Wedge excisions**
  • **V-shaped wedge excision and extended central wedge (hockey-stick extension) excision** (Alter[6]) (Box 63-4)

Box 63-4 *Wedge Excisions: Pros and Cons*

Pros	Cons
Versatile and allows lateral clitoral hood reduction by extension of dog-ears superiorly.	A scar runs from the base to the edge.
Debulks most protuberant portion of labia.[8]	May oppose dark pigmentation with light at wedge closure site.[37]
Applying posterior tension minimizes projection of the clitoral hood anteriorly.[2]	Posterior tension may cover more of the clitoral hood, potentially decreasing sensation.[3]

► Centered over the most prominent portions of the labia minora
► External edge or hockey-stick extension, curved anteriorly and laterally, allows removal of excess lateral clitoral hooding or dog-ears.
► **Markings** (Fig. 63-4)

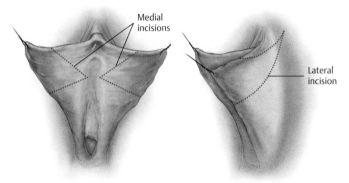

Medial incisions

Lateral incision

Fig. 63-4   Markings for a V-shaped wedge excision and extended central wedge excision described by Alter.

♦ The clitoral glans frenulum and lower clitoral hood converge, forming the labia minora. This point varies and is key element in resection pattern.
  – Anterior portion of the incision line is at or posterior to this convergence point.
♦ Medially, forceps are used to determine the amount of wedge excision to create a straight line without causing a tightened introitus or undue tension on the incision.
  – The wedge point must end just outside of the hymenal ring.
♦ Laterally, forceps are used to determine the extended lateral markings.
  – Markings are carried in a "hockey-stick" manner anteriorly to incorporate lateral clitoral hood or lateral hood folds.
♦ When creating the resection patterns, attention is given to the vaginal introitus to prevent tightening.
  – Two fingers should fit within the proposed resection pattern to prevent overtightening.

NOTE: The medial and lateral markings will be asymmetrical. Medial markings tend to extend from the edge of the labia and inward to a point toward the vaginal introitus. Lateral markings extend from the edge in a more anterior-type direction, toward the clitoral hood and prepuce, to address redundant skin.

► **Technique**[8] (Figs. 63-5 and 63-6)

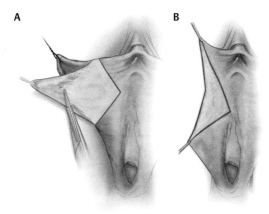

Fig. 63-5   A, Under gentle traction from a suture, the medial incision is made first, just through the mucosa, preserving the important subcutaneous tissue. A knife is used to remove the mucosa to the point of the traction suture. **B,** Completed excision of medial and lateral tissue, noting the preservation of the important subcutaneous tissue.

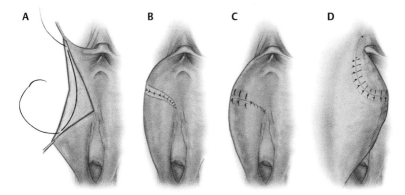

Fig. 63-6   A, Subcutaneous tissue is approximated using 5-0 Monocryl suture. Any excess, protruding medial or lateral subcutaneous tissue is removed. **B,** Completed approximation of subcutaneous tissue. Note the smooth transition of subcutaneous tissue following excess removal, to avoid dog-ears and thickened labia on closure. **C,** Skin closure from distal to proximal in vertical mattress fashion. The deep portions medially may be performed in a running fashion. **D,** Completed lateral incision line.

- ◆ Performing one labium at a time is critical, given the natural asymmetry that may exist.
- ◆ Medial incision first
  - – Placing traction on the labia, the incision is carefully carried just into the mucosa, preserving the thin, underlying subcutaneous tissue.
  - – The medial portion is removed carefully with a knife.
- ◆ Lateral incision
  - – On stretch, the lateral incision is made just through the dermis, preserving the underlying subcutaneous tissue.
- ◆ **Subcutaneous tissue approximation**
  - – 5-0 Monocryl suture on an atraumatic needle in two layers whenever possible

---

NOTE: Meticulous closure is essential to prevent wound dehiscence and eliminate fistula formation.[8]

- – Any excess, protruding subcutaneous tissue may be removed here to prevent dog-ears.
- ◆ **Skin closure** (see Fig. 63-6)
  - – Distal to proximal
  - – Interrupted vertical mattress sutures using 5-0 Monocryl
  - – The key point is the edge suture, bringing the medial and lateral edge points together. This should be the first suture, performed in meticulous fashion for proper eversion of the tissue.
  - – A running suture may be used in the deepest portions of the medial incision or occasionally on the lateral lines.
- ◆ Extended consideration[8]
  - – Attention must be given to the vaginal introitus both before and after resection.
    - ▲ A high posterior lip or overly tight introitus may lead to intercourse difficulty.
    - ▲ The posterior lip may need to be incised and vaginal mucosa sutured to the perineal skin.
  - – If vaginal tightening procedures are performed at the same time, they must be done before the labiaplasty.

- **Inferior wedge resection and superior pedicle flap reconstruction** (Munhoz et al[10]) (Box 63-5)

Box 63-5   *INFERIOR WEDGE RESECTION AND SUPERIOR PEDICLE FLAP: PROS AND CONS*

Pros	Cons
In correctly selected patients, the superior flap has a free margin with natural color and texture.	Posterior advancement of the superior flap may lead to a bulky labium. • Should this occur, less lateral clitoral hood skin is advanced posteriorly. The inferior edge of the labial resection is the thinnest and least protuberant portion of the minora.[35] • The transition sometimes results in a bulging contour with the more superior and bulky flap. • An unnatural transition, with a pulled-down appearance near the posterior fourchette, may result. The distal tip of the flap has poor vascularity with a less predictable result. Distal vascularization is more difficult to predict given the nonaxial nature of the flap.[38]

▶ **Superoanterior flap is created and advanced posteriorly.**
▶ **Indications**
   ◆ Moderate to large labia minora hypertrophy with dimensions >3 cm measured horizontally from the midline when placed on lateral traction with minimal tension
      – Important, because the superior flap in the reconstruction relies on the redundancy of skin and mucosa of the region, along with the dense network of perforating vessels near the midline of the perineum
▶ **Contraindication**
   ◆ Minimal hypertrophy or absence of skin laxity
▶ **Markings:** Pinch test using small forceps
   ◆ The middle portion of the labia minora is gently grasped and stretched inferiorly to the posterior portion of the vaginal introitus.
      – Simulates the amount of wedged tissue to be resected and the extension of the superior flap

- ◆ Tension is assessed.
  - – With too much tension, the marking is adjusted more anteriorly.
  - – With excess redundancy, this point is moved more posteriorly to resect more tissue.
- ◆ A wedge-shaped area is designed between this midlabial point and the posterior edge of the labia in the lithotomy position.
  - – The angle of the wedge will vary depending on tissue excess and cutaneous/mucosal laxity.
  - – Moderate hypertrophy designates a wedge more like an isosceles triangle located exclusively on the more posterior labia minora.
  - – With large hypertrophy, the resected area encompasses the more anterior region, with more curved borders and convex design to include excess tissue.

NOTE: Place two or three fingers inside the vaginal introitus and stretch the minora during this estimation to prevent postoperative tightness of the introitus secondary to excess tissue resection.

▶ **Technique** (Figs. 63-7 and 63-8)

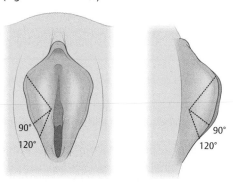

Fig. 63-7   Surgical plan showing the resected area and the superior flap design. For moderate hypertrophy, we prefer a small reduction with an angle between the two lines of 90 degrees. In the presence of severe hypertrophy, and if the patient desires more aggressive reduction, the angle can be 120 degrees.

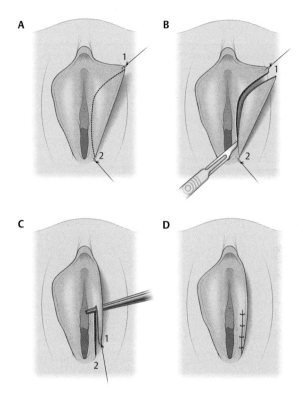

Fig. 63-8   A and **B,** The skin incision is carried down to the subcutaneous tissue on the medial layer. The complementary incision is performed on the lateral layer, and the total wedge-shaped area is resected. **C,** Point *1* is approximated to point *2*. **D,** The medial and lateral incisions are closed.

- Medial incision is made to the subcutaneous layer.
- Lateral incision is carried to the subcutaneous layer.
- Total wedge-shaped area is resected.
- Avoid undermining at the base of the flap, because the more anterior portion of the labia minora supplies the vascularity.
- Labial edge of the superior flap is approximated to the edge of the posterior labia.
- Medial and lateral borders are closed in layers with absorbable suture.

- **Modified double-wedge "star" labiaplasty** (Tepper et al[4]) (Box 63-6)

Box 63-6 *Modified Double-Wedge "Star" Labiaplasty: Pros and Cons*

Pros	Cons
Flexibility is increased over the vertical technique described by Alter and the inferior wedge technique described by Munhoz. An additional means of reduction is created, without the risk of widening the central vertical V excision.	Additional suture line and tissue dissection is involved.

- ▶ Takes advantage of the flexibility of the vertical wedge techniques by adding a horizontal V excision to the anterior and posterior flaps as needed
  - ◆ The angles of the horizontal edges are adjusted as well. Additional tissue resection is provided without the risk of widening the vertical V.
- ▶ **Indications**
  - ◆ Labial hypertrophy with skin laxity and excess skin
  - ◆ Labial hypertrophy not adequately addressed with a vertical wedge excision alone
- ▶ **Markings**
  - ◆ Lithotomy position
  - ◆ With labia gently stretched, vertical resection wedge is drawn, as per the Alter technique.[6]
  - ◆ Midway down the vertical limb, an additional horizontal wedge is designed, first on the anterior flap, then on the posterior flap.
- ▶ **Technique** (Fig. 63-9)

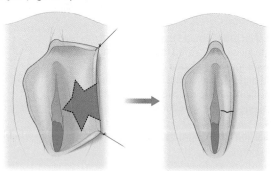

Fig. 63-9 Matarasso modification of a wedge excision using four limbs, also referred to as the *star technique*. This approach increases flexibility to preferentially excise the labia minora by altering the size or angle of the V and adding one or two horizontal wedge resections.

- ◆ Medial skin incision is made to the subcutaneous space.
- ◆ Lateral incision is made.
- ◆ Dimensions are adjusted for the horizontal wedge excisions.
- ◆ Closure is performed in layers with absorbable suture.

- **Posterior wedge resection** (Kelishada et al[26]) (Box 63-7)

Box 63-7   *POSTERIOR WEDGE RESECTION: PROS AND CONS*

Pros	Cons
The central wedge is an advantage, because it can be arranged to remove the most protuberant portion of each labium. The normal pigmentation of the outer surface of the minora is preserved.	The most undesirable portion of the labium is on the superior flap and is transposed more posteriorly.

► Creates a superiorly based flap which preserves the outer edge of much of the labia minora
► Differs from others with superiorly based pedicles
  ◆ Major part of the excision is posterior to the outer labium, between the inner and outermost labia minora.
    – Preserves the outermost edge or anterior edge, mainly at the most superior and inferior boundaries
    – Gives the results of a thinner-appearing superior pedicle by preserving the outer edge and theoretically decreasing the distance required to close the superior flap to the remnant minora base
    – Possibility of decreased tension and less bulk on the final flap
► **Markings**
  ◆ Must design a superior pedicle
  ◆ Lateral border of the labia minora first
    – Carried from posterior to anterior to end within 1 cm of the frenulum
    – Extended to the base and then posteriorly to within 1 cm of the fourchette
  ◆ Parallel markings made along the medial side
► **Technique** (Fig. 63-10)

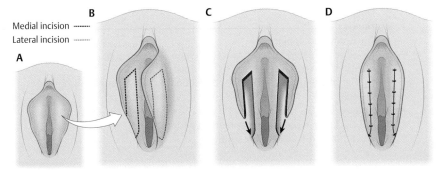

Fig. 63-10   A, The hypertrophic labia minora. **B,** Marks for posterior wedge resection. **C,** The *red arrows* indicate the superior pedicle flap. This is created from the remaining labia minora after resection and brought down toward the remaining labial base. **D,** The final appearance after placement of sutures.

- ◆ Multiple sutures are placed for traction.
- ◆ Sharp scissors are used to make full-thickness incisions through the resection patterns.
- ◆ Absorbable sutures are placed to imbricate the base of the labia minora.
- ◆ Excess labial tissue is trimmed using a "tailor-tacked" technique.
- ◆ The closure is completed in three layers using absorbable suture.
- ◆ How it differs from other superiorly[35]
    - – Thinner lateral edges of the minora are preserved and suture lines placed in natural creases.
    - – Base width of the minora is reduced by imbricating sutures to match the thinner lateral edge widths of the minora.
    - – Lateral edge trimming for symmetry is common.
- ◆ Allows concomitant clitoral hood and labia majora reductions
- • **Central wedge resection with a 90-degree Z-plasty** (Giraldo et al[31]) (Box 63-8)

Box 63-8   *CENTRAL WEDGE RESECTION WITH A NINETY-DEGREE Z-PLASTY: PROS AND CONS*

Pros	Cons
Z-plasty creates a nontense suture line, decreasing the likelihood of scar contracture and introital narrowing.[39] Because of thin labial mucosa, Alter[18-20] did not find this to be much of a problem. The base is not violated, thus preserving the site and entrance of the superficial perineal nerve and its distal branches so vital for sensation.[39]	The anterior and posterior surfaces have mismatched color.[39] The full-thickness resection pattern may increase the chance of postoperative fistula.

- ▶ Variation of the original Alter technique, with addition of two opposing Z-plasties to aid in closure
    - ◆ Z-plasties centered around only the most prominent portion of the bulky labia
- ▶ **Markings**
    - ◆ Traction suture is placed.
    - ◆ A wedge is created between two 90-degree Z-plasties. The apex of the wedge is designed to end just ventral to the urinary meatus.
        - – This marking is drawn on the corresponding lateral cutaneous border as well.
- ▶ **Technique** (Fig. 63-11)
    - ◆ Full-thickness resection of the marked patterns
    - ◆ Closure with 4-0 absorbable suture

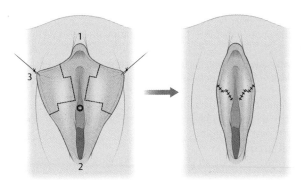

Fig. 63-11   Design of the technique. The bilateral paired 90-degree Z-plasties delimit the wedges of tissue to be resected, converging toward the ventral portion of the urinary meatus (*). (1, Clitoris; 2, vagina; 3, redundant tissue of the central third of the labia minora.)

- **Other methods**
  - ▶ **Lambda laser nymphoplasty**[9,34]
    - ◆ Central wedge V pattern of resection based on a lambda pattern
    - ◆ Creates superior flap
    - ◆ Asymmetrical V-type pattern (lambda design) with a rounded pattern to the shorter side
      - – Allows adjustment of the length of the two branches of the V resection at the base of the minora
      - – Theoretically, reduces the tension on closure of the wound
      - – Similar to other wedge resections, preserves the outer edge of the labia, reducing the color change[34]
    - ◆ Carbon dioxide laser used for excision
      - – Decreases bleeding
      - – Eliminates need for infiltration, possibly decreasing the effect of tissue distortion from local anesthetic injection
- ■ **Bilateral deepithelialization** (Choi and Kim[40]) (Box 63-9)

Box 63-9   *BILATERAL DEEPITHELIALIZATION: PROS AND CONS*

Pros	Cons
The entire edge of the labium is preserved. Demucosalization avoids injury to neurovascular supply. Postoperative tightness or pulling at the introitus may be less likely.	The anterior to posterior length of the minora is not addressed. A bulky labium with redundancy in the anterior and posterior portions may result.[35] The retained central parenchyma may create a bulge and increase the width at the base.[39]

- Central deepithelialization technique creating a vertical reduction
- Preserves the outer edge of the labia, benefiting both color and neurovascular supply
- Delicate technique involving partial-thickness resection
  - ▶ With a lack of full-thickness resection, more suitable for very mild hypertrophy[35]
- **Markings**
  - ▶ Under slight stretch, the medial and lateral areas to be deepithelialized are made.
  - ▶ A resection pattern is created to preserve a labial width of ~1 cm, with slight protrusion past the introitus.
- **Technique** (Fig. 63-12)

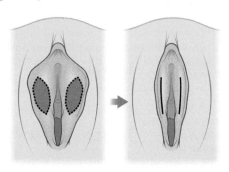

Fig. 63-12   Deepithelialization.

  - ▶ Medial incision made just to the subcutaneous tissue and deepithelialization performed.
  - ▶ Similarly done on the corresponding lateral edge
  - ▶ Margins of the raw surface reapproximated with running absorbable suture

CLITORIS AND CLITORAL HOOD
■ Excision of clitoral hood skin
- Addresses vertical and/or horizontal skin redundancy of the clitoral hood
  - ▶ Anterior hood redundancy, represented by excessive skin in the vertical dimension preoperatively, is best addressed with the lateral hockey-stick extension as a part of the Alter wedge resection (see Figs. 63-5 and 63-6).
    - ◆ Rarely, transverse folds of skin may be addressed as well.
- **Markings**
  - ▶ Redundant skin in the vertical dimension is marked in elliptical fashion.
    - ◆ Sagittal redundancy and coronal redundancy are labeled to be clear.
    - ◆ This is done on either the medial or lateral side of the clitoral hood.

- ◆ Incision is maintained along the length of the clitoral hood and parallel to the labia majora–clitoral hood sulci.
- ◆ Transverse skin excess that may need to be excised after the vertical resection is marked.
  - – An inverted-V pattern is designed for this.
  - – May be incorporated into a V-Y plasty to resuspend the clitoral glans[6,16]

NOTE: The glans must not be overexposed in aggressive hood reduction.

NOTE: When done in conjunction with labia minora procedures, the labia must be addressed first. Excess folds of the clitoral hood are addressed after the labia minora are treated.

- • **Clitoropexy**
  - ▶ Corrects the laxity of the clitoris and suspensory ligament, particularly in older patients with labia minora hypertrophy[16]
  - ▶ Descent of the clitoris more noticeable once labial hypertrophy has been addressed
  - ▶ Correcting the laxity with more superior and anterior suspension to match normal anatomic position provides a means of tightening the labia minora in the anteroposterior dimension.
  - ▶ A V-Y plasty anterior to the hood provides space for this movement, while providing access to the area of suspension.[16]
    - ◆ The pubic symphysis may be exposed.
    - ◆ Excess clitoral hood redundancy may be addressed.
  - ▶ Suspension is performed in the midline to achieve an anterosuperior lift.[16]
    - ◆ Area is delicate and may place the glans in jeopardy of neurovascular injury.
    - ◆ Laub[16] discussed the importance of remaining midline to avoid disrupting sensation from the deeper pudendal nerves, which are lateral.
    - ◆ Clitoropexy is performed first,[16] followed by assessment of excess hood skin and tissue. If needed, the Y may be extended to aid in movement of the glans.

CAUTION: Clitoropexy is technically difficult and may result in malposition of the clitoris. Strong consideration should be given to collaboration with a urologist.

- ▶ **Markings**
  - ◆ The outer edge is marked conservatively and the clitoral hood skin contoured (an inverted-V).
  - ◆ In the midline anteroposterior (AP) direction, a conservative Y extension is marked.
- ▶ **Technique** (Fig. 63-13)
  - ◆ Horizontal incision is carefully made, and, if needed, a conservative portion of the Y extension.
  - ◆ Remaining midline at all times, the dissection is very carefully carried down to expose the suspensory ligament of the clitoris and pubic symphysis.

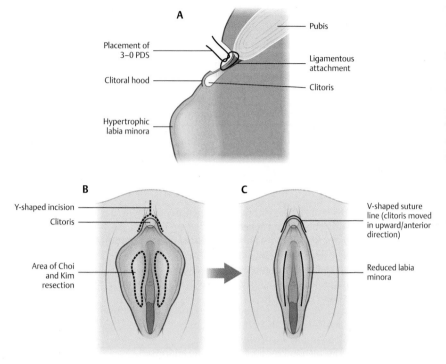

Fig. 63-13   A, Suture is placed in the midline, between the suspensory ligament of the clitoris and pubis. **B,** Markings of clitoropexy of Laub, along with labial reduction of Choi and Kim. **C,** Postoperative appearance.

> **NOTE: Deep dissection laterally will jeopardize sensory nerves.**

- A 3-0 PDS suture is placed first in the suspensory ligament.
- Movement in the anterosuperior direction is simulated, and a position of suspension in the midline is determined.
- The suture is anchored to the pubic symphysis in the midline.
  - Holds the potential V-Y clitoral hood reduction in place without tension[16]
- The Y may be extended to accommodate for movement.
- Closure is performed in layers in the standard described fashion.

LABIA MAJORA
- **Volume reduction**
  - Skin
  - Underlying fat
  - Skin and underlying fat

NOTE: **Regardless of method chosen, enough fat must be preserved to maintain normal contour and cushioning.**[20]

- **Excision**
  - Excess skin excision
  - Deeper fat excision
    - ▶ If needed, must be done conservatively to preserve the natural contour
    - ▶ May be performed from superiorly in the event of a pubic lift, although rare
      - ◆ Direct excision of both skin and fat
- **Suction-assisted reduction**
  - Liposuction
    - ▶ Can generally be done during pubic lift or even during liposuction of the abdomen
  - Some consider excision or liposuction performed from a superior position during pubic lift not as precise or effective.[22]

Direct Excision[7,20] (Box 63-10)

Box 63-10   *LABIA MAJORA DIRECT EXCISION: PROS AND CONS*

Pros	Cons
More effective and precise contouring by direct access to each component of the labia majora (skin, fat).	Overresection of labia majora fat and skin may cause a gaping introitus leading to vaginal dryness, discomfort in clothing, discomfort with activity, and an inability to completely abduct the legs
	May result in a perceived increased prominence of the clitoral hood or labia minora
	Contrast of skin color and hair pattern may occur

- **Markings**
  - Lithotomy position.
  - Mark medial thigh crease.
  - Mark lateral labial color differentiation.

- Mark the skin excess.
  - ▶ Crescent excision from the medial labium, extending from the anterior to posterior labial commissures
  - ▶ The patient is asked to stand.
    - ◆ Check the medial and lateral incision lines with a cotton swab.
  - ▶ The amount to be excised can be determined and demonstrated with the patient in preoperative holding area by using a cotton-tipped applicator to imbricate the tissue.
  - ▶ Segmental excision (*Hawaiian skirt*) is also a good option.
- Medial incision
  - ▶ Placed just lateral to the medial hairline of each labia majora
- Lateral incision
  - ▶ At least 2 cm of pigmented labium is preserved lateral to the lateral excision line.
    - ◆ Ensures preservation of enough skin to prevent gaping of the introitus while the legs are fully abducted
    - ◆ Important to test this with a cotton swab
  - ▶ Areas of possible fat excision are marked, if needed.

NOTE: Err on the conservative side and make markings while the patient's legs are fully abducted. Overresection may cause the introitus to gape on leg abduction.

- If patient has had a previous medial thigh lift[20,41]
  - ▶ *Probably should not have a pubic lift performed at the same time as a labia majora reduction through skin excision techniques, because the intervening vascular tissue may be in jeopardy*
  - ▶ If performed at the same time or recently performed, consider the possibility of a gaping introitus secondary to:
    - ◆ Overresection of skin
    - ◆ Relaxation of medial thigh lift Colles fascia tacking sutures leading to lateral pull on the labia majora[41]
- Important note
  - ▶ **The order of procedures is important.**
  - ▶ In conjunction with labia minora reduction:
    - ◆ The minora is treated first.
    - ◆ Reducing the labia majora will expose the labia minora.
  - ▶ In conjunction with a pubic lift:
    - ◆ The lift is performed first.
    - ◆ The lift will elevate the anterior labial commissure. An adequate amount of tissue deep must be maintained to preserve lymphatics.

NOTE: Patients must be informed that reducing the labia majora may cause the labia minora to appear longer.

■ **Technique** (Fig. 63-14)

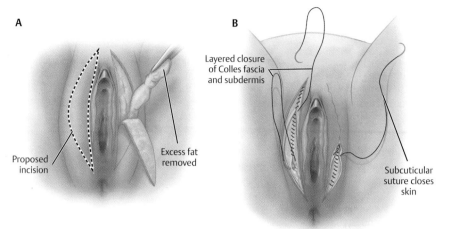

Fig. 63-14   Labia majora reduction. **A,** A crescent of skin is removed from the medial labium majus. The shape depends on the amount of excess skin. The two incision lines should not meet in the midline. Fat is excised. **B,** Closure is performed in layers. A subcuticular closure is performed on the skin, and a deep drain is placed only if significant fat is removed.

- Skin incision
- Fat excision (if needed)
  - ▶ Through the superficial Colles fascia
  - ▶ Resection with electrocautery
  - ▶ Clitoral hood should be identified and palpated during the process.
    - ◆ No injury to the clitoral hood will be noted if the resection is lateral to the pubic symphysis and superficial to the ischium.
- Tailor-tacking of the skin edges to adjust for symmetry
- Closure
  - ▶ If fat is excised, the superficial Colles fascia is closed with 4-0 or 5-0 Monocryl.
  - ▶ Subdermal layer is performed with running 5-0 Monocryl, incorporating the deeper Colles fascia to eliminate dead space.
  - ▶ Intracuticular running 5-0 Monocryl suture
    - ◆ Drains are only used for major fat excisions.

Liposuction of Labia Majora (Box 63-11)

Box 63-11   *LIPOSUCTION OF LABIA MAJORA: PROS AND CONS*

Pros	Cons
Less invasive technique to address labial protrusion May be combined with other contouring procedures such as mons liposuction/lift, or during abdominoplasty	Liposuction performed to the area may lead to significant firmness for weeks to months after the procedure. Considered to be less precise than direct excision

- ▪ **Markings**
  - • Topographic marking of fat protrusion
  - • Access incisions
    - ▸ Within a planned skin excision site
    - ▸ Suprapubic location in conjunction with adjunct contouring
    - ▸ Through suprapubic incision in conjunction with mons lift/abdominoplasty
- ▪ **Technique**
  - • Tumescent infiltration
  - • Suction assistance using 3 mm Mercedes-tip cannula
    - ▸ Do not overresect.
    - ▸ Cannula positions maintained lateral to the midline to prevent sensory nerve issues.
- ▪ **Patient and physician expectations**
  - • Labial swelling will usually start to resolve within a week.
  - • Patients should expect significant clitoral hood edema that **may persist for several months.**
    - ▸ Especially true if the pubic lift is performed at the same time
  - • Firmness of the labia majora may persist for several months.

MONS AND MONS PUBIS
- ▪ Mons remodeling to tighten and lift, addressing[21,41]:
  - • Subcutaneous fat and/or skin
  - • Volume reduction
  - • Correction of ptosis

Excision, Liposuction, Lift, or a Combination[42,43] (Box 63-12)

Box 63-12   *Mons Pubis Contouring, Combined Excision, Liposuction, and Lift: Pros and Cons*

Pros	Cons
Natural transition is created from the abdomen and ptotic mons skin.	Excessive resection of fat may lead to concavity of the mons.
The anterior labial commissure is returned to a more anatomic position.	Aggressive removal of underlying fat and/or skin can create an unnatural anterior labial commissure position and possible shortened escutcheon.[7]
Mons lift raises the ptotic labia majora; decreasing protrusion, effectively elongating the tissue	Urinary stream may be altered.[43]
Elevated genitalia is seen in >75% of patients.[43]	Liposuction may contribute to genital lymphedema.[22,43]
Hygiene and sex life are improved in >50% of patients.[43]	
Bladder incontinence is improved.[43]	

- Vertical excision, if needed, can be used for tightening.[21]
  - Midline skin excision may give an unsightly vertical scar.[22]
    - Combination transverse and vertical excision
      - Inverted triangle of skin and subcutaneous tissue excised with minimal undermining[35,42]
        - Severe deformities affecting the labia majora may extend this inverted triangle incision to include reduction of the labia majora.[35,42]
      - Results in an inverted-T incision on the skin
    - Consider the modest contraction of skin with underlying fat removal when planning amount of skin to resect.[20]
- **Liposuction**
  - Most often done in concert with abdominoplasty or pubic lift
  - Isolated liposuction will probably not address the excess skin or subsequent ptosis.
- **Technical pearls**
  - Perform direct undermining or liposuction of mons fat pad for optimal contour
  - Secure into position to prevent pubic descent[21,22,43,44]
- **Markings**
  - Patient is standing in front of a mirror and then in the lithotomy position.[20]
  - While the patient is standing, have them assist in strongly elevating the skin to determine the amount of pubic skin above the hairline that will need to be excised with the lift.
    - Positioning the anterior labial commissure at the pubic symphysis aids in this step.

NOTE: The actual amount of skin to be removed may be less than expected, given the modest amount of retraction that occurs after fat removal.[7,21]

- ▶ This represents the position of the scar.
- ▶ With massive horizontal skin excess, an upper inverted wedge of skin and subcutaneous tissue may be designed.[20]
- • If only mons is to be treated, this may be done with patient in the supine position, otherwise lithotomy.
  - ▶ Isolated lift
  - ▶ Conservative markings to best conceal the scar
- • Combination with existing abdominoplasty incision
- ▪ **Technique** (Figs. 63-15 and 63-16)
  - • Local anesthetic containing epinephrine is injected into the incision lines.
  - • A tumescent solution containing dilute lidocaine and epinephrine may also be injected.
  - • Upper incision is made and carried down to the rectus fascia.
    - ▶ Dissection just superficial to the rectus fascia is carried down to near the pubic symphysis.
    - ▶ Fat may be excised at this time, tapering its thickness in triangular fashion down toward the pubic symphysis.

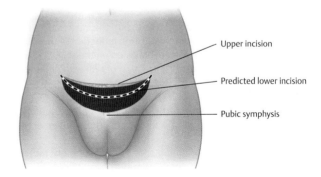

Fig. 63-15   The upper incision is made to the rectus fascia. The flap is undermined to the pubic symphysis and laterally to the inguinal canals and external rings.

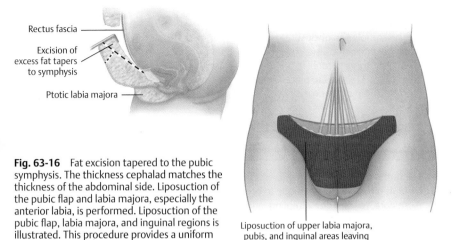

Fig. 63-16   Fat excision tapered to the pubic symphysis. The thickness cephalad matches the thickness of the abdominal side. Liposuction of the pubic flap and labia majora, especially the anterior labia, is performed. Liposuction of the pubic flap, labia majora, and inguinal regions is illustrated. This procedure provides a uniform flap without a pubic concavity.

Liposuction of upper labia majora, pubis, and inguinal areas leaving 1-2 cm of fat on the skin flap

Mons Lift[7,41,44] (Fig. 63-17)

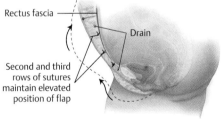

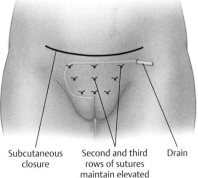

Fig. 63-17   Three rows of tacking sutures are usually placed. Significant dimpling should be prevented. The labia majora and anterior labial commissure are pulled up. A closed suction drain is placed from the pubic symphysis around the right side, then under the deep closure.

Subcutaneous closure

Second and third rows of sutures maintain elevated position of flap

Drain

- Three rows of tacking sutures, suspending the fibrofatty tissue to the superior rectus fascia
- No. 1 Ethibond sutures on a CTX needle (large taper)
- First row (the most caudal row)
  - Begins 1-2 cm cephalad to the anterior labial commissure with grasping of the dense fibrofatty tissue.

- The next bite of tissue should secure the lift to the rectus fascia just cephalad to the pubic symphysis, between the external inguinal rings.
- The completion of closure should incorporate the superficial fascial system (SFS) layer.
- At least three sutures in the row should be placed.
▪ Rows two and three are placed from inferior to superior in similar fashion.
▪ The upper flap of tissue may need to be liposuctioned to match tissue thickness with closure.

> **NOTE:** Resuspension using the SFS is essential in achieving long-lasting results and improving early and late wound-healing complications.[43]

▪ The remainder of the tissue is closed over a drain.
- Multiple attempts are made to prevent an abnormal, pulled appearance of the labia majora, to minimize dimpling, and to achieve symmetry.

POSTOPERATIVE CARE

▪ Ice packs and antibiotic ointment for postoperative days 1 and 2
▪ Cephalexin prophylactically for 2-3 days[7] (controversial)
▪ Some advocate preoperative antibiotic prophylaxis only, thinking that postoperative antibiotics only increase the risk of yeast vaginitis.[41]
▪ Restrictions
- Exercise is restricted for 3 weeks.
  ▶ Specific activities such as horseback riding and yoga are restricted for 8 weeks.
- Sexual intercourse is restricted for 6 weeks.
▪ 80% of swelling will resolve within 6 weeks.
  ▶ Most swelling and induration resolves in 4 weeks.
▪ Moderate discomfort lasts for about 2 weeks.[3]
▪ Absorbable suture irritation may occur.

COMPLICATIONS

▪ Rare

LABIA MINORA

▪ Alter[6] central wedge with extension technique
- Significant complication in 4%
- Stretching of labial scar in 4%
- Slight separation of the labial edge in 2% (most common issue)[7]
  ▶ Most resolve in 4-6 months without the need for revision.
- <1% have fistula or major wound dehiscence.[7]
▪ **Wound dehiscence** most common with all techniques.[3,38]
▪ Asymmetry of the minora and lateral clitoral hood
▪ Stretched, widened, or painful scars
▪ Revisions best delayed for a **minimum of 4 months**
- Allows time for healing and, more important, resolution of induration

- Persistent discomfort several months after treatment
  - Can be treated with several-week course of a potent cortisone cream like clobetasol 0.05%[7]
- Hematoma
- Infection
- Skin retraction
- Distal flap necrosis
  - 4.7% distal tip necrosis seen in Munhoz superior flap techniques[10,36]
- Transient dyspareunia
- Labial and vaginal mucosal dryness

LABIA MAJORA
- Hematoma (rare, but more common with excessive fat removal)
- **Inadequate reduction or asymmetry** of either skin or fat is most common[7]
  - Can be adjusted in 6 months
- Color issue or pain and sexual dysfunction rare
- Most concerning[7,22]:
  - Excessive skin excision leading to a gaping introitus
    - ▶ Aesthetic deformity
    - ▶ Discomfort in clothing
    - ▶ Vaginal dryness
  - Most often associated if medial thigh lift has been performed or will be performed at the same time[7]
    - ▶ Thigh lift Colles fascia tacking sutures loosen, causing posterior migration of the thigh skin, pulling the labia majora, and opening the introitus
    - ▶ Prevented by planning conservative resection of tissue in situations of recent or concomitant thigh lift

MONS PUBIS[7,20,22,43,45]
- Concavity with contour irregularities
- Altered urinary stream
- Skin necrosis
  - Prevent by delaying majoraplasty

OUTCOMES

LABIAPLASTY
- Alter study[6]
  - 407-patient study
  - Significant complication rate 4%
    - ▶ Revisions, patients wanting revisions, and chronic discomfort
  - Reoperation 2.9%
  - Average patient satisfaction score **9.2/10**
  - **98%** would undergo procedure again.
- Minor complication rate 24%[38]
- **Satisfaction rate 95%**[3,6,38,44-46]

MONS PUBIS
- Appearance
  - Significant improvement of patient satisfaction surveys
- Functional improvements
  - 75% increase in ability to visualize the genitalia postoperatively
  - >50% improvement in hygiene and sex life
    - 61.3 % hygiene
    - 51.6% improvement in sex life
    - 32.3% improvement in genital sensitivity
  - Improvement in bladder incontinence[45]

OTHER GENITAL PROCEDURES FOR MAINLY FUNCTIONAL CONCERNS[23]
- Vaginal tightening
- Hymenoplasty
- Perineoplasty
- G-spot (Gräfenberg-spot) amplification

TOP TAKEAWAYS
➤ Although aesthetic and functional ideals are being established, it is critical to review patient desires before surgery and point out how changes to one portion of the genitalia may affect other areas.
➤ The genital region is an aesthetic unit that must be viewed in total.
➤ Reducing the labia minora alone in women with other complex genital issues, regardless of the technique used, may result in an unnatural, imbalanced appearance of the external genitalia.[17]
➤ A prominent clitoral hood, for instance, appearing proportional to enlarged labia minora before reduction will become more prominent if not addressed.[17]
➤ Surgeons should be familiar with reduction techniques of the labia minora from each category to tailor specific anatomy to the patient population.
➤ Careful preoperative planning must include prior and planned procedures to decrease postoperative complications.
➤ Detailed postoperative expectations should be thoroughly reviewed with the patient including significant discomfort, swelling, and edema, which generally resolve in a few weeks but may persist for months.
➤ Thorough review of activity restrictions postoperatively is critical.

REFERENCES
1. Hamori CA. Postoperative clitoral hood deformity after labiaplasty. Aesthet Surg J 33:1030, 2013.
2. Dobbleleir JM, Van Landuyt KV, Monstrey SJ. Aesthetic surgery of the female genitalia. Semin Plast Surg 25:130, 2011.
3. Koning M, Zeijlmans IA, Bouman TK, et al. Female attitudes regarding labia minora appearance and reduction with consideration of media influence. Aesthet Surg J 29:65, 2009.

4. Tepper OM, Wulkan M, Matarasso A. Labioplasty: anatomy, etiology, and a new surgical approach. Aesthet Surg J 31:551, 2011.
5. Voracek M, Fisher ML. Shapely centerfolds? Temporal change in body measures: trend analysis. BMJ 325:1447, 2002.
6. Alter G. Female genital aesthetic surgery. In Nahai F, ed. The Art of Aesthetic Surgery: Principles and Technique, ed 2. New York: Thieme Publishers, 2011.
7. Mirzabeigi JN, Jandali S, Mettel RK, et al. The nomenclature of "vaginal rejuvenation" and elective vulvovaginal plastic surgery. Aesthet Surg J 31:723, 2011.
8. Felicio Yde A. Labial surgery. Aesthet Surg J 27:322, 2007.
9. Murariu D, Chun B, Jackowe DJ, et al. Comparison of mean labial width in patients requesting labioplasty to a healthy control: an anatomical study. Plast Reconstr Surg 129:214e, 2012.
10. Munhoz AM, Filassi JR, Ricci MD, et al. Aesthetic labia minora reduction with inferior wedge resection and superior pedicle flap reconstruction. Plast Reconstr Surg 118:1237, 2006.
11. Chavis WM, LaFerla JJ, Niccolini R. Plastic repair of elongated, hypertrophic labia minora. A case report. J Reprod Med 34:373, 1989.
12. Hodgkinson DJ, Hait G. Aesthetic vaginal labioplasty. Plast Reconstr Surg 74:414, 1984.
13. Capraro VJ. Congenital anomalies. Clin Obstet Gynecol 14:988, 1971.
14. Rouzier R, Louis-Sylvestre C, Paniel BJ, et al. Hypertrophy of labia minora: experience with 163 reductions. Am J Obstet Gynecol 182:35, 2000.
15. Kato K, Kondo A, Gotoh M, et al. Hypertrophy of labia minora in myelodysplastic women. Labioplasty to ease clean intermittent catheterization. Urology 31:294, 1988.
16. Laub DR. A new method for aesthetic reduction of labia minora (the deepithelialized reduction labioplasty) [discussion]. Plast Reconstr Surg 105:423, 2000.
17. Hunter JG. Commentary on: Labioplasty: anatomy, etiology, and a new surgical approach. Aesthet Surg J 31:519, 2011.
18. Alter GJ. Labia minora reconstruction using clitoral hood flaps, wedge excisions, and YV advancement flaps. Plast Reconstr Surg 127:2356, 2011.
19. Alter GJ. Pubic contouring after massive weight loss in men and women: correction of hidden penis, mons ptosis, and labia majora enlargement. Plast Reconstr Surg 130:936, 2012.
20. Alter GJ. Aesthetic labia minora and clitoral hood reduction using extended central wedge resection. Plast Reconstr Surg 122:1780, 2008.
21. Gray H, Pick TP, Howden R, eds. Gray's Anatomy (1901 Edition). Philadelphia: Rounding Press, 1974.
22. Moore KL, Dalley AF. Clinically Oriented Anatomy, ed 4. Philadelphia: Lippincott Williams & Wilkins, 1999.
23. Malinovsky L, Sommerova J, Martincik J. Quantitative evaluation of sensory nerve endings in hypertrophy of the labia minora pudenda in women. Acta Anat (Basel) 92:129, 1975.
24. Puppo V. Anatomy and physiology of the clitoris, vestibular bulbs, and labia minora with a review of the female orgasm and the prevention of female sexual dysfunction. Clin Anat 26:134, 2013.
25. Hwang WY, Chang TS, Sun P, et al. Vaginal reconstruction using labia minora flaps in congenital total absence. Ann Plast Surg 15:534, 1985.
26. Kelishadi SS, Elston JB, Rao AJ, et al. Posterior wedge resection: a more aesthetic labiaplasty. Aesthet Surg J 33:847, 2013.
27. Radman HM. Hypertrophy of the labia minora. Obstet Gynecol 48(1 Suppl):78s, 1976.
28. Maas SM, Hage JJ. Functional and aesthetic labia minora reduction. Plast Reconstr Surg 105:1453, 2000.
29. Martin-Alguacil N, Schober JM, Sengelaub DR, et al. Clitoral sexual arousal: neuronal tracing study from the clitoris through the spinal tracts. J Urol 180:1241, 2008.

30. Martin-Alguacil N, de Gaspar I, Schober JM, et al. Somatosensation: end organs for tactile sensation. In Pfaff DW, ed. Neuroscience in the 21st Century: From Basic to Clinical. Heidelberg: Springer, 2012.
31. Giraldo F, González C, de Haro F. Central wedge nymphectomy with a 90-degree Z-plasty for aesthetic reduction of the labia minora. Plast Reconstr Surg 113:1820; discussion 1826, 2004.
32. Bloom JM, Kouwenberg EV, Davenport M, et al. Aesthetic and functional satisfaction after monsplasty in the massive weight loss population. Aesthet Surg J 32:877, 2012.
33. Motakef S, Rodriguez-Feliz J, Chung MT, et al. Vaginal labiaplasty: current practices and a simplified classification system for labial protrusion. Plast Reconstr Surg 135:774, 2015.
34. Hunstad JP, Repta R. Atlas of Abdominoplasty. Philadelphia: Elsevier, 2009.
35. Smarrito S. Lambda laser nymphoplasty: retrospective study of 231 cases. Plast Reconstr Surg 133:231e, 2014.
36. Hunter JG. Commentary on: Postoperative clitoral hood deformity after labiaplasty. Aesthet Surg J 33:1037, 2013.
37. Maas SM, Hage JJ. Functional and aesthetic labia minora reduction. Plast Reconstr Surg 105:1453, 2000.
38. Schober J, Cooney T, Pfaff D, et al. Innervation of the labia minora of prepubertal girls. J Pediatr Adolesc Gynecol 23:352, 2010.
39. Martin-Alguacil N, Aardsma N, Litvin Y, et al. Immunocytochemical characterization of pacinian-like corpuscles in the labia minora of prepubertal girls. J Pediatr Adolesc Gynecol 23:352, 2010.
40. Choi HY, Kim KT. A new method for aesthetic reduction of labia minora (the deepithelialized reduction labioplasty). Plast Reconstr Surg 105:419, 2000.
41. Schober J, Aardsma N, Mayoglou L, et al. Terminal innervation of the female genitalia, cutaneous sensory receptors of the epithelium of the labia minor. Clin Anat 28:392, 2015.
42. Rubin JP, Matarasso A. Aesthetic Surgery after Massive Weight Loss. Philadelphia: Elsevier, 2007.
43. Pardo J, Solà V, Ricci P, et al. Laser labioplasty of labia minora. Int J Gynaecol Obstet 93:38, 2006.
44. Alter GJ. Management of the mons pubis and labia majora in the massive weight loss patient. Aesthet Surg J 29:432, 2009.
45. Michaels J V, Friedman T, Coon D, et al. Mons rejuvenation in the massive weight loss patient using superficial fascial system suspension. Plast Reconstr Surg 126:45e, 2010.
46. Goodman MP, Placik OJ, Benson RH III, et al. A large multicenter outcome study of female genital plastic surgery. J Sex Med 7(4 Pt 1):1565, 2010.

64. Noninvasive Body Contouring

Michael Bykowski, Derek Ulvila, Spero J. Theodorou, Christopher T. Chia

PREOPERATIVE EVALUATION

- History of weight loss and gain; type of exercise routine and current diet regimen, if any
- History of skin laxity disorders and previous procedures
- Physical examination: Pinch test, caliper measurement, skin laxity, body mass index, visceral fat assessment

INFORMED CONSENT

- Expectations of minor procedural discomfort and postprocedural erythema/edema
- The risk of temporary sensory deficits: Numbness and hyperesthesia
- The potential for undercorrection or overcorrection of fat areas, possible contour deformities, and overlying skin changes; no guarantee of aesthetic outcome

METHODS OF NONOPERATIVE TREATMENT

- Cryolipolysis (e.g., CoolSculpting)
- High-intensity focused ultrasound (HIFU) (e.g., Liposonix)
- Low-level laser therapy (e.g., Zerona)
- Radiofrequency energy (e.g., Vanquish)

CRYOLIPOLYSIS

- Application of cooling panels to localized areas of adiposity resulting **in apoptosis-mediated cell death and subsequent inflammatory response.**[1]
- Preclinical studies showed **33%** reduction in thickness of superficial fat layer[2] with maximal relative loss of nearly **80%.**[1]
- A systematic review of human studies showed average reduction in caliper measurement of **14.7%-28.5%** and average reduction by ultrasound **10.3%-25.5%.**[3]

SENIOR AUTHOR TIP: Changes seen as early as 3 weeks after treatment but most dramatic results seen after 2 months.

Indications

- Treatment of visible fat bulges of the submental area, upper arm, bra line fat, back fat, abdomen, flank, banana roll, and thighs in individuals with a body mass index (BMI) <30

Contraindications

- Pregnancy
- History of cold-induced dermatologic syndromes (e.g., cryoglobulinemia, paroxysmal cold hemoglobinuria, or cold urticaria)

- Large-volume weight loss in obese patients
- Patients with excessive skin laxity

Equipment
- Cooling applicator with attached mild vacuum
- One- or two-panel devices can be used (Fig. 64-1).
- Conduction gel applied between cooling device and treatment area

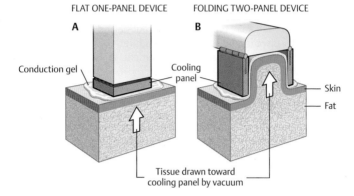

FLAT ONE-PANEL DEVICE   FOLDING TWO-PANEL DEVICE

Fig. 64-1   Various cryolipolysis applicators are available to contour to specific anatomic areas. **A,** Flat applicator for relatively flat surfaces (e.g., back or inner thigh). **B,** Concave applicator for curved surfaces ("muffin top" or "love handles").

Technique
- **Markings:** Markings depend on specific anatomic structure and focal area of adiposity.
- Conduction gel is placed on the area to be treated.
- Tissue is drawn into the cooling panel with the vacuum to create a seal (see Fig. 64-1).
- Cooling panels are set to an energy extraction rate ~60-70 mW/cm^2 and held in place for 30-60 minutes' exposure time.

> **TIP:**   Temperature and time of application are both important to induce selective cryolipolysis of fatty tissue.

Postoperative Care
- Postoperative dressings are not needed but may be applied for patient comfort.
- Topical and oral analgesics are used as needed.

Complications
- **Minor**
  - Minor discomfort during procedure[4]
  - Temporary (several days) edema and/or erythema to treated area[1,4]
  - Temporary (1-6 weeks) decreased light-touch sensitivity, temperature sensitivity, pain sensitivity to treated area[4]
- **Major**
  - Paradoxical adipose hyperplasia (incidence: 0.52%).[5]

- **Incidence**
  - 100% of patients had erythema, which resolved within 1 week.
  - 67% of patients developed postprocedural sensory deficits to treated area (all deficits were resolved by 2 months).[4]
- **Common treatments**
  - Pain is adequately controlled with topical and oral analgesics.
  - All minor complications are self-limited.

HIGH-INTENSITY FOCUSED ULTRASOUND (HIFU)

- High-intensity focused ultrasound is focused energy used to **thermally ablate subcutaneous adipose tissue and to induce neocollagenesis.**
- HIFU increases the local temperature within the midlamellar fat layer leading to coagulative necrosis of adipocytes and subsequent reduction of fat layer.
  - Two case series have been reported of 282 and 85 patients treated with HIFU to the abdomen and flank resulting in an average waist circumference decrease of **4.4 and 4.7 cm,** respectively.[6,7]
  - A multicenter, randomized, sham-controlled, single-blinded trial of 180 patients studying HIFU in trunk aesthetics showed a decrease of **2.5 cm** in the treatment group compared with 1.2 cm in the sham group.[8]
  - A multicenter, randomized, nonblinded study of 118 patients treated with a single HIFU treatment to the abdomen resulted in a decrease of **2.3 cm** in waist circumference.[9]

SENIOR AUTHOR TIP: Results typically seen 8-12 weeks after treatment.

Indications

- Noninvasive waist circumference reduction
- Ideal candidate for HIFU body contouring has >2.5 cm of tissue on caliper pinch and a BMI <30 kg/m²

Contraindications

- Pregnancy
- Lactating women
- <1 cm subcutaneous tissue at treatment area
- Hernia at treatment area
- Cancer
- Implanted electrical stimulation devices
- Large-volume weight loss in obese patients

Equipment

- HIFU transducer device (see Fig. 64-2)

Technique

- **Markings:** Markings depend on specific anatomic structure and focal area of adiposity and are done in the standing position.
- Patient is placed supine on the treatment table, exposing the area to be treated.
- Topical anesthetic is applied to the treatment area.
- The "nodes of treatment" are identified.

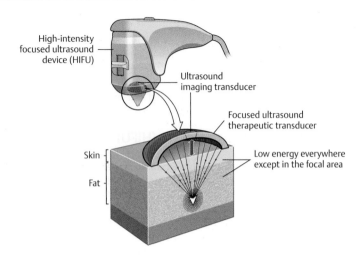

Fig. 64-2   The HIFU transducer focally delivers the beam to the treatment nodes to thermally ablate fat. The low-energy beams pass through skin over a wider area (with minimal damage) to converge at a focal depth within the fat.

> **TIP:**   Marking a grid within the treatment area helps to guide duration of treatment to specific nodes.

- The HIFU transducer is aimed at the nodes of treatment and calibrated to deliver a total energy dose of 100-150 J/cm^2 at a focal depth of 1.1-1.6 cm (Fig. 64-2).
- Multiple passes are made with the HIFU transducer to deliver the appropriate amount of energy.
- Treatment duration is typically <1 hour.

> **TIP:**   The focal depth is determined by the thickness of the adipose tissues being treated.

Postoperative Care
- Postoperative dressings are not needed but may be applied for patient comfort.
- Topical and oral analgesics as needed

Complications
- **Minor**
  - Tenderness, edema, ecchymosis, and hard lumps to treated area that resolves over 1-2 weeks[8]
- **Incidence**
  - 10%-15% that resolve within 1-2 weeks[8]
- **Common treatments**
  - Pain is adequately controlled with topical and oral analgesics.
- All complications are self-limited.

LOW-LEVEL LASER THERAPY (LLLT)

■ Low-level laser therapy (635 nm laser), is a noninvasive, nonthermal approach to fat reduction.
  • The proposed mechanism is that **LLLT induces a transitory pore into an adipocyte, resulting in release of lipids and resultant adipocyte deflation.**[10]
■ Controversy exists over efficacy
  • Depth of penetration of laser light depends on wavelength, power output, and biologic parameters of the target tissue
    ▶ 0.3% of photons penetrate to depth of <2 cm for a 635 nm laser at 50 cmW/cm^2.[11,12]
  • No consistent observations of adipocyte disruption were observed in histologic or electron-scanning microscopy photographs in a study of LLLT on cultured human preadipocytes, porcine Yucatan model, or lipoaspirates from human subjects with exposure to LLLT.[12]
■ Nonetheless, several studies report six treatments of LLLT decreases total combined circumference measurements.
  • Low sample size, no postprocedure BMI control, diet and exercise encouraged, dietary supplements permitted but use not recorded[13-15]
  • Six treatments over 2 weeks
    ▶ A double-blind, sham-controlled trial of 67 patients demonstrated a statistically significant reduction **(3.5 inches)** in **total combined circumference of waist, hip, and thigh measurements** after LLLT when compared with the sham-treated control group (0.6 inches) at 2 weeks posttreatment (four combined measurements).[13]
    ▶ A retrospective review of 660 patients, combined from 50 private practice sites demonstrated a total circumference reduction of 3.3 inches 1 week after completion of LLLT utilizing combined circumference measurements of waist, hips, and thighs (four combined measurements)[14]
    ▶ A double-blind, sham-controlled study involving 40 patients demonstrated significantly greater combined arm circumference reduction (three combined arm measurements) with LLLT than with sham treatment group (3.7 cm versus 0.2 cm, respectively) at 2 weeks posttreatment.[15]
  • Six consecutive weekly treatments
    ▶ Fifty-four patients had a mean combined circumference reduction of 5.4 inches utilizing measurements at the upper abdomen, waist, hip, and thighs, 1 week after completion of treatment (five combined measurements).[16]

Indications
■ Circumference reduction of upper arms, waist, hips, and thighs

Contraindications
■ Pregnancy
■ Cancer
■ Large-volume weight loss in obese patients

Equipment
■ Low-level laser device

Technique
- **Markings:** Markings depend on specific anatomic structure and focal area of adiposity.
- Patient is placed supine on the treatment table, exposing the area to be treated.
- The laser diode modules are suspended ~15 cm above the anterior and then the posterior aspect of the treatment area.
- Transdermal delivery of the 635 nm laser

> **TIP:** Specific distances, wattage, wavelength, and delivery duration vary depending on the device used.

Postoperative Care
- Postoperative dressings are not needed but may be applied for patient comfort.
- Topical and oral analgesics are given as needed.

Complications
- Mild warming sensation during procedure, prolonged erythema (>24 hours), and skin ulceration

Incidence
- Rare when laser-diode panel suspended ~15 cm above skin[13,14,16]
- When laser-diode panel applied directly to skin: Erythema >24 hours (12%) and erythema progressed to skin ulceration (12%).[17]
- **Common treatments**
  - Most complications are self-limited or resolve with local wound care.

TOP TAKEAWAYS
- ➤ An American Society of Plastic Surgeons report from 2010 states the number of patients seeking minimally invasive aesthetic procedures increased from 5.5 to 11.5 million from 2000 to 2010.[18]
- ➤ Noninvasive body contouring modalities are not a replacement for liposuction, healthy lifestyle, or a treatment to lose weight.
- ➤ Noninvasive treatment offers ease of use and limited patient downtime but often requires multiple treatments to achieve modest results.
- ➤ Noninvasive body contouring results are typically seen approximately 2 months after treatment.

REFERENCES
1. Manstein D, Laubach H, Watanabe K, et al. Selective cryolysis: a novel method of non-invasive fat removal. Lasers Surg Med 40:595, 2008.
2. Zelickson B, Egbert BM, Preciado J, et al. Cryolipolysis for noninvasive fat cell destruction: initial results from a pig model. Dermatol Surg 35:1462, 2009.
3. Ingargiola MJ, Motakef S, Chung MT, et al. Cryolipolysis for fat reduction and body contouring: safety and efficacy of current treatment paradigms. Plast Reconstr Surg 135:1581, 2015.
4. Coleman SR, Sachdeva K, Egbert B, et al. Clinical efficacy of noninvasive cryolipolysis and its effects on peripheral nerves. Aesthetic Plast Surg 33:482, 2009.

5. Karcher C, Katz B, Sadick N. Paradoxical hyperplasia post cryolipolysis and management. Dermatol Surg 43:467, 2017.
6. Fatemi A. High-intensity focused ultrasound effectively reduces adipose tissue. Semin Cutan Med Surg 28:257, 2009.
7. Fatemi A, Kane MA. High-intensity focused ultrasound effectively reduces waist circumference by ablating adipose tissue from the abdomen and flanks: a retrospective case series. Aesthetic Plast Surg 34:577, 2010.
8. Jewell ML, Baxter RA, Cox SE, et al. Randomized sham-controlled trial to evaluate the safety and effectiveness of a high-intensity focused ultrasound device for noninvasive body sculpting. Plast Reconstr Surg 128:253, 2011.
9. Robinson DM, Kaminer MS, Baumann L, et al. High-intensity focused ultrasound for the reduction of subcutaneous adipose tissue using multiple treatment techniques. Dermatol Surg 40:641, 2014.
10. Neira R, Arroyave J, Ramirez H, et al. Fat liquefaction: effect of low-level laser energy on adipose tissue. Plast Reconstr Surg 110:912; discussion 923, 2002.
11. Friedmann DP. A review of the aesthetic treatment of abdominal subcutaneous adipose tissue: background, implications, and therapeutic options. Dermatol Surg 41:18, 2015.
12. Brown SA, Rohrich RJ, Kenkel J, et al. Effect of low-level laser therapy on abdominal adipocytes before lipoplasty procedures. Plast Reconstr Surg 113:1796, 2004.
13. Jackson RF, Dedo DD, Roche GC, et al. Low-level laser therapy as a non-invasive approach for body contouring: a randomized, controlled study. Lasers Surg Med 41:799, 2009.
14. Jackson RF, Stern FA, Neira R, et al. Application of low-level laser therapy for noninvasive body contouring. Lasers Surg Med 44:211, 2012.
15. Nestor MS, Zarraga MB, Park H. Effect of 635nm low-level laser therapy on upper arm circumference reduction. J Clin Aesthet Dermatol 5:42, 2012.
16. Thornfeldt CR, Thaxton PM, Hornfeldt CS. A six-week low-level laser therapy protocol is effective for reducing waist, hip, thigh, and upper abdomen circumference. J Clin Aesthet Dermatol 9:31, 2016.
17. Jankowski M, Gawrych M, Adamska U, et al. Low-level laser therapy (LLLT) does not reduce subcutaneous adipose tissue by local adipocyte injury but rather by modulation of systemic lipid metabolism. Lasers Med Sci 32:475, 2017.
18. American Society of Plastic Surgeons. National Clearinghouse of Plastic Surgery Statistics: 2010 Report of the 2009 Statistics. Arlington Heights, IL: American Society of Plastic Surgeons, 2010.

65. Aesthetics of Gender Affirmation Surgery

Juan L. Rendon, Christopher J. Salgado

- The World Professional Association for Transgender Health (WPATH) promotes a multidisciplinary approach for the care of transgender patients.
- According to the WPATH, transgender patients should be under the care of primary care physicians, mental health services, and endocrinologist and surgical specialists.
- Although hormone and nonsurgical interventions may help in the transition of transgender patients, surgical interventions play a significant role in achieving psychological well-being and self-fulfillment.
- Surgeons who have received specialized training in transgender surgery may address the unique aesthetic and functional concerns of transgender patients.

FACIAL FEMINIZATION

- Facial feminization surgery (FFS) is primarily based on the modification of bone structures to soften masculine facial features.
- A comprehensive history and physical examination are necessary to appropriately diagnose a patient and to adapt specific surgical options rather than proceeding with a standardized approach.
- Goal is to use hidden approaches and protocolized surgical techniques to achieve a natural and aesthetic result, alleviating gender dysphoria and facilitating transition.

AESTHETIC EVALUATION (Fig. 65-1)
Craniofacial Skeleton
- **Upper third: Hairline and frontonasal-orbital complex**
  - Frontonasal-orbital complex: Greatest determinant of facial gender
    - ▶ Includes forehead, supraorbital ridge, orbit, frontal bossing, frontomalar region, temporal ridges, and frontonasal transition
    - ▶ Determines the position of the eyebrows and periorbital soft tissues, including the eyelids
    - ▶ Typically, more pronounced with greater bone volume in males versus females
- **Middle third: Nose, cheeks, and upper lip**
  - The male nose is generally larger than the female nose because of increased volume of bone and cartilage, most notable at **nasal dorsum and tip**.
  - Males have greater malar bone volume, resulting in well-defined cheeks. **Females have a greater concentration of fat in middle third of the face**, giving them prominent round cheeks, which are compatible with femininity.
  - In males, the distance between the upper lip and nose is longer than in females.
- **Lower third: Jaw and chin**
  - In males
    - ▶ The mandibular angle area is usually squared with well-defined corners.

▶ The mandibular body has greater bone volume, which produces a wider lower facial third and gives greater vertical height.

▶ The chin tends to be squared, providing a more pronounced and defined transition between the chin and mandibular body.

Neck: Thyroid Cartilage (Adam's Apple)

▪ The **thyroid cartilage is among the most prominent hallmarks of male gender.**

▪ In males, the trachea has a greater volume and diameter.

CAUTION: Although the most prominent portion of the thyroid cartilage can be modified during FFS, the tracheal structure itself should never be surgically approached for facial feminization, because it carries unacceptable and unnecessary risk for vocal cord damage and respiratory compromise.

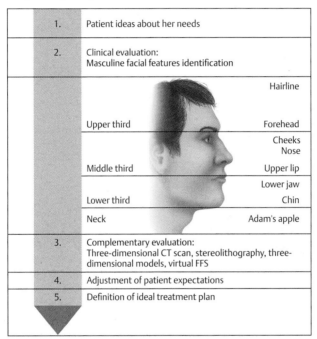

1.	Patient ideas about her needs
2.	Clinical evaluation: Masculine facial features identification
3.	Complementary evaluation: Three-dimensional CT scan, stereolithography, three-dimensional models, virtual FFS
4.	Adjustment of patient expectations
5.	Definition of ideal treatment plan

Fig. 65-1   Evaluation and diagnosis protocol. (*CT,* Computed tomography; *FFS,* facial feminization surgery.)

Secondary Traits

▪ Include the hair and hairline shape, facial hair, skin texture, and the distribution and volume of facial fat

▪ Males have M-shaped hairline with recession at temples, which may be affected by androgenic alopecia[1]; females usually have rounded hairline that extends slightly higher in the center than in men[2] (Fig. 65-2).

▪ Virtually all males have facial hair, which conditions skin to become thicker and rougher.

Hairline Pattern	Hairline Height	
	Normal	**High**
Rounded	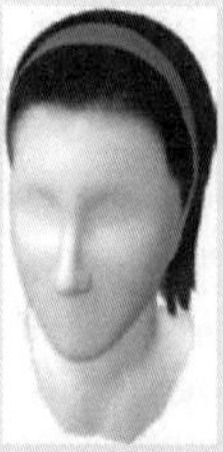 Type I: Ideal condition Percentage: 22% Treatment: None required	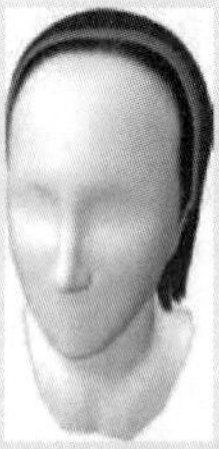 Type III: Naturally high Percentage: 4% Treatment: HLS or SHT*
M-shaped	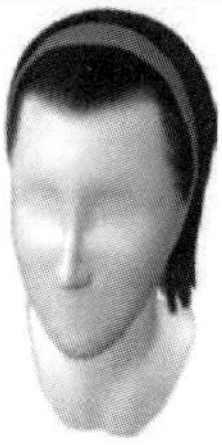 Type II: Receding hairline at temples Percentage: 43% Treatment: SHT Contraindications: HLS†	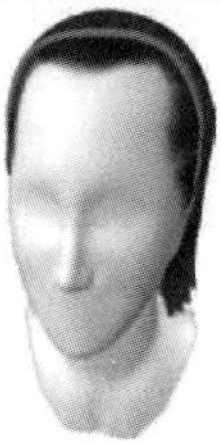 Type IV: Naturally high or caused by alopecia Percentage: 21% Treatment: SHT* Alternative: HLS + DHT
Undefined	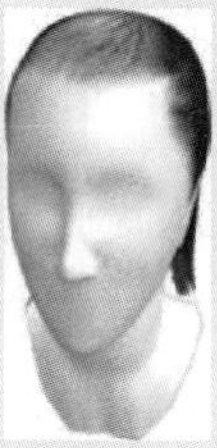 Type V: Advanced alopecia Percentage: 10% Treatment: SHT + DHT or untreated	*SHT is performed only if a small advancement (up to 1 cm) of the hairline is desired. †This does not improve or correct recessions.

Fig. 65-2 Hairline variations and possible treatments in male-to-female transgender patients. Based on the hairline analysis of transgender patients treated to date (N = 492) for any facial feminization procedure by our team. Both treatments, SHT (follicular unit strip surgery technique) and HLS, are performed in combination with a forehead reconstruction during the same surgery. A DHT treatment (follicular unit strip surgery or follicular unit extraction technique) is performed alone in a second session. (*DHT,* Deferred hair transplant; *HLS,* hairline lowering surgery; *SHT,* simultaneous hair transplant.)

- Largely influenced by hormones, females have a greater concentration and volume of facial fat within the middle third of the face (cheek).[3]
- Secondary features respond well to hormone therapy and should be addressed before FFS.[4]

SURGICAL CONSIDERATION FOR FACIAL FEMINIZATION SURGERY

- Facial CT with three-dimensional reconstructions should be obtained to assess anatomic features that can be addressed.
  - In cases of financial limitations, a Panorex and lateral cephalogram will often provide adequate information.
- Preoperative, intraoperative, and postoperative photographs (7 days, 6 months, and 1 year) should be maintained to provide an objective view of changes.

Upper Third
- **Forehead reconstruction**
  - Forehead reconstruction completely modifies the frontonasal-orbital region and softens and feminizes the patient's expression.
  - **Goal:** To reposition and remodel the forehead complex to soften frontal bossing, supraorbital rims, frontomalar buttresses, and temporal ridges
  - **Approach:** Osteotomy and repositioning of the anterior wall of the frontal sinus[5] or burring, depending on the anterior table thickness, to soften this region
  - Can be combined with hair transplantation to achieve upper-third feminization in one stage[6]
  - Hairline versus modified coronal incision should be determined by hairline position and patient desires.
    - ▶ If hairline is low, then coronal incision is used.

SENIOR AUTHOR TIP: If the anterior table of the frontal sinus is ≤3 mm, then a frontal bone setback will often be required to achieve a good result.

- **Hairline**
  - Hairline lowering surgery is recommended only in patients with a high hairline, and non-hair-bearing scalp is excised during the lowering procedure.

SENIOR AUTHOR TIP: Suturing of the posterior scalp flap to a cortical tunnel in the frontal bone or to titanium mesh or plates helps to maintain a lasting effect of hairline lowering.

- **Hair transplantation**
  - Should be performed after androgenic alopecia stabilizes
  - Recommended for patients with an M-shaped hairline and with sufficient hair density without active androgenic alopecia
  - **Goal:** To address the recessed corners of the hairline
    - ▶ Central section of the hairline can also be addressed if hair density here is an issue.
  - May be performed during forehead reconstruction or in a delayed fashion[6]
  - **Follicular unit strip (FUS):** Follicles are obtained from a strip of scalp removed in a small surgical procedure.
  - **Follicular unit extraction (FUE):** Individual follicles are obtained, without the need for a surgical procedure.

Middle Third
- **Cheeks**
  - Fixed **porous polyethylene implants** for augmentation, zygoma not commonly reduced in FFS
    - ▶ Placed using an intraoral approach
    - ▶ Results stable over time
  - Autologous fat
    - ▶ Deposited in supraperiosteal plane
    - ▶ Natural results but dependent on surgeon's experience
    - ▶ May require multiple sessions given graft resorption
- **Nose**
  - Standard rhinoplasty techniques are used to make nose smaller and compatible with surrounding facial features.
  - Reduction rhinoplasty is commonly performed immediately after forehead reduction when done as a combined procedure.
  - The final result is largely dependent on skin quality.
  - Reinforcement of nasal tip and dorsum with cartilage grafts to prevent collapse is recommended.
- **Upper liplift**
  - **Goal:** To reduce the vertical dimension between the upper lip and nose
  - **Approach:** Modified bullhorn technique to remove strip of skin and subcutaneous tissue without violating orbicularis oris[7]
  - *Performing the procedure in conjunction with an open rhinoplasty procedure is not recommended.*

Lower Third
- **Lower jaw and chin**
  - **Goals:** To modify width and height of the jaw, soften the jawline (including the transition between the mandibular angle and symphysis), and modify the size, shape, and position of the chin
  - **Intraoral approach is strongly advised.**
  - **Approaches**
    - ▶ Panorex or CT scan to evaluate both the course of inferior alveolar nerve and the third molar tooth roots and their relation to the mandibular angles
    - ▶ Burring: Used to reduce bone volume in parasymphysis, symphysis, mandibular body and angles
    - ▶ Standard osteotomies: Used to address chin position
    - ▶ Osteotomies with piezosurgery: Technique of choice for basal mandibular and chin bone resecting and for redesigning mandibular angles

Neck
- **Thyroid cartilage**
  - Recommended in the region of the cervicomental fold to conceal scar and prevent adhesions between thyroid cartilage and overlying soft tissues
  - Incision should not exceed 2 cm.
  - **Approach:** Burring, rongeuring, or sharp resection with scalpel
  - *Must avoid sculpting near vocal cords*

> **SENIOR AUTHOR TIP:**   Marking should be performed with the patient facing the surgeon; the surgeon should place the incision as cephalad as possible for maximal concealment.

TOP SURGERY

- For **transgender females,** this refers to **breast augmentation with implants and/or autologous tissue.**
  - Top surgery in transgender females may require a mastopexy because of the commonly low position of biologic male nipple on chest wall.
- For **transgender males,** this refers to **breast reduction/mastectomy.**
  - A double-incision mastectomy (free-nipple grafts) is the most common top surgery procedure for transgender males, with the most predictable results.
- Top surgery remains one of the most commonly performed surgeries in gender reassignment and one letter from a qualified mental health therapist recommending the patient for surgery should be obtained before performing the procedure in both transgender males and transgender females.
- Top surgery may significantly facilitate a patient's ability to live in a gender role congruent with their gender identity and is commonly performed before bottom surgery (vaginoplasty or metoidioplasty/phalloplasty).
- For some transgender people, top surgery will be the only surgical step during transition.

INDICATIONS
- Per WPATH[8]:
  - A persistent, well-documented history of gender dysphoria
  - The ability to make a fully informed decision and to give consent
  - Age of majority in a given country
    - ▶ A significant medical or mental health concern in a prospective patient for top surgery must be well controlled.
      - ◆ One letter from the patient's mental health therapist recommending the patient undergo the procedure is required.

ADDITIONAL RECOMMENDATIONS
- Transgender females should undergo feminizing hormone therapy for a **minimum of 1 year** before breast augmentation surgery to maximize breast growth and obtain superior aesthetic result.
- Usually, only a half to a full cup size is obtained in breast growth in transgender females on hormone therapy, and size will decrease if hormones are stopped.

MALE-TO-FEMALE TOP SURGERY
Aesthetic Considerations
- Hormone therapy promotes mammogenesis, which follows a pattern similar to female pubertal mammogenesis, resulting in a softly pointed breast, as seen in young girls, or the small conical form found in young adolescents (Tanner stage 2 or 3).[9]
  - Hormone effect is **not** dose dependent.

■ Males tend to have a wider chest, stronger pectoral fascia, more developed pectoralis muscles, and smaller nipple-areola complexes (NACs).

Surgical Considerations
■ Even with large volume and a wide implant, preventing wide cleavage between breasts is often not possible.
■ The NAC should always overlie the implant centrally.
■ Overly medial implant position can result in divergent nipple position and an unacceptable aesthetic result.[10]
■ **Implant selection**
  • Silicone gel–filled implants versus saline-filled implants
  • Use of textured implants may reduce the potential for capsular contracture.
  • Anatomic cohesive gel–filled implants provide additional lower pole projection.
■ **Incisions**
  • Axillary
  • Inframammary: Should be placed lower than preoperative inframammary fold because the inferior areolar margin and inframammary fold will expand after augmentation
  • Periareolar: Less popular because of smaller areola in transgender females
■ **Pocket**
  • Subglandar: Easier to perform; less pain with good aesthetic results in patients with more subcutaneous and glandular tissue (Tanner stage 4 or 5)
  • Subpectoral: More soft tissue coverage of implant, which is necessary in thin patients; lower risk for capsular contracture

Fat Grafting
■ Good alternative to implants in patients with some breast volume from hormone treatment
■ Can provide a small to moderate augmentation of the breast
■ Patients need to be informed that variable amounts of the injected fat will be resorbed.
  • May require multiple grafting sessions to achieve desired volume
■ May also be used as an adjunct to implants
  • Injected into subcutaneous plane
  • Decreased implant visibility
  • Helps to narrow wide cleavage between the breasts

FEMALE-TO-MALE TOP SURGERY
Aesthetic Considerations[11,12]
■ *Hormone therapy has minimal influence on breast size in transgender males.*

- Subcutaneous mastectomy (SCM) to create a male chest is the first surgery in transgender males.[13]
  - SCM helps patient live in gender role that is congruent with their gender identity, which is required before bottom surgery.
- Relative to males, the female chest has excess skin and glandular tissue, as well as abundant subcutaneous fat.
- In females the inframammary fold is well defined; in males the inferior margin of the pectoralis marks the inferior margin of the chest.
- During SCM, **the inframammary fold is often obliterated** to achieve aesthetic contouring.
- **Goals of SCM**
  - Removal of breast tissue and excess skin
  - Reduction and proper positioning of the NAC
  - Obliteration of the inframammary fold
  - Minimization of chest wall scars to achieve aesthetically pleasing male chest

Surgical Considerations

- Many techniques are similar to those used in the surgical treatment of gynecomastia in males (see Chapter 56).
- **Technique should be determined by amount of excess skin and skin elasticity, not by breast volume**[7,12] (Fig. 65-3).

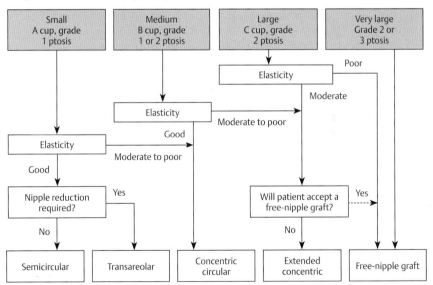

Fig. 65-3 Algorithm for choosing the appropriate subcutaneous mastectomy technique.

- Skin quality and elasticity may be affected by prior years of "breast binding" and should be carefully assessed before surgery.
- **Most commonly performed top surgery for transgender males is the double-incision mastectomy with free-nipple grafts** (Fig. 65-4).
- The lateral extent of the inframammary fold incision should be carried along the lateral border of the pectoralis major in a cephalad direction.
- Hormone therapy should be stopped 2-3 weeks before surgery.

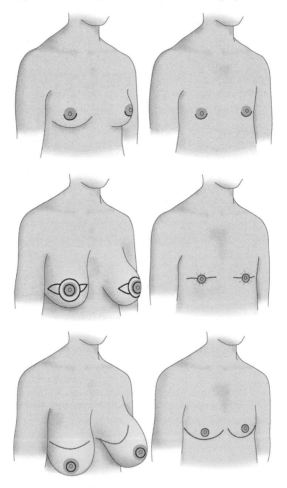

Fig. 65-4   Monstrey's schematic for choosing the appropriate SCM technique.

- **Liposuction**
  - Not recommended at the anterior aspect of breast
  - Good adjunct for addressing lateral excess fat
- **Incisions**[7,13]
  - **Semicircular** (Fig. 65-5)

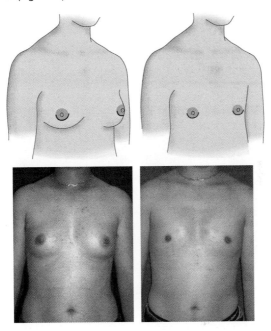

Fig. 65-5 Semicircular technique. Preoperative *(left)* and postoperative *(right)* images, with incisions and scars shown.

  - ▶ Ideal for patients with small breasts
  - ▶ Sufficient amount of glandular tissue must be preserved under NAC to prevent nipple depression.
  - ▶ Scar: Well-concealed, confined to periphery of lower half of areola
  - ▶ Technically challenging because of small operative window

• **Transareolar** (Fig. 65-6)

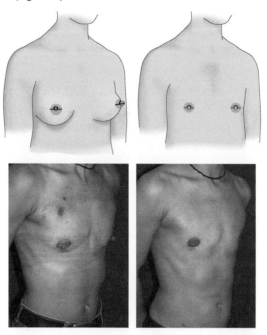

Fig. 65-6   Transareolar technique. Preoperative *(left)* and postoperative *(right)* images, with incisions and scars shown.

▶ Good approach for patients with small breast but large, prominent nipples
▶ Allows immediate subtotal resection of upper aspect of nipple (Fig. 65-7)
▶ Scar: Traverses the areola horizontally and passes around the upper aspect of the nipple, with optional extension medially and laterally. Approach is least common.
▶ Technically challenging because of small operative window

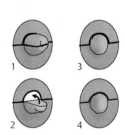

Fig. 65-7   Transareolar technique incisions.

- **Concentric circular** (Fig. 65-8)
  - ▶ Recommended in patients with medium-sized skin envelope (B cup) or smaller breast with poor skin elasticity
  - ▶ Concentric incision can be designed as circle or ellipse, allowing precise amount of deepithelialization.
  - ▶ Access to glandular tissue through inferior aspect of outer incision
  - ▶ Dermal pedicle to NAC; no need to leave excess glandular tissue beneath NAC
  - ▶ Permanent purse-string suture used to set desired areolar diameter
  - ▶ Scar: Confined circumferentially around NAC; may require scar revision if significant widening occurs
  - ▶ Can be extended with triangular excision of skin and subcutaneous tissue medially and laterally

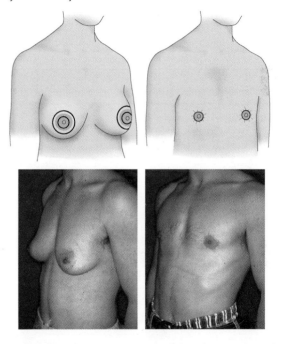

Fig. 65-8 Concentric circular technique. Preoperative *(left)* and postoperative *(right)* images, with incisions and scars shown.

- **Double-incision mastectomy with free-nipple grafts** (Fig. 65-9)
  - ▶ Optimal approach for large and ptotic breasts
  - ▶ NAC is harvested as full-thickness skin graft.
  - ▶ Horizontal incision is placed 1-2 cm above inframammary fold, taking care not to cross midline.
  - ▶ Liposuction may be used to smooth lateral and medial contour.
  - ▶ Lateral incision should be tapered superiorly along the border of the lateral pectoralis major to avoid dog-ear and to achieve superior aesthetic results.
  - ▶ NAC is grafted after closure with overlying bolster.
  - ▶ Nipple position: Placement along the existing vertical nipple line, approximately 2-3 cm above lower border of pectoralis major (usually at fourth or fifth intercostal segment), is recommended. Patient should always be positioned upright intraoperatively to confirm acceptable nipple position.[7]
  - ▶ Scar: Long horizontal scar
  - ▶ Free-nipple grafting increases risk for partial or complete NAC loss and pigment and sensory changes.

SENIOR AUTHOR TIP: The lateralmost aspect of the incision should be brought in a cephalad direction along the lateral aspect of the pectoralis major muscle.

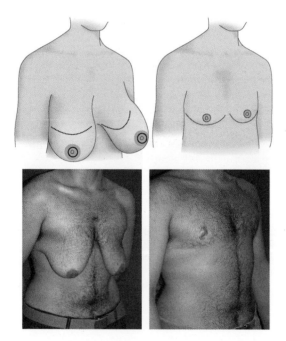

Fig. 65-9   Free-nipple technique. Preoperative *(left)* and postoperative *(right)* images, with incisions and scars shown.

COMPLICATIONS

- Contour abnormalities: Breast, inframammary fold, nipple
- NAC: Size, placement, viability
- Skin redundancy
- Poor scarring
  - Total laparoscopic or robotic hysterectomy and bilateral salpingo-oophorectomy may be safely performed in conjunction with SCM in female-to-male top surgery.[14,15]
- Highest risk of complications for top surgery in transgender males is 10.5% using periareolar approach; most commonly performed technique is the double-incision mastectomy, which carries the lowest risk of complications, including hematoma.[16]

TIPS FOR ACHIEVING AESTHETICALLY PLEASING SCM[7]

Preserving all subcutaneous fat during dissection of glandular tissue from skin flaps and pectoralis fascia during dissection of glandular tissue from chest wall will prevent tethering of flaps to chest wall.

The inframammary fold is released by extending the inferior skin flap onto the abdomen and carefully incising the tight band of tissue that exists inferiorly.

The lateral incision should be carried cephalad along the pectoralis major muscle to avoid a dog-ear and optimize the aesthetic result.

A drain is commonly placed during surgery and removed at the first postoperative visit.

A circumferential elastic bandage or chest compressive garment should be applied around the chest wall postoperative and worn for 4-6 weeks.

MALE-TO-FEMALE BOTTOM SURGERY

- Before gender reassignment surgery, patients and surgeons must adhere to the WPATH Standards of Care (SOC) documentation,[8] which requires two letters (as opposed to one for top surgery) from the patient's mental health therapist recommending the patient for surgery.
  - The letters must include:
    - ▶ Duration of the patient relationship with the therapist
    - ▶ Any associated diagnosis or diagnoses in addition to gender dysphoria
    - ▶ Length of time the patient has been living in their identified gender
    - ▶ Confirmation that the patient is mentally stable to undergo surgery
    - ▶ Statement that the therapist is familiar with WPATH SOC guidelines and recommends the patient for transition surgery
- **Goal:** To create a neovagina with satisfactory sexual function and aesthetic appearance, alleviating gender dysphoria
  - Neovagina must be of adequate depth and width.
- Several techniques are available employing a variety of skin grafts, penile/scrotal skin flaps, bladder/mucosal flaps, and intestinal segment flaps.[17,18]
- Results vary greatly and are influenced by:
  - Surgeon's experience
  - Skin elasticity and healing ability
  - Previous surgery

- Infection
- Nerve damage to neoclitoris during dissection of neurovascular pedicle
- Patient's pelvic anatomy
▪ Before surgery patients should undergo external genitalia examination (including preoperative length of outstretched phallus to determine need for scrotal graft if using penile skin inversion technique) and full hormone profile.[7]

AESTHETIC CONSIDERATIONS
▪ Neoclitoris size and position
▪ Hair growth over penile skin: Preoperative laser epilation is recommended to prevent hairy neovagina if using penile skin inversion technique.

PENILE SKIN–FLAP VAGINOPLASTY APPROACH[7]
▪ *The use of penile and scrotal skin to create a neovagina is the most commonly performed bottom surgery for transgender females.*
▪ **Advantages:** Penile skin has less tendency to contract, may preserve local innervation for sensibility of neovagina, can result in relatively hairless neovagina.
▪ **Disadvantages:** Scarring, eventual shrinkage and contracture, insufficient vaginal cavity, intravaginal hair growth, need for lubrication during intercourse, permanent need for dilation

Surgical Components
▪ **Bilateral orchiectomy**
▪ **Penile disassembly**
  - Dissection of penile skin, neurovascular bundle for neoclitoris from glans penis dorsally, in addition to urethra dissection ventrally
  - Corpora cavernosa must be dissected and removed at the level of attachment to the pubic rami. Short remnants of the corpora cavernosa are also destroyed to prevent postoperative erection.
▪ **Vaginoplasty**
  - The penile skin flap is fashioned into a vascularized island tube flap.
    ▸ *Preservation of the subcutaneous tissue is essential for formation of a long vascularized pedicle.*
    ▸ A hole is made at the base of the pedicle through which the urethra and neoclitoris are passed either individually or separately once the neovagina is inset.
    ▸ On the dorsal side of the skin tube flap, a superficial incision is made, leaving the subcutaneous layer intact; the urethral flap is then embedded along the tube and sutured in place.
    ▸ The distal end of the tube is closed before placement of the neovagina in the perineal space (Fig. 65-10).

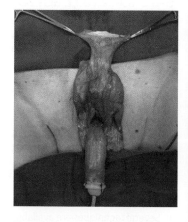

Fig. 65-10 Penile skin has been dissected off corporal tissues and inverted, preserving the dorsal neurovascular pedicle, which vascularizes the neoclitoris (not yet dissected).

- The urethra is separated from the remaining dorsal tissue, and blood supply is maintained through preservation of the corpus spongiosum.
- *Vascularized urethral flap has adequate length and is never a limiting factor.*
- Lining of the neovagina with the urethral flap
  - ▶ The urethra is spatulated to create the mucosal anterior portion of the neovagina.
  - ▶ *Bleeding in the urethra should be controlled with hemostatic sutures; use of electrocautery increases risk of vascular compromise.*
  - ▶ *Use of a urethral flap may provide more moisture postoperatively.*

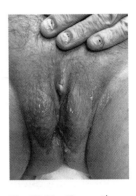

- ■ **Clitoroplasty**
  - The neoclitoris is formed from the remaining dorsal glans cap.
  - Later, it is fixed above the new urethral meatus with a U incision made in the penile skin flap (neovagina) to form a clitoral hood (Fig. 65-11).
  - A tunnel is created in the perineal cavity between the urethra, bladder, and rectum; the neovagina may be fixed to the sacrospinous ligament.
  - *Fixation to the sacrospinous ligament may avoid prolapse of the urethral part of the vagina.*

Fig. 65-11   Six months after an inverted penile skin technique vaginoplasty, this transgender female has erogenous sensation and successful penetrative vaginal intercourse with orgasm.

- ■ **Labioplasty**
  - Remaining penile skin is used to form the labia minora and sutured to deepithelialized areas of the neoclitoris, thus also creating a hood for the neoclitoris.
  - Scrotal skin is fashioned to create the labia majora, and the excess is removed.

POSTOPERATIVE MANAGEMENT
- ■ Drain care: Jackson-Pratt drain in perivaginal space for 3 days
- ■ Foley catheter: 10-14 days
- ■ Antibiotics: Cephalosporins and metronidazole for 5-7 days
- ■ Vaginal packing for 1 week, followed by vaginal stenting at night for 6 weeks, followed by dilation
  - Dilation of the neovagina once a day for 6 months; required unless daily vaginal penetrative intercourse
  - Five sizes
    - ▶ Diameters: 14-35 mm
    - ▶ Lengths: 70-163 mm

COLON VAGINOPLASTY APPROACH[7]
- ■ Total laparoscopic sigmoid vaginoplasty is a safe and effective technique for primary and revision vaginal reconstruction.
- ■ **Advantages:** Provides sufficient vaginal depth, self-lubricating, and less tendency to shrink
- ■ **Disadvantages:** Involvement of intestinal surgery and bowel anastomosis
- ■ **Indications**
  - Transgender females with insufficient penile skin for penile inversion vaginoplasty
  - Transgender females who have failed primary vaginoplasty (primary vaginoplasty with insufficient depth because of partial or complete stenosis)

■ **Contraindications**
  • Intestinal malignancy
  • Inflammatory bowel disease
  • Extensive abdominal surgery
  • Smoking
  • Obesity (BMI >30 kg/m^2)
■ HIV positive patients must have adequate CD4 count and undetectable viral load to avoid complications.
■ **Sigmoid colon** is most commonly used segment for vaginoplasty.
■ **Must be performed by two experienced surgeons:** Gastrointestinal surgeon with training in advanced laparoscopy and plastic surgeon with significant experience in gender affirmation surgery.

> **SENIOR AUTHOR TIP:**   Preference is given to a colon vaginoplasty in patients who desire less vaginal dilation and vaginal penetration without lubrication and who have an outstretched phallus length of ≤3.5 inches and have had no prior abdominal surgery.

Perineal Component
■ Dissection of the neovaginal tunnel
  • Caudally based perineoscrotal full-thickness triangular skin flap extending cranially to open into the perineal space
  • The levator ani muscle is partially dissected using bipolar cautery to provide sufficient width for the neovagina.
  • Blunt dissection above Denonvilliers fascia is carried up to the peritoneal fold where gauze is placed for visualization by the laparoscopic surgeon.
■ The blood supply to the corpus spongiosum is ligated, and the corporeal body is reduced.
■ Bilateral orchiectomy is performed.
■ The urethra is shortened and spatulated.
■ The penile skin is dissected as a proximally based skin flap.
■ A neoclitoris and labia minora are designed from glans penis and penile skin.
  • The neoclitoris is created similar to the method described in the penile inversion technique.
■ The corpora cavernosa are dissected and rami ligated individually from the pubic bone.
■ Fixing the neoclitoris and spatulated urethra together on a "throne," creates a pink, natural-looking and aesthetic infundibulum.
■ The penile skin is inverted.
■ A vertical incision is made in the inverted skin flap to bring out the clitoris, labia minora, infundibulum, and urinary meatus.
■ Scrotal skin is trimmed to form the labia majora.
  • Scars are placed in the inguinal fold.

Intraabdominal Component
■ A bowel prep is commonly performed before surgical intervention.
■ Sigmoid segment is mobilized from lateral peritoneal adhesions.
■ Sigmoid arteries/veins and surrounding vascular structures are identified.

■ To obtain a 6-inch segment of sigmoid colon, vasculature must be adequately mobilized.

CAUTION: Extreme care must be taken not to damage the sigmoid arteries and/or the common branch of Drummond, which supplies the distal sigmoid colon.

> **TIP:** Near-infrared fluorescence angiography may be used for intraoperative evaluation of vascular perfusion.

■ The mesosigmoid and sigmoid are divided using a linear bowel stapler/cutter just above the rectum.
  • Usually, the first distal or first and second distal sigmoid arteries must be divided to fully mobilize the sigmoid segment and achieve a tension-free perineal anastomosis.
■ In the pelvis, the peritoneal fold between the rectum and bladder is opened above the level of Denonvilliers fascia to the level of the gauze placed during the perineal component.
■ The patient is approached from the perineum and intraabdominally to adequately connect and bring the sigmoid segment through.
■ The mobilized sigmoid is passed into the perineum, with care to avoid vascular tension.
  • Superficial cuts can be made in the peritoneum to gain extra length.
  • If tension persists, further dissection of vascular structures is warranted.
■ The distal suture line of the sigmoid segment is opened and secured to the external neovagina.
■ The length of the neovagina may be determined by introducing a vaginal dilator into the sigmoid from the perineal opening and visualizing the desired length under transillumination.
  • A second linear stapler is used to transect at the appropriate level, usually 6 inches from the introitus.
■ The perineoscrotal and anterior penile inversion flaps are set into the sigmoid segment.
■ The neovagina may be fixed to the periosteum of the pelvic promontory to prevent future prolapse.
■ The proximal sigmoid and rectum are anastomosed using a stapled anastomosis.

Complications
■ Neovaginal stenosis
■ Neovaginal fistula
■ Neovaginal prolapse
■ Colon cancer risk
■ Bowel adhesions
■ Bowel leakage
■ Prolonged ileus
■ Intraabdominal infection

FEMALE-TO-MALE BOTTOM SURGERY[7]
■ Traditionally, bottom surgery for transgender males was relatively uncommon, compared with bottom surgery for transgender females and top surgery for transgender males.

- As more private insurers increase coverage for transgender patients, bottom surgery for transgender males is increasing.
- **Goals of female-to-male bottom surgery**
  - Male-appearing external genitalia and standing micturition
  - Ability to penetrate during sexual intercourse and have orgasm

AESTHETIC AND FUNCTIONAL CONSIDERATIONS
- Patient's primary concern for pursuing surgery:
  - Significant dysphoria with female genitalia
  - Desire to complete their transition to male
- Additional patient considerations:
  - Desire to retain receptive penetration (anal penetration option or metoidioplasty with vaginal canal preservation)
  - Single-stage surgery versus multistage surgeries
- Patient expectations will help to guide appropriate surgery: Metoidioplasty versus phalloplasty, with or without hysterectomy and salpingo-oophorectomy, vaginectomy and/or scrotoplasty

METOIDIOPLASTY
- Single-stage alternative to phalloplasty
- May be performed with or without vaginectomy, depending on desire for urethral lengthening and/or scrotoplasty
- Neophallus: 3-8 cm in length
- Aesthetically, provides a realistic-appearing microphallus capable of engorgement with erotic sensation
- Functionally, standing micturition is possible.
- **It is the only female-to-male bottom surgery that offers ability to retain reproductive potential.**
- Ideal for thin- to medium-build transgender males who lack significant mons pubis adiposity
- This approach takes advantage of hormone therapy–induced hypertrophy effects on the clitoris to allow surgical straightening of the hypertrophied clitoris.
  - The chordae are divided, releasing the corpora bodies from their attachment to the labia minora.
  - Urethral extension may be employed to elongate the short urethral plate when buccal mucosa is used.

Techniques[7]
- **Simple metoidioplasty**
  - Associated with minimal recovery
  - Based on transverse release of the chordae without manipulation of the urethra
    - ▶ Standing micturition is not possible postoperatively.
  - May be combined with a vaginectomy
  - Residual mucosa and Skene glands can result in persistent secretions after vaginectomy.
  - Complications: Malunion or malrotation of incisional closure

- **Ring metoidioplasty**
  - Involves release of chordae plus extension of the urethral plate
  - Standing micturition possible in some but not all patients
  - Associated with high sexual satisfaction rate
  - Complications: Urethral fistula (range 10%-26%), stricture (range 3%-5%), diminished orgasmic function
  - Reoperation rate: 30%
  - If desired, scrotoplasty can be performed in second stage.
- **Belgrade metoidioplasty**
  - Single-stage surgery to achieve removal of the vaginal mucosa, metoidioplasty, and creation of neourethra and scrotum
  - Standing micturition is possible in all patients.
  - Associated with high satisfaction in quality of erection, sensation of neophallus, and sexual arousal
  - Vaginectomy: Total removal of the vaginal mucosa, except for anterior vaginal wall adjacent to the urethra, which is used for urethral reconstruction
  - Urethral lengthening employs buccal mucosal and vaginal flaps.
  - Scrotoplasty includes implantation of testicular implants or fat grafting.

Complications

- **Minor:** Hematoma, wound infections, skin necrosis, urinary tract infections, dribbling, spraying, and urethral fistula. Most will resolve with conservative management.
- **Major:** Flap necrosis, wound dehiscence, urethral fistula, urethral strictures, and testicular implant displacement. Operative management is required.
- Urethral extension facilitates standing micturition.[19]
  - Various methods to elongate the *urethral plate and proximal* urethra
    - ▶ Buccal mucosa
    - ▶ Labial mucosa
    - ▶ Ring flap
  - The *distal urethra* is universally created from a labial mucosal island flap.
  - The *ventral portions* of the urethra are derived proximally from a vaginal pedicle flap.

PHALLOPLASTY

- **Goals:** To create a functional and aesthetic phallus to alleviate gender dysphoria
  - Normal, standing micturition
  - Phallic rigidity for penetration during sexual intercourse
- The preferred approach for patients desiring to live fully as a male
- Although several surgical techniques (i.e., radial forearm free flap, pedicled anterolateral thigh flap, and free latissimus dorsi flap) are used, a candid discussion regarding the patient's desired goals from surgery, including the length and circumference of the neophallus, is required to guide surgical approach.
- *Surgeons should understand the patient's preoperative ability to achieve an orgasm so that it can be matched postoperatively.*
  - A reduction in dysphoria is expected, and having an orgasm after surgery will remain difficult in patients who had difficulty before surgery.
- The radial forearm free flap is the most frequently used surgical phalloplasty technique and may be performed using either a prelaminated urethra or a tube within a tube technique.[20]

■ **Advantages**
  • Superior to other techniques because it meets the goal of creating an aesthetically pleasing and sensate neophallus with a functioning neourethra
  • Provides thin, malleable, and sensate tissue (at least two sensory nerves can be included in the flap) with a long pedicle
  • Can be harvested as an osteocutaneous flap, or a penile prosthesis can be placed in the flap at a later stage
  • Donor site scar does not produce functional or significant sensory losses.
■ **Disadvantages**
  • Requires advanced microsurgical techniques
  • Noticeable donor site morbidity
  • Multistage procedure
  • Frequent urethral complications
  • Penile prosthesis, as with any soft tissue flap option, often requires a revision procedure at 5 years because of implant malfunction, extrusion, or infection.

Aesthetic Considerations
■ For the tube within a tube technique, preoperative laser depilation is recommended on the ulnar aspect of the flap.
■ If the forearm flap will have a prelaminated urethra with mucosa, laser depilation is not necessary.
■ The mons region of a transgender male has abundant hair from exogenous testosterone therapy.
  • An abrupt transition from a mons full of hair to a hairless penile shaft may lead to a poor aesthetic outcome.
  • Superior aesthetic results may be achieved with depilation of the mons and penile shaft postoperatively.
■ **Aesthetic Contraindications**
  • Patient refusal to accept donor site scar on their body
  • Patient refusal to accept transfer of the nondominant hand forearm tattoo to the neophallus

SENIOR AUTHOR TIP: The glans creation may be performed safely during the flap transfer, or the surgeon may delay it if distal flap compromise is a concern.

COMMON SURGICAL SEQUENCING
■ **Stage 1:** Mastectomy
■ **Stage 2:** Hysterectomy and oophorectomy, vaginectomy, scrotoplasty, and reconstruction of the lengthened part of the urethra (similar to a metoidioplasty), prelamination of radial forearm with skin or mucosa
■ **Stage 3:** Phalloplasty

COMPLICATIONS
■ Partial/complete flap loss
■ An insensate flap
■ Anorgasmia/dyspareunia
■ Urinary complications (41%-80%)[21]: urethrocutaneous fistulas (decreased with concomitant gracilis muscle flap wrapped around urethral anastomosis[22]) or urinary stricture

- Radius fracture, if an osteocutaneous flap is harvested (risk very small if plate and screws used on radius)
- Bone or implant extrusion, implant infection

TESTICULAR AND ERECTILE IMPLANTS
- Testicular implants are usually the last stage of reconstruction.
  - Typically performed at least 12 months after phalloplasty to allow vascular integration of the phallus and to decrease the risk of vascular compromise during implantation
- Testicular implants
  - Silicone gel–filled implants are available off the shelf in small, medium, and large sizes.
    - ▶ Fat grafting is a good option to prevent implant-related complications.
  - In patients who elect to have an inflatable erectile device placed, only one testicular implant may be needed.
- Erectile implants
  - Readily available in many formats, lengths, and sizes
  - In transgender males, erectile implants are placed in fatty tissue with low blood supply and without the protection of corporeal bodies found in biologic men.
  - **Major complication in transgender males**: Infection, complete or partial flap loss
  - A plastic surgeon should be present during implant placement to facilitate surgery.

TOP TAKEAWAYS
- ➤ A suprapubic tube is strongly recommended during microsurgical phalloplasty.
- ➤ A pericatheter retrograde cystourethrogram approximately 2-3 months after phalloplasty is recommended to ensure no fistulas exist before penile Foley catheter removal and a voiding trial.
- ➤ Anterolateral thigh flaps are not recommended in obese patients because of resulting significant contour abnormalities at the donor site and flap manipulation during the flap transfer.
- ➤ Surgeons performing phalloplasty must ensure female reproductive organs have been removed, because they are often forgotten and can be carcinogenic.
- ➤ If performing neural anastomosis to clitoral nerve end to end, only one clitoral nerve should be used. Sensory nerves can be used for the remaining donor nerve anastomosis.
- ➤ Coronaplasty may be performed at the flap transfer or delayed; clitoral hood tissue may be used for coronaplasty skin.

REFERENCES
1. Norwood OT. Male pattern baldness: classification and incidence. South Med J 68:1359, 1975.
2. Nusbaum BP, Fuentefria S. Naturally occurring female hairline patterns. Dermatol Surg 35:907, 2009.
3. Wan D, Amirlak B, Rohrich R, et al. The clinical importance of the fat compartments in midfacial aging. Plast Reconstr Surg Glob Open 1:e92, 2014.
4. Hembree WC, Cohen-Kettenis P, Delemarre-van de Waal HA, et al; Endocrine Society. Endocrine treatment of transsexual persons: an Endocrine Society clinical practice guideline. J Clin Endocrinol Metab 94:3132, 2009.

5. Capitán L, Simon D, Kaye K, et al. Facial feminization surgery: the forehead. Surgical techniques and analysis of results. Plast Reconstr Surg 134:609, 2014.

6. Capitán L, Simon D, Meyer T, et al. Facial feminization surgery: simultaneous hair transplant during forehead reconstruction. Plast Reconstr Surg 139:573, 2017.

7. Salgado CJ, Monstrey SJ, Djordjevic ML, eds. Gender Affirmation Medical & Surgical Perspectives. Stuttgart, Germany: Thieme Publishers, 2017.

8. Coleman E, Bockting W, Botzer M, et al. Standards of care for the health of transsexual, transgender, and gender-nonconforming people, version 7. Int J Transgenderism 13:165, 2012.

9. Kanhai RC, Hage JJ, Karim RB, et al. Exceptional presenting conditions and outcome of augmentation mammaplasty in male-to-female transsexuals. Ann Plast Surg 43:476, 1999.

10. Laub DR, Fisk N. A rehabilitation program for gender dysphoria syndrome by surgical sex change. Plast Reconstr Surg 53:388, 1974.

11. Hage JJ, van Kesteren PJ. Chest-wall contouring in female-to-male transsexuals: basic considerations and review of the literature. Plast Reconstr Surg 96:386, 1995.

12. Hage JJ, Bloem JJ. Chest wall contouring for female-to-male transsexuals: Amsterdam experience. Ann Plast Surg 34:59, 1995.

13. Monstrey S, Selvaggi G, Ceulemans P, et al. Chest-wall contouring surgery in female-to-male transsexuals: a new algorithm. Plast Reconstr Surg 121:849, 2008.

14. Ergeneli MH, Duran EH, Ozcan G, et al. Vaginectomy and laparoscopically assisted vaginal hysterectomy as adjunctive surgery for female-to-male transsexual reassignment: preliminary report. Eur J Obstet Gynecol Reprod Biol 87:35, 1999.

15. O'Hanlan KA, Dibble SL, Young-Spint M. Total laparoscopic hysterectomy for female-to-male transsexuals. Obstet Gynecol 110:1096, 2007.

16. Bregten-Escobar P, Bouman MB, Buncamper ME, et al. Subcutaneous mastectomy in female-to-male transsexuals: a retrospective cohort-analysis of 202 patients. J Sex Med 9:3148, 2012.

17. Karim RB, Hage JJ, Mulder JW. Neovaginoplasty in male transsexuals: review of surgical techniques and recommendations regarding eligibility. Ann Plast Surg 37:669, 1996.

18. Selvaggi G, Ceulemans P, De Cuypere G, et al. Gender identity disorder: general overview and surgical treatment for vaginoplasty in male-to-female transsexuals. Plast Reconstr Surg 116:135e, 2005.

19. Djordjevic ML, Bizic M, Stanojevic D, et al. Urethral lengthening in metoidioplasty (female-to-male sex reassignment surgery) by combined buccal mucosa graft and labia minora flap. Urology 74:349, 2009.

20. Garaffa G, Christopher NA, Ralph DJ. Total phallic reconstruction in female-to-male transsexuals. Eur Urol 57:715, 2010.

21. Hu ZQ, Hyakusoku H, Gao JH, et al. Penis reconstruction using three different operative methods. Br J Plast Surg 58:487, 2005.

22. Salgado CJ, Nugent AG, Moody AM, et al. Immediate pedicled gracilis flap in radial forearm flap phalloplasty for trangender male patients to reduce urinary fistula. J Plast Reconstr Aesthet Surg 69:1551, 2016.

Credits

Chapter 1

Fig. 1-1 From Gorney M. Recognition and management of patient unsuitable for aesthetic surgery. Plast Reconstr Surg 126:2268, 2010.

Chapter 2

Fig. 2-1 Photograph courtesy of Phillip Pikart. Available at WikimediaCommons.

Fig. 2-3, *A* Photograph courtesy of brewbooks. Available at WikimediaCommons.

Fig. 2-3, *B* Photograph courtesy of Jitze Couperus. Available at WikimediaCommons.

Fig. 2-4, *B* Photograph courtesy of Georges Jansoone. Available at WikimediaCommons.

Fig. 2-5 Photograph courtesy of Shawn Lipowski. Available at WikimediaCommons.

Chapter 4

Fig. 4-1 Data from Jena AB, Seabury S, Lakdawalla D, et al. Malpractice risk according to physician specialty. N Engl J Med 365:629, 2011.

Fig. 4-2 Data from Rohrich RJ, Broughton G II, Horton B. The key to long-term success in liposuction: a guide for plastic surgeons and patients. Plast Reconstr Surg 114:1945; discussion 1953, 2004.

Chapter 5

Fig. 5-2 From Friedburg BL. Anesthesia in Cosmetic Surgery. New York: Cambridge University Press, 2007.

Fig. 5-3 Data from Mallampati SR, Gatt SP, Gugino LD, et al. A clinical sign to predict difficult tracheal intubation: a prospective study. Can Anaesth Soc J 32:429, 1985.

Table 5-1 Data from Saklad M. Grading of patients for surgical procedures. Anesthesiology 5:281, 1941.

Table 5-2 Data from American Society of Anesthesiologists Committee. Practice guidelines for preoperative fasting and the use of pharmacologic agents to reduce the risk of pulmonary aspiration: application to healthy patients undergoing elective procedures: an updated report by the American Society for Anesthesiologists Committee on Standards and Practice Parameters.

Table 5-3 Data from Bennett GD. Anesthesia for aesthetic surgery. In Shiffman MA, Di Giuseppe A, eds. Cosmetic Surgery. Berlin Heidelberg: Springer, 2013.

Table 5-4 Data from ASA continuum of depth of sedation: definition of general anesthesia and level of sedation/analgesia. Available at *www.asahq.org.*

Chapter 6

Fig. 6-1 From Chung F, Yegneswaran B, Liao P, et al. STOP questionnaire: a tool to screen patients for obstructive sleep apnea. Anesthesiology 18:812, 2008.

Chapter 9

Fig. 9-1 Data from Hynson JM, Sessler DI, Moayeri A, et al. The effects of preinduction warming on temperature and blood pressure during propofol/nitrous oxide anesthesia. Anesthesiology 79:219, 1993.

Fig. 9-2 and Table 9-4 From Davison SP, Venturi ML, Attinger CE, et al. Prevention of venous thromboembolism in the plastic surgery patient. Plast Reconstr Surg 114:43e, 2004.

Table 9-1 Based on ASA Physical Status Classification of the American Society of Anesthesiologists. A copy of the full text can be obtained from ASA, 161 American Lane Schaumburg, IL 6173-4973 or online at *www.asahq.org.*

Table 9-2 Data from Grazer FM, DeJong R. Fatal outcomes from liposuction: census survey of cosmetic surgeons. Plast Reconstr Surg 15:436, 2000.

Table 9-3 Data from Young VL, Watson ME. The need for venous thromboembolism (VTE) prophylaxis in plastic surgery. Aesthet Surg J 26:157, 2006; and Geerts WH, Pineo GH, Heit JA, et al. Prevention of venous thromboembolism: the Seventh ACCP Conference on Antithrombotic and Thrombolytic Therapy. Chest 126 (3 Suppl):S338, 2004.

Table 9-5 Data from Hatef DA, Kenkel JM, Nguyen MQ, et al. Thromboembolic risk assessment and the efficacy of enoxaparin prophylaxis in excisional body contouring surgery. Plast Reconstr Surg 122:269, 2008.

Tables 9-7 and 9-8 From Steinberg JP, Braun BI, Hellinger WC, et al; Trial to Reduce Antrimicrobial Prophylaxis Errors (TRAPE) Study Group. Timing of antimicrobial prophylaxis and the risk of surgical site infections: results from the Trial to Reduce Antimicrobial Prophylaxis Errors. Ann Surg 250:10, 2009.

Box 9-1 Data from Iverson RE, Lynch DJ. Practice advisory on liposuction. Plast Reconstr Surg 113:1478, 2004.

Box 9-2 Data from Colwell AS, Borud LJ. Optimization of patient safety in post-bariatric body contouring: a current review. Aesthet Surg J 28:437, 2008.

Chapter 10

Table 10-2 Data from Venturi ML, Davison SP, Caprini JA. Prevention of venous thromboembolism in the plastic surgery patient: current guidelines and recommendations. Aesthet Surg J 29:421, 2009.

Box 10-2 Data from Bogan V. Anesthesia and safety considerations for office-based cosmetic surgery practice. AANA Journal 80:299, 2012.

Box 10-4 Data from World Alliance for Patient Safety. Surgery Saves Lives: Second Global Patient Safety Challenge. Geneva: World Health Organization, 2008.

Chapter 11

Fig. 11-1 Reprinted from Disease of the Month, Vol. 51, Caprini JA, Thrombosis risk assessment as a guide to quality patient care, 2005, with permission from Elsevier.

Chapter 12

Table 12-2 Data from American Association for Accreditation of Ambulatory Surgery Facilities. Procedural Standards and Checklist for Accreditation of Ambulatory Facilities.

Chapter 13

Table 13-1 Data from Fitzpatrick TB. The validity and practicality of sun-reactive skin types I through VI. Arch Dermatol 124:869, 1988.

Chapter 15

Table 15-1 Data from Fitzpatrick TB. The validity and practicality of sun-reactive skin types I through VI. Arch Dermatol 124:869, 1988.

Chapter 16

Table 16-1 Data from Fitzpatrick TB. The validity and practicality of sun-reactive skin types I through VI. Arch Dermatol 124:869, 1988.

Chapter 19

Fig. 19-1 From Tonnard PL, Verpaele AM, Bensimon RH, eds. Centrofacial Rejuvenation. New York: Thieme Publishers, 2018.

Table 19-1 Data from Fitzpatrick TB. The validity and practicality of sun-reactive skin types I through VI. Arch Dermatol 124:869, 1988.

Table 19-2 Data from Glogau RG. Aesthetic and anatomic analysis of the aging skin. Semin Cutan Med Surg 15:134, 1996.

Chapter 20

Table 20-1 Data from Fitzpatrick TB. The validity and practicality of sun-reactive skin types I through VI. Arch Dermatol 124:869, 1988.

Table 20-2 Data from Glogau RG. Aesthetic and anatomic analysis of the aging skin. Semin Cutan Med Surg 15:134, 1996.

Boxes 20-1 and 20-2 Data from Hruza GJ. Dermabrasion. Facial Plast Surg Clin North Am 9:267, 2001.

Box 20-3 Data from Holck DE, Ng JD. Facial skin rejuvenation. Curr Opin Ophthalmol 14:246, 2003.

Chapter 22

Fig. 22-2 From Pu LLQ, Chen YR, Li QF, et al. Aesthetic Plastic Surgery in Asians: Principles and Techniques. New York: Thieme Publishers, 2015.

Fig. 22-3 From Tonnard PL, Verpaele AM, Bensimon RH, eds. Centrofacial Rejuvenation. New York: Thieme Publishers, 2018.

Chapter 23

Figs. 23-2 through 23-6 and 23-9 through 23-14 From Coleman SR, Mazzola, RF, Pu LLQ, eds. Fat Injection: From Filling to Regeneration, ed 2. New York: Thieme Publishers, 2018.

Figs. 23-7 and 23-8 Photography by Taylor Maulin & Associates.

Chapter 26

Table 26-1 Data from V-Loc™ Wound Closure Devices Product Overview. Available at http://www.medtronic.com/content/dam/covidien/library/us/en/product/wound-closure/v-loc-wound-closure-devices-product-overview.pdf.

Table 26-2 Data from Knotless Tissue-Closure Device. Available at http://www.quilldevice.com/material-guide-hp.

Chapter 28

Fig. 28-1 From Pollock H, Pollock T. Progressive tension sutures: a technique to reduce local complications in abdominoplasty. Plast Reconstr Surg 105:2583; discussion 2587, 2000.

Chapter 29

Figs. 29-1, 29-2, 29-5, 29-6, 29-9 through 29-14 and 29-16 through 29-26 From Codner MA, McCord CD Jr, eds. Eyelid & Periorbital Surgery, ed 2. New York: Thieme Publishers, 2016.

Chapter 30

Fig. 30-7 Data from Moss JC, Mendelson BC, Taylor GI. Surgical anatomy of the ligamentous attachments in the temple and periorbital regions. Plast Reconstr Surg 105:1475, 2000.

Fig. 30-9 From Feldman JJ. Neck Lift. New York: Thieme Publishers, 2006.

Chapter 31

Fig. 31-1 From Bashour M. History and current concepts in the analysis of facial attractiveness. Plast Reconstr Surg 118:741, 2006.

Figs. 31-2, 31-3, 31-5 through 31-7 From Rohrich RJ, Adams WP Jr, Ahmad J, Gunter JP, eds. Dallas Rhinoplasty: Nasal Surgery by the Masters, ed 3. New York: Thieme Publishers, 2014.

Fig. 31-4 From Codner MA, McCord CD Jr, eds. Eyelid & Periorbital Surgery, ed 2. New York: Thieme Publishers, 2016.

Table 31-1 Data from Fitzpatrick TB. The validity and practicality of sun-reactive skin types I through VI. Arch Dermatol 124:869, 1988.

Table 31-2 Data from Glogau RG. Aesthetic and anatomic analysis of the aging skin. Semin Cutan Med Surg 15:134, 1996.

Chapter 32

Figs. 32-1, 32-4, 32-6, 32-7 From Barrera A, Uebel CO. Hair Transplantation: The Art of Follicular Unit Micrografting and Minigrafting, ed 2. New York: Thieme Publishers, 2014.

Fig. 32-2 From Norwood OT, Shiell RC. Hair Transplant Surgery, ed 2. Springfield, IL: Charles C Thomas, 1984.

Fig. 32-3 From Ludwig E. Classification of the types of androgenic alopecia (common baldness) arising in the female sex. Br J Dermatol 97:247, 1977.

Chapter 33

Fig. 33-2 Data from Knize DM. An anatomically based study of the mechanism of eyebrow ptosis. Plast Reconstr Surg 97:1321, 1996.

Fig. 33-3 From Nahai F, Saltz R. Endoscopic Plastic Surgery, ed 2. New York: Thieme Publishers, 2008.

Fig. 33-5 From Guyuron B, Lee M. A reappraisal of surgical techniques and efficacy in forehead rejuvenation. Plast Reconstr Surg 134:426, 2014.

Boxes 33-1 and 33-2 Data from Knize DM. Anatomic concepts for brow lift procedures. Plast Reconstr Surg 124:2118, 2009.

Chapter 34

Figs. 34-2 through 34-4 and 34-6 From Nahai F, ed. The Art of Aesthetic Surgery: Principles & Techniques, ed 2. New York: Thieme Publishers, 2011.

Fig. 34-5 From Codner MA, McCord CD Jr, eds. Eyelid & Periorbital Surgery, ed 2. New York: Thieme Publishers, 2016.

Fig. 34-11 From Rohrich RJ, Coberly DM, Fagien S, et al. Current concepts in aesthetic upper blepharoplasty. Plast Reconstr Surg 113:32e, 2004.

Chapter 35

Figs. 35-4 through 35-6 From Barton FE. Facial Rejuvenation. New York: Thieme Publishers, 2008.

Chapter 36

Figs. 36-1; 36-4, C, D; 36-10 From Pu LLQ, Chen YR, Li QF, et al, eds. Aesthetic Plastic Surgery in Asians: Principles and Techniques. New York: Thieme Publishers, 2015.

Fig. 36-7 From Codner MA, McCord CD Jr, eds. Eyelid & Periorbital Surgery, ed 2. New York: Thieme Publishers, 2016.

Chapter 37

Fig. 37-2 From Nahai F, ed. The Art of Aesthetic Surgery: Principles & Techniques, ed 2. New York: Thieme Publishers, 2011.

Figs. 37-3 and 37-4 From Barton FE. Facial Rejuvenation. New York: Thieme Publishers, 2008.

Table 37-1 Data from Barton FE, Ha R, Awada M. Fat extrusion and septal reset in patients with the tear trough triad: a critical appraisal. Plast Reconstr Surg 113:2115, 2004.

Chapter 38

Figs. 38-3, 38-5, 38-6 From Barton FE. Facial Rejuvenation. New York: Thieme Publishers, 2008.

Fig. 38-4 From Hamra ST. The zygorbicular dissection in composite rhytidectomy: an ideal midface plane. Plast Reconstr Surg 102:1646, 1998.

Figs. 38-7 through 38-9 From Codner MA, McCord CD Jr, eds. Eyelid & Periorbital Surgery, ed 2. New York: Thieme Publishers, 2016.

Chapter 39

Figs. 39-1 and 39-6 From Codner MA, McCord CD Jr, eds. Eyelid & Periorbital Surgery, ed 2. New York: Thieme Publishers, 2016.

Fig. 39-3 From Bentz ML, Bauer BS, Zuker RM, eds. Principles and Practice of Pediatric Plastic Surgery, ed 2. New York: Thieme Publishers, 2016.

Table 39-3 Data from Liu MT, Totonchi A, Katira K, et al. Outcomes of mild to moderate upper eyelid ptosis correction using Müller's muscle-conjunctival resection. Plast Reconstr Surg 130:799e, 2012.

Chapter 40

Fig. 40-2 Data from Moss JC, Mendelson BC, Taylor GI. Surgical anatomy of the ligamentous attachments in the temple and periorbital regions. Plast Reconstr Surg 105:1475, 2000.

Figs. 40-3 and 40-9 From Codner MA, McCord CD Jr, eds. Eyelid & Periorbital Surgery, ed 2. New York: Thieme Publishers, 2016.

Fig. 40-4 From Blondeel PN, Morris SF, Hallock GG, Neligan PC, eds. Perforator Flaps: Anatomy, Technique, and Clinical Applications, ed 2. New York: Thieme Publishers, 2013.

Fig. 40-7 From Nahai F, ed. The Art of Aesthetic Surgery: Principles & Techniques, ed 2. New York: Thieme Publishers, 2011.

Chapter 41

Fig. 41-2 From Ponsky D, Guyuron B. Comprehensive surgical aesthetic enhancement and rejuvenation of the perioral region. Aesthet Surg J 31:382, 2011.

Fig. 41-3 From Pu LLQ, Chen YR, Li QF, et al, eds. Aesthetic Plastic Surgery in Asians: Principles and Techniques. New York: Thieme Publishers, 2015.

Fig. 41-5 From Tonnard PL, Verpaele AM, Bensimon RH, eds. Centrofacial Rejuvenation. New York: Thieme Publishers, 2018.

Fig. 41-6 From Barton FE. Facial Rejuvenation. New York: Thieme Publishers, 2008.

Chapter 42

Fig. 42-1 From Tonnard PL, Verpaele AM, Bensimon RH, eds. Centrofacial Rejuvenation. New York: Thieme Publishers, 2018.

Chapter 43

Figs. 43-3 and 43-4 From Nahai F, ed. The Art of Aesthetic Surgery: Principles & Techniques, ed 2. New York: Thieme Publishers, 2011.

Figs. 43-5 and 43-7 From Barton FE. Facial Rejuvenation. New York: Thieme Publishers, 2008.

Chapter 44

Fig. 44-2 Data from Rohrich RJ, Rios JL, Smith PD, et al. Neck rejuvenation revisited. Plast Reconstr Surg 118:1251, 2006.

Fig. 44-3 From Barton FE. Facial Rejuvenation. New York: Thieme Publishers, 2008.

Figs. 44-4 through 44-7 From Nahai F, ed. The Art of Aesthetic Surgery: Principles & Techniques, ed 2. New York: Thieme Publishers, 2011.

Chapter 45

Figs. 45-1, 45-2, 45-5, 45-8 through 45-21, 45-23, 45-24, D; 45-27, 45-29, 45-31 through 45-33, 45-37 From Rohrich RJ, Adams WP Jr, Ahmad J, Gunter JP, eds. Dallas Rhinoplasty: Nasal Surgery by the Masters, ed 3. New York: Thieme Publishers, 2014.

Chapter 46

Fig. 46-1 From Rohrich RJ, Adams WP Jr, Ahmad J, Gunter JP, eds. Dallas Rhinoplasty: Nasal Surgery by the Masters, ed 3. New York: Thieme Publishers, 2014.

Fig. 46-3 From Nahai F, ed. The Art of Aesthetic Surgery: Principles & Techniques, ed 2. New York: Thieme Publishers, 2011.

Figs. 46-4 through 46-7 From Rohrich RJ, Adams WP Jr, Ahmad J, Gunter JP, eds. Dallas Rhinoplasty: Nasal Surgery by the Masters, ed 3. New York: Thieme Publishers, 2014.

Chapter 48

Fig. 48-9, B From Ozturk CN, Li Y, Tung R, et al. Complications following injection of soft-tissue fillers. Aesthet Surg J 33:862, 2013.

Chapter 49

Figs. 49-1 and 49-8 Data from Cohen SR. Genioplasty. In Achauer BH, Eriksson E, Guyuron B, et al, eds. Plastic Surgery: Indications, Operations, and Outcomes, vol 5. St Louis: Mosby-Elsevier, 2000.

Figs. 49-4 and 49-7 From Nahai F, ed. The Art of Aesthetic Surgery: Principles & Techniques, ed 2. New York: Thieme Publishers, 2011.

Table 49-1 Data from Guyuron B, Michelow BJ, Willis L. Practical classification of chin deformities. Aesthetic Plast Surg 19:257, 1995.

Chapter 50

Fig. 50-4 From Bentz ML, Bauer BS, Zuker RM, eds. Principles and Practice of Pediatric Plastic Surgery, ed 2. New York: Thieme Publishers, 2016.

Chapter 51

Figs. 51-1, 51-3, 51-8 From Hall-Findlay EJ. Aesthetic Breast Surgery: Concepts & Techniques New York: Thieme Publishers, 2010.

Figs. 51-5 and 51-6 From Jones GE. Bostwick's Plastic & Reconstructive Breast Surgery, ed 3. New York: Thieme Publishers, 2010.

Chapter 52

Fig. 52-1 Data from Kirwan L. Augmentation of the ptotic breast: simultaneous periareolar mastopexy/breast augmentation. Aesthet Surg J 19:34, 1999.

Fig. 52-3 From Fisher J, Handel N, eds. Problems in Breast Surgery: A Repair Manual. New York: Thieme Publishers, 2014.

Table 52-1 From Adams WP Jr, Mallucci P. Breast augmentation. Plast Reconstr Surg 130:598e, 2012.

Table 52-2 From Hidalgo DA. Breast augmentation: choosing the optimal incision, implant, and pocket plane. Plast Reconstr Surg 105:2202, 2000.

Chapter 53

Fig. 53-1 Data from Kirwan L. Augmentation of the ptotic breast: simultaneous periareolar mastopexy/breast augmentation. Aesthet Surg J 19:34, 1999.

Fig. 53-4 Data from Rohrich RJ, Thornton JF, Jakubietz RG, et al. The limited scar mastopexy: current concepts and approaches to correct breast ptosis. Plast Reconstr Surg 114:1622, 2004.

Table 53-1 Data from Rohrich RJ, Beran SJ, Restifo RJ, et al. Aesthetic management of the breast following explanation: evaluation and mastopexy options. Plast Reconstr Surg 101:827, 1998.

Chapter 54

Fig. 54-2 From Hall-Findlay EJ. Aesthetic Breast Surgery: Concepts & Techniques New York: Thieme Publishers, 2010.

Table 54-1 Data from Stevens WG, Freeman ME, Stoker DA, et al. One-stage mastopexy with breast augmentation: a review of 321 patients. Plast Reconstr Surg 120:1674, 2007; and Calobrace MB, Herdt DR, Cothron KJ. Simultaneous augmentation/mastopexy: a retrospective 5-year review of 332 consecutive cases. Plast Reconstr Surg 131:156, 2013.

Table 54-2 Data from Lee MR, Unger JG, Adams WP Jr. The tissue-based triad: a process approach to augmentation mastopexy. Plast Reconstr Surg. 134:215, 2014.

Chapter 55

Fig. 55-4 From Nahai F, ed. The Art of Aesthetic Surgery: Principles & Techniques, ed 2. New York: Thieme Publishers, 2011.

Chapter 57

Fig. 57-1 From Nahai F, ed. The Art of Aesthetic Surgery: Principles & Techniques, ed 2. New York: Thieme Publishers, 2011.

Fig. 57-3 Data from Rohrich RJ, Smith PD, Marcantonio DR, Kenkel JM. The Zones of Adherence: Role in Minimizing and Preventing Contour Deformities in Liposuction. Plast Reconstr Surg 107:1562, 2001.

Chapter 58

Fig. 58-2 From Appelt EA, Janis JE, Rohrich RJ. An algorithmic approach to upper arm contouring. Plast Reconstr Surg 118:237, 2006.

Fig. 58-7 From Aly A, ed. Body Contouring After Massive Weight Loss. New York: Thieme Publishers, 2006.

Table 58-1 From Rohrich RJ, Beran SJ, Kenkel JM, eds. Ultrasound-Assisted Liposuction. New York: Thieme Publishers, 1998.

Chapter 59

Fig. 59-1 From Aly A, ed. Body Contouring After Massive Weight Loss. New York: Thieme Publishers, 2006.

Figs. 59-3 and 59-4 From Mendieta CG. The Art of Gluteal Sculpting. New York: Thieme Publishers, 2011.

Chapter 60

Fig. 60-7 From Pollock H, Pollock T. Progressive tension sutures: a technique to reduce local complications in abdominoplasty. Plast Reconstr Surg 105:2583; discussion 2587, 2000.

Fig. 60-8 Data from Heller JB, Teng E, Knoll BI, et al. Outcome analysis of combined lipoabdominoplasty versus conventional abdominoplasty. Plast Reconstr Surg 121:1821, 2008.

Fig. 60-12 Reprinted from Disease of the Month, Vol. 51, Caprini JA, Thrombosis risk assessment as a guide to quality patient care, 2005, with permission from Elsevier.

Box 60-1 Data from Rosenberger LH, Politano AD, Sawyer RG. The surgical care improvement project and prevention of post-operative infection, including surgical site infection. Surg Infect (Larchmt) 12:163, 2011.

Chapter 61

Table 61-3 From Song AY, O'Toole JP, Jean RD, et al. A classification of contour deformities after massive weight loss: application of the Pittsburgh rating scale. Semin Plast Surg 20:24, 2006.

Chapter 62

Fig. 62-7 From Aly A, ed. Body Contouring After Massive Weight Loss New York: Thieme Publishers, 2006.

Fig. 62-8 From Rubin JP, Toy J. Mastopexy and breast reduction in massive-weight-loss patients. In Nahai F, ed. The Art of Aesthetic Surgery: Principles & Techniques, 2nd ed. New York: Thieme Publishers, 2011.

Fig. 62-9 From Nahai F, ed. The Art of Aesthetic Surgery: Principles & Techniques, ed 2. New York: Thieme Publishers, 2011.

Table 62-1 Data from National Institutes of Health. Classification of overweight and obesity by bmi, waist circumference, and associated disease risks.

Chapter 63

Figs. 63-1 and 63-14 through 63-17 From Nahai F, ed. The Art of Aesthetic Surgery: Principles & Techniques, ed 2. New York: Thieme Publishers, 2011.

Table 63-1 Data from Mirzabeigi JN, Jandali S, Mettel RK, et al. The nomenclature of "vaginal rejuvenation" and elective vulvovaginal plastic surgery. Aesthet Surg J 31:723, 2011.

Table 63-2 Data from Felicio Y. Labial surgery. Aesthet Surg J 27:322, 2007.

Chapter 65

Fig. 65-1 From Salgado CJ, Monstrey SJ, Djordjevic ML. Gender Affirmation: Medical and Surgical Perspectives. New York: Thieme Publishers, 2017.

Fig. 65-2 From Capitán L, Simon D, Meyer T, et al. Facial feminization surgery: simultaneous hair transplant during forehead reconstruction. Plast Reconstr Surg 139:573, 2017.

Figs. 65-3 through 65-9; Table 65-1 From Monstrey SJ, Ceulemans P, Hoebeke P. Sex reassignment surgery in the female-to-male transsexual. Semin Plast Surg 25:229, 2011.

Several Figs. and Chapters 31, 39 and 54 were previously published in Janis JE, ed. Essentials of Plastic Surgery, ed 2. New York: Thieme Publishers, 2014.

Index

A

Abdominal wall, anatomy of, 837-840
Abdominoplasty
    aesthetic aspects of, 840
    after massive weight loss, 874-876
    anesthesia guidelines for, 98-100
    common malpractice claims and, 53
    complications of, 852-853
    contraindications for, 841
    indications for, 840-841
    infection and, 177
    informed consent for, 844-845
    postoperative care after, 851-852
    preoperative evaluation for, 842-843
    relevant anatomy for, 837-840
    techniques for
        fleur-de-lis abdominoplasty, 850, 874
        high-lateral-tension abdominoplasty, 849-850
        lipoabdominoplasty, 848
        miniabdominoplasty, 848-849
        progressive tension sutures, 847
        reverse abdominoplasty, 851
        traditional abdominoplasty, 845-847
    using progressive tension sutures, 344
    and venous thromboembolism, 99, 162, 164, 165
Ablative laser resurfacing
    anesthesia for, 214-216
    complications of, 218-220
    general characteristics of, 206
    goals of, 212
    markings for, 214
    postoperative care after, 217-218
    for rejuvenation of perioral region, 535-536
    safety, 214
    using carbon dioxide laser
        physics, 212-213
        technique, 216
    using erbium:yttrium aluminum garnet laser
        physics, 213
        technique, 216-217
    using fractional laser, 213-214

Abrading tips, 262-263
    diamond fraise, 262
    serrated wheel, 263
    wire brush, 263
Absorption, lasers and, 206
Accupoint electrostimulation, as antiemetic therapy, 79
Acellular dermal graft, micronized, 648
Acetaminophen, for analgesia, 111-112
Acetone, as a degreasing agent, 242
Acid aspiration prophylaxis, 67
Acne
    after carbon dioxide laser therapy, 220
    treatment, 199
Acneiform eruptions, after chemical peels, 255
Acrocordon, 188
Actinic keratosis, 187
Adipocyte transplantation, complications of, 311-312
Adnexal structures of skin, 181
Aesthetic evaluation
    of Asian eyelid, 466
    of breast, 719-721
    for facial feminization, 934-937
    of lower eyelid, 452
    of upper eyelid, 438-440
Aesthetic medicine, goals of, 13
Aesthetic surgeon, role of, 3
Aesthetics, defined, 13
Affirm laser, 224
Aging skin, causes of, 191
AHAs; see Alpha-hydroxy acids
AICD; see Automated implantable cardioverter defibrillator
Airway management, general principles, 71-72
Alar base, correction of, 610-612
Alar rim deformities, correction of, 611-612
Alcohol, and surgical complications, 148
All-trans-retinoic acid, 240
Alloderm, 338

Allogeneic materials
  bilaminate neodermal natrix, 338
  general characteristic of, 337
  homologous bone, 337
  homologous cartilage, 337
  homologous dermis, 338
  lyophilized fascia, 337
Alloplasts
  expanded polytetrafluoroethylene,
    341
  gelatin film, 342
  high-density porous polyethylene,
    339
  hydroxyapatite, 339-340
  metals, 338-339
  polydioxanone, 342
  polyglactin 910, 342
  polylactic acid derivatives, 341
  silicone, 340-341
Aloe vera, 195
Alopecia, 73, 402
Alpha-hydroxy acids, 193-194, 250
Ambulation, and venous thromboembolism
    prophylaxis, 153-154
Ambulatory surgery centers
  accreditation of, 174
  and cosmetic procedures, 176
  defined, 171
  federal regulations for, 175
  and Medicare, 175
  patient selection, 177
  standards for, 175
  state regulations for, 175-176
Ambulatory surgery, decision-making for,
    88-91
American Society for Aesthetic Plastic
    Surgery logo, 14
American Society of Anesthesiologists
    physical status classification,
    121-122
American Society of Plastic Surgeons seal,
    18
Aminolevulinic acid, as treatment for skin
    cancer, 187
Anagen, 182, 402
Analgesia; see Multimodal analgesia; opioids
  analgesic options for, 111-112
Anchor blepharoplasty, 444
  and total intravenous anesthesia, 60

Anesthesia
  ablative laser therapy and, 214-215
  airway management for, 71-72
  American Society of Anesthesiologists
    physical status classification,
    65-66
  for blepharoptosis repair, 502-503
  for chemical peel procedures, 241
  considerations with administration of, 61
  critical preoperative patient information,
    62
  fasting guidelines for, 66-67
  functional status and metabolic equiva-
    lents, 67-68
  general principles of, 59-61
  identifying risk factors for, 62-63
  for lip augmentation with injectable fill-
    ers, 650
  malignant hyperthermia and, 79-81
  for massive-weight-loss patients, 883-
    884
  model of provider(s), 61
  monitored anesthesia care, 68-71
  nonablative laser therapy and, 225
  postanesthesia recovery unit care, 81
  patient selection for, 61-62
  perioperative considerations for
    ambulatory surgery, 88-91
    cardiovascular diseases, 85-86
    herbal supplements, 91-92
    hypothermia, 74-76
    obstructive sleep apnea, 87-88
    pulmonary diseases, 86-87
  positioning for, 73-74
  postoperative and postdischarge nausea
    and vomiting, 76-79
  preoperative evaluation for, 61-62
  preoperative screening for, 61-62
  preoperative testing for, 63-65
  procedure-specific guidelines
    abdominal procedures, 98-100
    body contouring after massive weight
      loss, 98-100
    botulinum toxin injection, 272
    breast procedures, 98-100
    facial laser resurfacing, 97-98
    facial plastic surgery, 95-97
    fat grafting, 299, 304, 305, 307
    hair transplantation, 405

liposuction, 98-100
  soft tissue fillers, 285
  upper blepharoplasty, 442
pulmonary aspiration prevention, 66-67
Angiomas, 188
Anguloplasty, 672-673
Anterior jugular vein, 382
Anterior triangle of neck, 387
Antibiotic prophylaxis, for methicillin-resistant *Staphylococcus aureus*, 149
Anticoagulation, and laser therapy, 210
Antiemetic therapy, for postoperative nausea and vomiting, 78-79
  drugs most commonly used for, 79
Antifungals, laser therapy and, 210
Antiinflammatory agents, effects on wound healing, 185
Antineoplastic agents, effects on wound healing, 185
Antioxidants, 193, 194
Antivirals, laser therapy and, 210
Aortic stenosis, perioperative anesthesia considerations for, 85
Apfel stratified risk score, 78
Aphrodite of Milo; *see* Venus de Milo
Apnea-hypopnea index, 87
Apnea, defined, 87
Applicators, for chemical peel agents, 242
  approach for proper management of, 110-111
Arbutin, 199
Arcuate expansion, 363
Arms, photographic series for, 34
Arnica montana, 146, 294, 446
ASCs; *see* Ambulatory surgery centers
Aspiration prophylaxis medications, 67
Aspirin, for venous thromboembolism prophylaxis, 165
Asthma, perioperative anesthesia considerations for, 86
Asymmetry, after soft tissue filler injection, 294
Atypical melanocytic nevi, 188
Aufricht, Gustave, 18
Augmentation-mastopexy
  special considerations for, 759
    algorithm for selecting, 766
    alternatives to, 764
    complications of, 767

indications for, 764
    outcomes of, 765, 767
    postoperative care after, 767
    surgical planning and treatment, 765-767
    techniques for
      single-stage procedure, 764-765
      two-stage procedure, 765
Augmentation; *see* Augmentation-mastopexy; breast augmentation; lip augmentation
Autoaugmentation, 833
Autografts
  bone, 336
  cartilage, 336
  defined, 335
Autologous fat augmentation, 833-834
Automated implantable cardioverter defibrillator, 85
Averageness, defined, 18
Avobenzone, 189
Azelaic acid, 199

B
Baker classification of capsular contracture, 743
Balanced technique, for general anesthesia, 60
Baldness, patterns of, 403-404
Bariatric surgery, techniques for, 870-871
Barr, Mark, 15
Barton classification of nasolabial fold, 556
Basal cell cancer, 186
BCC; *see* Basal cell cancer
Beam shape, lasers and, 206
Beauty
  ancient concepts, 13-14
  classical concepts, 17-18
  golden ratio, 14-15
  Vitruvian Man, 16-17
Belotero products, 287
Belt lipectomy, 874-876
Benzodiazepine reversal, 71
Beta-lipohydroxy acid, 239
BIA-ALCL; *see* Breast implant-associated anaplastic large cell lymphoma
Bilopancreatic diversion, 871
Biomaterials, nonbreast
  allogeneic materials, 337-338
  alloplastic materials, 338-341

Biomaterials, nonbreast—cont'd
  autografts, 336
  biologic reactions to, 335
  defined, 335
  ideal properties of, 335
  resorbable types of, 341-342
Biooclusive dressings, 217
Bispectral index, 60
Blepharochalasis, defined, 436, 451
Blepharoplasty
  Asian
    complications of, 479-480
    preoperative evaluation for, 466-468
    techniques, 468-471
  common malpractice claims and, 52
  comparison of Asian and white eyelids,
    462-466
  of lower eyelid
    anatomy, 451-453
    complications, 458
    for correction of tear trough deformity,
      487-488
    postoperative care, 458
    techniques, 454-457
  of upper eyelid
    anatomy, 429-435
    equipment, 441
    indications, 429-435
    informed consent, 440-441
    postoperative care, 445-449
    preoperative evaluation, 436-440
    techniques, 441-445
Blepharoptosis
  anesthesia for, 502-503
  defined, 436, 498
  etiologic factors for
    acquired ptosis, 500
    congenital ptosis, 499-500
    pseudoptosis, 499
    true ptosis, 499
  preoperative evaluation for, 501
  algorithm for procedure selection, 503
  relevant anatomy for, 498-499
  techniques for
    external levator resection, 506-507
    Fasanella-Servat procedure, 503-504
    frontalis suspension, 507
    levator aponeurosis advancement,
      504-506
    levator reinsertion, 507
    Müller muscle-conjunctival resection,
      504

Blood glucose, preoperative testing for, 64
Blood loss, recommendations based on an-
    ticipated amount of, 123
BMI; see Body mass index
Body contouring
  after massive weight loss
    anesthesia guidelines for, 100-102
    for back, 877-878
    for breasts, 879-881
    for buttocks, 877
    complications of, 884-885
    for face and neck, 882-883
    liposuction, 871
    medial thigh lift technique, 862-863
    for medial thighs, 878-879
    preoperative evaluation for, 872, 873
    safety concerns for, 883-884
    staging considerations for, 873
    for trunk/abdomen, 874-876
    for upper arms, 882
    for waist and lateral thighs, 876
  noninvasive techniques for
    cryolipolysis, 927-929
    high-intensity focused ultrasound,
      929-930
    low-level laser therapy, 931
Body dysmorphic disorder
  characteristics of, 7
  incidence of, 7
  medicolegal considerations, 45
  recognizing patients with, 3
Body language, medicolegal considerations
    and, 47
Body mass index
  ASA physical status classification and, 122
  liposuction and, 124
  obesity and, 90-91, 869
  office-based surgery and, 91
  postbariatric body contouring and, 132,
    133
Body, photographic series for
  for massive weight loss, 35-36
  standard male series, 34-35
  standard series, 32-33
  supplemental views, 33-34
Bone graft, 336, 337
Botanicals, 194
Bottom surgery
  female-to-male surgery
    metoidioplasty, 952-953
    phalloplasty, 953-955
    testicular and erectile implants, 955

male-to-female surgery
   colon vaginoplasty approach, 949-951
   penile skin-flap vaginoplasty approach,
      948-949
Bottoming out, 742
Botulinum toxin, injection of
   anesthesia for, 272
   complications of, 278
   contraindications to, 270
   defined, 269
   history of, 269-270
   immunogenicity, 272-273
   indications for, 270
   informed consent for, 271-272
   patient evaluation for, 271
   physiology, 269-270
   postoperative care after injection of, 277
   precautions for using, 270-271
   reconstitution of, 272
   storage of, 272
   syringe and needles for using, 272
   technique, 273
      for chin, 276-277
      for forehead, 274-275
      for glabellar complex, 273-274
      for lateral periorbital region, 275
      for masseter, 277
      for nasal region, 274
      for necklift, 569
      for perioral region, 275-276
Boxy nasal tip, types of, 610
Brachioplasty
   after massive weight loss, 882
   equipment for, 821
   indications for, 818
   informed consent for, 820-821
   operative procedure for, 824-825
   postoperative care after, 826
   preoperative evaluation for, 819-820
   relevant anatomy for, 818-819
   techniques for
      liposuction, 825-826
      markings, 821-822
      two-ellipse technique, 823
Brag books, 53
Breast
   arterial supply to, 713-714
   development of, 711-712
   effects of menopause on, 713
   effects of menstrual cycle on, 712
   effects of pregnancy on, 712-713
   embryology of, 711

   examination of, 720-721
      photographic views, 721
   footprint, 720
   hypertrophy of, 769
   innervation of, 714-715
   lymphatic drainage of, 718-719
   muscles of, 717-718
   shape and aesthetics of, 719-720
   skin and parenchyma of, 716, 751
   venous drainage of, 714
Breast augmentation
   complications of, 739-745
   contraindications for, 724
   history of implants, 723-724
   implant filler material, 727-728
   implant shape/dimension, 729-730
   implant size, 730
   implant texture, 729
   implant volume, 728
   indications for, 724
   informed consent for, 726-727
   instrumentation for, 727
   photographic series for, 38
   postoperative care after, 739-740
   and postoperative pain, nausea, and vom-
      iting, 177
   preoperative evaluation for, 724-726
   technical point, 738-739
   techniques for
      incision location, 735-738
      markings, 730
      pocket position, 731-734
Breast implant-associated anaplastic large
      cell lymphoma, 746-747
Breast reduction
   in adolescents, 777
   after irradiation, 779
   common malpractice claims and, 52
   complications of, 783-785
   and free-nipple grafting, 782-783
   indications for, 769-770
   and infiltration, 779-780
   informed consent for, 771
   outcomes, 782
   and pedicle transection, 779
   photographic series for, 39
   postoperative care after, 783
   postoperative drains for, 781
   preoperative evaluation for, 770-771
   preoperative mammography for, 782
   secondary surgery, 777-778
   technical refinements for, 780-781

Breast reduction—cont'd
   techniques for
      excisional reduction, 772-777
      suction lipectomy, 771-772
Breast-feeding, after breast reduction, 784
Broadband light, 224
Bromelain, 146, 294, 446
Brow
   assessment of, 394
   effects of position changes, 411
   innervation of, 366
   photographic series for, 27-28
Browlift
   complications of, 426-427
      alopecia, 427
      contour deformities, 427
      facial nerve injury, 427
      overelevation, 427
   dissection planes for flap elevation, 422-423
   goals of, 418
   muscle modification, 425
   patient evaluation for, 416-418
   postoperative care after, 426
   preoperative planning for, 418
   techniques for
      custom coronal incisions, 416, 417
      fixation, 329-333, 424
      incision options, 418-422
      progressive tension sutures, 345
Browpexy, direct, 444
Buttock augmentation
   complications of, 834-835
   contraindications for, 828
   equipment for
      autologous fat grafting, 830
      silicone implants, 830
   indications for, 828
   informed consent for, 830
   postoperative care after, 834
   preoperative evaluation for, 829
   techniques for
      autologous fat augmentation, 833-834
      autologous fat grafting, 830-832
      silicone implants, 832-833

C
Calcium hydroxyapatite filler, 288-291, 649
Cancer detection, preoperative and postoperative, 747
Cancer, of skin, 186-187

Cannulas
   for fat grafting, 298, 302
   for liposuction, 804
Canons, neoclassical, 18-19, 391
Caprini risk assessment model for venous thromboembolism, 160-162, 853
Capsular calcification, 742
Capsular contracture, 742-745
Capsulopalpebral fascia, 362
Carac, 187, 189
Carbon dioxide laser
   equipment, 212-213
   for perioral rejuvenation, 535
   postoperative care after, 217-218
Cardiac arrhythmias, as complication of chemical peels, 254
Cardiac implantable electronic device, 85
Cardiff Scales of Reproduction, 22
Cardiovascular testing, advanced preoperative, 65
Carotenoids, 194
Cartilage graft, 336, 337
Catagen, 182, 402
Cavernous sinus thrombus, 563
Cellulite, 800-801
Centralizing genioplasty, 686
Cephalometric points, for genioplasty, 677
Cerebrovascular disease, perioperative anesthetic considerations for, 85
Cervical spinal nerves, 377-378
Cervicomental angle, 681
Chamomile, 195
Characteristics of aesthetic surgery patients, 3
Cheek
   assessment of, 399, 542
   fat compartment of, 373
Chemical peel
   agents
      beta-lipohydroxy acid, 239
      croton oil, 237-238
      glycolic acid, 235-236
      Jessner solution, 236
      Phenol-croton oil and TCA, 238
      salicylic acid, 238-239
      trichloroacetic acid, 237
   anesthesia for office-based procedures, 241
   choice of applicator, 242

combination peels, 248-249
  Glycolic acid and thrichloroacetic acid, 248-249
  Jessner solution and trichloroacetic acid, 248
complications of, 253-255
  early postoperative, 254
  intraoperative, 253-254
  late postoperative, 255
considerations for ethnic skin, 239-240
contraindications for, 231
degreasing the skin before, 242
depth of, 232, 235
dilution of agent, 242-243
facelift and, 252
indications for, 231
informed consent for, 234-235
nonfacial peeling, 234
occlusion, 243
order of areas to peel, 243
photograph series for, 28-29
postpeel care and instructions, 250-252
preoperative evaluation for, 231-235
results, 252-253
safety check, 240-241
taping versus petrolatum, 249
for perioral area, 244-245, 534
for periorbital area, 243-244
Chemodenervation
  for crow's-feet, 282
  for perioral rejuvenation, 530
Chemoprophylaxis for venous thromboembolism, 165
Chemoreceptor trigger zone, and postoperative nausea and vomiting, 77
Chemosis, 459
Chin
  anatomy of, 676-677
  assessment of, 400, 678-682
  assessment using Riedel plane, 400, 680
  classification of deformity and correction, 681-682
  dimpling, correction with soft tissue fillers, 282
  injection with botulinum toxin, 276
  projection, correction with and soft tissue fillers, 283
Chin pad analysis, 681
Chronic obstructive pulmonary disease, perioperative anesthesia considerations for, 86
Cleansers, 191-192

Clitoris and clitoral hood reduction, 912-914
Clostridium botulinum, 269-270
CO_2 laser; see Carbon dioxide laser
Coagulation studies, preoperative, 64
Coenzyme Q10, 193
Collagen
  aging and, 183
  augmentation with, 648
  monopolar radiofrequency effects on, 207
  nonablative laser effects on, 206-207
  topical retinol therapy and, 189
  vitamin C and, 147
Colles fascia, 856
Combination surgical procedures, 126-127
Commissures, alignment for photography, 25, 26
Communication, preoperative, 9
Comorbidities, affecting wound healing, 184
Compartment syndrome, patient positioning and, 73
Congenital nevi, 188
Congestive heart failure, perioperative anesthetic considerations for, 85
Conjunctiva, anatomy of, 369
Consults, medicolegal considerations and, 50
Contact dermatitis
  after CO_2 laser therapy, 220
Contamination, endogenous sources, 134
Converse-Wood-Smith otoplasty technique, 696, 701-703
Core principles for outpatient office-based surgery, 120-121
Corneal abrasion, 73-74
Corner mouthlift, 672-673
Coronary artery disease, perioperative anesthesia considerations, 85
Corticosteroids, 155
Cosmeceuticals
  cleansers, 191-192
  defined, 191
  moisturizers, 192-195
  for pigmented skin, 195
  for pigmented skin treatment, 195
  surfactants, 191, 192
Cosmetic procedures
  annual cost of, 3
  considerations for nonphysician providers, 176
  in medi spas, 171
Cosmetic surgery, defined, 3
Cottle test, 588
COX-2 inhibitors, and pain control, 111-112

Creases, evaluation of, 284
Cross-hatching, technique for, 288
Cross-radial, technique for, 288
Croton oil peel
    general features, 237-238
    postpeel care, 251-252
Crow's-feet
    chemodenervation for, 282
    defined, 275
    and soft tissue fillers, 282
Cryolipolysis, 927-929
Cryosurgery, 187
Cutis laxa, 184
Cyanoacrylates, 325-326

D

da Vinci, Leonardo, 16, 17
Dantroline as treatment for malignant hy-
        perthermia, 80
Davison-Caprini risk assessment model,
        130
De Architectura, 16
De Devina Proportione (The Divine
        Proportion)
Debulking of preaponeurotic tissues, 471-
        474
Decision-making for patient selection for
        ambulatory surgery, 88-90
Decolonization, staphylococcus and, 137,
        149
Deep venous thrombosis
    Caprini Risk Assessment Model, 149
    comorbidities affecting incidence of, 127
    in hospitalized patients, 127
    incidence of, 127, 129
Defibrillators, 86
Demographics of aesthetic surgery
        patients, 3
Depression
    description of patients with, 6
    recognizing signs of, 3
Dermabrasion
    complications of, 267-268
    contraindications for, 261
    equipment for, 262-263
    indications for, 261
    informed consent for, 262
    manual spot dermabrasion, 263
    microdermabrasion technique, 265-267
    for perioral rejuvenation, 535
    physical examination for, 262

preoperative evaluation for, 259-260
    preparation for, 262-263
    preprocedure details, 263-264
    technique for, 263-265
Dermal suspension autoaugmentation-
        mastopexy, 881
Dermatochalasis, defined, 435, 451
Dermatofibroma, 188
Dermis anatomy, 182
Dermis, homologous, 338
Dexamethasone, and pain control, 112
Diabetes, perioperative anesthesia consid-
        erations, 89
Diet
    after soft tissue filler injection, 293
    surgical complication and, 148-149
    wound healing and, 184
Digital single-lens reflex camera, use of, 23
Dilution, of chemical peel agents, 242-243
Dimethicone, 192-193
Dimorphism, sexual, and relationship to at-
        tractiveness, 18
Diode laser, 223
Direct liplift, 670-671
Distances for photography, 22-23
Diver's test, 842, 843
Documentation, medicolegal considerations
        and, 47-51
    defensive documentation, 50-51
    informed consent, 51
    legal defenses, 48-49
    legibility, 49
Donor site dominance for hair transplanta-
        tion, 404
Dorsal augmentation, 602-604
Dorsal hump reduction, 599-600
Double-bubble deformity, 742
Dry-eye syndrome, 459
Dual plane pocket dissection, 732-734
Dyschromia
    chemical peels for, 232
    erbium-doped fractionated laser for, 223
    nonablative laser resurfacing for, 226
Dyspigmentation, laser therapy for, 209
Dysplastic nevi, 188

E

Ear
    anatomy and development of, 691-693
    causes of abnormal morphology of, 69
    normal aesthetic proportions of, 399, 693

Ear, anatomy of, 399, 691-693
Ecchymosis, after soft tissue filler injection, 295
Ectropion
    after CO$_2$ laser therapy, 219
    defined, 451
Edema curve, 11
Efudex, 187, 189
Ehlers-Danlos syndrome, 184
Elastoderma, 184
Electrodessication and curettage (ED&C), 187
Elements, 14
Embrace, for scar management, 156
Embryology
    of breast, 711-712
    of ear, 691
Emetic zone, role in postoperative nausea and vomiting, 77
Endoscopic necklift, 573
Endotine ribbon, 330, 332
Endotine tack, 329, 332
Entropion, defined, 451
Epicanthoplasty, 468, 478-479
Epicanthus, types of, 464-465
Epidermal peels, 234
Epidermis, anatomy of, 181
ePTFE; see Expanded polytetrafluoroethylene
Erbium-doped fractional laser, 223
Erbium-yttrium aluminum garnet laser
    equipment, 213
    for perioral rejuvenation, 536
    and postoperative care, 217-218
Ethnic rhinoplasty
    anatomic variations of, 635-636
    complications of, 643
    grafting materials for, 636-637
    informed consent for, 635
    postoperative care after, 643
    preoperative evaluation for, 634-635
    technique for
        base reductions, 643
        closure, 642
        dorsal grafting, 640
        managing the bony vault, 638
        managing the middle third, 638
        managing the nasal base, 639
        opening the nose, 637-638
        tip contouring, 640-642
Ethnic skin, 197-200
    acne and, 199

chemical peels for, 239-240
dyschromia, 198-199
evaluation for hydration, 198
Fitzpatrick skin types, 197-198
general characteristics of, 197
hair removers for, 200
soft tissue fillers for, 200
sunscreen for, 200
Euclid, 14
Excitation mechanism of lasers, 205
Exogenous sources of wound contamination, 134
Expanded polytetrafluoroethylene, 341, 658
External carotid system, 364, 365, 381
External jugular vein, 382
External lower blepharoplasty and orbicularis suspension, 455-456
External lower blepharoplasty with orbicularis suspension and septal reset, 456-457
Eye protection, 97
Eyelashes, 369
Eyelid
    aesthetic evaluation of, 438-440
    anatomy of
        blood supply, 364-365
        deformities of, 435-436, 491-492
        fat, 370
        glands, 369
        margin, 369
        muscles, 357-364, 430-431
        nerves, 366-367
        skin, 356, 357-364
        upper eyelid, 429-435
    Asian
        comparison of Asian and white, 462-466
        assessment of, 394-395, 542
        normal versus ptotic, 498
        pathology of, 435-436
        photography of, 27-28

F
Face and neck
    anatomy of
        anterior triangle of neck, 387
        bones, 383
        danger zones, 380, 549
        facial bones, 383
        filaments, 386

Face and neck—cont'd
    anatomy of—cont'd
        motor nerves, 378-379
        nerves, 376-379
        retaining ligaments, 384-387
        sensory nerves, 376-378
        soft tissue layers, 372-376
        vessels, 381-382
    photography of, 23-27
    treatment after massive weight loss,
        882-883
Facelift
    anesthesia for, 547
    and bleeding risk, 165
    common malpractice claims and, 52
    complications of, 548-549
    intraoperative care during, 547
    postoperative care after, 547-548
    postoperative skin maintenance, 549
    preoperative evaluation for 540-543
    and progressive tension sutures, 345
    techniques for, 544-546
Facial analysis
    of cheek, 399
    of chin, 400
    for classifying rhytids, 390
    of divine proportion, using neoclassical
        canons, 391-392
    of ears, 399
    for Fitzpatrick skin type, 390
    of forehead, 394
    on frontal view, 392, 393
    of globe, 395
    on lateral view, 392, 393
    of lower eyelid, 395
    of mouth, 400
    of neck, 400
    of nose, 395-399
    for photoaging, 390
    for skin texture and thickness, 390
    of upper eyelid, 394-395
Facial expression for photography, 40
Facial feminization surgery, 934-939
Facial nerve, 367, 378-379
Facial plastic surgery
    anesthesia guidelines for, 95-97
Facial vein, 382
Factor Xa inhibitors for chemoprophylaxis,
        165
Fanning technique, 288
Farkas, 18, 19
Fasanella-Servat procedure, 503-504

Fascia
    of face, 374, 375
    lyophilized, 337
    of neck, 375-376
    parotidomasseteric, 375
    SMAS, 374
Fasciocutaneous retaining ligaments,
        385
Fasting guidelines, preoperative, 66
Fat
    of abdominal wall, 837
    of midface, 483-484
    periorbital compartments of, 370
    subcutaneous layers of, 799-800
    zones of adherence and, 800
Fat grafting
    complications of, 310-312
    equipment for, 298
    for facelift, 546
    informed consent for, 297
    for male-to-female top surgery, 940
    postoperative care after, 303
    preoperative evaluation for, 297
    preparation for
        harvest site selection, 297-298
        incisions for harvest, 297-298
    of selected areas
        cheek, 307-310
        lips, 305-307
        marionette grooves, 303-306
        nasolabial folds, 303-304
        tear trough, 307-310
    of tear trough deformities, 486
    technique for
        component separation, 300-301
        fat placement, 301-302
        harvest, 299
Federal regulations for ambulatory surgery
        centers, 175
Feet, positioning for photographing body
        series, 32-34
Female genital aesthetic surgery
    complications of, 922-923
    for functional problems, 924
    general considerations for, 887-888
    goals of, 891-892
    informed consent for, 897
    labia minora enlargement, 888-889
    outcomes, 923-924
    postoperative care after, 922
    preoperative evaluation for, 896-897
    relevant anatomy for, 892-895

techniques for
  clitoris and clitoral hood, 912-914
  labia majora, 915-918
  labia minora reduction, 898-912
  mons and mons pubis, 918-922
Female pattern baldness, 404
Femoral triangle, 856
Festoon, 453, 484
Feverfew, 195
FFS; see Facial feminization surgery
Fibrin glue, 323-325, 333
Fibonacci, 15
Fibonacci sequence, 15
Fibrous papules, 187
Fillers, soft tissue
  aesthetic evaluation for
    lines/furrows/creases, 284
    lips, 283
    lower lid/tear trough, 284
    midface/malar region, 284
  calcium hydroxyapatite, 288-291
    Radiesse, 288-291
  for chin dimpling, 282
  complications of, 294-295
  contraindications for, 282-283
  for crow's-feet, 282
  equipment for, 285-286
  for ethnic skin, 200
  for forehead, 280
  hyaluronic acid, 286-288
    FDA approved, 287
    indications for, 287
    injection techniques, 287-288
    nonanimal stabilized, 286-287
  ideal characteristics of, 286
  indications for, 282-283
  informed consent for, 284-285
  for labiomental groove, 282
  for lips, 281, 648-657
  for lower face, 281
  for midface, 280-281
  for nasal contouring, 282
  for perimental hollows, 282
  for perioral rejuvenation, 280, 530-533
Fire, and laser therapy, 220
First impression, 4
Fishtail excision, modified, 704
Fitzpatrick skin types
  chemical peels and, 233
  dermabrasion and, 259
  ethnic skin evaluation and, 197-198
  facial analysis and, 390

hyperpigmentation and, 185
laser therapy and, 208-209
5-fluorouracil, 187, 189, 226
Fixation devices
  advantages of, 332
  background of, 329
  complications of, 333
  direct needle sutures, 329
  disadvantages of, 332
  Endotine ribbon, 330
  Endotine tack, 329
  Mitek anchor, 330-331
  outcomes, 332-333
  quill suture, 331-332
  Ultratine tack, 330
  V-Loc barbed suture, 331
Flaps
  for epicanthoplasty, 478-479
  forehead, dissection planes, 422-423
Flash sterilization, 152
Flavonoids, 194
Fleur-de-lis abdominoplasty, 850, 874
FlexHD, 338
Fluence, and lasers, 206
Fluid management, for liposuction, 125
Flumazenil for benzodiazepine reversal, 71
Focal lengths, 22-23
Follicles, 182
Follicular unit extraction, 408
Forehead
  anatomy of
    blood supply, 364
    bones, 412-413
    fat compartment, 373
    galea aponeurosis, 412
    muscles, 413-415
    nerves, 415-416
    retaining structures, 412-413
    soft tissue layers, 412
    surface, 355
    zones of fixation, 412-413
  assessment of, 394, 416, 541
  ideal aesthetics of, 411
  injection with botulinum toxin, 274-275
  injection with soft tissue fillers, 280
  treatment algorithm for, 417
Fork-in-the-road legal defense, 48
Fractional lasers
  complications of, 220
  equipment, 207, 213-214

Frankfort plane, as reference for head positioning, 23
Fraxel, 223
Free-nipple grafting, 782-783
Frontal bone, 383
Frontal branch of facial nerve, course of, 379
Frontalis muscle, 357, 359, 414, 425
Frontalis suspension, 507
Full-scar facelift and necklift, 574
Functional capacity for anesthesia, 67-68
Functional status for anesthesia, 67-68
Furnas otoplasty, 696, 698-700
Furrows, evaluation of, 284

G

Gabapentin/pregabalin, for pain control, 112
Gabapentinoids, and pain control, 114
Galea aponeurosis, 412
Gastric emptying, comorbidities that affect, 67
Gelatin film, 342
Gender affirmation surgery
    facial feminization, 934-939
    female-to-male bottom surgery, 951-955
    male-to female bottom surgery, 947-951
    top surgery, 939-947
Genetic skin disorders, 184
Genioplasty
    complications of, 689-690
    contraindications for, 677
    equipment for
        alloplastic augmentation, 683-684
        biologic augmentation, 684
        osseous genioplasty, 684
    indications for, 677
    informed consent for, 682
    postoperative care after, 688
    preoperative evaluation for, 678-682
    relevant anatomy for, 676-677
    techniques for
        implant genioplasty, 687-688
        osseous genioplasty, 684-686
Genital aesthetic surgery; see Female genital aesthetic surgery
Giant congenital nevi, 188
Ginseng, 195
Glabellar complex, injection of, 273-274

Glide plane space, 412
Globe, assessment of, 395
Glogau photoaging scale, 233, 260, 390
Glycolic acid
    for chemical peels, general features, 235-236
    combined with trichloroacetic acid, 248-249
    as moisturizing agent, 193, 194
    perioral peeling technique, 244-245
Golden mean; see Golden ratio
Golden proportion; see Golden ratio
Golden ratio
    defined, 14
    and Fibonacci numbers, 15
    and golden rectangle, 15
    and Vitruvian explanation of proportion, 16
Golden rectangle, 14-15
Governance in office-based surgical facilities, 119
Grafts
    for lip augmentation, 660-664
    for nasal tip, 608-609
Granulomas, after soft tissue filler injection, 295
Great auricular nerve, 377, 378, 549
Greater occipital nerve, 377
Gull-wing liplift, 670-671
Gynecomastia
    complications of treating, 794
    contraindications for treating, 789
    demographics of, 789
    etiologic factors for, 789
    indications for treating, 789
    informed consent for treating, 791
    outcomes of treating, 794-795
    postoperative care after treating, 793-794
    preoperative evaluation of, 790
    staging of, 790
    techniques for treating
        combined/staged approach, 793
        nonoperative, 791
        operative, 791
        suction-assisted liposuction, 793
        surgical excision, 792
        ultrasound-assisted liposuction, 792-793
Gynoid lipodystrophy, 800-801

H

Hair color, considerations for transplantation, 404
Hair density, normal, 404
Hair growth, phases of, 182, 402
Hair reduction, and nonablative laser resurfacing, 226-227
Hair transplantation
  complications of, 409-410
  contraindications for, 403
  equipment for, 405
  for facial feminization, 937
  for facial feminization surgery, 937
  goals of, 402
  indications for, 403
  informed consent for, 404
  postoperative care after, 408-409
  preoperative care for, 404
  preoperative considerations for, 404
    donor site dominance, 404
  preoperative evaluation for
    Ludwig classification for female pattern baldness, 404
    Norwood classification for male pattern bladness, 403
  reasons for, 402
  technique for
    anesthesia, 405
    combined follicular unit extraction and transplantation, 408
    donor site harvesting, 405-406
    follicular unit extraction, 408
    graft dissection, 406
    graft insertion, 406-408
Hairline, 416-417, 935-936
Handpiece, control of
  for dermabrasion, 264
  for microdermabrasion, 266-267
Hatch suture, 705
Hatef risk assessment model, 131
Healing curve, 10
Health history, as component of patient consultation, 4
Health Insurance Portability and Accountability Act guidelines for photography, 40-41
Hematoma
  after facelift, 548
  after soft tissue filler injections, 295

peribulbar, 458
retrobulbar, 458
statistics from ambulatory surgery centers, 178
Herbal supplements
  after soft tissue filler injection, 294
  after upper blepharoplasty, 446
  discontinuation before laser therapy, 210
  negative effects of, 91
  perioperative anesthesia considerations for, 91-92
High-density porous polyethylene, 339
High-intensity focused ultrasound, 929-930
High-lateral-tension abdominoplasty, 849-850
Histrionic patients, 6
HIV infection, and poly-L-lactic acid, 291
Horizontal lower lid shortening, 495
Huger vascular zones, 838
Humectant, 193
Hutchinson-Gifford syndrome, 184
Hyaluronic acid fillers
  for correction of tear trough deformity, 485-486
  indications for, 287
  for lip augmentation, 648-649
  technique for, 287-288
Hyaluronidase, 294
Hydroquinone
  for ethnic skin, 240
  laser therapy and, 209-210
  mechanism of action, 189, 199
  treatment for pigmented skin, 195
Hydroxyapatite, 339-340
Hyperpigmentation
  after chemical peels, 255
  after dermabrasion, 267
  after erbium-yttrium aluminum garnet therapy, 220
  after sclerotherapy, 316
  postinflammatory, after carbon dioxide laser therapy, 219
  prevention after laser resurfacing, 218
Hypersensitivity reaction
  to botulinum toxin, 278
  to soft tissue fillers, 295

Hypertension
    and hematoma after facial rejuvenation, 4
    perioperative anesthesia considerations
        for, 85
Hypervascularity, laser therapy for, 209, 226
Hypopigmentation
    after carbon-dioxide laser therapy, 218
    after chemical peels, 255
    after dermabrasion, 267
    after erbium-yttrium aluminum garnet
        therapy, 220
Hypopnea, defined, 87
Hypothermia
    causes of, 122
    complications of, 75, 123
    contributing factors, 75
    defined, 74, 122, 152
    incidence of, 122
    PACU recovery, 76
    patient-associated risk factors for, 75
    perioperative, 74-76
    prevention of, 76, 123
    warming maneuvers for, 75-76
    wound healing and, 152

I

Imiquimod, as treatment for skin cancer, 187
Implant genioplasty, 687-688
Implants
    for breast augmentation, 727-730
    for buttock augmentation, 830, 832-833
    for female-to-male bottom surgery, 955
    nonbreast, 335-342
In situ squamous cell cancer, 186
In-line canthopexy, 493
Incision options, for browlift
    anterior hairline, 420
    coronal, 419-420
    direct forehead skin excision, 418-419
    endoscopic-assisted, 422
    limited incision, 420-421
    transblepharoplasty, 419
Incisional blepharoplasty, 467, 468-474
Inferior ligament of Schwalbe, 363
Inferior tarsal muscle, 361
Informed consent, 726-727
Inframammary fold, considerations for
    treating, 739
Inframammary incision, 735, 736
Infrared A, 199
Injection sites for facial nerve block, 241

Intense pulsed light, 207, 224, 226
Intermittent pneumatic compression, 164,
    165
Interpositional bone grafts, for genioplasty,
    685
Intralipid 20%, for treatment of local anes-
    thetic system toxicity, 105

J

Jessner solution
    combined with trichloroacetic acid, 248
    general features, 236
    perioral peeling technique, 245-246
    postpeel care, 250
Jowling, and retaining ligaments, 387
Jumping genioplasty, 685
Juvéderm products, 287

K

Keratinolytic agents, 189
Keratoacanthoma, 186
Ketamine, and pain control, 112
Kohl, 14
Kojic acid, 195, 199
Kybella, 570

L

L-ascorbic acid, 193
Labia majora reduction
    direct excision, 915-917
    liposuction, 918
Labia minora volume reduction
    bilateral deepithelialization, 911-912
    edge resection, 900-901
    wedge resection, 901-911
Labiaplasty; see Female genital aesthetic
    surgery
Labiomental groove, soft tissue fillers for, 282
Laboratory tests, preoperative, 64
Lacrimal apparatus, 434-435
Lacrimal function test, 438
Lacrimal glands, anatomy of, 369
Lactation, effects on breast, 712-713
Lactic acid, 193, 199
Lagophthalmos, 460
Landmarks
    for genioplasty, 676
    of patient identification for photograph
        series, 41
    of perioral region, 528
    of periorbital skeleton, 355

Laparoscopic adjustable gastric band, 870
Laser peel, photographic series for, 28-29
Laser resurfacing
    ablative, 212-220
    nonablative, 223-228
Laser therapy, 205-211
    anesthesia guidelines for, 97-98
    contraindications for, 208
    indications for, 207-208
    informed consent for, 210-211
    physics of, 205-206
    preoperative evaluation and preparation
        for, 208-210
    for prominent veins, 316-318
    types of lasers
        ablative, 206
        fractional, 207
        nonablative, 206-207
Lasers
    diode, 223
    erbium-doped fractional, 223-224
    intense pulsed light, 224
    midinfrared, 223
    ND:YAG, 223
    Q-switched ND:YAG, 223
    radiofrequency, 224-225
    visible light, 224
LAST; see Local anesthetic system toxicity
Lateral canthopexy
    complications of, 497
    defined, 490
    indications for, 491
    postoperative care, 497
    preoperative evaluation for, 491
    special anatomic considerations for
        deep-set eyes, 495-496
        prominent eyes, 496
    techniques for
        horizontal lower lid shortening, 495
        in-line canthopexy, 493
        orbicularis suspension, 493-494
        superficial retinacular lateral cantho-
            pexy, 492
        tarsal strip release, 495
        transcantho-canthopexy, 493
        transosseous canthopexy, 494-495
Lateral orbital thickening, 363, 385
Lathyrogens, wound healing and, 185
Lawsuits; see Malpractice
Legibility of documentation, 49
Length of surgical procedure, safety and, 123

Lentigo, 188
Leonardo of Pisa; see Fibonacci
Lesions, of skin, 185-189
Levator reinsertion, 507
Liber Abaci, 15
Licorice, 195, 199
Lid invagination, 444
Lidocaine
    liposuction and, 103-104, 805-806
    toxicity of, 104, 214, 806
Liedl, Charles, 18
Lifestyle, and surgical complications, 147-149
Lighting for photography, 21
Linear threading, 288
Lines, evaluation of, 284
Lip augmentation
    goals of, 645
    preoperative evaluation for, 646-648
    techniques for
        anguloplasty, 672-673
        bullhorn liplift, 667-669
        corner mouthlift, 672-673
        direct liplift, 670-671
        grafts, 660-664
        gull-wing liplift, 670-671
        implants, 657-660
        indirect liplift, 667-669
        injectable fillers, 648-657
        lip suspension, 669-670
        subnasal lift, 667-669
        V-Y advancement, 664-666
        vermilion liplift, 670-671
Lip suspension, 669-670
Lipectomy, suction-assisted, 53-54
Liplift, 536
Lipoabdominoplasty, 848
Liposuction
    anesthesia guidelines for, 102-104
    techniques for
        laser-assisted, 808
        power-assisted, 807
        radiofrequency-assisted, 809
        suction-assisted, 806
        ultrasound-assisted, 806-807
        water-assisted, 808
Lips
    ideal dimensions of, 646-647
    rejuvenation with implants, 537-538
    aesthetic evaluation of, 283, 400, 528-
        529
    augmentation with fat, 305-306

Lips—cont'd
  rejuvenation with implants—cont'd
    enhancement of, 283
    fat grafting of, 305-307
    photograph series of, 29-30
    rejuvenation with soft tissue fillers, 531
    youthful characteristics of, 281
Listener, defined, 3
Local anesthetic infiltration, 112-113
Local anesthetic system toxicity
  EMS and transfer protocols for, 105
  intralipid administration for, 105
  management of, 104-105, 816
Low-level laser therapy, 931
Lower lid-cheek junction, and soft tissue
    fillers, 280
Lower lid/tear trough, evaluation of, 284
Ludwig classification for female pattern
    baldness, 404
Lumpiness, after soft tissue filler injection,
    294
Lunchtime peel, 193-194
Lux 1540 fractional laser, 224
Lymphatics
  of breast, 718-719
  function of, 182
  massage of, 155
  of periorbita, 365

M
MAC; see Monitored anesthesia care
Maintenance counseling, 11
Malar bag, 453
Malar region, and soft tissue fillers, 280-281
Male pattern baldness, 404
Malignant hyperthermia
  basic considerations for, 79
  Malignant Hyperthermia Association of
      the United States (MHAUS), 81
  management of, 80-81
  North American Malignant Hyperthermia
      Registry, 81
  signs of, 80
  and total intravenous anesthesia, 60
Malignant Hyperthermia Association of the
    United States, 81
Mallampati airway classification, 72
Malposition of lower lid, postoperative, 460
Malpractice
  common claims, 52-54
  documentation and, 47-51
  frequency of claims by specialty, 43

patient communication and, 45-47
patient selection and, 44-45
Marionette grooves
  fat grafting of, 303-304
  rejuvenation with soft tissue fillers, 532-
      533
Masseter muscle, injection with botulinum
    toxin, 277
Massive weight loss
  photography after, 35-37
  techniques for body contouring after,
      862-863, 874-883
  tissue characteristics after, 874, 876, 877,
      878, 882
Mastopexy
  after explantation, 759
  after massive weight loss, 880, 881
  and augmentation, 759
  complications of, 758-759
  contraindications for, 752
  indications for, 752
  informed consent for, 753
  outcomes, 760-761
  photographic series for, 39
  postoperative care after, 758
  preoperative evaluation for, 752-753
  techniques for
    periareolar, 753-755
    vertical and horizontal scar, 757-758
    vertical scar, 755-757
  for tuberous breast deformity, 760
Mastopexy, photographic series for, 39
Medi spa
  ambulatory surgery center (ASC) and,
      171, 174-175
  defined, 171
  financial considerations for, 173-174
  marketing and advertising for, 173
  postoperative complications, 177-178
  practice settings for, 172
  services offered in, 171
  staffing for, 172
Medi-speak, medicolegal considerations
    and, 46
Medial thigh lift
  after massive weight loss, 878-879
  classification systems
    massive-weight-loss patients, 858
    non-massive-weight-loss patients,
        858
    Pittsburgh rating scale, 858
  contraindications for, 857

equipment for, 859-860
indications for, 857
informed consent for, 859
postoperative care after, 865-866
preoperative evaluation for, 857-859
relevant anatomy for, 856
techniques for
    after massive weight loss, 862-863
    classic technique with transverse skin
        excision/upper thigh crescent ex-
        cision, 860-862
    fasciofascial suspension technique,
        864
    spiral lift, 864-865
Medical clearance, 9
Medication storage and disposal, 108, 109
Medicolegal considerations
    common claims, 52-54
    documentation, 47-51
    patient communication, 45-47
    patient selection, 44-45
Meibomian glands, 369
Melanoma, 186-187
Menopause, effects on breast, 713
Menstrual cycle, effects on breast, 712
Metabolic equivalents, assessment for func-
    tional status, 67-68
Methicillin-resistant Staphylococcus aureus,
    antibiotic prophylaxis for, 149
Microdermabrasion, 263, 265-267
Micrografts, defined, 406
Microthermal zones of ablation, 213
Midcheek, defined, 482
Midface lift, fixation for, 329-333
Midface-malar region, evaluation of, 284
Midface, morphology classification for, 483
Midinfrared laser, 223
Mimetic muscles, 374-375
Miniabdominoplasty, 848-849
Minigrafts, defined, 406
Mitek anchor, 330-331, 333-334
Modiolus, 552
Mohs micrographic surgery, 187
Moisturizers, 192-195
Monitored anesthesia care
    agent reversal, 71
    goals of, 68
    medications for, 68-69
    sedation continuum, 70
    tools of airway continuum, 70
Monopolar radiofrequency, 207
Mons and mons pubis techniques, 918-922

Morbid obesity
    classification of, 869
    comorbidities of, 869
Motivation for aesthetic surgery, 6
Mouth, assessment of, 400
Moving needle technique, 112, 113
Müller muscle-conjunctival resection, 504
Multilevel filling, 281
Multimodal analgesia; see also Opioids
    addiction after surgery, 108-109
    local anesthetics and, 112-113
    medications for, 111-112
    and opioid use, 107-111
    recommendations for surgeons, 109-110
    regimen for, 113-115
    surgeon's role in, 108
Muscle necrosis, patient positioning and,
    73
Mushroom extract, 195
Mustardé otoplasty, 696, 698-700

N
Nahai classification of nasolabial fold, 556-
    557
Naloxone for reversal of narcotics, 71
Narcissistic patients, 6
Nasal contouring, soft tissue fillers for, 282
Nasal deviation, correction of, 613
Nasal obstruction, correction of, 587-588,
    614
Nasal region, botulinum toxin injection of,
    274
Nasojugal groove, defined, 482
Nasolabial fold
    algorithm for treatment options, 558-
        559
    anatomy of, 551
    causes of deepening, 554-555
    classification of, 556-557
    complications of treating, 563
    dynamics of, 553
        smiling, 553-554
    fat grafting of, 303-304
    histologic observations, 552
    informed consent for treating, 558
    observations after dissection, 551-552
    postoperative care after, 562
    rejuvenation with soft tissue fillers, 532
    relationship to SMAS, 552-553
    soft tissue fillers for, 281
    techniques for
        dermal fat grafting, 560

Nasolabial fold—cont'd
  techniques for—cont'd
    facelift, 561-562
    injections, 559
    nasolabial lipectomy, 561
    primary excision, 562
ND:YAG laser, 223
Neck
  assessment of, 400, 543
  injection with botulinum toxin, 276-277
  qualities of aging, 565
  qualities of youthful appearance, 400, 565
Necklift
  anesthesia guidelines for, 95-97
  complications of, 578-579
  component evaluation of
    chin, 568
    digastric muscles, 568
    fat, 566-567
    mandibulocutaneous ligament, 568
    platysma, 567
    skin, 566
    submandibular gland, 568
  fixation for, 329-333
  informed consent for, 568
  nonsurgical options for rejuvenation,
    569-570
    botulinum toxin, 569
    medication, 570
    ultrasonography, 569
  postoperative care of, 577-578
  surgical options for rejuvenation, 570-571
    endoscopic necklift, 573
    full-scar facelift and necklift, 574
    liposuction, 570-571
    platysmal procedures, 575-577
    short-scar facelift and necklift, 573-574
    skin flap procedures, 575
    submental anterior necklift, 571-573
Nefertiti, 13-14
Negative psychological indicators (red
  flags), 5
Neodermal matrix, bilaminate, 338
Neoteny, defined, 18
Nerves, facial danger zones for, 380, 549
Neurotic patients, 7
Nevi, 187
Nicotine metabolites, 148
Nipple sensation
  after breast augmentation, 740
  after breast reduction, 784

Nipple-areola complex, vascular compromise of, 783
Nodules, after soft tissue filler injections,
  295
Nonablative laser resurfacing
  anesthesia for, 225
  applications for, 226-227
  complications of, 227
  equipment for, 223-225
  postoperative care after, 227
  safety considerations for, 225
  side effects of, 227-228
  techniques for, 225-226
Nonablative lasers
  mechanism of action, 206-207
  risks of, 210-211
Nonanimal stabilized hyaluronic acid products, 286-287
Nonendothermal endovenous ablation, for
  prominent veins, 319
Nonincisional blepharoplasty, 474-478
Normothermia, 152
North American Malignant Hyperthermia
  Registry, 80
Norwood classification for male pattern
  baldness, 403
Nose
  anatomy of, 581-586
  assessment of, 395-399
  ethnic variations of, 398-399, 636
NSAIDs, 111-112, 114
Nutrition, and wound healing, 184

O
Obesity
  body mass index and, 90-91
  and clinical correlations, 90
  obstructive sleep apnea and, 87
Obstructive sleep apnea
  background information, 87
  perioperative anesthesia considerations
    for, 87-88
  physiologic derangement with, 87
  preoperative assessment for, 87-88
Occlusion classification, Angle, 678-679
Occlusives, 192-193
Ocular damage and blindness, 220
Ocular examination, 437
Office-based surgery
  administrative issues and, 119-120
  anesthesia evaluation for, 121

contraindications for, 147
core principles of, 120-121
liposuction and, 124-125
postoperative pain and nausea and, 123-124
preoperative evaluation for, 121
risk stratification of patients, 121
safety considerations for, 119
Oils, 192
Operative and follow-up care
day of surgery, 9-10
maintenance counseling, 11
postoperative care, 10
recovery after cosmetic surgery, 10-11
revisions, 12
Opioids; see also Multimodal analgesia
addiction to, 108-109
adverse effects of, 110-111
diversion and, 108
epidemic of, 107-108
and Medicaid patients, 108
prescribing patterns for, 107
risk factors for abuse of, 109
statistics, 107-108
storage and disposal of, 108
surgeon's role, 108
Orbera weight loss balloon, 870
Orbicularis suspension, 493-494
Orbit, fat compartment of, 373
Orbital anesthesia for ablative laser resurfacing, 215
Osteotomies, 601-602
Otoplasty
contraindications for, 695
preoperative evaluation for, 694-695
relevant anatomy for, 691, 692-693
equipment for, 696
goals of, 694
indications for, 695
informed consent for, 695
techniques for
Converse-Wood-Smith, 701-703
for Darwin tubercle, 705
Furnas, 698-700
for mastoid prominence, 705
Mustardé, 696-698
prominent helical root correction, 705
prominent lobule correction, 704
for Stahl ear, 705
Overcorrection, using soft tissue fillers, 294

P
P6-accupressure, as antiemetic therapy, 79
Pacemakers, 85, 86
Pacioli, Luca, 15
Pain management; see also multimodal analgesia; opioids
complication reduction with, 153
effects of inadequate management, 110
nonopioid options for, 110
Palpebromalar groove, defined, 482
Paranoid patients, 7
Parotidomasseteric fascia, 375
Patient communication
listening behaviors to avoid, 45-46
listening skills, 46
speaking habits, 46-47
Patient consultation
health history, 4
introduction and first impression, 4
motivation, 5-6
physical evaluation, 7-8
preparing for surgery, 9
psychology, 5, 6-7
rejection, 8
Patient positioning
for anesthesia, 73-74
complications of, 74
and venous thromboembolism prevention, 153-154
Patient safety in medi spas, 177-178
Patient selection
and medi spa procedures, 177
and medicolegal considerations, 44-45
PDT; see Photodynamic therapy
Pedicles, for breast reduction, 772-774
Peels; see Chemical peels
Periareolar incision, 736-737
Perimental hollows, soft tissue fillers for, 282
Perioral lines, soft tissue fillers for, 281
Perioral region
anatomy of, 528
assessment of, 543
injection with botulinum toxin, 275-276
Perioral rejuvenation
complications of, 538
techniques for
ablative laser resurfacing, 535-536
chemical peels, 534
chemodenervation, 530
dermabrasion, 535
fat grafting, 533-534

Perioral rejuvenation—cont'd
    techniques for—cont'd
        lip implants, 537-538
        soft tissue fillers, 530-531
        subnasal liplift, 536-537
Periorbital region
    anatomy of
        blood supply, 364-365
        conjunctiva, 369
        eyebrow, 355
        eyelashes, 369
        eyelid surface, 356-357, 369
        fat, 370
        glands, 369
        ligamentous framework, 361-364
        lymphatic, 367
        muscles, 357-364
        nerves, 366-367
        orbital septum, 367-368
        skeletal, 355
        skin, 357
        soft tissue, 355-370, 413
        tarsus, 368-369
    botulinum toxin injection of, 275
    characteristics of aging, 452
    measurements of, 357
    soft tissue fillers for, 280
Peripheral neuropathy, patient positioning
    and, 73, 74
Peripheral vascular disease, perioperative
    anesthetic considerations for, 86
Perlane products, 287
Personality disorders
    histrionic patients, 6
    narcissistic patients, 6
    neurotic patients, 7
    paranoid personality, 7
    schizoid patients, 6
Petrolatum, 192
Phenol-croton oil and TCA peels, 238
Phi, 15
Phidias, 15
Photoaging, 194
Photodynamic therapy, 187, 224
Photography
    background, 40
    for botulinum toxin injection, 271
    elements of standardization overview, 21
    focal lengths and distances, 21, 22-23
        Cardiff Scales of Reproduction, 22
        sensors, 22

for genioplasty, 679
informed consent for, 40-41
lighting, 40
preoperative planning and, 9
preparation of patient for, 40
series
    body, 32-34
    breast, 35-37
    brow and eyelids, 27-28, 418
    face and neck, 23-27
    laser/chemical peel, 28-29
    lip, 29-30
    male body, 34-35
    rhinoplasty, 30-32
Physical evaluation, 7-8
Physical status classification of American
        Society of Anesthesiologists, 122
Physics of lasers, 205
Pigmentation
    in ethnic skin, 198-199
    inhibitors, 199
    treatment with cosmeceuticals, 195
Pinch blepharoplasty, 454
Pitanguy line, 379
Plaintiffs fault legal defense, 48
Planner, defined, 3
Plastic and Reconstructive Surgery logo, 18
Platonic solids, 15
Platysmal banding
    botulinum treatment for, 276-277
    photography of, 27
Platysmal procedures, for necklift
    corset platysmaplasty, 576-577
    platysmal flap cervical rhytidoplasty, 575
    platysmal muscle sling, 576
Plutarch, 14
Poly-L-lactic acid, 291-292, 341, 649
Polydioxanone, 342
Polyglactin 910, 342
Polylactide derivatives, 341
Polymethylmethacrylate, 292
    indications for using, 292
    lip augmentation with, 649-650
    technical considerations for, 292
Polyphenols, 194
Polysomnography, and obstructive sleep
        apnea, 87
PONV; see Postoperative nausea and vomit-
        ing
Positioning, after soft tissue filler injection,
        293

Postanesthesia recovery unit care, 81
Postanesthetic shivering, 76
Postbariatric body contouring
    consensus guidelines for, 134
    preoperative laboratory testing, 133
    safety issues for, 132-134
    solo versus team approach for, 133
    surgical staging, 133
Postbariatric surgery
    involving liposuction, 131, 132
    and venous thromboembolism, 131-132
Postdischarge nausea and vomiting
    incidence, 76
    PACU rescue therapy for, 79
    risk factors and management, 77-78
Postoperative nausea and vomiting
    ambulatory surgery and, 90
    incidence of, 123-124
    in medi spa patients, 177
    multimodal management of, 124
    neurotransmitters and, 77
    in office-based procedures, 123-124
    PACU rescue therapy for, 79
    risk factors and management, 77-78
Pregnancy
    effects on breast, 712-713
    preoperative testing for, 63-64
Prejowl sulcus, soft tissue fillers for, 282
Premature peeling, 254
Preparing for surgery, 9
Preseptal fat, 433
Pressure ulcers, as complication of patient
        positioning for anesthesia, 73
Priming, before chemical peels, 239-240
Progeria, 184
Progressive tension sutures
    for abdominoplasty, 847
    complications of, 351
    contraindications for, 345
    defined, 344
    equipment for, 346
    indications for, 344-345
    informed consent for, 345-346
    outcomes, 350-351
    postoperative care, 349-350
    preoperative elevation for, 345
    technique, 346-349
Proportion of man; see Vitruvian Man
Proportion, facial, 391-393
Protected Health Information, 41
Pseudoblepharoptosis, defined, 436

Pseudofolliculitis barbae, 200
Pseudoptosis, 499
Pseudoxanthoma elasticum, 184
Psychological factors in patient evaluation,
        5, 6-7
Ptosis
    acquired, 500
    congenital, 499-500
    degrees of, 501
    of eyelids, 278
    glandular, 763-764
    involutional, algorithm for treatment, 505
    Regnault classification of, 751, 763
    true, 499
Ptosis adipose, defined, 436
Pull-away test, 453
Pulmonary aspiration prevention, 66, 67
Pulmonary hypertension, perioperative an-
        esthesia considerations for, 86
Pulse duration, and lasers, 206
Pulse width, and lasers, 206
Pulsed dye laser, 224, 226
Putterman procedure; see Müller muscle-
        conjunctival resection
Pythagoras, 14

Q
Q-switched ND:YAG laser
    general characteristics, 223
    for tattoo removal, 226
Q-switching, defined, 205
Qualifications of physicians in office-based
        surgical facilities, 119
Quality assessment and safety, 119
Quill suture, 331-332

R
Radiation, UVA and UVB, 194
Radiesse, 288-291
Radiofrequency, 224-225
Radiofrequency ablation, for prominent
        veins, 318
Radiotherapy, 187
Rayleigh scattering, 285
RCRI; see Revised Cardiac Risk Index
Reading view, photographic positioning
        for, 27
Recovery after cosmetic surgery
    edema curve, 11
    emotional response, 11
    healing curve, 10-11

Reduction genioplasty, 685
Reduction mammaplasty; *see* Breast reduc-
    tion
Reduction, of breast
    common malpractice claims and, 52
    photographic series for, 39
Reflection, lasers and, 205
Regional anesthesia, 61
Regnault classification of breast ptosis, 751,
    763
Rejection of patients for aesthetic surgery, 8
ReliefBand, for antiemetic therapy, 79
Reoperation, after breast augmentation,
    747
Restylane products, 287
Resurfacing modalities, 207
Retaining ligaments
    of anterior triangle, 387
    of cheek and mandible, 385, 386
    defined, 384
    of neck, 386-387
    of periorbital area, 384, 385
    of temporal area, 384
Retinoid therapy, 189, 193, 199
Retraction, defined, 452
Retroorbicularis oculi fat pads, anatomy of,
    370
Reverse abdominoplasty, 851
Revised Cardiac Risk Index, 65
Revision policy, 12
Rhinoplasty
    aesthetic indications for, 589
    anesthesia guidelines for, 98
    complications of
        aesthetic, 616-617
        functional-medical, 615-616
    corticosteroids and, 155
    equipment for, 596-597
    functional indications for, 589-590
    informed consent for, 596
    photographic series for, 30-32
    postoperative care after, 615
    preoperative evaluation for, 590-595
    relevant anatomy for, 581-586
    techniques for
        alar base and nostrils, 610-612
        closed (endonasal) approach, 598-599
        nasal airway obstruction, 614
        nasal deviation, 613
        nasal dorsum, 599-604
        nasal tip, 604-610

    open approach, 597-598
    septoplasty, 604
Rhytidectomy, anesthesia guidelines for,
    95-97
Rhytids
    after dermabrasion, 267
    classification of, 209, 390
    dynamic, defined, 411, 541
    erbium-doped fractionated laser for, 224
    nonablative laser resurfacing for, 226
    static, defined, 411, 541
Riedel line, 400, 680
Riedel plane, 400
Right of refusal, documentation of, 51
Rosacea
    defined, 189
    heat and, 200
    and intense pulsed light, 224
Roux-en-Y gastric bypass, 871
Ryanodex, for malignant hyperthermia, 80

S
SAFElipo; *see* Separation, aspiration, and fat
    equalization liposuction
Safety
    chemical peels and, 240-241
    laser therapy and, 214, 225
    office-based surgery and
        administrative issues, 119-120
        clinical issues, 121-122
        combination surgical procedures and,
            126-127
        core principles, 120-121
        liposuction, 124-125
        physiologic stresses, 122-123
        postoperative pain and nausea, 123-
            124
        postbariatric body contouring and, 132-
            134
        risk assessment and, 129-131
        supplements and, 146-147
        surgical site infections and, 134-137
        venous thromboembolism and
            postbariatric procedures, 131-132
Saline, for lip augmentation, 658
Scarring
    after chemical peels, 255
    after CO_2 laser therapy, 219
    after dermabrasion, 268
    as common malpractice claim, 52
    laser therapy for, 209, 226

postoperative management of, 155-156
and soft tissue fillers, 282
Scatter, lasers and, 205
SCC; see Squamous cell cancer
Schirmer test, 438
Schizoid patients, 6
Scleral show, 453
Sclerosing agents, 314
Sclerotherapy, for prominent veins, 313-316
Screening duplex ultrasound, and venous thromboembolism, 165
Sculptra, 291-292
Seal of American Society of Plastic Surgeons, 18
Sebaceous hyperplasia, 187
Seborrheic keratosis, 188
Secondary breast reduction, 777-778
Secondary rhinoplasty
complications of, 632
endonasal/closed approach for, 621
external/open approach for, 621
grafts for, 630-631
indications for, 620
postoperative care after, 631
preoperative evaluation for, 621-625
surgical obstacles, 621
technique
for contour irregularities, 630
for displaced/deviated structures, 625-626
for overresection, 628-629
for prosthetic complications, 630
for underresection, 626-628
treatment planning for, 625
Selective thermolysis, 206
Selenium, 195
Self-image versus true image, 5
Separation, aspiration, and fat equalization liposuction, 809-810
Septoplasty, 604
Septorhinoplasty, common malpractice claims and, 52-53
Serial puncture technique, 288
Seroma, and progressive tension sutures, 350-351
Shopper, defined, 3
Short-scar facelift and necklift, 573-574
Sign in, 150
Sign out, 150

Silicone
defined, 340
for lip augmentation, 649, 658
for nonbreast applications, 340-341
for scar management, 155-156
Skin
analysis of
for aging, 185, 540
for Fitzpatrick skin type, 185, 197-198, 208-209, 233, 259, 390
for quality, 185, 390, 540
anatomy of
and chemical peel depth, 235
normal, 181-182, 372
benign lesions of, 187-188
cancer, 186-187
basal cell cancer, 186
melanoma, 186-187
squamous cell cancer, 186
treatment, 187
common therapies for, 189
ethnic skin care, 197-200
genetic disorders of, 184
physiology of, 182-184
premalignant lesions of
actinic keratosis, 187
redundancy, 869
wound healing of, 183-185
Skin antisepsis protocol, 149
Skin flap procedures, for necklift, 575
Skin resurfacing
and facelift, 546
for lower blepharoplasty, 454
Skin tag; see Acrocordon
Skin-only blepharoplasty, 454
Sliding genioplasty, 685
SMAS; see Superficial musculoaponeurotic system
Smiling, stages of, 553
Smoking
patient history, 4
surgical complications of, 148
Smoking, perioperative anesthesia considerations for, 86
Snap test, 209
Snap-back test, 453
Soemmering ligaments, 364
Soft tissues of face and neck
Solar lentigo, 188
Spider angioma, 188
Spider veins; see Telangiectasias

Spot size, and lasers, 206
Squamous cell cancer, 186
Squinch test, 453
Squint test, 453
Standard of care legal defense, 48
Staphylococcus colonization, general considerations for, 137
State regulations for ambulatory surgery centers, 175-176
Statistics of aesthetic surgery patients, 3
Steatoblepharon, defined, 435, 452
Sterile technique, 134
Steroids, 184, 293
Stick and place technique for graft insertion, 406-407
STOP-BANG questionnaire, 87-88
Strobe flashes, 21
Sub-SMAS facelift, 545
Subcutaneous facelift, 545
Subcutaneous mastectomy, for female-to-male top surgery, 941-946
Subglandular/subfascial pocket dissection, 731
Submandibular triangle, 387
Submental anterior necklift
    indications, 571
    technical considerations, 571-573
Submental triangle, 387
Subnasal liplift, 536-537
Suborbicularis oculi fat pads, anatomy of, 370
Subpectoral pocket dissection, 731-732
Subperiosteal facelift, 545
Suction lipectomy, for breast reduction, 771-772
Sunscreen, 189, 194
Superficial musculoaponeurotic system, 374, 552-553
Superficial retinacular lateral canthopexy, 492
Supraorbital ligamentous adhesion, 384
Supraperiosteal facelift, 545
Surface cooling, and lasers, 206
Surfactants, 191, 192
Surgeon-patient communication, effects on outcomes, 147
Surgical Care Improvement Project, 845
Surgical drains, management of, 137
Surgical eligibility, 8
Surgical safety checklist from World Health Organization, 150-151

Surgical site infections, 134-137
Surgiholic patients, medicolegal considerations for, 45
Sutures
    barbed, 153
    continuous, for abdominoplasty, 349
    interrupted, for abdominoplasty, 346-348
    for umbilicus inset, 348
Symbolism of beauty, 14
Synmastia, 740
Symmetry, defined, 18
Syringomas, 187

T
Talker, defined, 3
Taping, after chemical peels, 243, 249
Tarsal strip release, 495
Tarsoligamentous complex, 431-432
Tarsus, anatomy of, 368-369
Tattoos, laser therapy and, 208, 226
TCA; see Trichloroacetic acid
Tear trough
    defined, 482
    grafts, 488
    and lower blepharoplasty, 453, 487-488
    soft tissue fillers for, 280, 485-486
Tear trough deformity
    anatomic considerations for
        central fat pad, 484
        festoons, 484
    contraindications for correction of, 484-485
    grading system for, 482-483
    indications for correction of, 484-485
    informed consent for, 485
    nonsurgical treatment of
        with hyaluronic acid filler, 485-486
    nonvascularized fat grafting for, 486
    preoperative evaluation for, 485
    surgical treatment of
        blepharoplasty midface lift, 488
        lower blepharoplasty and orbicularis suspension, 487
        lower blepharoplasty with orbicularis suspension and septal reset, 487-488
        tear trough grafts, 488
Tear trough triad, defined, 482
Tears, 435, 438
Telangiectasias, 188, 313

Telangiectatic matting, after sclerotherapy, 315
Telogen, 182, 402
Temporal ligamentous adhesion, 384
Tessari method, of sclerotherapy, 315
ThermaCool, 224
Thermal injuries resulting from suboptimal patient positioning for anesthesia, 73
Thermal injuries, and suboptimal patient positioning, 73
Thermal relaxation time, and lasers, 206
Time out, 150
Tip projection, correction of, 604-610
Tissue adhesives; see Tissue glues
Tissue glues
 cyanoacrylates, 325-326
 fibrin sealants, 323-325
 principles of, 323
Tissue manipulation, soft tissue fillers for, 293
Top surgery
 complications of, 947
 female-to-male surgery, 940-946
 indications for, 939
 male-to-female surgery, 939-940
Topical therapy for skin cancer, 187
Total intravenous anesthesia, 60
Transaxillary incision, 737
Transblepharoplasty midface lift, 488
Transcantho-canthopexy, 493
Transconjunctival fat removal, 454-455
Transepidermal water loss, 198
Transgender surgery; see Gender affirmation surgery
Transmission, lasers and, 205
Transosseous canthopexy, 494-495
Transpalpebral corrugator supercilii resection, 445
Transumbilical incision, for breast augmentation, 738
Tretinoin, 193
Trichloroacetic acid
 application technique, 246-247
 combined with glycolic acid, 248-249
 combined with Jessner solution, 248
 general characteristics, 237
 postpeel care, 250-251
True osteocutaneous retaining ligaments, 385
Tuberous breast deformity, 760

Tumescent anesthesia for ablative laser resurfacing, 215
Turmeric, 195
Tyndall effect, 285

U
Ulceration, after sclerotherapy, 315
Ultrasonography, for necklift, 569
Ultratine tack, 330, 332
Umbilicus
 anatomy of, 840
 suture technique for insetting, 348
Upper lip lines, and soft tissue fillers, 281
Urine cotinine test, 148

V
V-Loc barbed suture, 331, 333
V-Y advancement for lip augmentation, 664-666
Varicose veins, 188, 313-319
Veins
 prominent
  conservative management of, 313, 319
  endovenous laser ablation (EVLA) for, 318
  goals of treating, 313
  laser therapy for, 316-318
  nonendothermal endovenous ablation for, 319
  risk factors for, 313
  sclerotherapy for, 313-316
  surgery for, 319
 varicose
  defined, 313
  surgery for, 319
 sentinel, 381, 382
 of skin, 182
Venous lake, 188
Venous thromboembolism
 abdominoplasty and, 162
 algorithm for preventing, 129
 Caprini risk assessment model, 160-161, 161-162
 guidelines for prevention of, 160-161
 intraoperative risk reduction for, 164-165
 patients at risk for, 162
 and postbariatric surgery, 131-132
 postoperative risk reduction for, 165
 preoperative risk modification for, 163-164
 preoperative risk stratification for, 163

Venous thromboembolism—cont'd
    prophylaxis, 153-154
    statistics, 160, 178
Venus de Milo, 17-18
Vermilion liplift, 670-671
Vertical banded gastroplasty, 870
Vessels
    of abdominal wall, 838
    of face and neck, 381-382
    of periorbital region, 365
Visible light laser, 224
Vision loss, patient positioning and, 74
Vitamin A, 147, 193
Vitamin B, 147
Vitamin C, 147, 193
Vitamin E, 193
Vitruvian Man, 16-17
Vitruvian Triad, 16
Vitruvius Polio, Marcus, 16
Volume restoration, soft tissue fillers for, 283

W

Wavelength, and lasers, 206
Wicking, of fat, 300
Witch's-chin deformity, 681
Wood lamp
    for determining depth of dyschromia,
        232
World Health Organization surgical safety
        checklist, 150
Wound healing
    factors affecting, 184-185
    stages of, 183-184

X

Xenograft, defined, 335

Z

Zones of adherence, 800
Zuffrey classification of nasolabial fold,
        556